Textbook of
Erectile
Dysfunction

Textbook of Erectile Dysfunction

Edited by

Culley C. Carson III MD
Professor and Chief, Division of Urology, Department of Surgery,
University of North Carolina School of Medicine, USA

Roger S. Kirby MA MD FRCS(Urol) FEBU
Consultant Urologist, Department of Urology, St. George's Hospital, London, UK

and

Irwin Goldstein MD
Professor of Urology, Boston University School of Medicine, Boston, USA

I S I S
MEDICAL
MEDIA
Oxford

© 1999 by Isis Medical Media Ltd.
59 St Aldates
Oxford OX1 1ST, UK

First published 1999

British Library Cataloguing in Publication Data.
A catalogue record for this title is available from
the British Library.

ISBN 1 899066 96 9

Carson, C. C. (Culley)
Textbook of Erectile Dysfunction
Culley C. Carson, Roger S. Kirby, Irwin Goldstein (eds)

Always refer to the manufacturer's Prescribing
Information before prescribing drugs cited in this book.

Commissioning Editor: John Harrison
Senior Editorial Controller: Catherine Rickards
Production Controller: Geoff Holdsworth

Typeset by
Creative Associates Ltd., UK

Colour reproduction by
Track Direct, UK

Printed by,
Book Print, S.L. Spain

Distributed in the USA by
Books International, Inc., PO Box 605,
Herndon, VA 20172, USA

Distributed in the rest of the world by
Plymbridge Distributors Ltd., Estover Road,
Plymouth PL6 7PY, UK

Contents

List of contributors

Michael A. Adams
Professor of Pharmacology and Toxicology, Department of Urology, Kingston General Hospital, 76 Stuart Street, Kingston, Ontario K7L 2VY, Canada

Jan Adolfsson
Associate Professor of Urology, Karolinska Institute, Department of Urology, Huddinge University Hospital, S-141 86, Huddinge, Sweden

P. Allen
Clinical Nurse Specialist (Urology), Department of Urology, Royal Hallamshire Hospital, Glossop Road, Sheffield S10 2JF, UK

Stanley E. Althof
Associate Professor, Department of Urology, Case Western Reserve University School of Medicine, University Hospitals of Cleveland, Cleveland, Ohio; Co-director, Center for Sexual and Marital Health, Beachwood, Ohio, USA

Karl-Eric Andersson
Department of Urology, Box 422, University of Virginia Health Sciences Center, Charlottesville, VA 22902-0422, USA

Tricia Barnes
Director, Sexual and Relationship Therapy, Psychiatric and Psychological Consultant Services (PPCS), 14 Devonshire Place, London W1N 1PB, UK

Rupert Beck
Consultant Urologist, Princess Margaret Hospital, Swindon, UK

Jennifer R. Berman
Department of Urology, Boston University School of Medicine, 720 Harrison Avenue, Boston MA 02778, USA

Pierre-Marc G. Bouloux
Reader in Endocrinology, Royal Free Hospital, Pond Street, London NW3 2QG, UK

Peter Boyle
Division of Epidemiology and Biostatistics, European Institute of Oncology, Via Ripamonti 435, 20141 Milan, Italy

Gregory A. Broderick
Associate Professor of Surgery in Urology, Director of the Center for Male Sexual Dysfunction, University of Pennsylvania Health System, 3400 Spruce Street, Philadelphia, PA 19104, USA

Nicholas Burns-Cox
Research Fellow, Bristol Urological Institute, Southmead Hospital, Westbury-on-Trym Bristol BS10 5NB, UK

Culley C. Carson III
Professor and Chief, Division of Urology, UNC School of Medicine, 427 Burnett-Womack Bld, Chapel Hill, NC 27599-7235, USA

Ajay Chavan
Department of Radiology, Medizinische Hochschule Hannover, D-30623, Hannover, Germany

Timothy J. Christmas
Consultant Urological Surgeon, Department of Urology, Charing Cross Hospital, Fulham Palace Road, London W6 8RF, UK

Alex T. Chuang
Department of Urology, University of Virginia School of Medicine, Health Sciences Center, Box 422, Charlottesville VA 22908, USA

Brian Daines
Director, Share Psychotherapy Agency, 176 Crookesmoor Road, Sheffield S6 3FS, UK

Rina M. Davison
Senior Registrar, Department of Endocrinology, Royal Free Hospital, Pond Street, London SW3 2QG, UK

William D. Dunsmuir
Department of Urology, St. George's Hospital, London SW17 0QT, UK

Ian Eardley
Consultant Urologist, Department of Urology, St. James' University Hospital, Becket Street, Leeds, UK

Christine Evans
Consultant Urologist, Ysbyty Glan Clwyd Hospital, Rhyl, Clwyd LL18 5UJ, Wales

Riad N. Farah
Senior Staff Urologist and Vice Chairman, Department of Urology, Henry Ford Hospital, 2799 W. Grand Blvd, Detroit, MI 48202, USA

John M. Fitzpatrick
Professor of Surgery and Consultant Urologist, Mater Misericordiae Hospital and University College Dublin, 47 Eccles Street, Dublin 7, Ireland

Mark M. Foreman
University of Pennsylvania Health System, 3400 Spruce Street, Philadelphia, PA 19104, USA

Clare J. Fowler
Consultant in Uro-Neurology, National Hospital for Neurology and Neurosurgery, UCL Hospitals, Queen Square, London WC1N 3BG, UK

J. Clive Gingell
Consultant Urological Surgeon, Department of Urology, Southmead Hospital, Bristol BS10 5NB, UK

Francois Giuliano
Assistant Professor of Urology, Hôpital de Bicêtre, Service d'Urologie, 78 rue du Général Leclerc, 94275 Le Kremlin Bicêtre, Cedex, France

Irwin Goldstein
Professor of Urology, Boston University School of Medicine, 720 Harrison Avenue, Boston MA 02778, USA

Nestor F. Gonzalez-Cadavid
Department of Surgery, Division of Urology, Urology Research Laboratory, Harbor/UCLA Medical Center, 1000 West Carson Street, Building F-6, Torrance, CA 90506, USA

Jorn Hagemann
Department of Urology, Medizinische Hochschule Hannover, D-30623, Hannover, Germany

Jeremy P. W. Heaton
Professor of Urology, Department of Urology, Queen's University, Kingston General Hospital, 76 Stuart Street, Kingston, Ontario K7L 2V7, Canada

William F. Hendry
Consultant Urologist, St. Bartholomew's and Royal Marsden Hospitals, London, UK

U. Jonas
Professor and Chairman, Department of Urology, Medizinische Hochschule Hannover, D-30623, Hannover, Germany

Gerald H. Jordan
Professor, Department of Urology, Eastern Virginia Medical School, Norfolk; Director, Devine Fiveash Urology Ltd, Genito-urinary Reconstructive Surgery, Norfolk General Hospital, Norfolk, Virginia, USA

Klaus-Peter Jünemann
Associate Professor of Urology, Department of Urology, Klinikum Mannheim gGmBH, Universitätsklinikum, Fakultät für Klinische Medizin Mannheim der Universität Heidelberg, Theodor-Kutzer-Ufer 1, 68135 Mannheim, Germany

Michael G. Kirby
Family Practitioner, The Surgery, Nevells Road, Letchworth, Hertfordshire SG6 4TS, UK

Roger S. Kirby
Consultant Urologist, St. George's Hospital, London SW17 0QT, UK

Robert J. Krane
Department of Urology, Boston University School of Medicine, Boston University Medical Center, 720 Harrison Avenue, Boston MA 02778, USA

R. Krishnan
Chief Resident, Division of Urology, University of North Carolina School of Medicine, Chapel Hill, NC 27599-7235, USA

Michael D. LaSalle
Fellow – Erectile Dysfunction, Department of Urology, Boston University School of Medicine, Boston University Medical Center, 720 Harrison Avenue, Boston MA 02778, USA

William R. Lees
Professor of Radiology, Department of Radiology, The Middlesex Hospital, University College Hospitals London Group, Mortimer Street, London, UK

Laurence A. Levine
Associate Professor of Urology, Rush Medical College; Director of the Male Sexual Function and Fertility Program, Rush Presbyterian–St. Luke's Medical Center, 1725 W Harrison Street, Chicago, IL 60612, USA

Ronald W. Lewis
Professor and Chief of Urology, Medical College of Georgia, 1120 15th Street, Augusta, GA 30912, USA

Joseph LoPiccolo
Professor of Psychology, University of Missouri-Columbia, 210 McAlester Hall, Columbia, MO 65211, USA

Tom F. Lue
Professor of Urology, Department of Urology, University of California, San Francisco School of Medicine, San Francisco, CA 94143-0738, USA

Martina Manning
Department of Urology, Klinikum Mannheim gGmBH, Universitätsklinikum, Fakultät für Klinische Medizin Mannheim der Universität Heidelberg, Theodor-Kutzer-Ufer 1, 68135 Mannheim, Germany

Lesley Marson
University of North Carolina, Division of Urology, 427 Burnett Womack Building Chapel Hill, NC 27599-7235, USA

Jack W. McAninch
Professor and Vice Chairman, Department of Urology, University of California School of Medicine, 1001 Potrero Avenue, Rm 3A20, San Francisco, CA 94110, USA

Kevin E. McKenna
Associate Professor, Department of Physiology, Northwestern University Medical School, 5-755 Tarry Building M211, 303E Chicago Avenue, Chicago, IL 60611, USA

Arnold Melman
Chairman, Department of Urology, Montefiore Medical Center, Henry and Lucy Moses Hospital, 11 E 210th Street, Bronx, NY 10467, USA

Thomas M. Mills
Professor of Physiology and Endocrinology, Medical College of Georgia, Augusta, GA 30912, USA

Suks Minhas
Registrar in Urology, Department of Urology, St. James' University Hospital, Beckett Street, Leeds, UK

Kenneth T. H. Moore
Consultant Urological Surgeon, Clinical Director of Urology, Royal Hallamshire Hospital
Glossop Road, Sheffield S10 2JF, UK

Alvaro Morales
Professor of Urology, Department of Urology, Queen's University, Kingston General Hospital, 76 Stuart Street,
Kingston, Ontario K7L 2V7, Canada

Robert B. Moreland
Assistant Research Professor of Urology and Physiology, Department of Urology, Room W607A, Boston University
School of Medicine, 700 Albany Street, Boston, MA 02118-2394, USA

Ignacio Moncada Iribarren
Jose Jara Rascón, Hospital General Universitario Gregario Marañon, Madrid, Spain

John J. Mulcahy
Professor of Urology, Department of Urology, Indiana University Medical Center, Wishard Memorial Hospital,
1001 W. 10th Street, Indianapolis, IN 46202, USA

John P. Mulhall
Director, Center for Male Sexual Health, Department of Urology, Loyola University Medical Center, Stritch School
of Medicine, 2160 S First Avenue, Maywood IL 60153, USA

Alasdair M. Naylor
Head, Urogenital Diseases, Department of Discovery Biology, Central Research, Pfizer Limited, Sandwich, Kent
CT13 9NJ, UK

Ajay Nehra
Senior Associate Consultant, Mayo Clinic Foundation and Assistant Professor of Urology, Mayo Medical School,
200 First Street SW, Rochester, Minnesota 55905, USA

Don W. W. Newling
Department of Urology, Academic Hospital Vrije Universiteit, P.O. Box 7057, Amsterdam 1007 MB, The
Netherlands

Kenneth S. Nitahara
Chief Resident in Urology, Department of Urology, University of California, San Francisco, CA 94143-0738,
USA

Neil Oakley
Specialist Registrar in Urology, Department of Urology, Royal Hallamshire Hospital, Glossop Road, Sheffield S10
2JF, UK

Ian H. Osterloh
Global Candidate Teamleader, Pfizer Ltd, Ramsgate Road, Sandwich, Kent, CT13 9NJ, UK

Harin Padma-Nathan
Clinical Professor of Urology, Department of Urology, USC School of Medicine, 2025 Zonal Avenue, GH 5900,
Los Angeles; Director, The Male Clinic, Santa Monica, California, USA

Uday Patel
Consultant Radiologist, Department of Diagnostic Radiology, St. George's Hospital, Blackshaw Road, London
SW17 0QT, UK

Tim Pohlemann
Professor of Trauma Surgery, Medizinische Hochschule Hannover, D-30623, Hannover, Germany

John P. Pryor
Consultant Uro-andrologist, The Lister Hospital, Chelsea Bridge Road, London SW1 8RH, UK

Rudolph Raab
Consultant, Department of Abdominal and Transplant Surgery, Medizinische Hochschule Hannover, D-30623, Hannover, Germany

Jacob Rajfer
UCLA Medical Center, Division of Urology Box 5, 1000 W Carson Street, Torrance, CA 90502, USA

David J. Ralph
Consultant Urologist, St. Peter's Hospital; Senior Lecturer, The Institute of Urology, 48 Riding House Street, London W1P 7PN, UK

Olivier Rampin
Lab. Neurobiologie des Fonctions Végétatives, Institut National de la Recherche Agronomique 78352 Jouy-en-Josas Cedex, France

Harpal S. Randeva
Senior Registrar in Endocrinology, The Royal Free Hospital, Pond Street, London NW3 2QG, UK

Jonathan L. Richenberg
Senior Registrar, Department of Radiology, The Middlesex and St. Peters Hospitals, Mortimer Street, London W1N 8AA, UK

David Rickards
University College Hospitals London; The Middlesex Hospital, London W1N 8AA, UK

Raymond C. Rosen
Center for Sexual and Marital Health, Department of Psychiatry, UMDNJ-Robert Wood Johnson Medical School, 675 Hoes Lane, Piscataway, NJ 08854, USA

Iñigo Sáenz de Tejada
Fundacion para la investigacion y el desarrollo en Andrologia, Madrid and Departamento de Investigacion, Hospital Ramon y Cajal, Madrid, Spain

Allen D. Seftel
Assistant Professor, Department of Urology, Case Western University School of Medicine, University Hospitals of Cleveland, 11100 Euclid Avenue, Cleveland, Ohio 44106-5046, USA

Scott Serels
Department of Urology, Montefiore Medical Center, Henry and Lucy Moses Hospital, 11 E 210th Street, Bronx, NY 10467, USA

Pir J. R. Shah
Senior Lecturer and Honorary Consultant Urologist, Academic Unit, Institute of Urology, 48 Riding House Street, London W1P 7PN and St. Peters Hospital UCLH, London; Consultant Urologist to the Spinal Cord Injuries Unit, Royal National Orthopaedic Hospital, Stanmore, Middlesex, UK

Sugandh D. Shetty
Chief Resident in Urology, Henry Ford Hospital, 2799 W. Grand Blvd, Detroit, MI 48202, USA

Jason M. Shuker
Department of Urology, Boston University School of Medicine, 720 Harrison Avenue, Boston MA 02778, USA

Gillian L. Smith
Research Fellow, Department of Urology, Charing Cross Hospital, Fulham Palace Road, London W6 8RF, UK

Martin Spahn
Department of Urology, Klinikum Mannheim gGmBH, Universitätsklinikum, Fakultät für Klinische Medizin Mannheim der Universität Heidelberg, Theodor-Kutzer-Ufer 1, 68135 Mannheim, Germany

William D. Steers
Department of Urology, Box 422, University of Virginia School of Medicine, Health Sciences Center, Charlottesville, VA 22908, USA

Christian G. Stief
Professor of Urology, Department of Urology, Medizinische Hochschule Hannover, D-30623 Hannover, Germany

Justin A. Vale
Consultant Urological Surgeon, St. Mary's Hospital, Praed Street, London W2, UK

Eric Wespes
Department of Urology, University Clinic of Brussels and CHU Charleroi, Brussels, Belgium

Hunter Wessells
Assistant Professor, Section of Urology, University of Arizona College of Medicine, Tucson, Arizona 85724, USA

Christopher R. J. Woodhouse
Reader in Adolescent Urology, Institute of Urology and Nephrology, University College London Medical School, 48 Riding House Street, London W1P 7PN, UK

Michael G. Wyllie
Urodoc Ltd., Maryland, Ridgeway Road, Herne, Kent CT6 7LN, UK

Forewords

Erectile dysfunction affects many millions of men around the world. I suppose that I have been asked to write a foreword for this important book because I have worked all my scientific life on chemical mediators, with a special reference to the circulation. Those mediators that are usually released by the autonomic nervous system, such as acetylcholine and noradrenaline, have long been manipulated by preventing their release, or their activity, or by increasing their effects through inhibition of their breakdown.

In recent years, we have learned that the endothelial cell also exerts a highly important influence over the circulation through the release of mediators such as prostaglandins, nitric oxide (NO) and endothelin-1 (ET-1). Just as important was the subsequent discovery that non-adrenergic, non-cholinergic (NANC) transmission is largely mediated by NO. NANC NO is synthesized by parasympathetic neurons present in cavernous nerves and acts directly on guanylate cyclase in the vascular smooth muscle fibres. Other pro-erectile mediators, such as acetylcholine, calcitonin gene-related peptide or substance P, act by promoting the synthesis of NO in endothelial cells. Even the endothelial vasoconstrictor endothelin-1 has been implicated, working through ET-B-receptor stimulation and endothelial NO release.

The relevance of these chemical mediators to erectile dysfunction is thoroughly explored in this volume. Erection depends on vasodilatation and, as new endogenous vasodilators have been discovered, so they have been explored in erectile dysfunction. Intracavernosal injection of prostaglandin E1 is one of the more successful treatments, but the discovery, in 1986, that endothelium-derived relaxing factor is NO dramatically shifted the focus of attention towards this simple gaseous mediator. The fact that NO is also released by the nitro-vasodilators explains nicely the 'street' reputation of amyl nitrate as an aphrodisiac.

To overcome inadequate NO release, several pharmacological strategies are available. Replacement therapy, either locally or systemically with an NO donor, is possible. At the forefront is the insertion of a pessary into the urethra. NO relaxes smooth muscle by activating guanylate cyclase, leading to the formation of cyclic guanosine monophosphate (cGMP). Inhibition of the phosphodiesterase (PDE) enzyme specific for cGMP (PDE5) is another promising approach, especially as inhibitors are available for oral administration. Chapter 26 describes the clinical efficacy and safety of an orally available PDE5 inhibitor, sildenafil, which is now being marketed highly successfully around the world.

The textbook as a whole is comprehensive; each chapter is written by experts in the field. The basic science covers the history, epidemiology, anatomy and physiology, with good chapters on the chemical mediators involved. Clinical methods of evaluation include psychological and physical assessments. The promise of orally available or non-indictable techniques is fully covered, as is the use of surgery and surgically implanted prostheses.

This volume is most timely in that the problem of erectile dysfunction is clearly now more and more susceptible to pharmacological solutions. I commend it to the reader.

Sir John Vane
Honorary President, William Harvey Research Institute, London

Our understanding of erectile physiology has progressed rapidly in recent years, with the determination of the mechanisms involved at both cellular and molecular levels. Research has also unravelled the complex microscopic anatomy of the penis and has elucidated how messages are relayed between cells to bring about erection. This wealth of information has had important consequences for the many millions of men with impotence, or erectile dysfunction (ED), as it is more commonly known today. Clinicians can now understand the complex process of erectile dysfunction and appreciate that the patient's problems may be due not only to organic causes but also to psychological elements. Added to this knowledge is a vast array of treatment options that are available to the patient. We have even progressed to the point where a pill can potentially be used to overcome ED.

This book provides a comprehensive overview of all aspects of ED and includes contributions from a broad array of experts in the field. The initial section focuses on the history of ED, how widespread the condition is and the risk factors involved in its occurrence. Erectile physiology is reviewed at the vascular, neurological and endocrinological levels. Accurate diagnosis is essential and the progressive stages involved in this process are detailed. Initially, a patient history and sexual inventory is taken, followed by a physical examination and routine laboratory tests; psychological assessment may also be carried out at this stage. On the basis of these results, a number of tests may be appropriate, including nocturnal penile tumescence testing, Doppler imaging and pharmacavernosometry/cavernosography. Therapeutic options based on the diagnosis are reviewed in depth and range from simple vacuum devices to inflatable penile prostheses. Medical therapy may be administered via a number of routes, including cavernosal injection, urethral deposition and orally. Importantly, the complications that may be associated with the particular therapies are included. Of interest to the practising clinician are those patients who present with particular conditions that can give rise to ED, such as diabetes, pelvic injuries, cardiovascular problems and renal failure. These, as well as specific anatomical conditions that cause ED (such as Peyronie's disease, congenital anomalies and phalloplasty), are discussed.

This *Textbook of Erectile Dysfunction* provides an invaluable source of up-to-date information for the clinician treating patients with ED. It is hoped that it will help them not only to pinpoint the correct diagnosis but also to initiate the appropriate therapy. In this way, the quality of life may be improved, not only of the many sufferers of ED but also of their partners.

Gorm Wagner MD PhD
Department of Medical Physiology,
University of Copenhagen, Denmark

Preface

Erectile dysfunction has replaced the term impotence and is defined as the inability to obtain and maintain an erection satisfactory for sexual activity. Erectile dysfunction (or impotence) has plagued men for thousands of years. It has been described since the ancient times in both art and literature. Erectile dysfunction appears in Greek cup paintings, the works of Ovid, the Old Testament of the Bible and the writings of Hippocrates and the Hindus. Opinions regarding its aetiology and risk factors, as well as treatment alternatives, are described in these ancient writings, including cures involving recipes for magical potions and aphrodisiacs. Early physicians and healers were intrigued by the medical treatment of erectile dysfunction using a variety of agents including bifurcated roots of certain plants resembling the human body such as mandrake and ginseng. Although their effectiveness was widely proclaimed, it appears that their effectiveness, as today, was primarily placebo. Masters and Johnson in *Human Sexual Inadequacy*, published in 1970, wrote 'true biophysical dominance in the etiology of impotence is not a frequent occurrence in any reasonably representative clinical series, the incidence of primary physiological influence of impotence is indeed of minor consideration'.

Because sexual function has long been submerged in social and cultural taboos, research into the physiology, pathophysiology and treatment of erectile dysfunction has lagged behind other medical endeavours. Over the past two decades, however, clinical and basic science research has elucidated the physiology of erectile dysfunction in the penis and central nervous system and has led to an improved understanding of this essential bodily function. Similarly, advances in pharmacology, material sciences, surgery, and psychological counselling have combined to improve treatment modalities for restoring erection. In the past two decades, basic research into smooth muscle physiology has progressed and neurotransmitters have been identified to clarify the mechanisms for erectile function. Similarly, new drugs and surgical procedures as well as penile prostheses have been designed for treatment of this major medical condition. With the advent of new oral agents specifically designed to manipulate neurotransmitters in the corpus cavernosum and central nervous system, a revolution in the treatment of erectile dysfunction has begun.

In this textbook, the Editors have assembled an international group of authors whose contributions of recognized authority have been carefully chosen for each chapter in this volume. Each author has been able to bring to the subject significant experience in their area of erectile dysfunction, and to share with the readership this experience and skill in a particular area of reporting. Although the reader will notice some repetition in subject matter, this overlap will serve to demonstrate differences among various authors in approaching the evidence of erectile dysfunction and its management. The clear, concise and complete discussion of erectile dysfunction in this textbook has been made possible by the fine work of the individual contributors, each of whom has provided material that is instructional and valuable to all scientists, physicians and health care providers interested in erectile dysfunction, whether at the beginning of their practice or experts in the field of erectile dysfunction. Owing to the rapid increase in research, knowledge and changes in management of erectile dysfunction, the authors have been able to place skilfully newer technologies for the investigation and management of erectile dysfunction into their proper perspective. This textbook is organized to take the reader in a logical fashion from basic science, epidemiology, clinical evaluation, to treatment of basic and subtle causes of erectile dysfunction. Currently available management techniques are included, as well as discussion of specific clinical problems in erectile dysfunction requiring the expertise, care and skill of urologic surgeons, specialist physicians and psychotherapists.

The Editors hope that the *Textbook of Erectile Dysfunction* will serve its readership by reviewing the science of erectile dysfunction; by discussing controversies in its basic science, diagnosis and management; and by carefully reviewing the field of knowledge of erectile dysfunction for those at all levels of accomplishment in this new and rapidly advancing field.

The Editors would like to acknowledge the efforts of the individual contributors, each of whom has synthesized complex subjects and provided material that will be instructional and valuable to all interested in erectile dysfunction. They also express their sincere appreciation to John Harrison at Isis and to Christine McKillop, medical writer and Heather Russell, copy editor, for their assistance, encouragement and enthusiasm in completing the *Textbook of Erectile Dysfunction*.

C. Carson, R. Kirby, I. Goldstein

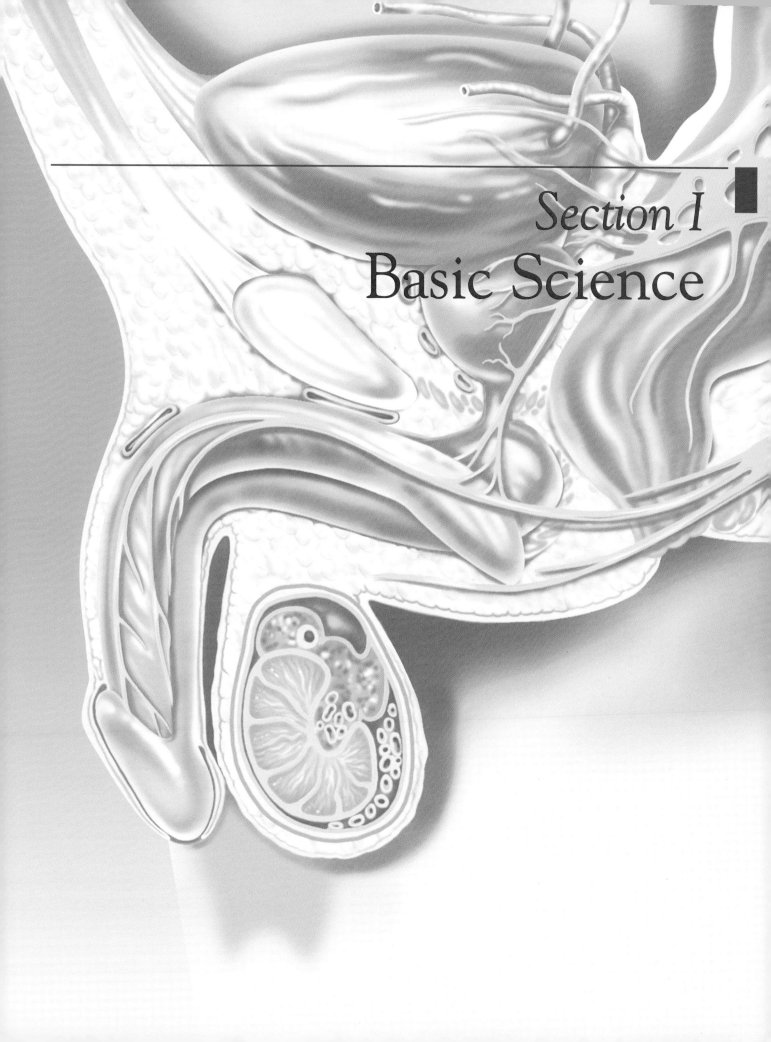

Section I
Basic Science

Chapter 1
History of erectile dysfunction

W. D. Dunsmuir

■ INTRODUCTION

The ability to maintain an erection is something fairly special to the human male. In the vast majority of animals, the act of copulation is quick and the need to maintain an erection for a prolonged period is unnecessary. In the rat, for instance, erection and ejaculation are more or less simultaneous reflex events. For the dog, the average length of the copulation period is about 20 seconds. Even the African ostrich, renowned for his ostentatious display during sexual courtship, has completed the act within a minute.[1]

Throughout the Animal Kingdom, various strategies have evolved to facilitate the entrance of the male phallus into the female genital orifice. Certain mammals, such as the walrus, whale, gibbon and orang-outang, have a degree of ossification within the penile shaft. This bone, or 'os penis', eases vaginal penetration. However, for a few species, survival does not depend on the frenetic deposition of sperm within the female genital tract. Indeed, the *protraction* of sex for pleasure is a feature of copulation that has evolved, perhaps solely, in humans. We can, therefore, assume that erectile failure has been an ever-present problem throughout man's evolutionary history. Furthermore, strategies to deal with impotence are probably as old as man himself and will have included potions, ointments and prayers. This chapter examines the impact of impotence through the ages and traces the development of theory and treatment, from antiquity to the present day.

■ THE IMPACT OF IMPOTENCE THROUGH THE AGES

Throughout history, impotence has influenced society in two major ways. First, unlike many other stigmatized diseases, there has often been an immense associated sense of humiliation. Second, it has had a major impact on determining the validity of marriage in law. In the days when divorce was difficult to obtain, claims of 'non-consummation' were frequently used to 'annul' a marriage. Impotence — a condition difficult to prove — was often levelled at the male party to validate this claim. Furthermore, humiliation has always been a powerful form of social control, and many men have been ridiculed and destroyed by the public exposure of their impotence.

Indeed, the medieval Church took full advantage of this terror and, by the 16th century, ecclesiastic trials for impotence were widespread. Embittered women, and people with inheritance claims based on paternity disputes, would frequently bring victims to the Church Courts for trial. Juries comprising theologians, physicians and midwives demanded that the accused 'prove' himself with a public display of erection and ejaculation. The gallery delighted at these civic displays of voyeurism and the trial reports were printed and distributed in their thousands. So great was the public exhilaration, and so great was the fear generated in men, that these courts bestowed tremendous power to the Church[2] (Fig. 1.1). Indeed, it was in response to the struggle for power between the Church and the State, that the High Court of Paris abolished these shameful Court rituals in 1677.[3]

However, the problem remained very real and the interface between the Law, the Church and the medical profession remained unclear. In 1896, when the Illinois Supreme Court annulled a marriage on the grounds of impotence, a doctor was called to give evidence.[4] This raised an ethical dilemma: when a condition is difficult to prove, then it may require a doctor to break his professional code of confidence. This was the very situation that arose in Illinois. The doctor testified that the cause of the impotence was excessive masturbation. This bizarre case led to the Court ruling that the doctor

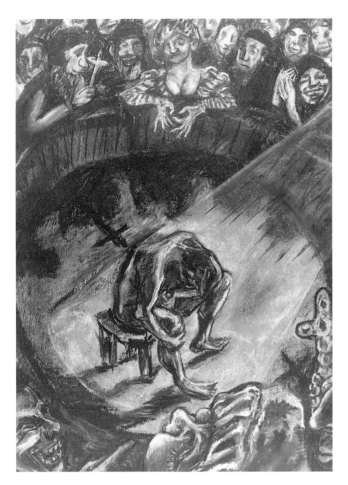

Figure 1.1. Medieval Church Court trial. (Reproduced courtesy of Wilma Cluness.)

must 'over-see' the defendant's attempt at self-restraint in order to test the curability of the condition. The law subsequently changed to introduce the term 'naturally impotent' to the statute. This meant that the cause of the impotence was immaterial but, to this day, impotence remains grounds for annulment of marriage.

Nevertheless, the fear of humiliation has long remained a reason for men to conceal their problem. Since ancient times, this theme of humiliation has coloured the literature. In the *Satyricon* by Petronius, the author describes the fate of Encolpius who was damned to impotence for desecrating the rites of Priapus (the god of fertility). Having been rendered impotent, he was then further humiliated by being forced to undergo a public orgy with the priestess Quartilla.[5] Indeed, exposing the afflicted has for ever been of great public interest. An example can be provided by the case of John Ruskin, the famous 19th century English writer and reformer. Following the public dissolution of his marriage on the

grounds of non-consummation, Ruskin suffered a mental breakdown, retreated from public life and lived his remaining years in isolation.[6] Like so many men, both before and since, the loss of potency led to the crumbling of all feelings of self-worth. It is not surprising that so much time and energy has been spent in finding a cure.

■ FROM ANTIQUITY TO ENLIGHTENMENT

In ancient times, agriculture, animal husbandry and human fertility were all linked by religious ritual. The gods of harvest were worshipped with phallic icons and impotent men turned to the priesthood for help. Gods were invoked to explain and cure impotence. The Ancient Greeks prayed to Aphrodite, and the Bible describes cases of impotence as divine retribution for adultery. In Genesis, God rendered Abimelech impotent for sleeping with Abraham's wife.[7] It is also said that God allowed the Devil power only over the genitals. Indeed, if a witch tied a knot in a strip of leather, the Devil was empowered to strike a man impotent.[8] In medieval times this belief was so widely held that we can only guess as to how many women were burned at the stake in response to men's sexual failings.

The teachings of Hippocrates (~ 400 BC) pervaded Western medical thinking until the Renaissance. Hippocrates stated that erections were generated by *pneuma* (air) and 'vital spirits' flowing into the penis. Any illness, or imbalance between the four humours (blood, phlegm, yellow bile and black bile) and the four elements (earth, air, fire and water), could lead to impotence. Furthermore, as semen was the most potent fraction of male bodily fluid, it was not surprising that a man, having lost vital fluid, should be weakened after ejaculation. Hippocrates believed that sexual excess could reduce potency — a theme that has been re-explored many times over the last 2000 years. Hippocrates also believed that the testes were connected to the penis by fine erectile cords that facilitated erection — rather like a system of 'pulleys'. Damage to these cords (such as would occur with castration) would profoundly affect man's erectile capability.[9]

During the Renaissance, these 'classical' models were challenged by Leonardo da Vinci. He had observed that men executed by hanging, frequently developed reflex erections. When he cut the penises from such men, he found them to be full of blood, not air.[3] Later, in 1677,

Reiner de Graaf demonstrated that erection could be generated in a human cadaver following the injection of water into the internal iliac artery.[10] In 1863, Eckhard demonstrated that erection was a neurovascular phenomenon and, by applying electrical stimulation to the pelvic nerves (nervi erigentes), he was able to induce tumescence in a dog.[11]

THE 19TH TO MID-20TH CENTURY

During the 19th century three main schools of thought developed: first, there were those who believed that impotence had an endocrine cause; second, there were those who believed that the problem could be explained by local genital pathology; third, there was the 'psychogenic' school, whose adherents firmly believed that the problem was rooted in the mind. The manner in which these schools evolved, clashed and fused, is explored in turn below.

The endocrine debate

The association between the testis, male behaviour, potency and fertility, has probably been recognized since man started to practise castration. There is evidence that Neolithic tribes in Asia Minor castrated animals for domestication as early as 4000 BC. The practice in humans probably originated in Babylon in the second millennium BC as a measure against adultery.[12] However, castration has also been practised for many other reasons. For instance, the early Christian priesthood (about the 3rd century AD) practised voluntary castration to help them maintain their self-imposed religious celibacy. In addition, many civilizations would regularly castrate slaves to suppress rebellion. This practice was widespread in the early Eastern Roman Empire, where both the effects on potency and libido and the critical timing of the castration were well understood. Boys castrated before puberty would grow with the recognizable 'eunuchoid' proportions and usually developed a relatively docile personality. Furthermore, as castration made them infertile, they became the ideal guardians for the harems where any carnal transgressions could not result in an illicit pregnancy.

However, the notion that castration would ensure impotence was far from true. The females of the Roman harems often found the eunuchs to be novel playmates: their contraception was guaranteed, and their sexual prowess often intact (Fig. 1.2). In addition, early Christian choirboys, who had been gelded in their youth to ensure the maintenance of their soprano voice, frequently lived sexually active lives. Indeed, Italian literature is replete with stories of these 'castrati' and their sexual cavortings.

In more recent times, the effects of castration on potency have been more clearly defined. The practice still occurs in parts of India, the Middle East and China. For example, the *Hijaras* are an Indian sect of biological males who have been convinced (or coerced) to undergo voluntary castration. They function as transvestite male prostitutes and are ready to indulge in all manner of sexual paraphilia, many being fully potent.[13] Castration for sex crimes was practised until very recently in many European countries; Heim reported that 31% of such men remained potent following emasculation and that rapists were more likely to be sexually active than homosexuals or paedophiles.[14] It is also known that up to 19% of older men who undergo surgical or chemical castration for the treatment of prostate cancer will retain their potency.[15] It has become apparent that castration, performed for whatever reason, will not necessarily render a man impotent.

However, the influence of the testis on sexual behaviour is more complex. Even the most ancient civilizations realized that the testes exert some form of control, not only influencing potency but in some respect affecting libido as well. Not surprisingly, the testes have frequently been the focus for impotence cures. Indeed, Susruta of India (500 BC) advocated the ingestion of

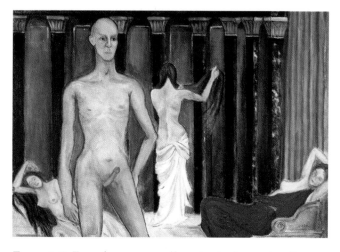

Figure 1.2. Eunuchs were sexually active in the ancient Roman harems. (Reproduced courtesy of Paula Day.)

testicular tissue for the treatment of impotence[12] and, in 1889, Brown-Séquard reported himself to be both 'rejuvenated' and cured of impotence, following the self-injection of an aqueous testicular extract from a dog.[16]

A clear androgenic role for the testis was first shown by Berthold in 1849. His experiments showed that castration of the rooster caused regression of both the comb and wattle and this regression could be prevented by transplanting the testis back into the abdominal cavity.[17] However, defining testicular function was difficult and confusion prevailed for the next 100 years. The problem was twofold: first, methodologies were crude; second, man's desperation to find a solution for both ageing and impotence led to many erroneous conclusions and practices. For example, in spite of sound scientific work by Astley Cooper in 1823, showing that ligation of the vas deferens had no effect on spermatogenic or testicular function,[18] Ancel and Bouin reported different results for the same experiments in 1904. They claimed that vasoligation caused sperm cell atrophy with concomitant Leydig cell hyperplasia and they suggested that ligating the vasa might increase the endogenous male hormone production, resulting in benefits to both potency and well-being[19] (Fig. 1.3).

The excitement generated by these observations led many doctors to explore this idea as a method to cure

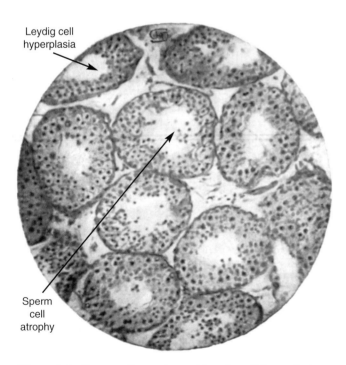

Figure 1.3. Sperm cell atrophy and Leydig cell hyperplasia as described in ref. 19.

(labels on figure: Leydig cell hyperplasia; Sperm cell atrophy)

impotence. In 1917, the Austrian surgeon Professor Steinach conducted many vasal ligations on ageing rams. His studies seemed to provide clear evidence that these animals were markedly 'rejuvenated'. Encouraged by his findings, he applied the principle to humans, and numerous vasoligations were performed on impotent men.[20] Even more alarming were the transplantation techniques of Voronoff[21] in France and Lespinasse[22] in Chicago (Fig. 1.4), both of whom performed transplantations of testicular grafts from apes, either directly into the human testis, or into the subtunical space (Fig. 1.5b,c). However, despite initial claims of success, this procedure did not restore the 'fountain of youth' nor did it cure impotence. The credibility of the proponents was called into question and, by the early 1930s, many clinicians were beginning to challenge the work of the 'rejuvenationists'.[23] One of the most eloquent and ferocious challenges was published by T.E. Hammond in the *British Journal of Urology*, in 1934.[24] He questioned the role of the testis in erection physiology. He reviewed a series of his own adult castrates; these were men who had lost both testes through accident or tuberculosis, and he reported that they all had retained their potency. Furthermore, the early 20th century was also a time when many urologists were practising castration to cure the symptoms of prostatic enlargement. Naturally, they were keen to stress that impotence was an infrequent consequence of this procedure.[25,26] Vasoligations were also being performed for prostatic enlargement and the lack of efficacy in terms of both prostatic shrinkage and improved erectile function had been well documented long before the 'rejuvenating' operations became fashionable.[27] Clearly, the medical profession was in a mess.

Fortunately, careful scientific studies gradually clarified male genitourinary and reproductive physiology.[28] In 1934, W.E. Lower cleverly demonstrated the pituitary gonadotrophic control of the testis. By creating a peritoneal anastomosis between two rabbits (coelenteral fusion), he was able to develop an experimental model whereby he could selectively ablate the endocrine system at many different levels. In doing so, he conclusively showed that the maintenance of prostatic, erectile and testicular function was under pituitary control[29] (Fig. 1.6).

Another great contemporary advance came in 1931 when Butenandt succeeded in isolating 15 mg of androsterone from 25 000 litres of policemen's urine.[30] This was followed by the synthesis of testosterone from

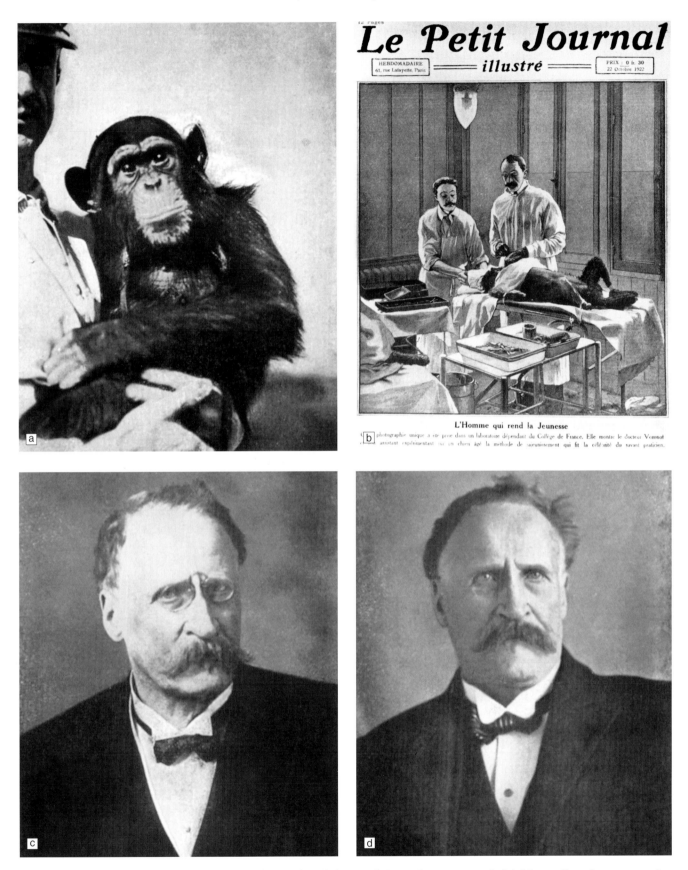

Figure 1.4. (a) Voronoff with his monkey. (Reproduced from ref. 21 with permission.) (b) Voronoff performs testicular transplantation from a monkey to a man. (c,d) As witnessed by his countenance, an elderly man is rejuvenated and has his potency restored following testicular transplantation. (Reproduced from ref. 21 with permission.)

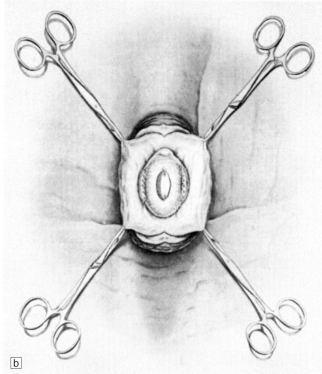

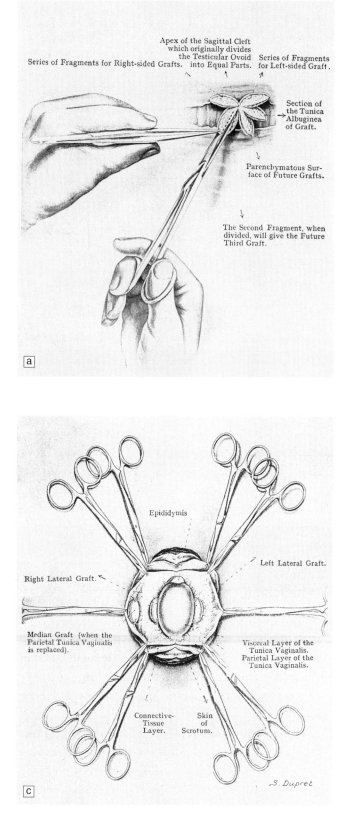

Figure 1.5. (a,b) Direct grafting into the tunica albuginea. (c) Grafting into the subtunical space. (Reproduced from ref. 21 with permission.)

consumption of anabolic–androgenic steroids, both legally and illegally. The expansion of this industry has enabled a greater understanding of how endocrine agents can affect both erectile and sexual function. The effects vary, depending on the dose, administration and circumstances of both use and abuse but, in general, hormone supplementation rarely improves erectile function.[9] Even to this day, the roles of androgens in the maintenance of erectile function remain poorly understood. However, for the impotent man at the beginning of the 20th century, the endocrine confusions served only to cloud the other two great controversies of the day.

The 'organic' versus 'psychogenic' debate

During the late 19th and early 20th century, proponents of the 'organic' and the 'psychogenic' schools frequently clashed in acrimonious debate. Sigmund Freud had founded the discipline of psychoanalysis in the late 19th century. His followers sought to explain impotence in terms of regression of unresolved conflicts into the unconscious mind. Freud had believed that healthy

cholesterol by Ruzicka in 1935.[31] In 1939, both men shared the Nobel prize for chemistry, following which a whole industry spawned with the development and

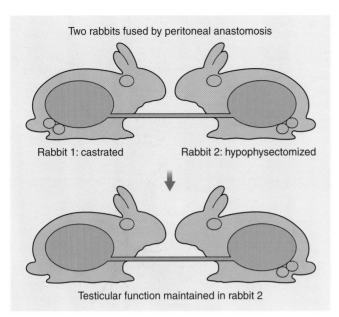

Figure 1.6. The ingenious coelenteral fusion model of W.E. Lower.[29]

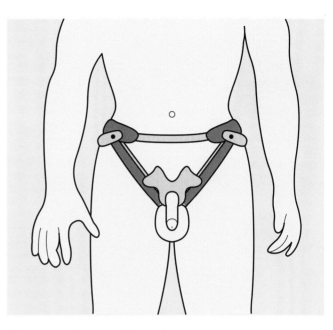

Figure 1.7. Antimasturbatory device.

psychological development required the experience of an Oedipus complex — a stage in infant sexual development constituting the erotic attachment of the child to the parent of the opposite sex. This coincided with hostile feelings towards the other parent. Freud's disciples believed that in later adult life, transference of these feelings to a new sexual partner could result in inner conflict, and this often resulted in impotence.

The psychoanalytic approach was championed by many influential psychiatrists but, realistically, treatment was available only to the rich. For most men who did seek medical help, the general advice was to 'resensitize' the erectile mechanism by abstaining from sex for long periods. Excess masturbation was blamed by many doctors and great anxieties were generated among the youth, who feared they would 'fail' in later married life, if they continued to masturbate.[32] Indeed, in 1927, the psychoanalytic school reported that repressed sexuality was responsible for at least 95% of cases of impotence[33] and specially designed antimasturbatory devices were constructed and prescribed (Fig. 1.7). In 1934, a joint statement was made by a group of New York psychiatrists, which effectively declared 'open war' with the urologists of the day. In this statement, they urged general practitioners not to refer their patients to urologists, and so fuelled a bitter debate that raged in the medical literature of the day. Psychiatrists accused urologists of charlatanism, and urologists defended their practice with

elaborate descriptions of the many pathologies that they claimed to observe.[34]

Thomas Curling's classic publication in 1878 summarized the many factors that were thought to be important.[35] He described a wide range of identifiable pathologies, venereal disease in particular, and he was probably one of the first people to associate impotence with both diabetes and Peyronie's disease. However, of greater contemporary significance was his description of the cystoscopic appearances of the verumontanum. Many urologists believed that they frequently observed inflamed swellings of this posterior urethral structure in patients with erectile failure. Indeed, Wolbarst, reviewing 300 cases of impotence, claimed that 87% of patients had pathological posterior urethral changes.[36] The significance of all this was most eloquently summarized in 1936 by Max Huhner, who mounted a sterling defence of contemporary urological practice.[37] Huhner defined a model of perpetual prostatic 'irritation' caused by these urethral swellings. The result was a constant desire ('like an itch') for sexual excess. Men would, therefore, indulge too frequently in either coitus or masturbation and so desensitize their central erectile centres, leading to impotence[37] (Fig. 1.8). Treatment was aimed at reducing this itch. Cauterization of the posterior prostatic urethra along with the urethral instillation of cantharides was common urological practice.[37] Many practitioners, including both psychiatrists (such as W.A. Hammond)[38]

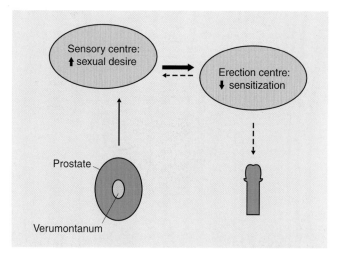

Figure 1.8. Perpetual prostatic irritation resulting in desensitization of the erectile centres. (Adapted from ref. 37 with permission.)

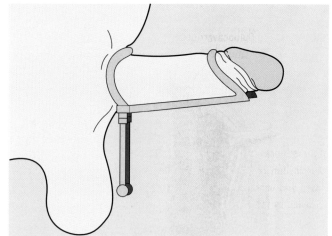

Figure 1.10. Penile 'scaffold'.

and urologists (such as Curling),[35] applied faradic electrical current to the penis, prostatic urethra and spinal cord in an attempt to reduce the central nervous system 'bombardment' and so resensitize the erection centre (Fig. 1.9).

However, all treatment was disappointing. Psychoanalysis, aphrodisiacs, vasoligation, testicular grafting, forced abstention and desensitization by whatever method, helped but a few. More practical devices, such as suction pumps and penile supports (scaffolds), were introduced early in the 20th century (Fig. 1.10). Many devices were patented, and some sold by the thousand.[39]

Various other surgical manoeuvres were tried, including dorsal vein ligation to retard the outward flow of blood from the penis. This was first advocated by Wooten in 1902[40] and then championed by Lilienthal in the 1930s.[37] Further attempts to impede the venous outflow included the ischiocavernosal muscle plication of Lowsley and Bray (1936)[41] (Fig. 1.11). Despite claims of great success, the latter procedure has passed into obscurity and the former has drifted in and out of fashion ever since.

■ THE POST-WAR PERIOD

By the end of the Second World War, many pilots and soldiers had lost their genitalia through burn injuries and land mines, respectively. The early post-war period saw the development of plastic surgical penile reconstruction. In 1948 Bergman fashioned a new penis over an autografted rib cartilage[42] (Fig. 1.12). Such techniques were later extended to treat impotence, but, unfortunately, they were limited by the fact that eventually reabsorption of the cartilage occurred. However, it paved the way for prosthetic implant surgery and, by 1964, Loeffler had reported on the insertion of acrylic rods into the penis to treat impotence.[43] Subsequently, numerous and more sophisticated devices have been designed and are now in common use.

The post-war period was also a time of changing attitudes towards impotence. Before the war, male sexual dysfunction was taboo and free discussion was largely repressed. Indeed, as remarked by Lesley Hall, even the sad heroes of the great early 20th century literary works — Hemingway's Jake Barnes in *The Sun Also Rises*, and

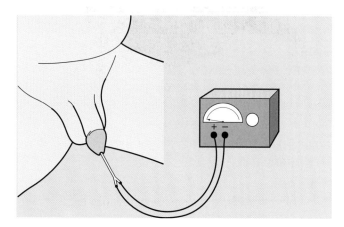

Figure 1.9. Faradic electrical desensitization of the verumontanum.

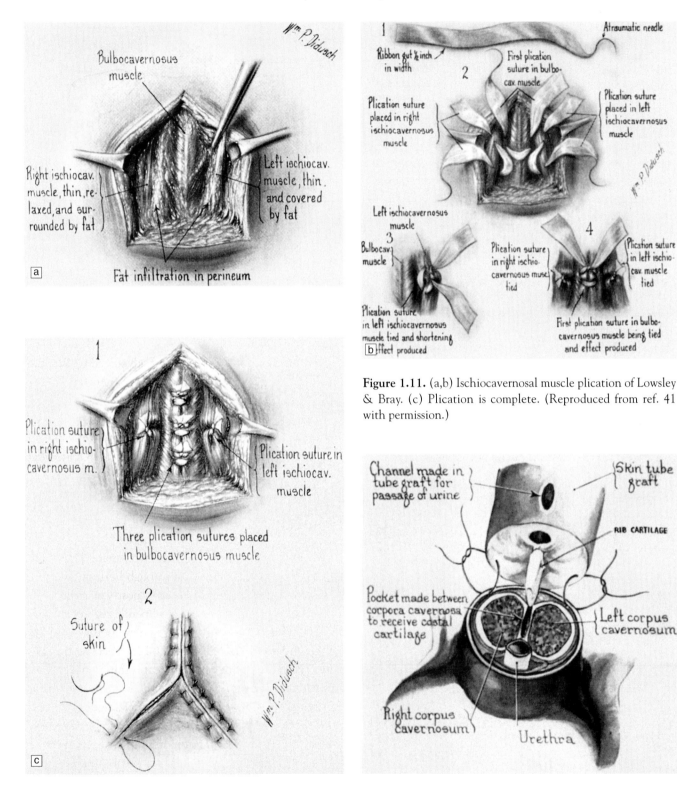

Figure 1.11. (a,b) Ischiocavernosal muscle plication of Lowsley & Bray. (c) Plication is complete. (Reproduced from ref. 41 with permission.)

Figure 1.12. Autograft of rib cartilage. (Reproduced from ref. 42 with permission.)

D.H. Lawrence's Clifford Chatterley in *Lady Chatterley's Lover* — had sustained their impotence as unfortunate victims of war.[6] People did not feel comfortable identifying with men who were deficient through lack of their 'manliness'. However, with the publication of the Kinsey report in 1948, the widespread prevalence of the problem was realized.[44] Changes in attitudes have been slow but, gradually, a greater openness has evolved and more men are prepared to seek help from their doctors.

The 1960s and 70s heralded the arrival of Masters and Johnson,[45] Helen Kaplan[46] and a renaissance from which were born the 'new sexual therapies'. In 1982, Virag[47] and Brindley[48] introduced the effective intracavernosal agents papaverine and phentolamine, respectively. Prostaglandins and other agents have recently been added to the therapeutic options and, with the development of erectile tissue-specific phosphodiesterase inhibitors, an effective oral erectogenic agent is now a reality. Increasingly, psychologists, physicians and surgeons work together with a multidisciplinary approach and the many competing factors are recognized.

A great deal has been achieved since the days when men first prayed to the goddess Aphrodite for deliverance. Many causes of erectile failure have been identified and the underlying pathology defined. Furthermore, attitudes have changed and effective remedies are often available. However, for those who are affected the feeling of destruction remains the same and still the solutions are imperfect. The many causes of erectile dysfunction are still not fully understood; treatments remain crude, and patient and doctor alike hope that the current strategies will soon be replaced with something even better.

■ REFERENCES

1. Sambraus H H. The sexual behavior of the African ostrich (Struthio camelus). Tierarztl Prax 1994; 22: 538–541

2. Darmon P. Damning the innocent. A history of the persecution of the impotent in pre-revolutionary France. New York: Viking Penguin, 1986: 1–234

3. Van Driel M F, Van de Wiel H B M, Mensink H J A. Some mythologic, religious and cultural aspects of impotence before the present modern era. Int J Impot Res 1994; 6: 163–169

4. Editorial Panel. Impotence and the law. JAMA 1896; 27: 1074

5. Johnson J. Literary and historical aspects of disorders of sexual potency. In: Johnson J (ed) Disorders of sexual impotence in the male. London: Pergamon Press, 1968: 1–9

6. Hall L A. 'The most miserable of all patients': male sexual problems in the consulting room. In: Hall L A (ed) Hidden anxieties. Cambridge: Polly Press, 1991: 114–122

7. The Bible. Gen 20: 3

8. Trethowan W H. The demonopathology of impotence. J Ment Sci 1963; 109: 341–346

9. Hippocrates. Airs, waters and places. In: Chadwick A J, Mann W N (eds) Hippocratic writings. London: Penguin, 1987: 47–64

10. de Graaf R. Tractatus de Virorum Organis. In: Opera Omnia. Ex Officina Hackiana 1667: 1–53

11. Eckhard C. Untersuchungen uber die erection des penis beim hunde. Beitr Anat Physiol 1863; 3: 123–150

12. Newerla G J. The history of the discovery and isolation of the male hormone. N Engl J Med 1943; 228: 39–47

13. Jani S, Rosenberg L A. Systematic evaluation of sexual functioning in eunuch-transvestites: a study of 12 cases. J Sex Marital Ther 1990; 16: 103–110

14. Heim N. Sexual behaviour of castrated sex offenders. Arch Sex Behav 1981; 10: 11–19

15. Rousseau L, Dupont A, Labrie F, Couture M. Sexuality changes in prostate cancer patients receiving antihormonal therapy combining the anti-androgen flutamide with medical (LHRH agonist) or surgical castration. Arch Sex Behav 1988; 17: 87–98

16. Brown-Séquard E C. The effects produced in man by subcutaneous injections of a liquid obtained from the testicles of animals. Lancet 1889; 2: 105–107

17. Berthold A A. Transplantation des Hoden [Transplantation of testicles]. Arch Anat Physiol Wiss Med 1849; 16: 42–46

18. Cooper A P. Observations on the structure and diseases of the testis. London: S. McDowall, Leadenhall Street, 1830: 51

19. Bouin, Ancel. Tractus genital et testicule chez le pore cryptorchide. CR Soc Biol (Paris) 1904; 56: 281–282

20. Thorek M. Steinach's vasoligation experiments and so-called rejuvenation operation. In: The human testis. Philadelphia: Lippincott, 1942: 285–297

21. Voronoff S. Rejuvenation by grafting. London: George Allen and Unwin 1925: 1–67

22. Lespinasse V D. Impotency: its treatment by transplantation of the testicle. Surg Clin Chicago 1918; 2: 281–288

23. Walker K M. Surgical treatment of impotence. In: Difficulties in the male. London: Jonathan Cape, 1934: 92–97

24. Hammond T E. The function of the testis after puberty. Br J Urol 1934; 6: 128–141

25. O'Neill T. Castration for prostate problems in the 1900's. Br J Sex Med 1995: 16–17

26. White J W. The results of double castration in hypertrophy of the prostate. Ann Surg 1895; 22: 1–80

27. Wood A C. The results of castration and vasectomy in hypertrophy of the prostate gland. Ann Surg 1900; 32: 309–350

28. Parkes A S. The rise of reproductive endocrinology, 1926–1940. J Endocrinol 1966; 34: 20–32

29. Lower W E. The exocrine and endocrine functions of the testis. J Urol 1934; 31: 391–396

30. Butenandt A, Tscherning K. Uber Androsteron, ein Krystallisiertes Mannliches Sexualhormon I. Isoliereng und Reindarstellung aus Mannerharn [Androsterone, a crystalline male sex hormone I. Isolation and purification of urine.] Z Physiol Chem 1934; 229: 167–184

31. Ruzicka L, Wettstein A. Uber die Krystalliche Herstellung des Testikelhormons, Testeron (Androsten-3-on-17-ol) [The crystalline production of the testicle hormone, testosterone (Androsten-3-on-17-ol)]. Helv Chim Acta 1935; 18: 986–994

32. Hammond W A. Some remarks on sexual excesses in adult life as a cause of impotence. Va Med Mon 1883; 10: 145–150

33. Stekel W. Impotence in the male. New York: Liveright, 1927: 100–125

34. Ballenger E G, Elder O F, McDonald P H. Impotence. J Urol 1936; 36: 250–254

35. Curling T B. Functional disorders of the testicle: impotency. In: Diseases of the testis, spermatic cord and scrotum. London: Churchill, 1878: 429–465

36. Wolbarst A L. Urological aspects of sexual impotence. J Urol 1933; 29: 77–82

37. Huhner M. Masturbation and impotence from a urological standpoint. J Urol 1936; 36: 770–784

38. Meyer M. Electricity in its relation to medical practice. New York: Appleton, 1874: 91–108

39. Loewenstein J. History and literature of mechanotherapy. In: The treatment of impotence: with special reference to mechanotherapy. London: Hamish Hamilton, 1947: 13–21

40. Wooten J S. Ligation of the dorsal vein of the penis as a cure for atonic impotence. Tex State Med J 1902; 18: 325–327

41. Lowsley O S, Bray J L. The surgical relief of impotence: further experiences with a new operative procedure. JAMA 1936; 107: 2029–2035

42. Bergman R T, Howard A H, Barnes R W. Plastic reconstruction of the penis. JAMA 1948; 59: 1174–1180

43. Loeffler R A, Sayegh E S, Lash H. The artificial os penis. Plast Reconstr Surg 1964; 34: 71–74

44. Kinsey A C, Pomeroy W B, Martin C E, Gebhard P H. Sexual behaviour in the human male. Philadelphia: Saunders, 1948: 120–167

45. Masters W H, Johnson V E. Human sexual inadequacy. London: Churchill, 1970: 3–97

46. Kaplan H. The new sex therapy. New York: Brunner/Mazel, 1974: 10–27

47. Virag R. Intracavernous injection of papaverine for erectile failure. Lancet 1982; 2: 938

48. Brindley G S. Cavernosal alpha-blockade: a new technique for investigating and treating erectile impotence. Br J Psychiatry 1983; 143: 332–337

Chapter 2

Epidemiology of erectile dysfunction

P. Boyle

■ INTRODUCTION

There is a centuries-old tradition that 'impotence' is a consequence of witchcraft or satanic magic.[1] In European culture, the issue is of masculinity with the capacity for a strong erection symbolic of the strong man. Bancroft[2] reviews the history of impotence and the historical literature. The frequency of impotence has not been well investigated until recently and one of the major difficulties is the sensitivity of the information, with respondents tending to give unreliable replies.[3] For example, Marsey et al.[4] investigated the occurrence of impotence in a large cohort of men who had undergone vasectomy, together with an equally large control group. Hidden among questions about many aspects of health and well-being were questions about impotence. These produced incidence estimates of approximately 17 new cases per 100 000 man-years.[4] This is slightly lower than the incidence rate of bladder cancer in the same community and difficult to believe. The epidemiological investigation of impotence has also been held back by the lack of a clear and common definition of the condition.

Impotence is the persistent failure to develop and maintain erections of sufficient rigidity for penetrative sexual intercourse. The disorder is common enough, from all accounts, but there are few reliable data available about the population prevalence. Many patients, and even their doctors, are still very reluctant to discuss such problems and, consequently, a large proportion of both the public and the medical profession are ignorant about available treatment options.[5]

The general terminology used to describe this condition has been moving away from the highly emotive term impotence towards a more widely descriptive term erectile dysfunction (ED). Today it is recognized that the causes of ED are frequently multiple, with psychological, neurological, endocrinological, vascular, traumatic and iatrogenic components described. Very little high-quality epidemiological investigation of ED has been undertaken and completed, so that the relative importance of each of these groups of causes to the overall burden of impotence in the community is unknown at present. There are incomplete indications of a precise role of environmental or lifestyle factors in the development of impotence, although smoking, hypertension, hyperlipidaemia, diabetes mellitus and the presence of vascular disease have been proposed as potential risk factors.[5] Research on ED proceeded for many years in parallel among the psychological community and the medical community and it was only after the two groups began serious interaction that true progress was made. Neither group would admit the importance of issues in the other's domain as a cause of this problem: surgeons pronounced that 80–90% of impotence is caused by physical, not psychological, problems,[6] whereas sex therapists have to come to terms with the fact that many men with erectile dysfunction, possibly as many as 50%, have physical abnormalities that contribute to their erectile problems.[1]

The epidemiology of ED is so poorly understood that to entitle a chapter 'Epidemiology of erectile dysfunction', giving the indication that there was some certainty about any statements, is a little presumptuous. In this chapter, the author discusses some of the epidemiological data available, puts it in some perspective and outlines the basic requirements necessary to understand more completely the epidemiological picture.

■ ERECTIONS AND THE CAUSES OF DYSFUNCTION

Sexual arousal is a function of great evolutionary antiquity and is often best understood by specialists in research on human nature, such as sociobiologists. Sexual arousal in men is, in some important respects, quite different from sexual arousal in women, particularly with regard to the stimuli and experiences that are optimally exciting.[7] Sexual arousal to erotic stimuli diminishes as initially highly exciting stimuli lose their ability to create arousal with habituation. This has also been shown in laboratory animals, where the male quickly tires of the same partner but whereby rates of intercourse are quickly restored if a fresh partner is found.[8] Farm animals, such as bulls and rams, have a marked preference for novel females: for example, rams introduced to the same partner have a much longer time to ejaculation (around 17 minutes) compared with rams introduced to different partners at the same rate (around 2 minutes).[9] Thus, it could be possible that factors such as habituation could play a part in the development of ED although there are physiological mechanisms as well as psychological mechanisms that must be kept in mind in the potential aetiology of erectile dysfunction.

In simple terms, erection of the penis depends on the adequate filling of the paired corpora cavernosa with blood at systolic pressure (or even slightly above).[5] Erection occurs when the tonically contracted cavernosal and helicine arteries relax, increasing blood flow to the lacunar spaces and resulting in engorgement of the penis. Relaxation of the trabecular smooth muscle of the corpora cavernosa is mediated by acetylcholine, which acts on endothelial cells causing them in turn to release a further non-adrenergic non-cholinergic carrier of the relaxation signal. The strongest suspect for this second carrier is currently nitric oxide, although other candidates, particularly vasoactive intestinal polypeptide, cannot be entirely ruled out at present.[10]

Thus, the search for aetiological factors in erectile dysfunction has certain clues to begin with: factors that interfere with the filling of the corpora cavernosa, with the blood flow to the lacunar spaces, or with the production and regulation of nitric oxide (or other carriers of the relaxation signal) are prime suspects for any aetiological investigation.

Erectile dysfunction is not always, however, the failure of some mechanical or biochemical process: sexual function cannot be considered on its own without bearing in mind the concept of sexuality. The human sexual response is a complex, multifaceted phenomenon that is not completely, or nearly, understood by anyone at present. Problems with potency are frequently multifactorial in origin.

In nervous or anxious men, increased sympathetic tone and raised circulating catecholamine concentrations may interfere with the mechanisms of smooth muscle relaxation underlying erection. Psychogenic impotence is self-perpetuating: each failure increases the associated anxiety levels and frequently can lead to the continual failure to have erections. This is the commonest cause of intermittent erectile dysfunction in young men, although it is usually secondary to organic dysfunction from middle age onwards.[11]

Free serum testosterone concentrations fall progressively with age, while erectile dysfunction increases in frequency. Falling testosterone levels are associated with a loss of libido and reduced frequency of erections,[5] although the straightforward restoration of circulating androgen levels often does not restore sexual function. This underlines, once again, the complex nature of male sexual function and the interplay with sexuality.

Although endocrinological impotence frequently is a consequence of poorly understood processes, neurogenic impotence often can have a precise cause attributed. Several neurological disorders can impair erectile function, although it is unusual — but not completely unknown — for impaired erectile function to be the sole manifestation of diseases or disorders of the nervous system. Peripheral neuropathies, most frequently associated with alcoholism or diabetes, are associated with impotence.

Probably the most important causes of erectile dysfunction are impaired blood flow to the penis or excessive leakage from the penis; frequently, both are present. In older men, reduced blood flow into the penis due to atherosclerotic lesions of the internal iliac, pudendal and cavernosal arteries is the most common cause.[11,12] With large increases taking place in the ageing population,[13] vascular impotence will take on ever-increasing importance in urological practice.

■ BASIC EPIDEMIOLOGICAL CONSIDERATIONS

The most useful definition of epidemiology is that it is the scientific study of the distribution and determinants of disease in humans.[14] From this evolves the two components of descriptive epidemiology — the description of disease incidence, mortality and prevalence by persons, place and time — and analytical epidemiology — the search for determinants of disease risk that may serve to increase prospects for prevention.

Determination of disease frequency, the first step towards geographical and temporal comparisons, relies on a definition (or at least on a working epidemiological definition) of the disease or condition under investigation. ED shares with the other common urological condition of benign prostatic hyperplasia (BPH)[15] the absence of a unifying definition of which the sensitivity and specificity can be determined. This is a fundamental problem that requires resolution. It should also be a priority to establish a system of classification, after determination of the severity and 'cause' of erectile dysfunction.

Many questionnaires have been developed in the hope of achieving this (among other goals),[16] although many have suffered from being too long and fussy with detail. Recently, two questionnaire-based symptom scales have been developed[17,18] that employ modern concepts of psychometric methodology and that attempt to overcome the inherent difficulties experienced with earlier attempts. The brief Sexual Function Index (SFI)[17] covers the domains of sexual drive, erection, ejaculation, perceptions of problems in each of these areas and overall satisfaction in a total of nine questions. The International Index of Erectile Dysfunction (IIEF)[18] has been developed and covers in 15 questions the domains of erectile function, orgasmic function, sexual desire, intercourse satisfaction and overall satisfaction. The similarity of these two instruments, both developed on the basis of detailed statistical analysis, is very reassuring. Time is necessary to observe which comes into the forefront of international usage, although the shorter version of O'Leary and his colleagues[17] has its attractions, if all other things are equal (i.e. if the questionnaires perform similarly).

A particular problem surrounds the probability of a man declaring his impotence and, to a large extent, this can be influenced by aspects of sexuality. There will be couples who accept the reduction in sexual activity and potency as a natural consequence of ageing (and many may, in fact, be pleased and relieved). In similar circumstances, others will be extremely concerned and upset. Such facets of sexuality will have a strong influence on who comes to the doctor or who admits to the interviewer that they have erectile dysfunction. Frequency of self-reports is not to be trusted and consequently will bias any epidemiological study that would investigate the aetiology of the phenomenon. Solstad and Hertoft[19] interviewed 100 men who had previously completed a questionnaire regarding erectile dysfunction: whereas less than 4% of all men who completed the questionnaire (16 of 439) reported erectile dysfunction, among the 100 men from the initial sample who were subsequently interviewed, nearly 40% reported some kind of sexual dysfunction. Interestingly, only 7% found their problems abnormal for their age and only 5% indicated that they would seek treatment for their problems.[19]

◼ DESCRIPTIVE EPIDEMIOLOGY OF ERECTILE DYSFUNCTION

The reported frequency of erectile problems in completely unrepresentative samples is very similar. For example, Sanders[20,21] reports an analysis of responses to two surveys published in *Woman* magazine: 7% of men reported themselves to have erectile problems compared with 8% of women who made the same report. Frank et al.[22] studied 100 married couples and reported that 7% had difficulty in getting an erection; the same figure (in a study of 58 men) was reported by Nettelbladt and Uddenberg.[23] Even although the figures are all so similar, this may just reflect the effects of the same major biases that have been outlined above.

Many of these (and similar previous) reports on the frequency of erectile dysfunction are of very limited value, being based on poor epidemiological methodology and likely to be biased in directions that are frequently difficult for the reader to determine; these should be discarded immediately. Even in many recent reports, the methods for obtaining study populations have differed, the definitions of impotence have varied widely from study to study, and stratified information of prevalence by age has frequently been omitted completely or has been unreliable owing to the small numbers of subjects in each of the age classes. These are catastrophic failures from the point of view of comparison of rates. However, some limited data are available regarding the occurrence of ED.

Among 1180 men attending a medical outpatient clinic, Slag et al.[24] observed that 34% reported impotence to their interviewers. These were attendees at a medical outpatient clinic and may differ from the general population in having over-representation of diabetes, hypertension and other vascular diseases.

Erectile dysfunction is the most common presenting symptom among men attending sexual problem clinics. For example, in Edinburgh, over a 3-year period, over one-half of all men presenting at this clinic reported erectile dysfunction as their main complaint. The next most common complaint was premature ejaculation,[25] which was reported by 13% of the men. Of these men, over one-half (52%) had some other condition that contributed to their erectile dysfunction: 32% arterial, 21% neurological, 29% urological and 19% diabetes mellitus.[25] In a similar clinic in Singapore, 72.5% of men attending the Sexual Dysfunction Clinic at Toa Payoh Hospital had erectile dysfunction due to organic causes with the remaining 27.5% of patients having erectile dysfunction due to psychogenic causes.[26] Of the patients with organic impotence, in 81% of cases this could be attributed to the effects of diabetes and vascular disease.[27]

In a small study (212 family practice patients) with a young mean age (37 years), 27% of men, on detailed questioning, reported being impotent.[27] The small sample and the young average age argue strongly against the representativeness of these findings to a community, however.

Morley[28] determined the prevalence of impotence to be 27% in men of more than 50 years of age undergoing a general health screening. In terms of size of the sample and the mean age of the men, this sample is better than most. However, it is still hindered by the lack of definition of the term impotence and is potentially biased, for reasons associated with the discussion in the previous section.

Diokno and colleagues included questions about sexual activity and its correlates in a clinic examination, whose participants were identified by a household survey of a probability sample of Washtenaw County, Michigan, USA. Men were aged 60 years and over and were questioned with regard to medical, epidemiological and social aspects of ageing.[29] Of married men, 73.8% reported that they were sexually active (whereas the corresponding figure for married women was 55.8%), with levels decreasing with age. Overall, 35.3% of men included in this sample reported that they were impotent.

Feldman and his colleagues conducted the most useful and comprehensive study of the epidemiology of impotence until the present time.[30] The study sample

consisted of respondents to the Massachusetts Male Ageing Study (MMAS): this was a cross-sectional, random sample survey of health status and related issues in men aged between 40 and 70 years. The MMAS was conducted between 1987 and 1989 in 11 randomly selected towns in the Boston area of Massachusetts, USA. Of 1709 respondees, 1209 men provided complete responses and constitute the sample on which the findings were based. Although the 419 men excluded did not differ from the study sample with respect to all essential variables, a 2/3 non-response rate to sexual questions should be a cause for some hard cynical questioning. A total of 291 men did not respond because they had no sexual partner, and this could bias the prevalence downward. Discriminant analysis was employed to create an impotence scale of nil, minimal, moderate and complete impotence, which was accorded to each individual in the survey.[30]

Between the fifth and seventh decades, the probability of complete impotence almost tripled, from 5.1% to 15% (Fig. 2.1); 60% of men were potent in their fifth decade, whereas only 33% were potent at 70 years.[30]

Of 1680 men who participated in the (free) Prostate Cancer Awareness Week and who were invited to complete a self-administered questionnaire containing questions on urinary symptoms, impotence, quality of life and age, 1517 answered the questionnaire, a response rate of 90.3%.[31] A total of 129 men (7.7%) had not had any erections during the previous 12 months. Of subjects who

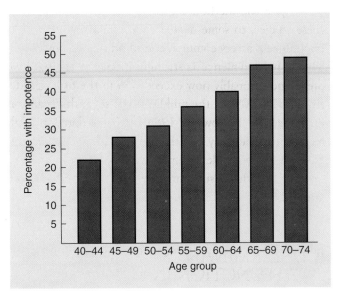

Figure 2.1. Probability of complete or moderate impotence in Massachusetts Male Ageing Survey.[30]

reported that they had experienced erections during the previous 12 months, 12.4% had had erections on less than one occasion in five when sexually stimulated during the last month. There was a striking association between the frequency of varying degrees of impotence and age.

Sexual function was assessed in the prospective Olmsted County Study of Urinary Symptoms and Health Status Among Men, involving a random sample of men living there.[32] The prevalence of sexual problems and erectile dysfunction increased with age. Comparison of men aged 70–79 years with men aged 40–49 years indicated that older men were more worried about sexual function (46.6% vs 24.9%), had worsened performance compared with a year ago (30.1% vs 10.4%), expressed extreme dissatisfaction with sexual performance (10.7% vs 1.7%), had an absence of sexual drive (25.9% vs 0.6%) and reported complete erectile dysfunction when sexually stimulated (27.4% vs 0.3%).[32] Age did not appear to be an independent determinant of this dissatisfaction; rather, this could be accounted for primarily by the age-related increase in erectile dysfunction, decreased libido and their interaction.

Prior to Jonler et al.[31] and Feldman et al.,[30] Kinsey et al.[33] had found impotence to be an age-dependent disorder with a prevalence of 1.9% at 40 years and 25% at age 65.[33] All three studies share the common feature of being based on selected population subgroups. The trends with age, and the high prevalences at older ages, are comfortingly similar, not only to themselves but also compared with other surveys of this area.[22,34–38]

Despite the methodological inadequacies in each of these studies, to some degree or another, it is clear that impotence is a very common condition in men and one in which the prevalence is strongly linked to ageing. The prevalence probably now exceeds 2% in the fifth decade, rising to 25–30% by the middle of the seventh decade, as estimated by Furlow in 1985.[39] Good data are still required, particularly by ethnic group and at older ages. No data are available for impotence among men aged 75 or over, of whom substantially over one-half may be affected.[5]

■ DETERMINANTS OF ERECTILE DYSFUNCTION IN MEN

Until the early 1980s, it was commonly held that psychogenic causes were the aetiology in up to 90% of cases of erectile dysfunction.[40–42] Current thinking favours arterial changes as the key factor in the largest proportion of impotence,[5,12,24,43] with alterations in the flow of blood to and from the penis the single most important cause. Some studies have indicated that there may be evidence of a role for certain cardiovascular risk factors in determining the risk of impotence, including tobacco, hypertension, diabetes mellitus and hyperlipidaemia.

Cigarette smoking has been implicated as an independent risk factor for (vascular) impotence.[44] In the MMAS, among subjects with treated heart disease the age-adjusted probability of complete impotence was 56% for current smokers, compared with 21% in current non-smokers.[30] Among treated hypertensives, those who currently smoked cigarettes had an elevated probability of complete impotence (20%), whereas the non-smokers (8.5%) were comparable to the general sample (9.4%). Feldman et al.[30] also found that drug effects were exacerbated by current smoking, which increased the age-adjusted probability of complete impotence in those taking cardiac medication (from 14 to 41%), using antihypertensive medications (from 7.5 to 21%) and using vasodilators (from 21 to 52%). However, in this study an overall effect of current smoking was not noted,[30] with complete impotence present in 11% of smokers and 9.3% of non-smokers. Among current smokers, the probability of impotence demonstrated no dose dependency with current smoking or lifetime cigarette consumption.

Diabetes is widely recognized to be associated with impotence. A review of seven prevalence surveys found rates of erectile dysfunction ranging from 35% to 59% among diabetics.[45] The association with increasing prevalence with age is also found. For example, Figure 2.2 contrasts the prevalence of erectile dysfunction in diabetic and non-diabetic men,[1] and clearly demonstrates the differences between diabetic and non-diabetic men in terms of prevalence of erectile dysfunction as well as the striking association with age in both groups. Similar prevalences have been reported recently[46,47] and, additionally, erectile dysfunction in diabetic men has been associated with the presence of severe diabetic retinopathy, a history of peripheral neuropathy, amputation, cardiovascular disease, a higher glycosylated haemoglobin, use of antihypertensive drugs and a higher body mass index.[46] It would appear that tighter glycaemic control and careful selection of antihypertensive

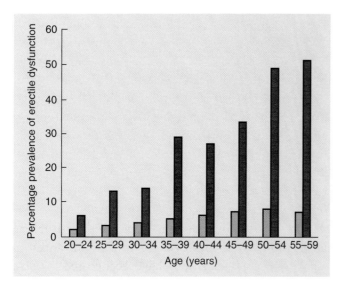

Figure 2.2. Prevalence of erectile dysfunction in diabetic ■ and non-diabetic ■ men. Data have been abstracted from ref 1.

medication could prove beneficial in the avoidance of erectile dysfunction in diabetic patients.[46]

In the MMAS, the age-adjusted probability of complete impotence was three times higher in men who reported having treated diabetes than in those without diabetes. In studies of diabetic patients, there have been consistent findings of high prevalences of impotence, with estimates ranging between one-third and one-half and, occasionally, up to three-quarters.[48,49] It has been reported that impotence in diabetics increases from 15% at age 30–34 to 55% at age 60 years.[50] It has been reported that impotence occurs at an earlier age in men with diabetes than in men in general, both in type I and type II diabetes.[51,52]

Vascular disease is the aspect of diabetes most widely held to be responsible for associated impotence. The association of impotence with vascular disease appears to be quite consistently reported. Impairment in the haemodynamics of erection has been demonstrated in men with a number of vascular diseases: in a group of men aged 31–86 with myocardial infarction, 64% were impotent,[53] and 57% of men in a study of coronary bypass surgery were found to be impotent.[54] Similar excesses of impotence have been demonstrated in men with peripheral vascular disease[55] and cerebrovascular accidents.[56] It has also been reported that impotence was increased among patients with arthritis,[57] although Feldman noted that the same association in the MMAS study was confined to smokers.[30]

The effect on sexual function of lifestyle factors related to cardiovascular disorders such as alcohol consumption has been reported to be either slight[30] or unclear.[58,59] There is no consistent evidence suggesting that obesity per se is associated with impotence.[30,58,59] A high level of total cholesterol or low level of high-density-lipoprotein cholesterol (HDL-C) may result in arteriosclerosis and induce erectile dysfunction by arterial insufficiency. Wei et al.[60] reported the relation between serum cholesterol and erectile dysfunction among blood samples obtained from the Cooper Clinic in Dallas, Texas, USA. The study included a total of 3250 men aged 26–83 years (mean age reported to be 51 years) without erectile dysfunction at the first visit and who had a further clinic visit between 6 and 48 months following.[60] Erectile dysfunction was reported by 71 men (2.2%) during this period and every mmol/litre increase in total cholesterol was associated with 1.32 times the risk of erectile dysfunction (95% confidence interval [CI] 1.04, 1.68). Men with an HDL-C measurement over 1.55 mmol/litre (60 mg/dl) had 0.30 times the risk (95% CI 0.09, 1.03). Men with total cholesterol over 6.21 mmol/litre (240 mg/dl) had 1.83 times the risk (95% CI 1.00, 3.37) of that of men with less than 4.65 mmol/litre (180 mg/dl). These differences remained essentially unchanged after adjustment for potential confounding factors (Fig. 2.3).[60]

Feldman et al.[30] reported that the probability of impotence varied inversely with HDL-C. For younger men, aged 40–55 years, the age-adjusted probability of moderate impotence increased from 6.7% to 25% as HDL-C decreased from 90 to 30 mg/dl. In older subjects, aged 56–70 years, the probability of complete impotence increased from near zero to 16% as HDL-C decreased from 90 to 30 mg/dl. No association with total cholesterol was found in this study.[30]

Impotence is often reported following radical prostatectomy, although preservation of the neurovascular bundles helps to reduce the frequency of the condition. Quinlan et al.[61] reported 600 radical retropubic prostatectomies from the Johns Hopkins Hospital of which 503 men were potent preoperatively.[61] Three factors were found to be related to the return of sexual function postoperatively, namely age, clinical stage of the tumour and surgical approach — i.e. whether the neurovascular bundles were preserved or excised. In young men, aged less than 50 years, potency was similar in patients who had both neurovascular bundles preserved (90%) and in those

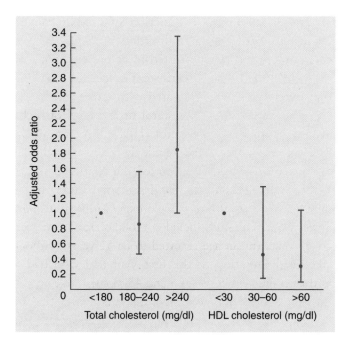

Figure 2.3. Relative (and 95% confidence interval) risk of erectile dysfunction by levels of total cholesterol and high density lipoprotein (HDL) cholesterol. Data abstracted from ref. 60.

who had one neurovascular bundle widely excised (91%). In men over 50 years, sexual function was better in men who had both bundles preserved than in men in whom one neurovascular bundle was widely excised ($p < 0.05$). When the relative risk of impotence was adjusted for age, the risk of postoperative impotence was twofold greater if there was capsular penetration or seminal vesicle invasion, or if one neurovascular bundle was excised ($p < 0.05$). In contrast, the proportion of men who stated that they were impotent following transurethral resection of the prostate (TURP) for BPH (24%) was essentially similar to the preoperative impotence rate (22%).[62] Previous anecdotal reports of an association between TURP and erectile dysfunction may have arisen because of patients' confusion in equating retrograde ejaculation with erectile dysfunction.[63]

Of 40 patients with aorto-iliac occlusive disease (AIOD) scheduled for surgery, 31 were given questionnaires and penile dynamic colour Doppler ultrasonography.[64] Five of the 31 who volunteered were found to be potent (16%) and the remaining 26 (84%) were found to have erectile dysfunction. This was found to be entirely arteriogenic in 8% of cases, purely venogenic in 23% of cases and a combination of arteriogenic and venogenic in 53%. Following surgery, 20 patients returned for evaluation and erectile function was found to have improved in seven patients. Of these patients, six (of nine) had undergone endarterectomy and one (of 11) had undergone reconstruction.[64]

The association between impotence and taking medication is still controversial in many instances, as many of these associations have been based on case reports and personal case series. Morley[28] noted that 16 of the 200 most widely prescribed drugs in the United States were associated with impotence and that 1/4 men in a medical outpatient population were reported to have drug-induced erectile dysfunction.[24] The frequency of erectile dysfunction was found to be slightly elevated in men receiving finasteride, a 5-alpha-reductase inhibitor used in the treatment of BPH.[65,66] Erectile dysfunction has been associated with a wide range of antihypertensive preparations, including diuretics, sympatholytics, beta-adrenoceptor-blocking agents and vasodilators.[67,68] Unfortunately, many of these reports are from studies where the presence of impotence was not ascertained before the trial began and, in most of the studies, it is difficult to separate the effect of the treatment from the effect of the disease. The one exception appears to be doxazosin, an alpha-adrenergic receptor blocker used in the treatment of hypertension and BPH, which was shown in a four-arm study to enhance sexual function.[69]

Psychological factors directly involved in the development of impotence have been very poorly studied from the aetiological point of view. It has not been common practice to include psychological assessments in prospective studies and, in retrospective surveys, it is difficult to avoid the effect similar to confounding by indication, wherein men who become impotent then become depressed and exhibit other psychological traits.

CONCLUSIONS AND RECOMMENDATIONS

With the 20th century has come a wide range of diseases of affluence and ageing, including appendicitis, myocardial infarction, osteoporosis and old age. Prior to age 40, impotence is a relatively uncommon disorder but the prevalence rises in such a way that the majority of men over 70 years of age may suffer from erectile dysfunction. Although 100 years ago this was of little consequence in public health terms, today life expectancy approaches 80 years in the most developed countries. Although ED does not kill, it is a major contributor to a reduced quality of life and to the consequent psychological sequelae of many ageing men.

The epidemiology of erectile dysfunction is very poorly researched and incompletely understood, although several aspects of the epidemiology are clear, at least in qualitative terms. Most importantly, despite the presence of all possible methodological failings in the available studies, the prevalence of the disease in ageing men is very high. The aetiology of erectile dysfunction is classified into several major subheadings; whereas psychogenic impotence was held, only 20 years ago, to account for over 80% of cases, today it is widely accepted that the commonest cause, and the explanation for the majority of cases, is the vascular changes commonly found in ageing men. In particular, erectile dysfunction appears to be common in diabetic patients and in men with clearly defined, serious vascular disease. A number of risk factors for vascular disease appear to be related to the risk of impotence, including cigarette smoking and serum cholesterol levels, particularly HDL-C. Erectile function also appears to be very sensitive to unrelated drug therapy effects.

Smoking is the largest single source of preventable mortality worldwide today. Smokers have great difficulty in stopping the habit, although it is very tempting to speculate that if it could be demonstrated that smoking cessation reduced the probability of becoming impotent, then men might be more motivated to give up this noxious habit and improve the expected duration as well as the quality of their lives.

There are a number of priorities in epidemiological research on erectile dysfunction. First, it is necessary to develop standard instruments to determine with certain sensitivity and specificity the presence, frequency and nature of erectile dysfunction in men; there have been important developments in this field in the recent past. Subsequently, this should be used to determine variations in the occurrence of erectile dysfunction, be it internationally, temporally or in special groups of the population; this is now ongoing. There is an urgent need to have a better understanding of the aetiology of erectile dysfunction: risk factors need to be identified more clearly so that prevention possibilities can be investigated. In this line, it would be interesting and useful to have urgent information on whether the cessation of cigarette smoking or lowering HDL-C levels could lead to a reduction in the probability of developing impotence. A positive effect of cholesterol-lowering drugs on nocturnal penile tumescence has been observed and, given the association now developing between cardiovascular disease and decreased nocturnal penile tumescence,[70] this could lead to the prioritization of this research line as one important way forward towards prevention. However, this line of aetiological and preventive research appears to have stalled and is developing only very slowly at present.

ACKNOWLEDGEMENTS

This work was conducted within the framework of support from the Associazione Italiana per la Ricerca sul Cancro.

REFERENCES

1. Bancroft J. Human sexuality and its problems, 2nd edn. Edinburgh: Churchill Livingstone, 1989

2. Bancroft J. Impotence in perspective. In: Gregoire A, Pryor J P (eds) Impotence: an integrated approach to clinical practice. Edinburgh: Churchill Livingstone, 1993

3. Clement U. Surveys of heterosexual behaviour. Annu Rev Sex Res. 1990; 1: 45–74

4. Marsey F J, Bernstein G S, O'Fallon W M et al. Vasectomy and health: results from a large cohort study. JAMA 1984; 252: 1023–1029

5. Kirby R S. Impotence: diagnosis and management of male erectile dysfunction. Br Med J 1994; 308: 957–961

6. Goldstein I, Rothstein L. The potent male: facts, fiction and future. Los Angeles: Body Press, 1990

7. Wilson G D. The psychology of male sexual arousal. In: Gregoire A, Pryor J P (eds) Impotence: an integrated approach to clinical practice. Edinburgh: Churchill Livingstone, 1993

8. Michael R P, Zumpe D. Potency in male rhesus monkeys: effects of continuously receptive females. Science 1978; 200: 451–453

9. Beamer W, Bermant G, Clegg M. Copulatory behaviour of the ram, Ovis aires II: Factors affecting copulatory satiation. Anim Behav 1969; 17: 706–711

10. Lerner S E, Melman A, Christ G J. Review of erectile dysfunction: new insights and more questions. J Urol 1993; 149: 1246–1255

11. Krane R J, Goldstein I, Saenz De Tejada I. Medical Progress: impotence. N Engl J Med 1989; 321: 1648–1659

12. Michael V. Arterial disease as a cause of impotence. Baillières Clin Endocrinol Metab 1982; 11: 725–748

13. Brody J. Prospects for an ageing population. Nature 1985; 315: 463–466

14. MacMahon B, Trichopoulos D. Epidemiology: basic principles and methods. Boston: Little Brown, 1996

15. Barry M J, Boyle P, Garraway M et al. Epidemiology and natural history of benign prostatic hyperplasia. In: Cockett A T K, Khoury S, Aso Y et al. (eds) Proceedings, The 2nd International Consultation on Benign Prostatic Hyperplasia (BPH), Paris, June 27–30, 1993. Jersey, Channel Islands: Scientific Communication International Ltd, 1994: 144–147

16. Gregoire A. Questionnaires and rating scales. In: Gregoire A, Pryor J P (eds) Impotence: an integrated approach to clinical practice. Edinburgh: Churchill Livingstone, 1993

17. O'Leary M P, Fowler F J, Lenderking W R et al. A brief sexual function inventory for Urology. Urology 1995; 46: 697–706

18. Rosen R C, Riley A, Wagner G et al. The International Index of Erectile Dysfunction (IIEF): a multidimensional scale for the assessment of erectile dysfunction. Urology 1997; 49: 822–830

19. Solstad K, Hertoft P. Frequency of sexual problems and sexual dysfunction in middle-aged Danish men. Arch Sex Behav 1993; 22: 51–58

20. Sanders D. The *Woman* book of love and sex. London: Sphere, 1985

21. Sanders D. The *Woman* report on men. London: Sphere, 1987

22. Frank E, Anderson C, Rubinstein D. Frequency of sexual dysfunction in 'normal' couples. New Engl J Med 1978; 299: 111–115

23. Nettelbladt P, Uddenberg N. Sexual dysfunction and sexual satisfaction in 58 married Swedish men. J Psychosom Res 1979; 23: 91–100

24. Slag M F, Morley J E, Elson M K et al. Impotence in medical clinic outpatients. JAMA 1983; 249: 1736–1742

25. Warner P, Bancroft J and members of the Edinburgh Human Sexuality Group. A Regional Service for Sexual Problems: a three-year study. J Sex Marital Ther 1987; 2: 115–125

26. Lim P H, Ng F C. Erectile dysfunction in Singapore men: presentation, treatment and results. Ann Acad Med Singapore 1992; 21: 248–253

27. Schein M, Zyzanski S J, Levine S et al. The frequency of sexual problems among family practice patients. Fam Pract Res J 1988; 7: 122–134

28. Morley J E. Impotence in older men. Hosp Pract 1988; 23: 139–142

29. Diokno A C, Brown M B, Herzog A R. Sexual function in the elderly. Arch Intern Med 1990; 150: 197–200

30. Feldman H A, Goldstein I, Hatzichristou D G et al. Impotence and its medical and psychological correlates: results of the Massachusetts Male Ageing Study. J Urol 1994; 151: 54–61

31. Jonler M, Moon T, Brannan W et al. The effect of age, ethnicity and geographical location on impotence and quality of life. Br J Urol 1995; 75: 651–655

32. Panser L A, Rhodes T, Girman C J et al. Sexual function of men ages 40 to 70 years: the Olmsted County Study of urinary symptoms and health status among men. J Am Geriatr Soc 1995; 43: 1107–1111

33. Kinsey A C, Pomeroy W, Martin C E. Age and sexual outlet. In: Kinsey A C, Pomeroy W, Martin C E (eds) Sexual behaviour in the human male. Philadelphia: Saunders, 1948

34. Pearlman C K, Kobashi L J. Frequency of intercourse in men. J Urol 1972; 107: 298–301

35. Morley J E. Impotence. Am J Med 1986; 80: 897–905

36. Pfeiffer E, Davis G C. Determinants of sexual behaviour in middle and old age. J Am Geriatr Soc 1972; 20: 151–158

37. Mulligan T, Retchin S M, Chinchilli V M, Bettinger C B. The role of ageing and chronic disease in sexual dysfunction. J Am Geriatr Soc 1988; 36: 520–524

38. Keil J E, Sutherland S E, Knapp R G et al. Self-reported sexual functioning in elderly blacks and whites: the Charleston heart study experience. J Aging Health 1992, 4: 112

39. Furlow W L. Prevalence of impotence in the United States. Med Aspects Hum Sex 1985; 19: 13–16

40. Kinsey A C, Pomeroy W B, Martin C E. Sexual behaviour in the human male. Philadelphia: Saunders, 1948

41. Bishop M W H. Ageing and reproduction in the male. J Reprod Fertil Suppl 1970; 12: 68–87

42. Butler R N. Psychologic aspects of reproductive ageing. In: Scheidner E L (ed) The ageing reproductive system. New York: Raven Press, 1978

43. Mulligan T, Katz P G. Why aged men become impotent. Arch Intern Med 1989; 149: 1365–1366

44. Rosen M P, Greenfield A J, Walker T G et al. Cigarette smoking — an independent risk factor for atherosclerosis in the hypogastric–cavernous arterial bed of men with arteriogenic impotence. J Urol 1991; 145: 759–763

45. Fairbairn C G, McCulloch D K, Wu F C. The effects of diabetes on male sexual function. Baillières Clin Endocrinol Metab 1982; 11: 749–784

46. Klein R, Klein B E, Lee K E et al. Prevalence of self-reported erectile dysfunction in people with long-term IDDM. Diabetes Care 1996; 19: 135–141

47. Brunner G A, Pieber T R, Schattenberg S et al. Erectile dysfunction in patients with type I diabetes mellitus. Wien Med Wochenschr 1995; 145: 584–586

48. Zemel P. Sexual dysfunction in the diabetic patient with hypertension. Am J Cardiol 1988; 61: 27H–33H

49. Rubin A et al. Impotence and diabetes mellitus. JAMA 1958; 168: 496

50. Smith A D. Causes and classification of impotence. Urol Clin North Am 1981; 8: 79–89

51. Whitehead E D, Klyde B J. Diabetes- related impotence in the elderly. Clin Geriatr Med 1990; 6: 771–795

52. McCulloch D K, Campbell I W, Wu F C et al. The prevalence of diabetic impotence. Diabetologia 1980; 18: 279–283

53. Wabrek A J, Burchell R C. Male sexual dysfunction associated with coronary heart disease. Arch Sex Behav 1980; 9: 69–75

54. Gundle M J, Reeves B R, Tate S et al. Psychological outcome after aortocoronary artery surgery. Am J Psychiatry 1980; 137: 1591–1594

55. Ruzbarski V, Michal V. Morphologic changes in the arterial bed of the penis with ageing: relationship to the pathogenesis of impotence. Invest Urol 1977; 15: 194–199

56. Agarwal A, Jain D C. Male sexual dysfunction after stroke. J Assoc Physicians India 1989; 37: 505–507

57. Blake D J, Maisak R, Koplan A et al. Sexual function among patients with arthritis. Clin Rheumatol 1988; 7: 50–60

58. Kosch S G, Curry R W, Kuritzky L. Evaluation and treatment of impotence: a pragmatic approach addressing organic and psychogenic components. Fam Pract Res J 1988; 7: 162–174

59. Fried L P, Moore R D, Parson T A. Long-term effects of cigarette smoking and moderate alcohol consumption on coronary artery diameter. Mechanism of coronary artery disease independent of atherosclerosis or thrombosis? Am J Med 1986; 80: 37–44

60. Wei M, Macera C A, Davis D R et al. Total cholesterol and high density lipoprotein cholesterol as important predictors of erectile dysfunction. Am J Epidemiol 1994; 140: 930–937

61. Quinlan D M, Epstein J L, Carter B S, Walsh P C. Sexual function following radical prostatectomy: influence of preservation of neurovascular bundles. J Urol 1991; 145: 998–1002

62. Doll H A, Black N A, McPherson K et al.. Mortality, morbidity and complications following transurethral resection of the prostate for benign prostatic hyperplasia. J Urol 1992; 147: 1566–1573

63. Soderdahl D W, Knight R W, Hansberry K L. Erectile dysfunction following transurethral resection of the prostate. J Urol 1996; 156: 1354–1356

64. Cormio L, Edgren J, Lepantalo M et al. Aortofemoral surgery and sexual function. Eur J Vasc Endovasc Surg 1996; 11: 453–457

65. Gormley G J, Stoner E, Bruskewitz R C et al. The effect of finasteride in men with benign prostatic hyperplasia. New Engl J Med 1992; 327: 1185–1191

66. Finasteride Study Group. Finasteride (MK-906) in the treatment of benign prostatic hyperplasia. Prostate 1993; 22: 291–299

67. Segraves R T, Madsen R, Corter C S. Erectile dysfunction associated with pharmaceutical agents. In: Segraves R T, Schoenber H W (eds) Diagnosis and treatment of erectile disturbances. A guide for clinicians. New York: Plenum Press, 1985: 22–63

68. Wein A J, van Arsdalen K N. Drug-induced male sexual dysfunction. Urol Clin North Am 1988; 15: 23–31

69. Treatment of Mild Hypertension Research Group. A randomized, placebo-controlled, trial of a nutritional–hygienic regime along with various drug monotherapies. Arch Intern Med 1991; 151: 1413–1423

70. Rosen R C, Weiner D N. Cardiovascular disease and sleep-related erections. J Psychosom Res 1997; 42: 517–530

Chapter 3
Anatomy of erectile function

S. D. Shetty and R. N. Farah

■ INTRODUCTION

The penile erectile apparatus consists of paired vascular spongy organs (corpora cavernosa) that are closely attached to each other except in the proximal third. The corpus spongiosum with the urethra is related to the ventral aspect of the penile shaft and expands distally to form the glans penis. The pendulous part of the penis is 4–6 inches (≈10.2–15.2 cm) long. The penile skin is continuous with that of the lower abdominal wall and continues over the glans penis to form the prepuce; it then folds on itself to reattach at the coronal sulcus. The penile skin envelopes the shaft and can be moved freely over the erect organ. The underlying fascial layer or dartos fascia (Colles' fascia) is continuous with Scarpa's fascia of the lower abdominal wall; inferiorly, it continues as the dartos fascia of the scrotum and Colles' fascia of the perineum and attaches to the posterior border of the perineal membrane. The superficial dorsal vein is seen in this layer of the fascia. Buck's fascia is the deep layer of the penile fascia that covers both the corpora cavernosa and the corpus spongiosum in separate fascial compartments (Fig. 3.1). Proximally, Buck's fascia is attached to the perineal membrane; distally, it is tightly attached to the base of the glans penis at the coronal sulcus, where it fuses with the ends of the corpora. The ischiocavernosus and the bulbospongiosus muscles lie beneath Colles' fascia, but superficial to Buck's fascia, to which their intrinsic fascia is loosely attached. Buck's fascia has a dense structure and is composed of longitudinally running fibres; it is firmly attached to the underlying tunica albuginea and encloses the deep dorsal vein, dorsal arteries and dorsal nerves.

The fundiform ligament is a thickening of the superficial penile fascia, deep to which is the suspensory ligament which is in continuity with Buck's fascia. The attachment of the ligament to the pubic symphysis maintains the penile position during erection. Severance of this ligament will lead to a lower angulation of the penile shaft during erection.

The tunica albuginea forms a thick fibrous coat to the spongy tissue of the corpora cavernosa and corpus spongiosum. It consists of two layers, the outer longitudinal and the inner circular. The tunica albuginea becomes thicker ventrally where it forms a groove to accommodate the corpus spongiosum. As the crura diverge proximally, the circular layer provides the support. The corpora are separated in the centre by an intercavernous septum. The septum is incomplete distally, perforated on its dorsal margin by vertically orientated openings in the pectiniform septum that provides communication between the corpora. Along the inner aspect of the tunica albuginea, numerous flattened columns or sinusoidal trabeculae composed of fibrous tissue, elastin fibres and smooth muscle surround the endothelium-lined sinusoids or cavernous spaces. In addition, a row of structural trabeculae arises near the junction of the three corporal bodies and inserts in the wall of the corpora about the midplane of the circumference.[1] The tunica albuginea provides a tough uniform backing for the engorged sinusoidal spaces. The tunica albuginea of the corpus spongiosum is thinner and contains smooth muscles that aid ejaculation. The glans is devoid of tunica albuginea. The corpus spongiosum becomes bulbous where it is covered by the bulbospongiosus to form the urethral bulb.

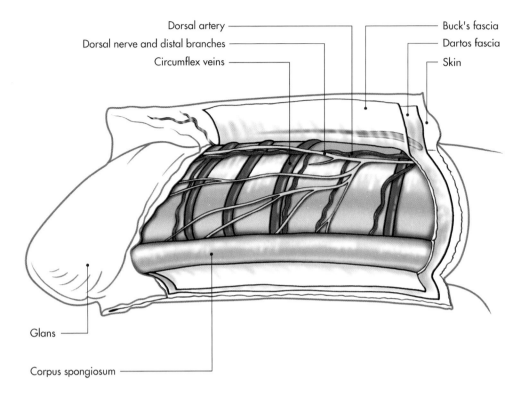

Dorsal artery
Dorsal nerve and distal branches
Circumflex veins
Buck's fascia
Dartos fascia
Skin
Glans
Corpus spongiosum

a

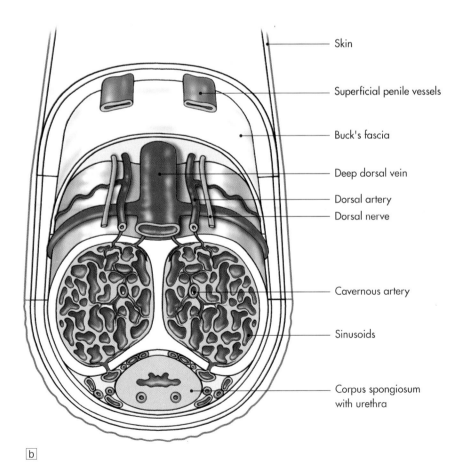

Skin
Superficial penile vessels
Buck's fascia
Deep dorsal vein
Dorsal artery
Dorsal nerve
Cavernous artery
Sinusoids
Corpus spongiosum with urethra

b

Figure 3.1. (a) Fascial layers; (b) cross-section at mid-shaft.

■ MUSCLES OF ERECTILE FUNCTION

The ischiocavernosus is a paired muscle that arises from the inner surface of the ischial tuberosity and inserts into the medial and inferior surface of the corpora. These muscles increase penile turgor during erection beyond that attainable by arterial pressure alone. They are supplied by the perineal branch of the pudendal nerve (S3–4).

The bulbospongiosus muscle invests the bulb of the urethra and distal corpus spongiosum. It arises from the central tendon of the perineum. The fibres run obliquely upwards and laterally on each side of the bulb and insert in the midline dorsally. The muscle is supplied by a deep branch of the perineal nerve and helps to empty the last few drops of urine and to ejaculate semen.

■ ARTERIAL SUPPLY

The arterial supply to the erectile apparatus originates from superficial and deep arterial systems. The superficial arterial system arises as two symmetrically arranged vessels arising from the inferior external pudendal artery (a branch of the femoral artery). Each of these vessels divides into a dorsolateral and ventrolateral branch, which supply the skin of the shaft and prepuce. At the coronal sulcus there is communication with the deep arterial system. The deep arterial system arises from the internal pudendal artery, which is the final branch of the anterior trunk of the internal iliac artery. This passes dorsal to the sacrospinous ligament at the level of the ischial spine and passes through Alcock's canal. As it emerges, it divides into the perineal and penile arteries, running deep to the superficial transverse perineal muscle and pubic symphysis (Fig. 3.2). It pierces the urogenital diaphragm medial to the inferior ramus of the ischium close to the bulb of the urethra and then divides into three branches — the bulbo-urethral artery, the urethral artery and the cavernous artery or deep artery of the penis; it terminates as the deep dorsal artery of the penis. An accessory internal pudendal artery may arise from the obturator, inferior vesical or superior vesical and may be damaged during radical prostatectomy in as many as 50% of patients. The bulbo-urethral artery supplies the bulb of the urethra, the corpus spongiosum and the glans penis. It may arise from cavernous, dorsal or accessory pudendal arteries. The urethral artery commonly arises as a separate branch from the penile artery, but may

arise from the artery to the bulb, the cavernous or the dorsal artery. It runs on the ventral surface of the corpus spongiosum beneath the tunica albuginea.

The cavernous artery (deep artery of the penis) usually arises from the penile artery, but may originate from the accessory pudendal. It runs lateral to the cavernous vein along the dorsomedial surface of the crura to enter the erectile tissue where the two corpora fuse; it then continues in the centre of the corpora cavernosa.

The dorsal artery of the penis is the termination of the penile artery; it runs over the respective crus and then along the dorsolateral surface of the penis as far as the glans between the dorsal vein medially and dorsal nerve of the penis laterally. This artery has a tortuous configuration to accommodate for elongation during erection. It may arise from the accessory internal pudendal artery within the pelvis, and thus may be at risk during radical pelvic surgery. On its way to the glans, it gives off circumflex arteries to supply the corpus spongiosum. Distally, the dorsal artery runs in a ventrolateral position near the sulcus prior to entering the glans. The frenular branch of the dorsal artery curves around each side of the distal shaft to enter the frenulum and glans ventrally.

■ INTRACORPORAL CIRCULATION

Arterial blood is conveyed to the erectile tissue in the deep arterial system by means of dorsal, cavernous and bulbo-urethral arteries. The cavernous artery (deep artery of the penis) gives off multiple helicine arteries among the cavernous spaces within the centre of the erectile tissue. Most of these open directly into the sinusoids bounded by trabeculae, but a few helicine arteries terminate in capillaries that supply the trabeculae. The pectiniform septum distally provides communication between the two corpora. The emissory veins at the periphery collect the blood from the sinusoids through the subalbugineal venous plexuses and empty it into the circumflex veins which drain into the deep dorsal vein. With erection, the arteriolar and sinusoidal walls relax secondary to neurotransmitters and the cavernous spaces dilate, enlarging the corporal bodies and stretching the tunica albuginea. The venous tributaries between the sinusoids and the subalbugineal venous plexus are compressed by the dilating sinusoids and the stretched tunica albuginea.[2] The direction of blood flow could be summarized as follows: cavernous artery → helicine

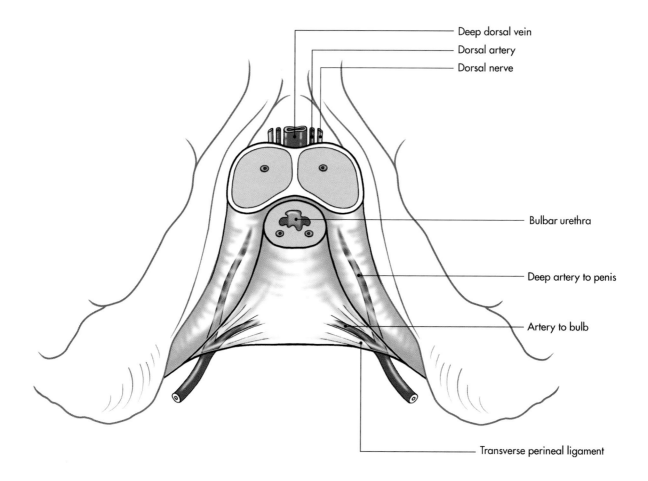

Figure 3.2. Arterial and venous supply of the penis at the level of the perineal membrane.

arteries → sinusoids → post-cavernous venules → subalbugineal venous plexus → emissary vein.

■ VENOUS DRAINAGE

The venous drainage system consists of three distinct groups of veins — superficial, intermediate and deep. The superficial drainage system consists of venous drainage from the penile skin and prepuce which drain into the superficial dorsal vein that runs under the superficial penile fascia (Colles') and joins the saphenous vein via the external pudendal vein. The intermediate system consists of the deep dorsal vein and circumflex veins that drain the glans, corpus spongiosum and distal two-thirds of the corpora cavernosa. The veins leave the glans via a retrocoronal plexus to join the deep dorsal vein that runs in the groove between the corpora. Emissary veins from the corpora join the circumflex veins; the latter communicate with each other at the side by lateral veins and corresponding veins from the opposite side, and run under Buck's fascia before emptying obliquely into the deep dorsal vein. The latter passes through a space in the suspensory ligament and between the puboprostatic ligament and drains into the prostatic plexus, which drains into the internal iliac veins. The deep drainage system consists of the cavernous vein, bulbar vein and crural veins. Blood from the sinusoids from the proximal third of the penis, carried by the emissary veins, drains directly into cavernous veins at the periphery of the corpora cavernosa. The two cavernous veins join to form the main cavernous vein that lies under the cavernous artery and nerves. The cavernous vein runs between the bulb and the crus to drain into the internal pudendal vein; it forms the main venous drainage of the corpora cavernosa.[3] The crural veins arise from the dorsolateral surface of each crus and unite to drain into the internal pudendal vein. The bulb is drained by the bulbar vein, which drains into the prostatic plexus.

LYMPHATIC DRAINAGE

The lymphatics from the penile skin and prepuce run proximally towards the presymphyseal plexus and then divide to right and left trunks to join the lymphatics from the scrotum and perineum. They run along superficial external pudendal vessels into the superficial inguinal nodes, especially the superomedial group. Some drainage occurs through the femoral canal into Cloquet's node. The lymphatics from the glans and penile urethra drain into deep inguinal nodes, presymphyseal nodes and, occasionally, into external iliac nodes.

NERVES

Somatic innervation arises from sacral spinal segments S2–4 via the pudendal nerve. The perineal branch of the pudendal nerve supplies the posterior part of the scrotum and the rectal nerve to the inferior rectal area. The pudendal nerve continues as the dorsal nerve of the penis, which runs over the surface of obturator internus under the levator, runs deep to the urogenital diaphragm, and passes through the deep transverse perineal muscle to run along the dorsum of the penis accompanied by the dorsal vein and dorsal artery. In epispadias and exstrophy the dorsal nerves are displaced laterally in the middle and distal portion of the penile shaft. Cutaneous nerves to the penis and scrotum arise from the dorsal and posterior branch of the pudendal nerve. The anterior part of the scrotum and proximal penis is supplied by the ilio-inguinal nerve after it leaves the superficial inguinal ring. The pudendal nerve supplies the ischiocavernosus and bulbocavernosus muscles. It branches into the inferior

rectal nerve and the scrotal nerve and continues as the dorsal nerve of the penis.

Autonomic nerves consist of sympathetics that arise from lumbar segments L1 and L2 and parasympathetics from S2–4 (nervi erigentes or pelvic nerve). Lumbar splanchnic nerves join the superior hypogastric plexus over the aortic bifurcation, left common iliac vein and sacral promontory. From this plexus, right and left hypogastric nerves travel medial to the internal iliac artery to the inferior hypogastric plexus. The pelvic plexus adjacent to the base of the bladder, prostate, seminal vesicles and rectum contain parasympathetic fibres as well. Nerves from the inferior pelvic plexus supply the prostate, seminal vesicles, epididymis, membranous and penile urethra and bulbo-urethral gland.

Cavernous nerve neurovascular bundles

The cavernous nerves arise from the pelvic plexus from the lateral surface of the rectum. These nerves run posterolateral to the apex, mid-portion and base of the prostate anterior to Denonvilliers' fascia between the posterolateral surface of the prostate and the rectum to lie between the lateral pelvic fascia and the prostatic fascia.[4,5] The branches from the cavernous nerve accompany the branches of the prostatovesicular artery and provide a macroscopic landmark for nerve-sparing radical prostatectomy. The cavernous nerve leaves the pelvis between the transverse perineal muscles and membranous urethra before passing beneath the pubic arch to supply each corpus cavernosum; it also supplies the corpus spongiosum and penile urethra, and terminates in a delicate network around the erectile tissue.

REFERENCES

1. Hinman F. Penis and male urethra. In: Hinman F (ed) Atlas of urosurgical anatomy. Philadelphia: Saunders, 1993: 417–448
2. Lue T F, Tanagho E A. Physiology of erection and pharmacological management of impotence. J Urol 1987; 137: 829–836
3. Aboseif S R, Breza J, Lue T F, Tanagho E A. Penile venous drainage in erectile dysfunction. Anatomical, radiological and functional considerations. Br J Urol 1989; 64(2): 183–190
4. Lepor H, Gregerman M, Crosby R et al. Precise localization of the autonomic nerves from the pelvic plexus to the corpora cavernosa: a detailed anatomical study of the adult male pelvis. J Urol 1985; 133: 207–212
5. Lue T F, Zeineh S J, Schmidt R A, Tanagho E A. Neuroanatomy of penile erection: its relevance to iatrogenic impotence. J Urol 1984; 131(2): 273–280

Chapter 4
Microscopic anatomy of the penis

K. S. Nitahara and T. F. Lue

■ INTRODUCTION

Gross anatomy of the penis

The penis is divided into three anatomical components: the root is that part of the erectile tissue that lies infrapubically in the superficial perineal pouch; the body is composed of three cylindrical tubes all covered by fascia and skin; the glans is the continuation of the corpus spongiosum.

The erectile tissue is housed within the paired corpora cavernosa and single corpus spongiosum, which are enveloped by the tunica albuginea. The paired corpora cavernosa lie side by side on the dorsal aspect of the penis. Along the body of the penis there is some connection by the septum penis. More proximally, towards the perineum, the corporal bodies diverge bilaterally to form the crura of the penis. Each crus is anchored to the pubic arch at the level of the ischial tuberosity, where it is surrounded by the fibres of the ischiocavernosus muscles.

The corpus spongiosum is a single cylindrical tube that lies just ventral to the paired cavernosal bodies. It surrounds the urethra in its pendulous and bulbar portions. The distal portion of the spongiosum expands and covers the distal portion of the corporal bodies; this is the glans of the penis.

The tunica albuginea is a tough layer surrounding the corpora cavernosa. It also covers the corpus spongiosum but there it is thinner. The skin of the penis is redundant near its distal end and forms the prepuce, which covers the glans. The superficial dartos fascia of the penis comprises of loosely arranged areolar tissue and no fat. Buck's fascia is thicker and completely surrounds all erectile bodies and the neurovascular bundles. Support for the penis is by two ligamentous structures: the fundiform ligament is continuous with the linea alba and splits to surround the body of the penis, then fuses with the septa of the scrotum. The suspensory ligament is a triangular condensation of fascia that suspends the penis from the front of the symphysis pubis.

Vascular components of the penis

Most of the penile arterial blood flow originates from the hypogastric artery, which gives off the internal pudendal artery. After passing through Alcock's canal, the internal pudendal artery becomes the common penile artery, which branches to the three end arteries — the bulbo-urethral, cavernosal and dorsal penile arteries (Fig. 4.1). The cavernosal artery extends through the cavernosal bodies after entering at the inferomedial aspect of the hilum of the penis where the crura merge. At the base of the penis the cavernosal arteries are close to the septum; more distally, they are in the centre of each cavernosal body. Along its course the cavernosal arteries give off multiple helicine branches which supply the erectile tissue; in the flaccid state they are tortuous and contracted whereas during erection they become straight and larger in calibre. There may be accessory arteries, the accessory pudendal from the vesical or external pudendal, which may serve as the main blood supply to the erectile tissue. The paired dorsal arteries course within the neurovascular bundles at the 11 o'clock and 1 o'clock positions to supply the more superficial components of the penis, and may provide blood flow to the erectile bodies.

Venous drainage of the penis may occur at three levels (Fig. 4.2). The superficial system drains the skin and superficial tissues. It consists of the superficial dorsal vein between Colles' and Buck's fasciae on the dorsal aspect of the penis. This system drains into the saphenous veins via the external pudendals. The intermediate system consists of the deep dorsal and circumflex veins. The deep dorsal vein originates from the retrocoronal plexus, and receives

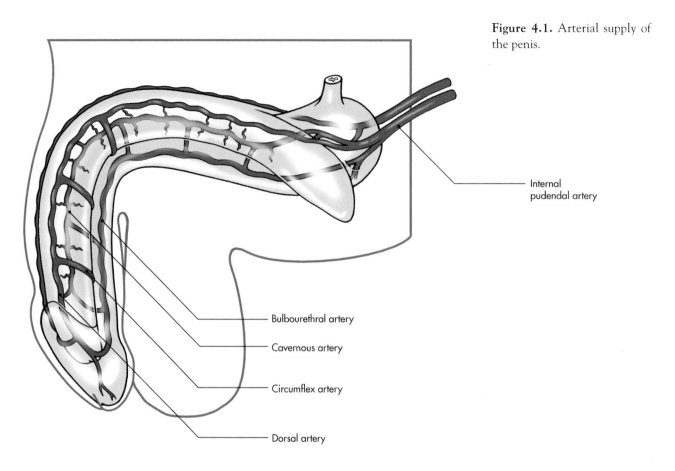

Figure 4.1. Arterial supply of the penis.

Internal pudendal artery

Bulbourethral artery

Cavernous artery

Circumflex artery

Dorsal artery

blood from emissary veins and circumflex veins in the distal half of the penis. This blood drains into the periprostatic plexus and then into the internal pudendal vein. The deep drainage system includes the crural and cavernosal veins, which empty into the internal iliac veins via the internal pudendals.

Penile lymph drainage is via the superficial and deep inguinal nodes, which in turn drain into the external and common iliac nodes.

Neuro-anatomy of the penis

The innervation of the penis may be divided into autonomic (sympathetic and parasympathetic) and somatic (sensory and motor). The penile nerves may contain various amounts of each of these components, which originate at various levels within the spinal cord and peripheral nerves. Sympathetic preganglionic nerve fibres to the penis arise from preganglionic neurons in intermediolateral grey matter from the 11th thoracic to the second lumbar spinal cord segments. Variations have been described in which fibres may originate from as high as the ninth thoracic or as low as the fourth lumbar cord

segments.[1] These preganglionic fibres pass to the sympathetic chain ganglia (paravertebral), where they make synaptic connections with ganglion cells at various levels. The ganglion cells are located in the sacral and caudal lumbar ganglia[1] and send postganglionic fibres to the urogenital tract via the pelvic, cavernous and pudendal nerves. Postganglionic fibres leave the chain ganglia and pass along the lumbar splanchnic nerves to prevertebral ganglia in the superior hypogastric plexus, which overlies the great vessels at the level of the third lumbar to first sacral vertebrae. The superior hypogastric plexus (presacral nerve) divides into the left and right hypogastric nerves as the sympathetic fibres extend toward the pelvic plexus.

Parasympathetic fibres originate from the second, third and fourth sacral vertebral segments (Fig. 4.3). Sacral preganglionic nerves (pelvic nerves or nervi erigentes) travel towards the pelvic plexus, or inferior hypogastric plexus. The pelvic plexus serves as a relay and integration centre within which preganglionic axons make synaptic connections with postganglionic neurons innervating the penis. The cavernous nerves

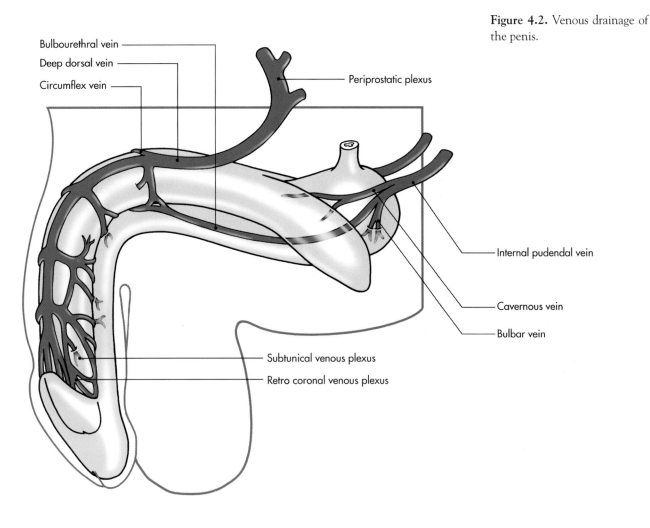

Figure 4.2. Venous drainage of the penis.

Bulbourethral vein

Deep dorsal vein

Circumflex vein

Periprostatic plexus

Internal pudendal vein

Cavernous vein

Bulbar vein

Subtunical venous plexus

Retro coronal venous plexus

project from the pelvic plexus; they are located in the pelvic fascia before it fuses with the prostatic capsule, then travel along the posterolateral aspect of the prostate at the 5 and 7 o'clock positions. At the level of the membranous urethra the nerves are at the 3 and 9 o'clock positions. Distal to that, some of the fibres penetrate the tunica albuginea of the corpus spongiosum; some of the remaining fibres, lying at the 11 and 1 o'clock positions, enter the penile crura along with terminal branches of the pudendal artery and exiting cavernous veins. The remainder use the dorsal nerve as a scaffold to innervate the distal portion of the penis.

Somatic sensory pathways begin at the sensory receptors in the penile skin, glans and urethra. The nerve fibres from these receptors converge to form bundles of the dorsal nerve of the penis; this joins other nerves to become the internal pudendal nerve. These fibres then ascend via the dorsal roots of the second, third and fourth

nerves of the spinal cord. Activation of these receptors sends messages of pain, temperature and touch via the dorsal and pudendal nerves, spinal cord and spinothalamic tract to the thalamus and sensory cortex for sensory perception.

The motor pathway to the penis lies within the sacral nerves to the pudendal nerve to innervate the bulbocavernosus and ischiocavernosus muscles. Contraction of the ischiocavernosus muscles produces a rigid erection phase by compression of the engorged corpora cavernosa which, along with venous outflow restriction, can increase the intracavernous pressure to several hundred millimetres of mercury (mmHg). Rhythmic contraction of the bulbocavernosus muscle expels the semen down the narrowed urethral lumen and results in external ejaculation from the meatus. The centre of somatomotor penile innervation is Onuf's nucleus in the second, third and fourth sacral segments of the spinal cord.

33

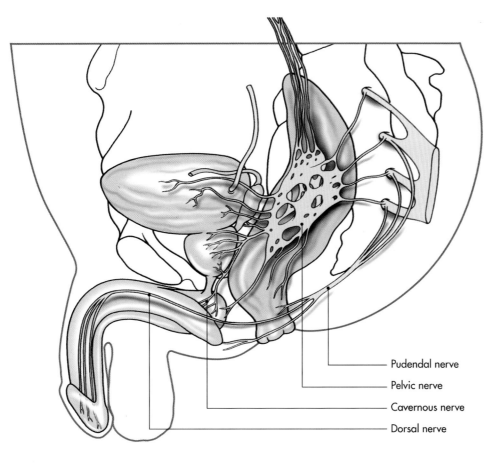

Figure 4.3. Somatic and autonomic innervation of the penis.

Pudendal nerve
Pelvic nerve
Cavernous nerve
Dorsal nerve

■ FUNCTIONAL MICROSCOPIC PENILE ANATOMY

Tunica albuginea

The tunica albuginea offers great flexibility, rigidity and tissue strength to the penis[2] and is composed of two layers (Fig. 4.4). The inner layer bundles of the corpora cavernosa are circular and support and contain the cavernous tissue. Intracavernosal pillars radiate from the inner layer and act as struts to augment the septum. The outer layer bundles are orientated in a longitudinal orientation and extend from the glans penis to the proximal crura. Between the 5 and 7 o'clock positions there is no outer layer tunic; this is the location where most prostheses are extruded. By contrast, the tunica over the corpus spongiosum lacks an outer layer or intracorporal struts, to ensure low pressures during erection.

The tunica is composed of elastic fibres that form an irregular, latticed network on which the collagen fibres rest. This microstructure provides strength and allows the tissue to return to its baseline configuration after moderate stretch (i.e. erection).

Emissary veins travel between the inner and outer layers of the tunica and often pierce the outer bundles in an oblique manner. Branches of the dorsal artery traverse the outer layer in a perpendicular fashion and are surrounded by a periarterial fibrous sheath. The outer tunical layer also serves as a backboard for the compression of the emissary veins when the penis becomes engorged with blood. This venous compression minimizes the amount of penile blood that is able to drain, and thus allows an erect penis.

Corpora cavernosa

The corpora cavernosa are two spongy cylinders on the dorsal aspect of the penis. Their proximal ends, the crura, originate at the undersurface of the pubo-ischial rami as two separate structures; these merge under the pubic arch and

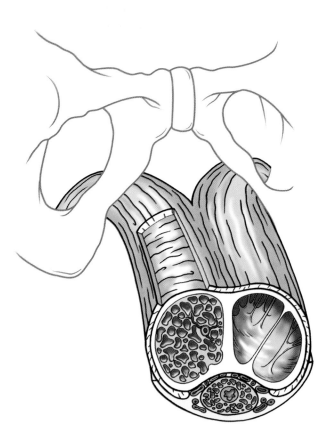

Figure 4.4. Structure of the tunica albuginea.

remain attached up to the glans. Each cylinder is contained within the tough tunical covering; an incomplete septum allows blood to flow from one side to the other.

The corpora are supported by a fibrous skeleton that includes the tunica albuginea, intracavernous pillars, intracavernous fibrous network and the peri-arterial and perineural fibrous sheath.[3] It has been suggested that the intracavernous framework also adds strength to the tunica albuginea. Within the tunica are the interconnected sinusoids separated by smooth muscle trabeculae and surrounded by elastic fibres, collagen and loose areolar tissue. The terminal cavernous nerves and helicine arteries are intimately associated with smooth muscle. Each corpus cavernosum is a conglomeration of sinusoids, which are larger in the centre and smaller at the periphery. In the flaccid state, the blood slowly diffuses from the central to the peripheral sinusoids and the blood gas levels are similar to those of venous blood. During erection, the rapid entry of arterial blood to the central and peripheral sinusoids increases the oxygen tension level to approximately that of arterial blood.

The structure of the corpus spongiosum is similar to that of the corpora cavernosa except that the sinusoids are larger and the outer layer of tunica is non-existent. The glans has no tunical covering at all.

Microscopic vascular supply and drainage
The majority of the arterial supply to the erectile tissue is via the cavernosal artery, although there may be accessory arterial supply. The cavernosal artery enters the corpus cavernosum at the hilum of the penis where the crura converge. Multiple helicine arterial branches are given off the cavernosal artery to supply the trabecular erectile tissue and sinusoids. The helicine arteries are contracted and tortuous in the flaccid state and become straight and dilated during erection.

The venous drainage from the erectile tissue originates in the venules starting from the peripheral sinusoids immediately beneath the tunica albuginea. They travel in the trabeculae between the tunica and the peripheral sinusoids, and form the subtunical venular plexus prior to exiting as the emissary veins.

■ MICROSCOPIC ANATOMICAL AND PHYSIOLOGICAL CHANGES DURING ERECTION

Corpora cavernosa
As part of a complex system, the cavernosal bodies have an essential role in the erectile process. In the flaccid state, the smooth muscle fibres are tonically contracted under the control of sympathetic discharge. Only a small amount of arterial inflow is permitted, to supply nourishment to this tissue.

During erection, relaxation of smooth muscles in the trabeculae and the arterial wall allows the following cascade of events to occur[4] (Fig. 4.5):

1. Dilatation of the arterioles and arteries increases blood flow;
2. Expansion of sinusoids causes trapping of blood;
3. Subtunical venular plexuses are compressed between the tunica albuginea and the peripheral sinusoids, reducing the venous outflow;
4. The tunica albuginea is stretched to its capacity and the emissary veins are choked, to decrease further the venous outflow;

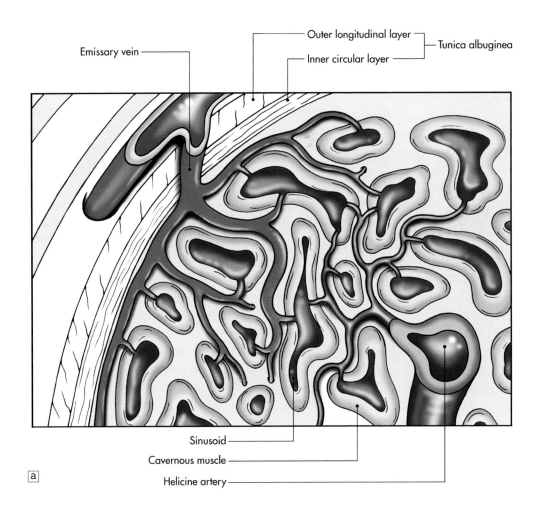

Emissary vein

Outer longitudinal layer
Inner circular layer
Tunica albuginea

Sinusoid

Cavernous muscle

Helicine artery

a

Figure 4.5. Microscopic changes during penile erection. In the flaccid state (a) the arteries, arterioles and sinusoids are contracted. The inter-sinusoidal and subtunical venular plexuses are open, allowing free flow to the emissary veins.

5. Intracavernous pressure is increased to about 100 mmHg to achieve the full erection state;
6. Contraction of the ischiocavernosus muscles further increases the intracavernosal pressure to several hundred mmHg (rigid erection phase).

Detumescence has been described to occur in three phases.[5] First, gradual smooth muscle contraction against a closed venous system causes a transient increase in intracavernous pressure. The venous channels then slowly open with resumption of the basal level of arterial flow and a slow pressure decrease. Finally, there is a rapid pressure decrease with fully restored venous outflow capacity.

Corpus spongiosum and glans penis

During erection, the blood flow to the corpus spongiosum increases in a manner similar to that of the cavernosal bodies. However, the intraspongiosal pressure reaches only one-half to one-third that of the cavernosa because of its thinner, less constraining tunical layer which provides less venous occlusion. The natural advantage is that minimal increases in pressure will not cause occlusion of the urethra which could, in turn, prevent ejaculation. During the full erection phase, partial compression of the deep dorsal and circumflex veins between Buck's fascia and the engorged corpora cavernosa contribute to glanular tumescence, although the spongiosum and glans essentially function as a large arteriovenous shunt during this phase. In the rigid erection phase, the spongiosum and penile veins are forcefully compressed by the ischiocavernosus and bulbocavernosus muscles to increase engorgement and pressure further in the glans and spongiosum.

Neurotransmitters and receptors found in the penis

Adrenergic nerve fibres and receptors have been identified in the cavernous trabeculae and surrounding

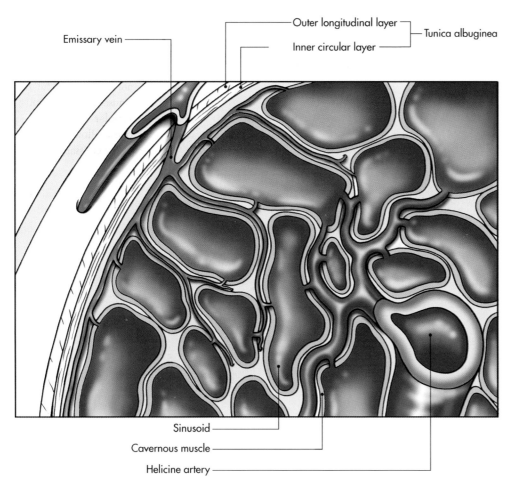

Emissary vein

Outer longitudinal layer

Inner circular layer

Tunica albuginea

Sinusoid

Cavernous muscle

Helicine artery

b

Figure 4.5. In the erect state (b), the muscles of the sinusoidal wall and the arterioles relax, allowing maximal flow to the compliant sinusoidal spaces. Most of the venules are compressed between the expanding sinusoids. The larger intermediary venules are sandwiched and flattened by distended sinusoids and the tunica albuginea; this effectively reduces the venous flow to a minimum.

the cavernous arteries, with noradrenaline being the major neurotransmitter controlling flaccidity and tumescence.[6,7] Receptor-binding studies have demonstrated that there are ten times the number of alpha-adrenoceptors as beta-adrenoceptors in erectile tissue.[8] Sympathetic contraction is thought to be mediated by activation of postsynaptic alpha-1a, -1b, and -1c-adrenergic receptors[9,10] and modulated by presynaptic alpha-2-adrenergic receptors.[11]

Acetylcholine is required for ganglionic transmission (by nicotinic receptors) and vascular smooth muscle relaxation (by muscarinic receptors). Cholinergic nerves have been demonstrated within the human cavernous smooth muscle and surrounding penile arteries, and ultrastructural examination has identified terminals containing cholinergic vesicles in the same area. The muscarinic receptors of human corpus cavernosal tissue are suggested to be of the M2 or M3 subtype; however, this has not been conclusively demonstrated.[12]

Nitric oxide (NO) appears to be the most likely principal neurotransmitter causing penile erection. Non-adrenergic, non-cholinergic (NANC) neurons have been found to release NO; this increases the production of cyclic guanosine monophosphate (cGMP) which in turn relaxes cavernosal smooth muscle.[13–15] NO-mediated responses are progressively inhibited as a function of decreasing oxygen tension;[16] reverting to normal oxygen tension restores endothelium-dependent and neurogenic relaxation. NO can also be synthesized and released by endothelial cells and released by either electrical or chemical stimulation.

There is some suggestion that vasoactive intestinal peptide (VIP) is one of the neurotransmitters responsible for erection. VIP-immunoreactive nerve fibres have been identified within the cavernous trabeculae and surrounding penile arteries, and neurostimulation-induced cavernous smooth muscle relaxation has been shown to be blocked by a VIP antagonist or anti-VIP serum.[17,18] VIP may also be found with acetylcholine in parasympathetic fibres; they may act synergistically to induce erection through inhibition of alpha-1 activity by acetylcholine and release of NO by VIP.

Other neurotransmitters that may have a role in modulating penile erection include calcitonin gene-related peptide (CGRP),[19] peptide histidine methionine,[20] pituitary adenylate cyclase-activating polypeptide[21] and prostaglandins.[11,22] Prostaglandin E1 receptor density was found to be lower in impotent men than in controls.[23] The role of these many neurotransmitters is not well established. Because of their identification in the erectile tissue and perivascular nerves, further investigation is needed to elucidate the interactions between neurotransmitters and neuromodulators at the neuromuscular junction, as well as between the neural and endothelial control of vascular tone.[24]

Intercellular communication

During the process of penile erection and detumescence, some coordinating mechanism among the cavernous smooth muscle fibres allows synchronized relaxation and contraction.[25] Although the electromyographic activity in the cavernous tissue of patients with normal erectile function is synchronous,[26] the relatively sparse neuronal innervation of cavernous smooth muscle cannot explain this. It has been suggested that there are gap junctions in the membrane of the adjacent muscle cells that allow exchange of ions such as calcium and second-messenger molecules. The major component of gap junctions is connexin 43, a membrane-sparing protein of less than 0.25 μm that has been identified between smooth muscle cells of human corpus cavernosum.[27] Cell-to-cell communication through these gap junctions probably explains the synchronized erectile response, although their pathophysiological impact is still unclear.

■ PENILE ERECTILE DYSFUNCTION IN DISEASED STATES

Erectile dysfunction has had an increasing impact on our society, with an estimated 10–20 million men affected,[28] most of whom are more than 65 years old. Over the past two decades, great strides have been made in understanding and integrating the normal anatomy and physiology of penile erection. Equally important, a better understanding of the pathophysiology of erection has offered new treatment to patients with such afflictions.

Psychogenic impotence had been considered the most common type of impotence,[29] but many of these patients are considered to have significant physiological or anatomical contributing features. Direct inhibition of the spinal erection centre by the brain as an exaggeration of the normal suprasacral inhibition is one proposed mechanism.[30] It has also been proposed that excessive sympathetic outflow or elevated peripheral catecholamines, which may increase penile smooth muscle tone, may be a contributing factor. Diederichs et al. reported that activation of sympathetic nerves or administration of adrenaline causes detumescence of the erect penis.[31] Clinically, higher levels of serum noradrenaline have been reported in patients with psychogenic erectile dysfunction than in normal controls or patients with vasculogenic erectile dysfunction.[32]

Neurological causes of impotence may occur as a result of any abnormality of the brain, spinal cord, cavernous and pudendal nerves, or receptors in the terminal arterioles. Iatrogenic damage to the nerves to the penis may occur by surgical procedures in the pelvic area. The incidence of such iatrogenic impotence has been reported to be as follows: radical retropubic prostatectomy 43–100%;[33,34] perineal prostatectomy 25%;[33] abdomino-perineal resection of the rectum, 15–100%;[35] and external sphincterotomy, 2–49%.[36] An improved understanding of the neuroanatomy of the pelvic and cavernous nerves has resulted in modified surgery for retroperitoneal and pelvic areas, resulting in lowered rates of impotence.[35] For example, use of nerve-sparing radical prostatectomy has allowed the preservation of sexual function in many patients.[37] Following pelvic fracture, nerve fibres to the penis may be injured. If the nerve is partially damaged, there may be replenishment of neurons with potential recovery. Using nitric oxide synthase (NOS) staining as a marker, it has been shown that regeneration of the cavernous nerves is more likely a result of sprouting from the remaining non-injured bundles than of re-innervation from the severed ones.[38]

Neurotransmitter deficiency may cause impotence as a result of alcoholism, vitamin deficiency or diabetes. In diabetic subjects, impairment of neurogenic and endothelium-dependent relaxation results in inadequate NO release.[39] Diabetes may also cause a change in the cavernous arteries and cavernous erectile tissue.[39] In a polysomnographic study, impotent men with diabetes were found to have fewer sleep-related erections, less tumescence time, diminished penile rigidity, decreased heart-rate response to deep breathing, and lower penile blood pressure than age-matched non-diabetic men.[40]

Atherosclerotic or traumatic arterial occlusive disease of the hypogastric–cavernous–helicine arterial tree may decrease the perfusion pressure and arterial flow to the sinusoidal spaces; this increases the time to maximal erection and decreases the rigidity of the erect penis. Common risk factors for arterial insufficiency from atherosclerosis include hypertension, hyperlipidaemia, cigarette smoking, diabetes mellitus and pelvic irradiation.[41] This correlates clinically with arteriographic findings of diffuse, bilateral stenosis of internal pudendal, common penile, and cavernous arteries in men with impotence. Focal stenosis of the common penile or cavernous artery is most often seen in young patients who have sustained blunt perineal or pelvic trauma.[42] Nicotine may adversely affect erectile function by decreasing arterial flow to the penis and blocking corporal smooth muscle relaxation, thus preventing normal venous occlusion.[43,44] Chronic hypertension causes stenotic microarterial lesions, which are thought to contribute to erectile dysfunction.[45]

Inadequate venous occlusion has been proposed as one of the more common causes of erectile dysfunction.[4] This may be caused by any of several factors:

1. The presence of large venous channels draining the corpora cavernosa;
2. Degenerative changes or traumatic injury to the tunica albuginea, resulting in inadequate compression of the subtunical and emissary veins;
3. Abnormal communication between the corpus cavernosum and spongiosum, allowing blood to drain from the cavernosum. The latter may occur from any of several causes, such as penile fracture or internal urethrotomy for pendulous urethral stricture;
4. Structural alterations in the fibroelastic components of the trabeculae, cavernous smooth muscle and endothelium;
5. Insufficient trabecular smooth muscle relaxation from inadequate neurotransmitter release.

■ OTHER CHANGES IN PENILE ARCHITECTURE

Loss of compliance of the penile sinusoids may be the result of ageing associated with increased deposition of collagen. Hypercholesterolaemia-related altered collagen synthesis may cause loss of compliance.[46] Prostaglandin E1 has been shown to suppress collagen synthesis induced by transforming growth factor beta-1 (TGF-β1) in human cavernous smooth muscle.[47]

The amount of smooth muscle in impotent men may be decreased,[48] especially in those with arteriogenic and venogenic erectile dysfunction in whom the muscle content corresponds to the severity of vascular disease and the failure of erectile response to intracavernous injection. Hypercholesterolaemia may also affect the smooth muscle component: rabbits fed a high-cholesterol diet had significant smooth muscle degeneration, with loss of cell-to-cell contact.[49] Cavernous nerve injury may affect cavernous smooth muscle relaxation, as demonstrated in neurotomized dogs.[50]

Damaged smooth muscle fibres from vasculogenic and neurogenic causes of impotence have some similar ultrastructural changes suggesting a variety of pathological mechanisms.[51] In this study, patients who underwent prosthesis placement for a variety of aetiological causes of impotence were found to have any of a combination of (1) decreased number of smooth muscle cells, (2) decreased cell-to-cell contacts, (3) sinusoidal endothelial changes, (4) degenerative changes in nerve fibres, and (5) increase in interstitial collagen.

Cellular electrical activity may also be important in impotence. In a study of different potassium-channel subtypes in cultured cavernous smooth muscle cells, there was found to be an alteration of the 'Maxi-K' channel in cells from impotent patients.[52] Gap junctions allow the synchronized and coordinated erectile response, although their impact is not fully understood. In severe arterial disease, a loss or reduction of membrane contact is seen because of the presence of collagen fibres between cellular membranes.[53] This may suggest that the loss of normal gap-junction function may alter the coordinated smooth muscle activity.

■ REFERENCES

1. de Groat W C, Steers W D. Neuroanatomy and neurophysiology of penile erection. In: Tanagho E A, Lue T F, McClure R D (eds) Contemporary Management of Impotence and Infertility. Baltimore: Williams & Wilkins, 1988: 3–27

2. Hsu G L, Brock G, Martinez-Pineiro L et al. The three dimensional structure of the human tunica albuginea: anatomical and ultrastructural levels. Int J Impot Res 1992; 4: 117–129

3. Goldstein A M B, Padma-Nathan H. The microarchitecture of the intracavernosal smooth muscle and the cavernosal fibrous skeleton. J Urol 1990; 144: 1145–1146

4. Lue T F, Broderick G. Evaluation and nonsurgical management of erectile dysfunction and priapism. In: Walsh P C, Retik A B, Vaughan E D Jr, Wein A. (eds) Campbell's Urology, 7th edn. Philadelphia: Saunders 1997, 1181–1214

5. Bosch R J, Benard F, Aboseif S R et al. Penile detumescence: characterization of three phases. J Urol 1991; 146: 867–871

6. Hedlund H, Andersson K. Comparison of the responses to drugs acting on adrenoreceptors and muscarinic receptors in human isolated corpus cavernosum and cavernous artery. J Auton Pharmacol 1985; 5: 81–88

7. Diederichs W, Stief C G, Lue T F, Tanagho E A. Norepinephrine involvement in penile detumescence. J Urol 1990; 143: 1264–1266

8. Levin R M, Wein A J. Adrenergic alpha receptors outnumber beta receptors in human penile corpus cavernosum. Invest Urol 1980; 18: 225–226

9. Christ G J, Maayani S, Valcic M, Melman A. Pharmacologic studies of human erectile tissue: characteristics of spontaneous contractions and alterations in alpha-adrenoreceptor responsiveness with age and disease in isolated tissues. Br J Pharmacol 1990; 101: 375–381

10. Traish A M, Netsuwan N, Daley J et al. A heterogeneous population of alpha 1 adrenergic receptors mediates contraction of human corpus cavernosum smooth muscle to norepinephrine. J Urol 1995; 153: 222–227

11. Saenz de Tejada I, Kim N, Lagan I et al. Regulation of adrenergic activity in penile corpus cavernosum. J Urol 1989; 142: 1117–1121

12. Steif C, Benard F, Bosch R et al. Acetylcholine as a possible neurotransmitter in penile erection. J Urol 1989; 141: 1444–1448

13. Ignarro L J, Bush P A, Buga G M et al. Nitric oxide and cyclic GMP formation upon electrical field stimulation causes relaxation of corpus cavernosum smooth muscle. Biochem Biophys Res Commun 1990; 170: 843–850

14. Kim N, Azadzoi K M, Goldstein I, Saenz de Tejada I. A nitric oxide-like factor mediates nonadrenergic-noncholinergic neurogenic relaxation of penile corpus cavernosum smooth muscle. J Clin Invest 1991; 88: 112–118

15. Holmquist F, Steif C G, Jonas U, Anderson K E. Effects of the nitric oxide synthase inhibitor NG-nitro-L-arginine on the erectile response to cavernous nerve stimulation in the rabbit. Acta Physiol Scand 1991; 143: 299–304

16. Kim N, Vardi Y, Padma-Nathan H et al. Oxygen tension regulates the nitric oxide pathway. Physiological role in penile erection. J Clin Invest 1993; 91: 437–442

17. Ottesen B, Wagner G, Virag R, Fahrenkrug J. Penile erection: possible role for vasoactive intestinal peptide as a neurotransmitter. Br Med J 1984; 288: 9–11

18. Kim Y C, Kim J H, Davies M G et al. Modulation of vasoactive intestinal peptide (VIP)-mediated relaxation by nitric oxide and prostanoids in the rabbit corpus cavernosum. J Urol 1995; 153: 807–810

19. Steif C G, Benard F, Bosch R J et al. A possible role of calcitonin-gene-related peptide in the regulation of the smooth muscle tone of the bladder and penis. J Urol 1990; 143: 392–397

20. Kirkeby H J, Fahrenkrug J, Holmquist F, Ottesen B. Vasoactive intestinal peptide (VIP) and peptide histidine methionine (PHM) in human penile corpus cavernosum tissue and circumflex veins: localization and in vitro effects. Eur J Clin Invest 1992; 22: 24–30

21. Hedlund P, Alm P, Hedlund H et al. Localization and effects of pituitary adenylate cyclase-activating polypeptide (PACAP) in human penile erectile tissue. Acta Physiol Scand 1994; 150: 103–104

22. Adaikan P G, Ratnam S S. Pharmacology of penile erection in humans. Cardiovasc Intervent Radiol 1988; 11: 191–194

23. Aboseif S, Riemer R K, Stackl W et al. Quantification of prostaglandin E1 receptors in cavernous tissue of men, monkeys, and dogs. Urol Int 1993; 50: 450–459

24. Andersson K-E, Holmquist F. Regulation of tone in penile cavernous smooth muscle. Established concepts and new findings. World J Urol 1994; 12: 249–261

25. Christ G J, Moreno A P, Parker M E et al. Intercellular communication through gap junctions: a potential role in pharmacomechanical coupling and syncytial tissue contraction in vascular smooth muscle isolated from the human corpus cavernosum. Life Sci 1991; 49: PL195–PL200

26. Steif C G, Djamilian M, Anton P et al. Single potential analysis of cavernous electrical activity in impotent patients: a possible diagnostic method for autonomic cavernous dysfunction and cavernous smooth muscle degeneration. J Urol 1992; 148: 1437–1440

27. Campos de Calvalho A C, Roy C, Moreno A P et al. Gap junctions formed of Connexin 43 are found between smooth muscle cells of human corpus cavernosum. J Urol 1993; 149: 1568–1575

28. Shabsigh R, Fishman I J, Scott F B. Evaluation of erectile impotence. Urology 1988; 32: 83–90

29. Masters W H, Johnson V. Human sexual response. Boston: Little, Brown, 1970

30. Steers W D. Neural control of penile erection. Semin Urol 1990; 8: 66–70

31. Diederichs W, Stief C G, Lue T F, Tanagho E A. Sympathetic inhibition of papaverine induced erection. J Urol 1991; 146: 195–198

32. Kim S C, Oh M M. Norepinephrine involvement in response to intracorporeal injection of papaverine in psychogenic impotence. J Urol 1992; 147: 1530–1532

33. Finkle A L, Taylor S P. Sexual potency after radical prostatectomy. J Urol 1981; 125: 350

34. Walsh P C, Donker P J. Impotence following radical prostatectomy: insight into etiology and prevention. J Urol 1982; 128: 492–497

35. Yeager E S, van Heerdan J A. Sexual function following proctocolectomy and abdominoperineal resection. Ann Surg 1980; 191: 169

36. McDermott D W, Bates R J, Heney N M, Althausen A. Erectile impotence as complication of direct vision cold knife urethrotomy. Urology 1981; 18: 467–469

37. Catalona W J, Bigg S W. Nerve-sparing radical prostatectomy: evaluation of results after 250 patients. J Urol 1990; 143: 538–543

38. Carrier S, Zvara P, Nunes L et al. Regeneration of nitric oxide synthase-containing nerves after cavernous nerve neurotomy in the rat. J Urol 153: 1722–1727

39. Saenz de Tejada I, Kim N, Lagan I et al. Regulation of adrenergic activity in penile corpus cavernosum. J Urol 1989; 142: 1117–1121

40. Hirshkowitz M, Karacan I, Rando K C et al. Diabetes, erectile dysfunction, and sleep related erections. Sleep 1990; 13: 53–68

41. Goldstein I, Feldman M I, Deckers P J et al. Radiation associated impotence. A clinical study of its mechanism. JAMA 1984; 251: 903–910

42. Levine F J, Greenfield A J, Goldstein I. Arteriographically determined occlusive disease within the hypogastric–cavernous bed in impotent patients following blunt perineal and pelvic trauma. J Urol 1990; 144: 1147–1153

43. Rosen M P, Greenfield A J, Walker T G et al. Cigarette smoking: an independent risk factor for atherosclerosis in the hypogastric–cavernous arterial bed of men with arteriogenic impotence. J Urol 1991; 145: 759–763

44. Junemenn K P, Lue T F, Luo J A et al. The effect of cigarette smoking on penile erection. J Urol 1987; 138: 438–441

45. Hsieh J T, Muller S C, Lue T F. The influence of blood flow and blood pressure on penile erection. Int J Impot Res 1992; 4: 117–129

46. Hayashi K, Takamizawa K, Nakamura T et al. Effects of elastase on the stiffness and elastic properties of arterial walls in cholesterol fed rabbits. Atherosclerosis 1987; 66: 259–267

47. Moreland R B, Traish A, McMillan M A et al. PGE1 suppresses the induction of collagen synthesis by transforming growth factor beta 1 in human corpus cavernosum smooth muscle. J Urol 1995; 153: 826–834

48. Wespes E, Goes P M, Schiffman S et al. Computerized analysis of smooth muscle fibers in potent and impotent patients. J Urol 1991; 146: 1015–1017

49. Junemann K P, Aufenanger J, Konrad T et al. The effect of impaired lipid metabolism on the smooth muscle cells of rabbits. Urol Res 1991; 19: 271–275

50. Paick J S, Goldsmith P C, Batra A K et al. Relationship between venous incompetence and cavernous nerve injury: ultrastructural alteration of cavernous smooth muscle in the neurotomized dog. Int J Impot Res 1991; 3: 185–195

51. Mersdorf A, Goldsmith P C, Deiderichs W et al. Ultrastructural changes in impotent penile tissue: a comparison of 65 patients. J Urol 1991; 145: 749–758

52. Fan S F, Brink P R, Melman A, Christ G J. An analysis of the Maxi-K+ (KCa) channel in cultured human corporal smooth muscle cells. J Urol 1995; 153: 818–825

53. Perrson C, Diederichs W, Lue T F et al. Correlation of altered penile ultrastructure with clinical arterial evaluation. J Urol 1989; 142: 1462–1468

Chapter 5

Animal models used in the study of erectile dysfunction

F. Giuliano, O. Rampin and K. E. McKenna

◼ INTRODUCTION

Erectile dysfunction (ED) is now recognized as a significant disease, and its aetiology and treatments have been debated at an NIH Consensus Conference.[1] Although the dysfunction can have multifactorial aetiology, invariably this translates as an aberrant erectile response. Owing to the 'greying' of the population and an increased awareness of the disease and treatment options, there has been a resurgence of interest in basic research designed to increase our understanding of the erectile process under normal and abnormal conditions.

Penile erection is the vasculo-tissue response to an integrated complex series of physiological processes subserving reproductive behaviour. Ultimately, erection depends on the tone of smooth muscle fibres in both erectile and vascular tissue and relies upon coordinated neural and humoral responses at many levels. Although research into the neurophysiology of erection began in the 19th century,[2,3] knowledge of the integrated control is still somewhat superficial. However, experiments using isolated organs or tissues have given us some insight into some discrete aspects of the 'erectile' process. However, to exploit these findings fully, it is necessary (and will become increasingly so in the future) to determine the relevance in the whole animal. This chapter describes the value of available animal models and the potential utility in understanding the pathophysiology of the erectile process and erectile dysfunction. Apart from situations where in vitro pharmacological experiments have helped the understanding of differences between normal and aberrant situations, this type of study, which may involve tissue of animal origin, is described in more detail elsewhere in this book (Chapter 7).

◼ MODELS USED TO STUDY THE ERECTILE PROCESS

The understanding of the basic neurophysiology of erection owes much to pioneering work of, among others, Langley and Anderson, Eckhard, Gaskell and Goltz in anaesthetized animals.[2,3] In several species, electrical stimulation of sacral nerves, anterior sacral roots or the lumbosacral spinal cord was found to increase blood leakage from the sectioned penis, which was considered to be a surrogate endpoint for the erectile response. These experiments also demonstrated that anti-erectile fibres were carried within the lumbosacral paravertebral sympathetic chain, reaching the penis via the pudendal nerve. A synergistic erectile response between the autonomic and somatic nerves was also described at an early stage.[3,4]

Using the new technique of penile plethysmography to measure overall penile volume, Sjöstrand and Klinge[5] demonstrated that the sympathetic innervation carried within the pudendal nerve was responsible for penile vasoconstriction and retraction. The role of the sympathetic nervous system was further reinforced by the penile protrusion observed in response to sympathetic nerve section or pudendal nerve anaesthesia.

More recently, the measurement of intracavernosal pressure changes as an index of penile erection has greatly enhanced our understanding of basic erectogenic pathways and systems. In anaesthetized dogs and monkeys, erection was shown to be accompanied by increases in penile pressure, reaching levels equivalent to systolic blood pressure.[6,7] In these and other studies a combination of intracorporal drug administration and selective nerve stimulation or ablation has greatly increased understanding of the neurophysiology and neuropharmacology of erection.[6–10]

Studies in both conscious and anaesthetized animals have also played a pivotal role in the determination of the spinal and supraspinal control of erection. On the basis of such studies and from observations in spinal cord patients and in men with impotence after neurosurgical lesioning, penile erection was originally considered to be initiated by two distinct pathways, reflexogenic and psychogenic (Chapter 7). However, although reflex and centrally activated pathways may exist, there is considerable synergy and their consideration as two independent systems may be too facile.[11] Nevertheless, it is apparent that the overall control of erection is based on integration of local, spinal and supraspinal neural activity.

Animal studies have also helped to determine the interrelationship between local vascular changes and erection. Early studies used morphological approaches and selective nerve trunk stimulation on which to base conclusions regarding the temporal association of local haemodynamics and penile erection in several species.[3,4,12] In dogs, the observed increase in arterial blood flow was considered to be sufficient to account for cavernosal engorgement.[13] Pelvic nerve stimulation induced a tenfold increase in arterial inflow in dogs and monkeys, which was independent of cholinergic mechanisms.[6,14] In anaesthetized dogs and monkeys, Lue and colleagues demonstrated that cavernosal nerve stimulation produced a transient increase in internal pudendal arterial flow, which was followed by a sustained increase in intracavernosal pressure.[7,15]

These and other studies have unequivocally demonstrated the obligatory role of a transient and dramatic increase in arterial flow to the penis in the generation of the erectile response. Similar studies (described later) are being used to determine the effect of vascular impairment on the development of erectile dysfunction. It is known, for example, that diseases such as atherosclerosis cause reduction in blood flow to the penis. Potentially, an animal model could be developed to be used in the identification of novel treatment strategies for atherosclerosis-associated erectile dysfunction (see below).

■ PHARMACOLOGICAL STUDIES

Although much has been learned about the control of erection from studies in vitro of isolated tissue (Chapter 7),[16] animal studies are invariably required to determine the functional significance of such observations and the potential therapeutic application. The hierarchy of experimentation is often as follows: in relatively simple experimental situations, potential neurotransmitters/neuromodulators are routinely identified using immunohistochemical localization or radioligand-binding studies. Functional activity is then determined by application of agents to cavernosal tissue isolated from several species, including humans. There are now several criteria that must be satisfied before any endogenous substance can be considered to be an endogenous neurotransmitter. Finally, the contribution to the overall physiological homeostasis is confirmed in anaesthetized or conscious animals. Using a combination of in vitro and in vivo techniques, the key role of the major neurotransmitters noradrenaline and acetylcholine was established at an early stage.[16] Subsequently, using similar techniques, the potential contribution from other neuromodulators, e.g. vasoactive intestinal peptide (VIP), calcitonin gene-related peptide (CGRP), angiotensin II (AII), prostanoids and endothelins has been investigated (Chapter 6). A major focus of this type of research is now obviously into the synaptic dynamics of nitric oxide (NO) (see Chapter 11). It is likely that 'gene knockout' studies, involving animals in which relevant NO genes have been disrupted,[17,18] will be at the forefront of these evaluations and may provide the ultimate proof of physiological function.

Iatrogenic sexual dysfunctions are increasingly listed with drug precautions. The identification of such sexual side effects of drugs, along with studies of mechanism of action and characterization in animals, now forms the basis for strategies directed towards the medical management of sexual dysfunction. In this context, the use of animal models is a key component of basic research within the pharmaceutical industry. Several pharmacological agents, e.g. apomorphine, amantadine, N-n-propyl-norapomorphine, LY 17155, LY 163502, lisuride, pilocarpine, RDS-127, fluoxetine, m-chlorophenylpiperazine and D1/D2 or D2 agonists, have been shown to induce penile erection in several species.[19–26] It is anticipated that a more complete analysis of the erectogenic action of these agents may facilitate the development of novel therapeutic compounds.

■ ANIMAL MODELS OF ERECTILE DYSFUNCTION

Not unexpectedly, owing to the multifactorial nature of erectile dysfunction, many diverse potential models have been described. A major focus has been on models based on associated risk factors, especially ageing, diabetes, atherosclerosis and other vascular disorders.[27]

Diabetic models

Erectile dysfunction is a common and devastating consequence of diabetes in adult men. In an attempt to understand the diabetes-induced changes, several strategies have been developed. The most common has been to analyse neural, vascular and biochemical changes subsequent to streptozotocin-induced (hyperglycaemia-dependent) diabetes in rats or rabbits.[28–31] Several indices of neural function were found to be altered: compared with control animals, the reflex increase in corpus cavernosal pressure elicited by dorsal penile nerve activation was attenuated,[32] as was the erectile response to intracerebroventricular VIP.[31] Histomorphometric analysis has shown selective changes in specific nerve tracts, e.g. rat dorsal nerve in streptozotocin-treated animals,[33] and additional evidence, based on noradrenergic varicosity neurotransmitter content[34] and nitric oxide synthase,[35] has been observed.

In contrast to the morphological deterioration, there is no evidence of a reduction in levels of cyclic guanosine or adenosine monophosphates (cGMP or cAMP), the second messengers primarily involved in cavernosal smooth muscle relaxation, subsequent to streptozotocin-induced diabetes in rodents and lagomorphs.[36,37] One possibility is that this represents an adaptive change to compensate for reduced efficiency of the neuronal processing of the erectile response. The observed augmented erectogenic response to locally applied VIP in diabetic rats, in comparison to control animals,[38] would be consistent with this hypothesis.

The BB/WOR rat represents a model of type I diabetes in which a spontaneous autoimmune destruction of pancreatic beta cells, and associated diabetes, occurs. The animal is insulin dependent for survival and prone to ketoacidosis, but without microangiopathy. However, as diabetic neuropathy is present, it may represent a useful model for examining the neural components of diabetes in the absence of confounding vascular changes. As in the case of streptozotocin-diabetic animals, there is substantial electrophysiological, histomorphological and biochemical evidence of diabetes-induced changes in erectile function.[28,39–41] However, it is not known whether these changes reflect selective changes in the neuronal architecture or result from the metabolic sequelae of the hyperglycaemia.

In addition to these neural changes, diabetes-induced changes in penile vascular reactivity may also contribute to the overall deficit in erectile dysfunction[36] and contributions from endocrine factors cannot be ruled out. Circulating testosterone, which plays a key role in sexual behaviour and reflexes, is reduced in diabetic animals.[28]

Overall, the animal data indicate that the erectile dysfunction associated with diabetes results from a selective, though generalized, neuropathy. This is likely to involve spinal cord processing, afferent–efferent reflex activity and activity within efferent autonomic pathways.

Atherosclerotic models

The appreciation that corpus cavernosal trabecular smooth muscle can be affected by vascular disorders (Chapter 10)[1] has led to the search for relevant animal models. In particular, in an attempt to reproduce the structural and morphometric changes within the cavernosal tissue, atherosclerotic models have been developed and characterized.[42–44] In essence, these are based on feeding rabbits with a diet enriched with cholesterol and other additives to produce a functional hypercholesterolaemia.[42] This, by analogy to changes induced in other blood vessels, is thought to induce collagen synthesis and deposition within the penile vasculature. Impairment of arterial inflow will in turn lead to reduced oxygenation of erectile tissue and the metabolic consequences thereof.[44] Under these conditions, not surprisingly, malfunctions of endothelium-dependent relaxation and general smooth muscle contractile properties have been demonstrated.[42,43]

It is likely that, in the future, this type of model will be used in the identification of agents that affect the underlying disease progression rather than of agents to produce acute symptomatic relief.

Ageing models

Epidemiological studies suggest a close association between impotence and increasing age.[27] Ageing certainly causes changes in penile responsiveness to mechanoreceptor activation, and conduction velocity within the dorsal penile nerve is reduced.[45] Under anaesthesia, old rats (20 months) display a smaller erectile response to cavernosal nerve stimulation than young animals (5 months); this can be rectified by chronic androgen treatment.[46] Changes become more dependent of major changes in the NO–cGMP pathway, as age increases, which has led to the suggestion that ageing has not only a direct myogenic action, reducing the response and sensitivity to pro-erectile neurotransmitters/neuromodulators.[46] This would be consistent with the observed reduction in response to in vitro or intracavernosal administration of papaverine[47,48] and the reduced amplitude and filling rate of the corpora of old rats (27 months). Interpretation of the results is complicated, as the magnitude and direction of the age-induced changes can be dependent on the age of the animals.[47,48] An additional complication is that changes may be secondary to those induced elsewhere on the overall animal homeostasis rather than reflecting a direct action on corporal tissue per se.

Spinal cord injury and other trauma

Comparative studies in anaesthetized and conscious animals have played a key role in understanding the spinal and supraspinal control of erectile function (Chapter 8). In particular, they have led to our current knowledge on the independence and synergy between the reflexogenic and psychogenic control processes. In addition, it has been possible to demonstrate that there are both inhibitory and facilitatory influences at spinal and higher centres.

There are several examples but, in particular, spinal trauma has been shown, in as little as 4 weeks, to increase the magnitude of the erectile response to papaverine, minoxidil and nitroglycerine when delivered locally to lightly anaesthetized rats, and papaverine was more potent in rats with spinal cord injury.[49] Further evidence of spinal inhibition comes from rodent studies where reflexogenic activity was enhanced by spinalization at T8.[50,51] Spinal cord transection has also been shown to augment activity in other urogenital reflex arcs.[52] In conscious dogs and rats, a supraspinal inhibitory pathway on penile erection has been demonstrated by thoracic transection.[53–55] Following cauda equina lesioning, stimulation of the hypothalamic medial pre-optic area (paradoxically for a sympathetic pathway) elicits penile erection in conscious rats; this is consistent with the development of a compensatory pathway via the sympathetic thoracolumbar outflow.[56]

Similar adaptive or compensatory phenomena have been described subsequent to section of peripheral nerves. Several days after unilateral section of the pelvic nerve, hypogastric nerve stimulation applied to the lesioned side produces a rise in intracavernosal pressure. In contrast, corporal pressure is unaffected when the stimulus is applied to the hypogastric nerve on the intact side.[57] Similarly, section of the paravertebral sympathetic chain at the L4–L5 level influences the rise in intracavernosal pressure induced by stimulation of the medial pre-optic nuclei, suggesting that at a supraspinal level the sympathetic paravertebral outflow plays a regulatory role in the erectile process.[58] Finally and intriguingly, 6 months after unilateral cavernosal nerve section, evidence of nerve regeneration within the previously denervated cavernosal tissue has been reported.[59] There is a corresponding increase in nerve-induced intracavernosal pressure over this period.[59]

There is only limited information on the impact of tissue irradiation on erectile function. In one series of experiments by Carrier and colleagues, this was measured in the rat.[60] Over the radiation dose range 100–2000 cGy, several indices of erectile function were changed. In conscious rats the erectile response to systemic apomorphine was reduced. In anaesthetized animals, there were attenuated intracorporal pressure increases on intracavernosal papaverine and cavernosal nerve stimulation. It is likely, therefore, that penile irradiation may affect penile innervation and smooth muscle function as well as the penile vascular supply.

Androgen-dependent models

The role of androgens in the development ('organization') and maintenance ('activation') of sexual function is well known.[61] In several species, castration substantially altered sexual reflexes — a condition that could be reversed by androgen, but not oestrogen, replacement.[61] For several years, androgens have been hypothesized to have permissive actions on penile afferents and sensory receptors and on spinal motor neurons innervating the perineal muscles.[62,63] More recent support for androgen dependency comes from studies of cavernosal nerve stimulation in anaesthetized rats, where the effect of castration on cavernosal pressure and nitric oxide synthase (NOS) was measured.[64–67] Both pressure and enzyme activity were reduced by castration. There is, however, an apparent paradox in that there are few cavernosal androgen receptors in the adult rat[68] and the relaxant response of isolated rabbit cavernosal tissue is unaffected by castration. On this basis it has been hypothesized that the site of action of androgens was not myogenic and within the autonomic nervous system. Consistent with this assumption is the demonstration of androgen receptors on penile parasympathetic postganglionic neurons.[69] Overall, therefore, a precise role for androgens in generation of erectile dysfunction has yet to be demonstrated. However, should a key role for androgens be identified subsequently, androgen-dependent animal models have the advantage in so far as they are relatively easily produced surgically.

ANIMAL MODELS: FUTURE PERSPECTIVES

Within this decade, molecular biology has come of age and is now being used even in animal research in transgenic and/or gene knockout experiments. Although the ultimate goal of this type of research, i.e. gene therapy directed to rectification of aberrant gene activity, may be some way off, important contributions have already been made towards understanding of the pathophysiology of various disease processes. Particularly relevant to impotence is the translation of transgenic technology directed towards an increased understanding of NO–cGMP-dependent systems.[17,18,70,71] However, interpretation of data is often complicated. For example, transgenic mice lacking neuronal NOS (nNOS) are able to generate and maintain erections,[17] which would appear to be at variance with pharmacological and biochemical studies which unequivocally link this NOS isoform to corporal smooth muscle (Chapter 11). This anomaly may be reconciled on the basis of a compensatory induction of other NOS isoforms present in penile vasculature and sinusoidal epithelium.

Although animal models have already considerably advanced understanding of the neurophysiology of erection, interpretation — of necessity — is often compromised by the presence of anaesthesia. Traditionally, only data from sexual behavioural experiments have been available. More recently, using telemetric techniques, it has become possible to accrue information from conscious animals in social groups[72] or in isolation.[73–75] In the case of the latter it has even been possible to measure intracavernosal and intraspongiosal pressure in conscious rodents.

CONCLUSIONS

Tremendous advances in our understanding of the integrated neurophysiology of erection and the pathophysiology of erectile dysfunction have been made over the last 15 years. Although major contributions have been made by the pharmacologist and molecular biologist, ultimately the piecing together of the jigsaw has involved studies in animals. Further, with the advent of transgenic technology, it is likely that an increasingly important contribution will be made to basic penile research.

However, although several models, e.g. diabetic, atherosclerotic and spinal injury, have been developed that display some of the characteristics of the underlying human disease condition, there is no validated model of erectile dysfunction. In general, these models have successfully been directed by the pharmaceutical industry towards the identification of agents for the acute medical management of the symptoms of male erectile dysfunction. Increasingly, it is likely that this type of basic and applied animal research will be targeted towards treatment of the underlying aetiology and disease progression. Correspondingly, animal models will play an ever-increasing role in these endeavours.

REFERENCES

1. National Institutes of Health Consensus Conference: Impotence. NIH Consensus Development Panel on Impotence. JAMA 1993; 270: 83–90

2. Eckhard C. Untersuchungen über die Erection des Penis beim Hunde. Beitr Anat Physiol 1863; 3: 123–150

3. Langley J N, Anderson H K. The innervation of the pelvic and adjoining viscera. J Physiol (Lond) 1895; 19: 71–130

4. Henderson V E, Roepke M H. On the mechanisms of erection. Am J Physiol 1933; 106: 441–448

5. Sjöstrand N O, Klinge E K. Principal mechanisms controlling penile retraction and protrusion in rabbits. Acta Physiol Scand 1979; 106: 199–214

6. Carati C J, Creed K E, Keogh E J. Vascular changes during penile erection in the dog. J Physiol (Lond) 1988; 400: 75–88

7. Lue T F, Takamura T, Schmidt R A et al. Hemodynamics of erection in the monkey. J Urol 1983; 130: 1237–1241

8. Lue T F, Umraiya M, Takamura T et al. Animal model for penile erection studies. Neurourol Urodyn 1983; 2: 225–231

9. Giuliano F, Rampin O, Bernabé J, Rousseau J P. Neural control of penile erection in the rat. J Auton Nerv Syst 1995; 55: 36–44

10. Jünemann K P, Persson-Jünemann C, Lue T F et al. Neurophysiological aspects of penile erection: the role of the sympathetic nervous system. Br J Urol 1989; 64: 84–92

11. Sachs B D. Placing erection in context: the reflexogenic–psychogenic dichotomy reconsidered. Neurosci Biobehav Rev 1995; 19: 211–224

12. Christensen G C. Angioarchitecture of the canine penis and the process of erection. Am J Anat 1954: 95: 227–261

13. Dorr L D, Brody M J. Hemodynamic mechanisms of erection in the canine penis. Am J Physiol 1967; 213: 1526–1531

14. Andersson P O, Bloom S R, Mellander S. Haemodynamics of pelvic nerve induced penile erection in the dog: possible mediation by vasoactive intestinal polypeptide. J Physiol (Lond) 1984; 350: 209–224

15. Lue T F, Takamura T, Umraiya M et al. Hemodynamics of canine corpora cavernosa during erection. Urology 1984; 24: 347–352

16. Andersson K E. Pharmacology of lower urinary tract smooth muscles and penile erectile tissues. Pharmacol Rev 1993; 45: 254–308

17. Huang P L, Dawson T M, Bredt D S et al. Targeted disruption of the neuronal nitric oxide synthase gene. Cell 1993; 75: 1273–1286

18. Huang P L, Huang Z, Mashimo H et al. Hypertension in mice lacking the gene for endothelial nitric oxide synthase. Nature 1995; 377: 239–242

19. Baraldi M, Benassi-Benelli A, Lolli M. Penile erection in rats after fenfluramine administration. Riv Farmacol Ther 1977; 8: 375–379

20. Benassi-Benelli A, Ferrari F, Pellegrini Quarantotti B. Penile erection induced by apomorphine and N-n-propyl-norapomorphine in rats. Arch Int Pharmacodyn Ther 1979; 241: 128–134

21. Berendsen H H G, Jenck F, Broekkamp C L E. Involvement of 5-HT1C receptors in drug-induced penile erections in rats. Psychopharmacology 1990; 101: 57–61

22. Gower A J, Berendsen H H G, Proncen M M, Broekkamp C L E. The yawning–penile erection syndrome as a model for putative dopamine autoreceptor activity. Eur J Pharmacol 1984; 103: 81–89

23. Maeda N, Matsuoka N, Yamaguchi I. Septohippocampal cholinergic pathway and penile erections induced by dopaminergic and cholinergic stimulants. Brain Res 1990; 537: 163–168

24. Maeda N, Matsuoka N, Yamaguchi I. Possible involvement of the septo-hippocampal cholinergic and raphe–hippocampal serotonergic activations in the penile erection induced by fenfluramine in rats. Brain Res 1994; 652: 181–189

25. Szele F G, Murphy D L, Garrick N A. Effects of fenfluramine, m-chlorophenylpiperazine, and other serotonin-related agonists and antagonists on penile erection in non-human primates. Life Sci 1988; 43: 1297–1303

26. Millan M J, Peglion J L, Lavielle G, Perrin-Monneyron S. 5-HT2C receptors mediate penile erections in rats: actions of novel and selective agonists and antagonists. Eur J Pharmacol 1997; 325: 9–12

27. Benet A E, Melman A. The epidemiology of erectile dysfunction. Urol Clin North Am 1995; 22: 699–709

28. Murray F T, Johnson R D, Sciadini M et al. Erectile and copulatory dysfunction in chronically diabetic BB/WOR rats. Am J Physiol 1992; 263: E151–E157

29. Olsson Y, Save-Soderbegh J, Sourander P, Angerdall Z A. Pathoanatomical study of the central and peripheral nervous system in diabetes of early onset and long duration. Pathol Eur 1968; 3: 62–79

30. Leedom L J, Meehan W R. The psychoneuroendocrinology of diabetes mellitus in rodents. Psychoneuroendocrinology 1989; 14: 275–294

31. Yamaguchi Y, Kobayashi H. Effects of apomorphine, physostigmine and vasoactive intestinal peptide on penile erection and yawning in diabetic rats. Eur J Pharmacol 1994; 254: 91–96

32. Italiano G, Marin A, Pescatori E S et al. Effect of streptozotocin-induced diabetes on electrically evoked erection in the rat. Int J Impot Res 1993; 5: 27–35

33. Italiano G, Petrelli L, Marin A et al. Ultrastructural analysis of the cavernous and dorsal penile nerves in experimental diabetes. Int J Impot Res 1993; 5: 149–160

34. Felten D L, Felten S Y, Melman A. Noradrenergic innervation of the penis in control and streptozotocin-diabetic rats: evidence of autonomic neuropathy. Anat Rec 1983; 206: 49–59

35. Elabbady A A, Gagnon C, Hassouna M M et al. Diabetes mellitus increases nitric oxide synthase in penises but not in major pelvic ganglia of rats. Br J Urol 1995; 76: 196–202

36. Miller M A, Morgan R J, Thompson C S et al. Adenylate and guanylate cyclase activity in the penis and aorta of the diabetic rat: an in vitro study. Br J Urol 1994; 74: 106–111

37. Miller M A, Morgan R J, Thompson C S et al. Effects of papaverine and vasoactive intestinal peptide on penile and vascular cAMP and cGMP in control and diabetic animals: an in vitro study. Int J Impot Res 1995; 7: 91–100

38. Gozes I, Reshef A, Salah D et al. Stearyl-norleucine-vasoactive intestinal peptide [VIP]: a novel VIP analog for noninvasive impotence treatment. Endocrinology 1994; 134: 2121–2125

39. McVary K T, Rathnau C, McKenna K E. Sexual dysfunction in the diabetic BB/WOR rat: a role of central neuropathy. Am J Physiol 1997; 272: R259–R267

40. Vernet D, Cai L, Garban H et al. Reduction of penile nitric oxide synthase in diabetic BB/WOR^{dp} [Type I] and BB/WOR^{dp} [Type II] rats with erectile dysfunction. Endocrinology 1995; 136: 5709–5717

41. Brannigan R E, McVary K T, McKenna K E. Nitric oxide synthase levels in chronic diabetic rats. Soc Neurosci Abstr 1996; 22: 1052

42. Azadzoi K M, Saenz de Tejada I. Hypercholesterolemia impairs endothelium-dependent relaxation of rabbit corpus cavernosum smooth muscle. J Urol 1991; 146: 238–240

43. Kim J H, Klyachkin M L, Svendsen E et al. Experimental hypercholesterolemia in rabbit induces cavernosal

atherosclerosis with endothelial and smooth muscle cell dysfunction. J Urol 1994; 151: 198–205

44. Azadzoi K M, Siroky M B, Goldstein I. Study of etiologic relationship of arterial atherosclerosis to corporal veno-occlusive dysfunction in the rabbit. J Urol 1996; 155: 1795–1800

45. Johnson R D, Murray F T. Reduced vibrotactile sensitivity of penile mechanoreceptors in aging rats with sexual dysfunction. Brain Res Bull 1992; 28: 61–64

46. Garban H, Marquez D, Cai L et al. Restoration of normal adult penile erection response in aged rats by long-term treatment with androgens. Biol Reprod 1995; 53: 1365–1372

47. Garban H, Vernet D, Freedman A et al. Effect of aging on nitric oxide mediated penile erection in rats. Am J Physiol 1995; 268: H467–H475

48. Calabro A, Italiano G, Pescatori E S et al. Physiological aging and penile erectile function: a study in the rat. Eur Urol 1996; 29: 240–244

49. Rivas D A, Chancellor M B, Huang B, Salzman S K. Erectile response to topical, intraurethral and intracorporal pharmacotherapy in a rat model of spinal cord injury. J Spinal Cord Med 1995; 18: 245–250

50. Steers W D, Mallory B, DeGroat W C. Electrophysiological study of neural activity in penile nerve of the rat. Am J Physiol 1988; 254: R989–R1000

51. Pescatori E S, Calabro A, Artibani W et al. Electrical stimulation of the dorsal nerve of the penis evokes reflex tonic erections of the penile body and reflex ejaculatory responses in the spinal rat. J Urol 1993; 149: 627–632

52. McKenna K E, Chung S K, McVary K T. A model for the study of sexual function in anesthetized male and female rats. Am J Physiol 1991; 261: R1276–R1285

53. Hart B L. Testosterone regulation of sexual reflexes in spinal male rats. Science 1967; 155: 1283–1284

54. Sachs B D, Garinello L D. Spinal pacemaker controlling sexual reflexes in male rats. Brain Res 1979; 171: 152-156

55. Hart B L, Kitchell R L. Penile erection and contraction of penile muscles in the spinal and intact dog. Am J Physiol 1966; 210: 257–262

56. Courtois F J, MacDougall J C, Sachs B D. Erectile mechanisms in paraplegia. Physiol Behav 1993; 53: 721–726

57. Dail W G, Walton G, Olmsted M P. Penile erection in the rat: stimulation of the hypogastric nerve elicits increases in penile pressure after chronic interruption of the sacral parasympathetic outflow. J Auton Nerv Syst 1989; 28: 251–258

58. Giuliano F, Bernabé J, Brown K et al. Erectile response to hypothalamic stimulation in rats: role of peripheral nerves. Am J Physiol 1997; 273: R1990–R1997

59. Carrier S, Zvara P, Kour N W et al. The effect of cavernous nerve neurotomy on erectile function and nitric oxide synthase containing nerves in the rat. Int J Impot Res 1994; 6(suppl1): A6

60. Carrier S. Baba K, Hricak H et al. Radiation induced decrease in nitric oxide synthase-containing nerves in the rat penis. J Urol 1995; 153(Suppl): 507A

61. Meisel R L, Sachs B D. The physiology of male sexual behaviour. In: Knobil E, Neill J D (eds) The physiology of reproduction, 2nd edn. New York: Raven Press, 1994; ch 35: 3–105

62. Sachs B D. Potency and fertility: hormonal and mechanical causes and effects of penile actions in rats. In: Balthazart J, Pröve E, Gilles R (eds) Hormones and behaviour in higher vertebrates. Springer-Verlag: Berlin, 1983; 86–110

63. Arnold A P, Jordan C L. Hormonal organization of neural circuits. In: Martini L, Ganong W F (eds) Frontiers in neuroendocrinology. New York: Raven Press, 1988; 10: 185–214

64. Mills T M, Wiedmeyer V T, Stopper V S. Androgen maintenance of erectile function in the rat penis. Biol Reprod 1992; 46: 342–348

65. Giuliano F, Rampin O, Schirar A et al. Autonomic control of penile erection: modulation by testosterone in the rat. J Neuroendocrinol 1993; 5: 677–683

66. Lugg J A, Rajfer J, Gonzalez-Cadavid N F. Dihydrotestosterone is the active androgen in the maintenance of nitric oxide-mediated penile erection in the rat. Endocrinology 1995; 136: 1495–1501

67. Chamness S L, Ricker D D, Crone J K et al. The effect of androgen on nitric oxide synthase in the male reproductive tract of the rat. Fertil Steril 1995; 63: 1101-1107

68. Rajfer J, Namkung P C, Petra P H. Identification, partial characterization and age-related changes of a cytoplasmic androgen receptor in the rat penis. J Steroid Biochem 1980; 13: 1489–1492

69. Schirar A, Chang C, Rousseau J P. Localization of androgen receptor in nitric oxide synthase- and vasoactive intestinal peptide-containing neurons of the major pelvic ganglion innervating the rat penis. J. Neuroendocrinol 1997; 9: 141–150

70. Ignarro L J, Bush P A, Buga G M et al. Nitric oxide and cyclic GMP formation upon electrical field stimulation cause relaxation of corpus cavernosum smooth muscle. Biochem Biophys Res Commun 1990; 170: 843–850

71. Holmquist F, Stief C G, Jonas U, Anderson K E. Effects of the nitric oxide synthase inhibitor NG-nitro-L-arginine on the erectile response to cavernous nerve stimulation in the rabbit. Acta Physiol Scand 1991; 143: 299–304

72. Giuliano F, Bernabé J, Rampin O et al. Telemetric monitoring of intracavernous pressure in freely moving rats during copulation. J Urol 1994; 152: 1271–1274

73. Schmidt M H, Valatx J L, Schmidt H S et al. Experimental evidence of penile erections during paradoxical sleep in the rat. Neuroreport 1994; 5: 561–564

74. Bernabé J, Rampin O, Giuliano F, Benoit G. Intracavernous pressure changes during reflexive penile erections in the rat. Physiol Behav 1995; 57: 837–841

75. Schmidt M H, Valatx J L, Sakai K et al. Corpus spongiosum penis pressure and perineal muscle activity during reflexive erections in the rat. Am J Physiol 1995; 269: R904–R913

Chapter 6
Vascular physiology of penile erection

I. Moncada Iribarren and I. Sáenz de Tejada

■ INTRODUCTION

Penile erection is a complex series of integrated vascular events culminating in the accumulation of blood under pressure and end-organ rigidity. Fundamentally involved in the intrapenile response are the paired corpus cavernosa, which contain the erectile components and are surrounded by a thick fibroelastic sheath, the tunica albuginea. As there is vascular connectivity along three-quarters of the length of the corpora, in physiological terms they function as a single-compartment blood or hydraulic system. The erectile tissue comprises multiple interconnecting sinusoidal spaces or lacunae. The lacunar walls or trabeculae contain the fibromuscular contractile elements, consisting of smooth muscle, elastin and collagen, attached to the inner surface of the tunica. The tone of the smooth muscle, which can represent up to 45% of the trabecular tissue, is the prime physiological determinant of organ flaccidity or erection. In the flaccid state, the trabecular smooth muscle is tonically contracted by discharge within the sympathetic noradrenergic nervous system. Under these conditions, only basal arterial inflow sufficient for maintenance of cellular metabolism is present. In this state blood gas levels are equivalent only to those found in venous blood.

During erection there is a considerable (up to eightfold) increase in the effective intrapenile blood volume, with corresponding expansion of trabecular walls and lacunar spaces. As a result, intracorporal pressure approaches systemic blood pressure, producing both an increase in penile volume (tumescence) and rigidity.

The autonomic nervous system provides the integrated control of most of these smooth muscle-dependent changes in local vascular reactivity.

■ ARTERIAL CONTROL

Increase in intracorporal blood flow has several consequences. First, the resultant increase in volume and pressure in the corpus cavernosum establishes a full erection. Failure of the arterial supply to provide adequate inflow results in incomplete erection. In addition, the supply of freshly perfused, highly oxygenated blood is required to support the enhanced cellular metabolism associated with erection. Furthermore, there is a local homoeostatic role as oxygen alters the synthesis of local erectogenic vasodilator substances.[1,2]

Blood supply to the deep structures of the penis is derived from the internal pudendal artery, which is the final branch of the anterior trunk of the internal iliac artery. The former becomes the common penile artery which in turn branches into three — the bulbo-urethral, cavernosal and dorsal penile end arteries. The cavernosal artery is the most important determinant of intracavernosal pressure; along its length this artery gives off mutiple helicine branches which encompass the lacunar spaces. During the flaccid state the vascular smooth muscle in these resistance vessels is contracted, allowing only limited blood flow into the lacunar spaces. On activation of the appropriate component of the autonomic system the vascular smooth muscle relaxes and the arteries lengthen and relax, increasing intracorporal blood flow and pressure. Although only relatively low local blood flow is required to maintain erection, flow rate into the lacunar spaces determines the rate of filling of the corporal bodies.[3,4] On this basis it can be concluded that, under normal conditions, penile rigidity will be more dependent on arterial pressure than on flow. Occasionally the cavernosal arteries divide into two or three branches inside the corpus cavernosum and in 30% of cases there are communications between both cavernosal arteries; in some instances, connections with dorsal arteries are also present.[5] This would represent a compensatory mechanism in cases of cavernosal arteriopathy.

ROLE OF THE VEINS: THE CORPOROVENO-OCCLUSIVE MECHANISM

The accumulation of blood inside the corpora cavernosa determines the establishment of an erection. Arterial inflow must enter a closed space to expand the lacunae and the trabecular walls against the tunica albuginea, enabling the transmission of the arterial pressure to the tunica albuginea. The mechanism that traps the pressurized blood within the corpora is known as the corporoveno-occlusive mechanism[3,6] (Fig. 6.1).

The lacunae are intercommunicating vascular spaces lined by endothelium. The communication allows blood flow and transmission of pressure from proximal to distal zones of the corpora and from one to the other corpus cavernosum. Lacunar spaces have a greater diameter in the central zone surrounding the cavernosal artery in each corpus cavernosum and this diameter decreases progressively towards the most peripheral areas next to the tunica albuginea, from where the drainage of the corpora takes place. The progressively decreasing proportions of the lacunar spaces probably represent the first obstacle that limits the drainage from the corpora, as resistance is inversely proportional to the radius of the vessel. Nevertheless, in the flaccid penis, inasmuch as there is a wide drainage plexus, emptying of the penis occurs easily and, globally, at low resistance. Venules, forming a network under the tunica albuginea, drain the peripheral lacunae and coalesce to form the emissary veins, which pierce the tunica and drain either directly into the deep dorsal vein or by way of the circumflex veins.

The current hypothesis is that the veno-occlusive mechanism relies, mainly, on the subtunical venules whose conformational change, induced by the expansion of the penis from flaccidity to tumescence, provokes an increase in the resistance to the drainage of corpora. When the penis increases its volume, the venules stretch out, diminishing their diameter. The

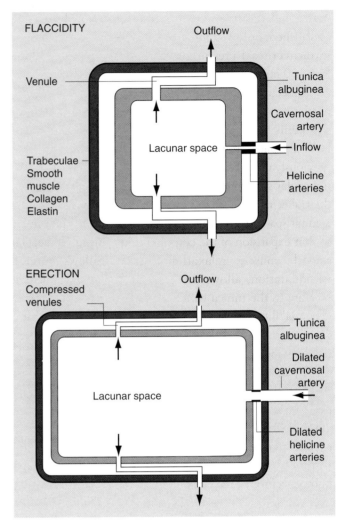

Figure 6.1. The penile corporoveno-occlusive mechanism. In flaccidity (above), constrictor tone causes a low-flow, low-pressure state in lucunar spaces. In erection (below), arterial dilatation, through cavernosal and helicine arteries, leads to relaxation of trabecular muscles with additional expansion of lacunar spaces against the tunica albuginea. Subtunical venules stretch, leading to an increase in the resistance to arterial outflow.

channels now, being longer and narrower, offer a higher resistance to the passage of blood.[7] Alternatively, there is the probable presence of collapsible venules (most of them), through which no flow would be possible and, at the same time, non-collapsible venules (very few), which would be open during erection. The veno-occlusive mechanism, eventually, allows the maintenance of high intracavernosal pressure (ICP) with a low maintenance flow and is so efficient that outflow resistance increases one hundredfold compared with the flaccid state.[4] Once erection has been established, only 1–5 ml of blood are needed to maintain intracavernosal pressures within a physiological range (60–100 mmHg).[3]

Trabecular smooth muscle plays a crucial role in the regulation of the veno-occlusive mechanism. In order for the penis to change its volume, pressure within the lacunar spaces must be transmitted to the tunica, as previously mentioned.[8] Compliance of the tunica and the trabecular structures allow expansion of the penis. When the trabecular smooth muscle is contracted, pressure in the lacunar spaces is not transmitted effectively to the tunica, so that expansion of the corpora is only partial. Trabecular smooth muscle relaxation, which follows arterial vasodilatation, allows the transmission of intralacunar pressure to the tunica which expands to reach its limit of expandability, from which point compliance of the tunica diminishes dramatically, reaching levels next to zero; that is the moment at which rigidity occurs.

Expansion of cavernosal bodies may also generate partial compression of venules piercing the tunica. The crossing-over architecture of the different layers that compose the tunica albuginea would give anatomical support to this mechanism, which would be activated, for instance, when the skeletal muscles (ischio- and bulbocavernosal) have stretched the tunica to which they are attached. Voluntary or reflex contraction (bulbocavernosal reflex) of those muscles cause the ICP to rise.[9] In addition to the above-mentioned mechanism of coarctation of the emissary veins, contraction of the ischio- and bulbocavernosal muscles decreases the volume of the cavernosal bodies. As the penis is rigid, lacking the tunica compliance, any external compression produces a major increase in ICP, over the systolic perfusion pressure. This temporary increment in ICP may contribute to increased penile rigidity at moments when it is most necessary, as during penetration.

■ PHASES OF ERECTION AND ITS HAEMODYNAMIC CORRELATES

The vascular process of erection and detumescence takes place in several different phases (Fig. 6.2).

Phase 0
Phase 0 is the flaccid phase. During flaccidity, the penis is mainly under adrenergic control. The presence of

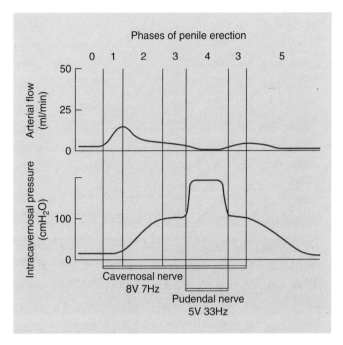

Figure 6.2. Phases of penile erection: (0) flaccidity; (1) filling; (2) tumescence; (3) full erection; (4) rigid erection; (5) detumescence. (Modified from ref. 15 with permission.)

adrenergic nerves has been demonstrated in cavernosal and helicine arteries, as well as in cavernosal smooth muscle of humans. Endothelin 1, a potent vasoconstrictor synthesized by the corpus cavernosum, contributes to the maintenance of penile flaccidity by providing a sustained tone to the smooth muscle.[10,11] The tone provided by nerves and endothelium maintains the smooth muscle of the cavernous and helicine arteries in a state of tonic contraction, allowing the passage of only a few millilitres of blood per minute, creating a large pressure gradient between the cavernosal artery and the lacunar spaces. The subtunical venules, in turn, freely drain this scant amount of blood to the emissary veins. Thus, a state of low flow and low pressure exists in the penis.

Haemodynamic correlates
In the flaccid state, ICP is close to that of the venous system (5–7 mmHg) and the partial pressure of O_2 is also like that of the veins (~60 mmHg). Colour or duplex Doppler ultrasound under these circumstances shows an inner diameter of the cavernosal arteries of 0.5 mm or less at the base of the penis, and this is frequently measurable only with the help of colour. The peak flow velocity of the blood in the cavernosal artery is usually below 15 cm/s and the end-diastolic velocity of the blood is very low.

The resistance index is close to 1, indicating a high peripheral resistance.

Phase 1

Phase 1 is the latent or filling phase. When the erection mechanism is initiated by any stimulus, a sacral parasympathetic and nitrergic nerve input occurs. Recent studies[12,13] have shown that the main neurotransmitter mediating erection is a non-adrenergic, non-cholinergic (NANC) neurotransmitter identified as nitric oxide (Fig. 6.3). It is probable, however, that more than one neurotransmitter is released (e.g. also vasoactive intestinal peptide [VIP]). After the neurogenic stimulus has taken place, the arterial and trabecular smooth muscle relaxes, increasing the blood inflow and decreasing the peripheral resistance to blood outflow.

The consequence of the relaxation of arterial smooth muscle is the dilatation of the cavernosal and helicine arteries (the resistance vessels of the corpora). There is increased blood flow into the corpora cavernosa during the diastolic and systolic phases of the pulse wave, causing filling of the lacunar spaces.

Haemodynamic correlates

In this phase, the ICP is still close to that of the venous system (5–7 mmHg or even lower) but the partial pressure of O_2 increases rapidly, becoming like that of the arteries (~ 90–100 mmHg). In a healthy potent man, colour or duplex Doppler ultrasound shows a twofold dilatation of the cavernous artery to 1 mm in diameter at the base of the penis. The peak flow velocity of the blood in the cavernosal artery is over 30 cm/s.[14] In addition, end-diastolic velocity increases to 10–15 cm/s and the resistance index decreases rapidly, approaching 0.6, which indicates an easy passage of blood flow through the dilated arteries.

Phase 2

Phase 2 is the tumescence phase. Neurotransmitters released from nerve endings and endothelium-derived substances produce relaxation of the smooth muscle of the trabecular walls. The stream of blood beating against the endothelium lining the lacunar spaces produces mechanical forces (shear stress), and vasodilator substances in blood (e.g. bradykinin) stimulate the release of endothelial nitric oxide that diffuses to the underlying smooth muscle, causing its relaxation. This paracrine mechanism for the control of the vascular tone was described by Furchgott, in 1980, in the aorta of the rabbit.[1] By means of all these mechanisms relaxation of the trabecular smooth muscle takes place, constituting the second main event of penile erection.

In this phase the penis changes in volume, elongating and expanding with scant increase of the ICP. There is a great increase in the resistance to the passage of flow as a consequence of the elongation and compression of

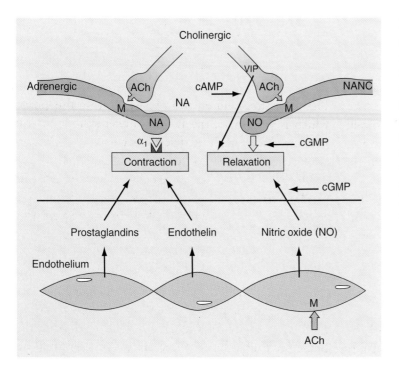

Figure 6.3. Schematic representation of the mechanisms that control trabecular penile smooth muscle contractility. Neurogenic mechanisms involve three neuro-effector systems — adrenergic, cholinergic and non-adrenergic/non-cholinergic (NANC; nitrergic). Vasoactive substances such as endothelium-derived nitric oxide, endothelin and prostaglandins may also contribute to the control of trabecular smooth muscle tone. (ACh, acetylcholine; VIP, vasoactive intestinal polypeptide; M, muscarinic receptor; NANC, non-adrenergic, non-cholinergic; NO, nitric oxide; NA, noradrenaline.) (From ref. 26 with permission.)

subtunical venules that follows the change in penile volume; in other words, the corporoveno-occlusive mechanism is activated.[7,13,15] This mechanism is regulated by the tone of the trabecular smooth muscle: when the smooth muscle is contracted there is low resistance to outflow, allowing for the easy evacuation of the corporal bodies and contributing to the maintenance of penile flaccidity. Conversely, following smooth muscle relaxation there is a major increase in outflow resistance. This phase of erection is very short, leading rapidly to the next phase.

Haemodynamic correlates

In this phase, the ICP rises rapidly to reach an equilibrium level, at approximately the mean systolic arterial pressure. The partial pressure of O_2 is like that of the arteries (~100 mmHg). Colour or duplex Doppler ultrasound shows a complete dilatation of the cavernous artery to a diameter of 1 mm at the base of the penis. The peak flow velocity of the blood in the cavernosal artery is over 30 cm/s.[14] During this phase, end-diastolic velocity is high but begins to decrease as the ICP increases. When the ICP exceeds the diastolic pressure, inflow occurs only during the systolic phase. The resistance index follows the inverse profile to end-diastolic velocity, increasing as the ICP rises, close to 0.8–0.9, indicating a progressively more difficult passage of blood flow through the arteries.

Phase 3

Phase 3 is the full erection phase. When the corporoveno-occlusive mechanism is fully activated, the penis expands and elongates to its maximal capacity. When the limit of compliance for the fibro-elastic elements of the penis has been reached, the ICP then increases rapidly. When it rises above the diastolic pressure, inflow occurs only in the systolic phase.[16] The ICP levels off at a pressure approximating the cavernosal artery systolic occlusion pressure minus the pressure loss from corporal drainage, which depends on the integrity of the veno-occlusive mechanism. In this phase the penis is usually at 90 degrees to the vertical in the standing position and moves rhythmically with the heart beat. This movement represents a minor fall in ICP that occurs in the diastolic phase and the immediate rise in ICP during the systolic phase of the pulse.

Haemodynamic correlates

It is during this phase that most of the analysis of the haemodynamics of erection can be achieved. Probably the most useful tool in the study of the haemodynamics of erection is dynamic infusion cavernosometry and cavernosography (DICC).[4,17] The ICP during this phase is in dynamic equilibrium at a point that is close to the mean systolic pressure. A gradient not longer than 40 mmHg between brachial and cavernosal systolic pressure is considered normal. During dynamic cavernosometry a physiological leak (flow to maintain a normal ICP) can be measured; in normal conditions it should not be over 6 ml/min. Larger such flows would indicate a pathological venous leak that could be moderate (7–12 ml/min) or severe (over 13 ml/min). Before this leak can be measured, it is necessary to ensure that the patient has attained complete smooth muscle relaxation and hence has a constant resistance to the outflow. Once the state of complete smooth muscle relaxation has been assessed, the ICP can be set at 150 mmHg — a suprasystolic pressure — and the fall in ICP in 30 seconds is calculated. The fall should be less than 55 mmHg in 30 seconds to be considered within the normal limits. The arterial factor also may be explored during DICC. The ICP at which the cavernosal artery flow ceases can be studied with a continuous Doppler device. This represents the cavernosal artery occlusion pressure (CAOP). Bearing in mind that erection is the accumulation of blood under pressure and that this pressure should be donated by the cavernosal artery, the calculation of CAOP is of great help in the diagnosis of erectile dysfunction. At this stage, colour or duplex Doppler ultrasound shows that peak systolic velocity is still high, but tends to diminish as the ICP rises, owing to the high resistance. End-diastolic velocity is very low, next to zero, or even negative.

Phase 4

Phase 4 is the rigid erection phase. During this phase, which is very short, the ICP rises over systolic arterial pressure and complete rigidity occurs.[18–20] Voluntary contraction (or the reflex contraction that follows stimulation of the glans penis (bulbocavernosal reflex) or penile skin) of the ischio- and bulbocavernosal muscles is responsible for this change in ICP. In the full erection phase the tunica albuginea was at the limit of its compliance; in this state, any external compression (for example, that due to contraction of the ischio- and bulbocavernosal muscles) produces a major rise in ICP. This increase in ICP may help to increase the penile rigidity necessary for vaginal penetration. During this phase no arterial inflow takes place. Although ICP has been recognized as the main component for penile rigidity, the widely varying magnitude of ICPs associated with penile rigidity has made it clear that there are additional contributory factors. The importance of the architecture and the geometry of the penis to penile rigidity has been demonstrated in several studies.[21–23] The major factors associated with penile rigidity are (a) high ICP values (pressure is related to rigidity in an exponential fashion), (b) high values of the ratio between length and diameter of the penis or relatively large diameter and short length penile geometry, and, finally, (c) high expandability of erectile tissue, implying the ability to achieve maximal volume at low pressure values during pressure loading.

Haemodynamic correlates

During this phase, owing to its short duration, it is very difficult to perform any diagnostic technique. The ICP during this phase is at a suprasystolic level; no maintenance flow is recorded and the cavernosal arteries are occluded, so no flow can be registered. Colour or duplex Doppler ultrasound shows an undetectable peak systolic velocity of the cavernosal arteries due to the aforementioned occlusion of the artery. End-diastolic velocity is also undetectable, and the resistance index is close to 1[24,25] (Fig. 6.4).

Phase 5

Phase 5 is the detumescence phase. Penile detumescence takes place with the contraction of the penile smooth muscle. Contraction of the arteries leads to a decrease of the blood inflow to the lacunar spaces. Contraction of the trabecular muscle leads to collapse of the lacunar spaces, causing decompression of the subtunical venules that drain the corpora. These events allow the penis to regain the state of flaccidity.

At the end of this phase, the haemodynamic findings are very similar to those in the flaccid phase.

■ REFERENCES

1. Furchgott R F, Zawadzki J V. The obligatory role of endothelial cells in the relaxation of arterial smooth muscle by acetylcholine. Nature 1980; 288: 373–376
2. Kim N, Azadzoi K M, Goldstein I, Saenz de Tejada I. Oxygen tension regulates the nitric oxide pathway. Physiological role in penile erection. J Clin Invest 1993; 91: 437–442
3. Saenz de Tejada I, Moroukian P, Tessier J et al. Trabecular smooth muscle modulates the capacitor function of the penis. Studies on a rabbit model. Am J Physiol 1991; 260: H1590–H1595
4. Hatzichristou D G, Saenz de Tejada I, Kupferman S et al. In vivo assessment of trabecular smooth muscle tone, its application in pharmaco-cavernosometry and analysis of intracavernous pressure determinants. J Urol 1995; 153: 1126
5. Wegner H E H, Andersen R, Knispel H H et al. Evaluation of penile arteries with color-coded duplex sonography: prevalence and possible therapeutic implications of conections between dorsal and cavernous arteries in impotent men. J Urol 1995; 153: 1469–1471
6. Lue T F, Tanagho E A, Functional anatomy and mechanism of penile erection. In: Tanagho E A, Lue T F, McClure R D (eds) Contemporary management of impotence and infertility. Baltimore: Williams and Wilkins, 1988: 39–50
7. Saenz de Tejada I. The physiology of erections. Signposts to impotence. Contemp Urol 1992; 4(7): 52–65
8. Wespes E, Schulman C C. Rôle hémodynamique de l'albuginée dans l'érection. In: VI Curso de Andrología para postgraduados. Barcelona: Fundación Puigvert, 1986: 199–206
9. Lue T F. Physiology of erection and pathophysiology of impotence. In: Walsh P, Retik A, Stamey T, Vaughan E D Jr (eds) Campbell's Urology, 6th edn. Philadelphia: Saunders, 1992: 709–728
10. Saenz de Tejada I, Carson M P, de las Morenas A et al. Endothelin: localization, synthesis, activity and receptor types in the human penile corpus cavernosum. Am J Physiol 1991; 261 (Heart Circ Physiol 30): H1078
11. Holmquist F, Andersson K E, Hedlund H. Actions of endothelin on isolated corpus cavernosum from rabbit and man. Acta Physiol Scand 1990; 139: 113
12. Burnett A L, Lowenstein C J, Bredt D S et al. Nitric oxide: a physiologic mediator of penile erection. Science 1992; 257: 401–403

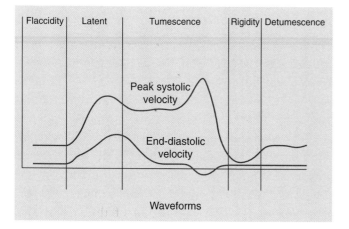

Figure 6.4. Diagrammatic representation of arterial flow waveforms showing normal progression of blood flow in the cavernosal artery during the erection process, from flaccidity to rigidity. (Modified from ref. 27 with permission.)

13. Kim N, Azadzoi K M, Goldstein I, Saenz de Tejada I. A nitric oxide-like factor mediates nonadrenergic-noncholinergic neurogenic relaxation of penile corpus cavernosum smooth muscle. J Clin Invest 1991; 88: 112–118

14. Lue T F, Tanagho E A. Physiology of erection and pharmacological management of impotence. J Urol 1987; 137: 829–836

15. Aboseif S R, Lue T F. Hemodynamics of penile erection. Urol Clin North Am 1988; 15: 1–8

16. Fournier G R, Junemann K P, Lue T F, Tanagho E A. Mechanisms of venous occlusion during canine penile erection: an anatomic demonstration. J Urol 1987; 137: 163–167

17. Wespes E, Delcour C, Struyven S. Pharmacocavernosometry–cavernosography in impotence. Br J Urol 1986; 58: 429–433

18. De Groat W C, Steers W D. Neuroanatomy and neurophysiology of penile erection. In: Tanagho E A, Lue T F, McClure R D (eds) Contemporary management of impotence and infertility. Baltimore: Williams and Wilkins, 1988: 39–50

19. Holmquist F, Hedlund H, Andersson K E. Characterization of inhibitory neurotransmission in the isolated corpus cavernosum from rabbit and man. J Physiol 1992; 449: 295–311

20. Holzmann S. Endothelium-induced relaxation by acetylcholine associated with large rises in cyclic GMP in coronary arterial strips. J Cyclic Nucl Res 1982; 8: 409–419

21. Udelson D, Nehra A, Hatzichristou G et al. Penile rigidity determinants: engineering analysis of penile buckling forces as a function of corporal soft tissue characteristics, corporal geometry and intracavernosal pressure. Int J Impot Res 1994; 6 (S1): P56

22. Penson D F, Seftel A D, Krane R J et al. The hemodynamic pathophysiology of impotence following blunt trauma to the erect penis. J Urol 1992; 148: 1171

23. Moncada I, Lledó E, Jara J et al. Correlation of penile geometry, intracavernosal pressure and penile axial rigidity. Eur Urol 1996; 30(suppl2): P33

24. Rhee E, Osborn A, Witt M. The correlation of cavernous systolic occlusion pressure with peak velocity using color duplex doppler ultrasound. J Urol 1995; 153: 358–360

25. Knispel H H, Andresen R. Color-coded duplex sonography in impotence: significance of different flow parameters in patients and controls. Eur Urol 1992; 21: 22–26

26. Saenz de Tejada I. Mechanisms for the regulation of penile smooth muscle contractility. In: Lue T (ed) World book of impotence. London: Smith-Gordon, 1992: 39–48

27. Fitzgerald S W, Erickson S J, Foley W D et al. Color Doppler sonography in the evaluation of erectile dysfunction: patterns of temporal response to papaverine. Radiographics 1992; 12: 3–17

Chapter 7

Neurophysiology of penile erection

A. T. Chuang and W. D. Steers

■ INTRODUCTION

Penile erection is an integrated component of a complex series of physiological processes that encompass male sexual behaviour. Erection is a vascular event associated with tumescence of the cavernous bodies, which relies upon integration of neural and humoral mechanisms at various levels of the neuroaxis. It is unique among visceral functions in that it absolutely requires central neural input for proper function: any disturbance of neural pathways can produce erectile dysfunction. An appreciation of the organization of, and neurotransmitters within, neural pathways to and from the penis offers insight into the mechanisms responsible for penile erection and processes causing impotence. This knowledge may lead to better understanding of the neurophysiological basis for impotence associated with anxiety and depression (formerly often classified under 'psychogenic' impotence), development of centrally directed pharmacotherapies for the treatment of impotence, and a refinement of diagnostic testing for neurogenic erectile dysfunction. This chapter discusses current concepts in the neural control of penile erection, focusing on the organization of central and peripheral neural networks and interplay of neurotransmitters at various levels. Familiarity with these concepts provides clinicians with a rational framework to understand the aetiologies of erectile dysfunction and ultimately to improve its treatment.

■ ORGANIZATION OF PATHWAYS

Peripheral neuro-anatomy

The penis receives innervation from sacral parasympathetic (pelvic), thoracolumbar sympathetic (hypogastric and lumbar sympathetic chain) and somatic (pudendal) nerves (Figs. 7.1, 7.2).[1] Erection requires participation of all three systems.

Parasympathetic pathways

The parasympathetic nervous system provides the major excitatory input to the penis, responsible for vasodilatation of the penile vasculature and erection.[2] Its preganglionic input originates within segments 2–4 of the sacral spinal cord (Fig. 7.1).[3] These preganglionic neurons are found in the intermediolateral cell column and project to laminae V, VII, IX and X of the spinal cord.[4] The sacral spinal cord receives sensory information from both visceral and somatic structures such as the bladder and genital skin.[5] Preganglionic neurons communicate with descending inputs from supraspinal centres, such as the hypothalamus, reticular formation, midbrain, and other sites in the brain. These diverse sites coordinate the autonomic networks responsible for other sexual responses.[6]

The sacral preganglionic fibres to the pelvic plexus travel in the pelvic nerve.[7] The pelvic nerve also contains sympathetic fibres (Figs. 7.1, 7.2).[8] The cavernous nerves exiting the pelvic plexus (Figs. 7.1, 7.2) reside in the pelvic fascia before it fuses with the prostatic capsule and travel along the posterolateral aspect of the prostate.[9] At the prostatic apex, the nerves are only a few millimetres from the urethral lumen. The cavernous nerves exit the pelvis by two routes: one group of fibres lies between the fascia of the levator ani and urethra en route to the penis while other branches enter the striated urethral sphincter.[4] At the membranous urethra, the cavernous nerves are located at the 3 and 9 o'clock positions. More distally, some fibres penetrate the tunica albuginea of the corpus spongiosum, whereas the remaining fibres, lying at the 1 and 11 o'clock positions, enter the penile crura with the branches of the pudendal artery and cavernous veins.[10]

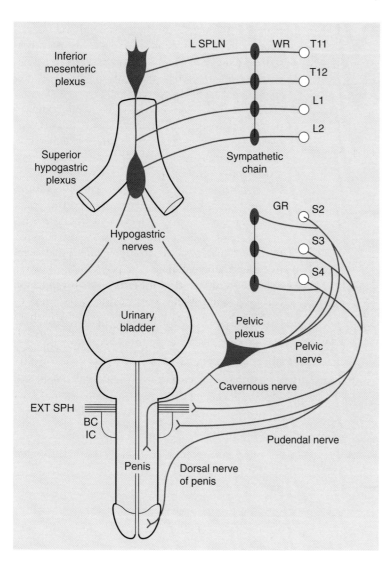

Figure 7.1. Diagram showing the parasympathetic, sympathetic and somatic efferent pathways to the penis. Sacral parasympathetic preganglionic axons arise in the S2–S4 segments of the spinal cord and pass from the pelvic nerve to the pelvic plexus. Ganglion cells in the pelvic plexus send axons into the cavernous nerve which passes in close proximity to the prostate gland en route to the penis. The thoracolumbar sympathetic pathway emerges primarily from the T11 (may be as high as T9) to L2 segments of the cord and passes via the white rami (WR) to the sympathetic chain ganglia and then via the lumbar splanchnic nerves (L SPLN) to the prevertebral ganglia in the inferior mesenteric and superior hypogastric plexuses, from which fibres travel in the hypogastric nerves to the pelvic plexus. Sympathetic preganglionic fibres also descend in the sympathetic chain to the sacral ganglia, from which postganglionic fibres pass in the grey rami (GR) to the sacral nerves, at which point they join the pelvic or pudendal nerves. Branches of the pudendal nerve innervate the external sphincter (EXT SPH) and the bulbocavernosus (BC) and ischiocavernosus (IC) muscles, as well as providing sensory fibres to the dorsal nerve of the penis. The pudendal nerve arises in the S2–S4 segments of the spinal cord. (Reproduced from ref. 13 with permission.)

The cavernous nerves contain parasympathetic and sympathetic fibres (Fig. 7.2), providing the vasodilator and vasoconstrictor input to penile smooth muscle. The course of the cavernous nerves is clinically relevant. Bulbous or membranous urethral injury — as well as prostatic, rectal, or bladder surgery — can disrupt these nerves and cause impotence.[9]

Sympathetic pathways

The sympathetic nervous system is responsible for detumescence, yet sympathetic pathways also maintain erections after injury to parasympathetic pathways. Sympathetic preganglionic nerve fibres to the penis originate from neurons in the intermediolateral cell column and intercalated nucleus of the ninth thoracic to the second lumbar spinal cord segments (Fig. 7.1).[11] These preganglionic neurons receive input from the supraspinal centre and pelvic viscera.[12]

Preganglionic fibres pass from the ventral roots via the white rami to the sympathetic chain ganglia (paravertebral), where they make synaptic connections with sacral and caudal lumbar ganglion cells. These cells send postganglionic axons into the gray rami and then to the urogenital tract via the pelvic, cavernous and pudendal nerves (Fig. 7.2).[13]

Somatic pathways

In addition to an autonomic innervation, the penis also receives somatic afferents from sensory branches of the pudendal nerve as the dorsal nerve of the penis (DNP) (Figs. 7.1, 7.2). The DNP enters the urogenital diaphragm before passing through the suspensory ligament to enter the dorsum of the penis. The sensory innervation of the glans penis is unique compared with other cutaneous regions: 80–90% of afferent terminals in the glans are free nerve endings with few corpuscular-type endings. These

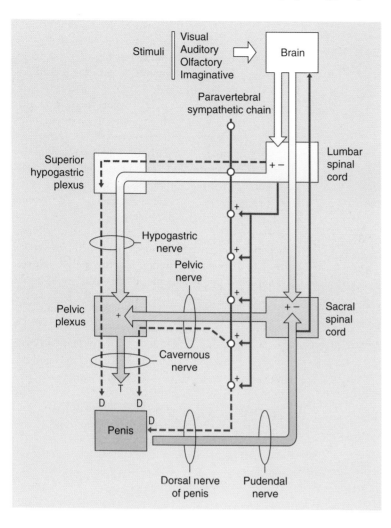

Figure 7.2. Diagram of the peripheral and central neural pathways controlling penile erection. Reflexogenic erections are initiated by a spinal parasympathetic reflex pathway organized in the sacral spinal cord. The afferent limb of this pathway is composed of the dorsal nerve of the penis/pudendal nerve, whereas the efferent limb consists of preganglionic axons that travel in the pelvic nerve to the pelvic plexus. Ganglion cells in the pelvic plexus send axons to the penis via the cavernous nerve. Psychogenic erections can be initiated by various stimuli received by, or generated within, the brain. The brain also receives sensory input from the penis via ascending spinal pathways. Descending pathways from the brain control lumbar sympathetic and sacral parasympathetic outflow to the penis. Both pathways are involved in the initiation of psychogenic erections. Sympathetic vasoconstrictor pathways to the penis arise in the paravertebral sympathetic chain ganglia and travel to the penis in the pudendal, hypogastric and pelvic nerves; the former two pathways are the most important. D, penile detumescence; T, penile tumescence. Synaptic excitatory and inhibitory mechanisms are indicated by + and –, respectively. (Reproduced from ref. 13 with permission.)

nerves are C-fibres or A-delta fibres.[14] These somatic afferents project to spinal centres in close proximity to dendrites from sacral preganglionic neurons. Afferent input from the penile skin, prepuce and glans conveyed by the DNP initiates and maintains reflexogenic erections. Ageing and diabetes affect axons in the DNP and cause impotence.[15,16]

Somatic efferents in the pudendal nerve arise from Onuf's nucleus located in the second, third and fourth segments of the sacral spinal cord[17] (Fig. 7.1). Pudendal motor fibres innervate bulbocavernous and ischiocavernous muscles as well as other striated muscles of the pelvis and perineum. Contraction of these muscles occurs during ejaculation, and augments penile rigidity during erection. Pudendal motor neurons receive supraspinal input and influence the activity of preganglionic neurons. Synaptic connections between somatic and visceral neurons could facilitate coordination between autonomic (penile erection) and somatic (ejaculation) events.[4]

Central control and pathways

Insight into the central control of erection (see Chapter 8) is based mainly on animal models (see Chapter 5) and from observations made in patients with spinal cord injury or impotence due to neurosurgical lesioning.[18] Penile erection can be induced by at least two distinct control mechanisms, predominantly involving reflexogenic and psychogenic stimuli and involving both spinal and supraspinal reflex arcs (Figs. 7.2 and 7.3).

Tactile-evoked or reflexogenic erections are mediated by a reflex arc exclusively at the spinal level; supraspinal cord transection preserves and can even enhance erection. In contrast, destruction of sacral spinal cord or its outflow via pelvic or pudendal nerves abolishes tactile dependent erections. Psychogenic erections induced by visual, imaginative, olfactory and tactile inputs undoubtedly involve higher supraspinal centres (Fig. 7.3). The efferent limb of this reflex pathway follows the thoracolumbar or the sacral autonomic outflow. It is probable under normal circumstances that the psychogenic and reflexogenic arcs act

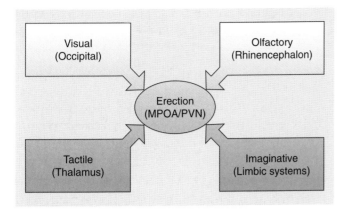

Figure 7.3. Central processing of stimuli. Psychogenic erections occur in response to various stimuli. Sensory inputs are processed in higher centres and integrated in the medial–pre-optic and anterior hypothalamic regions (MPOA) and paraventricular nucleus (PVN). The higher centres thus provide the anatomical substrates for the complex cerebral modulation of sexual behaviour.

synergistically to determine the erectile response via a final common path involving a sacral parasympathetic route.

The individual components and integration of the supraspinal control of erection are poorly understood. However, most studies indicate that hypothalamic and limbic pathways play a key role. In particular, the medial pre-optic and anterior hypothalamic regions (MPOA) are fundamentally involved in the erectile response (Fig. 7.4).[19,20] It is at this level that co-ordination of the autonomic events associated with sexual responses occurs with afferent responses being relayed from the forebrain. A variety of supraspinal mechanisms can influence sexual behaviour and erectile response. These include visual, olfactory, auditory, tactile and imaginary stimuli. These inputs from thalamic nuclei that process somatosensory and visual sensory information, the rhinencephalon that receives olfactory information and limbic structure and the hippocampus jointly responsible for emotion and memory, together provide the anatomical substrates for the complex central control of sexual behaviour (Fig. 7.3).[13] Subsequent to integration an appropriate erectile response is relayed to the target organ via the pathways described above and shown in Figures 7.2 and 7.3.

■ NEUROCHEMICAL REGULATION

Traditionally, it is thought that erection is regulated by opposing inputs from the sympathetic and parasympathetic divisions of the autonomic nervous system.

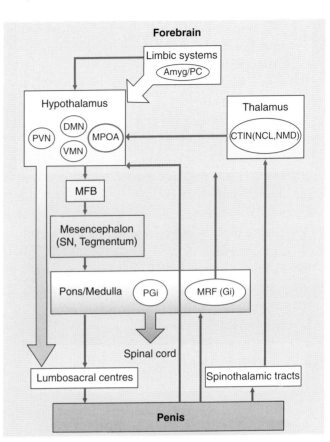

Figure 7.4. Supraspinal pathways involved in erectile function. Sensory information is processed in the forebrain and then relayed to the MPOA (medial–pre-optic and anterior hypothalamic regions). The efferent pathways from the MPOA enter the medial forebrain bundle (MFB), then pass caudally to the mesencephalon, pons/medulla and subsequently the spinal cord. Note that the lumbosacral autonomic centres and sacral ventral horn (Onuf's nucleus) receive direct projections from hypothalamic nuclei (PVN, paraventricular nucleus). The inhibitory pathways are denoted by arrowheads. DMN, dorsomedial nucleus; VMN, ventromedial nucleus; Amyg, amygdaloid complex; PC, pyriform cortex; CTIN (NCL, NMD), caudal thalamic intralaminar nuclei (nucleus centralis lateralis, nucleus medialis dorsalis); SN, substantia nigra; PGi, nucleus paragigantocellularis; MRF (Gi), medullary reticular formation (nucleus reticularis gigantocellularis).

These two inputs release transmitters with antagonistic actions (e.g. acetylcholine from parasympathetic cholinergic nerves and noradrenaline from sympathetic adrenergic nerves). In 1863, Eckhard elicited penile erections in dogs by stimulation of the pelvic nerves;[7] his work was later duplicated in other species. However, acetylcholine failed to relax the corpus cavernosum consistently. Likewise, atropine, a muscarinic cholinergic antagonist, had little if any effect on penile erections in several species, including human.

In 1895, Langley and Anderson[1] elicited vasoconstriction in the genital organs by electrical stimulation of the lumbar sympathetic chain. Subsequent work by Semans and Langworthy[21] established that detumescence was clearly a sympathetic phenomenon. It is now realized that psychogenic erections may also be mediated through the sympathetic pathway under certain circumstances.

The traditional view on neurochemical regulation of penile erection was simplistic and incomplete. It is now clear that certain parasympathetic and sympathetic pathways to the penis can act synergistically. Non-adrenergic, non-cholinergic (NANC) neurotransmitters such as nitric oxide (NO), vasoactive intestinal peptide (VIP) and neuropeptide Y (NPY) play an important role in the control of penile function (Table 7.1) (for reviews, see refs. 18, 22). These substances are synthesized, stored and released from the same neurons that release either cholinergic or adrenergic transmitters.[23,24] Co-transmission thus adds to the complexity of neural control

mechanisms and appears to be a critical aspect to regulation of penile function.

Peripheral neurotransmitters (Table 7.1)
Acetylcholine
Acetylcholine acts at cholinergic synapses in autonomic ganglia and at various parasympathetic postganglionic neuroeffector junctions. In ganglia, acetylcholine has an excitatory action mediated primarily by nicotinic receptors, whereas in vascular smooth muscle it works at muscarinic receptors, of M_2 or M_3 subtype in human corpus cavernosum, to elicit vasodilatation (Figs. 7.5, 7.6). Although morphological data[25,26] clearly support the presence of cholinergic nerves in the penis, and physiological studies implicate the parasympathetic nervous system as the primary effector of penile erection, conflicting pharmacological data refute the concept that only acetylcholine works at neuroeffector junctions in the penis.[18] It is likely that acetylcholine acts synergistically

Table 7.1. Effects of peripheral transmitters and drugs on erection

Transmitter	Receptor	Effect on erection	Drugs and effects
Acetylcholine	M_2, M_3	Facilitate	
Noradrenaline	alpha-1, alpha-2	Inhibit	Trazodone (alpha-blocker)
NO		Facilitate	NTG/SNP (NO donor) MB (GC inhibitor) Sildenafil (PDEI(V))
VIP		Facilitate	
NPY		Inhibit	
CGRP		Afferent/sensory	
Substance P		Afferent/sensory	
Serotonin		Inhibit	

M, muscarinic; NO, nitric oxide; NTG/SNP, nitroglycerine/sodium nitroprusside; MB, methylene blue; GC, guanylate cyclase; PDEI(V), type V phosphodiesterase inhibitor; VIP, vasoactive intestinal peptide; NPY, neuropeptide Y; CGRP, calcitonin gene-related peptide.

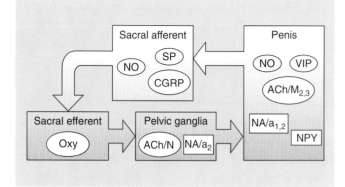

Figure 7.5. Neuropharmacology of penile erection: peripheral neurotransmitters. Diagram based on immunohistochemical and pharmacological investigations. Neurotransmitters (not depicted) that interact with the receptors (shown) produce either an excitatory (depicted with an oval) or inhibitory (square) action. NO, nitric oxide; ACh/N, acetylcholine/ nicotinic receptor; ACh/M, acetylcholine/ muscarinic receptor; VIP, vasoactive intestinal peptide; NA, noradrenaline; NPY, neuropeptide Y; CGRP, calcitonin gene-related peptide; SP, substance P. Oxy (oxytocin) is a central neurotransmitter that acts at the brain/spinal cord level.

with other vasodilators that are released by nerves or contained within vascular tissues.

It is important to note that sympathetic pathways may also produce penile erection via a cholinergic mechanism,[27] as preganglionic axons in the hypogastric nerve synapse with neurons innervating the penis in the rat, and that these neurons stain for acetylcholinesterase, NO and VIP.[28]

Noradrenaline

Histological and pharmacological studies indicate that adrenergic fibres and receptors are present in human corporal tissue and blood vessels. Radioligand receptor-binding studies show a greater density (10:1) of alpha-adrenergic receptors than beta-adrenergic receptors in penile smooth muscle.[29] Furthermore, there is an increase in alpha-adrenergic tone with ageing and disease states.[30] Therefore, alpha-adrenergic vasoconstriction may be the predominant adrenergic response over beta-adrenergic vasodilatation to sympathetic nerve stimulation. Both phenylephrine (selective for alpha-1) and clonidine (selective for alpha-2) contract corpus cavernosum tissue (Figs. 7.5, 7.6). However, clonidine is less potent than phenylephrine and noradrenaline, favouring a functional predominance of alpha-1 adrenoceptors.[18]

Alpha-2 receptors are present on cholinergic nerve terminals in human penile tissue. This is important in

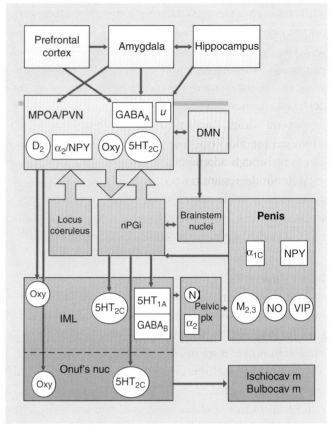

Figure 7.6. Neuropharmacology of penile erection: central neurotransmitters. Diagram is based on immunohistochemical and pharmacological investigations. Neurotransmitters (not depicted) that interact with the receptors (shown) produce either an excitatory (depicted with an oval) or inhibitory (square) action. 5-HT, serotonin; Oxy, oxytocin; GABA, gamma-aminobutyric acid; u, opioids; D, dopamine; α_2, noradrenaline; NPY, neuropeptide Y; NO, nitric oxide. MPOA, medial–pre-optic and anterior hypothalamic regions; PVN, paraventricular nucleus; DMN, dorsomedial nucleus; nPGi, nucleus paragigantocellularis; IML, thoracolumbosacral autonomic centres; plx, plexus.

detumescence, as prejunctional noradrenaline action reduces vasodilator transmitter release in addition to producing post-junctional vasoconstriction of vascular smooth muscles.[31,32] Conversely, activation of muscarinic in addition to alpha-2 receptors on adrenergic terminals decreases the release of noradrenaline in human cavernous tissues.[32] Thus, communication between adrenergic and cholinergic nerves, termed 'cross-talk', occurs during penile erection or detumescence and serves as a form of neuromodulation to increase both detumescence or erectile mechanisms when activated.

Uncertainty exists regarding the physiological role of the adrenergic pathways to the human penis. Patients who had extensive sympathectomies do not have persistent erections.[33] On the other hand, intracavernosal injection of alpha-adrenergic blocking agents induced erections. Whether an active and tonic sympathetic vasoconstrictor input is necessary to maintain detumescence remains unclear.

Several drugs, not primarily classified as alpha-adrenoceptor blockers, influence, at least partly, penile erection through adrenergic mechanisms. Thus the non-tricyclic antidepressant trazodone, which causes priapism, in addition to possible central effects as a serotonergic agent (see section on Central Neurotransmitters, p. 66), is shown to have marked alpha-adrenoceptor-blocking properties.[34]

Nitric oxide

As previously mentioned, acetylcholine may depend on endothelium-derived factors to induce relaxation of human cavernosal tissue,[35] and it is not the sole neurotransmitter responsible for erections. The biological actions of endothelium-derived relaxing factor (EDRF) can be accounted for by NO, which acts as a neurotransmitter and is synthesized from L-arginine by NO synthase (NOS). The presence of NOS has been demonstrated in human, rat and rabbit corpus cavernosum.[36–38] Furthermore, NOS inhibitors prevent electrically induced erections in vivo at peripheral and central sites. These findings implicate NO as a potential neurotransmitter in both peripheral and central neurons (Figs. 7.5, 7.6). It also suggests that the most important source of NO in penile tissue is neuronal. In support of this view, isolated cavernous tissue responded with relaxation to electrical stimulation of nerves after destruction of the endothelium, while responses to acetylcholine were abolished.[39,40] NO acts via stimulation of guanylate cyclase, resulting in increased levels of cyclic guanosine monophosphate (cGMP) in the smooth muscle cells.[41] This in turn leads to decrease in cytosolic calcium and relaxation. In support of this view, neuronally evoked relaxation of bovine retractor penis smooth muscle is associated with an increase in cGMP.[42]

Vasodilators such as nitroglycerine, currently used to produce erection following intracavernosal injection, act via this mechanism. Methylene blue, a guanylate cyclase inhibitor, has been used successfully to treat priapism.[43] Sildenafil, a type V phosphodiesterase inhibitor specific to the corpus cavernosum (see Chapter 26), is an oral agent currently undergoing clinical trials for the treatment of impotence. Sildenafil presumably exerts its action by preventing degradation of cGMP, thereby raising its tissue concentration. The synthesis of NO can also be altered by hypertension, arteriosclerosis, or diabetes contributing to vascular impotence.[35]

Vasoactive intestinal peptide

VIP is found in postganglionic nerves in the penis and is released during penile erection. Exogenous VIP produces vasodilatation and relaxes penile smooth muscle; when VIP is administered locally to the penis of humans, monkeys and dogs, it increases penile volume (Figs. 7.5, 7.6).[13] This effect is presumed to be mediated by an increase in cyclic adenosine monophosphate (cAMP) levels in the smooth muscle cells, which in turn leads to a reduction in cytosolic calcium concentrations and decreased contractility.[41] VIP might also facilitate muscarinic cholinergic transmission. It has been identified as a co-transmitter with acetylcholine in some parasympathetic postganglionic neurons.[44] Ultrastructural studies in human and animal penile tissue demonstrated a co-localization of large VIP-immunoreactive vesicles within varicosities containing small, clear, presumably cholinergic vesicles.[45] These may act synergistically in penile tissue to initiate or maintain erection.

Tissue levels of VIP in the human penis are decreased in diabetic impotence.[46] However, the inability of VIP to produce erection when injected intracavernosally in healthy volunteers[47] and in impotent men,[48,49] and the demonstration of the effects of NO on penile erectile tissues, indicates that VIP is probably not the main NANC mediator of penile erection. However, it is of interest that substances that act via two separate transduction pathways[5] — cGMP (NO) and cAMP (VIP) — have the same net effects. This redundancy may be important in disease states.

Neuropeptide Y

Electrical field stimulation of nerves in human cavernosal arteries and corpus cavernosal strips in vitro elicits biphasic contractions.[50] The second component of the evoked contractions can be abolished by adrenergic antagonists, but the initial contractile response is resistant. This suggests that contractile transmitters other than noradrenaline are released from the nerve terminal. Neuropeptides might be involved in neurotransmission in the penis since they are co-localized with noradrenaline in adrenergic postganglionic neurons and can participate with noradrenaline in the initiation of vasoconstriction in various vascular beds.[24] One of the likely candidates is NPY, which has been identified in the human penis.[51] It weakly contracts corporal smooth muscle (Figs. 7.5, 7.6),[52] although its effects are inconsistent.[18]

Calcitonin gene-related peptide

CGRP is a potent vasodilator, and is believed to produce an endothelium-dependent relaxation.[53] CGRP-like immunoreactivity has been demonstrated in human corpus cavernosum,[54] and CGRP binding sites are numerous in rat penile tissue extracts.[55] In the sacral nerves, CGRP is exclusively found in sensory fibres. Its role in normal penile physiology is probably related to the afferent limb of erectile reflexes (Fig. 7.5).

Substance P

Available information does not suggest that substance P has any direct effects on corpus cavernosum smooth muscle or penile vessels of importance for erection. Like CGRP, substance P probably participates in the sensory innervation from the penis (Fig. 7.5).[56,57]

Serotonin

Serotonin exerts an inhibitory action on penile erection by a peripheral mechanism involving the 5-HT_{1D} subtype, although it probably plays a more important role as a central neurotransmitter.

Central neurotransmitters

Animal studies have provided insights into the central neurotransmitters involved in the control of male sexual function (Table 7.2) (see refs. 18, 22 for reviews). A variety of transmitters distributed throughout supraspinal and spinal centres are essential for sexual behaviour (Fig. 7.7). However, the role of these substances is difficult to determine because of the wide range of sexual parameters affected, species differences, dose dependence, conflicting results depending on the site in the central nervous system where the transmitter acts, and the existence of receptor subtypes. Despite these challenges, understanding these mechanisms may lead to centrally targeted therapy for impotence.

Serotonin (5-hydroxytryptamine)

Serotonin (5-HT) inhibits copulation behaviour,[18] but the effects of drugs that directly activate specific 5-HT receptor subtypes are less certain. The multiplicity of 5-HT receptors may translate into functional heterogeneity with regard to sexual behaviour. In general, activation of 5-HT_{1A} receptor inhibits, and activation of 5-HT_{2C} facilitates erection (Fig. 7.6).[58,59] 5-HT drugs act at the level of the spinal cord, since responses are similar in both intact and chronic spinal rats. The antidepressant trazodone, whose main metabolite by-product is mCPP (*m*-chlorophenylpiperazine; a 5-HT_{2C} agonist), has the side effect of priapism. It is used anecdotally for treatment of impotence.

Dopamine

Dopamine released from supraspinal neurons facilitates male copulatory behaviour.[18] L-Dopa enhances libido and penile erections in humans,[60,61] and levels of dopamine in cerebrospinal fluid increase during copulation. Intracerebroventricular administration of L-dopa (a precursor of dopamine) or apomorphine (a dopamine receptor agonist) increased sexual responses (Figs. 7.6, 7.7).[62,63] Furthermore, selective administration of apomorphine within the paraventricular nucleus produces erection.[64] However, high doses of intrathecally administered dopamine agonists inhibit penile erection. Conversely, lesions in the substantia nigra,[65] or the administration of dopamine receptor-blocking agents in doses that did not impair other motor behaviours, depressed copulatory behaviour in rats;[62] furthermore, parkinsonian patients often have erectile dysfunction.

The central action of dopamine may depend upon activation of specific dopamine receptor subtypes. The facilitatory effects of specific D_2 receptor agonists such as quinelorane on sexual behaviour in animals suggest that low doses of dopamine agonists, possibly acting at autoreceptors, may be of clinical use.[66]

Clinically, dopamine agonists enhance sexual desire rather than directly activating erection.

Noradrenaline

The noradrenergic neurons in the brain may exert an inhibitory influence on penile erection. Clonidine, an alpha-2 adrenergic receptor agonist and an antihypertensive, inhibits erections in rats (Figs. 7.6, 7.7).[67] Moreover, impotence and decreased libido are common side effects of this medication. Conversely, yohimbine, an alpha-2-adrenergic receptor antagonist, reverses the effects of clonidine and increases sexual activity in rats but not primates, suggesting that sexual response is tonically inhibited by a central noradrenergic pathway,[68] at least in some species. Yet the clinical

Table 7.2. Effects of central transmitters and drugs on erection

Transmitter	Receptor	Site of action	Effect on erection	Drugs and effects
Serotonin	$5\text{-}HT_{1A, 1B}$	Brain	Inhibit	8OH-DPAT (+)
	$5\text{-}HT_{1C, 2C}$	Spinal cord	Facilitate	mCPP/Trazodone (+)
Dopamine	D_1, D_2	Brain/spinal cord	Facilitate	L-Dopa (+)
				Apomorphine (+)
Noradrenaline	alpha-1	Brain/spinal cord	Inhibit	
	alpha-2	Brain	Inhibit	Clonidine (+)
				Yohimbine (−)
Opioids	mu	Brain	Inhibit	Morphine (+)
				Naloxone (−)
Oxytocin		Brain/spinal cord	Facilitate	
GABA	$GABA_A$	Brain	Inhibit	Muscimol (+)
				Bicuculline (−)
	$GABA_B$	Spinal cord	Inhibit	Baclofen (+)
Prolactin		Brain	Facilitate	
ACTH		Brain	Facilitate	

5-HT, 5-hydroxytryptamine; 8OH-DPAT, 8-hydroxy-2-(di-n-propylamino) tetralin; mCPP, m-chlorophenylpiperazine; GABA, gamma-aminobutyric acid; ACTH, adrenocorticotrophic hormone. Receptor agonists are designated by (+), antagonists by (−).

efficacy of yohimbine in the treatment of impotence is poor, suggesting the existence of cross-species differences.[69,70]

Opioids

Administration of opiate receptor agonists to the central nervous system inhibits, whereas administration of opiate receptor antagonists facilitates, copulatory behaviour in rats (Figs. 7.6, 7.7).[67] Impotence, decreased libido and anorgasmia are common with narcotic abuse.[71,72] Spontaneous erections, priapism and ejaculation occur during narcotic withdrawal,[72] and are associated with opiate antagonists (such as naloxone). It is of interest that similarities exist between postulated mechanisms regarding the development of narcotic addiction and the central pathways and transmitters involved in sexual function. Clinically, endogenous opiates may contribute to impotence associated with pain disorders.

Interestingly, the combination of naloxone with yohimbine was reported to cause sustained and full erection in healthy volunteers,[73] suggesting a functional relationship between central opioid and noradrenergic systems in erection.

Oxytocin

Oxytocin is localized in descending pathways from the hypothalamus to brain stem and spinal autonomic centres (Fig. 7.6). Moreover, oxytocin induces penile erections in rats.[74,75] When injected into the lateral cerebral ventricle, the paraventricular nucleus or hippocampus, oxytocin triggers penile erections.[74] Following sexual activity,

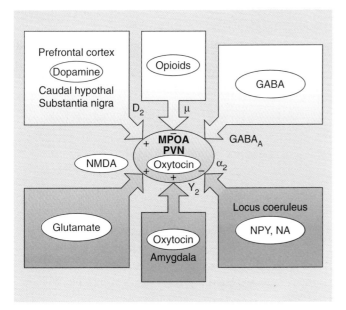

Figure 7.7. Diagram depicting the interaction of various central (supraspinal) neurotransmitters and their putative regions of action. MPOA, medial–pre-optic and anterior hypothalamic regions; PVN, paraventricular nucleus; GABA, gamma-aminobutyric acid; D, dopamine; ACTH, adrenocorticotrophic hormone; NPY, neuropeptide Y; NA, noradrenaline; NMDA, N-methyl-D-aspartate.

serum and cerebrospinal fluid levels of oxytocin are elevated.[76,77] These results suggest that oxytocin functions as an excitatory transmitter in the hypothalamic regulation of erections.[76] The action of oxytocin on neurons appears to be dependent on NO, since NOS inhibitors prevent oxytocin-induced penile erection in male rats.[78]

Interactions occur between dopaminergic and oxytocinergic mechanisms in the control of erectile function (Fig. 7.7). PVN neurons have both dopaminergic and oxytocinergic receptors. Dopamine neurons in the PVN are located mainly in the proximity of oxytocinergic neurons.[79,80] D$_2$-agonists elicit a rise in oxytocin during penile erection in primates.[12] Furthermore, the facilitatory effect of apomorphine on penile erection can be blocked by either dopamine or oxytocin antagonists.[3] Some investigators speculate that dopaminergic neurons activate oxytocinergic neurons in the PVN and that oxytocin released by these neurons produces erection.[81–83]

Morphine microinjected into the PVN can prevent oxytocinergic effects, suggesting that endogenous opioids can exert an inhibitory control on central oxytocinergic transmission.[81]

Gamma-aminobutyric acid

High concentrations of gamma-aminobutyric acid (GABA) have been measured in the MPOA of male rats.[84,85] Administration of GABA$_A$ receptor agonists (e.g. muscimol) to the central nervous system inhibit, and administration of GABA$_A$ receptor antagonists (e.g. bicuculline) facilitate, copulatory behaviour in rats.[18] Intrathecal baclofen (a GABA$_B$ agonist) reduces or abolishes tactile or reflexogenic erections, but is associated with preservation of psychogenic and nocturnal erections in humans.[12] These observations suggest that GABA functions as an inhibitory transmitter in the central nervous system with regard to erections (Figs. 7.6, 7.7). In support of this, the levels of GABA in the cerebrospinal fluid of freely moving rats increased by over 1000% during the postejaculatory interval, at a time when the rats are completely refractory to sexual stimuli.[86]

Both GABAergic fibres and GABA$_B$ receptors have been demonstrated in the spinal dorsal horn, as well as in the vicinity of the sacral parasympathetic and bulbocavernosal motor nuclei.[87,88] GABA has a direct inhibitory effect on sacral preganglionic neurons.[89,90] This suggests that GABA may be an inhibitory modulator in the autonomic and somatic reflex pathways involved in penile erection.[91]

Prolactin

Long-term exposure to increased levels of prolactin suppresses sexual behaviour and reduces potency in men.[92–94] Prolactin also disrupts genital reflexes, leading to decreased frequency of erections in rats.[95,96] This reduction of the number of erections is counteracted by spinal transection,[95] implying that the disruption of genital reflexes is exerted at a supraspinal site. Ultimately, the mechanism through which prolactin inhibits sexual behaviour may originate in alterations in brain dopamine (Fig. 7.7).[22] Independent of these observations, prolactin also reduces testosterone levels, which, in turn, may affect neural mechanisms.

Adrenocorticotrophic hormone

Adrenocorticotrophic hormone (ACTH) induces penile erection in animals.[97,98] The hypothalamus and areas of the brain surrounding the third ventricle are probably sites of action, as MPOA lesions abolish ACTH-induced erections.[97] ACTH may act as an endogenous antagonist of opiates (Fig. 7.7), as exemplified by the withdrawal syndrome seen in morphine-dependent rats.[99] Similarly, the effects of ACTH are completely antagonized by morphine.[97] The sexual response to ACTH is also abolished by castration, which indicates a permissive role for testicular androgens.[97]

It is clear that a broad spectrum of neurotransmitters at various levels of the neuroaxis are involved in the control of male sexual behaviour (Figs. 7.5–7.7). Certain transmitter systems are also influenced by the levels of sex hormones. This diversity of neurochemical regulation undoubtedly contributes to the susceptibility of sexual function to a wide range of drugs, chemicals and neurological disorders.

■ CONCLUSIONS

Penile erection is a complex behaviour response that is dependent on the coordination of neural and humoral mechanisms at various levels of the neuroaxis. The diverse central and peripheral neural pathways controlling erection employ a variety of putative neurotransmitters, including acetylcholine, monoamines, neuropeptides and others for effective synaptic transmission. A refined understanding of these neurohumoral mechanisms will help to facilitate the development of new diagnostic methods and therapies for erectile dysfunction.

■ REFERENCES

1. Langley J N, Anderson H I. The innervation of the pelvic and adjoining viscera. J Physiol 1895; 19: 71–130
2. Lue T F, Takamura T, Schmidt A R et al. Hemodynamics of erection in the monkey. J Urol 1983; 130: 1237–1241
3. de Groat W C, Steers W D. Autonomic regulation of the urinary bladder and sexual organs. In: Spyer R M, Loewy A (eds) Central regulation of autonomic functions. Oxford: Oxford University Press, 1990: 310–333
4. Steers W D. Neural innervation of the cavernous tissue. In: Jonas U et al. (eds) Impotence. Heidelberg: Springer-Verlag, 1991: 16–33
5. Nunez R, Gross G H, Sachs B D. Origin and central projections of rat dorsal penile nerve: possible direct projection to autonomic and somatic neurons by primary afferents of nonmuscle origin. J Comp Neurol 1986; 247: 417–429
6. Marston L, McKenna K E. The identification of a brainstem site controlling spinal sexual reflexes in male rats. Brain Res 1990; 515: 303–308
7. Eckhard C. Untersuchungen uber die erection des penis beim hunde. Beitr Anat Physiol 1863; 3: 123–150
8. Pick J, Sheehan D. Sympathetic rami in man. J Anat 1946; 80: 12–20
9. Lepor H, Gregerman M, Crosby R et al. Precise localization of the autonomic nerves from the pelvic plexus to the corpora cavernosa: a detailed anatomical study of the adult male pelvis. J Urol 1985; 133: 201–212
10. Steers W D. Neural control of penile erection. Semin Urol 1990; 8(2): 66–79
11. Learmonth J R. A contribution to the neurophysiology of the urinary bladder in man. Brain 1931; 54: 147–176
12. Steers W D. Neuroanatomy and neurophysiology of erection. Sex Disabil 1994; 12: 17–26
13. de Groat W C, Steers W D. Neuroanatomy and neurophysiology of penile erection. In: Tanagho E R, Lue T F, McClure R D (eds) Contemporary management of impotence and infertility. Baltimore: Williams and Wilkins, 1988: 3–27
14. Halata Z, Munger B. The neuroanatomical basis for the protopathic sensibility of the human penis. Brain Res 1986; 371: 205–230
15. Steers W D, Mackway A, de Groat W C. Electrophysiological properties of the cavernous nerve in the streptozotocin diabetic rat. Int J Impot Res 1991; 3: 197–205
16. Johnson R D, Murray F T. Reduced sensitivity of penile mechanoreceptors in aging rats with sexual dysfunction. Brain Res Bull 1992; 28: 61–64
17. Onuf (Onufrowicz) B. On the arrangement and function of the cell groups of the sacral region of the spinal cord in man. Arch Neurol Psychopathol 1900; 3: 387–411
18. Andersson K-E, Wagner G. Physiology of penile erection. Physiol Rev 1995; 75(1): 191–236
19. Herbert J. The role of the dorsal nerve of the penis in the sexual behavior of the male rhesus monkey. Physiol Behav 1973; 10: 292–300
20. MacLean P D, Denniston R H, Dua S. Further studies on cerebral representation of penile erection: caudal thalamus, midbrain, and pons. J Neurophysiol 1963; 26: 274–293
21. Semans J H, Langworthy O R. Observation on the neurophysiology of sexual function in the male cat. J Urology 1938; 40: 836–846
22. Meisel R L, Sachs B D. The physiology of male sexual behavior. In: Knobil E, Neill J D (eds) The physiology of reproduction. New York: Raven Press, 1994: 3–105
23. Hokfelt T. Nonadrenergic, noncholinergic autonomic neurotransmission mechanisms. Neurosci Res Prog Bull 1979; 17: 424–443
24. Burnstock G. The changing face of autonomic neurotransmission. Acta Physiol Scand 1986; 126: 67–91
25. Shirai M, Sasaki K, Rikimaru A. Histochemical investigation on the distribution of adrenergic and cholinergic nerves in human penis. Tohoku J Exp Med 1972; 107: 403–404
26. McConnell J, Benson G S, Wood J. Autonomic innervation of the mammalian penis: a histochemical and physiological study. J Neural Trans 1979; 45: 227–238

27. Andersson P O, Bloom S R, Mellander S. Hemodynamics of pelvic nerve induced penile erection in the dog: possible mediation by vasoactive intestinal polypeptide. J Physiol (Lond) 1984; 350: 209–224

28. Ottsen B, Wagner G, Virga R et al. Penile erection: possible role for vasoactive intestinal polypeptide as a neurotransmitter. Br Med J 1984; 288: 9–11

29. Levin R M, Wein A J. Adrenergic alpha receptors outnumber beta receptors in the human penile corpus cavernosum. Invest Urol 1980; 18: 225–226

30. Christ G J, Maayani S, Valcic M. Pharmacological studies of human erectile tissue: characteristics of spontaneous contractions and alterations in alpha-adrenoceptor responsiveness with age and disease in isolated tissues. Br J Pharmacol 1990; 101: 375

31. Hedlund H, Andersson K-E. Comparison of the responses to adrenoreceptor and muscarinic receptor active drugs in isolated human corpus cavernosum and cavernous artery. J Auton Pharmacol 1985; 5: 81–88

32. Saenz de Tejada I, Kim N, Logan I et al. Regulation of adrenergic activity in penile corpus cavernosum. J Urol 1989; 142: 1117–1121

33. Kedia K R, Markland C, Fraley E E. Sexual function following high retroperitoneal lymphadenectomy. J Urol 1975; 114: 237–239

34. Abber J C, Lue T F, Luo J A et al. Priapism induced by chlorpromazine and trazodone: mechanism of action. J Urol 1987; 137: 1039–1042

35. Saenz de Tejada I, Goldstein I, Azadzoi K et al. Impaired neurogenic and endothelium-mediated relaxation of penile smooth muscle from diabetic men with impotence. N Engl J Med 1989; 320: 1025–1030

36. Burnett A L, Lowenstein C J, Bredt D S et al. Nitric oxide: a physiologic mediator of penile erection. Science 1992; 257: 401–403

37. Bush P A, Gonzalez N E, Ignarro L J. Biosynthesis of nitric oxide and citrulline from L-arginine by constitutive nitric oxide synthase present in rabbit corpus cavernosum. Biochem Biophys Res Commun 1992; 186: 308–314

38. Hung A, Vernet D, Kic Y et al. Expression of inducible nitric oxide synthase in smooth muscle cells from rat penile corpora cavernosa. J Androl 1995; 16(6): 469–481

39. Azadzoi K M, Kim N, Brown M L et al. Endothelium-derived nitric oxide and cyclooxygenase products modulate corpus cavernosum smooth muscle tone. J Urol 1992; 147: 220–225

40. Saenz de Tejada I, Blanco R, Goldstein I et al. Cholinergic neurotransmission in human corpus cavernosum. I. Responses of isolated tissue. Am J Physiol 1988; 254 (Heart Circ Physiol 23): H468–H472

41. Hoffman F. The molecular basis of second messenger systems for regulation of smooth muscle contractility: state of the art lecture. J Hypertens 1985; 3: 53–58

42. Bowman A, Gillespie J S. Neurogenic vasodilatation in isolated bovine and canine penile arteries. J Physiol 1983; 341: 603–616

43. Steers W D, Selby J B Jr. Use of methylene blue and selective embolization of the pudendal artery for high flow priapism refractory to medical and surgical treatments. J Urol 1991; 146: 1361–1363

44. Dail W G. Autonomic control of penile erectile tissue. Exp Brain Res 1987; 16: 340–344

45. Steers W D, McConnell J, Benson G. Anatomical localization and some pharmacological effects of vasoactive intestinal polypeptide in human and monkey corpus cavernosum. J Urol 1984; 132: 1048–1053

46. Crowe R, Lincoln J, Blackley P F et al. Vasoactive intestinal polypeptide-like immunoreactive nerves in the diabetic penis. Diabetes 1983; 32: 1075–1079

47. Wagner G, Gerstenberg T. Intracavernous injection of vasoactive intestinal polypeptide (VIP) does not induce erection in man per se. World J Urol 1987; 5: 171–177

48. Adaikan P G, Kottegod S R, Ratnam S S. Is vasoactive intestinal polypeptide the principal transmitter involved in human penile erection? J Urol 1986; 135: 638–640

49. Roy J B, Petrone R L, Said S. A clinical trial of intracavernous vasoactive intestinal polypeptide to induce penile erection. J Urol 1990; 143: 302–304

50. Stief L, Bernard F, Bosch R et al. Acetylcholine as a possible neurotransmitter in penile erection. J Urol 1989; 141: 1444–1448

51. Gu J, Polak J M, Probert L et al. Peptidergic innervation of human male genital tract. J Urol 1983; 130: 386–391

52. Wespes E, Schiffman S, Vanderhaeghen J J et al. Light and electron microscopic demonstration of NPY in the human penis with pharmacological aspects. Proc Int Symp Corpus Cavernosum Revascularization Boston, MA, 6–9 Oct 1988: 44

53. Crossman D, McEwan J, MacDermot J et al. Human calcitonin gene-related peptide activates adenylate cyclase and releases prostacycline from human umbilical vein endothelial cells. Br J Pharmacol 1987; 92: 695–701

54. Stief C G, Wetterauer U, Schaebsdau F H et al. Calcitonin gene-related peptide: a possible role in human penile erection and its therapeutic application in impotent patients. J Urol 1991; 146: 1010–1014

55. Wimalawansa S J, Emson P C, MacIntyre I. Regional distribution of calcitonin gene-related peptide and its specific binding sites in rats with particular reference to the nervous system. Neuroendocrinology 1987; 46: 131–136

56. Keast J R, de Groat W C. Immunohistochemical characterization of pelvic neurons which project to the bladder, colon, or penis in rats. J Comp Neurol 1989; 288: 387–400

57. Keast J R, de Groat W C. Segmental distribution and peptide content of primary afferent neurons innervating the urogenital organs and colon of male rats. J Comp Neurol 1992; 319: 615–623

58. Ahlenius S, Larsson K, Arvidsson L E. Effects of stereoselective $5HT_{1A}$ agonists on male rat sexual behavior. Pharmacol Biochem Behav 1989; 33: 691–695

59. Steers W D, de Groat W C. Effects of m-chlorophenylpiperazine on penile and bladder function in rats. Am J Physiol 1990; 257: 1441–1449

60. Benkert O, Crombach G, Kockott G. Effects of L-dopa on sexually impotent patients. Psychopharmacology 1972; 23: 91–95

61. Lal S, Laryea E, Thavundayil J X et al. Apomorphine-induced penile tumescence in impotent patients–preliminary findings. Neuropsychopharmacol Biol Psychiatry 1987; 1: 235–242

62. Tagliamonte A, Fratta W, del Fiacco M et al. Possible stimulatory role of brain dopamine on the copulatory behavior of male rats. Pharmacol Biochem Behav 1974; 2: 257

63. Malmnas C O. The significance of dopamine versus other catecholamines for L-dopa induced facilitation of sexual behavior in the castrated male rat. Pharmacol Biochem Behav 1976; 4: 521–526

64. Pehek E A, Thompson J T, Hull E M. The effects of intracranial administration of the dopamine agonist apomorphine on penile reflexes and seminal emission in the rat. Brain Res 1989; 500: 325–332

65. Brackett N L, Iuvone P M, Edwards D A. Midbrain lesions, dopamine and male sexual behavior. Behav Brain Res 1986; 20: 231–240

66. Foreman M, Hall J. Effects of D_2-dopaminergic receptor stimulation on male rat sexual behavior. J Neural Transm 1987; 327: 153–170

67. Bitran D, Hull E M. Pharmacological analysis of male rat sexual behavior. Neurosci Bio Behav Rev 1987; 11: 365–389

68. Chambers K C, Phoenix C H. Apomorphine, deprenyl, and yohimbine fail to increase sexual behavior in rhesus males. Behav Neurosci 1989; 103: 816–822

69. Morales A, Surridge D H C, Marshall P G et al. Nonhormonal pharmacologic treatment of organic impotence. J Urol 1982; 128: 45–47

70. Davidson J M, Smith E R, Clark J T. Endocrine and neuropharmacologic approaches in animal models and their relevance to systemic pharmacologic intervention in male sexual dysfunction. In: Striker G E, Rodgers C H (eds) Abstracts of a conference on the scientific basis of sexual dysfunction. Sponsored by the NIH and National Kidney Foundation, Baltimore, Maryland, June 1986. Bethesda, MD: National Institutes of Health, 1986

71. Mintz J. Sexual problems of heroin addicts. Arch Gen Psychiatry 1974; 31: 700–707

72. Cushman P. Sexual behavior in heroin addiction and methadone maintenance. NY State J Med 1978; 72: 1262–1263

73. Charney D S, Heninger G R. Alpha$_2$-adrenergic and opiate receptor blockade: synergistic effects on anxiety in healthy subjects. Arch Gen Psychiatry 1986; 43: 1037–1041

74. Melis M R, Argiolas A, Gessa G L. Oxytocin-induced penile erection and yawning: site of action in the brain. Brain Res 1986; 398: 259–265

75. Dornan W A, Malsbury C W. Neuropeptides and male sexual behavior. Neurosci Bio Behav Rev 1989; 13: 1–15

76. Carmichael M S, Humbert R, Dixen J et al. Plasma oxytocin increases in the human sexual response. J Clin Endocrinol Metab 1987; 64: 27–34

77. Hughes A M, Everitt B J, Lightman S L et al. Oxytocin in the central nervous system and sexual behavior in male rats. Brain Res 1987; 414: 133–137

78. Melis M R, Argiolas A. Nitric oxide synthase inhibitors prevent apomorphine- and oxytocin-induced penile erection and yawning in male rats. Brain Res Bull 1993; 32: 71–74

79. Theodosis D T. Oxytocin-immunoreactive terminals synapse on oxytocinergic neurons in the supraoptic nuclei. Nature 1985; 313: 682–684

80. Theodosis D T, Poulain D A. Neuronal-glial and synaptic plasticity in the adult paraventricular nucleus. Brain Res 1989; 484: 361–366

81. Argiolas A. Oxytocin stimulation of penile erection. Pharmacology, site, and mechanism of action. Ann N Y Acad Sci 1992; 652: 194–203

82. Argiolas A, Melis M R, Stancampiano R. Role of oxytocinergic pathways in the expression of penile erection. Regul Pept 1993; 45: 139–142

83. Melis M R, Stancampiano R, Argiolas A. Effect of excitatory amino acid receptor antagonists on apomorphine-, oxytocin- and ACTH-induced penile erection and yawning in male rats. Eur J Pharmacol 1992; 220: 43–48

84. Elekes I, Patthy T, Lang T et al. Concentrations of GABA and glycine in discrete brain nuclei. Stress-induced changes in the levels of inhibitory amino acids. Neuropharmacology 1986; 25: 703–709

85. Tappaz M L, Brownstein M J, Kopin I F. Glutamate decarboxylase (GAD) and GABA in discrete nuclei of hypothalamus and substantia nigra. Brain Res 1977; 125: 109–121

86. Qureshi G A, Sodersten P. Sexual activity alters the concentration of amino acids in the cerebrospinal fluid of male rats. Neurosci Lett 1986; 70: 374–378

87. Bowery N G, Hudson A L, Price G W. GABA$_A$ and GABA$_B$ receptor site distribution in the rat central nervous system. Neuroscience 1987; 20: 365–383

88. Magoul R, Oteniente B, Geffard M et al. Anatomical distribution and ultrastructural organization of the GABA-ergic system in the rat spinal cord. An immuncytochemical study using anti-GABA antibodies. Neuroscience 1987; 20: 1001–1009

89. de Groat W C. The actions of glycine, GABA and strychnine on sacral parasympathetic preganglionic neurons. Brain Res 1970; 18: 542–544

90. de Groat W C. The actions of γ-aminobutyric acid and related amino acids on mammalian autonomic ganglia. J Pharmacol Exp Ther 1970; 172: 384–396

91. de Groat W C, Booth A M. Neural control of penile erection. In: Maggi C A (ed) The autonomic nervous system. Nervous control of the urogenital system. London: Harwood, 1993; 6: 465–513

92. Bancroft J, O'Carroll R, McNeilly A et al. The effects of bromocriptine on the sexual behavior of hyperprolactinemic man: a controlled case study. Clin Endocrinol 1984; 21: 131–137

93. Perryman R L, Thorner M O. The effects of hyperprolactinemia on sexual and reproductive function in men. J Androl 1981; 2: 233–242

94. Schwartz M F, Banman J E, Masters W H. Hyperprolactinemia and sexual dysfunction in men. Biol Psychiatry 1982; 17: 861–876

95. Doherty P C, Baum M J, Todd R B. Effects of chronic hyperprolactinemia on sexual arousal and erectile function in male rats. Neuroendocrinology 1986; 42: 368–375

96. Clark J T, Kalra P S. Effects on penile reflexes and plasma hormones of hyperprolactinemia induced by MITW15 tumors. Horm Behav 1985; 19: 304–310

97. Bertolini A, Gessa G L. Behavioral effects of ACTH-MSH peptides. J Endocrinol Invest 1981; 4: 241–251

98. Bertolini A, Poggioli R, Vergoni V. Cross-species comparison of the ACTH-induced behavioral syndrome. Ann N Y Acad Sci 1988; 525: 114–129

99. Bertolini A, Poggioli R, Fratta W. Withdrawal symptoms in morphine-dependent rats intracerebroventricularly injected with $ACTH_{1-24}$ and with β-MSH. Life Sci 1981; 29: 249–252

Chapter 8

Central nervous system control

L. Marson

■ INTRODUCTION

Several reviews that focus on the behavioural and neuroendocrine aspects of sexual function have been published.[1–5] The major emphasis of this chapter is on the neural control of erectile and ejaculatory reflexes in males, focusing on neuro-anatomical and neurophysiological studies, primarily performed in the rat. Although present knowledge of spinal and brain-stem circuits is not complete, an attempt has been made to provide an updated view of the excitatory and inhibitory central nervous system (CNS) regions involved. Studies have been focused on the rat, which has become, over the last decade, the most common animal model for neurobiological studies of sexual function. In addition, many of the autonomic and somatic changes seen during sexual reflexes in the rat, are similar to those reported in humans.[6–11]

Initial studies attempting to understand the CNS organization of erectile and ejaculatory process were based on the results of studies of fairly large lesions that took place in the 1960s, and their resultant effect on sexual behaviour. With the development of more sophisticated techniques, an effort has been made to identify and characterize subgroups of neurons that are involved in various aspects of sexual behaviour. Most of the work has focused on the forebrain or the spinal/peripheral systems involved.[1,2,4] This chapter summarizes these findings and outlines the use of more recent technical advances in neuroanatomy that have allowed visualization of the CNS cell groups that may be involved in the regulation of sexual reflexes.

Frank Beach proposed, over 30 years ago,[12] a general framework for the central nervous organization of sexual function in the male, which was based on his concepts and published research at that time. Beach proposed that

hormonal and sensory inputs regulating sexual behaviour were integrated in the forebrain. Forebrain nuclei relayed through the brain stem to the spinal cord and thus controlled the lower genital reflexes. The higher brain regions could initiate sexual behaviour. There is evidence of the excitatory influence of sexual reflexes in nocturnal erections and psychogenic erections. Beach also proposed that genital reflexes, such as erection and ejaculation, could be produced in response to genital stimulation even if the connections from the brain were severed from the spinal cord; thus, the spinal cord contains the necessary circuitry for producing sexual reflexes. Evidence for this hypothesis came from spinal cord injured patients, in which genital stimulation could still produce erections, and from spinalized experimental animals in which genital stimulation more easily produced sexual reflexes.[6–8,12–17] These studies also implied that spinal sexual reflexes were primarily under inhibitory control from the brain stem (Fig. 8.1).

This framework still stands today and, until recently, the brain region controlling the tonic inhibition of spinal cord sexual reflexes remained elusive. This chapter presents information concerning the brain regions that are known to be involved in both the excitatory and inhibitory control of erectile and ejaculatory reflexes.

■ MODELS OF ERECTION AND EJACULATION

Study of male sexual behaviour and reflexes has necessitated the development of several models that exemplify various aspects of male sexual reflexes. Undoubtedly, the most complete way of examining male sexual reflexes is to monitor sexual contacts with a female, in the awake state. Many laboratories have used,

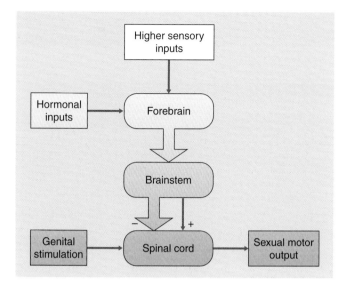

Figure 8.1. Schematic drawing of the hierarchical control of sexual reflexes. Higher sensory inputs are integrated with hormonal inputs in the forebrain, which then relays information through the brain stem to the spinal cord. The brain stem provides primarily an inhibitory input to the spinal cord circuits regulating sexual reflexes. Genital stimulation can also initiate motor output by activating spinal cord systems directly.

and currently are using, this approach to examine the influence of putative neurotransmitters and the role of brain regions on male sexual behaviour. In addition to monitoring mounts, intromissions and ejaculations, aspects of motivational behaviour, aggression and reward systems can be assessed. This chapter focuses on more reflex aspects of sexual function, i.e. the neurophysiology and neuroanatomy of genital reflexes, and in so doing outlines the CNS regions involved in the actual processing of these reflexes. Neurophysiological and neuroanatomical techniques require surgical interventions and may also require anaesthesia to monitor the autonomic and somatic components of sexual reflexes; thus, complete parallelism with sexual behaviour cannot necessarily be confirmed. However, data gained from these types of studies not only have supported that obtained from behavioural studies but also have been paramount in elucidating for the first time the brain region involved in tonically inhibiting spinal sexual reflexes.[18]

Ex copula reflexes

Hart[19–21] and Sachs[22,23] have described a preparation for eliciting penile reflexes in male awake rats, in the absence of females. Male rats were lightly restrained in a supine position and the penile sheath retracted. This elicited, within a few minutes, clusters of penile reflexes, including erection of the penile body and glans. This response is greatly facilitated by spinal transection, indicative of a descending inhibition of sexual reflexes.

Intracavernous pressure

Intracavernous pressure (ICP) recordings have been used as an index of penile erection.[24] When the ICP is increased, an erection occurs due to vasodilatation within the penis. This model, therefore, measures erection but does not account for skeletal muscle contractions, which are required to provide a full, rigid erection.

The urethrogenital reflex

The urethrogenital (UG) reflex model was developed by McKenna and colleagues, in an attempt to develop a model of erection in which neurophysiological recordings could be made and examined in relationship to activation of genital reflexes.[10,17] The model comprises urethral stimulation which reliably evokes a coordinated response that consists of clonic contractions of the perineal muscles (ischiocavernosus and bulbocavernosus muscles), an increase in ICP, rhythmic firing in the cavernous nerve, penile erections and expulsion of the urethral contents (ejaculation) (Fig. 8.2). This response can be initiated in the spinalized, anaesthetized male rat by increasing intra-urethral pressure (20–60 mmHg) and then suddenly releasing the pressure. The perineal muscles were all activated simultaneously during ejaculation of the urethral contents, as is seen in human climax.[21,25–27] These perineal muscle bursts (which are due to bursts of pudendal motor nerve activity) resulted in penile erections and increases in ICP (Fig. 8.2). The skeletal muscle activity was synchronized with firing in the cavernous nerve. The cavernous nerve activity was driven by both the pelvic (parasympathetic) and hypogastric (sympathetic) nerves. Ischiocavernosus and bulbospongiosus muscle activity has also been recorded during copulation in male rats: these muscles fired in synchrony during mounting and intromission, and sometimes during ejaculation.[22,28]

The UG reflex was present after transection of peripheral efferent nerves or complete paralysis with ganglionic and neuromuscular blocking drugs.[10,17] The UG reflex, therefore, was centrally generated and triggered by a spinal pattern generator that involves

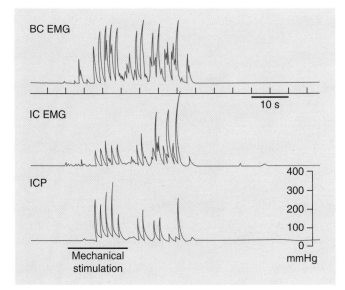

Figure 8.2. Recording of the UG reflex demonstrating the synchrony of penile muscle activity and penile erections, recorded as intracavernosal pressure (ICP). The UG reflex was elicited in the spinalized anaesthetized rat, by mechanical stimulation of the urethral bulb with a fine catheter at the period indicated by the bar (mechanical stimulation). This resulted in rhythmic bursting of the muscles. The UG reflex was elicited at the termination of the stimulus. Electromyographic recordings were obtained from the bulbospongiosus (BC) and ischiocavernosus (IC) muscles. Both recordings were rectified and integrated with a 200 ms time constant. ICP showed large increases coincident with penile muscle contractions and erections. (Modified from ref. 10 with permission.)

multiple spinal segments which coordinate somatic, sympathetic and parasympathetic efferents innervating the sexual organs.[10,17,29] The UG reflex can be evoked only by urethral stimulation or by electrical stimulation of the afferent fibres in the pudendal sensory nerve branch. A build-up of seminal fluids in the urethra of the dog can also lead to ejaculatory contractions.[30]

The UG reflex is believed to represent the neural concomitants of sexual climax in males. The peripheral activity seen during the UG reflex strongly resembles that seen during sexual climax, especially the clonic contractions of the perineal muscles, and forceful expulsion from the urethra (ejaculation). There are many other similarities between the UG reflex and sexual climax: they are relatively insensitive to gonadal hormones;[30,31] both are the product of spinal generators;[6,14,15,32–35] both require coordinated autonomic and somatic neural mechanisms, and the UG reflex and climax is similar in males and females.[7,10] To date there

have been only a few neurophysiological recordings of sexual climax in men[8,25–27,36] and in male rats.[11,28] More studies of neural activity in sexually active animals are needed to understand further the neural mechanisms that control ejaculation and climax.

■ FOREBRAIN REGIONS INVOLVED IN MALE SEXUAL REFLEXES

As previously mentioned, lesions studies in the early 1960s confirmed that a region of the forebrain was essential for male sexual behaviour. In rodents, the olfactory system is important in sexual motivation. The olfactory–vomeronasal system sends direct inputs to the medial amygdala, and studies have been performed to demonstrate the importance of the amygdala in sexual behaviour.[37–39] The medial pre-optic area (MPOA) receives inputs from the amygdala and many studies have shown that the MPOA is necessary for the execution of male sexual behaviour.[40–43] Lesions of the MPOA and adjacent anterior hypothalamus caused copulation deficits in several species,[4,38,44–46] whereas stimulation of the MPOA induced or facilitated sexual behaviour.[40,42,43,47] The MPOA contains a high density of neurons that concentrate gonadal androgens[48] and is extensively interconnected with many other brain regions, including the limbic system and lower autonomic brain-stem nuclei.[49–53] The MPOA is therefore capable of integrating sensory and hormonal signals that initiate sexual reflexes in males.

Since the MPOA does not project directly to the preganglionic neurons and motor neurons in the spinal cord that coordinate the sexual output, facilitation of sexual reflexes must relay through sites within the brainstem for the appropriate response to occur. Preliminary data from the author's laboratory suggests that the periaqueductal grey matter is a strong candidate for one of these relay sites.

The effect of hypothalamic stimulation on the UG reflex was examined in intact anaesthetized male rats.[54] Electrical stimulation of areas including the MPOA induced rhythmic firing of the pudendal motor nerve, indicative of the UG reflex. This response could be initiated in either the presence or absence of urethral distension (Fig. 8.3). Moreover, microinjections of excitatory amino acids, which activate cell bodies and not fibres of passage, into the MPOA also initiated the UG reflex (Fig. 8.4). This study suggests that neurons in the

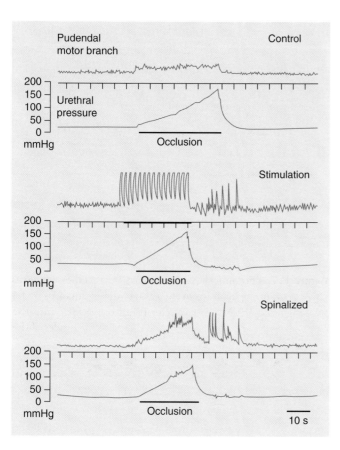

Figure 8.3. Polygraph tracing demonstrating the effect of bilateral electrical stimulation of the hypothalamus on the UG reflex. Male rats spinally intact and anaesthetized. Top trace: prior to stimulation, perfusion and brief occlusion of the urethral meatus failed to elicit the UG reflex ('control'). Bilateral electrical stimulation of the MPOA [250 μA/0.2 ms pulses at 50 Hz, 1 s on, 1 s off, indicated by the black bar in the timer trace ('stimulation')] in combination with urethral stimulation initiates the UG reflex. Following spinal transection, the UG reflex can still be initiated by urethral distension alone ('spinalized'). Note that the UG reflex is the coordinated rhythmic firing of the pudendal motor nerve at the termination of the stimulus. (From ref. 54 with permission.)

MPOA are responsible for activating the UG reflex. Behavioural studies have demonstrated that MPOA stimulation facilitates sexual behaviour. The observation that activation of neurons in the MPOA initiates the UG reflex not only agrees with the published work but also supports usefulness of the UG reflex model in elucidating the excitatory pathways involved in sexual function. In addition to activation of the UG reflex, changes in blood pressure and respiration were noted; as cardiovascular and respiratory changes accompany sexual climax, this was not surprising.

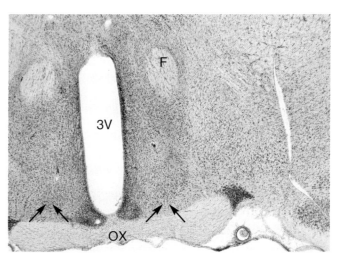

Figure 8.4. Photomicrograph illustrating the location of a bilateral injection of DL-homocysteic acid (DLH; 0.05 M, 100 nl each side) into the medial pre-optic area, which was successful in eliciting the UG reflex. Arrows indicate the position of the tip of the micropipette. The injected DLH spread approximately 225 μm in diameter. 3V, third ventricle; F, fornix; OX, optic chiasma. (From ref. 54 with permission.)

C-fos studies

Immunohistochemical staining for the transcription factor encoded by the immediate early gene c-fos have been used to identify brain neurons that are trans-synaptically activated in the CNS.[55–57] A wide variety of stimuli, including visceral and sensory stimuli, specific behaviours, and noxious and non-noxious activation, have been shown to induce c-fos expression at specific sites in the CNS.[58–61] Studies published to date have identified neurons, in particular in the forebrain, that are activated in response to mating behaviour. More recently, studies have differentiated the cell groups that are activated in response to mounting, intromissions and ejaculations.[60–63] These studies cannot dissociate between neurons that are active in response to, or those that are involved in, the initiation of sexual function. However, the data from these studies have confirmed the importance of the MPOA in ejaculatory reflexes. In addition, other areas within the forebrain have been identified that demonstrate increases in c-fos activity that correlate to specific stages of sexual behaviour. In summary, the bed nucleus of the stria terminalis (BSTN) and the medial amygdala are thought to receive chemosensory signals that are processed through the accessory olfactory bulb. In addition, the BSTN has been shown to be involved in the regulation of sexual behaviour related to previous sexual experiences.[64] Consummatory behaviour increases neural activity in the MPOA and the subparafascicular thalamic nucleus (SPFp), which is located dorsal to the substantia nigra. The SPFp projects to the MPOA and posterior nucleus of the amygdala, where neural activity is abundant after copulation.[60,61,63]

Transneuronal tracing studies

Pseudorabies virus (PRV) is an alpha herpes virus that has been shown to be trans-synaptically transported within the CNS.[65–68] The virus crosses synapses and is self-amplifying (owing to its replication in the nucleus) and therefore is extremely useful in mapping the CNS circuits that innervate a variety of peripheral organs.[69] When the virus is injected into a peripheral organ it is retrogradely transported through the ganglia and spinal cord to the brain; in this way, the CNS circuits innervating a particular organ can be elucidated. Recent studies have demonstrated that injection of PRV results in specific labelling of efferent first-order neurons, presumptive spinal interneurons and descending brain neurons.[67,70] The author and colleagues have used this technique to map the CNS circuits that project to the penis and perineal muscles of male rats.[70,71] After the longest survival times (3–4 days), PRV-labelled neurons can be visualized in the forebrain. At shorter survival times, PRV neurons were found in the spinal cord and lower brain stem (see below).

Similar labelling patterns were seen in the brain after injections of the penis and perineal muscles, suggesting a common hierarchical control over these pelvic organs. Neurons consistently labelled in the forebrain included the paraventricular nucleus of the hypothalamus (PVN), MPOA, lateral hypothalamic area and the ventral tegmental region (Fig. 8.5).[70,71] In animals that received the heaviest labelling, PRV-containing cells were also found in the BSTN and cortex (frontal and parietal regions, Fig. 8.6). The PVN projects directly to the pudendal motor neurons and the PVN may modulate oxytocin-induced penile erections.[72–75] In addition, the PVN projects to other brain stem regions involved in sexual function, for example, the periaqueductal grey (PAG, also termed the central grey) and the ventral medulla. Further caudal in the brain stem, areas constantly labelled with PRV included the PAG, Barrington's nucleus (pontine micturition centre), A5

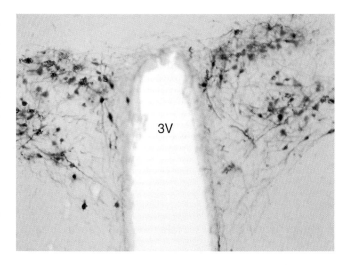

Figure 8.5. Photomicrograph illustrating pseudorabies virus (PRV)-containing neurons in the paraventricular nucleus of the hypothalamus (PVN), 4 days after injection of PRV into the bulbocavernous muscle. Note the PRV cells on both sides of the midline. 3V, third ventricle.

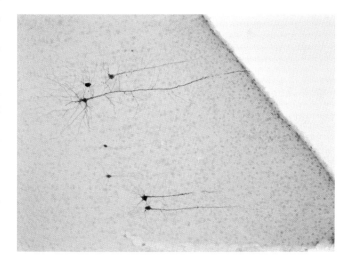

Figure 8.6. Photomicrograph illustrating pseudorabies virus (PRV)-containing cells in the dorsal cortex, 4 days after injection of PRV into the bulbocavernous muscle.

noradrenergic cell group, nucleus paragigantocellularis (nPGi) and the raphe pallidus and magnus. All of these areas are known to project to pelvic efferents and the nPGi has been shown to play an important role in controlling spinal sexual reflexes.[18] These results further suggest that the PRV labelling method has potential in identifying circuits controlling specific organs. Obviously, correlative functional studies are needed to establish the role of the neurons identified in the viral tracing studies with respect to sexual function.

Summary

The forebrain regions identified to date appear to regulate the initiation and execution of sexual function. The MPOA is important for the integration of sensory and hormonal signals related to sexual function; other forebrain regions, such as the amygdala, BSTN and SPFp, appear to play a role in the execution and reward aspects of sexual function. Whether sexual function is initiated by separate excitatory pathways or via disinhibition of neurons that tonically inhibit sexual reflexes remains unknown. In order to understand further the relay pathways from the forebrain that govern sexual reflexes, it was important to isolate the brain region that controlled the descending inhibition.

■ BRAINSTEM REGIONS CONTROLLING SEXUAL REFLEXES

The UG reflex could not be elicited by genital stimulation in animals with intact spinal cords; the UG reflex, therefore, must be inhibited from a supraspinal site.[10,17] This made the UG reflex model the ideal model in which to isolate the inhibitory brain neurons. In a series of physiological, anatomical and pharmacological studies, the author and colleagues have identified the source of the descending inhibition of sexual reflexes in males.[18,70,76–78] Initially, brain transections were performed to isolate the brain level that contained the inhibitory neurons. Cuts rostral to the rostral medulla were ineffective in releasing the inhibition; however, cuts of the caudal medulla consistently exposed the UG reflex (Fig. 8.7).

Electrolytic and neurotoxic lesions were performed to define more precisely the inhibitory region. Lesions of the rostral pole of the ventral medulla were equivalent to spinal transections in removing the descending inhibition. Use of neurotoxic substances to create lesions indicated that the elimination of the inhibition was due to destruction of cell bodies in this region, not of axons of passage (Fig. 8.8). The effective lesion site was localized in the rostral nPGi, which lies just rostral to the inferior olives, medial to the caudal facial nucleus and immediately lateral to the pyramids (Fig. 8.9). Lesions had to be made bilaterally in order to be effective.

A series of conventional anatomical tracing studies suggested that the nPGi contains bulbospinal cells that project to the lumbosacral spinal cord. Injection of

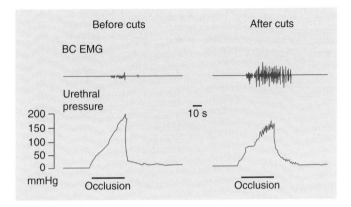

Figure 8.7. Polygraph tracings of the UG reflex before and after cuts through the rostral medulla. Cuts rostral to the medulla did not evoke the UG reflex ('before cuts'). However, cuts at the level of the facial nucleus, in the rostral medulla, allowed the UG reflex to be exposed ('after cuts'). The UG reflex was evoked by infusion of saline into the urethra and brief occlusion of the urethral meatus ('occlusion'). On release of the occlusion, the UG reflex can be seen as rhythmic firing of the bulbocavernosus muscle (BC EMG activity).

retrograde tracers into the region of pelvic efferents in the L6 spinal cord labelled a discrete population of neurons in the nPGi (Fig. 8.10).[18,76,77] Injection of anterograde tracers into the nPGi resulted in labelling of presumptive terminals in the lumbosacral spinal cord in the region of pudendal motor neurons in dorsolateral (DL) and dorsomedial (DM) nuclei, in the area containing the sympathetic and parasympathetic preganglionic neurons (PGNs) and in the medial spinal cord, the site of presumptive interneurons that modulate pelvic reflexes.[70,76,78] These studies indicate that the descending inhibition of spinal sexual reflexes may be mediated by a direct projection from bulbospinal neurons in the nPGi to pelvic efferents and interneurons in the lumbosacral spinal cord.

In order to confirm the role of the nPGi in sexual function, the author and colleagues examined the effect of bilateral nPGi lesions on ex copula sexual reflexes. Ex copula penile reflexes were examined prior to, and 3–11 days following, bilateral nPGi lesions.[79] In rats that received nPGi lesions there was a significant reduction in the time to onset of penile reflexes (i.e. a reduction in the latency to onset) and an increase in the number of dorsiflexions of the penile body (flips). These results are consistent with an inhibitory control of spinal sexual reflexes by the nPGi. Further studies examining the effect of nPGi lesions on male sexual behaviour have also confirmed that removal of this brain site led to

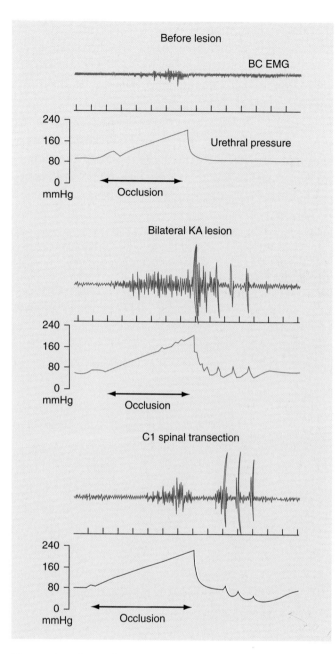

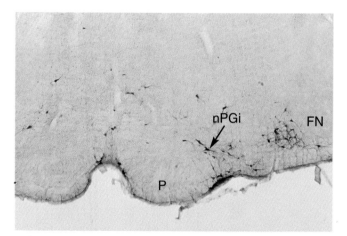

Figure 8.9. Schematic diagram showing the location of effective (left) and ineffective (right) electrolytic and kainic acid lesions. All lesions were made bilaterally, only one side is shown. Lesions are delineated by the thin solid lines. The large midline lesion was ineffective. V, trigeminal nucleus; VII, facial nucleus; pyr, pyramids. (From ref. 18 with permission.)

Figure 8.10. Photomicrograph of pseudorabies virus (PRV) cells in the nucleus paragigantocellularis (nPGi) after injection of PRV into the corpus cavernosum of the penis. P, pyramids; FN, facial nucleus; nPGi, nucleus paragigantocellularis.

Figure 8.8. Recordings demonstrating the UG reflex after bilateral kainic acid (KA) lesion of the rostral pole of the nucleus paragigantocellularis (middle panel). The reflex could not be elicited by elevations of intra-urethral pressure prior to the lesion (top panel, 'occlusion'). The bottom panel shows that the kainic acid lesion was as effective in abolishing the descending inhibition as was spinal transection. Top trace in each panel shows electromyographic activity of the bulbospongiosus muscle (BC EMG). (From ref. 18 with permission.)

facilitation of male sexual behaviour.[80] Male rats that received bilateral nPGi lesions were more likely to copulate to ejaculation during their first exposure to a receptive female than were males without lesions. In addition, rats with nPGi lesions showed an increased number of ejaculations prior to sexual exhaustion.[80]

Following injection of PRV into the penis or perineal muscles, the nPGi was consistently transneuronally labelled.[70,71] In addition to receiving inputs from the MPOA and PVN, the nPGi receives dense projections from the midbrain central grey.[53,81-83] The midbrain central grey has been shown to be an important component of the control of sexual function, and may be an important relay region for forebrain inputs as they descend to the spinal cord.[5,84]

The nPGi has long been thought to be involved in the regulation of cardiovascular systems and pain.[85,86] This may give rise to some concern about its role in sexual function. However, this area has been shown to contain excitatory and inhibitory neurons that respond to genital stimulation and manipulations of the pelvic, pudendal and dorsal nerves of the penis.[87–89] This area also contains neurons responsive to genital stimulation in the female rat.[90] This area projects to, and receives projections from, the lumbosacral spinal cord.[18,77,78,90–92] Although changes in cardiovascular activity, respiration and nociception accompany sexual function, the nPGi may coordinate the homoeostatic responses to behavioural activation of many types.[86,88,93]

Serotonergic involvement in descending inhibition

Pharmacological and immunohistochemical studies were performed to identify the neurotransmitter that mediates the descending inhibition of spinal sexual reflexes. Evidence for the involvement of 5-hydroxytryptamine (5HT, serotonin) was examined, because CNS injections of 5HT alter sexual function and neurons in the nPGi contain 5HT.[18,92,94,95] Both facilitatory[96–98] and inhibitory[99,100] effects have been reported. Some of the confusion of the role of 5HT is due to the large number of receptor subtypes and potential sites of action. The author's studies focused on the role of the descending serotonergic projection in controlling spinal sexual reflexes.

Serotonergic nerves innervate the pudendal motor neurons and intermediate grey matter of the lumbar spinal cord.[77,101,102] Tracing studies showed that 78% of the ipsilateral cells (15% contralateral) in the nPGi that project to the lumbar cord were immunoreactive for serotonin.[77]

Intrathecal application of 5HT caused complete inhibition of the UG reflex in male rats.[77] The inhibition was blocked by pre-administration of methysergide, a general 5HT antagonist. In addition, removal of

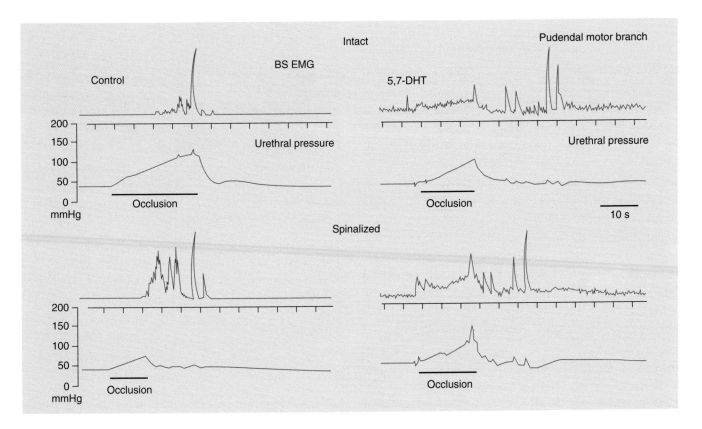

Figure 8.11. Polygraph tracings illustrating the effects of intrathecal 5,7-DHT (5,7-dihydroxytryptamine) and spinal cord transection on the UG reflex. Distension of the urethra was accomplished by saline infusion and brief occlusion of the urethral meatus. The UG reflex consists of rhythmic firing of the bulbospongiosus muscle (BS EMG) and the pudendal motor branch (rectified and integrated signal with a 200 ms time constant) on release of the occlusion. In the intact control (top panel) the UG reflex cannot be evoked; however, pretreatment with 5,7-DHT exposed the UG reflex (top panel). After spinal cord transection at C1 ('spinalized') the UG reflex is present in both control and 5,7-DHT-treated rats (bottom panels). (From ref. 76 with permission.)

descending spinal serotonergic inputs, by intrathecal or intracerebroventricular injections of the 5HT neurotoxin 5,7-dihydroxytryptamine (5,7-DHT), allowed the UG reflex to be exposed in the non-spinalized rat (Fig. 8.11).[76]

The physiological, behavioural, pharmacological, neuroanatomical and immunohistochemical data together strongly support the hypothesis that a localized centre in the rostral ventral medulla (in the region of the nPGi) mediate tonic descending inhibition of spinal sexual reflexes. It is highly likely that this inhibition is mediated by a direct descending serotonergic pathway. However, the possibility that other neurotransmitters, which are co-localized with 5HT, may also modulate this inhibition, has not been examined. Questions concerning control of the tonic inhibitory activity in the nPGi and the pathways and mechanism by which sexual reflexes are modulated from forebrain sites remain to be answered.

Other brain-stem regions that were labelled from the PRV tracing study include the noradrenergic cell groups — A5, A6 (locus coeruleus) and sub-coeruleus.[70,71] These areas are the only noradrenergic groups that project directly to the lumbosacral cord.[103-105] The functional significance of these cell groups remains unknown. However, pelvic efferent neurons receive a dense noradrenergic innervation that is sexually dimorphic, suggesting a role in sexual behaviour.[102,106,107] In addition, the ventral tegmental region in the ventral midbrain has been shown to have a role in sexual behaviour.[108-110] Lesions of the midbrain raphe facilitate male sexual behaviour.[111,112] This region was not often labelled in the transneuronal tracing studies and therefore may modulate sexual function via forebrain pathways. However, the caudal raphe, including raphe magnus and raphe pallidus, was labelled after injection of PRV into the penis and perineal muscles.[70,71] These areas project directly to the spinal cord[92,113,114] and may regulate nociception during sexual function. In addition, the PAG may play a pivotal role in regulating the forebrain and lower brain-stem nuclei with respect to spinal sexual reflexes.

Barrington's nucleus in the dorsal pons also was consistently labelled after injection of PRV into the penis and perineal muscles.[70,71] Neurons in this area project to the preganglionic parasympathetic neurons of the pelvic nerve.[115,116] This area has for a long time been known to regulate micturition and may mediate a variety of straining reflexes.[117,118] To date, a role for Barrington's nucleus in sexual reflexes has not been established.

■ SPINAL AND PERIPHERAL INNERVATION

Details of the autonomic and somatic innervation of the pelvic organs have been reviewed elsewhere[119-126] and thus are summarized only briefly in this chapter. The autonomic innervation of the pelvic organs in the rat is derived primarily from the major pelvic ganglion. This triangular structure is located on the lateral margin of the lateral prostate in males. The pelvic ganglion receives input from both the hypogastric and pelvic nerves. Numerous postganglionic nerves exit the ganglion to innervate the pelvic organs, including the bladder, urethra, accessory sex glands and penis. The largest of the nerves, the cavernous nerve (also termed the penile nerve and which is a mixed sympathetic and parasympathetic nerve), provides innervation to the penis, as well as to the bulbo-urethral gland and anococcygeus muscle.[126,127] The somatic innervation of the pelvic organs arises from the pudendal nerve.[125] During sexual function the autonomic and somatic nerves are often activated in synergy to regulate vasodilatation of the penis, prostatic sections and ejaculation.[125,126,128-133] Erection is due to vasodilatation of the penis, which is mediated primarily by sympathetic and parasympathetic mechanisms, as well as contraction of the perineal skeletal muscles.[10,17,22,23,131,134-136] Ejaculation also requires coordination of the sympathetic, parasympathetic and somatic nerves in such a way that seminal fluids are infused into the urethra and expelled with the aid of perineal muscle contractions.[10,25,131,134] These sexual reflexes are regulated by spinal and peripheral circuits that are under tonic descending inhibition from the nPGi and can be evoked by stimulation of forebrain regions, as described earlier.

Somatic control

The pudendal nerve provides efferent innervation of the striated perineal muscles — the ischiocavernosus, bulbospongiosus (previously referred to as bulbo-cavernosus) and ischio-urethralis — and the external anal and urethral sphincters.[125,137-140] The pudendal nerve also provides the major somatic sensory innervation of the pelvis. In the rat, the sensory and motor branches of the pudendal nerve travel in two distinct nerves, the sensory and motor nerves.[125] The major portion of the pudendal sensory branch becomes the dorsal nerve of the penis. Branches also distribute to the perineal skin, including the prepuce and perineal area, and extending almost to the edge of the thigh and the urethra.

Pudendal motor neurons (the DL and DM nuclei, the DM is also called the spinal nucleus of the bulbocavernosus) in the rat are located in the L5 and L6 segments of the spinal cord.[125,140,141] The DL nucleus in the male consists of motor neurons innervating the external urethral sphincter and the ischiocavernosus muscle. The DM nucleus innervates the bulbospongiosus muscle and the external anal sphincter.[125] The pudendal motor neurons in non-rodent species that have been examined to date are located in Onuf's nucleus.[142]

The afferent spinal innervation of the pudendal sensory branch arises from the dorsal root ganglion (DRG) neurons in segments L6 and S1. These primary afferents terminate in the medial edge of the dorsal horn, on both sides of the spinal cord, and the midline dorsal grey commissure (DGC).[125]

Autonomic control

The PGNs of the pelvic nerve are located in the intermediolateral column (IML, also called the sacral parasympathetic nucleus) in segments L6–S1 of the spinal cord.[143,144] Dendrites of the PGNs extend medially, into the lateral funiculus and dorsally along the lateral edge of the dorsal horn. The afferent, sensory, fibres of the pelvic nerve are found in Lissauer's tract and along the medial and the lateral edge of the dorsal horn. The lateral afferent input extends within the region of the PGNs, suggesting the possibility of monosynaptic connections between pelvic nerve afferents and PGNs.[144,145]

The sympathetic PGNs of the hypogastric nerve are located bilaterally in the IML and in the DGC, in spinal segments T13–L3.[146–148] Only a few hypogastric afferent fibres have been recorded and these were located in the superficial lateral and medial margins of the dorsal horn.

The cavernous nerve is important in the mediation of the vasodilatory component of erection in several species, including humans.[149–152] Electrical stimulation of the cut peripheral end of the cavernous nerve produces an increase in penile volume that causes engorgement of the penis (tumescence) but not a rigid erection, confirming that contraction of the penile muscles is also required for a full erection.[22,151] Recent studies have identified nitric oxide as the mediator of penile vasodilatation.[153–155]

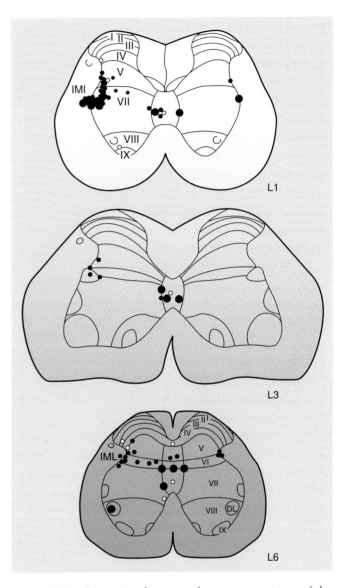

Figure 8.12. Composite drawings of transverse sections of the spinal cord after injection of pseudorabies virus into the ischiocavernosus muscle. Small filled circles, 1–4 virus-labelled neurons; large filled circles, 5–10 virus-labelled neurons. (From ref. 71 with permission.)

Transneuronal labelling studies with pseudorabies virus

Following injection of PRV into the penis, labelled neurons were identified in the major pelvic ganglion.[70] The number and location of these neurons were consistent with labelling seen after injection of conventional tracers into the penis. Sympathetic and parasympathetic PGNs were labelled in the spinal cord. The virus was transneuronally transferred from the penile postganglionic neurons to PGNs in a specific manner. At longer survival times, spinal interneurons were also labelled in addition to the PGNs. These consisted of presumptive interneurons in the region of, and dorsal to, the IML and DGC around the central canal, extending throughout the lumbosacral and lower thoracic cord. Some of these were located within the terminal field of afferents from the pelvis.

Injections of PRV into either the bulbospongiosus or ischiocavernosus muscles retrogradely labelled the pudendal motor neurons in the DM and DL nuclei, respectively.[71] After longer survival times, spinal interneurons were found in the region of the IML, intermediate and DGC of segments T13–S1 (Fig. 8.12). Double labelling of PGNs demonstrated that less than 5% of the PRV cells in the region of the IML and DGC were, in fact, PGNs, suggesting that the pudendal motor neurons do not directly synapse onto PGNs of the pelvic and hypogastric nerves but, rather, that information may be integrated in spinal interneurons in the medial grey and dorsal to the PGNs. Interneurons were also documented in these regions after injection of wheatgerm agglutanin-horse radish peroxidase (WGA-HRP) into the bulbospongiosus muscle.[156] Studies mapping the location of c-*fos*-activated neurons, in response to the UG reflex, have also documented the presence of activated cells in the DGC and dorsal to the IML (unpublished observations).

■ SUMMARY

In this chapter, an attempt has been made to summarize what is currently known about the CNS regions that regulate erectile and ejaculatory reflexes. Although much research has demonstrated a primary role for the medial pre-optic area in integrating and eliciting sexual reflexes, how this information is relayed through the brain to the spinal cord remains unknown. Although several candidate regions have been postulated, including the periaqueductal grey, midbrain tegmentum and ventral medulla, the exact pathways governing neural activity that allows activation of sexual reflexes are still undefined. Recently, the brain region that tonically inhibits spinal cord sexual reflexes has been elucidated and it has been shown that serotonin may have an important role in this inhibition. However, whether there are separate excitatory and inhibitory pathways to the spinal cord, or whether sexual reflexes occur in part via disinhibition of descending inputs, is unknown. In addition, other neurotransmitters may also be involved. Recent transneuronal tracing techniques have enabled 'visualization' of the putative neurons that innervate the pelvic organs, and immunohistochemical identification of the intermediate early gene c-*fos* has allowed documentation of the neurons that are activated directly as a result of erections and ejaculations. A summary of the hierarchical organization is depicted in Figure 8.13.

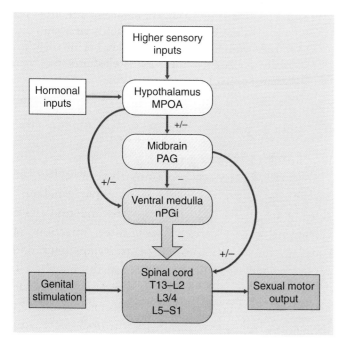

Figure 8.13. Schematic drawing of the hierarchical control of sexual reflexes. Higher sensory inputs are integrated with hormonal inputs in the medial pre-optic area (MPOA), which then relays information through the brainstem to the spinal cord. The brainstem inputs onto the spinal cord circuits regulating sexual reflexes are primarily inhibitory. Neurons in the nucleus paragigantocellularis (nPGi) control this inhibition. Excitatory pathways may relay through the midbrain periaqueductal grey (PAG) to the spinal cord or via disinhibition of nPGi neurons. Genital stimulation can initiate motor output by activating spinal cord systems directly. Sympathetic, parasympathetic and somatic systems are interconnected by spinal interneurons that regulate spinal motor output.

■ ACKNOWLEDGEMENTS

The authors wish to thank Dr Kevin E. McKenna for his support and for introducing us to this research and our colleagues who assisted in the experiments described: Marsha List, Cynthia Polchow, Anne M. Peternel and Jennifer Bradley. The research described was supported in part by NIH Grants NS 23659, NS 29420 and an award to L. Marson from the New York Academy of Medicine, Edwin Beer Foundation.

■ REFERENCES

1. Eberhart J A. Neural and hormonal correlates of primate sexual behavior. Comp Primate Behav 1988; 4: 675–705

2. Hart B L, Leedy M G. Neurological bases of male sexual behavior: a comparative analysis. In: Adler N, Pfaff D, Goy R W (eds) Handbook of Behavioral Neurobiology, Vol. 7, Reproduction. New York: Plenum Press, 1975: 373–422

3. Marberger H. Mechanisms of ejaculation. In: Coutinho E M, Fuchs F (eds) Physiology and Genetics of Reproduction. New York: Plenum Press, 1974: 99–110

4. Sachs B D, Meisel R L. The physiology of male sexual behavior. In: Knobil E, Neill J (eds) The Physiology of Reproduction, Vol 2. New York: Raven Press: 1994: 1393–1485

5. Rose J D. Brainstem influences on sexual behavior. In: Klemm W R, Vertes R P (eds) Brainstem Influences on Sexual Behavior. New York: Wiley, 1990: 407–463

6. Riddoch G. The reflex functions of the completely divided spinal cord in man, compared with those associated with less severe lesions. Brain 1917; 40: 264–402

7. Masters W H, Johnson V E. Human Sexual Response. Boston: Little, Brown, 1966

8. Kollberg S, Petersen I, Stener I. Preliminary results of an electromyographic study of ejaculation. Acta Chir Scand 1962; 123: 478–483

9. Kinsey A C, Pomeroy W B, Martin C E. Sexual Behavior in the Human Male. Philadelphia: Saunders, 1948

10. McKenna K E, Chung S K, McVary K T. A model for the study of sexual function in anesthetized male and female rats. Am J Physiol 1991; 261: R1276–1285

11. Holmes G M, Sachs B D. The ejaculatory reflex in copulating rats: normal bulbospongiosus activity without urethral stimulation. Neurosci Lett 1991; 125: 195–197

12. Beach F A. Cerebral and hormonal control of reflexive mechanisms involved in copulatory behavior. Physiol Rev 1967; 47: 289–316

13. Henderson V E, Roepke M H. On the mechanism of erection. Am J Physiol 1933; 106: 441–448

14. Hart B L, Odell V. Elicitation of ejaculation and penile reflexes in spinal male rats by peripheral electric shock. Physiol Behav 1981; 26: 623–626

15. Griffith E R, Tomko M A, Timms R J. Sexual function in spinal cord injured patients: a review. Arch Phys Med Rehabil 1973; 54: 539

16. Sachs B D, Bitran D. Spinal block reveals roles for brain and spinal cord in the mediation of reflexive penile erections in rats. Brain Res 1990; 528: 99–108

17. Chung S K, McVary K T, McKenna K E. Sexual reflexes in male and female rats. Neurosci Lett 1988; 94: 343–384

18. Marson L, McKenna K E. The identification of a brainstem site controlling spinal sexual reflexes in male rats. Brain Res 1990; 515: 303–308

19. Hart B L. Testosterone regulation of sexual reflexes in spinal male rats. Science 1967; 155: 1283–1284

20. Hart B L. Sexual reflexes and mating behavior in the male rat. J Comp Physiol Psychol 1968; 65: 453–460

21. Hart B L. Reflexive mechanism in copulatory behavior. In: McGill T E, Dewsbury D A, Sachs B D (eds) Sex and Behavior. New York: Plenum Press, 1978

22. Sachs B D. Role of striated penile muscles in penile reflexes, copulation, and induction of pregnancy in the rat. J Reprod Fertil 1982; 66: 433–443

23. Sachs B D. Potency and fertility. Hormonal and mechanical causes and effects of penile actions in rats. In: Balthazart J, Prove E, Gilles R (eds) Hormones and Behavior in Higher Vertebrates. Berlin: Springer-Verlag, 1983: 87–110

24. Giuliano F, Rampin O, Bernabe J, Rousseau J P. Neural control of penile erection in the rat. J Auton Nerv Sys 1995; 55: 36–44

25. Gerstenberg T C, Levin R J, Wagner G. Erection and ejaculation in man. Assessment of the electromyography activity of the bulbocavernosus and ischiocavernosus muscles, Br J Urol 1990; 65: 395–402

26. Rattner W H, Gerlaugh R L, Murphy J J, Erdman W J II. The bulbocavernosus reflex. I. Electromyographic study of normal patients. J Urol 1958; 80: 140

27. Petersen I, Stener I. An electromyographical study of the striated urethral sphincter, the striated anal sphincter, and the levator ani muscle during ejaculation. Electromyography 1970; 1: 23–68

28. Holmes G M, Chapple W D, Leipheimer R E, Sachs B D. Electromyographic analysis of male rat perineal muscles during copulation and reflexive erections. Physiol Behav 1991; 49: 1235–1246

29. Kimura Y. On peripheral nerves controlling ejaculation. Tohoku J Exp Med 1970; 105: 177–190

30. Davidson J M, Kwan M, Greenleaf W J. Hormonal replacement and sexuality in men. Clin Endocrinol Metab 1982; 11: 599–623

31. Sanders D, Bancroft J. Hormones and the sexuality of women—the menstrual cycle. Clin Endocrinol Metab 1982; 11: 639–659

32. Bors E, Comarr A E. Neurological disturbances of sexual function with special reference to 529 patients with spinal cord injury. Urol Surv 1969; 10: 191–222

33. Brindley G S. Sexual and reproductive problems of paraplegic men. In: Clarke J R (ed) Oxford Reviews of Reproductive Biology. Oxford: Clarendon Press,1986: 214–222

34. Sarkarati M, Rossier A B, Fam B A. Experience in vibratory and electroejaculation techniques in spinal cord injury patients: a preliminary report. J Urol 1987; 138: 59–62

35. Bergman B, Nilsson S, Petersen I. The effect on erection and orgasm of cystectomy, prostatectomy and vesiculectomy for cancer of the bladder: a clinical and electromyographic study. Br J Urol 1979; 51: 114–120

36. Bohlen J G, Held J P, Anderson M O. The male orgasm: pelvic contractions measured by anal probe. Arch Sex Behav 1980; 9: 503–521

37. De Jonge F H, Oldenburger W P, Louwerse A L, Van de Poll N E. Changes in male copulatory behavior after sexual exciting stimuli: effects of medial amygdala lesions. Physiol Behav 1992; 52: 327–332

38. Giantonio G W, Lund N L, Gerall A A. Effect of diencephalic and rhinencephalic lesions on male rat's sexual behavior. J Comp Physiol Psychol 1970; 73: 38–46

39. Kondo Y. Lesions of the medial amygdala produce severe impairment of copulatory behavior in sexually inexperienced male rats. Physiol Behav 1992; 51: 939–943

40. Hughes A M, Everitt B J, Herbert J. Comparative effects of preoptic area infusions of opioid peptides, lesions, and castration on sexual behavior in male rats: studies of instrumental behavior, conditioned place preference and partner preference. Psychopharmacology 1990; 102: 243–256

41. Malsbury C W. Facilitation of male rat copulatory behavior by electrical stimulation of the medial preoptic area. Physiol Behav 1971; 7: 797–805

42. Merari A, Ginton A. Characteristics of exaggerated sexual behavior induced by electrical stimulation of the medial preoptic area in male rats. Brain Res 1975; 86: 97–108

43. Paredes R G, Agmo A. Facilitation of sexual behavior shortly after electrolytic lesion of the medial preoptic area. What does it mean? Brain Res 1992; 29: 125–128

44. Hanson S, Kohler C, Goldstein M, Steinbusch H V M. Effects of ibotenic acid-induced neural degeneration in the medial preoptic area and the lateral hypothalamic area on sexual behavior in the male rat. Brain Res 1982; 239: 213–232

45. Shimura T, Yamamoto T, Shimokochi M. The medial preoptic area is involved in both sexual arousal and performance in male rats: re-evaluation of neuron activity in freely moving animals. Brain Res 1994; 640: 215–222

46. Stefanick M L, Davidson J M. Genital responses in noncopulators and rats with lesions in the medial preoptic area or midthoracic spinal cord. Physiol Behav 1987; 41: 439–444

47. Giuliano F, Rampin O, Brown K et al. Stimulation of the medial preoptic area of the hypothalamus in the rat elicits increases in intracavernous pressure. Neurosci Lett 1996; 209: 1–4

48. Sar M, Stumf W. Cellular localization of androgen in the brain and pituitary after the injection of tritiated testosterone. Experientia 1972; 28(11): 1364–1366

49. Finn P D, De Vries G J, Yahr P. Efferent projections of the sexually dimorphic area of the gerbil hypothalamus: anterograde identification and retrograde verification in males and females. J Comp Neurol 1993; 338: 491–520

50. Maillard-Gutekunst C A, Edwards D A. Preoptic and subthalamic connections with the caudal brainstem are important for copulation in the male rat. Behav Neurosci 1993; 108: 758–766

51. Chiba T, Murata Y. Afferent and efferent connections of the medial preoptic area in the rat: a WGA–HRP study. Brain Res 1985; 14: 261–272

52. Simerly R B, Swanson L W. The organization of neural inputs to the medial preoptic nucleus of the rat. J Comp Neurol 1986; 246: 312–342

53. Simerly R B, Swanson L W. Projections of the medial preoptic nucleus. A Phaseolus vulgaris leucoagglutinin anterograde tract-tracing study in the rat. J Comp Neurol 1988; 270: 209–242

54. Marson L, McKenna K E. Stimulation of the hypothalamus initiates the urethrogenital reflex in male rats. Brain Res 1994; 638: 103–108

55. Morgan J I, Cohen D R, Hempstead J L, Curran T. Mapping patterns of c-fos expression in the central nervous system after seizure. Science 1987; 237: 192–196

56. Baum M J, Everitt B J. Increased expression of c-fos in the medial preoptic area after mating in male rats: role of afferent inputs from the medial amygdala and midbrain central tegmental field. Neuroscience 1992; 71: 1063–1072

57. Traub R J, Pechman P, Iadarola M J, Gebhart G F. Fos-like proteins in the lumbosacral spinal cord following noxious and non–noxious colorectal distention in the rat. Pain 1992; 49: 393–403

58. Birder L A, de Groat W C. Increased C-fos expression in spinal neurons after irritation of the lower urinary tract in the rat. J Neurosci 1992; 12: 4878–4889

59. Birder L A, de Groat W C. Induction of C-fos expression in spinal neurons by nociceptive and non-nociceptive stimulation of LUT. Am J Physiol 1993; 265: R326–333

60. Coolen L M, Peters H J P W, Veening J G. Fos immunoreactivity in the rat brain following consummatory elements of sexual behavior: a sex comparison. Brain Res 1996; 738: 67–82

61. Coolen L M, Peters H J P W, Veening J G. Distribution of fos immunoreactivity following mating versus anogenital investigation in the male rat brain. Neuroscience 1997; 77(4): 1151–1161

62. Heeb M M, Yahr P. C-Fos immunoreactivity in the sexually dimorphic area of the hypothalamus and related brain regions of male gerbils after exposure to sex related stimuli or performance of specific sexual behaviors. Neuroscience 1996; 72: 1049–1071

63. Kollack S S, Newman S W. Mating behavior induces selective expression of Fos protein within the chemosensory pathways of the male Syrian hamster brain. Neurosci Lett 1992; 143: 223–228

64. Claro F, Segovia S, Guilamon A, Del Abril A. Lesions in the medial posterior region of the BST impair sexual behavior in sexually experienced and inexperienced male rats. Brain Res Bull 1995; 36: 1–10

65. Kuypers H G J M, Ugolina G. Viruses as transneuronal tracers. Trends Neurosci 1990; 13: 71–75

66. Strack A M, Loewy A D. Pseudorabies virus: a highly specific transneuronal cell body marker in the sympathetic nervous system. J Neurosci 1990; 10: 2139–2147

67. Strack A M, Sawyer W B, Hughes J H et al. A general pattern of CNS innervation of the sympathetic outflow demonstrated by transneuronal pseudorabies viral infections. Brain Res 1989; 491: 156–162

68. Strack A M, Sawyer W B, Platt K B, Loewy A D. CNS cell groups regulating the sympathetic outflow to adrenal gland as revealed by transneuronal cell body labeling with pseudorabies virus. Brain Res 1989; 491: 274–296

69. Card J P, Rinaman L, Lynn R B et al. Pseudorabies virus infection of the rat central nervous system: ultrastructural characterization of viral replication, transport and pathogeneses. J Neurosci 1993; 13: 2515–2539

70. Marson L, Platt K B, McKenna K E. CNS innervation of the penis as revealed by the transneuronal transport of pseudorabies virus. Neuroscience 1993; 55: 263–280

71. Marson L, McKenna K E. CNS cell groups involved in the control of the ischiocavernosus and bulbospongiosus muscles: a transneuronal tracing study using pseudorabies virus. J Comp Neurol 1996; 374: 161–179

72. Wagner C K, Clemens L G. Projections of the paraventricular nucleus of the hypothalamus to the sexually dimorphic lumbosacral region of the spinal cord. Brain Res 1991; 539: 254–262

73. Argiolas A, Melis M R, Mauri M R, Gessa M R. Paraventricular nucleus lesion prevents yawning and penile erection induced by apomorphine and oxytocin but not ACTH in rats. Brain Res 1987; 421: 349–352

74. Hosoya Y. The distribution of spinal projecting neurons in the hypothalamus of the rat: studied with the HRP method. Exp Brain Res 1980; 40: 79–87

75. Luiten P G M. The course of paraventricular hypothalamic efferents to autonomic structures in medulla and spinal cord. Brain Res 1985; 329: 374–378

76. Marson L, McKenna K E. Serotonergic neurotoxic lesions facilitate male sexual reflexes. Pharmacol Biochem Behav 1994; 47(4): 883–888

77. Marson L, McKenna K E. A role for 5-hydroxytryptamine in mediating spinal sexual reflexes. Exp Brain Res 1992; 88: 313–320

78. Peternel A M, Marson L, McKenna K E. Projections of the rostral nPGi: a region involved in modulation of sexual function. Soc Neurosci Abstr 1991; 17: 1001

79. Marson L, List, M, McKenna K E. Lesions of the nucleus paragigantocellularis alter ex copula penile reflexes. Brain Res 1992; 592: 187–192

80. Yells D P, Hendricks S E, Prendergast M A. Lesions of the nucleus paragigantocellularis: effects on mating behavior in male rats. Brain Res 1992; 596: 73–79

81. Andrezik J A, Chan-Palay V, Palay S L. The nucleus paragigantocellularis lateralis in the rat. Demonstration of afferents by the retrograde transport of horseradish peroxidase. Anat Embryol 1981; 161: 373–390

82. Holstege G, Griffiths D, De Wall H, Dalm E. Anatomical and physiological observations on supraspinal control of bladder and urethral sphincter muscles in the cat. J Comp Neurol 1986; 250: 449–461

83. Van Bockstaele E J, Pieribone V, Aston-Jones G. Diverse afferents converge on the nucleus paragigantocellularis in the rat ventrolateral medulla: retrograde and anterograde tracing studies. J Comp Neurol 1989; 290: 561–584

84. Pfaff D W, Schwartz-Giblin S. Cellular mechanisms of female reproductive behaviors. In: Knobil E, Neill J (eds) The Physiology of Reproduction, Vol 2. New York: Raven Press, 1994: 1487–1568

85. Azami J, Wright D H, Roberts M H T. Effects of morphine and naloxone on the responses to noxious stimulation of neurons in the nucleus reticularis paragigantocellularis. Neuropharmacology 1981; 20: 869–876

86. Brown D L, Guyenet P G. Cardiovascular neurons of the brainstem with projection to spinal cord. Am J Physiol 1984; 247: R1009–R1016

87. Hubscher C H, Johnson R D. Responses of medullary reticular formation neurons to input from the male genitalia. J Neurophysiol 1996; 76(4): 2474–2482

88. Hornby J B, Rose J D. Responses of caudal brain stems neurons to vaginal and somatosensory stimulation in the rat and evidence of genital–nociceptive interactions. Exp Neurol 1976; 51: 363–376

89. Rose J D. Response properties and anatomical organization of pontine and medullary units responsive to vaginal stimulation in the cat. Brain Res 1975; 96: 79–93

90. Holstege J C, Kuypers H G J M. Brainstem projection to lumbar motoneurons in rat. I. An ultrastructural study using autoradiography and the combination of autoradiography and horseradish peroxidase histochemistry. Neuroscience 1987; 21: 345–367

91. Martin G F, Vertes R P, Waltzer R. Spinal projections of the gigantocellular reticular formation in the rat. Evidence for projections from different areas to laminae I and II and lamina IX. Exp Brain Res 1985; 58: 154–162

92. Marson L. Evidence for colocalization of substance P and 5-hydroxytryptamine in spinally projecting neurons in the cat medulla oblongata. Neurosci Lett 1989; 96: 54–59

93. Feldman J. Neurophysiology of breathing in mammals. In: Bloom F E (ed) Handbook of Physiology: The Nervous System IV. 1986: 463–524

94. Ahlenius S, Larsson K, Svensson L et al. Effects of a new 5-HT receptor agonist on male rat sexual behavior. Pharmacol Biochem Behav 1981; 15: 785–792

95. Larsson K, Fuxe K, Everitt B J et al. Sexual behavior in the male rat after intracerebroventricular injection of 5,7-dihydroxytryptamine. Brain Res 1978; 141: 293–303

96. Ahlenius S, Larsson K, Arvidsson L E. Effects of stereoselective 5-HT1A agonists on male rat sexual behavior. Pharmacol Biochem Behav 1989; 33: 691–695

97. Lee R L, Smith D R, Mas M, Davidson J M. Effects of intrathecal administration of 8-OH-DPAT on genital reflexes and mating behavior in male rats. Physiol Behav 1990; 47: 665–669

98. Schnur S L, Smith E R, Lee R L et al. A component analysis of the effects of DPAT on male rat sexual behavior. Physiol Behav 1989; 45: 897–901

99. Fernandez-Guasti A, Escalante A, Agmo A. Inhibitory action of various 5-HT1B receptor agonists on rat masculine sexual behavior. Physiol Biochem Behav 1989; 34: 811–816

100. Foreman M M, Hall J L, Love R L. The role of the 5HT2 receptor in the regulation of sexual performance of male rats. Life Sci 1989; 45: 1263–1270

101. Kojima M, Sano Y. Sexual differences in the topographical distribution of serotonergic fibers in the anterior column of rat lumbar spinal cord. Anat Embryo 1984; 170: 117–121

102. Micevych P E, Coquelin A, Arnold A P. Immuno-histochemical distribution of substance P, serotonin and methionine-enkephalin in sexually dimorphic nuclei of the rat lumbar spinal cord. J Comp Neurol 1986; 248: 235–244

103. Loewy A D, Marson L, Parkinson D et al. Descending noradrenergic pathways involved in the A5 depressor response. Brain Res 1986; 386: 313–324

104. Monaghan E P, Breedlove S M. Brain sites projecting to the spinal nucleus of the bulbocavernosus. J Comp Neurol 1991; 307: 370–374

105. Proudfit H K, Clark F M. The projections of locus coeruleus neurons to the spinal cord. Prog Brain Res 1991; 88: 123–141

106. McKenna K E. The catecholaminergic innervation of the lumbosacral spinal cord of male and female rats. Soc Neurosci Abstr 1986; 12: 1056

107. Schroder H D, Skagerberg G. Catecholamine innervation of the caudal spinal cord in the rat. J Comp Neurol 1985; 242: 358–368

108. Barfield R J, Wilson C, McDonald P G. Sexual behavior: extreme reduction of postejaculatory refractory period by midbrain lesions in male rats. Science 1975; 189: 147–149

109. Hansen S, Gummersson B M. Participation of the lateral midbrain tegmentum in the neuroendocrine control of sexual behavior and lactation in the rat. Brain Res 1982; 251: 319–325

110. Clark T K, Caggiula A R, McConnell R A, Antelman S M. Sexual inhibition is reduced by rostral midbrain lesions in the male rat. Science 1975; 190: 169–171

111. Albinsson A, Andersson G, Andersson K et al. The effects of lesions in the mesencephalic raphe systems on male rat sexual behavior and locomotor activity. Behav Brain Res 1996; 80: 57–63

112. Monaghan E P, Arjomand J, Breedlove S M. Brain lesions affect penile reflexes. Horm Behav 1993; 27: 122–131

113. Holstege G, Kuypers H G J M, Boer R C. Anatomical evidence for direct brain stem projections to the somatic motoneuronal cell groups and autonomic preganglionic cell groups in cat spinal cord. Brain Res 1979; 171: 329–333

114. Loewy A D. Raphe pallidus and raphe obscurus projections to the intermediolateral cell column in the rat. Brain Res 1981; 222: 129–133

115. Loewy A D, Saper C B, Baker R P. Descending projections from the pontine micturition center. Brain Res 1979; 172: 533–538

116. Holstege G, Tan J. Supraspinal control of motoneurons innervating the striated muscles of the pelvic floor including urethral and anal sphincters. Brain 1987; 110: 1323–1344

117. Morrison J F B. Central nervous control of the bladder. In: Jordan D (ed) Central Nervous Control of Autonomic function, Vol 11. The Netherlands: Harwood 1997: 129–149

118. Fukuda H, Fukai K. Location of the reflex centre for straining elicited by activation of pelvic afferent fibers of decerebrate dogs. Brain Res 1986; 380: 287–286

119. Bell C. Autonomic nervous control of reproduction: circulatory and other factors. Pharmacol Rev 1972; 24: 657–736

120. Janig W, McLachlan E M. Organization of lumbar spinal outflow to distal colon and pelvic organs. Physiol Rev 1987; 67: 1332–1403

121. Langley J N, Anderson H K. The innervation of the pelvic and adjoining viscera. Part III. The external generative organs. J Physiol 1885; 19: 85–121

122. Langley J N, Anderson H K. The innervation of the pelvic and adjoining viscera. Part IV. The internal generative organs. J Physiol 1885; 19: 122–130

123. Langworthy O R. Innervation of the pelvic organs of the rat. Invest Urol 1965; 2: 491–511

124. Purinton P T, Fletcher T F, Bradley W E. Innervation of pelvic viscera in the rat. Invest Urol 1976; 14: 28–32

125. McKenna K E, Nadelhaft I. The organization of the pudendal nerve in the male and female rat. J Comp Neurol 1986; 248: 532–549

126. Dail W G. Autonomic control of penile erectile tissue. Exp Brain Res Ser 1987; 16: 340–344

127. Dail W G, Trujillo D, de la Rosa D, Walton G. Autonomic innervation of reproductive organs: analysis of the neurons whose axons project in the main penile nerve in the pelvic plexus of the rat. Anat Rec 1989; 224: 94–101

128. Dail W G, Manzanares K, Moll M A, Minorsky N. The hypogastric nerve innervates a population of penile neurons in the pelvic plexus. Neuroscience 1985; 16: 1041–1046

129. Bruschini H, Schmidt R A, Tanagho E A. Neurologic control of prostatic secretion in the dog. Invest Urol 1978; 15: 288–290

130. Farnsworth W E, Lawrence M H. Regulation of prostatic secretion in the rat. Proc Soc Exp Biol Med 1965; 119: 373–376

131. Beckett S D, Purohit R C, Reynolds T M. The corpus spongiosum penis pressure and external penile muscle activity in the goat during coitus. Biol Reprod 1975; 12: 289

132. Wang J, McKenna K E, Lee C. Determination of prostatic secretion in rats; effect of neurotransmitters and testosterone. Prostate 1991; 18: 289–301

133. Root W S, Bard P. The mediation of feline erection through sympathetic pathways with some remarks on sexual behavior after deafferentation of the genitalia. Am J Physiol 1947; 151: 80–90

134. Dail W G, Minorsky N, Moll M A, Manzanares K. The hypogastric nerve pathway to penile erectile tissue. Histochemical evidence supporting a vasodilator role. J Auton Nerv Syst 1986; 15: 341–349

135. Lavoisier P, Courtois F, Barres D, Blanchard M. Correlation between intracavernous pressure and contraction of the ischiocavernosus muscle in man. J Urol 1986; 136: 936–939

136. Lavoiser P, Proulx J, Courtois F et al. Relationship between perineal muscle contractions, penile tumescence, and penile rigidity during nocturnal erections. J Urol 1988; 139: 176–179

137. Breedlove S M, Arnold A P. Sexually dimorphic motor nucleus in the rat lumbar spinal cord: response to adult hormone manipulation, absence in androgen insensitive rats. Brain Res 1981; 225: 297–307

138. Jordan C L, Breedlove S M, Arnold A P. Sexual dimorphism and the influence of neonatal androgen in the dorsolateral motor nucleus of the rat lumbar spinal cord. Brain Res 1982; 249: 309–314

139. Dail W G, Sachs B D. The ischiourethralis muscle of the rat: anatomy, innervation and function. Anat Rec 1991; 229: 203–208

140. Ueyama T, Arakawa H, Mizuno N. Central distribution of efferent and afferent components of the pudendal nerve in the rat. Anat Embryol 1987; 177: 37–49

141. Schroder H D. Organization of the motoneurons innervating the pelvic muscles of the male rat. J Comp Neurol 1980; 192: 567–587

142. Schroder H D. Anatomical and pathoanatomical studies on the spinal efferent systems innervating pelvic structures. J Auton Nerv Syst 1985; 14: 23–48

143. Hancock M B, Peveto C A. Preganglionic neurons in the sacral spinal cord of the rat: An HRP study. Neurosci Lett 1979; 11: 1–5

144. Nadelhaft I, Booth A M. The location and morphology of the preganglionic neurons and the distribution of visceral afferents from the rat pelvic nerve: a horseradish peroxidase study. J Comp Neurol 1984; 226: 238–245

145. Mawe G M, Bresnahan J C, Beattie M S. Primary afferent projections from dorsal and ventral roots to autonomic preganglionic neurons in the cat sacral cord: light and electron microscopic observations. Brain Res 1984; 290: 152–157

146. Nadelhaft I, McKenna K E. Sexual dimorphism in sympathetic preganglionic neurons of the rat hypogastric nerve. J Comp Neurol 1987; 256: 308–315

147. Hancock M B, Peveto C A. A preganglionic autonomic nucleus in the dorsal gray commissure of the lumbar spinal cord of the rat. J Comp Neurol 1979; 183: 65–72

148. Neuhuber W. The central projections of visceral primary afferent neurons of the inferior mesenteric plexus and hypogastric nerve and the localization of the related sensory and preganglionic sympathetic cell bodies in the rat. Anat Embryol 1982; 163: 413–425

149. Lue T F, Takamura T, Schmidt R A et al. Hemodynamics of erection in the monkey. J Urol 1983; 130: 1237–1241

150. Lue T F, Takamura T, Umraiya M et al. Hemodynamics of canine corpora cavernosa during erection. Urology 1984; 24: 347–352

151. Quinlan D M, Nelson R J, Partin A W et al. The rat as a model for the study of penile erection. J Urol 1989; 14: 28–32

152. Bowman A, Gillespie J S. Neurogenic vasodilation in isolated bovine and canine penile arteries. J Physiol 1983; 341: 603–616

153. Burnett A L, Lowenstein C J, Bredt D S et al. Nitric oxide: a physiological mediator of penile erection. Science 1992; 257: 401–403

154. Holmquist F, Hedlund H, Andersson K E. Characterization of inhibitory neurotransmission in the isolated corpus cavernosum from rabbit and man. J Physiol 1992; 449: 295–311

155. Pickard R S, Powell P H, Zar M A. The effect of inhibitors of nitric oxide biosynthesis and cyclic GMP formation on nerve-evoked relaxation of human cavernosal smooth muscle. Br J Pharmacol 1991; 104: 755–759

156. Collins W F, Erichsen J T, Rose R D. Pudendal motor and premotor neurons in the male rat: a WGA transneuronal study. J Comp Neurol 1991; 308: 28–41

Chapter 9
Endocrinology

H. S. Randeva, R. M. Davison and P. -M. G. Bouloux

■ INTRODUCTION

Optimal male sexual and reproductive capability depends upon a complex interrelationship between psychological, emotional, neurological, vascular and endocrine factors. Endocrine disturbances are an important and potentially treatable cause of sexual dysfunction, and include disorders of the hypothalamic–pituitary–testicular (HPT) axis, hyperprolactinaemia (both associated with hypogonadism) and diabetes mellitus. Disturbances of thyroid, adrenal and calcium disorders may also result in subtle but adverse disturbances of sexual function. The commonest endocrinopathy causing impotence is diabetes mellitus, prevalence studies suggesting that up to 50% of patients with both insulin-dependent and non-insulin-dependent diabetes mellitus suffer from sexual dysfunction.[1] Endocrinopathies have been estimated to account for 5–35% of cases of impotence. If diabetes mellitus is included, the higher figure is probably accurate. The predominant focus of this chapter is on the physiology and pathophysiology of the HPT axis and prolactin secretion in so far as they are relevant to the understanding of sexual dysfunction. It also reviews recent advances in the pathophysiology of diabetic impotence.

■ THE HYPOTHALAMIC–PITUITARY–TESTICULAR (HPT) AXIS

Endocrinology of the HPT axis

The endocrine function of the testicle involves a complex, finely regulated interaction between the central nervous system (CNS), the anterior pituitary and the testis. The hypothalamus forms the most important part of the axis in the CNS, secreting gonadotrophin-releasing hormone (GnRH), which stimulates pituitary production of luteinizing and follicle-stimulating hormones (LH and FSH), which in turn stimulate the testes. The latter contain two functionally distinct compartments, each of which subserves a different role:

1. The seminiferous tubules house the Sertoli cells and spermatogonia; their function is to produce spermatozoa;
2. The Leydig or interstitial cells produce and secrete sex steroids, notably testosterone, dihydrotestosterone and, to a lesser extent, oestradiol.

Testosterone is responsible for the initiation, development and maintenance of primary and secondary sexual characteristics, as well as having a role in normal male sexual behaviour and potency. Testosterone also has an intratesticular paracrine (local) role in the initiation and maintenance of spermatogenesis. Testicular function is regulated by the pituitary gonadotrophins, luteinizing hormone (LH) and FSH. These glycoprotein hormones are made up of an alpha and beta subunit. The alpha subunit is common to all glycoprotein hormones (thyroid-stimulating hormone [TSH], human chorionic gonadotrophin [HCG]), biological activity and specificity being conferred by the beta subunit. LH acts on a specific Leydig cell receptor which is coupled to the adenyl cyclase enzyme. The ensuing intracellular cyclic adenosine monophosphate (cAMP) generation initiates the cascade of effects leading to testosterone, dehydrotestosterone (DHT) and, to a much lesser extent, oestradiol biosynthesis and secretion. The biosynthesis of testosterone requires the activities of four enzymes — cholesterol side-chain cleavage enzymes (P450scc), 3-beta-hydroxysteroid dehydrogenase/delta-4-isomerase (3 β-HSD), 17-alpha-hydroxylase/C17–20 lyase (P450-17-alpha), and 17-ketosteroid reductase. The expression of these enzymes appears to be regulated by different mechanisms; with the recent isolation of the mouse cDNAs and structural genes that encode these enzymes, studies of the replication of gene expression are currently under way.[2]

Testosterone feeds back to the hypothalamus and pituitary to regulate LH secretion. Hypothalamic feedback on GnRH secretion is thought to be via the intermediary oestradiol, which is formed from CNS testosterone aromatization. FSH stimulates Sertoli cells predominantly, and possibly the developing spermatogonia. Stimulation also results in intracellular cAMP generation, leading to the synthesis of proteins important in spermatogenesis. These include androgen-binding protein (ABP) and transferrin. In the rat germ cell, proliferation is at its peak when ABP production is maximal, and this physiological steroid-binding protein may well be a paracrine regulator of spermatogenic DNA synthesis.[3]

Recent insight into the regulation of FSH secretion

Inhibins and activins are structurally related dimeric proteins mainly produced by the Sertoli cells under FSH stimulation. Inhibins are 32 kD glycoproteins consisting of an alpha subunit and one of two beta subunits (beta A or beta B). Activins consist of two beta subunits, either identical (activin A or B) or not (activin AB).[4] Inhibins decrease and activins stimulate pituitary FSH selectively. Follistatin is a structurally unrelated peptide that binds activin and may act indirectly through modulation of inhibin–activin effects.[5] These three peptides are thus involved in an endocrine feedback loop affecting FSH release. Besides their endocrine action they act as paracrine factors, being involved in the regulation of spermatogenesis.[6] In addition to the endocrine control of Leydig cell function by LH, FSH indirectly contributes to testosterone production through paracrine mechanisms. Inhibin, activin, insulin-like growth factor (IGF-1), transforming growth factor beta (TGF-beta), as well as interleukins, have trophic effects regulating the LH receptor number and thus responsiveness of Leydig cells to LH.[7]

Regulation of gonadotrophin secretion

Both LH and FSH are released in a pulsatile manner from pituitary gonadotrophs. The periodicity of pulsatility for LH is about 90 minutes. Pulsatile gonadotrophin secretion is secondary to pulsatile secretion of hypothalamic GnRH, which is produced in the hypothalamic arcuate nucleus and reaches the anterior pituitary via portal vessels in the pituitary stalk. GnRH interacts with specific gonadotroph receptors which are coupled to adenyl cyclase. Generation of intracellular cAMP is necessary for both synthesis and secretion of gonadotrophins. Continuous exposure of these receptors to GnRH is associated with a desensitization process (downregulation) and loss of responsivity to GnRH. A similar process follows administration of superactive analogues of GnRH. Therapeutic suppression of GnRH secretion by such analogues to produce medical castration is in current use in the management of androgen-dependent prostatic cancers and in the suppression of precocious puberty. Secretion of GnRH is under the influence of central catecholamines and neuropeptides, including opioids. The roles of the newly described leptins and neuropeptide Y (NPY) are currently under investigation.

■ BIOLOGICAL ACTIONS OF TESTOSTERONE

In most androgen-responsive tissues, testosterone is reduced to its active metabolite DHT by the enzyme 5-alpha-reductase. The genes encoding the two isoenzymes of 5-alpha-reductase — 5AR1 and 5AR2 — have been cloned, and are located on chromosomes 5 and 2, respectively.[8] Mutations in 5AR2 result in androgen insensitivity, causing an autosomal recessive form of male pseudohermaphroditism. Increased 5-alpha-reductase activity (possibly mediated through 5AR1) can result in idiopathic hirsutism or benign prostatic hyperplasia.[9] In other tissues (hypothalamus and some peripheral tissues), testosterone may also be converted to oestradiol.

Testosterone has both paracrine (local) actions and systemic effects. In the circulation it is bound to the plasma beta-globulin, sex-hormone-binding globulin (SHBG, derived from the liver) and, to a lesser extent, albumin. SHBG has one androgen-binding site per molecule and also binds oestradiol. It binds DHT with two to three times greater affinity than testosterone; however, androstenedione and oestrogen binding are only about 40% that of testosterone. In the blood, about 42% testosterone is bound to SHBG (low capacity, high affinity) and 54% is bound to albumin and other proteins (high capacity, low affinity). SHBG production is depressed by pharmacological doses of androgens and stimulated by pharmacological doses of oestrogens. Insulin may also play a role in its control by suppressing it, as in obesity. Only the non-protein-bound steroid (3%) is biologically active. Factors that determine the SHBG concentration and hence the total testosterone level are listed in Table 9.1. In men with an intact HPT axis the consequences of alteration in SHBG levels and hence in free testosterone are few, since the system merely resets to establish a normal steady-state level of free testosterone. In disturbances of HPT function, alterations in SHBG can have a profound effect on the level of free sex steroids, particularly the free testosterone/oestrogen ratio.

Androgen action

In androgen-dependent tissues, testosterone and DHT bind to androgen receptors to produce the androgen–receptor complex which interacts within the nucleus with regulatory elements of the genome. The androgen receptor, AR, is a member of a group of four closely related steroid receptors, the other members of which are the glucocorticoid, mineralocorticoid and progesterone receptors. The AR gene, a single-copy X chromosomal gene that spans 75–90 kilobases of genomic DNA, encodes a receptor protein of molecular weight 110–114 kDa, comprising 910–919 amino acids. AR is a single (modular) polypeptide comprising three relatively discrete functional domains — a transcription-regulating N-terminal domain, a DNA-binding domain and a steroid-binding domain; there is also a hinge region. Androgen binding induces a conformational change in the AR that facilitates receptor dimerization, nuclear transport and interaction with target DNA, and that culminates in regulation of target-gene transcription.[10] The AR has the highest affinity for DHT, followed by testosterone. It has relatively low affinity for adrenal androgens such as dihydroepiandrosterone and androstenedione and for non-androgenic steroids such as progesterone and oestradiol. AR has been demonstrated in the nuclei of a wide variety of tissues, including sweat glands, hair follicles, cardiac muscle, vascular and gastrointestinal smooth muscle cells, thyroid follicular cells and adrenal cortical cells. Regulation of AR is mediated by hormones such as androgens and FSH via cAMP, but also by polypeptide growth factors such as IGF-1 and EGF (epidermal growth factor), possibly by protein kinase activation.[11] Mutations in the AR gene leading to qualitative and quantitative changes in the AR are associated with androgen-insensitivity syndromes causing phenotypic abnormalities of male sexual development that range from a female phenotype (complete testicular feminization) to that of undervirilized or infertile men.[12] Androgens may also exert their effects through activation independent of genomic interaction. This may be responsible for the progression of prostate tumours to the rapidly proliferating androgen-independent state.[13]

The effects of testosterone deficiency differ according to the stage of development at which it occurs. In utero, it leads to the development of varying degrees of ambiguous genitalia, ranging from phenotypic females to near-normal males. Testosterone deficiency before puberty causes failure of secondary sexual development, with infantile genitalia, eunuchoidism, lack of androgen-dependent hair growth, high-pitched voice and persistence of prepubertal body fat distribution. In adults, testosterone deficiency is associated with reduced libido and potency, infertility, lethargy, fatigue and a number of behavioural changes. The hypogonadal male characteristically also has smooth, youthful-looking skin, lack of temporal hair recession and sparse facial and corporal hair (Fig. 9.1). A decrease in ejaculatory volume (or absence thereof) is an early feature of loss of libido

Table 9.1. Factors influencing circulating levels of sex-hormone-binding globulin (SHBG)

Causes of raised SHBG	Causes of reduced SHBG
Thyrotoxicosis	Androgens
Oestrogens	Acromegaly
Cirrhosis of the liver	Obesity
Hypogonadism	Hypothyroidism
Pre-puberty	Chronic liver failure
Alcohol	Insulin-like growth factor 1 (IGF1)
Anticonvulsants	
Any liver-enzyme-inducing drug	
Free fatty acids	

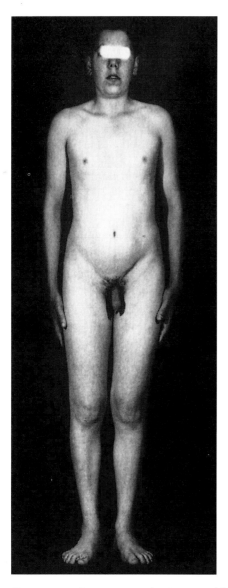

Figure 9.1. Appearance of a 21-year-old hypogonadal male. Note the bilateral inguinal scars, female hair line and habitus, paucity of body hair and eunuchoid segments.

caused by hypogonadism. This is because stimulation of prostatic and seminal vesicular secretions requires high levels of testosterone. In general, the presence of a normal seminal volume indicates that a hormonal cause for the sexual dysfunction is unlikely.

Actions of testosterone on sexual behaviour

Three lines of evidence support the importance of androgens in male sexual activity:

1. Male castrates report a decline in sexual interest and ability, though potency is not lost in all.[14]
2. Hypogonadal males have decreased sexual interest which is reversed by androgen administration.[15]

3. Both anti-androgens such as cyproterone acetate, spironolactone or flutamide and the superactive GnRH agonists will suppress sexuality in man. In the case of GnRH superactive agonists, impotence may become complete, although sexual awareness and interest may persist.

Although it is recognized that low circulating testosterone levels adversely affect the whole gamut of male sexual behaviour (libido, sexual thoughts and fantasies, potency), the precise mechanisms whereby androgens exert these effects are largely unknown. In the human male, prepubertal castration uniformly prevents the development of normal sexual behaviour; orchiectomy in adults causes decline in sexual activity, with only occasional castrated males continuing to have intercourse over a period of years.[14,16] In such individuals it is possible that the small quantities of testosterone and oestrogen formed by the adrenal may be adequate to sustain libido and potency. Androgen replacement to physiological levels in such men rapidly and reliably restores male sexual activity.[15,17] In men, raising the circulating testosterone level above the normal range by exogenous testosterone administration has little effect on sexual function, although pharmacological doses of androgens — as, for example, taken by body-builders — have been reported in some (but not all) studies to increase aggressive behaviour. The latency from administration of androgen to onset of sexual effect in the treatment of the hypogonadal male, particularly between the different components of sexual behaviour (sexual thoughts, fantasies, the capacity to respond to sexual stimuli, potency, orgasm and ejaculation frequency), has been poorly investigated. However, hypogonadal males receiving replacement treatment with intramuscular testosterone preparations usually describe peak erectile responsiveness as occurring 2–6 days after injection. Priapism not infrequently results in the androgen-'naïve' individual; for this reason, testosterone replacement should be built up gradually to the full dose over a number of months in such individuals.

Effect of age

There is a tendency for local and peripheral concentrations of testosterone to fall slightly with advancing age in the male, although true male 'climacteric' is exceedingly rare. As SHBG also increases with age, bioavailable testosterone decreases to an even greater extent. There is also evidence for loss of the testosterone circadian rhythm with advancing age (usually highest at 0900 hours with a 20–30% fall in the afternoon). Reduced LH pulsatility also occurs, but cross-sectional studies on LH levels give varying results (some show the expected rise with the fall in testosterone by feedback; others show no change). Chronic illnesses, common in older age-groups, depress circulating testosterone levels, which are also reduced as a consequence of massive obesity (depressing SHBG levels) and alcohol consumption. However, despite lower mean concentrations, many elderly men continue to maintain plasma testosterone within the young adult normal range, with normal sexual function although, by the age of 65 years, 25% of males experience erectile failure.[18] Low testosterone levels are associated with decreased sexual activity, and studies have shown that older men with high testosterone levels tend to be sexually more active than men with lower values. However, the association is modest and does not support a causal relationship; in general, testosterone therapy in this age-group has rarely been followed by improved sexual function.

CLINICAL AND LABORATORY EVALUATION OF THE IMPOTENT MALE

In the younger patient the history should focus on developmental milestones, progression through puberty and development of secondary sexual characteristics. This will include questions on axillary, pubic and facial hair and shaving frequency, growth, change in voice and body habitus and phallic enlargement, frequency of morning erections and masturbation. A complaint of reduced libido or potency after puberty may be the earliest clue to hypogonadism, antedating changes in shaving habits, loss of axillary or pubic hair, or development of gynaecomastia or galactorrhoea. Clinical examination may reveal anosmia, suggesting Kallmann's syndrome (olfactogenital dysplasia) and eunuchoidism (defined as an arm span of 5 cm or more in excess of height, or sole-to-pubis length exceeding crown-to-pubis length by more than 2 cm), indicative of delayed fusion of the long bone epiphyses. Regression of secondary sexual characteristics may be present, as well as gynaecomastia and galactorrhoea. The latter is characterized by increased retroareolar glandular tissue rather than adipose tissue and is often seen in primary testicular failure secondary to a fall in testosterone/

oestradiol ratios. Testicular size should be measured using a Prader orchidometer and the testes carefully examined for evidence of nodularity that would suggest a possible Leydig cell oestrogen-secreting tumour (gynaecomastia and loss of libido are invariably present in such cases). In Klinefelter's syndrome the testes are pea-sized; the patients are tall and eunuchoid; gynaecomastia is usually present, and the buccal smear is positive with an XXY karyotype. Other signs of systemic illness should be sought. In suspected prolactinoma, visual field and fundal examination should be carried out, and galactorrhoea sought. A classification of hypogonadism according to cause is given in Table 9.2.

BIOCHEMICAL EVALUATION

If hypogonadism is present, the next step is to determine whether it is due to testicular or hypothalamopituitary disease. Total testosterone level, SHBG, LH, FSH, oestradiol and prolactin levels should be measured at 0900 hours. Blood glucose, ferritin and total iron-binding capacity (TIBC) levels are required to rule out haemochromatosis. Low testosterone levels associated with high gonadotrophin levels and elevated oestrogen levels suggest primary gonadal failure. Provocative testing with human chorionic gonadotrophin (LH-like) in a dose of 4000 units intramuscularly for 4 days will fail to give the normal 2.5-fold increase in testosterone level in this situation; however, it is rarely necessary to perform this test as it does not usually add information to the basal studies. Low gonadotrophin and testosterone but elevated oestradiol levels suggest the presence of an oestrogen-secreting testicular or adrenal tumour. The finding of low gonadotrophin levels associated with low testosterone levels should prompt a search for hypothalamopituitary disease. A skull radiograph should be performed to detect an abnormal pituitary fossa or suprasellar calcification (this may signify the presence of a craniopharyngioma) together with magnetic resonance imaging (MRI) scanning of the hypothalamic–pituitary region. Measurement of other basal hormones (thyroxine, cortisol), plasma and urine osmolality should be performed. A GnRH test (100 µg GnRH i.v.) with measurement of LH and FSH at 0, 30 and 60 min will evaluate the pituitary gonadotrophin reserve. The clomiphene test (50 mg clomiphene twice daily for 10 days) will test the integrity of the hypothalamic–pituitary axis (normal response is a doubling or more of the basal LH level). A positive response to GnRH but non-

Table 9.2. Causes of hypogonadism

GnRH deficiency
    Hypothalamic lesions (tumours; encephalitis; granulomas; craniopharyngioma)
    Isolated GnRH deficiency (idiopathic; associated with Kallmann's)
    Prader–Willi syndrome (massive obesity, neonatal hypotonia, hyperphagia, mental retardation)
    Laurence–Moon–Biedl syndrome (growth retardation, obesity, syndactyly, retinitis pigmentosa)
    Alstrom's syndrome (obesity, nephropathy, hypertriglyceridaemia, hyperuricaemia, acanthosis nigricans and
        hypogonadotrophic hypogonadism)
    Familial cerebellar syndrome (cerebellar ataxia, nerve deafness, short fourth metacarpal)
    Hyperprolactinaemia (functional)
    Haemochromatosis
    Neurosarcoid
Pituitary disorders (gonadotrophin deficiency)
    Isolated LH deficiency (Pasqualini syndrome; eunuchoidism, absent secondary sexual characteristics,
        oligospermia)
    Tumours (functioning and non-functioning)
    Pituitary infarction
    Pituitary apoplexy
    Empty sella syndrome
    Haemochromatosis

Testicular disorders (primary gonadal failure)
    Undescended testes
    Bilateral torsion of testes
    Orchitis
    Seminiferous tubule dysgenesis (Klinefelter's syndrome)
    Haemochromatosis
    Impaired Leydig cell activity:
    (a) Inborn errors of testosterone biosynthesis:
        (i)   3,3-hydroxysteroid dehydrogenase
        (ii) 17-alpha-hydroxylase
        (iii) 17, 20-desmolase
        (iv) 17-alpha-hydroxysteroid dehydrogenase
    (b) Leydig cell hypoplasia

Androgen-resistant states and enzyme defects
    Testicular feminization (absence of androgen receptors)
    Incomplete androgen insensitivity
    5-alpha-reductase deficiency

response of LH and FSH to clomiphene suggests GnRH deficiency (hypothalamic disease). A high gonadotrophin level with elevated testosterone level is compatible with an androgen-insensitivity state or, alternatively, a gonadotrophin-secreting pituitary tumour.

■ HYPERPROLACTINAEMIA

Unlike other anterior pituitary hormones, the dominant regulation of prolactin secretion in humans is inhibitory, mediated by hypothalamic dopamine originating in the tubero-infundibular neurons of the arcuate nucleus. Minor prolactin secretagogues are thyrotrophin-releasing hormone (TRH), vasoactive intestinal peptide (VIP) and peptide histidine isoleucine (PHI). In animals, the neuropeptides galanin and pituitary adenylate cyclase-activating peptide (PACAP) have been implicated in the physiological regulation of lactotroph function, both stimulating prolactin release to a similar maximal extent. The most important signalling pathway for prolactin release activated by both peptides is via phospholipase C, although they also regulate cAMP levels, which are increased by PACAP and decreased by galanin.[19] In man, galanin increases prolactin release only slightly and therefore may not be responsible for physiological prolactin release.[20] Hyperprolactinaemia ensues if, for any reason, hypothalamic dopamine fails to reach the pituitary lactotroph and bind to the lactotroph membrane receptor, where it acts to suppress both cAMP generation and the phosphoinositide pathways.

Prolactin (and growth hormone) receptors belong to a superfamily of receptors including those of cytokines, the genes of which are located on the short arm of chromosome 5 in the human genome. The suppressible action of dopamine forms the basis for the therapeutic effect of the longer-acting dopamine agonist bromocriptine in hyperprolactinaemic disorders. However, bromocriptine has some adverse effects (nausea, vomiting, postural hypotension) and, for patients who are unable to tolerate oral bromocriptine, newer dopamine agonists are used. Cabergoline is a synthetic ergoline that shows high specificity and affinity for the dopamine D2 receptor. It is a potent and very long-acting inhibitor of prolactin secretion, administered once or twice weekly.[21] This drug has been shown to be significantly more effective than bromocriptine in suppressing prolactin secretion in hyperprolactinaemic patients, and is better tolerated, particularly in terms of nausea and vomiting.[22] Hypothalamic disturbances with destruction of dopaminergic neurons, stalk lesions with impaired dopamine transport to the anterior pituitary, and compression of portal vessels by a pituitary tumour impairing the delivery of dopamine (pseudoprolactinoma) are all associated with hyperprolactinaemia. Drugs that block the dopamine receptor (e.g. metoclopramide and phenothiazines) have a similar effect. Prolactin-secreting tumours (prolactinomas) are among the commonest pituitary tumours seen in women, but are more rare in men. A number of medical conditions may also lead to hyperprolactinaemia (Table 9.3).

Table 9.3. Causes of hyperprolactinaemia

Disorders of dopamine synthesis

Hypothalamic disease
  Tumours (craniopharyngioma; third ventricular tumour; glioma; hamartoma; metastases)
  Granulomas (sarcoidosis; histiocytosis X; tuberculoma)

Pituitary disorders
  Tumours (prolactinoma; acromegaly; non-functioning tumours [pseudoprolactinomas])
  Stalk section (surgical; traumatic; meningioma)
  Drugs (dopamine antagonists, e.g. phenothiazines and metoclopramide; methyldopa; reserpine; oestrogens; opiates; intravenous cimetidine)

Miscellaneous disorders
  Primary hypothyroidism
  Chronic renal failure
  Cirrhosis
  Chest wall lesions (neurogenic mechanisms)
  Stress
  Idiopathic

Hyperprolactinaemia and sexual dysfunction in men

Severe hyperprolactinaemia (prolactin >2000 mμ/l) may cause hypogonadism and is almost invariably associated with sexual dysfunction in the male. In one cohort of 850 impotent males screened systematically for hyperprolactinaemia there were ten with hyperprolactinaemia (prolactin >700 mμ/l; 1.2%), of whom six showed evidence of a pituitary adenoma; 17 patients with mild hyperprolactinaemia (360–700 mμ/l) were also found.[23] Of 124 patients with premature ejaculation, 10% had mild hyperprolactinaemia. However, it is unlikely that the association is causal. Friedman and colleagues[24] have reported a cohort of 49 unselected men (age range 19–69 years) presenting with erectile failure of a year's duration, and in whom other endocrinopathy and hepatic dysfunction had been excluded; the prolactin level was raised in only one subject, and that only mildly. Although hyperprolactinaemia is a rare cause of impotence, it remains a remediable cause and therefore estimation of prolactin level should feature in the investigative work-up of all impotent men.

Clinical features

Men with hyperprolactinaemia usually have gonadal dysfunction of gradual onset and, unless impotence is complete, patients may minimize symptoms, attributing them to ageing or stresses. Similarly, the physician may easily invoke a psychogenic cause in a 40–50-year-old man with declining libido and elect to treat empirically with testosterone. The mean age for men at diagnosis of hyperprolactinaemia is about ten years greater than that for women.[25] This delay in diagnosis may account for the greater incidence of macroadenomas, visual field defects and hypopituitarism in men at the time of presentation. The level of hyperprolactinaemia does not always correlate with the presence of symptoms.

About 40% of men with a prolactinoma have a visual field defect of some sort and headache is not infrequent. Men with hyperprolactinaemia tend to have not only reduced libido and erectile dysfunction but also a small ejaculatory volume. Some 14–33% of men with hyperprolactinaemia have galactorrhoea,[26] and this important physical sign has to be carefully sought in the impotent male, although its absence does not rule out hyperprolactinaemia. Hyperprolactinaemia is also a cause of infertility.[27] In a survey of 171 infertile men, seven (4%) had hyperprolactinaemia, which was reversed by bromocriptine.

Measurement of serum prolactin

Because of the pulsatile nature of prolactin release and the rise that may follow stress (fear, pain, venepuncture), a minimum of three measurements are required before confirming the presence of hyperprolactinaemia. Once drugs and systemic disease (see Table 9.3) have been excluded, prolactin-secreting pituitary micro- or macroadenomas are the usual underlying cause, although levels of up to 2000 mμ/l are often seen in apparently functionless tumours due to interference with dopamine delivery to the lactotroph. The patient should then be referred to an endocrinologist for further work-up: this will include lateral skull radiography, scanning by computed tomography (CT) or MRI, formal plotting of visual fields, and full basal and dynamic anterior pituitary function tests.

Mechanism of hyperprolactinaemic hypogonadism

Hyperprolactinaemia may lead to hypogonadism, as well as exerting behavioural effects. The mechanism of hypogonadism is complex.

Actions of prolactin on the hypothalamus

In the rat, hyperprolactinaemia causes an increase in tubero-infundibular dopamine content, leading to disruption of the normal pulsatility of GnRH and hence of LH and FSH secretion. Similar mechanisms are believed to operate in the hyperprolactinaemic man, where levels of LH and testosterone tend to be lower as a group than in normal subjects. As the LH and FSH response to exogenous GnRH is frequently normal or frankly excessive in these patients, suggesting a normal pituitary gonadotrophin reserve, the defect is likely to reside in the hypothalamus and is generally thought to be a functional and potentially reversible alteration in GnRH secretion.

Increased hypothalamic dopamine content is thought to cause inhibition of LH and FSH release in men.[28] A defect in GnRH pulsatility in hyperprolactinaemia has been suggested by some studies. A rise in portal vein dopamine has been inferred from the excessive response of TSH to dopamine receptor blockade in this situation,[29] as well as the stimulation of LH and FSH secretion following dopamine antagonists reported in some (but not all) studies.[30] Failure of LH pulsatility,[31] with a decreased 24 h urinary LH secretion, has been recorded in male prolactinoma patients. In these studies, pulsatile administration of GnRH restored LH pulsatility and normal testosterone levels in four males with hyperprolactinaemia. Prolactin-induced increases in hypothalamic opioid tone may also contribute to the decrease in amplitude and pulsatility of GnRH secretion.

Pituitary actions

A destructive or invasive pituitary tumour not only may impair GnRH delivery to the gonadotroph but also may compress or destroy the gonadotrophs, leading to hypogonadotrophic hypogonadism. In such situations, gonadotrophins and testosterone levels are low, and the LH/FSH response to exogenous GnRH is impaired.

Peripheral actions of hyperprolactinaemia

Several abnormalities of testosterone metabolism have been demonstrated in hyperprolactinaemia. A direct effect of prolactin on the gonad was suggested in two studies demonstrating a blunted testosterone response to exogenous HCG in hyperprolactinaemia.[32,33] In contrast, Ambrosi and colleagues[34] reported an enhanced testosterone response to HCG stimulation in males with drug-induced hyperprolactinaemia. Martikainen and Vinko[35] found a blunted response of plasma 17-beta-oestradiol to HCG stimulation in hyperprolactinaemia, suggesting an inhibition of testicular aromatase activity. Magrini and colleagues[36] failed to demonstrate an alteration in testosterone response to HCG, but found a diminished rise in the testosterone metabolite 5-alpha-dihydrotestosterone, suggesting an inhibitory effect of hyperprolactinaemia on 5-alpha-reductase activity in peripheral tissues. Clearly, both central and peripheral mechanisms may be operating, although the variability of the above results suggest that other factors — for example, the severity of hyperprolactinaemia and its origin (tumour versus drug) — may represent confounding factors.

Prolactin and libido

Diminished testosterone levels, in themselves, appear to be rather less important in the mechanism of sexual dysfunction than hyperprolactinaemia per se. Thus, increasing plasma testosterone by intramuscular injections does not appear to improve potency consistently in hyperprolactinaemic patients. In contrast, administration of the dopamine agonist bromocriptine, which rapidly lowers prolactin, produces a rapid improvement in potency even when the testosterone level remains subnormal.[37,38] The suggestion implicit in this finding is that hyperprolactinaemia, in some way, acts centrally to depress the mechanisms responsible for libido and potency.

■ THYROID DYSFUNCTION AND IMPOTENCE

Both hyper- and hypothyroidism may be associated with decreased potency. Hyperthyroidism has been associated with decreased libido in 71% of men affected.[39] Gynaecomastia is present in 40–83% and is probably due to increased circulating oestrogens and SHBG, which may reflect increased peripheral conversion of androgen to oestrogen.[40] In hyperthyroid men, basal levels of gonadotrophins are normal, with LH and FSH responses to exogenous GnRH significantly greater in the untreated than in euthyroidism after treatment, suggesting a direct effect of thyroid hormone on gonadotroph sensitivity to GnRH. Hyperthyroidism may lead to a decrease in testicular volume and a lower sperm count, with normal motility.

Patients with hypothyroidism frequently complain of lethargy, loss of libido and erectile failure. Hypothyroid males may show decreased or normal SHBG serum levels, low total serum testosterone concentrations with an elevated biological/immunological LH ratio, and normal levels of oestradiol. The metabolic transformation of testosterone is shifted towards aetiocholanolone rather than androsterone.[41] Studies strongly indicate the Sertoli cell as the target of thyroid hormone action in the testis. In vivo or in vitro administration of 3,5,3'-triiodothyronine (T3) increases, at RNA and/or at protein level, glucose carrier units, IGF-1, and inhibin, while it decreases the aromatase activity and the production of ABP, the latter needed to maintain a high local androgenic environment for developing germ cells. Hypothyroidism reduces oxidative capacity and increases inhibin levels. Finally, hyperprolactinaemia may also contribute to impotence in such individuals. Thyroid function should be evaluated in cases of unexplained impotence.

■ ADRENAL AND CALCIUM DISORDERS

These can produce sexual dysfunction by non-specific effects. Impotence is usually rectified on correction of the underlying defect.

■ DIABETES MELLITUS AND IMPOTENCE

Diabetes mellitus is one of the most common causes of organic impotence. Some 15% of diabetic men below the age of 35 years and 65% of diabetic men aged 60 years or above are impotent, the incidence being threefold and twofold higher than in the general population, respectively. Ejaculatory problems occur in up to 30% of diabetic men. Factors that are associated with erectile dysfunction in diabetes are listed in Table 9.4. Both vasculogenic and neurogenic causes are among the major aetiological factors in diabetic impotence. Libido is usually preserved, and testosterone and gonadotrophin levels are almost invariably within the normal range.

Clinical features

Erectile dysfunction in diabetics is usually gradual in onset, and develops late in the disease. However, it may sometimes be the presenting symptom in impotent men with previously unrecognized diabetes.[42] A decrease in penile rigidity is followed by a decline in the frequency of early morning erections; nocturnal, masturbatory and coital erections become similarly impaired. Although libido is usually preserved, several studies have reported a decreased libido and frequency of sexual arousal among diabetic men, and have implicated a 'central' autonomic neuropathy as a cause of erectile dysfunction.[43] Psychological stress may occur secondarily or reactively in patients with organic impotence, complicating the clinical picture and exacerbating the impairment. Thus, men with partial erectile failure may achieve sufficient rigidity to permit penetration and coitus when unstressed, but experience total erectile failure under stress, presumably due to increased sympathetic anti-erectile activity. Associated risk factors for developing erectile dysfunction are early age of onset, and insulin-dependent diabetes, poor glycaemic control, heavy alcohol intake, smoking, claudication, retinopathy and clinical neuropathy.

As with spinal cord injury, transverse myelitis and multiple sclerosis, ejaculatory disturbances also occur in diabetes — particularly retrograde ejaculation, whereby the patient experiences the rhythmic pumping action associated with ejaculation without semen emerging from the penis (anejaculation). A similar problem may arise following guanethidine and phenoxybenzamine therapy and, in diabetes, it is thought that the competence of the alpha-adrenergically innervated internal sphincter of the bladder is compromised. Problems with ejaculation are thought to be secondary to autonomic neuropathy.

Recent insights into the mechanism of diabetic impotence

Normal erectile physiology relies on an 'intact' penile vasculature and is mediated through both parasympathetic and sympathetic autonomic nerve fibres. It is heavily dependent on a delicate balance between the effects of various neurotransmitters, neuromodulators and locally (endothelial) synthesized vasoactive agents on the tone of the corporal smooth muscle.

Vascular factors

Studies in animal models of diabetes, as well as in humans, have revealed penile arterial narrowing and arteriolar closure leading to 'penile hypotension' and cavernous arterial insufficiency. Veno-occlusive dysfunction caused by lack of control of smooth muscle relaxation (organic) and morphological alteration of the corporeal tissue (functional) may coexist and is rarely the sole aetiology for impotence.[44]

Neurogenic factors

Somatic and autonomic nerve dysfunction can be demonstrated in those patients who have longer latencies

Table 9.4. Causes of diabetic erectile dysfunction

Neurogenic factors

Vasculogenic factors
  Arterial insufficiency
  Veno-occlusive dysfunction

Psychological components

Target organ (erectile tissue) changes
  Biochemical
  Structural

Endocrine

Drugs

of somatosensory evoked potentials of the posterior tibial and pudendal nerves, and of the bulbocavernous and urethro-anal reflexes,[45,46] and of cerebral evoked potentials following stimulation of the dorsal penile nerve.[47] Further, it has been suggested that patients with a penile sensory neuropathy may have difficulty in sustaining an erection during coitus,[48] as continuous tactile or erogenous stimulation to maintain an erection is lost. Finally, the long parasympathetic nerves to the pelvic organs are the most vulnerable of the autonomic nerves, which may, perhaps, explain why erectile failure may be the earliest and most common feature of diabetic autonomic neuropathy. Like the pathological changes in penile arteries, these morphological alterations in penile nerves are likely to relate to the effects of atherosclerosis, hypertension and hyperlipidaemia associated with diabetes mellitus.

Local biochemical and neuro-effector dysfunction

Tumescence is controlled locally by both parasympathetic cholinergic and non-adrenergic, non-cholinergic fibres and their neurotransmitters, as well as by the vascular endothelium. Recently, both in vitro and in vivo studies have suggested that nitric oxide (NO), an endothelium-derived relaxing factor, is the major neurotransmitter mediating smooth muscle relaxation in the penis.[49] NO, synthesized from L-arginine by the enzyme nitric oxide synthase (NOS), stimulates the enzyme guanylate cyclase, which converts guanosine monophosphate to 3, 5-cyclic guanosine monophosphate (cGMP). This results in an intracellular depletion of calcium ions, leading to muscle relaxation. Animal studies have demonstrated that, despite increased NOS activity,[50] diabetic rats were impotent, suggesting that blockage of action of NO may be due to impaired receptors or transduction mechanisms for second-messenger or increased catabolism. VIP, which induces vasodilatation by activating adenylate cyclase, like acetylcholine, is released as a co-transmitter and facilitates presynaptic events. A reduction in VIP immunoreactivity has been demonstrated in human diabetic erectile tissue. Recently, a defect at the level of the VIP receptor or associated G-protein has been associated with erectile dysfunction in the diabetic rat.[51] Local production of erectogenic endogenous prostaglandins (PGs) such as PGE-1, PGE-2 and PGI 2 (prostacyclins), and noradrenaline, have also been shown to be reduced. In addition, substance P and calcitonin gene-related peptide (CGRP), which are involved in the sensory innervation of the penis, have been shown to be reduced in human diabetic men.

Detumescence is mediated by alpha-adrenergic sympathetic activity, and smooth muscle contraction by intracellular second-messenger cAMP. A number of vasoconstrictor peptides have been found in corpora cavernosal tissue, such as thromboxane A2, prostaglandin F-2-alpha and NPY. More recently, endothelins — of which there are three isoforms (types 1, 2 and 3) — have been identified as powerful vasoactive peptides. These act on two types of receptor (ETA and ETB), and both endothelin type 1 and 2 act via ETA receptors, found in cavernosal tissue, to induce detumescence. It has been shown that endothelin type 1 and ETA receptor binding is increased in diabetic rat cavernosal tissue, which may be of some significance.[52]

Drugs and endocrine factors

Certain drugs — such as cimetidine, anti-androgens and certain antihypertensives (betablockers, thiazide diuretics, methyldopa) — have been associated with erectile dysfunction. This was thought to be related to lowering of blood pressure and hence penile arterial blood flow, but the fact that certain antihypertensives cause less or no impotence (angiotensin-converting enzyme [ACE] inhibitors, calcium antagonists) would suggest a direct effect on erectile function and genital reflexes.

Hormonal alterations have been implicated in the development of impotence in diabetic patients. Some investigators have revealed increased urinary LH and diminished total and free testosterone in serum of diabetic men with organic impotence, implying primary gonadal dysfunction.[53] However, most other studies have not demonstrated this association and, of more importance, testosterone replacement therapy is not beneficial unless the person is profoundly hypogonadal. Finally, serum prolactin levels are similar in normal subjects and in diabetic patients with impotence.

Aetiology of diabetic neuropathy

Diabetic neuropathy is either metabolic or vascular in origin, or both.

Metabolic sequelae of hyperglycaemia

Much of what is known of the metabolic sequelae of hyperglycaemia is derived from observations in experimental diabetes mellitus. It is currently envisaged that the peripheral nerves of diabetic patients take up glucose from blood, this being converted to sorbitol by aldose reductase. Sorbitol is in turn converted to fructose by the enzyme sorbitol dehydrogenase, the whole reaction being in direct relationship to blood glucose level. Fructose accumulation leads to inhibition of sodium-dependent myoinositol uptake, depressed intraneural myoinositol and, consequently, reduced membrane phospholipid. Na^+/K^+ ATPase activity is thereby depressed, and this sets up a vicious circle further inhibiting sodium-dependent myoinositol uptake. In experimental diabetes the administration of aldose reductase inhibitors can reverse these metabolic changes with restoration of Na^+/K^+ ATPase activity and normalization of conduction velocities. Aldose reductase inhibitors (ARIs) prevent the deficiency in NO release or action and reduce vascular albumin permeation and microsphere entrapment by vasa nervosum. A recent meta-analysis of trials on ARIs in diabetic peripheral neuropathy in humans[54] seems to suggest a possible role of ARIs in diabetic neuropathy, but also suggests that the evidence is not sufficient to support their generalized use. No beneficial effects of these agents on impotence have, as yet, been reported.

Vascular effects

Vasa nervorum that are diseased in diabetic patients[55] have their own supply of small autonomic fibres. Loss of these fibres may be due to ischaemic damage itself, leading to impairment of regulation of flow, the development of arteriovenous shunts and imbalance between vasoconstriction and vasodilatation. Micro-neurography suggests that this damage occurs early in the disease process. It is recognized that human nerve is ischaemic from direct measurement of nerve oxygen tension and that flow of fluorescein is delayed and deficient.[56] A deficiency of gamma-linolenic acid (GLA), involving a potential shortfall of the enzyme delta-6-desaturase, leads to an imbalance and increase in the thromboxane A2/prostacyclin ratio, resulting in increased vasoconstriction and nerve ischaemia.

Tissue glycosylation

Advanced glycosylation end-products (AGEs) are glucose-derived moieties that form non-enzymatically and accumulate on long-lived tissue proteins. They have been implicated to impair the function of tunica albuginea and smooth muscles, and hence of vasodilatation, but also contribute to neuronal malfunction in diabetes. AGEs can react with and chemically inactivate NO[57] and lead to a deficiency of NO, which seems to be associated with increased effects of angiotensin II and endothelium I, which again cause vasoconstriction; this leads to nerve ischaemia, production of oxygen free radicals and so to more endothelial cell damage. Inhibition of advanced glycosylation with aminoguanidine prevents NO quenching and ameliorates the vasodilatory impairment.

Endothelium-dependent abnormalities in diabetes

Recent studies have shown impaired neural and endothelium-dependent mechanisms of corporal smooth muscle relaxation in specimens of tissue from diabetic patients with impotence.[58] Autonomic nerve relaxation of corporal smooth muscle is impaired (Fig. 9.2a), although autonomic mediated contractions are maintained, suggesting dysfunction of vasodilator nerves. Further, reduced endothelium-dependent relaxation of the trabecular smooth muscle in response to acetylcholine has been demonstrated (Fig. 9.2b). The relaxation response in vitro to sodium nitroprusside and papaverine is normal in this tissue (Fig. 9.2c), suggesting that diabetic men have a decreased synthesis or release of endothelium-derived relaxing factor rather than insensitivity of smooth muscle to its actions. These observations suggest that diabetes can fundamentally alter the properties of the trabeculae, thereby impairing their relaxation and thus the erectile process. These findings also form a rational basis for the use of intracavernosal smooth muscle relaxant drugs (phentolamine, papaverine) in the management of diabetic impotent men.

■ TREATMENT OF ENDOCRINE CAUSES OF IMPOTENCE

Hypothalamopituitary disorders require referral to an endocrinologist for assessment and treatment. The underlying condition will require investigation and treatment in its own right. Prolactinomas may be treated medically or surgically, with or without radiotherapy. The response of this tumour to the dopamine agonists, such as bromocriptine and cabergoline (the latter being more efficacious and with fewer side effects), can be dramatic, with significant shrinkage of the tumour and resumption of normal pituitary function where this had previously been defective (Fig. 9.3). Visual field defects due to

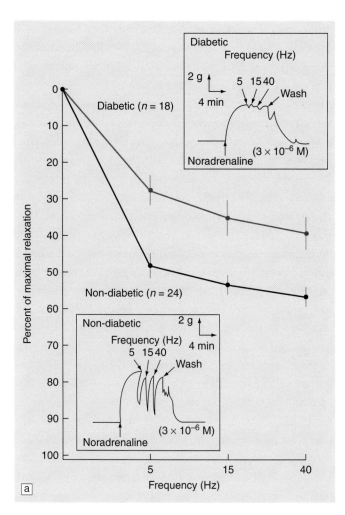

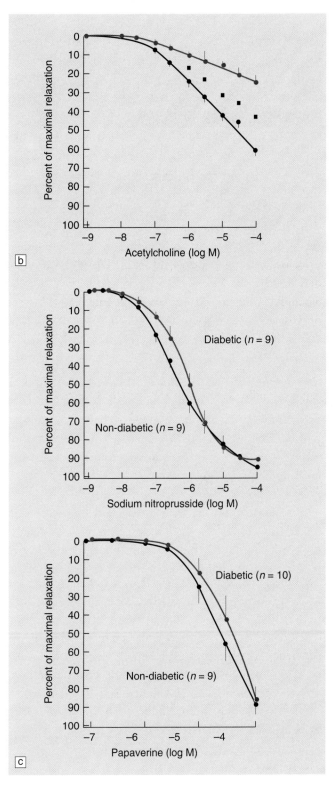

Figure 9.2. (a) Relaxation of a smooth muscle from the corpora cavernosa of diabetic and non-diabetic men, induced by transmural electrical stimulation of autonomic nerves; (b) relaxation of smooth muscle from the corpora cavernosa of 16 diabetic (●) and 22 non-diabetic (●) men induced by acetylcholine (results given as mean + s.e.m.); (c) relaxation of smooth muscle from the corpora cavernosa of diabetic and non-diabetic patients induced by sodium nitroprusside and papaverine. Tone was induced in each muscle strip by noradrenaline (3×10^{-6} M). There were no significant differences in the contraction caused by noradrenaline or in the relaxation induced by either endothelium independent diabetic and non-diabetic tissue. (Reproduced from ref. 58 with permission).

suprasellar extensions and potency may be rapidly restored to normal on treatment. However, the benefits of dopamine agonists are usually only maintained for as long as the patient remains on treatment; definitive therapy in the form of surgery and radiotherapy (or the combination) is usually required. When residual hypogonadism persists, long-term androgen replacement is indicated. This may be accomplished by administering the orally active compound testosterone undecanoate (Restandol) at a dose of 40–80 mg t.d.s. or testosterone enanthate (Primoteston Depot) i.m. 3–4-weekly at a dose of 250–500 mg. Testosterone implants every 3–6 months (400–600 mg) can also be used and, more recently,

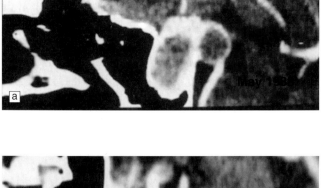

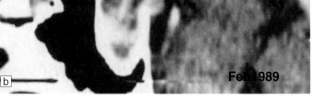

Figure 9.3. Contrast enhanced sagittal reconstructed CT scans showing macroadenoma (a) before and (b) after bromocriptine-induced shrinkage.

testosterone patches (Andropatch) have been used with variable success. The same doses are usually effective in the treatment of hypogonadism due to Leydig cell failure. It should be remembered that patients on testosterone should have yearly prostate-specific antigen measurements, as there is a risk of inducing prostatic dysplasia.

Endocrinologists are frequently referred patients with sexual dysfunction and mild hyperprolactinaemia (360–800 mµ/l). In these instances it is customary to repeat the measurements on two or more occasions to confirm the abnormality. In the absence of drug or other 'secondary' causes of hyperprolactinaemia (see Table 9.3), investigation with CT and MRI scanning rarely reveals a tumour. A therapeutic trial of a dopamine agonist should be given in such instances, although this is rarely successful.

■ TREATMENT OF DIABETIC IMPOTENCE

Diabetic impotence poses an altogether greater management problem. Specific therapeutic measures include sex therapy, psychotherapy, treatment for alcohol or tobacco dependency, androgen replacement therapy (if hypogonadal), treatment of hypercholesterolaemia,

replacement of offending medications (see above) and, importantly, improved glycaemic control. The effect of intensified insulin treatment was borne out in the Diabetes Control and Complications Trial,[59] in which intensive therapy (insulin pumps or three or more daily insulin injections) delayed the onset and slowed the progression of microvascular complications, including neuropathy.

As yet, there is no effective oral agent for erectile dysfunction, although yohimbine hydrochloride, an alpha-2-adrenergic blocking agent has been used, with limited efficacy. However, recently, sildenafil has been demonstrated as an effective oral therapy for erectile dysfunction of no established organic cause.[60] It competitively inhibits the phosphodiesterase type V enzyme, thereby increasing intracellular levels of cGMP in corporal smooth muscle. It is currently being evaluated in phase III clinical trials (see Chapter 26).

Injection of vasodilator agents directly into the corpora cavernosa (with papaverine, phentolamine and prostaglandin E1, alone or in combination) is effective in some 70% of diabetic patients. Although effective, it is invasive and local complications of therapy include fibrotic nodules (1.5–60%), infection and priapism (2.5–15%) which, if not treated urgently, may lead to pancavernosal scarring. The painless nodules can lead to penile curvature. Systemic side effects of treatment include vasovagal attacks and hepatotoxicity (associated with papaverine but reversible after cessation of therapy). The prostanoid prostaglandin E1 is not associated with prolonged erections or corporal fibrosis, although penile pain after injection is frequent. Other therapies include vacuum tumescence devices, constrictive bands and penile prostheses, but the latter have an increased incidence of failure, mainly due to infection.

Finally, antegrade ejaculation can occasionally be achieved with sympathomimetics (pseudoephrine), but these induce impotence. Rectal probe electrostimulation combined with assisted reproductive techniques, such as in vitro fertilization (IVF) and, more recently, intracytoplasmic sperm injection (ICSI), has provided diabetic men, and others with anejaculation (see above), with a means of producing their own biological offspring.

■ REFERENCES

1. McCulloch D K, Campbell I W, Wu F C et al. The presence of diabetic impotence. Diabetologia 1980; 18: 279–283
2. Payne A H, Youngblood G L. Regulation of expression of steroidogenic enzymes in Leydig cells. Biol Reprod 1995; 52(2): 217–225
3. Gerard A, Bedjou R, Clerc A et al. Growth response of adult germ cells to rat androgen-binding protein and human sex hormone binding globulin. Horm Res 1996; 45(3–5): 218–221
4. Pigny P, Dewailly D, Racadot A et al. Family of inhibins and activins: from endocrine to paracrine action. Ann Endocrinol (Paris) 1996; 57(5): 385–394
5. Halvorson L M, DeCherney A H. Inhibins, activin and follistatin in reproductive medicine. Fertil Steril 1996; 65(3): 459–469
6. Ying S Y, Zhang Z, Furst B. Activins and activin receptors in cell growth. Proc Soc Exp Biol 1997; 214: 114–122
7. Lejeune H, Chuzel F, Thomas T et al. Paracrine regulation of Leydig cells. Ann Endocrinol (Paris) 1996; 57(1): 55–63
8. Mowszowicz I, Berthault I, Mestayer C et al. 5,2-Reductases: physiology and pathology. Ann Endocrinol (Paris) 1995; 56(6): 555–559
9. Wilson J D. Role of dihydrotestosterone in androgen action. Prostate 1996; 6: 88–92
10. Quigley C A, De Bellis A, Marschke K B et al. Androgen receptor defects: historical, clinical and molecular perspectives. Endocr Rev 1995; 16(3): 271–321
11. Culig Z, Hobisch A, Cronauer M V et al. Activation of the androgen receptor by polypeptide growth factors and cellular regulators. World J Urol 1995; 13(5): 285–289
12. McPhaul M J, Marcelli M, Zoppi S et al. Genetic basis of endocrine disease. 4. The spectrum of mutations in the androgen receptor gene that causes androgen resistance. J Clin Endocrinol Metab 1993; 76(1): 17–23
13. Nazareth L V, Weigel N L. Activation of the human androgen receptor through a protein kinase: a signalling pathway. J Biol Chem 1996; 271: 19900–7
14. Bremer J. Asexualization: a follow-up study of 244 cases. New York: Macmillan, 1959: 63–117
15. Davidson J M, Camargo C A, Smith E R. Effect of androgens on sexual behaviour in hypogonadal men. J Clin Endocrinol Metab 1979; 48: 955–958
16. Beach F A. Hormonal control of sex-related behaviour: In: Human sexuality in four perspectives. Baltimore: John Hopkins Press, 1977: 247–267
17. Shakkebaek N E, Bancroft J, Davidson D W. Androgen replacement with oral testosterone undecanoate in hypogonadal men: a double controlled study. Clin Endocrinol 1981; 14: 49–61
18. Federman D D. Impotence: etiology and management. Hosp Pract 1982; 17: 155–159
19. Hammond P J, Smith D M, Akinsanya K O et al. Signalling pathways mediating secretory and mitogenic responses to galanin and pituitary adenylate cyclase – activating polypeptide in the 235-1 clonal rat lactotroph cell line. J Neuroendocrinol 1996; 8: 457–464
20. Arvat E, Gianotti L, Ramunni J et al. Effect of galanin on basal and stimulated secretion of prolactin, gonadotrophins, thyrotrophin, adreno-cortico trophin and cortisol in humans. Eur J Endocrinol 1995; 133(3): 300–304
21. Rains C P, Bryson H M, Fitton A. Cabergoline: a review of its pharmacological properties and therapeutic potential in the treatment of hyperprolactinaemia and inhibition of lactation. Drugs 1995; 49(2): 255–279
22. Webster J. A comparative review of the tolerability profiles of dopamine agonists in the treatment of hyperprolactinaemia and inhibition of lactation. Drug Safety 1996; 14(4): 228–238
23. Buvat J, Lemaire A, Buvat-Herbaut M et al. Hyperprolactinaemia and sexual function in males. Horm Res 1985; 22: 196–203
24. Friedman D E, Clare A W, Rees L H, Grossman A et al. Should impotent males who have no clinical evidence of hypogonadism have routine endocrine screening? Lancet 1986; (i): 1041
25. Franks A, Jacobs H S. Hyperprolactinaemia. Clin Endocrinol Metab 1983; 12: 641–668
26. Carter J N, Tyson J E, Tolis G. Prolactin secreting tumours and hypogonadism in 22 men. N Engl J Med 1978; 299: 847–852
27. Segal S, Jaffe H, Laufer S. Hyperprolactinaemic effects on infertility. Fertil Steril 1979; 32: 556–559
28. Yen S C C. Neuroendocrine aspects of regulation of cyclic gonadotrophin release in women. In: Martini L, Besser (eds) Clinical Neuroendocrinology. New York: Academic Press, 1977: 27–34
29. Scanlon M F, Rodriguez-Arnao M D, McGregor A M et al. Altered dopaminergic regulation of thyrotropin release in patients with prolactinomas: comparison with other tests of hypothalamic pituitary function. J Clin Endocrinol Metab 1980; 14: 133–143
30. Quigley M E, Judd S J, Gililand G B, Yen S C C. Effects of dopamine antagonist on the release of gonadotropin and prolactin in normal women and women with hyperprolactinaemic anovulation. J Clin Endocrinol Metab 1979; 48: 718–720
31. Bouchard P, Lagoguey M, Brailly S, Schaison G. Gonadotrophin releasing hormone pulsatile administration restores luteinizing hormone pulsatility and normal testosterone levels in males with hyperprolactinaemia. J Clin Endocrinol Metab 1985; 60: 258–262
32. Besser G M, Thorner M O. Bromocriptine in the treatment of the hyperprolactinaemia hypogonadism syndromes. Postgrad Med J 1976; 52 (suppl1): 64–70
33. Faglia G, Beck-Peccoz P, Travaglini P et al. Functional studies in hyperprolactinaemic states. In: Crosignani P G, Robyn C (eds) Prolactin and human reproduction. New York: Academic Press, 1977: 225–238
34. Ambrosi B, Traraglini P, Beck-Peccoz P et al. Effect of sulpiride-induced hyperprolactinaemia on serum testosterone

response to HCG in normal men. J Clin Endocrinol Metab 1976; 43: 700–703

35. Martikainen H, Vinko F. HCG stimulation of testicular steroidogenesis during induced hyper and hypoprolactinaemia in man. Clin Endocrinol 1982; 16: 227–234

36. Magrini G, Ebiner J R, Burchardt P, Felber J P. Study on the relationship between plasma prolactin levels and androgen metabolism in man. J Clin Endocrinol Metab 1976; 43: 944–947

37. Nagulesparen M, Ang V, Jenkins J S. Bromocriptine treatment of males with pituitary tumours, hyperprolactinaemia and hypogonadism. Clin Endocrinol 1978; 9: 73–79

38. Prescott R W G, Kendall Taylor P, Hall K et al. Hyperprolactinaemia in men: response to bromocriptine therapy. Lancet 1982; (i): 245–249

39. Kidd G S, Glass A R, Vigersky R A. The hypothalamo–pituitary–testicular axis in thyrotoxicosis. J Clin Endocrinol Metab 1979; 48: 798–801

40. Chopra I J, Tulchinsky D. Status of estrogen–androgen balance in hyperthyroid men with Graves' disease. J Clin Endocrinol Metab 1974; 38: 297–301

41. Hellman L, Bradlow H L. Recent advances in human steroid metabolism. Adv Clin Chem 1970; 13: 1–25

42. Deutsch S, Sherman L. Previously unrecognised diabetes mellitus in sexually impotent men. JAMA 1980; 244: 2430–2432

43. Nofzinger E A, Schmidt H S. An exploration of central dysregulation of erectile function as a contributing cause of diabetic impotence. J Nerv Ment Dis 1990; 178: 90–95

44. Petrou S, Lewis R W. Management of corporal veno-occlusive dysfunction. Urol Int 1992; 49: 48–55

45. Bemelmans B L, Meuleman E J, Doesburg W H et al. Erectile dysfunction in diabetic men: the neurological factor revisited. J Urol 1994; 151: 884–889

46. Jevitch M J, Edson M, Jarman W D et al. Vascular factors in erectile failure among diabetics. Urology 1982; 19: 163–168

47. Pickard R S, Powell P H, Schofield I S. The clinical application of dorsal penile nerve cerebral-evoked response recording in the investigation of impotence. Br J Urol 1994; 74: 231–235

48. Goldstein I, Saenz de Tejada I, Heeren T et al. Dorsal nerve impotence: a clinical study of the mechanism. J Urol 1985; 133: 000–000

49. Burnett A L, Lowenstein C J, Bredt D et al. Nitric oxide: a physiologic mediator of penile erection. Science 1992; 257: 401–403

50. Elabbady A A, Gagnon C, Hassouna M M et al. Diabetes mellitus increases nitric oxide synthase in penises but not in major pelvic ganglia of rats. Br J Urol 1995; 76: 196–202

51. Maher E, Bachoo M, Elabbady A A et al. Vasoactive intestinal peptide and impotence in experimental diabetes mellitus. Br J Urol 1996; 77: 271–278

52. Bell C R, Sullivan M E, Dashwood M R et al. The density and distribution of endothelial receptor subtypes in normal and diabetic rat corpus cavernosum. Br J Urol 1995; 76: 203–207

53. Murray F T, Wyss H U, Thomas R G et al. Gonadal dysfunction in diabetic men with organic impotence. J Clin Endocrinol Metab 1987; 65: 127–135

54. Nicolucci A, Carinici F, Cavaliere D. A meta-analysis of trials of aldose reductase inhibitors in diabetic peripheral neuropathy. Diabetic Med 1996; 13: 1017–1027

55. Dyck P J, Thomas P K, Asbury A K et al (eds). Diabetic neuropathy. Philadelphia: Saunders, 1987

56. Tesfaye S, Harris N, Jakubowski J J. Impaired blood flow and arterio-venous shunting in human diabetic neuropathy: a novel technique of nerve photography and fluorescein angiography. Diabetologia 1993; 36: 1266–1274

57. Bucala R, Tracey K J, Cerami A. Advanced glycosylation products quench nitric oxide and mediate defective endothelial-dependent vasodilation in experimental diabetes. J Clin Invest 1991; 87: 432–438

58. De Tejada I S, Goldstein I, Azadzoi K et al. Impaired neurogenic and endothelium-mediated relaxation of penile smooth muscle from diabetic men with impotence. N Engl J Med 1989; 320: 1025–1030

59. Diabetes Control and Complications Trial. The effect of intensive treatment of diabetics on the development and progression of long-term complications in insulin-dependent diabetes mellitus. N Engl J Med 1993; 329: 977–986

60. Boolell M, Gep-Attee S, Gingell J C et al. Sildenafil, a novel effective oral therapy for male erectile dysfunction. Br J Urol 1996; 78: 257–261

Chapter 10

Pathophysiology of erectile dysfunction: a molecular basis

R. B. Moreland and A. Nehra

■ INTRODUCTION

The field of erectile dysfunction underwent a revolution with the advent of intracavernosal pharmacotherapy. The pioneering work of Brindley[1] and Virag,[2] in conjunction with basic science research, has resulted in advances defining the peripheral mechanisms involved in erectile physiology and pathophysiology.[4–10] Numerous discoveries of neurotransmitters, autacoids and vasoactive factors that mediate trabecular smooth muscle tone and, hence, erectile function have been reported (reviewed in ref. 6). Another significant development has been the appreciation that vascular disease affects the corpus cavernosum trabecular smooth muscle.[4–10] This has led to a diagnosis of male sexual dysfunction in terms of cavernosal arterial insufficiency (failure to fill), structural and histomorphometric changes within the corpora cavernosa (a failure to store), or leakage of the draining venules from the corpora cavernosa (a failure to veno-occlude). Most recently, there has been progress in defining the molecular pathophysiology of erectile dysfunction.[6,11] In this chapter, the relationship between penile corpus cavernosal structure and erectile function is explored and the current state of the molecular pathology of erectile dysfunction is reviewed. Finally, the implications of these findings to therapeutic and surgical treatments of erectile dysfunction are examined.

■ ASSOCIATION OF ERECTILE DYSFUNCTION WITH VASCULAR DISEASE

There are an estimated 20–40 million American men with some form of impotence.[3,4,6–9] The National Institutes of Health Consensus Development Panel on Impotence concluded, in December 1992, that, although it is difficult to separate pyschogenic effects from organic disease, vasculogenic impotence accounts for ~75% of erectile dysfunction.[3] Epidemiological studies suggest an association between impotence and increasing age and/or peripheral vascular disease.[12,13] One recent study examined a random population of 1709 non-institutional men aged 40–70 in the Boston area. The overall probability of some degree of sexual dysfunction was 52%. After adjusting for age, impotence was correlated with heart disease (39%), diabetes (28%), and hypertension (15%), as well as with other vascular risk factors such as cigarette smoking. Treated heart disease (vasodilating drugs, 36%), use of cardiac drugs (28%), and antihypertensive agents were also strongly associated.[13] Correlations were also found with untreated medical conditions such as ulcers (18%), arthritis (15%) and allergies (12%).[13] Thus, erectile dysfunction is primarily an organic disorder that is associated with vascular disease. Clinically, vascular alterations in erectile haemodynamics — that is, abnormal regulation of the inflow and/or the outflow of blood to and from the penis — are thought to be the most frequent causes of organic impotence.[3,4,6–9]

■ PENILE ANATOMY AND PHYSIOLOGY: IMPLICATIONS OF THE ASSOCIATION OF STRUCTURE WITH FUNCTION

Before examining erectile dysfunction, it is helpful briefly to review penile anatomy and physiology, which is discussed in greater depth elsewhere in this volume. The penis is composed of three bodies of erectile tissue — the corpus spongiosum, which encompasses the urethra and terminates in the glans penis and the two corpora cavernosa, which provide the principal structure to the erect organ.[4,6–10] Anatomically, the corpora cavernosa are a unique vascular bed consisting of sinuses (the trabeculae), whose arterial blood supply arises from the resistant helicine arterioles; these, in turn, are fed from the cavernosal artery.[4,6–10] The trabeculae are drained by the emissary venules which, in turn, drain into the cavernosal veins. The trabeculae, while arterially fed, have measured blood P_{O_2} of 20–40 mmHg when the penis is in the flaccid state.[14] In contrast, during erection, the measured P_{O_2} of the corpora increases to arterial levels (90–100 mmHg).[14] These changes in corporal oxygen tension have been confirmed by other urology research groups.[15–17]

Since the penis is composed only of soft tissue, in order for sufficient rigidity to be attained at erection to accomplish vaginal penetration,[18] the penis must function as a rigid, blood-filled capacitor.[18,19] The two bodies of erectile tissue — the corpora cavernosa — that are integral to this function are composed of a specialized vascular tissue that has a high content (48–55%) of connective tissue.[4–8,11,18,20] Penile erection is the end result of smooth muscle relaxation. As the trabecular smooth muscles relax and fill with blood, intracavernosal pressure and volume increase. Veno-occlusion develops through stretching and compressive forces by 'expandable' trabecular tissue on subtunical venules.[4–8,11,18] The trabecular smooth muscle cells also synthesize connective tissue, which affects the structural integrity of the corpora (see below). It is this dual function of trabecular smooth muscle that contributes to the balance of connective tissue and smooth muscle (Fig. 10.1).

FUNCTIONAL TRABECULAR SMOOTH MUSCLE/CONNECTIVE TISSUE BALANCE

What molecular and structural alterations occur in the corpus cavernosum that precipitate vasculogenic impotence? Histological studies have shown an association between penile arterial insufficiency, collagen accumulation and erectile dysfunction.[21–25] In these studies, the notable ultrastructural features reported were smooth muscle cell hypoplasia and atrophy and the

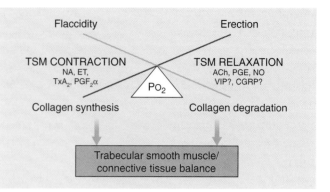

Figure 10.1. The seesaw of erectile (dys)function. At flaccidity, corpus cavernosal blood P_{O_2} is low (25–40 mmHg)[1], the trabecular smooth muscle (TSM) of the lacunar spaces is contracted by the action of neurotransmitters such as noradrenaline (NA), vasoactive factors such as endothelin (ET) and autacoids such as thromboxane A_2 (TxA_2) or prostaglandin $F_2 \alpha$ ($PGF_2 \alpha$). It is the authors' hypothesis that these conditions favour the production of growth factors, cytokines, and vasoactive factors which favour connective tissue synthesis. During erection, corpus cavernosal blood P_{O_2} increases and plateaus at 90–100 mmHg[11] and the trabecular smooth muscle of the lacunar spaces relaxes via the action of vasoactive factors such as nitric oxide (NO), acetylcholine (ACh) and possibly vasoactive intestinal peptide (VIP) and the calcitonin gene-related peptide (CGRP). The authors further hypothesize that these conditions favour connective tissue degradation. It is the sum of both processes which leads to the trabecular smooth muscle/connective tissue balance. (Adapted from ref. 5 with permission.)

accumulation of extracellular matrix composed primarily of collagen fibrils.[21–25] In one study, the severity of symptoms and clinical findings in impotent men was related to the number of altered corporal smooth muscle cells.[22] All of these studies retrospectively suggest that increase in collagen content (e.g. connective tissue) with a compensatory decrease in trabecular smooth muscle cells was related to erectile dysfunction.[21–25]

In a prospective study of men undergoing penile prosthesis insertion, the authors have found a direct correlation between erectile function and the ratio of trabecular smooth muscle to total erectile tissue.[10] Erectile function was defined by experimentally determined parameters of flow to maintain erection, resistance to filling, and pressure decay using dynamic infusion corpus cavernosography/cavernosometry[26] before penile implant insertion. Postoperatively, penile biopsies were examined by quantitative histomorphometry staining, with desmin (a smooth muscle selective marker) immunohistochemistry and Masson's trichrome staining (Fig. 10.2). Biopsies from potent men (with penile cancer, crural trauma and Peyronie's disease) had a range of smooth muscle from 40 to 45%, consistent with accepted 'normal' values of percentage smooth muscle. The correlation between flow to maintain erection and percentage trabecular smooth muscle per total erectile tissue area is shown in Figure 10.3a. Patients with the highest mean percentage of trabecular smooth muscle (41–43%) exhibited a narrow range of normal flow-to-maintain values (< 5 ml/min, group I), consistent with good veno-occlusion. Patients with intermediate values of mean percentage of trabecular smooth muscle (32–40%) displayed intermediate values of abnormal flow-to-maintain (15–30 ml/min, group II), and some venous leakage. Patients with the lowest mean percentage of trabecular smooth muscle (13–30%) revealed a wide range of high abnormal flow-to-maintain values (50–120 ml/min, group III) and substantial venous leakage. Similar relationships are found when outflow resistance and pressure decay are examined (Figs. 10.3b, c). Thus, flow to maintain erection increases owing to venous leakage; resistance falls as veno-occlusion mechanism fails; and pressure decay, a measure of both inflow and outflow, increases with decreased veno-occlusion. These results show clearly that there is a critical ratio of corporal smooth muscle per total erectile tissue necessary for successful veno-occlusion and that excessive connective tissue is correlated with a higher likelihood of venous leakage.[10] A defined understanding of the pathophysiology of erectile dysfunction requires a knowledge of the molecular and biochemical regulation of connective tissue synthesis and degradation in the corpus cavernosum.

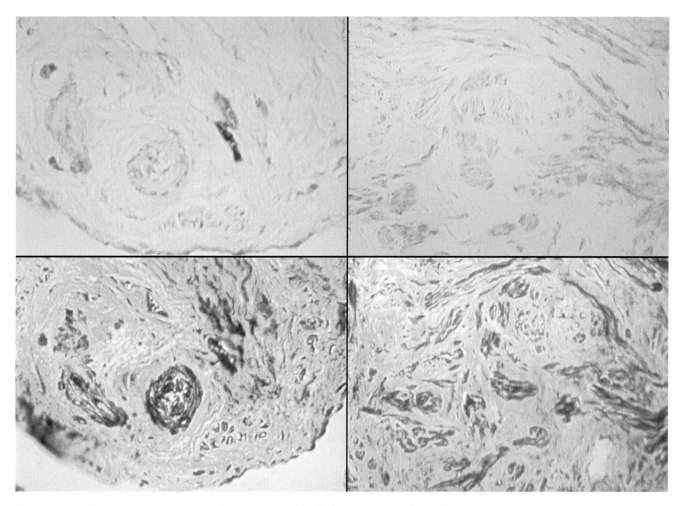

Figure 10.2. Human corpus cavernosum biopsies stained with desmin (a smooth muscle-specific marker) by immunohistochemistry or Masson's trichrome stain. Serial sections stained with either (top row) desmin or (bottom row) Masson's trichrome, which stains trabecular smooth muscle red and connective tissue blue. Magnification X 100. (From ref. 11 with permission.)

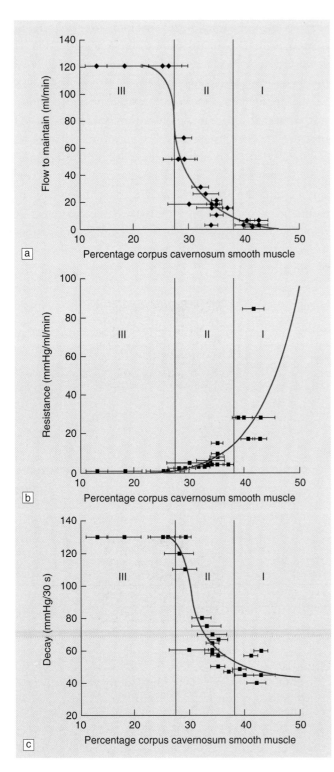

Figure 10.3. Relationships among (a) flow-to-maintain, (b) venous outflow resistance and (c) pressure decay values, obtained during repeat-dosing pharmacocavernos-ometry/ography with percentage trabecular smooth muscle determined histomorphometrically for 24 patients. Patients with the highest mean percentage of trabecular smooth muscle had the lowest flow-to-maintain (<5 ml/min; group I), highest venous outflow resistance, and lowest pressure decay values (r = –0.89, 0.82 and –0.85, respectively. (From ref. 11 with permission.)

SYNTHESIS AND DEPOSITION OF CONNECTIVE TISSUE BY VASCULAR SMOOTH MUSCLE CELLS

The trabecular smooth muscle cell, the predominant mesenchymal cell type in the corpus cavernosum, regulates vasoconstriction and vasodilatation, thus providing the state of erection of the corpora.[4–10,20] What is less recognized is that vascular smooth muscle cells synthesize collagen and connective tissue proteins.[27–37] It has been suggested that, in large and medium-sized arteries, the only cell type in the medial layer is a smooth muscle cell.[27,28] Thirty years ago, Wissler proposed that, by changing from a contractile to a synthetic phenotype, the vascular smooth muscle could accomplish both roles of muscle tone and connective tissue synthesis — in essence, as a multifunctional mesenchyme.[28] The collagen superfamily of proteins includes 19 different genes and ten related genes with collagen-like domains; the fibrillar collagens include types I, II, III, V and XI.[38] Pulmonary artery medial smooth muscle cells have been shown to express both $\alpha 1(I)$ procollagen mRNA and type I collagen in vivo.[28] Incorporation of radiolabelled precursors into collagen in developing aortas in the rat,[30,31] as well as histomorphometric and ultrastructural studies of collagen associated with medial aortic smooth muscle,[32] have been demonstrated. Aortic media explants in organ culture,[33] as well as smooth muscle cells in culture,[34–37] have also been shown to express fibrillar collagen (types I, III, V and XI). These cells synthesize the extracellular matrix proteins (collagen and other proteins) surrounding the individual smooth muscle cells, thus providing the structural integrity of the corpora. Human corpus cavernosum smooth muscle cells in culture express type I, III and V/XI fibrillar collagens.[39] Type IV collagen is involved in basement membrane assembly and has been reported in corpus cavernosum biopsies at the smooth muscle–endothelial cell boundary of the trabeculae, as well as between smooth muscle cells.[24,40] Collagen accumulation can be reversed by degradative enzymes secreted by the surrounding cells. The matrix metalloproteinases are a family of secreted zinc proteinases that degrade collagen and gelatin (denatured collagen).[41] These proteins are expressed as zymogens and activated by proteolysis. The normal processes of remodelling and deposition of extracellular matrix, as well as events leading to excess matrix accumulation, remain to be characterized fully in the corpus cavernosum.

POSSIBLE ROLE OF TGF-β_1 IN THE MOLECULAR PATHOLOGY OF ERECTILE DYSFUNCTION

It has been discussed how erectile dysfunction is associated with vascular disease and how the principal histopathology observed is a loss of trabecular smooth muscle and an increase in connective tissue. What molecular factors are involved in the molecular pathology of this disease? Cytokines and growth factors are thought to play key roles in the regulation of synthesis and assembly of connective tissue proteins. TGF-β_1 is a pleotrophic cytokine that induces extracellular matrix expression[42,43] and inhibits growth of vascular smooth muscle cells.[44] These are the two main changes observed in corpus cavernosum histopathology (e.g. increases in connective tissue and atrophy and death of smooth muscle cells).[19-24] TGF-β_1 alters the composition of extracellular matrix by inducing expression of collagens, fibronectin and proteoglycans, while inhibiting the activity and expression of collagenases and other proteases.[40,41] The growth-inhibitory effects of TGF-β_1 are mediated in normal rat kidney cells in culture, in part through fibrillar collagen accumulation.[45] Thus, an increase in collagen may have detrimental effects on smooth muscle growth, leading to atrophy and death.

What is the evidence for a role of TGF-β_1 in soft tissue fibrosis of other organs? In studies on pulmonary, hepatic and renal fibrosis, the severity of disease was correlated with increased expression of TGF-β_1.[42,43,46-49] In the vasculature, increased expression of TGF-β_1 has been correlated with diffuse intimal thickenings in human coronary arteries[49] and human restenosis lesions.[48] TGF-β_1 is expressed in human corpus cavernosum at the mRNA level by Northern blot analysis,[39] reverse-transcription–polymerase chain reaction (RT–PCR) of archival surgical specimens[11] (Fig. 10.4) and by immunohistochemical staining in corpus cavernosum biopsies.[50] TGF-β_1 induces a two- to fourfold increase in collagen synthesis in human corpus cavernosum smooth muscle cells in culture.[39] In order to establish an in vivo model for TGF-β_1-induced corporal fibrosis, TGF-β_1-impregnated slow-release pellets were introduced into the rabbit corpus cavernosum.[51] Within 72 hours, fibrotic

changes in the corpus cavernosum were observed. Controls included placebo time-release pellets and untreated controls. A significant increase ($p<0.002$) in connective tissue was observed compared with placebo by 3 days of treatment (35% smooth muscle per erectile tissue area versus 40% for placebo and 43% for untreated controls).[51] This induction of corporal fibrosis is comparable to that seen in 16-week atherosclerotic, ischaemic rabbits.[18] The expression of TGF-β_1 mRNA and protein in human corpus cavernosum, as well as induction of collagen synthesis in cell culture and

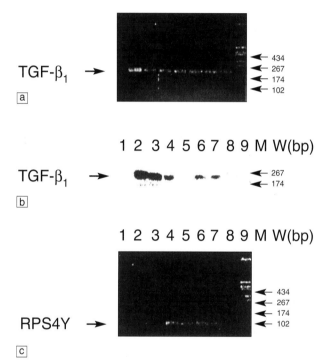

Figure 10.4. Detection of TGF-β_1 mRNA by RT–PCR from formalin-fixed, paraffin-embedded specimens from four representative patients. (a) RT–PCR for TGF-β_1: lane 1, minus RNA control; lane 2, WJ paraffin block (group III); lane 3, MA paraffin block (group II); lane 4, RK paraffin block (group I); lane 5, JF paraffin block (group II); lane 6, WJ HCCSMC (group III); lane 7, MA HCCSMC (group II); lane 8, WB HCCSMC (group I); lane 9, *Hae*III-digested pGEM3zf(-) molecular weight markers. (b) Southern blot hybridization for TGF-β_1. Note that lanes 2–8 show hybridization [lanes are the same as in (a)]. (c) RT–PCR for housekeeping gene RPS4Y [lanes are the same as in (a)]. A basal level of expression of TGF-β_1 mRNA was detected in all representative patient tissues (procured at the time of surgical harvest), independent of smooth muscle content. (From ref. 11 with permission.)

connective tissue in an animal model, suggests a role for TGF-β_1 in corpus cavernosum connective tissue synthesis.

The actions of TGF-β_1 are dependent on three different subclasses of cell surface receptors.[52] The high-affinity type I and type II receptors transmit signals via a threonine/serine kinase pathway, while the type III receptor is a low-affinity, non-signalling cell surface proteoglycan (betaglycan).[53] This low-affinity receptor may facilitate the concentration of TGF-β_1 on the cell surface and present it to the high-affinity receptors.[52,53] Human corpus cavernosum smooth muscle cells express all three types of TGF-β receptors, as determined by crosslinking to [125I]-TGF-β_1.[11,39] The type II receptor was expressed more than the type I, consistent with a smooth muscle phenotype.[54,55] The type III receptor was apparent as an abundant >200 kDa crosslinked complex.[11,39] The dose of TGF-β_1 that results in half-maximal stimulation of collagen synthesis in human corpus cavernosum smooth muscle cells[39] is consistent with the reported affinity constants for the high-affinity receptors (kD ~8pM).[52] While different roles have been ascribed to the type I (induction of extracellular matrix and connective tissue synthesis) and the type II (growth effects and dephosphorylation of the retinoblastoma gene product) receptors,[56,57] both high-affinity receptors are

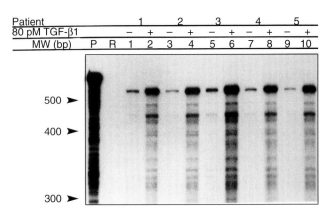

Figure 10.5. RNAase protection analysis of TGF-β_1 mRNA from human corpus cavernosum smooth muscle cells derived from five representative patients: P, undigested probe; C Control; T, treated with 80pM TGF-β_1. Patient 1: RO (group I); patient 2: WB (group I); patient 3: HH (group II); patient 4: LPC (group III); patient 5: WJ (group III). A basal level of expression of TGF-β_1 mRNA was detected in all representative patient tissues independent of corporal veno-occlusive function or smooth muscle content, implying that abnormal collagen regulation and not overexpression of TGF-β_1 is the basis for corporal fibrosis. (From ref. 11 with permission.)

required in a heterodimeric complex for effective signal transduction to occur.[52] Of particular interest, cells derived from each of the three groups in Figure 10.2 all

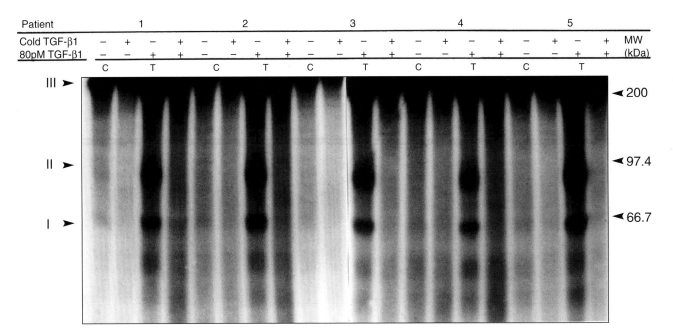

Figure 10.6. TGF-β receptors in HCCSMC. SDS-PAGE (sodium dodecyl sulphate–polyacrylamide gel electrophoresis; 7.5%) run under reducing conditions of [125I]-labelled TGF-β_1 crosslinked to HCCSMC derived from five representative patients with no addition (C), and 80pM TGF-β_1 (T). Competition with a 100 molar excess of TGF-β_1 is shown (cold TGF-β_1 +). Sample loads were normalized per cell number. Patient 1: RO (group I); patient 2: WB (group I); patient 3: HH (group II); patient 4: LPC (group III); patient 5: WJ (group III). (From ref. 11 with permission.)

express TGF-β_1 mRNA, and TGF-β_1 autoinduces its own mRNA (Fig. 10.5) as well as all three types of TGF-β receptors (Fig. 10.6).[11] Thus, TGF-β_1 can induce itself and its receptors, perpetuating a potential fibrotic response — consistent with what Border and Ruoslahti termed 'the dark side of fibrosis'.[42]

POSSIBLE ROLE OF PROSTAGLANDINS AND COLLAGEN SYNTHESIS

What is the potential 'off switch' for the TGF-β_1 response? It is known that prostaglandin E relaxes corporal smooth muscle strips in organ baths, while PGF2α, thromboxane A$_2$ and prostacyclin elicit corpus cavernosal contractions (reviewed in ref. 6). Interestingly, relaxation may not be the only effect of PGE: previous studies have shown that PGE$_1$[58,59] and PGE$_2$[60] suppress collagen synthesis in primary cultures of human lung fibroblasts; treatment with PGE$_1$ resulted in a 47% reduction in collagen biosynthesis with little or no effect on other secreted proteins.[58] TGF-β_1-induced collagen synthesis is suppressed by PGE$_2$.[60] It has been reported that cultured lung fibroblasts from patients suffering from idiopathic pulmonary fibrosis have a diminished capacity

to synthesize PGE$_2$.[61] The authors have reported that PGE$_1$, which elevates cAMP in human corpus cavernosum smooth muscle cells, suppresses TGF-β_1-induced collagen synthesis.[39] Human aortic smooth muscle cells actively synthesize PGE.[62] Both human[63] and rabbit[64] corpus cavernosum in organ culture synthesize PGE; in the rabbit,[64] low oxygen tension inhibits this production. Human corpus cavernosum smooth muscle cells also produce PGE and this process is inhibited by lower oxygen tensions.[50] Therefore, the interaction between PGE and TGF-β_1 pathways may be a key factor in determining connective tissue/smooth muscle balance in the corpus cavernosum. A working hypothesis accounting for the information above, and relating the molecular mechanisms within the trabecular smooth muscle cell, is presented in Figure 10.7.

ROLE OF NOCTURNAL PENILE TUMESCENCE IN MAINTAINING POTENCY

Prostaglandin synthesis,[50,64] as well as nitric oxide synthesis,[14] is dependent on oxygen tension. The corpus cavernosum is exceptional as a vascular bed in that oxygen tension changes, depending on whether the penis

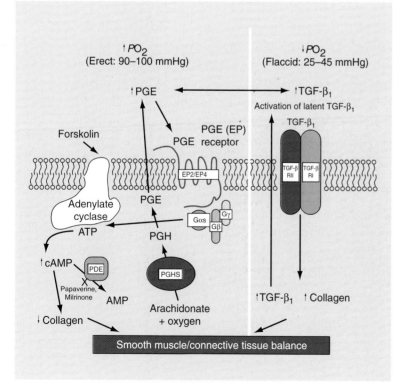

Figure 10.7. Working hypothesis of regulation of collagen synthesis in human corpus cavernosum smooth muscle. Left panel depicts activity of PGHS1/2 in the synthesis of PGE precursors and finally PGE at high oxygen tension associated with the erect state. PGE binds to specific EP2 and/or EP4 receptors which, through a Gs protein-coupled signal, activate adenylate cyclases to synthesize cAMP. cAMP inhibits collagen synthesis. Phosphodiesterases (PDE) terminate the cAMP signal by hydrolysis to AMP — a process inhibited by PDE inhibitors such as papaverine, or the type III PDE inhibitor, milrinone. Right panel depicts how, at low oxygen tension associated with the flaccid state, TGF-β_1 expression is increased and TGF-β_1 is secreted, activated and then binds to high-affinity type I and type II receptors (TGF-βRI and TGF-βRII). This increases TGF-β_1 expression and expression of TGF-β receptors, and induces collagen and connective tissue synthesis. Both pathways at high and low oxygen tension work together to yield the final connective tissue/smooth muscle balance, which may be altered in diseased states. (From ref. 5 with permission.)

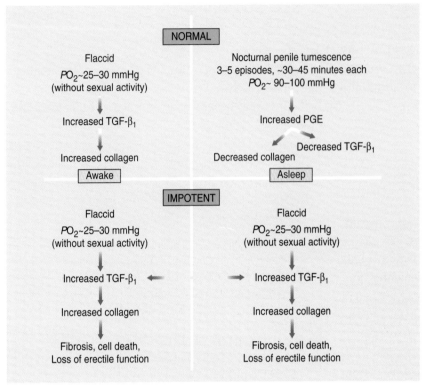

Figure 10.8. Hypothesized effects of circadian oxygenation on corpus cavernosal collagen regulation. Under normal circumstances, corpora in potent men are oxygenated by nocturnal penile tumescence every 18 hours per 24-hour period in the absence of sexual activity, resulting in synthesis of factors [for example prostaglandin E (PGE), which decreases collagen and transforming growth factor-β_1 (TGF-β_1) synthesis]. This circadian oxygenation is hypothesized to promote optimum connective tissue/corpus cavernosum smooth muscle ratios. In impotence, and in the absence of normal sexual functions, inhibitors of collagen synthesis are not produced and collagen accumulates, leading to fibrosis, cell death, and ultimate loss of erectile function. PO_2, oxygen partial pressure. (From ref. 11 with permission.)

is flaccid or erect.[14–17] A working hypothesis on the relationship of erection to maintenance of potency is shown in Figure 10.8. Oxygen tension consistent with flaccidity (20–40 mmHg) favours synthesis of TGF-β_1 in human corpus cavernosum smooth muscle cells in culture[50] and suppresses prostaglandin E synthesis both in cells in culture[50] and in rabbit corpus cavernosum in organ culture.[64] Men normally have three to five erectile episodes per night with a duration that typically ranges between 20 and 40 minutes for each of these episodes, during rapid eye movement sleep.[65] This 1–3.5 hours of erection exposes the corpus cavernosum to high (arterial) oxygen tension. This is in contrast to the awake state during which, unless engaged in sexual activity, the human corpus cavernosum would be continually exposed to low oxygen tension. In patients with insufficient penile blood flow, sleep-related erections are incomplete or absent.[10] It is possible that, during sleep-related erections, oxygenation of the corpora regulates the synthesis of cytokines, growth factors, and prostaglandins. These substances may control the structure of the trabecular wall through extracellular matrix remodelling.

What evidence supports such a hypothesis (Fig. 10.8)? Several examples that are consistent with this view are presented. Radical retropubic prostatectomy, even when performed by nerve-sparing techniques, often results in either a temporary or permanent loss of erectile

function.[66,67] Three recent reports of patients undergoing nerve-sparing radical prostatectomy showed that those patients on postoperative prophylactic PGE$_1$ were more likely to recover erectile function than those on placebo.[68–70] The cardiac glycoside digoxin has been proposed as an agent to treat unresolved veno-occlusive priapism, potentially by inhibiting Na$^+$/K$^+$ ATPase and causing trabecular smooth muscle contraction.[71] In healthy volunteers, subtherapeutic blood levels of digoxin resulted in altered nocturnal penile tumescence; this may explain the correlation of erectile dysfunction in males on cardiac medication.[13] It is curious that patients on high doses of non-steroidal anti-inflammatory drugs such as aspirin, paracetamol (acetaminophen) and ibuprofen, all of which inhibit prostaglandin synthase, report an incidence of sexual dysfunction (ulcers 18%; arthritis 15%).[13] Could this be due to lowered endogenous PGE production? Finally, while pyschogenic effects cannot be ruled out, up to 28% of patients in one study using intracorporal PGE$_1$ achieved improved spontaneous erections and less frequent need for intracorporal injections.[72] Taken together, the clinical prospective and retrospective studies, as well as the tissue culture studies, suggest a role for both PGE and TGF-β_1 in the maintenance of a functional trabecular smooth muscle/connective tissue ratio.

ACKNOWLEDGEMENTS

This work was supported in part by grants DK 49750, DK 39080, DK 40025, and DK 40487 from the National Institutes of Health, a grant from Upjohn-Pharmacia and a Dornier Fellowship from the American Foundation for Urologic Diseases (A.N.).

SUMMARY AND CONCLUSIONS

The study of the molecular pathology of erectile dysfunction has begun only within the last ten years. Basic research is still needed to address which other factors regulate a functional smooth muscle/connective tissue ratio. How is connective tissue turnover regulated in the corpus cavernosum? Can it be accelerated? What is the molecular basis of preservation of potency? Is nocturnal penile tumescence a key in maintaining potency, and how can it be enhanced? All these questions await discoveries. Clinically, there is a need for early and non-invasive diagnosis. Such testing has been recently suggested by an animal model.[18] If detected early, can treatment 'reverse' the condition? The issue of prophylaxis (e.g. preservation of potency) both after radical retropubic prostatectomy and with ageing, is one that awaits new studies. Finally, a working knowledge of the basic science of these processes promises to lead to rational design of effective therapeutic strategies for the treatment of vasculogenic impotence.

REFERENCES

1. Brindley G S. Cavernosal alpha-blockade: a new technique for investigating and treating erectile impotence. Br J Psych 1983; 143: 322–327
2. Virag, R. Intracavernous injection of papaverine for erectile failure. Lancet 1982; 2: 938
3. Impotence. National Institutes of Health Consensus Statement. JAMA 1993; 123: 23–27
4. Christ G J. The penis as a vascular organ. Urol Clin North Am 1995; 22: 727–745
5. Moreland R B. Is hypoxemia associated with penile fibrosis? Int J Impot Res: in press
6. Andersson K-E, Wagner G. Physiology of penile erection. Physiol Rev 1995; 75: 191–236
7. Porst H. The rationale for prostaglandin E1 in erectile failure: a survey of worldwide experience. J Urol 1996; 155: 802–815
8. Saenz de Tejada I, Moreland R B. Physiology of erection, pathophysiology of impotence and implications of PGE_1 in the control of collagen synthesis in the corpus cavernosum. In: Goldstein I, Lue T F (eds) The role of alprostadil in the diagnosis and treatment of erectile dysfunction. Princeton: Excerpta Medica, 1993: 1–33
9. Lerner S, Melman A, Christ G J. A review of erectile dysfunction: new insights and more questions. J Urol 1993; 149 (5 Part 2): 1246–1255
10. Krane R J, Goldstein I, Saenz de Tejada I. Impotence. Medical progress. N Engl J Med 1989; 321: 1648–1659
11. Nehra A, Goldstein I, Pabby A et al. Mechanisms of venous leakage: a prospective clinicopathological correlation of corporeal function and structure. J Urol 1996; 156: 1320–1329
12. Benet A E, Melman A. The epidemiology of erectile dysfunction. Urol Clin North Am 1995; 22: 699–709
13. Feldman H A, Goldstein I, Hatzichristou D G et al. Impotence and its medical and pyschosocial correlates: results of the Massachusetts Male Aging Study. J Urol 1994; 151: 54–61
14. Kim N, Vardi Y, Padma-Nathan H et al. Oxygen tension regulates the nitric oxide pathway: physiological role in penile erection. J Clin Invest 1993; 91: 437–443
15. Sattar A A, Salpigides G, Vanderhaeghen J J et al. Cavernous oxygen tension and smooth muscle fibers: relation and function. J Urol 1995; 154: 1736–1739
16. Brown S, Seftel A D, Strohl K et al. Cavernosal oxygen tension and corporal ischemia. J Urol 1997; 157: 179 (abstr 696)
17. Rosselló-Barbará M, Santiseban M. Corpus cavernosum fibrosis treated with oxygenated and pressurized arterial blood: encouraging preliminary results. New electronic vacuum plus treatment. J Urol 1997; 157: 202 (abstr 788)
18. Nehra A, Azadzoi K, Pabby A et al. The role of penile tissue mechanical parameters in the relationship between trabecular histology and hemodynamic function in vasculogenic impotence. J Urol 1996; 155: 465A (abstr 617)
19. Saenz de Tejada I, Moroukian P, Tessier J et al. The trabecular smooth muscle modulates the capacitor function of the penis. Studies on a rabbit model. Am J Physiol 1991; 250 (Heart Cir Physiol 29): H1590–H1595
20. Conti G, Virag R. Human penile erection and organic impotence: normal histology and histopathology. Urol Int 1989; 44: 303–308
21. Mersdorf A, Goldsmith P C, Diederichs W et al. Ultrastructural changes in impotent penile tissue: a comparison of 65 patients. J Urol 1991; 145: 749–758
22. Jevtich M, Khawand N Y, Vidic B. Clinical significance of ultrastructural findings in the corpus cavernosum of normal and impotent men. J Urol 1990; 143: 289–293
23. Wespes E, Goes P M, Schiffmann S et al. Computerized analysis of smooth muscle fibers in potent and impotent patients. J Urol 1991; 146: 1015–1017
24. Luangkhot R, Rutchik S, Agarwal V et al. Collagen alterations in the corpus cavernosum of men with sexual dysfunction. J Urol 1992; 148: 467–471

25. Wespes E, de Goes P M, Sattar A A, Schulman C. Objective criteria in the long-term evaluation of penile venous surgery. J Urol 1994; 152: 888–895

26. Hatzichristou D G, Saenz de Tejada I, Kupferman S et al. In vivo assessment of trabecular smooth muscle tone, its application in pharmacocavernosometry and analysis of intracavernosal pressure determinants. J Urol 1995; 153: 1126–1131

27. Pease D C, Paule W J. Electron microscopy of elastic arteries. The thoracic aorta of the rat. J Ultrastruct Res 1960; 3: 469–483

28. Wissler R H. The arterial medial cell, smooth muscle or multifunctional mesenchyme? J Atherosclerosis Res 1968; 8: 201–213

29. Botney M D, Liptay M J, Kaiser L R et al. Active collagen synthesis by pulmonary arteries in human primary pulmonary hypertension. Am J Pathol 1993; 143: 121–129

30. Gerrity R G, Adams E P, Cliff W J. The aortic tunica media of the developing rat. II. Incorporation by medial cells of ^{3}H-proline into collagen and elastin: autoradiographic and chemical studies. Lab Invest 1975; 32: 601–609

31. Gerrity R G, Cliff W J. The aortic tunica media of the developing rat. I. Quantitative stereological and biochemical analysis. Lab Invest 1975; 32: 585–601

32. Karrer H E. An electron microscope study of the aorta in young and adult mice. J Ultrastruc Res 1961; 5: 1–27

33. Jarmolych J, Daoud A S, Landau J et al. Aortic media explants, cell proliferation, and production of mucopolysaccharides, collagen, and elastic tissue. Exp Mol Pathol 1968; 9: 171–188

34. Stepp M A, Kindy M S, Franzblau C, Sonenshein G E. Complex regulation of collagen gene expression in cultured bovine aortic smooth muscle cells. J Biol Chem 1986; 261: 6542–6547

35. Ang D H, Tachas G, Campbell J H et al. Collagen synthesis by cultured rabbit aortic smooth-muscle cells. Alteration with phenotype. Biochem J 1990; 265: 461–469

36. Brown K E, Lawrence R, Sonenshein G E. Concerted modulation of $\alpha1(XI)$ and $\alpha2(V)$ collagen mRNAs in bovine vascular smooth muscle cells. J Biol Chem 1991; 266: 23268–23273

37. Lawrence R, Hartmann D J, Sonenshein G E. Transforming growth factor β stimulates type V collagen expression in bovine vascular smooth muscle cells. J Biol Chem 1994; 269: 9603–9609

38. Prockop D J, Kivirikko K I. Collagens: molecular biology, diseases, and potentials for therapy. Ann Rev Biochem 1995; 64: 403–434

39. Moreland R B, Traish A M, McMillin M A et al. PGE$_1$ suppresses the induction of collagen synthesis by transforming growth factor-$\beta1$ in human corpus cavernosum smooth muscle. J Urol 1995; 153: 826–834

40. Raviv G, Kiss R, Vanegas J P et al. Objective measurement of the different collagen types in the corpus cavernosum of potent and impotent men: an immunohistochemical staining with computerized-image analysis. World J Urol 1997; 15: 50–55

41. Woessner J F. Matrix metalloproteinases and their inhibitors in connective tissue remodeling. FASEB J 1991; 5: 2145–2154

42. Border W A, Ruoslahti E. Transforming growth factor-β in disease: the dark side of tissue repair. J Clin Inv 1992; 90: 1–7

43. Border W A, Noble N A. Transforming growth factor β in tissue fibrosis. N Engl J Med 1994; 331: 1286–1291

44. Majack R A. Beta-type transforming growth factor specifies organizational behavior in vascular smooth muscle cell cultures. J Cell Biol 1987; 105: 465–471

45. Nugent M A, Newman M J. Inhibition of normal rat kidney cell growth by transforming growth factor-$\beta1$ is mediated by collagen. J Biol Chem 1989; 264: 18069–18077

46. Raghow R, Irush P, Kang A H. Coordinate regulation of transforming growth factor β gene expression and cell proliferation in hamster lungs undergoing bleomycin-induced pulmonary fibrosis. J Clin Invest 1989; 84: 1836–1842

47. Castilla A, Prieto J, Fausto N. Transforming growth factor $\beta1$ and α in chronic liver disease. Effects of interferon alpha therapy. N Engl J Med 1991; 324: 933–940

48. Merrilees M J, Beaumont B. Structural heterogeneity of the diffuse intimal thickening and correlation with distribution of TGF-β_1. J Vasc Res 1993; 30: 293–302

49. Nikol S, Isner J M, Pickering J G et al. Expression of transforming growth factor-$\beta1$ is increased in human vascular restenosis lesions. J Clin Invest 1992; 90: 1582–1592

50. Moreland R B, Nehra A, Watkins M et al. Oxygen tension modulates TGF-β_1-expression and PGE production in human corpus cavernosum smooth muscle cells. Mol Urol 1998; 2: 41–47

51. Nehra A, Nugent M, Pabby A et al. An in vivo model for transforming growth factor-$\beta1$ induced corporal fibrosis: implications for penile ischemia-associated fibrosis. J Urol 1996; 155: 622A (abstr 1243)

52. Massague J, Attisano L, Wrana J L. The TGF-β family and its composite receptors. Trends Cell Biol 1994; 4: 172–178

53. Lopez-Casillas F, Wrana J L, Massague J. Betaglycan presents ligand to the signaling receptor. Cell 1993; 73: 1435–1444

54. Goodman L V, Majack R A. Vascular smooth muscle cells express distinct transforming growth factor-β receptor phenotypes as a function of cell density. J Biol Chem 1989; 264: 5241–5244

55. Massague J, Like B. Cellular receptors for type β transforming growth factor. Ligand binding and affinity labeling of human and rodent cell lines. J Biol Chem 1985; 260: 2636–2645

56. Chen R H, Ebner R, Derynck R. Inactivation of the type II receptor reveals two receptor pathways for the diverse TGF-β activities. Science 1993; 260: 1335–1338

57. Brand T, Schneider M D. Inactive type II and type I receptors for TGF-β are dominant inhibitors of TGF-β-dependent transcription. J Biol Chem 1995; 270: 8274–8284

58. Baum B J, Moss J, Bruel S D, Crystal R G. Association in normal human fibroblasts of elevated levels of adenosine 3':5'-monophosphate with a selective decrease in collagen production. J Biol Chem 1978; 253: 3391–3394

59. Baum B J, Moss J, Bruel S D et al. Effect of cyclic AMP on the intracellular degradation of newly synthesized collagen. J Biol Chem 1980; 255: 2843–2847

60. Fine A, Poliks C F, Donahue L P et al. The differential effect of prostaglandin E2 on transforming growth factor-β and insulin-induced collagen formation in lung fibroblasts. J Biol Chem 1989; 264: 16988–16991

61. Wilborn J, Croffrod L J, Burdick M D et al. Cultured lung fibroblasts isolated from patients with idiopathic pulmonary fibrosis have a diminished capacity to synthesize prostaglandin E2 and to express cyclo-oxygenase-2. J Clin Inv 1995; 95: 1861–1868

62. Alexander R W, Gimbrone M A. Stimulation of prostaglandin E synthesis in human umbilical vein smooth muscle cells. Proc Natl Acad Sci, USA 1976; 73: 1617–1620

63. Roy A C, Tan S M, Kottegoda S R, Ratnam S S. Ability of human corpus cavernosum to generate prostaglandins and thromboxanes in vitro. IRCS Med Sci 1984; 12: 608

64. Daley J T, Brown M L, Watkins M T et al. Prostanoid production in rabbit corpus cavernosum I. Regulation by oxygen tension. J Urol 1996; 155: 1482–1487

65. Fischer C, Gross J, Zuch J. Cycle of penile erections synchronous with dreaming (REM) sleep: preliminary report. Arch Gen Psychiatry 1965; 12: 29–45

66. Walsh P C, Donker P J. Impotence following radical prostatectomy: insight into etiology and prevention. J Urol 1982; 128: 492–503

67. Eggleston J C, Walsh PC. Radical prostatectomy with preservation of sexual function: pathologic findings in the first 100 cases. J Urol 1985; 133: 1146–1157

68. Montorsi F, Guazzoni G, Strambi F et al. Intracavernosal alprostadil after nerve sparing radical prostatectomy: one year follow-up objective analysis of successes and failures in recovering spontaneous erectile activity. J Urol 1997; 157: 364 (abstr 1423)

69. Padma-Nathan H, Linet O, Sheu W P. The impact on return of spontaneous erections of short term alprostadil therapy post nerve sparing radical prostatectomy. J Urol 1997; 157: 363 (abstr 1422)

70. Costabile R A, Govier F E, Ferrigni R G et al. Efficacy and safety of transurethral alprostadil in patients with erectile dysfunction following radical prostatectomy. J Urol 1997; 157: 364 (abstr 1424)

71. Gupta S, Daley J, Pabby A et al. A new mechanism for digoxin-associated impotence: in vitro and in vivo study. J Urol 1996; 155: 621A (abstr 1239)

72. Basile G, Goldstein J, Malkevich D et al. Can self-injection therapy "cure" impotence? In: Goldstein I, Lue T F (eds) The role of alprostadil in the diagnosis and treatment of erectile dysfunction. Princeton, NJ: Excerpta Medica, 1993: 109–116

Chapter 11

Nitric oxide as a neurotransmitter in the corpus cavernosum

A. M. Naylor

■ INTRODUCTION

Nitric oxide (NO) is a labile gas that is synthesized throughout the nervous system, immune system and vascular system, and which is involved in mediating a large number of varied biological actions.[1] Thus, NO is a key component of a signal transduction process with roles as a vasodilator, antiplatelet aggregator, neurotransmitter and cytotoxic agent.[1] In addition to the many biological functions attributed to NO, much evidence exists to suggest that NO acts as a neurotransmitter involved in the autonomic control of the lower urinary tract,[2] especially the corpus cavernosum. The purpose of this review is to describe evidence implicating NO as a transmitter in the corpus cavernosum and to postulate that NO is the key endogenous mediator of penile erection in the peripheral nervous system.

■ NEUROTRANSMITTER ROLE FOR NITRIC OXIDE IN THE CORPUS CAVERNOSUM

The identity of non-adrenergic, non-cholinergic (NANC) neurotransmitters in autonomic nerves and their function have been the subject of much debate over the years. Purines, neuropeptides and, more recently, NO have all been implicated in various tissues throughout the autonomic nervous system. However, in the corpus cavernosum, NO appears to fulfil the role of the NANC inhibitory neurotransmitter mediating relaxation of the corpus cavernosum.

Synthesis of nitric oxide

Nitric oxide is synthesized from L-arginine by a reaction catalysed by nitric oxide synthase (NOS), resulting in the formation of citrulline as a by-product[3] (Fig. 11.1). Three distinct forms of NOS derived from separate gene products have been identified.[4–7] These isoforms have been purified, cloned and designated as neuronal (nNOS), endothelial (eNOS) or inducible (iNOS). The neuronal form of the enzyme, nNOS, has been demonstrated throughout the autonomic nervous system including the penis.[8] Thus, NOS immunoreactivity has been localized to discrete neuronal endings including the pelvic plexus, cavernous nerves and nerve endings in the corpus cavernosum, as well as associated vasculature.[8] Immunohistochemical staining for nNOS and eNOS in human corpus cavernosum indicates differential localization: staining with nNOS and eNOS antibodies localized nNOS to nerves and eNOS to the endothelium and smooth muscle.[9] Both nNOS and eNOS are believed to play a role in corpus cavernosum smooth muscle relaxation (see later) but the presence of (and function of) iNOS in this process is less understood. Recently, iNOS has been localized to the endothelial surface of arteries and smooth muscle of the corporal smooth muscle in rats,[10] suggesting that all three isoforms may play a role in the erectile process. In addition, novel nNOS isoforms have been identified in tissues from the lower urinary tract, including the corpus cavernosum.[11] The high NOS activity in the penis has been shown by immunoblotting to be due to nNOS,[12] suggesting that the neuronal isoform is the most abundant NOS responsible for corpus cavernosum smooth muscle relaxation and erection.[13]

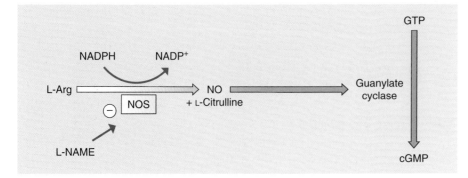

Figure 11.1. Calcium influx triggers the activation of nitric oxide synthase (NOS), initiating the conversion of L-arginine (L-Arg) to L-citrulline and nitric oxide (NO). NO diffuses to adjacent cells and activates soluble guanylate cyclase. Guanylate cyclase converts GTP to cGMP, a second messenger that initiates smooth muscle relaxation. L-NAME, L-nitro-arginine methyl ester.

Deficiencies in the activity of NOS could provide a pathological mechanism to explain some forms of erectile dysfunction. Indeed, animal models where a deficiency in NOS have been demonstrated include those for diabetes mellitus,[14] ageing,[15] cardiovascular risk factors[16] and low androgens,[17,18] all of which have been associated with erectile dysfunction. However, a direct link between deficiencies in NOS and specific types of erectile dysfunction in man remains to be demonstrated.

NO: functional actions on corpus cavernosum

The distribution of NOS in nerves, endothelium and smooth muscle of the corpus cavernosum suggests that NO plays a key role in modulating the tone of musculature in the penis. The functional effects of NO on corpus cavernosum smooth muscle are described below. For penile tumescence to occur, the smooth muscle of the corpus cavernosum and related arterioles relax, enabling increased blood flow into the trabecular spaces of the corpus cavernosum and leading to erection. The regulatory mechanisms governing corporal smooth muscle tone include adrenergic and nitrergic mechanisms, among others. The role of endogenous noradrenaline released from sympathetic terminals appears to be the maintenance of cavernosal and arterial tone in such a way that blood flow is low and tumescence does not occur.[19] This section describes the functional role of NO in relaxing smooth muscle of the corpus cavernosum and presents evidence suggesting that NO is the NANC transmitter responsible for mediating erection.

During sexual stimulation, NO is synthesized and released from NANC nerve terminals in the corpus cavernosum and also from endothelial cells (Fig. 11.2). Both nNOS and eNOS are believed to be important sources of NO, as relaxation responses[20] and erectile responses[21] were evident following removal or destruction of the endothelium. Nitric oxide activates soluble guanylate

cyclase, which converts 5-guanosine triphosphate (GTP) to 3,5 cyclic guanosine monophosphate (cGMP), which acts as an intracellular second-messenger molecule to elicit corpus cavernosum smooth muscle relaxation and erection.[22]

The pivotal role of NO in the erectile process can be demonstrated using animal and human tissue in vitro and animal models in vivo. Electrical field stimulation (EFS) or muscarinic receptor stimulation induces rapid relaxation responses in pre-contracted human corpus cavernosum.[19,20] The relaxant effects of acetylcholine are dependent on the presence of an intact endothelium and are secondary to release of NO. The relaxation responses induced by EFS persist in the presence of atropine and guanethidine and are blocked by tetrodotoxin, suggesting that NANC neurotransmission is involved. Moreover, inhibition of NOS completely blocked human corpus cavernosum smooth muscle relaxation in response to EFS

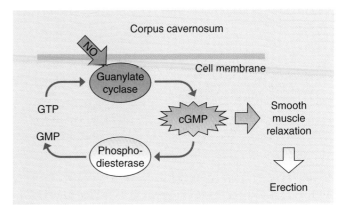

Figure 11.2. During sexual stimulation, nitric oxide (NO) is released from nerve endings and endothelial cells in the corpus cavernosum. NO stimulates the cytosolic enzyme guanylate cyclase to produce cGMP, resulting in a decrease in intracellular calcium and smooth muscle relaxation. The cGMP is metabolized by cyclic nucleotide phophodiesterases that terminate the biological activity of cGMP (see text for further details).

(Fig. 11.3).[22–26] The inhibition of the relaxant response to EFS by NOS inhibitors such as Nω-nitro-L-arginine (L-NOArg) can be reversed by the addition of increased amounts of the precursor to NO, L-arginine (not D-arginine) (Fig. 11.3), supporting the key neurotransmitter role of NO. Animal models where erectile responses are measured in vivo also identify the NO/cGMP pathway as a key component of the erectile process. Electrical stimulation of nerves to the corpus cavernosum of the rat[12] and rabbit[27] produced erectile responses. These effects were blocked by inhibition of NOS and reversed by exogenous administration of substrates of NO (L-arginine). In the anaesthetized dog, further evidence supports the neurotransmitter role for NO and activation of the cGMP system in mediating erection following stimulation of the pelvic nerves.[21] Thus, intracavernosal administration of an NOS inhibitor or an inhibitor of guanylate cyclase (methylene blue) prevented neurally mediated tumescence. Overall, these data suggest that activation of the NO/cGMP system in the corpus cavernosum plays a key, if not pivotal, role in initiating physiological responses responsible for penile erection.

Although there is substantial evidence implicating neuronally derived NO as the key neurotransmitter

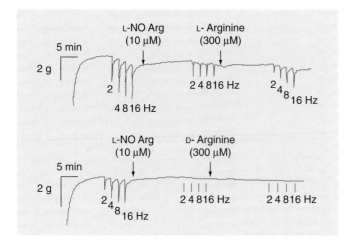

Figure 11.3. Human corpus cavernosum strips pre-contracted with phenylephrine in the presence of guanethidine and atropine. Electrical field stimulation (EFS) induced frequency-dependent relaxation responses that were inhibited by the NOS inhibitor Nω-nitro-L-arginine (L-NOArg). Addition of the precursor for NO synthesis, L-arginine (but not D-arginine), reversed the inhibitory response observed following L-NOArg confirming the key role of NO as an inhibitory NANC transmitter in the human corpus cavernosum. (From ref. 35 with permission.)

mediating corporal smooth muscle relaxation and, therefore, erection, some data do not fit within this hypothesis. Transgenic mice lacking nNOS are able to achieve erections and are fertile,[28] suggesting that, in these genetically altered animals, compensatory mechanisms have developed to ensure that the erectile process can occur in the absence of neuronally derived NO. Such evidence questions the hypothesis that neuronal NO is the key neurotransmitter mediating erection. However, further investigation of these animals revealed that these nNOS-deficient mice have a much greater amount of eNOS present in the penile vasculature and sinusoidal epithelium within the corpus cavernosum.[29] The erectile mechanisms in nNOS-deficient mice still involve NO, as they are prevented by NOS inhibitors such as L-nitro-arginine methyl ester (L-NAME) and reversed by L-arginine.[29] These data show that a compensatory mechanism of erection has emerged to restore erectile function in nNOS-deficient mice but that the same mediator (i.e. NO) is responsible, albeit from a different gene product (eNOS).

Nitric oxide is a key physiological mediator of penile erection. Activation of NANC nerves to the corpus cavernosum by sexual stimulation results in NO release, activation of guanylate cyclase and cGMP production leading to a series of downstream events culminating in relaxation of the corpus cavernosum. Other mediators may be important in modulating the actions of NO and may contribute to the physiological mechanisms underlying erection (see ref. 30). However, their physiological role in relation to NO is likely to be minor and remains to be proven.

Inactivation of the biological actions of nitric oxide in the corpus cavernosum

The biological actions of cGMP in the corpus cavernosum, elevated as a consequence of NO activation of guanylate cyclase, are terminated by cyclic nucleotide phosphodiesterase enzymes (PDEs). Currently, at least seven families of PDE can be characterized on the basis of substrate specificity, inhibitor profile and sensitivity to calmodulin[31] (Table 11.1). In the human corpus cavernosum, the presence of PDEs 2, 3 and 5 has been demonstrated,[32] together with that of PDE4.[33] The major cGMP metabolizing PDE in the human corpus cavernosum is cGMP-specific PDE5.[32] Agents that inhibit the breakdown of cGMP by inhibiting PDE5 have the ability to augment the normal physiological pathway mediating

Table 11.1. Classification of PDE isoenzymes by substrate specificity, inhibitor profile and sensitivity to calmodulin

Isoenzyme family	Substrate specificity	Effect of cGMP on cAMP hydrolysis	Effect of calcium calmodulin	Standard inhibitor
PDE1	cAMP/cGMP	–	Stimulation	Zaprinast
PDE2	cAMP/cGMP	Stimulation	No effect	–
PDE3	cAMP	Inhibition	No effect	Milrinone
PDE4	cAMP	No effect	No effect	Rolipram
PDE5	cGMP	–	No effect	Zaprinast, sildenafil
PDE6	cGMP	–	No effect	–
PDE7	cAMP	–	–	–

erection by increasing the amount of cGMP available for relaxing the corpus cavernosum (Fig. 11.2). Sildenafil, a potent and selective PDE5 inhibitor (Table 11.2),[34] enhanced the relaxation responses of the human corpus cavernosum induced by EFS, by acting in this way.[35] Animal models of penile erection can also be used to demonstrate the facilitatory role of PDE5 inhibitors on erectile function following NO-mediated relaxation of the corpus cavernosum. Thus, sildenafil[36] and zaprinast[21]

augment NO/cGMP-driven tumescence in the anaesthetized dog. Inhibition of PDE5 by sildenafil underlies the beneficial effects on erectile function observed in clinical trials in patients with erectile disorders (Chapter 26).[32,37]

Interactions of nitric oxide with other transmitters in the corpus cavernosum

In addition to NO, a large number of substances have been implicated as transmitters responsible for mediating relaxation of the corpus cavernosum and therefore penile erection (reviewed in ref. 30). Along with neural release of NO, several other neurotransmitters influence corporal tone by releasing NO from the endothelium. Bradykinin[38] and acetylcholine[39] function in this way, and VIP has been co-localized with NOS. Evidence supporting a significant role for these and other factors in corpus cavernosal smooth muscle relaxation and tumescence is required before a role in the physiology of penile erection can be attributed to agents other than NO. However, it is possible that some of these putative neurotransmitters may function alongside NO in the complex control of corporal smooth muscle tone. Indeed, a greater understanding of the pathological changes that occur in the corpus cavernosum and that contribute to erectile dysfunction may aid understanding of how the neural control of corporal smooth muscle tone changes under pathophysiological conditions.

Table 11.2. Selectivity of sildenafil for PDE5 over other known PDEs from human corpus cavernosum (PDEs 2 and 3) and other known PDEs

Compound	Sildenafil
PDE1	75
PDE2	> 7500
PDE3	4300
PDE4	1800
PDE5	1
PDE6	10

Potency of sildenafil for PDE5 (= IC_{50}) 3.9 nM. PDEs 2, 3 and 5 were isolated from corpus cavernosum, PDE1 from cardiac ventricle, PDE4 from skeletal muscle and PDE6 from bovine retina. (Adapted from ref. 34 with permission.)

SUMMARY AND CONCLUSIONS

There is a large body of evidence implicating NO as a neurotransmitter in the corpus cavernosum responsible for mediating penile erection. By activating guanylate cyclase, with resultant elevation of cGMP, NO results in a lowering of intracellular calcium and smooth muscle relaxation. nNOS has been located in neurons innervating the corpus cavernosum and related vasculature, suggesting that NO is the postganglionic neurotransmitter mediating relaxation of the corporal smooth muscle. Functional evaluation of these relaxation responses strongly supports a key role for NO in this process. Indeed, inhibition of NOS completely blocked the relaxation of the corpus cavernosum induced by EFS in vitro and prevented tumescence in vivo. Furthermore, preventing the breakdown of cGMP, the second-messenger effector of corporal smooth muscle relaxation, augmented the erectile process in patients with erectile dysfunction. Thus, in response to sexual stimulation, NO plays a pivotal neurotransmitter role in the physiological process whereby the corpus cavernosum relaxes and penile erection results. The physiological role, if any, of other neurotransmitters in the erectile process remains to be proven, although it is possible that other modulators may act together with NO in the process. Finally, whether an abnormality in NOS in the corpus cavernosum is responsible for certain forms of erectile dysfunction remains to be demonstrated conclusively.

REFERENCES

1. Moncada S, Palmer R M J, Higgs E A. Nitric oxide: physiology, pathophysiology, and pharmacology. Pharm Rev 1991; 43: 109–142

2. Burnett A L. Nitric oxide control of lower genitourinary tract functions: a review. Urology 1995; 45: 1071–1083

3. Palmer R M, Ferrige A G, Moncada S. Nitric oxide release accounts for the biological activity of endothelium-derived relaxing factor. Nature 1987; 327: 524–526

4. Bredt D S, Hwang P M, Glatt C E et al. Cloned and expressed nitric oxide synthase structurally resembles cytochrome P-450 reductase. Nature 1991; 351: 714–718

5. Lamas S, Marsden P A, Li G K et al. Endothelial nitric oxide synthase: molecular cloning and characterization of a distinct constitutive enzyme isoform. Proc Natl Acad Sci USA 1992; 89: 6348–6352

6. Lowenstein C J, Glatt C S, Bredt D S, Snyder S H. Cloned and expressed macrophage nitric-oxide synthase contrasts with the brain enzyme. Proc Natl Acad Sci USA 1992; 89: 6711–6715

7. Sessa W C, Harrison J K, Barber C M et al. Molecular cloning and expression of a cDNA encoding endothelial cell nitric oxide. J Biol Chem 1992; 267: 15274–15276

8. Burnett A L, Tillman S L, Chang T S K et al. Immunohistochemical localization of nitric oxide synthase in the autonomic innervation of the human penis. J Urol 1993; 150: 73–76

9. Seftel A D, Ganz M B, Block C et al. Activation of endothelial nitric oxide synthase in endothelium and corporal smooth muscle of human corpus cavernosum mediates relaxation via an NO–K conductance pathway. J Urol 1996; 155: 678A

10. Moceanu M C, Brannigan R E, McKenna K E et al. Localisation of nitric oxide synthase I, II and III in rat penile tissue. J Urol 1996; 155: 620A

11. Magee T, Fuentes A M, Garban H et al. Cloning of novel neuronal nitric oxide synthase expressed in penis and lower urinary tract. Biochem Biophys Res Commun 1996; 226: 145–151

12. Burnett A L, Lowenstein C J, Bredt D S et al. Nitric oxide: a physiologic mediator of penile erection. Science 1992; 257: 401–403

13. Burnett A L. Nitric oxide control of lower genitourinary tract functions: a review. Urology 1995; 45: 1071–1083

14. Vernet D, Cai L, Garban H et al. Reduction of penile nitric oxide synthase in diabetic BB/WORdp (type I) and BBZ/WORdp (type II) rats with erectile dysfunction. Endocrinology 1995; 136: 5709–5717

15. Garban H, Vernet D, Freedman A et al. Effect of aging on nitric oxide-mediated penile erection in rats. Am J Physiol 1995; 268: H467–H475

16. Xie Y, Garban H, Ng C et al. Effect of long-term passive smoking on erectile function and penile nitric oxide synthase in the rat. J Urol 1997; 157: 1121–1126

17. Chamness S L, Ricker D D, Crone J K et al. The effect of androgen on nitric oxide synthase in the male reproductive tract of the rat. Fertil Steril 1995; 63: 1101–1107

18. Garban H, Marquez D, Cai L et al. Restoration of normal adult penile erectile response in aged rats by long-term treatment with androgens. Biol Reprod 1995; 53: 1365–1372

19. Hedlund H, Andersson K E. Comparison of the responses to drugs acting on adrenoceptors and muscarinic receptors in isolated corpus cavernosum and cavernous artery. J Auton Pharmacol 1985; 5: 81–88

20. Azadzoi K M, Kim N, Brown M L et al Endothelium derived nitric oxide and cycloxygenase products modulate corpus cavernosum smooth muscle tone. J Urol 1992; 147: 220–225

21. Trigo-Rocha F, Hsu G L, Donatucci C F, Lue T F. The role of cyclic adenosine monophosphate, cyclic guanosine monophosphate, endothelium and nonadrenergic, noncholinergic neurotransmission in canine penile erection. J Urol 1993; 149: 872–877

22. Ignarro L J, Bush P A, Buga G M et al. Nitric oxide and cyclic GMP formation upon electrical field stimulation causes relaxation of corpus cavernosal smooth muscle. Biochem Biophys Res Commun 1990; 170: 843–850

23. Holmquist F, Hedlund H, Andersson K E. L-NG-nitro arginine inhibits non-adrenergic, non-cholinergic relaxation of human isolated corpus cavernosum. Acta Physiol Scand 1991; 141: 441–442

24. Pickard R S, Powell P H, Zar M A. The effect of inhibitors of nitric oxide biosynthesis and cyclic GMP formation on nerve evoked relaxation of human cavernosal smooth muscle. Br J Pharmacol 1991; 104: 755–759

25. Rajfer J, Aronson W J, Bush P A et al. Nitric oxide as a mediator of the corpus cavernosum in response to non cholinergic, non adrenergic neurotransmission. New Engl J Med 1992; 326: 90–94

26. Holmquist F, Andersson K E, Hedlund H. Characterisation of inhibitory neurotransmission in the isolated corpus cavernosum from rabbit and man. J Physiol 1992; 449: 295–311

27. Holmquist F, Stief C G, Jonas U, Andersson K E. Effects of the nitric oxide synthase inhibitor NG-nitro-L-arginine on the erectile response to cavernous nerve stimulation in the rabbit. Acta Physiol Scand 1991; 143: 299–304

28. Huang P L, Dawson T M, Bredt D S et al. Targeted disruption of the neuronal nitric oxide synthase gene. Cell 1993; 75: 1273–1286

29. Burnett A L, Nelson R J, Calvin D C et al. Nitric oxide dependent penile erection in mice lacking neuronal nitric oxide synthase. Mol Med 1996; 2: 288–296

30. Andersson K E, Wagner G. Physiology of penile erection. Physiol Rev 1995; 75: 191–236

31. Beavo J A, Conti M, Heaslip R J. Multiple cyclic nucleotide phosphodiesterases. Mol Pharm 1994; 46: 399–405

32. Boolell M, Allen M J, Ballard S A et al. Sildenafil: an orally active type 5 cyclic GMP specific phosphodiesterase inhibitor for the treatment of penile erectile dysfunction. Int J Impot Res 1996; 8: 47–52

33. Stief C G. Phosphodiesterase isoenzyme of the human cavernous tissue and its functional significance. Akt Urol 1995; 26: 22–24

34. Naylor A M, Ballard S A, Gingell J C et al. Sildenafil (Viagra): an inhibitor of cyclic GMP-dependent specific phosphodiesterase type 5 for the treatment of male erectile dysfunction. Eur Urol 1996; 30(suppl2): 567

35. Ballard S A, Gingell J C, Tang K et al. Effects of sildenafil on the relaxation of human corpus cavernosum tissue in vitro and on the activities of cyclic nucleotide phosphodiesterase isozymes. J Urol 1998; 159: 2164–2171

36. Carter A J, Ballard S A, Naylor A M. Effect of the selective phosphodiesterase type 5 inhibitor sildenafil on erectile function in the anaesthetised dog. J Urol 1997; 157: 1398

37. Buvat J, Gingell C J, Jardin A et al. Sildenafil (Viagra™), an oral treatment for erectile dysfunction: a 1 year open-label, extension study. J Urol 1997; 157: 793

38. Kimoto Y, Kessler R, Constantinou C E. Endothelium dependent relaxation of human corpus cavernosum by bradykinin. J Urol 1990; 144: 1015–1017

39. Knispel H, Goessl C, Beckmann R. Basal and acetylcholine stimulated nitric oxide formation mediates relaxation of rabbit cavernous smooth muscle. J Urol 1991; 146: 1429–1433

Chapter 12

Receptor pharmacology related to erectile dysfunction

K. -E. Andersson and M. G. Wyllie

■ INTRODUCTION

Penile erection requires a change of tone of corpus cavernosum and penile vascular smooth muscle cells from a state of contraction to relaxation. The required degree of relaxation could be achieved either by elimination of the contractant influences or by enhancement of the effects of relaxant factors. In all probability, both elimination of contractant and enhancement of relaxant factors are required.[1] It has been suggested that the aetiology of erectile dysfunction in some patients may be related to heightened corporal smooth muscle tone and/or impaired smooth muscle relaxation,[2] and experimental evidence supporting this has been presented by several investigators.[3,4] Fewer nitric oxide (NO)-containing neurons and less expression of NO synthase (NOS) mRNA were found in the corpora cavernosa of old compared with young rats, whereas the expression of alpha-1-adrenoceptor mRNA was unchanged. However, in human cavernosal tissue, ageing and disease produce an increase in alpha-mediated tone.[5] Even a subtle alteration in the balance between factors contributing to corporal relaxation (e.g. NO) and favouring contraction (e.g. alpha-1-adrenoceptors) may result in erectile dysfunction.

Many endogenous factors may be involved in the maintenance of tone and in relaxation of penile smooth muscles (Tables 12.1, 12.2), and their potential roles in penile physiology and pathophysiology have been the subject of several recent reviews.[1,6–12] However, new information is accumulating and, to add to our knowledge, recent results on the effects and possible importance of some contractant and relaxant factors acting through membrane receptors in penile tissues are briefly reviewed here. NO and NO-dependent mechanisms are not

Table 12.1. Agents that may increase tone in penile smooth muscle

- Noradrenaline
- Endothelins
- Prostanoids
- Angiotensin
- Vasopressin

Table 12.2. Agents that may relax penile smooth muscle

- Acetylcholine
- Nitric oxide
- Vasoactive intestinal peptide and related peptides
- Calcitonin gene-related peptide
- Prostaglandin E
- ATP, adenosine
- Adrenomedullin?
- Nociceptin?

discussed in detail as they are subject to more detailed review elsewhere in this book (Chapter 11).

■ CONTRACTION-MEDIATING TRANSMITTERS AND RECEPTORS

Noradrenaline and alpha-adrenoceptors

It is generally accepted that the penis is kept in the flaccid state mainly via tonic sympathetic nervous activity. Noradrenaline is released and stimulates alpha-

123

adrenoceptors in the penile vasculature contracting the helicine vessels, and in the corpus cavernosum, contracting the trabecular smooth muscle.[1] Noradrenaline can stimulate not only alpha, but also beta-adrenoceptors. However, in the human corpus cavernosum, receptor-binding studies have revealed that the density of alpha-adrenoceptors is almost ten times higher than that of beta-adrenoceptors:[13] the number of alpha-adrenoceptor binding sites per cell was estimated to be 650 000.[14] Not only the number of receptors but also the effect of endocrine and hormonal factors is of importance. In particular, androgens may regulate the alpha-adrenoceptor responsiveness of cavernous smooth muscle.[15] Compared with normal rats, castrated animals showed an enhanced reactivity to alpha-1 adrenoceptor stimulation.

Although both alpha-1 and alpha-2 adrenoceptors have been demonstrated in human corpus cavernosum tissue,[1,16,17] available information supports the view of a functional predominance of alpha-1 adrenoceptors. This may be the case also in the penile vasculature, although a contribution of alpha-2 adrenoceptors to the contraction induced by noradrenaline and electrical stimulation of nerves cannot be excluded (see below). In horse penile resistance arteries, noradrenaline activated predominantly alpha-1 adrenoceptors, whereas post-junctional alpha-2 adrenoceptors seemed to have a minor role.[18]

The role of alpha-adrenoceptor subtypes in the mediation of noradrenaline-induced cavernosal smooth muscle contraction has also been examined. The subtypes of alpha-1 adrenoceptor with high affinity for prazosin,[19] currently designated as alpha-1A, alpha-1B and alpha-1D (the cloned counterparts are termed alpha-1a, alpha-1b and alpha-1d), have been demonstrated in human corporal tissue. In a preliminary communication, Price and colleagues[20] reported that, in human corporal tissue, mRNAs for alpha-1a, alpha-1b and alpha-1d (current terminology) could be identified, the alpha-1a and alpha-1d adrenoceptors predominating. This was confirmed by other investigators.[21] However, it is known that the levels of mRNA expression do not always parallel the expression of a functional receptor protein. Traish and colleagues[16] characterized the functional alpha-1 adrenoceptor proteins in human corpus cavernosum tissue, using both receptor binding and classical isolated tissue contractions. This group demonstrated the presence of alpha-1A, alpha-1B and alpha-1D adrenoceptors, and hypothesized that two (or possibly three) receptor subtypes mediate the noradrenaline-induced contraction in this tissue.

Interpretation can be complicated by species variation. In the rabbit corpus cavernosum, Furukawa and colleagues[22] found that the alpha-1-adrenoceptor subtype mediating phenylephrine-induced contraction had the characteristics of the alpha-1B subtype. On the other hand, Tong and Chen[23] found alpha-1A adrenoceptors responsible for the methoxamine-induced contraction of rat cavernosal smooth muscle. Both the rabbit and the rat are frequently used models for human erectile mechanisms. It is essential, therefore, to understand better the magnitude and nature of interspecies differences in penile alpha-1-adrenoceptor subtypes before the species most relevant to man can be unequivocally determined.

There is increasing evidence that an additional alpha-1-adrenoceptor subtype with low affinity for prazosin (alpha-1L), which is not yet fully characterized, may occur in, for example, vascular smooth muscle.[24] However, the possibility that the alpha-1L-adrenoceptor subtype may be of importance in penile erectile tissues has apparently not been explored. Whether antagonists, selectively acting at any of the alpha-1-adrenoceptor subtypes, would offer any advantages over currently used drugs (phentolamine, moxisylyte) in the treatment of erectile dysfunction remains to be established.

Traish and colleagues[17] demonstrated expression of mRNA for alpha-2A, alpha-2B and alpha-2C adrenoceptors in whole human corpus cavernosum tissue. Radioligand-binding studies with a highly selective ligand for alpha-2 adrenoceptors revealed specific alpha-2-adrenoceptor binding sites, and functional experiments showed that the selective alpha-2-adrenoceptor agonist, UK 14,304, induced concentration-dependent contractions of isolated strips of corpus cavernosum smooth muscle. These results support previous data[1] suggesting the occurrence of post-junctional alpha-2 adrenoceptors in the human corpus cavernosum. However, whether these alpha-2 adrenoceptors are of importance for the normal physiological contractile regulation of tone in corpus cavernosum smooth muscle is still unclear. Consistent with other neuroeffector junctions, prejunctional alpha-2 adrenoceptors (autoreceptors) have been shown to modulate stimulus-evoked release of noradrenaline from noradrenergic nerves in the human corpus cavernosum, stimulation inhibiting the release of the amine.[25] However, stimulation of prejunctional alpha-2 adrenoceptors in horse penile resistance arteries was shown also to inhibit non-adrenergic, non-cholinergic

(NANC)-transmitter release.[26] This could suggest that noradrenaline, in addition to a direct contractile action on smooth muscle, could also act prejunctionally, via heteroreceptors, to maintain detumescence.

Endothelins and endothelin receptors

Several investigators have suggested that endothelins (ETs) may contribute to the maintenance of corporal smooth muscle tone.[1] Three distinct ET peptides (ET-1, ET-2 and ET-3) have been demonstrated, all widely distributed in the body. Two types of ET receptors have been cloned and expressed: these are the ET_A receptor, which is stimulated by ETs with the rank order potency ET-1 = ET-2 > ET-3, and the ET_B receptor, for which the rank order is ET-1 = ET-2 = ET-3. ET-receptors are G-protein coupled; they may use various transduction systems in mediating their actions.[27]

Saenz de Tejada and colleagues[28] showed that cultured endothelial cells from the human corpus cavernosum, but not non-endothelial cells, expressed ET-1 mRNA. In the endothelium of human cavernous tissue, intense ET-like immunoreactivity was observed; immunoreactivity was observed also in the cavernous smooth muscle.[28] Binding sites for ET-1 were demonstrated by autoradiography in the vasculature and cavernous tissue.[29.30] Both ET_A and ET_B receptors have been found in human corporal membranes, and it cannot be excluded that both receptor subtypes are functional.[31] In rat corpus cavernosum, ET-1 and ET_A receptor-binding sites were primarily localized to the endothelium lining the cavernosal lacunar spaces.[32]

ET-1 potently induces slowly developing, long-lasting contractions in different penile smooth muscles — in the corpus cavernosum, cavernous artery, deep dorsal vein and penile circumflex veins.[1] Contractions can be evoked in human corpus cavernosal tissue also by ET-2 and ET-3, although these peptides have a lower potency than ET-1.[28] In bovine retractor penis muscle and penile artery, the contraction induced by ET-1 was mediated primarily by ET_A-receptors.[33]

The contractions induced by ET-1 may be dependent on both transmembrane calcium flux (through voltage-dependent and/or receptor-operated calcium channels) and on the mobilization of inositol triphosphate (IP_3)-sensitive intracellular calcium stores.[29,34] ET-1 may function not only as a long-term regulator of corporal smooth muscle tone but also as a modulator of the contractile effect of other agents, e.g. noradrenaline,[29,31,35] or as a modulator of cellular proliferation and phenotypic expression.[36]

Ari and colleagues[37] found that, in the pithed rat, intravenously injected ET-1 had a vasodilator action (increase in corporal pressure) at low doses, but a vasoconstrictor action at high doses. ET-3 had mainly vasodilator effects. They suggested that activation of ET_B receptors on the endothelium and local release of NO mediated the vasodilator actions, since these actions were inhibited by N^ω-nitro-L-arginine methyl ester. Parkkisenniemi and Klinge[33] suggested that the ET_B receptors that could be demonstrated on the bovine retractor penis muscle, at least partly were located on the inhibitory nerves that mediate relaxation via activation of the L-arginine/NO/cGMP pathway.

Although much available in vitro information suggests that ETs may be of importance for erectile physiology and pathophysiology, the role of the peptides in vivo is unclear. Christ and colleagues[31] found no detectable age- or diabetes-related changes in contractile effects in human corpus cavernosum tissue. On the other hand, ET-1 and ET_A receptor binding was found to be increased in diabetic rat cavernosal tissue.[32] Francavilla and colleagues[38] found no differences in plasma concentrations of ET-1 in diabetic and non-diabetic patients with erectile dysfunction, and the concentrations of ET-1 in cavernous body blood were no different following intracavernosal injection of prostaglandin E1. Further studies are needed to define the role of ETs in erectile function and dysfunction.

Angiotensin and angiotensin receptors

Human corpus cavernosum was found to produce and secrete physiologically relevant amounts of angiotensin II.[39] In vitro, angiotensin II contracted canine corpus cavernosum smooth muscle, an effect that was increased by NOS inhibition.[40] Intracavernosal injection of angiotensin II caused contraction and terminated spontaneous erections in anaesthetized dogs, whereas administration of losartan, which selectively blocked angiotensin II receptors (type AT1), resulted in smooth muscle relaxation and erection.[39] Also in the rabbit corpus cavernosum, results were obtained suggesting involvement of the renin–angiotensin system in the regulation of corpus cavernosum smooth muscle tone, and that the angiotensin II receptor subtype AT1 is important for mediation of the response.[41]

Whether angiotensin II is an important regulator of tone in penile erectile tissues is unclear. Studies using angiotensin II-receptor antagonists, for example losartan, designed to answer this question, would be of interest.

RELAXATION-MEDIATING TRANSMITTERS AND RECEPTORS

Acetylcholine and cholinergic receptors

The importance of parasympathetic nerves for producing penile erection has been well established.[6] Penile tissues from humans and several animal species are rich in nerves staining for acetylcholine (ACh) esterase.[42] From these nerves, ACh can be released by transmural electrical field stimulation. Human corpus cavernosum contains a high density of muscarinic receptors: Costa and colleagues[14] calculated the number of binding sites on isolated corpus cavernosum smooth muscle cells to be 45 000, which was about 15 times less than the number of alpha adrenoceptors. In these cells, carbachol consistently produced contraction. The implication is that relaxation induced by ACh is subserved either by inhibition of release of a contractant factor, e.g. noradrenaline, and/or is produced by the release of a relaxation-producing factor, e.g. NO. Four muscarinic-receptor subtypes (m1–m4) were shown to be expressed in human corpus cavernosum tissue;[43] the receptor on smooth muscle appeared to be the m2 subtype,[43,44] whereas that on the endothelium was the m3 subtype.[43]

It is pertinent to note that parasympathetic activity is not equivalent to the actions of ACh, as other transmitters may be released from cholinergic nerves.[45] Thus, parasympathetic activity may produce penile tumescence and erection by inhibiting the release of noradrenaline through stimulation of muscarinic receptors on adrenergic nerve terminals,[46] and/or by releasing NO and, for example, vasodilating peptides from nerves and endothelium.

Vasoactive intestinal polypeptide (VIP) and VIP receptors

The penis of men as well as that of male animals is richly supplied with nerves containing VIP.[42] The majority of these nerves also contain immunoreactivity to NOS. In addition, co-localization of NOS and VIP within nerves innervating both the human and the animal penis has been demonstrated by many investigators.[47–54] It would appear that most of these NO- and VIP-containing neurons are cholinergic, since they also contain the vesicular ACh transporter (VAChT),[55] which is a specific marker for cholinergic neurons.[56] However, Tamura et al.[50] reported that, in the human penis, NOS could be found also in nerves containing tyrosine hydroxylase,

suggesting that NO may be generated within adrenergic neurons. As discussed by the investigators, the physiological significance of such a localization is not yet clear and the finding has to be confirmed.

VIP receptors (types 1 and 2), linked via stimulatory G-proteins to adenyl cyclase, are considered to mediate the actions of the peptide.[57] The importance of the different subtypes of VIP in penile tissues has not been clarified. VIP-related peptides, e.g. pituitary adenyl cyclase-activating peptide (PACAP), which has been found to be co-localized with VIP in penile nerves,[48] seem to act through one of the VIP receptors.

The stimulatory effect of VIP on adenylyl cyclase leads to an increase in cAMP, which in turn activates cAMP-dependent protein kinase. However, VIP may increase not only cAMP but also cGMP concentrations in various smooth muscles.[58] On the other hand, this does not seem to be the case in corporal tissue from humans,[48] or from rats and rabbits,[59] where VIP increased cAMP concentrations without affecting the cGMP levels.

In experimental diabetes in rats, Maher and colleagues[60] found that the VIP content of the major pelvic ganglion and penis was markedly increased, whereas intracavernous injection of VIP, which caused erection in control rats, had no effect in diabetic animals. Since forskolin, which directly activates adenyl cyclase, induced erection in both control and diabetic rats, it was concluded that there was a defect at the level of the VIP receptor or of the associated G-protein. This is in contrast to previous findings in diabetic rats, showing that VIP-stimulated cAMP generation was significantly increased.[59] It is also in contrast to observations in human diabetes[61,62] that showed that, in patients with concomitant impotence, there was a marked reduction of VIP-like immunoreactivity in nerves associated with the cavernous smooth muscle. However, the latter observation has not been confirmed by other investigators.[63]

Undeniably, VIP has an inhibitory and relaxant effect on strips of human corpus cavernosum tissue and cavernosal vessels in vitro, but it has been difficult to show convincingly that VIP released from nerves is responsible for relaxation of penile smooth muscle in vitro or in vivo.[1] VIP-antiserum[64] and alpha-chymotrypsin[65] reduced or abolished the relaxant effect of exogenous VIP on isolated human corpus cavernosum tissue, but had no effect on relaxation induced by electrical stimulation of nerves. Kim and colleagues[66] reported that, in rabbit corpus cavernosum, a VIP antagonist inhibited electrically-induced contractions, suggesting that the peptide was released from nerves during stimulation. The authors concluded that VIP appeared to contribute to NANC-mediated corpus cavernosum relaxation and that its mechanism of relaxation was dependent on prostanoids and involved the generation of NO. However, this is in contrast to the conclusion drawn by Hayashida and colleagues,[67] who found no evidence for a role of VIP in the regulation of tone in the canine corpus cavernosum.

As described previously, many penile nerves contain NO, VIP and ACh, and the possible interactions between these agents should be of particular interest. The effects of NO and the NO donor linsidomine (SIN-1) on human isolated cavernous artery and corpus cavernosum were studied:[68] non-synergistic, independent relaxant effects were found in both types of preparation. Suh and colleagues[69] investigated the effect of VIP and VIP combined with ACh given intracavernosally in rats: they found that VIP and ACh, individually or in combination, did not produce full erection, and concluded that neither VIP nor acetylcholine were likely to be principal transmitters.

Not only NOS but also other peptides seem to be co-localized with VIP. Peptide histidine methionine (PHM), which is derived from the same precursor as VIP,[70–73] and the VIP-related PACAP and helospectin,[48,72–74] have been found to be co-localized with VIP. Although Hedlund and colleagues[48] demonstrated some of these peptides to be effective relaxants of human corpus cavernosum preparations, a role for them as neurotransmitters and/or neuromodulators has yet to be demonstrated.

Thus, whether VIP has a role as a neurotransmitter or modulator of neurotransmission in the penis has not been established. This has been the subject of debate ever since the first reports on the occurrence of VIP in the penis and on its effects on isolated penile tissues.[1] Even if the physiological role of VIP in penile erection and in erectile dysfunction is equivocal, VIP receptors in the penis are considered to be a reasonable therapeutic target. In particular in combination with phentolamine, VIP has shown some promise in the treatment of erectile dysfunction.[75,76]

Prostanoids and prostanoid receptors
Prostaglandins (PGs) and thromboxanes are locally acting hormones derived from arachidonic acid by the action of cyclooxygenases. Human corpus cavernosum tissue has the ability to synthesize various prostanoids[77,78] and also the ability to metabolize them locally. The production of prostanoids can be modulated by oxygen tension and suppressed by hypoxia.[79,80] There are five primary active prostanoid metabolites — PGD2, PGE2, PGF2α, PGI2, and TXA2 — and it has been proposed that there are five major groups of receptors, corresponding to these metabolites, that mediate their effects, namely DP, EP, FP, IP and TP receptors.[81,82] cDNAs encoding representatives of each of these groups of receptors have been cloned, including several subtypes of EP receptors. The prostanoid receptors are G-protein-coupled receptors with differing transduction systems.[81]

Penile tissues may contain most of these receptor groups. However, their role in penile physiology is still far from established. Prostanoids may be involved in contraction of erectile tissues via PGF2α and thromboxane A2, stimulating TX and FP receptors and initiating phosphoinositide turnover, as well as in relaxation via PGE1 and PGE2, stimulating EP receptors (EP2/EP4) and initiating an increase in the intracellular concentration of cAMP. Recent data suggest that prostanoids and transforming growth factor beta-1 (TGFβ1) may have a role in modulation of collagen synthesis and in the regulation of fibrosis of the corpus cavernosum,[83] and thereby in the underlying aetiology of impotence.

PGE1, injected intracavernously or administered intraurethrally, is currently one of the most widely used drugs for treatment of erectile dysfunction,[78,84–86] and several aspects of its effects and clinical use have been reviewed recently.[78,84] PGE1 is metabolized in penile tissue to PGE0,[87] which is biologically active and may contribute to the effect of PGE1.[88] PGE1 may act partly by inhibiting the release of noradrenaline,[89] but the main action of PGE1 and PGE0 is probably to increase the intracellular concentrations of cAMP in the corpus cavernosum smooth muscle cells through EP receptor stimulation.[88,90–92]

Palmer and colleagues[90] found that forskolin, which directly stimulates adenylate cyclase, was a potent stimulant of intracellular cAMP formation in cultured human corporal smooth muscle cells. Threshold forskolin doses were found to increase significantly the production of cAMP by PGE1, which suggested a possible synergistic effect. Traish and colleagues[88] confirmed these synergistic effects of forskolin and PGE1 in cultured human corpus cavernosum cells. They also demonstrated that the augmentation of the forskolin-induced cAMP generation by PGE1 and PGE0 was mediated by EP receptors and attributable to interactions at the adenylyl cyclase and G-protein levels.

Both forskolin and PGE1 elicited concentration-dependent increases in the magnitude and duration of intracorporal pressure changes in dogs, without systemic effects.[92] A clinical correlate was observed by Mulhall and colleagues,[93] who reported that intracorporal administration of forskolin to patients with erectile dysfunction and who were not responding to triple-drug therapy, brought about a response when forskolin was added.

These results suggest that it is possible to enhance the relaxant corporal effects of PGE1 and, perhaps, of other vasodilators with forskolin and analogues,[94] and it cannot be excluded that this may provide new strategies for pharmacological treatment of erectile dysfunction.

FUTURE PERSPECTIVES

Adrenomedullin is a recently discovered vasodilator peptide isolated from human phaeochromocytoma cells.[95] It consists of 52 amino acids and has structural similarities to calcitonin gene-related peptide (CGRP). Adrenomedullin has been suggested to serve as a circulating hormone regulating systemic arterial pressure.[95] Champion and colleagues[96–98] showed that adrenomedullin, injected intracavernously in cats, caused an increase in intracavernosal pressure and in penile length. The increase in intracavernosal pressure at a concentration of 1 nM adrenomedullin amounted to 75% of that induced by a triple-drug combination of papaverine, phentolamine and PGE1, or with the response to CGRP at a dose ten times lower.[97] The erectile responses to adrenomedullin or CGRP were unaffected by NOS inhibition with L-NAME, or by K_{ATP}-channel inhibition with glibenclamide, suggesting that NO or K_{ATP} channels were not involved in the response. Since the CGRP antagonist CGRP (8–37), at doses having no effects on the adrenomedullin response, reduced CGRP responses, it was suggested that the peptides acted on different receptors. In the highest doses used, both adrenomedullin and CGRP (and the control triple combination) reduced blood pressure. These results with CGRP are in agreement with clinical experience and support the suggestion by Stief and colleagues[99] that CGRP may be useful in the treatment of erectile dysfunction. In patients, intracavernosal injection of CGRP induced dose-related increases in penile arterial

inflow, cavernous smooth muscle relaxation, cavernous outflow occlusion, and erectile responses. The combination of CGRP and PGE1 may be even more effective than PGE1 alone.[100,101]

Nociceptin is a 17-amino acid peptide that shares structural homology with the dynorphine family of peptides. It differs from other opioid peptides by not having the NH_2-terminal residue which is essential for activity at mμ, delta and kappa opioid receptors.[102] The drug is an endogenous ligand for the orphan opioid receptor that has been identified in several species: the human clone is called ORL1. Its function is not established; it may be involved in hyperalgesia or analgesia.[102]

Champion and colleagues[96] compared the erectile responses to intracavernosal nociceptin with those of a triple-drug combination (see above; VIP, adrenomedullin and an NO-donor) in cats. Nociceptin in doses of 0.3–3 nM elicited dose-related increases in intracavernosal pressure and penile length comparable to that of the triple-drug combination, but the duration of the response was shorter.

These data on previously unknown receptors in penile erectile tissues that, on stimulation, can induce erectile responses are exciting and show that the complex mechanisms involved in penile erection are far from clarified.

ACKNOWLEDGEMENTS

This work was supported by the Swedish Medical Research Council (grant no. 6837) and by the Medical Faculty, University of Lund, Sweden.

REFERENCES

1. Andersson K-E, Wagner G. Physiology of penile erection. Physiol Rev 1995; 75: 191–236
2. Taub H C, Lerner S E, Melman A, Christ G J. Relationship between contraction and relaxation in human and rabbit corpus cavernosum. Urology 1993; 42: 698–704
3. Carrier S, Nagaraju P, Morgan D M et al. Age decreases nitric oxide synthase-containing nerve fibers in the rat penis. J Urol 1997; 157: 1088–1092
4. Dahiya R, Lin A, Bakircioglu M E et al. mRNA and protein expression of nitric oxide synthase and adrenoceptor alpha 1 in young and old rat penile tissues. Br J Urol 1997; 80: 300–306
5. Christ G J, Maayani S, Valcic M. Pharmacological studies of human erectile tissue; characteristics of spontaneous contractions and alterations in alpha-adrenoceptor

responsiveness with age and disease in isolated tissues. Br J Pharmacol 1990; 101: 375

6. Andersson K-E. The pharmacology of lower urinary tract smooth muscles and penile erectile tissues. Pharmacol Rev 1993; 45: 253–308

7. de Groat W C, Booth A M. Neural control of penile erection. In: Maggi C A (ed) The autonomic nervous system, Vol. 6. London: Harwood Academic, 1993: 467–524

8. Argiolas A, Melis M R. Neuromodulation of penile erection: an overview of the role of neurotransmitters and neuropeptides. Progr Neurobiol 1995; 47: 235–255

9. Giuliano F A, Rampin O, Benoit G, Jardin A. Neural control of penile erection. Urol Clin North Am 1995; 22: 747–766

10. Giuliano F A, Rampin O, Benoit G, Jardin A. The peripheral pharmacology of erection. Prog Urol 1997; 7: 24–33

11. Klinge E, Sjöstrand N O. Smooth muscle of the male reproductive tract. In Pharmacology of smooth muscle. In: Szekeres L, Papp J G (eds) Handbook of experimental pharmacology, Vol 111. Berlin: Springer-Verlag, 1994: 533–573

12. Lerner S E, Melman A, Christ G J. A review of erectile dysfunction: new insights and more questions. J Urol 1993; 149: 1246–1255

13. Levin R M, Wein A J. Adrenergic alpha-receptors outnumber beta-receptors in human penile corpus cavernosum. Invest Urol 1980; 18: 225–226

14. Costa P, Soulie-Vassal M L, Sarrazin B et al. Adrenergic receptors on smooth muscle cells isolated from human penile corpus cavernosum. J Urol 1993; 150: 859–863

15. Reilly C M, Stopper V S, Mills T. Androgens modulate the α-adrenergic responsiveness of vascular smooth muscle in the corpus cavernosum. J Androl 1997; 18: 26–31

16. Traish A, Netsuwan N, Daley J et al. A heterogenous population of α1 adrenergic receptors mediates contraction of human corpus cavernosum smooth muscle to norepinephrine. J Urol 1995; 153: 222–227

17. Traish A M, Moreland R B, Huang Y H, Goldstein I. Expression of functional alpha2-adrenergic receptor subtypes in human corpus cavernosum and in cultured trabecular smooth muscle cells. Recept Signal Transduc 1997; 7: 55–67

18. Simonsen U, Prieto D, Hernandez M et al. Adrenoceptor-mediated regulation of the contractility in horse penile resistance arteries. J Vasc Res 1997; 34: 90–102

19. Hieble J P, Bylund D B, Clarke D E et al. International Union of Pharmacology X. Recommendation for nomenclature of a1-adrenoceptors: consensus update. Pharmacol Rev 1995; 47: 267–270

20. Price D T, Schwinn D A, Kim J H et al. Alpha-1 adrenergic receptor subtype mRNA expression in human corpus cavernosum. J Urol 1993; 149: 285A (abstr 287)

21. Traish A, Gupta S, Toselli P et al. Identification of α1-adrenergic receptor subtypes in human corpus cavernous tissue and in cultured trabecular smooth muscle cells. Receptor 1996; 5: 145–157

22. Furukawa K, Chess-Williams R, Uchiyama T. α_{1B}-Adrenoceptor subtype mediating the phenylephrine-induced contractile response in rabbit corpus cavernosum penis. Jpn J Pharmacol 1996; 71: 325–331

23. Tong Y-C, Chen J-T. Subtyping of α_1-adrenoceptors responsible for the contractile response in the rat corpus cavernosum. Neurosci Lett 1997; 228: 159–162

24. Muramatsu I, Ohmura T, Hashimoto S, Oshita M. Functional subclassification of vascular a1-adrenoceptors. Pharmacol Commun 1995; 6: 23–28

25. Molderings G J, Göthert M, van Ahlen H, Porst H. Noradrenaline release in human corpus cavernosum and its modulation via presynaptic alpha 2-adrenoceptors. Fundam Clin Pharmacol 1989; 3: 497–504

26. Simonsen U, Prieto D, Hernandez M et al. Prejunctional alpha 2-adrenoceptors inhibit nitrergic neurotransmission in horse penile resistance arteries. J Urol 1997; 157: 2356–2360

27. Rubanyi G M, Polokoff M A. Endothelins: molecular biology, biochemistry, pharmacology, physiology, and pathophysiology. Physiol Rev 1994; 46: 325–341

28. Saenz de Tejada I, Carson M P, de las Morenas A et al. Endothelin: localization, synthesis, activity, and receptor types in human penile corpus cavernosum. Am J Physiol 1991; 261: H1078–H1085

29. Holmquist F, Andersson K-E, Hedlund H. Actions of endothelin on isolated corpus cavernosum from rabbit and man. Acta Physiol Scand 1990; 139: 113–122

30. Holmquist F, Kirkeby H J, Larsson B et al. Functional effects, binding sites and immunolocalization of endothelin-1 in isolated penile tissues from man and rabbit. J Pharmacol Exp Ther 1992; 261: 795–802

31. Christ G J, Lerner S E, Kim D C, Melman A. Endothelin-1 as a putative modulator of erectile dysfunction: I. Characteristics of contraction of isolated corporal tissue strips. J Urol 1995; 153: 1998–2003

32. Bell C R W, Sullivan M E, Dashwood M R et al. The density and distribution of endothelin 1 and endothelin receptor subtypes in normal and diabetic rat corpus cavernosum. Br J Urol 1995; 76: 203–207

33. Parkkisenniemi U-M, Klinge E. Functional characterization of endothelin receptors in the bovine retractor penis and penile artery. Pharmacol Toxicol 1996; 79: 73–79

34. Holmquist F, Persson K, Garcia-Pascual A, Andersson K-E. Phospholipase C activation by endothelin-1 and noradrenaline in isolated penile erectile tissue from rabbit. J Urol 1992; 147: 1632–1635

35. Kim D C, Gondre C M, Christ G J. Endothelin-1-induced modulation of contractile responses elicited by an alpha 1-adrenergic agonist on human corpus cavernosum smooth cells. Int J Impot Res 1996; 8: 17–24

36. Zhao W, Christ G J. Endothelin-1 as a putative modulator of erectile dysfunction. II. Calcium mobilization in cultured human corporal smooth muscle cells. J Urol 1995; 154: 1571–1579

37. Ari G, Vardi Y, Hoffman A, Finberg J P. Possible role for endo-thelins in penile erection. Eur J Pharmacol 1996; 307: 69–74

38. Francavilla S, Properzi G, Bellini C et al. Endothelin-1 in diabetic and nondiabetic men with erectile dysfunction. J Urol 1997; 158: 1770–1774

39. Kifor I, Williams G H, Vickers M A et al. Tissue angiotensin II as a modulator of erectile function. I. Angiotensin peptide

content, secretion and effects in the corpus cavernosum. J Urol 1997; 157: 1920–1925

40. Comiter C V, Sullivan M P, Yalla S V, Kifor I. Effect of angiotensin II on corpus cavernosum smooth muscle in relation to nitric oxide environment: in vitro studies in canines. Int J Impot Res 1997; 9: 135–140

41. Park J K, Kim S Z, Kim S H et al. Renin angiotensin system in rabbit corpus cavernosum: functional characterization of angiotensin II receptors. J Urol 1997; 158: 653–658

42. Dail W G. Autonomic innervation of male reproductive genitalia. In: Maggi C A (ed) The autonomic nervous system, Vol. 6. London: Harwood Academic, 1993: 69–101

43. Traish A M, Palmer M S, Goldstein I, Moreland R B. Expression of functional muscarinic acetylcholine receptor subtypes in human corpus cavernosum and in cultured smooth muscle cells. Receptor 1995; 5: 159–176

44. Toselli P, Moreland R, Traish A M. Detection of m2 muscarinic acetylcholine receptor mRNA in human corpus cavernosum by in-situ hybridization. Life Sci 1994; 55: 621–627

45. Lundberg J M. Pharmacology of cotransmission in the autonomic nervous system: integrative aspects on amines, neuropeptides, adenosine triphosphate, amino acids and nitric oxide. Pharmacol Rev 1996; 48: 113–178

46. Klinge E, Sjöstrand N O. Suppression of the excitatory adrenergic neurotransmission; a possible role of cholinergic nerves in the retractor penis muscle. Acta Physiol Scand 1977; 100: 368–376

47. Ehmke H, Junemann K P, Mayer B, Kummer W. Nitric oxide synthase and vasoactive intestinal polypeptide colocalization in neurons innervating the human penile circulation. Int J Impot Res 1995; 7: 147–156

48. Hedlund P, Alm P, Ekström P et al. Pituitary adenylate cyclase-activating polypeptide, helospectin, and vasoactive intestinal polypeptide in human corpus cavernosum. Br J Pharmacol 1995; 116: 2258–2266

49. Hedlund P, Larsson B, Alm P, Andersson K-E. Distribution and function of nitric oxide-containing nerves in canine corpus cavernosum and spongiosum. Acta Physiol Scand 1995; 155: 445–455

50. Tamura M, Kagawa S, Kimura K et al. Coexistence of nitric oxide synthase, tyrosine hydroxylase and vasoactive intestinal polypeptide in human penile tissue — a triple histochemical and immunohistochemical study. J Urol 1995; 153: 530–534

51. Tamura M, Kagawa S, Tsuruo Y et al. Localization of NADPH diaphorase and vasoactive intestinal polypeptide-containing neurons in the efferent pathway to the rat corpus cavernosum. Eur Urol 1997; 32: 100–104

52. Vanhatalo S, Klinge E, Sjöstrand N O, Soinila S. Nitric oxide-synthesizing neurons originating at several different levels innervate rat penis. Neuroscience 1996; 75: 891–899

53. Dail W G, Galindo R, Leyba L, Barba V. Denervation-induced changes in perineuronal plexuses in the major pelvic ganglion of the rat: immunohistochemistry for vasoactive intestinal polypeptide and tyrosine hydroxylase and

histochemistry for NADPH-diaphorase. Cell Tissue Res 1997; 287: 315–324

54. Schirar A, Chang C, Rousseau J P. Localization of androgen receptor in nitric oxide synthase- and vasoactive intestinal peptide-containing neurons of the major pelvic ganglion innervating the rat penis. J Neuroendocrinol 1997; 9: 141–150

55. Hedlund P, Alm P, Andersson K-E. NO synthase in cholinergic nerves and NO-induced relaxation in the rat isolated corpus cavernosum. Br J Pharmacol; 1998: submitted

56. Arvidsson U, Reidl M, Elde R, Meister B. Vesicular acetylcholine transporter (VAChT) protein: a novel and unique marker for cholinergic neurons in the central and peripheral nervous systems. J Comp Neurol 1997; 378: 454–467

57. Fahrenkrug J. Transmitter role of vasoactive intestinal peptide. Pharmacol Toxicol 1993; 72: 354–363

58. Chakder S, Rattan S. Involvement of cAMP and cGMP in relaxation of internal anal sphincter by neural stimulation, VIP, and NO. Am J Physiol 1993; 264: G702–G707

59. Miller M A W, Morgan R J, Thompson C S et al. Effects of papaverine and vasointestinal polypeptide on penile and vascular cAMP and cGMP in control and diabetic animals: an in vitro study. Int J Impot Res 1995; 7: 91–100

60. Maher E, Bachoo M, Elabbady A A et al. Vasoactive intestinal peptide and impotence in experimental diabetes mellitus. Br J Urol 1996; 77: 271–278

61. Gu J, Polak J M, Lazarides M et al. Decrease of vasoactive intestinal polypeptide (VIP) in the penises from impotent men. Lancet 1984; ii: 315–318

62. Lincoln J, Crowe R, Blackley P F et al. Changes in the VIPergic, cholinergic and adrenergic innervation of human penile tissue in diabetic and non-diabetic impotent males. J Urol 1987; 137: 1053–1959

63. Haberman J, Valcic M, Christ G, Melman A. Vasoactive intestinal peptide and norepinephrine concentration in the corpora cavernosa of impotent men. Int J Impot Res 1991; 3: 21–28

64. Adaikan P G, Kottegoda S R, Ratnam S S. Is vasoactive intestinal polypeptide the principal transmitter involved in human penile erection? J Urol 1986; 135: 638–640

65. Pickard R S, Powell P H, Zar M A. Evidence against vasoactive intestinal polypeptide as the relaxant neurotransmitter in human cavernosal smooth muscle. Br J Pharmacol 1993; 108: 497–500

66. Kim Y C, Kim J H, Davies M G et al. Modulation of vasoactive intestinal polypeptide (VIP)-mediated relaxation by nitric oxide and prostanoids in the rabbit corpus cavernosum. J Urol 1995; 153: 807–810

67. Hayashida H, Okamura T, Tomoyoshi T, Toda N. Neurogenic nitric oxide mediates relaxation of canine corpus cavernosum. J Urol 1996; 155: 1122–1127

68. Hempelmann R G, Papadopoulos I, Herzig S. Non-synergistic relaxant effects of vasoactive intestinal polypeptide and SIN-1 in human isolated cavernous artery and corpus cavernosum. Eur J Pharmacol 1995; 276: 277–280

69. Suh J K, Mun K H, Cho C K et al. Effect of vasoactive intestinal peptide and acetylcholine on penile erection in the rat in vivo. Int J Impot Res 1995; 7: 111–118

70. Yiangou Y, Christofides N D, Gu J et al. Peptide histidine methionine (PHM) and the human male genitalia. Neuropeptides 1985; 6: 133–142

71. Kirkeby H J, Fahrenkrug J, Holmquist F, Ottesen B. Vasoactive intestinal polypeptide (VIP) and peptide histidine methionine (PHM) in human penile corpus cavernosum tissue and circumflex veins: localization and in vitro effects. Eur J Clin Invest 1992; 22: 24–30

72. Hauser-Kronberger C, Hacker G W, Graf A-H et al. Neuropeptides in the human penis: an immunohistochemical study. J Androl 1994; 15: 510–520

73. Hauser-Kronberger C, Hacker G W, Mack D et al. Pituitary adenylate cyclase-activating peptide (PACAP), helospectin, peptide histidine methionine (PHM) and vasoactive intestinal polypeptide (VIP) in the human penis: an immunocytochemical evaluation on the occurrence of VIP-related peptides. Cell Vision 1994; 1: 319–323

74. Hedlund P, Alm P, Hedlund H et al. Localization and effects of pituitary adenylate cyclase-activating polypeptide (PACAP) in human penile erectile tissues. Acta Physiol Scand 1994; 150: 103–104

75. Gerstenberg T C, Metz P, Ottesen B, Fahrenkrug J. Intracavernous self-injection with vasoactive intestinal polypeptide and phentolamine in the management of erectile failure. J Urol 1992; 147: 1277–1279

76. McMahon C G. A pilot study of the role of intracavernous injection of vasoactive intestinal peptide (VIP) and phentolamine mesylate in the treatment of erectile dysfunction. Int J Impot Res 1996; 8: 233–236

77. Miller M A W, Morgan R J. Eicosanoids, erections and erectile dysfunction. Prostaglandins Leukot Essent Fatty Acids 1994; 51: 1–9

78. Porst H. A rationale for prostaglandin E1 in erectile failure: a survey of worldwide experience. J Urol 1996; 155: 802–815

79. Daley J T, Brown M L, Watkins M T et al. Prostanoid production in rabbit corpus cavernosum: I. Regulation by oxygen tension. J Urol 1996; 155: 1482–1487

80. Daley J T, Watkins M T, Brown M L et al. Prostanoid production in rabbit corpus cavernosum: II. Inhibition by oxidative stress. J Urol 1996; 156: 1169–1173

81. Coleman R A, Smith W L, Narumiya S. International Union of Pharmacology classification of prostanoid receptors: properties, distribution, and structure of the receptors and their subtypes. Pharmacol Rev 1994; 46: 205–229

82. Pierce K L, Gil D W, Woodward D F, Regan J W. Cloning of human prostanoid receptors. Trends Pharmacol Sci 1995; 16: 253–256

83. Moreland R B, Traish A, McMillan M A et al. PGE1 suppresses the induction of collagen synthesis by transforming growth factor-β1 in human corpus cavernosum smooth muscle. J Urol 1995; 153: 826–834

84. Linet O I, Ogrinc F G. Efficacy and safety of intracavernosal alprostadil in men with erectile dysfunction. N Engl J Med 1996; 334: 873–877

85. Hellstrom W J G, Bennett A H, Gesundheit N et al. A double-blind, placebo-controlled evaluation of the erectile response to transurethral alprostadil. Urology 1996; 48: 851–856

86. Padma-Nathan H, Hellstrom W J G, Kaiser F E et al. Treatment of men with erectile dysfunction with transurethral alprostadil. N Engl J Med 1997; 336: 1–7

87. Hatzinger M, Junemann P, Woeste M et al. Pilot study on systemic plasma concentrations of prostaglandin E1, 15-keto PGE0 and PGE0 after intravenous injection in patients with chronic erectile dysfunction. J Urol 1995; 153: 367A

88. Traish A M, Moreland R B, Gallant C et al. G-protein-coupled receptor agonists augment adenylyl cyclase activity induced by forskolin in human corpus cavernosum smooth muscle cells. Recept Signal Transduc 1997; 7: 121–132

89. Molderings G J, van Ahlen H, Göthert M. Modulation of noradrenaline release in human corpus cavernosum by presynaptic prostaglandin receptors. Int J Impot Res 1992; 4: 19–26

90. Palmer L S, Valcic M, Giraldi A M et al. Characterization of cyclic AMP accumulation in cultured human corpus cavernosum smooth muscle cells. J Urol 1994; 152: 1308–1314

91. Lin J S-N, Lin J-M, Jou Y-C, Cheng J-T. Role of cyclic adenosine monophosphate in prostaglandin E$_1$-induced penile erection in rabbits. Eur Urol 1995; 28: 259–265

92. Cahn D, Melman A, Valcic M, Christ G J. Forskolin: a promising new adjunct to intracavernous pharmacotherapy. J Urol 1996; 155: 1789–1794

93. Mulhall J P, Daller M, Traish A M et al. Intracavernosal forskolin: role in management of vasculogenic impotence resistant to standard 3-agent pharmacotherapy. J Urol 1997; 158: 1752–1758

94. Laurenza A, Robbins J D, Seamon K B. Interaction of aminoalkylcarbamates of forskolin with adenylyl cyclase: synthesis of an iodinated derivative of forskolin with high affinity for adenylyl cyclase. Mol Pharmacol 1992; 41: 360–368

95. Kitamura K, Kangawa K, Kawamoto M et al. Adrenomedullin: a novel hypotensive peptide isolated from human pheochromocytoma. Biochem Biophys Res Commun 1993; 192: 553–560

96. Champion H C, Wang R, Hellstrom W J G, Kadowitz P J. Nociceptin, a novel endogenous ligand for the ORL1 receptor, has potent erectile activity in the cat. Am J Physiol 1997; 273: E214–E219

97. Champion H C, Wang R, Santiago J A et al. Comparison of responses to adrenomedullin and calcitonin gene-related peptide in the feline erection model. J Androl 1997; 18: 513–521

98. Champion H C, Wang R, Shenassa B B et al. Adrenomedullin induces penile erection in the cat. Eur J Pharmacol 1997; 319: 71–75

99. Stief C G, Benard F, Bosch R J L H et al. A possible role for calcitonin-gene-related peptide in the regulation of the smooth muscle tone of the bladder and penis. J Urol 1990; 143: 392–397

100. Stief C G, Wetterauer U, Schaebsdau F, Jonas U. Calcitonin-gene-related peptide: a possible role in human penile erection and its therapeutical application in impotent patients. J Urol 1991; 146: 1010–1014

101. Truss M C, Becker A J, Thon W F. Intracavernous calcitonin gene-related peptide plus prostaglandin E1: possible alternative to penile implants in selected patients. Eur Urol 1994; 26: 40–45

102. Henderson G, McKnight A T. The orphan opioid receptor and its endogenous ligand — nociceptin/orphanin FQ. Trends Pharmacol Sci 1997; 18: 293–300

Chapter 13

Treatment strategies for erectile dysfunction from CNS pharmacology

J. P. W. Heaton, M. A. Adams and A. Morales

■ INTRODUCTION

There has been a rapid advance in the understanding of the physiology of erection in the last 10 years and a marked increase in sophistication, as can be seen from the chapters in this section. Clinicians have been very involved in this rapid progress, perhaps because of the direct need to apply this new science in the diagnosis and management of patients, and of the lack of simple acceptable and effective therapies. This direct link between the science and the patient in the clinic is one of the interesting factors in erectile dysfunction (ED) and may contrast with some other disease complexes. Science provides an understanding of the physiology and pathophysiology but is less successful in its ability to specify, and hence to rectify, the exact aetiology of ED in an individual. Treatment, therefore, has come from an understanding of the factors that contribute to the normal physiology of erection rather than from an intimate understanding of the problems causing ED in an individual patient.

There has been great interest in evolving new treatment options for ED in the last few years. In general, the development of optimal therapeutic strategies involves an iterative process based on understanding and successful hypothesis-testing in both basic science and clinical application. The details of the relevant biology need to be worked out and the treatment formulated. The clinical response can then be observed and measured. The outcome of these patient–treatment–response interactions generates further knowledge and supplementary questions requiring additional scientific enquiry. The scope of the whole field advances with each new layer of study — so it is, in the study of ED now. The range and the upcoming availability of new drugs, acting through known central and peripheral mechanisms, will provide an essential ingredient in this progress towards optimal therapy for ED.

However, in the late 20th century we are still treating ED with agents that have little specificity of action. Ideally, it would be efficient to use a drug or treatment protocol designed around a patient-specific diagnosis with known pharmacological requirements. The status of the field at present is that we are still far from that ideal. In fact, route of delivery of a drug may influence drug choice in patients, more than the efficacy or appropriateness of a drug (observation based on reports from focus groups and other unpublished studies). In order to address the rapid change in available therapies, this chapter reviews the ways in which the understanding of the new pharmacology of ED can be harnessed and the rational link between drugs with known mechanisms and their use in clinically important subtypes of ED can be developed.

■ SCIENTIFIC UNDERSTANDING IN ERECTILE DYSFUNCTION: PHARMACOLOGY IN PRACTICE

In theoretical terms, optimal therapy, acting with some level of specificity, should normalize only the 'causative' abnormality, leaving normal tissue functions unaltered; i.e. there should be no adverse or side effects. An understanding of the local, neural and humoral physiological control systems involved in the initiation and maintenance of a normal erection, as described in preceding chapters, is essential to the identification of the potential for systems to experience dysfunction. In addition, recognition of the sites of action within these systems provides a more refined target for new therapeutic interventions.

Ultimately, the success of an intervention, with a known mechanism of action, in normalizing erectile function should also be harnessed as a diagnostic tool. Patients could be classified as responders to the known pharmacology. This does not define the specific nature of the actual dysfunction but it does add clear evidence that processes distal to the successful intervention are normal. This type of treatment-and-positive-response outcome would provide an important step in refining the diagnosis and would thereby point to a range of appropriate and inappropriate therapies. This important realization is developed later in this chapter. Using new treatment–response successes and failures in this way reinforces the interdependence of concepts developed in basic science and clinical practice. To summarize, an understanding of both the physiology and patho-physiology of erection, as well as of the mechanisms and site of drug action, will efficiently guide the development of useful and specific therapies.

Unfortunately, in ED only part of the normal and abnormal physiology is accessible to simple measurement and evaluation. It is reasonably easy to study penile function, but not events in the central nervous system (CNS). Vascular endpoints such as blood pressure, intracavernous pressure, blood flow, tumescence and rigidity are all measurable. In contrast, the ability to assess the changes in function of the CNS relevant to erection, despite being integral to the generation of penile erection, is vague and indirect (Fig. 13.1).

An instrument that is able to provide a diagnosis of CNS dysfunction would be invaluable in assessing the

nature of causality in certain forms of ED. The methodology that is currently available includes positron emission tomographic scanning, functional magnetic resonance imaging and cortical evoked potentials, all of which can provide indirect glimpses of CNS function. These techniques can be applied to ED but mean little without correlation with clearly defined clinical observations. Clinical observations in ED cover a wide range of quality-of-life and partner issues, as well as dimensions that are more amenable to quantification and rigorous analysis such as stress and anxiety. Here, again, one can see the necessity of the iterative cycle of basic mechanisms and clinical interpretation. Written questionnaires[1] provide scores that require similar correlation for full understanding and these are just beginning to attract the rigour that will be needed in the future. At the moment it is not possible to measure or observe in a practical way the pharmacological basis of CNS action in the clinical setting. In fact — far from the explicit molecular level explanations of receptors, neurotransmitters, neurons and pathways — the CNS is largely a 'black box' when it comes to clinical management — it is not possible to 'see in' but, sometimes, the overall shape is recognizable (e.g. depression, addiction).

In the assessment of patients there is an uneasy partnership between the physiological 'erection monitors', such as the RigiScan™ (Osbon Medical Systems, Augusta, GA, USA) and mercury strain gauges, and the 'soft' instruments (diaries, questionnaires and partner opinion). These are all used in the attempt to provide accurate assessment of new therapies, which points dramatically to the need for a wide range of skills, paradigms and specialty training in the detailed evaluation of ED.

Traditional 'successful' therapies have had little regard for target selectivity. Often, the treatment used has been termed a 'sledgehammer' approach (e.g. intracavernous injection (ICI) triple therapy in psychogenic patients). More recently there has been a trend to deliver pharmacologically 'cleaner' drugs[2,3] that are better understood in terms of mechanism of action. The next phase of agents promises to add greater pharmacological sophistication[4,5] and improved delivery characteristics, although there may be a risk of decreased selectivity for erectile systems. We are still a few years away from the first dedicated diagnostic drug. Until then, clinicians will exercise their expertise by first trying out drugs that have a low potential for causing irreversible changes. This can

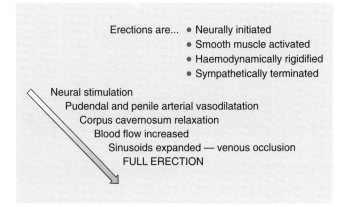

Erections are... • Neurally initiated
• Smooth muscle activated
• Haemodynamically rigidified
• Sympathetically terminated

Neural stimulation
Pudendal and penile arterial vasodilatation
Corpus cavernosum relaxation
Blood flow increased
Sinusoids expanded — venous occlusion
FULL ERECTION

Figure 13.1. The erection cascade: a coordinated action of systems.

be viewed as an important change in practice, as a permanent intervention 'now' could deny a patient access to 'better' future therapies. Ideally, treatment in the future will be individualized and directed at a unique and known property of the pathophysiology that is primarily causative for the patient's specific dysfunction. Selective therapies would become truly diagnostic and should have advantageous adverse effect profiles.

It has already been pointed out that a precise understanding of the mechanism of action of any successful therapeutic modality in ED will reveal characteristics of the physiological mechanisms involved in the erectile process itself. These details in understanding, therefore, may lead to more refined therapies directed at mechanisms specific for ED, that have little or no effect in similar mechanisms elsewhere in the body. An example of this line of thinking can be found in the 'mapping' of enzymes and receptors by anatomical location. Certain proteins, if identified to have an anatomically and functionally specific role, may be used as diagnostic (e.g. cardiac troponin T in the diagnosis of myocardial injury[6]) or therapeutic targets (angiotensin-converting enzyme inhibitors acting in hypertension). In fact, the selectivity of a common enzyme for a particular system depends entirely on anatomical localization of a particular function (e.g. creatine kinase is a ubiquitous muscle enzyme; the MB isoform is more localized to the anatomically and functionally distinct muscle fibres of the heart). The question that arises is how much of the erectile system is sufficiently distinct to have truly dedicated isotypes of enzymes, receptors, etc? An example is that a nitric oxide synthase that is relatively specific for the penis has been proposed.

The process of erection is multidimensional and complex, and deliberately exhibits pathway redundancy and overlap.[7] The initiation and maintenance of sexual erection involves components of the entire CNS and its transducer targets. Erectogenic roles have been found for neurons in the cortex,[8] midbrain[9] and interneurons[10] in the spine. There is strong evidence clinically that erotic imagery[11] and sensory reinforcement[12] play significant roles in normal sexual erections, but these are difficult to reduce to simple neurobiology at this time. Somatic[13] and autonomic[14] neural pathways are well known and documented to be involved, just as multiple vasoconstrictor[15] and vasodilator systems have been shown to have some activity. Furthermore, at the end organ, all known smooth muscle and endothelial functional control mechanisms have a potential role acutely and chronically (see chapter 5) including various neurotransmitter and second-messenger systems.

Erections, then, occur as a result of actions in complex systems at multiple levels and in various interdependent and parallel pathways. Most of the clinical (and even basic science) data inevitably come from observation of systems in isolation, and it is inevitable that integrated analysis, which examines components in context, is less common. In life, erections are multisystem phenomena with built-in overlap and multiplicity, since that is what is required to protect procreative potential.[16]

■ THERAPEUTIC STRATEGY BASED ON SYSTEMS ANALYSIS AND PHARMACOLOGICAL UNDERSTANDING

In the foregoing, an argument has been built up that emphasizes complexity in the systems subtending erectile function and dysfunction. It is a reasonable caveat to indicate that this complexity may, at present, be less of a problem of understanding in the periphery, where more is known, whereas, in the CNS, the complexity is so overwhelming that, after a few broad brush strokes of understanding and only a few precise details from experiments, the process remains largely a mystery. Therapeutic opportunities often come from a detailed understanding of function and anatomy. Further, this argument includes the concept that the detail can potentially be harnessed for use in therapeutic (or diagnostic) drug design. Most of the particulars that are useful for drug development will be based on anatomical and functional characteristics that are distinctive and can be harnessed (Fig. 13.2).

It is becoming clear that some of the most profound factors governing the specificity of growth and development of tissue come from the particular anatomical milieu in which it differentiates.[17] There develops an intimate relationship between structure and function that is privileged to the anatomical site of the system. In biochemical terms, there are a limited number of ways of doing things, so the broad principles of neurotransmitter–receptor interaction and second-messenger activation remain relatively constant. The specifics of enzyme structure may become structure/function specific, as with the prior example of creatine

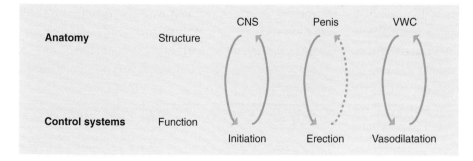

Figure 13.2. Structure–function relationships underlie all biological systems. CNS, central nervous system; VWC, vascular wall complex.

kinase isoenzymes. In this case, the distinction in functional roles between creatine kinases acting in skeletal muscle and the equivalent enzymes acting in cardiac muscle are profound. The differences between penile vascular tissue and other small vascular beds may not be as great, although penile-specific nitric oxide synthase isoenzymes[18] have been described. It is too early to be certain that other representations of this isoenzyme will not be found elsewhere.

The CNS has its own functional identity with respect to erectile function. It is the sole source of signalling that will generate a coordinated sexual penile erection. It acts through cortical pathways, midbrain coordination, neural activation and inactivation involving the autonomic nervous system and sensory afferents, detailed elsewhere in this chapter. The CNS erectogenic machinery controls mostly vascular tissue, and the primary effects are seen in the vasodilatation of pudendal and penile vessels.[19] Only CNS/nerve-mediated control could achieve the full recruitment of the various levels of the vasculature necessary to normal penile function.

The penis, as a functional system, has peculiar anatomy (e.g. helicine arteries, cavernous lacunae and venous occlusion) and functional control that is unique in that there is, as yet, no evidence for the provision of positive or negative neural feedback from tumescent tissue.

The vascular wall complex (VWC) has the most thoroughly researched pharmacology and biochemistry and has almost complete parallelism with normal vascular biology (see earlier sections of this chapter). Further, even the more complex interrelations in the VWC are becoming understood and the opportunities for drug intervention are great. One difficulty is that the multiplicity of control is likely to mask the subtleties of a dysfunction in a specific system. Most treatments available today act on the vasculature, despite the fact that there is good evidence that penile vascular tissue in men judged to be impotent may often be found to be fully functional in vitro.[20]

The anatomy and function of the specific system determines the locus of control for a drug designed to affect a system. The CNS clearly concentrates control above the brainstem — the more peripheral in the system, the more generalized will be the effects of a pharmacological intervention. The more central the locus of activity of a drug, the more closely it may mimic the endogenous system. The VWC, on the other hand, has many systems in balance but they are very focused anatomically; they are also very generalized in pharmacological properties — the anatomical location of the tissue provides the major means to produce a distinctive response.

Therefore, drugs that modulate processes in the CNS have a privileged position. An agent with action in the CNS can have the capacity to act at the start of a cascade and thereby control the onset and course of an erection (Fig. 13.1). Despite the fact that less is known about the structure–function relationships in the brain, there are advantages to this as a therapeutic strategy. Drugs acting in small groups of cells in the brain do so to create actions that will be amplified in the usual mode of CNS/peripheral interaction. Neural signals are intrinsically arranged to achieve effects through transduction into effector systems of greater power — a process of amplification that is efficient and often replicated in modern electronics, for example.

Drugs that act in the periphery do so, in general, by acting at endpoint effector sites. They act close to, or through, the mechanisms that actually change blood flow, modifying the tone of vascular walls against transmural forces deriving from pulsatile arterial pressures. Peripheral action restricts the direct influence of an agent to distal or downstream components of the system. Although not clear, feedback or other indirect actions would be very useful in influencing more proximal parts of the erection cascade. Even if this occurs, it is unlikely that this process would replicate the signalling patterns of normal CNS-generated erection. For example, a vasodilator given by ICI will cause local vasodilatation that will spread within the penis by local neural mechanisms and possibly by flow effects. As inflow increases, there may be some flow recruitment of the most distal supplying vessels. However, this sequence is quite different from the normal situation, where a strong coordinated neural signal concomitantly dilates feeder vessels with penile resistance vessels and corporal tissue.

A further ramification of the central/peripheral distinction can be found in the analysis of the clinical response to a drug. In general, normal activation of a system in response to a drug indicates that the system, and other supporting systems, distal to the site of action of the drug is intact. The same cannot be said of a negative or incomplete response. Thus, a failure to respond does not allow the observer to determine where in the complex of systems the remaining, blocking, dysfunction is sited. Drugs with central action have the potential to act as diagnostic agents as well as therapeutic agents. An effective centrally acting drug eliciting a full erectile response provides confirmation of the normality of the entire cascade distal to the site of action. An effective response, once properly documented, investigated and validated could then be used as a diagnostic indicator that agents acting more distally, although effective, may not be needed or justified. The logic of deficit-specific therapy pertains only if the adverse-effect profile and efficacy of the more specific agents lives up to the expectation of being superior. Such diagnostic sophistication also presumes that there will be agents available with robust central activity or deficit-specific action.

A final contrast between central and peripheral agents in ED refers back to the extent to which these agents may overlap in normal pathways. There is some evidence that there are several parallel and interdependent pathways within and leaving the CNS that serve to induce erections. Indeed, it would be illogical to insist on multiple pathways in the periphery ('to preserve procreative function') if this principle were to be abandoned in the CNS. Thus, it is unlikely that all the central processes are funnelled through one privileged but vulnerable neural pathway. There is evidence for a difference between visual-erotic and sexually induced erections.[21] Of interest is whether the recent clinical development of centrally acting dopaminergic compounds such as sublingual apomorphine[22] in man will more closely reproduce nocturnal erections, sexual erections or a component or amalgam of identifiable

pathways. For the moment it will not matter but, as the numbers and varieties of drugs increase the mechanistic details will become more critical in the appropriate selection of a drug for an individual patient.

DIAGNOSTIC STRATEGY BASED ON PHARMACOLOGICAL UNDERSTANDING

The discussion above has laid out many of the theoretical considerations that can go into designing or matching a drug to use in treating ED. The principles that distinguish central and peripheral action are logical, if not absolutely inviolable. For instance, a side effect of most vasoactive agents could be an action on other vessels such as intracerebral vessels (e.g. a headache induced by application of glyceryl trinitrate cream to the penis). These effects could have a positive or negative impact on erectile function via these 'non-specific' effects. However, if the preponderance of erectogenic activity is the result of effects in the penile vasculature at the chosen dose, and there are no other markers of clinically relevant CNS activity, then it is reasonable to define that agent as a peripheral agent.

The Matrix of Treatment Strategies (Table 13.1) has been proposed on the basis of much of the foregoing understanding.[23] The purpose of this classification is to clarify agents in this complex field in a way that has some intuitive logic and facilitates more accurate, or at least appropriate, comparison of therapeutic agents.

The distinction between initiating and conditioning is based as much on time-course issues for drugs as it is on an absolute consideration of mechanism of action. Many scientists are modelling the complex multisystem process as an issue of balance. In a system based on balance, adjustment of the force of action on one side of the

Table 13.1. Matrix of treatment strategies

	Initiator	Conditioner
Central	I	III
Peripheral	II	IV
		Other V

balance, as by the effective action of a drug, will cause the preponderance of effect to shift and other influences having the same direction of action will find their effects enhanced or facilitated. Thus, if penile vasculature is held in a relatively vasoconstricted state by some pathological process, incoming neural traffic trying to initiate an erection is relatively disadvantaged and erections are impaired. A drug that successfully corrects or antagonizes the pathological processes can re-establish the balance and facilitate an effective action of the neural traffic in causing its intended response. Thus, the distinction is with respect to drugs that initiate the neural traffic required for the erection. This class of agents, the prototype of which is apomorphine, are termed initiators (Table 13.2).

It is possible to place most of the therapies that are currently available or contemplated in the Matrix of Treatment Strategies (MATS) with little difficulty (Table 13.3). It is possible that a single drug could be placed in two categories if it were to be designed for use in two different doses and/or routes of delivery.

The MATS clarifies how the current inventory of erectogenic agents can be approached. It suggests strongly that there may be different patients who will be optimally treated by drugs from one class where drugs from another may be ineffective or inappropriate — the early stages of dysfunction-specific therapy. It also logically groups drugs by the type of effect that they should be able to create, so that within-class comparisons, taking account of the different routes of delivery, should be more reasonable than across-class comparisons. It also suggests that, if the drug effects cluster logically around some dysfunction-specific characteristics within a class, then the characteristics of patients themselves within a class may justify certain approaches to assessment as well as treatment. As a hypothetical example, patients requiring central conditioners may have more native erectile function and may be more prone to desire disorders. The instruments used to test drugs, and the endpoints sought, in this class should differ from the instruments and endpoints in, say, a group of men with ED after radical extirpative pelvic surgery.

This is not yet a fine-grained classification but it is a significant conceptual and clinically useful advance over the single mass of ED of mixed and multiple aetiologies — none of which have clear, sustainable, aetiological definitions. The next step will be to go round the cycle with the new generations of drugs and to use them and the responses that they create to define a new diagnostic classification — one based on true aetiology, buttressed by information from dysfunction-specific treatments.

Table 13.2. Definition of classes in the matrix of treatment strategies

Class	Definition
Central initiator (I)	Compounds that have their main site of action in the CNS to activate neural events which result in coordinated signalling that results in the initiation of a penile erection
Peripheral initiator (II)	Compounds that have their main site of action in the periphery to activate events that result in a penile erection
Central conditioner (III)	Compounds that act mainly to improve the internal milieu of the CNS so that penile erection is enabled or enhanced, they do not on their own initiate an erection
Peripheral conditioner (local or systemic) (IV)	Compounds that act mainly to improve the local or systemic internal milieu so that penile erection is enabled or enhanced
Other (V)	Other ways of promoting penile rigidity including devices and surgery

Table 13.3. Examples of compounds that have been used for the treatment of erectile dysfunction classified in the Matrix of Treatment Strategies

	Initiator	Conditioner
Central	Apomorphine MSH analogues	Testosterone
Peripheral	PGE1 VIP+PAP TT, SIN 1, K+	Sildenafil Phentolamine
		Other Prostheses, VED

(MSH, melanocyte-stimulating hormone; PGE1, prostaglandin E1; VIP, vasoactive intestinal polypeptide; PAP, papaverine; TT, triple therapy; SIN 1, an NO donor; K+, potassium channel openers; VED, vacuum erection device.) (From ref. 17 with permission.)

■ CONCLUSIONS

The endpoint of a logical and integrative analysis of the mechanisms of function and dysfunction in ED has been the creation of a simple two-by-two classification — the Matrix of Treatment Strategies. Inherent in that simplification has been the strong identification that central and peripheral processes have very different implications for drug action and delivery. It is becoming apparent that the patients who respond to drugs within a therapeutic class are themselves very different from those responding to drugs in other classes.

An unexpected and useful insight that comes from an examination of how treatments separate out in this classification is that multi-agent therapy can be logically based. Some patients may be tried on several alternative drugs from the same class, and some patients may require agents from two or more classes. In fact, it may become common practice to add peripheral conditioners to central initiators to achieve enhanced responses. Despite attempts at focusing drugs on righting putative deficits in an attempt to make patients functional, the treating professionals will be drawn to combining therapies to create the best effect for their patients.

■ ACKNOWLEDGEMENTS

JH and MA were partially supported in this work by grants from the Kidney Foundation of Canada and the MRC/HRF.

■ REFERENCES

1. Rosen R C, Riley A, Wagner G et al. The international index of erectile function (IIEF): a multidimensional scale for assessment of erectile dysfunction. Urology 1997; 49(6): 822–830

2. Linet O I, Ogrinc F G. Efficacy and safety of intracavernosal alprostadil in men with erectile dysfunction. New Engl J Med 1997; 334(14): 873–877

3. Padma-Nathan H, Hellstrome W J G, Kaiser F E et al. Treatment of men with erectile dysfunction with transurethral alprostadil. New Engl J Med 1997; 336(1): 1–7

4. Goldstein I, Lue T F, Padma-Nathan H et al. Oral sildenafil in the treatment of erectile dysfunction. Sildenafil Study Group. N Engl J Med 1998; 338: 1397–1404

5. Padma-Nathan H, Fromm-Freeck S, Ruff DD et al. Apomorphine SL Study Group. Efficacy and safety of apomorphine SL vs placebo for male erectile dysfunction (MED). J Urol 1998; 159: 241

6. Mair J. Progress in myocardial damage detection: new biochemical markers for clinicians. Crit Rev Clin Lab Sci 1997; 34: 1–66

7. Adams M A, Banting J D, Maurice D H et al. Vascular control mechanisms in penile erection: phylogeny and the inevitability of multiple and overlapping systems. Int J Impot Res 1997; 9: 85–91

8. Pfaus J, Everitt B. In: Kupfer F B A D (ed) Psychopharmacology: the fourth generation of progress. New York: Raven Press, 1995: 743

9. Melis M R, Succu S, Iannucci U, Argiolas A. Prevention by morphine of apomorphine- and oxytocin-induced penile erection and yawning: involvement of nitric oxide. Naunyn Schmiedebergs Arch Pharmacol 1997; 355(5): 595–600

10. Giuliano F A, Rampin O, Benoit G, Jardin A. Neural control of penile erection. Urol Clin North Am 1995; 22: 747–766

11. Rowland D L, Greenleaf W J, Dorfman L J, Davidson J M. Aging and sexual function in men. Arch Sex Behav 1993; 22: 545–557

12. Lavoisier P, Aloui R, Schmidt M H, Watrelot A. Clitoral blood flow increases following vaginal pressure stimulation. Arch Sex Behav 1995; 24(1): 37–45

13. Bird S J, Hanno P M. Bulbocavernosus reflex studies and autonomic testing in the diagnosis of erectile dysfunction. J Neurol Sci 1998, 154: 8–13

14. Rampin O, Giuliano F, Benoit G, Jardin A. [Central nervous system control of erection]. In French. Prog Urol 1997; 7: 17–23

15. Andersson K-E, Holmquist F. Regulation of tone in penile cavernous smooth muscle. Established concepts and new findings. World J Urol 1994; 12: 249–261

16. Heaton J P W, Adams M A, Morales A. A therapeutic taxonomy of treatments for erectile dysfunction: an evolutionary imperative. Int J Impot Res 1997; 9: 115–121

17. Murphy B C, Pienta K J, Coffey D S. Effects of extracellular matrix components and dihydrotestosterone on the structure and function of human prostate cancer cells. Prostate 1992; 20(1): 29–41

18. Garban H, Marquez D, Magee T et al. Cloning of rat and human inducible penile nitric oxide synthase. Application for gene therapy of erectile dysfunction. Biol Reprod 1997; 56(4): 954–963

19. Manabe K, Heaton J P W, Morales A et al. Pre-penile arteries are dominant in the control of penile vascular resistance. J Urol 1998; (in revision)

20. Rajfer J, Aronson W J, Bush P A et al. Nitric oxide as a mediator of relaxation of the corpus cavernosum in response to nonadrenergic, noncholinergic neurotransmission. N Engl J Med 1992; 326(2): 90–94

21. Rousseau L, Dupont A, Labrie F, Couture M. Sexuality changes in prostate cancer patients receiving antihormonal therapy combining the antiandrogen flutamide with medical (LHRH agonist) or surgical castration. Arch Sex Behav 1988; 17(1): 87–98

22. Heaton J P, Morales A, Adams M A et al. Recovery of erectile function by the oral administration of apomorphine. Urology 1995; 45: 200–206

23. Heaton J P W. Neural and pharmacological determinants of erection. Int J Impot Res 1998; 10(suppl. 2): 34–39

Chapter 14
Risk factors for impotence

R. W. Lewis and T. M. Mills

■ INTRODUCTION

The incidence of impotence increases with age.[1] Although age would, at first glance, appear to be a direct risk factor for erectile dysfunction, it is likely that those diseases that are seen more commonly as ageing occurs may actually be the risk factors responsible, as opposed to age itself. Such include vascular insufficiency, hormonal derangement, interruption of neural pathways, diabetes and psychogenic factors.[1] Erectile dysfunction is also clearly associated with many medical disorders that are not necessarily age related. Certain medical diseases such as insulin-dependent diabetes mellitus and chronic renal disease, particularly when associated with dialysis or transplant, have clearly been associated with increased risk for erectile dysfunction. Similarly, some conditions that produce hypogonadism are definite risk factors for erectile dysfunction. Since, erectile function in men is considered to be principally a neuro-hemodynamic event, the presence of cardiovascular disease or certain neurological disorders should be considered risk factors for erectile dysfunction as well. This chapter reviews the literature substantiating risk factors for erectile dysfunction and discusses some risk factors that have less rigorous scientific proof. It is important to remember that a risk factor does not imply cause and effect but implies only an association with impotence.

■ MEDICATION RISK FACTORS FOR ERECTILE DYSFUNCTION

Erectile dysfunction due to prescription medications is under-reported. This topic has been discussed summarily by Lundberg and Biriell.[2] Meinhardt and colleagues recently have reviewed the influence of medication on erectile dysfunction in some detail.[3] In Table 1 from that article, the authors list some 332 medications that have been associated with erectile dysfunction (Table 14.1). Major classes of prescription drugs that are commonly reported to have side effects of erectile dysfunction are psychotrophic drugs, cardiovascular drugs, histamine-2-receptor antagonists, hormones, anticholinergics and certain cytotoxic agents.

Certainly, antihypertensive drugs appear to represent a major risk factor for erectile dysfunction; Lundberg and Biriell report that this is more likely to be noted with alpha- and alpha/beta-blocking agents as well as guanidine derivatives than with calcium-blocking agents, angiotensin-converting enzyme (ACE) inhibitors or diuretics.[2] All antihypertensives are given to lower blood pressure and this action is probably the main reason that these agents lead to erectile dysfunction; however, reported decreases in libido with certain antihypertensives indicate that there may also be a central effect of these medications. On the basis of Lundberg and Biriell's commentary and the article by Meinhardt and colleagues, it would appear that beta-blocking agents, whether non-selective or selective, may be more likely than other antihypertensives to cause erectile dysfunction.[2,3] As suggested by Meinhardt and colleagues, this may be due to the change in balance between alpha and beta sympathetic influence, resulting in insufficient antagonism of alpha-1 vasoconstriction.[3] It has also been suggested that diuretics, particularly thiazide diuretics, are the most common cause of impotence resulting from prescription drugs because of their common usage.[4] Despite the expectations that calcium re-entry blocking drugs would be unlikely to cause erectile dysfunction, Lindberg and Biriell did report them as risk factors,

Table 14.1. Medications* associated with erectile dysfunction

acebutolol	buprenorphine	desmethylimipramine	flurazepam
acetazolamide	buserelin	dexamethasone	fluspirilene
alimemazine	buspirone	dexamphetamine	flutamide
allopurinol	busulphan (busulfan)	(dextroamphetamine)	fluvoxamine
alprazolam	butaperazine	dextromoramide	gemfibrozil
alprenolol	butobarbitone	dextropropoxyphene	gestagenen
alseroxylon	(butobarbital)	diazepam	gestonoron caproate
alufibrate	butizide	dibenzepin	glutethimide
amiloride	camazepam	dichlorphenamide	glycopyrrolate
amiodarone	camylofin	diclofenac	glycopyrronium bromide
amitriptyline	canrenoate-K	dicyclomine	goserelin
amoxapine	captopril	diethylpropion	guanabenz
amphetamine	carazolol	digoxin	guanadrel
anisotropine	carbamazepine	dihydralazine	guanethidine
atenolol	carteolol	dihydroergotamine	guanfacine
atropine	celiprolol	dimenhydrinate	guanidine
aurothioglucose	chlordiazepoxide	diphenhydramine	guanoclor
azathioprine	chloroquine	disopyramide	guanoxan
baclofen	chlorpromazine	disulfiram	haloperidol
bendrofluazide	chlorprothixene	dixyrazine	hexamethonium
(bendroflumethiazide)	chlorphentermine	dosulepin	homatropine
benperidol	chlorthalidone	doxepin	hydantoins
benzatropine	choline theofyllinate	doxylamine	hydralazine
benzbromarone	cimetidine	droperidol	hydrochlorothiazide
benzhexol	cinnarizine	ephedrine	hydrocortisone
benzphetamine	clobazam	enalapril	dimorphone
benztropine	clofibrate	ergotamine	(hydromorphone)
betamethasone	clomipramine	ethionamide	hydroxychloroquine
betaxolol	clonazepam	etofibrate	hydroxyprogesterone
bethanidine	clonidine	famotidine	hydroxyzine
bezafibrate	clopenthixol	felodipine	hyoscyamine
biperiden	clozepam	fenfluramine	imipramine
bisoprolol	cortisol	fenofibrate	indapamide
bopindolol	cortisone acetate	finasteride	indomethacin
bornaprine	cyclobarbitone	flecainide	interferon
bromazepam	(cyclobarbital)	fluanisone	iodide
bromocriptine	cyclobenzaprine	flunarizine	iproniazid
bromperidol	cyclosporin A	flunitrazepam	isocarboxazid
brotizolam	cyproterone	fluocortolone	isoniazid
bumetanide	dantrolene	fluoxetine	isopropamide
bunitrolol	deserpidine	flupentixol	itraconazole
bupranolol	desipramine	fluphenazine	ketamine

*Where UK and US drug names differ, the latter is shown in parentheses.
(Adapted from ref. 3 with permission.)

Table 14.1. (cont'd)

ketanserin	midazolam	phenelzine	rauwolfia
ketazolam	minoxidil	phenmetrazine	reserpine
ketoconazole	moclobemide	(phendimetrazine)	hyoscine (scopolamine)
labetalol	morphine	phenobarbitone	quinalbarbitone
leuprolide	nadolol	(phenobarbital)	(secobarbital)
levomepromazine	naltrexone	phenoxybenzamine	selegiline
lisinopril	naproxen	phenylephrine	simvastatin
lithium	nifedipine	phenytoin	sotalol
lofepramine	nitrazepam	phentermine	spironolactone
lorazepam	nitrendipine	phenylpropanolamine	stilboestrol
lormetazepam	nizatidine	pimozide	(diethylstilbestrol)
loxapine	nordazepam	pindolol	sulpiride
maprotiline	norethandrolone	pipamperone	tamoxifen
mazindol	norethisterone	pipoxolan	temazepam
mebanazine	(norethindrone)	pirenzepine	terazosin
mecamylamine	norlutin	piritramide	testosterone
medroxyprogesterone	nortriptyline	pizotifen	thiabendazole
melperon	oestrogens	poldine	thiazinamium
mepenzolate	omeprazole	polythiazide	thiethylperazine
mepindolol	opipramol	pramiverine	thioridazine
meprobamate	orphenadrine	prazepam	thiothixene
mesoridazine	oxazepam	prazosin	tilidine
mesterolone	oxazolam	prednisolone	timolol
metaclazepam	oxprenolol	prednisone	tranylcypromine
methadilazin	oxybutinin (oxybutynin)	prednylidene	trazodone
methadone	oxycodone	pridinol	triamcinolone
methamphetamine	oxymetazoline	primidone	triazolam
methantheline	oxypertine	probucol	trichlormethiazide
methaqualone	oxyphencyclimine	prochlorperazine	tridihexethyl
methazolamide	oxyphenonium	procyclidine	trifluoperazine
methotrexate	paramethasone	progesterone	trifluperidol
methyldopa	pargyline	proguanil	triflupromazine
methylphenobarbitone	paroxetine	prolonium iodide	trihexyphenidyl
(methylphenobarbital)	penbutolol	promazine	trimeprazine
methylprednisolone	pentazocine	promethazine	trimetaphan
methyltestosterone	pentobarbitone	propafenone	trimipramine
methysergide	(pentobarbital)	propanolol	triptorelin
metipranolol	perazine	propantheline	trospium chloride
metixene	perhexiline	prothipendyl	verapamil
metoclopramide	pericyazine	protionamide	vincristine
metoprolol	perphenazine	protriptyline	vinylbitone (vinylbital)
metronidazole	pethidine (meperidine)	pseudoephedrine	zopiclone
metyrosine	phencyclidine	ramipril	zuclopenthixol
mexiletine	phendimetrazine	ranitidine	

probably due to their action of lowering blood pressure.[2] Reserpine, alpha-methyldopa, and ACE antagonists may be risk factors for erectile dysfunction not only because of their blood-pressure-lowering effect but also because of hormonal influences;[3,4] there may be central effects of these agents as well.[2,4] Every clinician who deals with erectile dysfunction has anecdotal data to suggest that changing the type of antihypertensive for the patient will often reverse erectile dysfunction. Calcium-channel blockers and alpha-adrenergic blockers may, theoretically, be the best alternative therapy when erectile dysfunction results from other antihypertensive agents.

Patients on psychotrophic drugs such as phenothiazine and butyrophenone tranquillizers, antidepressants including tricyclics, monoamine oxidase inhibitors, lithium and fluoxetine (Prozac), benzodiazepines and antipsychotics are definitely at greater risk of erectile dysfunction. An antidepressant that is less likely to cause erectile dysfunction but instead has a risk for priapism is trazodone. This agent might be considered as an alternative antidepressant drug when others produce the side effect of erectile dysfunction.[3] In general, it is suggested that antipsychotics with strong alpha-1 receptor-affinity properties may be the best substitutes when other psychotrophic drugs are associated with erectile dysfunction.

Histamine-2-receptor antagonists have a high risk for causing erectile dysfunction, particularly cimetidine.[2] More modern anti-ulcer drugs do not appear to present the same risk factor. Hormones and enzymes affecting hormones, including estrogens, progesterone, cortico-steroids, cyproterone acetate, flutamide, finasteride, and gonadotrophin-releasing hormone agonists, as well as non-hormonal drugs such as spironolactone and ketoconazole, lower testosterone and thus have a significant risk factor for erectile dysfunction.[3,4] Digoxin may be associated with erectile dysfunction from a hormonal etiology; however it has been suggested recently that the underlying mechanism for digoxin-associated impotence is an inhibition of the Na^+/K^+ ATPase pump.[3,4]

■ DIABETES AS A RISK FACTOR FOR ERECTILE DYSFUNCTION

Erectile dysfunction occurs in at least 50% of men with diabetes mellitus.[4] The onset of impotence occurs at an earlier age in those with diabetes mellitus.[5] In more than 50% of patients with impotence and diabetes, the impotence is noted within ten years of the onset of diabetes;[5] it may present as the first sign of diabetes in 12% of patients.[5] Temporary impotence may be due to poorly controlled diabetes, although this point is debatable.[5] Impotence occurs at an earlier age in type I insulin-dependent diabetic patients than in type II non-insulin-dependent diabetic patients, although impotence probably occurs with equal frequency in the two types.[5] In the Massachusetts Male Ageing Study (MMAS) sample, the age-adjusted probability of complete impotence was three times greater in diabetic patients on treatment than in those without diabetes.[1] Each of the pathological effects of diabetes mellitus on tissue, such as effects on small arteries and arterioles, neurological demyelinization, and sinus smooth-muscle deterioration, has been implicated as the etiological factor associated with the erectile difficulty. It has been reported that diabetic macrovascular complications are related to age, whereas microvascular complications are affected by duration of diabetes and degree of glycemic control.[5] Impotence is present in almost all patients with diabetes who have other manifestations of diabetic neuropathy, such as bladder dysfunction or decreased testicular sensation.[5]

De Tejada and colleagues reported impaired autonomic nerve-mediated and endothelium-dependent relaxation of corporal smooth muscle in diabetic patients while autonomic nerve-mediated contraction was maintained.[6] The longer the duration of diabetes, the less pronounced the neurogenic relaxation; no difference was seen between men who were treated and those who were not treated with insulin, nor were there differences in diabetic patients when controlled for hypertension and smoking. Relaxation was normal in diabetic subjects when induced by endothelium-independent vasodilators, sodium nitroprusside and papaverine.[6] Sullivan and colleagues demonstrated a significant increase in endothelin B (ET-B) receptor-binding sites on the rabbit corpus cavernosum 6 months after the induction of diabetes mellitus by alloxan.[7] They suggested that this could represent a pathophysiological pathway in diabetic erectile dysfunction (upregulation of smooth muscle constriction and initiation of cellular proliferation) or a compensatory response to impaired nitric oxide (NO) or prostacyclin (PGI2) release that had been reported in diabetic animal models.[7] Indeed, plasma concentration of endothelin-1 (ET-1) in peripheral venous blood was significantly increased in non-diabetic and diabetic men with impotence, compared with control men, and also was significantly higher in diabetic patients than in non-diabetic patients.[8]

There is much to be learned about the pathological effects of diabetes on the corporal tissue and, with understanding of these processes, clues to the pathophysiology of erectile dysfunction in the ageing male may be forthcoming. As this is such a prevalent disorder in diabetic men, a major research effort for studying impotence in diabetic patients has recently been announced by the National Institutes of Health.

■ CARDIOVASCULAR DISEASE AS A RISK FACTOR FOR ERECTILE DYSFUNCTION

Vasculogenic impotence can result from a reduction in arterial supply to the penis due to occlusive vascular disease (arteriogenic impotence) and/or due to the inability of the penis to trap by the veno-occlusive mechanism (venous leak). Atherosclerotic plaque formation and the resultant vascular occlusion may result in (1) narrowing of penile and pelvic vessels, (2) vascular damage to erectile and endothelial tissues and (3) a secondary venous leak. Not surprisingly, erectile dysfunction is often associated with known cardiovascular risk factors including ischemic heart disease, hypertension, diabetes mellitus, peripheral vascular disease and hyperlipidemia.[1,9,10] In addition, cardiac surgery may also affect erectile function, although interpretation can be complicated. This is best illustrated by Heaton et al. who focus on the complexity of assessment of pre- and post-surgery in patients undergoing coronary artery bypass graft surgery.[11] The authors draw attention to the psychological factors affecting erection in cardiac patients, such as fear of angina or death during intercourse and concern over wound opening in patients post bypass surgery. In addition, significant physiological effects such as enhanced sympathetic drive observed in congestive heart failure patients or significant coronary artery disease will counteract the localized vasodilatation that is a prerequisite for erection.[11] Not surprisingly, the authors conclude that a prospective study will be required to define more precisely the relationship between cardiovascular risk factors and erectile dysfunction. Even

a relatively simple analysis of the relationship between hypertension and blood pressure showed equivocal results; in a long-term study of several antihypertensive agents, both positive and negative effects on impotence could be observed.[12]

It has become clear over the last twenty years that the major cause of erectile dysfunction in the majority of men presenting with impotence is of arteriogenic origin. In essence the penis is a modified vascular bed and the underlying basis of the dysfunction is an occlusive vascular disorder similar to that observed elsewhere in the vasculature. Information from the general circulation, corporal blood flow and studies on smooth muscle function has greatly increased our understanding of the underlying pathophysiology.

As our knowledge of the underlying etiology of erectile dysfunction increases, it is tempting to speculate that modification of many of the cardiovascular risk factors will be of benefit to the impotent patient. Thus, treatment of hypertension, hyperlipidemia, diabetes mellitus, hyperfibrinogenemia or cessation of smoking may directly or indirectly help to maintain or improve erections and thereby improve quality of life. However, carefully controlled double-blind studies will be required to establish benefit in the use of such strategies in the treatment of impotence.

■ OTHER CHRONIC DISEASE STATES AS RISK FACTORS FOR ERECTILE DYSFUNCTION

While spinal cord injury patients are at increased risk for erectile dysfunction, psychogenic-induced erections are possible in those with lower spinal cord injury and reflexogenic erection remains possible in those with upper cord injury. Chronic neurological diseases correlated with a high risk for impotence include cerebrovascular accidents, temporal lobe epilepsy, multiple sclerosis, Arnold–Chiari syndrome, Guillain–Barré syndrome, autonomic neuropathy associated with AIDS or diabetes mellitus, Alzheimer's disease, tumours and infection.[4] Vardi and others recently reported a 38% coincidence of polyneuropathy and impotence in diabetic and a 10% coincidence rate in non-diabetic patients.[13] The reported prevalence of erectile dysfunction in multiple sclerosis is highly variable but certainly is a concern for almost 40% of the males afflicted with the disease.[14] Impotence is rarely seen early in the disease but generally occurs a decade after disease onset, and there is approximately another 5 years from the time of the first symptom of erectile dysfunction until medical attention is sought.[14] The effect of this disease on erectile function can be predominantly central (psychogenic) or the result of a neurological lesion of the spinal cord. Certain tests, such as monitoring of nocturnal penile tumescence (NPT), often do not clearly distinguish the two.[14]

Men suffering from depression have a greater risk for impotence, which may be related to decreased testosterone level.[1,4] Medications used to treat depression also are a risk factor for impotence, as mentioned above. In the MMAS, the psychological factors strongly associated with impotence include depression, low levels of dominance, and anger, either expressed outward or directed inward.[1]

Chronic renal failure is associated with impotence in up to 40% of those affected.[4] Hyperprolactinemia, hypogonadism, hyperparathyroidism and zinc deficiency have been suggested as etiological factors in the face of renal disease.[4] An excellent review of the hemodyamic pathophysiology in impotence associated with renal failure was prepared in 1994 by Kaufman and associates.[15] In patients with hepatic failure there is an increased risk from impotence, particularly in those with alcoholic cirrhosis.[4]

Chronic obstructive lung disease (perhaps associated with oxygen dependency for nitric oxide synthase) has been implicated as a risk for erectile dysfunction.[16] In fact, three patients in this report by Fletcher and Martin were given home oxygen because of resting or nocturnal hypoxemia and two had improvement of erectile function on therapy.[16]

Other diseases that can account for an increased risk for erectile dysfunction include Peyronie's disease, and other diseases or injury leading to scarring or fibrosis of the tunica albuginea of the corpora, injury to the intracavernosal tissue itself (such as post-priapism seen with sickle-cell disease and other states), chronic brucellosis and other infective or parasitic diseases. The widower's syndrome (unresolved feelings about the death of the first wife) has also been reported to be associated with erectile dysfunction.[4] Scleroderma has been reported as a risk factor for erectile dysfunction, the latter being associated with 12–60% of cases.[17] Impotence has been the presenting symptom of systemic scleroderma in 12–21% of cases.[17]

ENDOCRINE DISORDERS AS A RISK FACTOR FOR ERECTILE DYSFUNCTION

Endocrine disorders commonly associated with impotence include hypopituitarism, prolactin-secreting and non-functioning pituitary tumours, hypo- or hyperthyroidism and hypogonadism.[4] A recent review of the association of androgens and erectile dysfunction put the risk of low androgens in perspective.[18] In the author's experience measurement of free (non-protein-bound) testosterone, or free plus loosely bound testosterone (bioavailable), obtained on at least two different mornings, gives a better indication of hypogonadism than measurement of total testosterone alone. This is a more reliable predictor of response to exogenous testosterone therapy in the patient with partial erectile dysfunction, thus adding some degree of precision to the management of patients with hypogonadism as a risk factor for impotence. This has been substantiated recently by Govier and colleagues.[19] In some patients treated with bromocriptine for prolactin-secreting pituitary tumours, testosterone may not become normal despite the decrease of prolactin to normal levels; testosterone supplementation may also be necessary for these patients.[20]

SURGICAL AND TRAUMATIC RISKS FOR ERECTILE DYSFUNCTION

Surgery or trauma that may affect any level of neurological control of erection or interfere with the arterial supply to the corpora cavernosa are unquestionably risk factors for erectile dysfunction; these include head trauma and brain surgery. Spinal cord injury (as mentioned above), lumbar disc surgery, non-nerve-sparing retroperitoneal lymph node dissection, and abdominal aneurysmectomy all are risk factors for erectile dysfunction.[4] Certainly, pelvic trauma and surgery (particularly radical bowel and genitourinary cancer surgery) are likely to be risk factors for erectile dysfunction. The use of nerve-sparing surgery for radical genitourinary cancer has received impetus for avoiding the high incidence of impotence previously reported from this type of surgery. The variability of the reports of successfully preserving sexual function with the nerve-sparing techniques has been well discussed by Benet and

Melman.[4] Radiation therapy for prostate malignancy is a risk factor for erectile dysfunction; symptoms are usually delayed compared with the immediate presentation of symptoms seen with surgery.[21] Both membranous urethral injury and surgical procedures designed to repair the strictures resulting from such injury are risk factors for erectile dysfunction. Transurethral resection of the prostate (TURP) for benign prostatic hyperplasia and stricture disease have been reported as minor risk factors for erectile dysfunction. However, in a recent excellent prospective study, erectile dysfunction after TURP has been seriously questioned, possibly because previous reports have been tainted by patients equating retrograde ejaculation with erectile dysfunction.[22]

DePalma has recently reviewed the impact of vascular surgery on impotence.[9] Aortic and aorto-inguinal bypass surgery are certainly procedures that carry a risk for the development of erectile dysfunction; however, techniques for aorto-iliac surgery have been improved to lessen this possibility. In some cases, erection was restored in patients who were impotent preoperatively with large-vessel reconstructive procedures; approximately 60% of 23 men obtaining spontaneous erections in that author's own series.[9]

◼ LIFESTYLE-RELATED RISK FACTORS FOR ERECTILE DYSFUNCTION

The use of tobacco is clearly a risk factor for erectile dysfunction;[23] this has been substantiated in animal models.[24,25] Cigarette smoking has been reported as an independent risk factor in the development of atherosclerotic lesions in the internal pudendal and common penile arteries of young impotent men.[10] In the MMAS group of patients, cigarette smoking exacerbated the risks of impotence associated with cardiovascular diseases and medication.[1] In a small group of patients, NPT measurements showed improvement in patients avoiding cigarettes for 24 hours.[26] Another report showed that smoking interfered with the erection response to intracavernosal papaverine injection.[27]

Other lifestyle risk factors for erectile dysfunction that are less well established include chronic alcoholism and the chronic use of marijuana, codeine, meperidine, methadone and heroin.[4] A recent case report describes how a chronic alcoholic, who was suffering from vitamin

B1 deficiency, had a reversal of his erectile dysfunction 2 weeks after receiving daily oral doses of 25 mg thiamine.[28]

Certain sports-related activities such as bicycle riding, gymnastics involving bars or projections on gymnastic equipment, water-ski and water-jet-ski accidents, as well as football-related trauma, which cause site-specific blunt trauma to the perineum, may lead to erectile dysfunction.[29] Reports from the same institution have also recently been published in the lay press suggesting that the current designs of bicycle saddle may be a source of chronic injury to the perineum and thus a risk factor for erectile dysfunction; however, to date this has not been reported in peer-reviewed scientific literature.

◼ REFERENCES

1. Feldman H A, Goldstein I, Hatzichristou D G et al. Impotence and its medical and psychosocial correlates: results of the Massachusetts Male Aging Study. J Urol 1994; 151: 54–61

2. Lundberg P O, Biriell C. Impotence — the drug risk factor. Int J Impot Res 1993; 5: 237–239

3. Meinhardt W, Kropman R F, Vermeij P et al. The influence of medication on erectile function. Int J Impot Res 1997; 9: 17–26

4. Benet A E, Melman A. The epidemiology of erectile dysfunction. Urol Clin North Am 1995; 22: 699–709

5. Whitehead E D, Klyde B J. Diabetes-related impotence in the elderly. Clin Geriatr Med 1990; 6: 771–795

6. Saenz de Tejada I, Goldstein I, Azadzoi K et al. Impaired neurogenic and endothelium-mediated relaxation of penile smooth muscle from diabetic men with impotence. N Engl J Med 1989; 320: 1025–1030

7. Sullivan M E, Dashwood M R, Thompson C S et al. Alterations in endothelin B receptor sites in cavernosal tissue of diabetic rabbits: potential relevance to the pathogenesis of erectile dysfunction. J Urol 1997; 158: 1966–1972

8. Francavilla S, Properzi G, Bellini C et al. Endothelin-1 in diabetic and non-diabetic men with erectile dysfunction. J Urol 1997; 158: 1770–1774

9. DePalma R G. Vascular surgery for impotence: a review. Int J Impot Res 1997; 9: 61–67

10. Rosen M P, Greenfield A J, Walker T G et al. Cigarette smoking: an independent risk factor for atherosclerosis in the hypogastric–cavernous arterial bed of men with arteriogenic impotence. J Urol 1991; 145: 759–763

11. Heaton J P W, Evans H, Adams M A et al. Coronary artery graft surgery and its impact on erectile dysfunction: a preliminary retrospective study. Int J Impot Res 1996; 8: 35–39

12. Grimm R H, Granditis G A, Pineas R J et al. Long-term effects on sexual function of five antihypertensive drugs and nutritional hygenic treatment in hypertensive men and women. Hypertension 1997; 29: 8–14

13. Vardi Y, Sprecher E, Kanter Y et al. Polyneuropathy in impotence. Int J Impot Res 1996; 8: 65–68

14. Staerman F, Guiraud P, Coeurdacier P et al. Value of nocturnal penile tumescence and rigidity (NPTR) recording in impotence patients with multiple sclerosis. Int J Impot Res 1996; 8: 241–245

15. Kaufman J M, Hatzichristou D G, Mulhall J P et al. Impotence and chronic renal failure: a study of the hemodynamic pathophysiology. J Urol 1994; 151: 612–618

16. Fletcher E C, Martin R J. Sexual dysfunction and erectile impotence in chronic obstructive pulmonary disease. Chest 1982; 81: 413–421

17. Nehra A, Hall S J, Basile G et al. Systemic sclerosis and impotence: a clinicopathological correlation. J Urol 1995; 153: 1140–1146

18. Mills T M, Reilly C M, Lewis R W. Androgens and penile erection: a review. J Androl 1996; 17: 633–638

19. Govier F E, McClure R D, Kramer-Levien D. Endocrine screening for sexual dysfunction using free testosterone determinations. J Urol 1996; 156: 405–408

20. Leonard M P, Nickel C J, Morales A. Hyperprolactinemia and impotence: why, when and how to investigate. J Urol 1989; 142: 992–994

21. Goldstein I, Feldman M I, Deckers P J et al. Radiation-associated impotence. A clinical study of its mechanism. JAMA 1984; 251: 903–910

22. Soderdahl D W, Knight R W, Hansberry K L. Erectile dysfunction following transurethral resection of the prostate. J Urol 1996; 156: 1354–1356

23. Condra M, Surridge D H, Morales A et al. Prevalence and significance of tobacco smoking in impotence. Urology 1986; 27: 495–498

24. Juenemann K-P, Lue T F, Luo J-N et al. The effect of cigarette smoking on penile erection. J Urol 1987; 138: 438–441

25. Xie Y, Garban H, Ng C et al. Effect of long term passive smoking on erectile function and penile nitric oxide synthase in the rat. J Urol 1997; 157: 1121–1126

26. Guay A, Heatley G. Cessation of smoking produces rapid improvement in erectile function. J Androl (21st Annual Meeting Program) 1996; abstract 068: 39

27. Glina S, Reichelt A C, Puech Leao P, Marcondes dos Reis J M S. Impact of cigarette smoking on papaverine-induced erection. J Urol 1988; 140: 523–524

28. Tjandra B S, Janknegt R A. Neurogenic impotence and lower urinary tract symptoms due to vitamin B1 deficiency in chronic alcoholism. J Urol 1997; 157: 954–955

29. Munarriz R M, Yan R Q, Nehra A et al. Blunt trauma: the pathophysiology of hemodynamic injury leading to erectile dysfunction. J Urol 1995; 153: 1831–1840

Iatrogenic erectile dysfunction: pharmacological and surgical therapies that alter male sexual behaviour and erectile performance

G. A. Broderick and M. M. Foreman

■ INTRODUCTION

Until recently, iatrogenic sexual dysfunction was rarely listed with drug precautions; such effects were considered to be unfortunate, but predictable, complications of pelvic surgery, especially of that for malignancy. Although these effects were viewed as relatively unimportant compared with the primary therapeutic benefits, actual or anticipated male sexual dysfunction caused patient non-compliance with drug therapies and reluctance to undergo surgical procedures. These events produced significant changes in pharmaceutical marketing, research and clinical practice. First, the limited profitability of drug therapies that produced sexual disorders led to an appreciation of quality-of-life issues. This, in turn, led to the development of new drug therapies with fewer side effects. The identification of sexual side effects of drugs in humans, coupled with concomitant characterization in animals, provided a foundation for pharmacological strategies to treat sexual disorders. Judicious exploitation of side effects (e.g. drug-induced anorgasmia) is being employed to treat different types of sexual complaints, such as premature ejaculation. Finally, within the urologic community, patients' complaints generated an increased interest in the neuro-urological mechanisms regulating sexual response in the male. Subsequently, anatomical refinements in surgical procedures dramatically reduced the risks of postoperative male sexual dysfunction. This overview provides examples of iatrogenic sexual dysfunction associated with drug treatments and surgical procedures.

■ CLASSIFYING DRUG-INDUCED SEXUAL DISORDERS

Drug-induced effects include changes in the behavioural, erectile and ejaculatory functions, each of which are segments of a sequential response cascade.[1–3] The incidence and type of sexual side effects elicited by drugs depend on pharmacological, therapeutic and patient response variables: the pharmacological variables include the biological effects of the drug; the therapeutic variables include dosage and duration of therapy; the patient variables include the pharmacological sensitivity of the selected patient population and the predisposition of the patient to sexual response disorders. When considering the adverse effects of pharmacotherapies it must be acknowledged that the majority of men in the United States complaining of sexual dysfunction are aged 65 years or older. The ratio of organic to psychological male sexual dysfunction is directly proportional to age, with the estimate that 85% of men over the age of 50 complaining of sexual dysfunction have some organic basis for complaints. Diabetes, hypertension and atherosclerosis should each be regarded as modifiable para-ageing phenomena that affect normal sexual function and sensitivity to iatrogenic sexual dysfunction. Unfortunately, most of the clinical information about sexual side effects of drug therapy is derived from case reports or the incidence of sexual disorders in trials, and baseline sexual function is never established. The list of sexual side effects in this review represents a summary of these observations (Table 15.1).

Table 15.1. Reported sexual side effects of drugs

Drug type	Sexual side-effects reported* On libido	On erection	On ejaculation
Sympatholytics			
Bethanidine	Suppression	Suppression	Suppression
Debrisoquine	Suppression	Suppression	Suppression
Guanethidine	Suppression	Suppression	Suppression
Guanadrel	Suppression	Suppression	Suppression
Alpha-methyldopa	Suppression	Suppression	Suppression
Reserpine	Suppression	Suppression	Suppression
Adrenergic			
Alpha-1 agonists			Enhancement
Ephedrine			Enhancement
Phenylpropanolamine			Enhancement
Pseudoephedrine			Enhancement
Alpha-2 agonists			
Clonidine	Suppression	Suppression	
Alpha-1 antagonists			
Phenoxybenzamine		Mixed	Suppression
Phentolamine		Mixed	Suppression
Prazosin		Mixed	Suppression
Alpha-2 antagonists			
Yohimbine	Enhancement	Enhancement	
Beta-adrenergic antagonists			
Atenolol		Suppression	
Labetalol		Suppression	Suppression
Metoprolol	Suppression	Suppression	
Oxyprenolol	Suppression	Suppression	
Pindolol		Suppression	
Propranolol	Suppression	Suppression	Suppression
Timolol	Suppression	Suppression	
Diuretics			
Acetazolamide		Suppression	
Amiloride	Suppression	Suppression	
Bendroflumethiazide		Suppression	
Chlorthalidone	Suppression	Suppression	
Dichlorphenamide	Suppression	Suppression	
Methazolamide	Suppression	Suppression	
Spironolactone	Suppression	Suppression	

Table 15.1. (cont'd)

Drug type	Sexual side-effects reported*		
	On libido	On erection	On ejaculation
Parkinsonian drugs			
Apomorphine	Enhancement	Enhancement	
Bromocriptine	Enhancement	Enhancement	
Deprenyl	Enhancement		
L-Dopa	Enhancement	Enhancement	Enhancement
Lisuride	Enhancement	Enhancement	
Pergolide	Enhancement	Enhancement	Enhancement
Anticholinergics			
Anisotropine		Suppression	
Clidinium		Suppression	
Dicyclomine		Suppression	
Glycopyrrolate		Suppression	
Hexocyclium		Suppression	
Homatropine		Suppression	
Mepenzolate		Suppression	
Methantheline		Suppression	
Oxybutinin		Suppression	
Propantheline		Suppression	
Tridihexethyl		Suppression	
Antipsychotics			
Benperidol	Suppression	Suppression	
Butaperazine	Suppression	Suppression	Suppression
Chlorpromazine	Suppression	Suppression	Suppression
Chlorprothixene	Suppression	Suppression	Suppression
Fluphenazine	Suppression	Suppression	Suppression
Haloperidol	Suppression	Suppression	
Mesoridazine	Suppression	Suppression	
Molidone		Priapism	
Perphenazine	Suppression	Suppression	Suppression
Pimozide	Suppression	Suppression	Suppression
Sulpiride	Suppression	Suppression	
Thiothixene	Suppression	Suppression	
Thioridiazine	Suppression	Suppression	Suppression
Trifluoperazine	Suppression	Suppression	Suppression

*Suppression, mixed and enhancement, indicate the types of disorders reported. †(Priapism) denotes an infrequent observation of sustained erection. (Data from refs. 4–8, 10–12 and 15.)

Table 15.1. (cont'd)

Drug type	Sexual side-effects reported*		
	On libido	On erection	On ejaculation
Anxiolytics			
Benzodiazepines			
Alprazolam			
Chlordiazdepoxide			Suppression
Diazepam			Suppression
Flurazepam	Enhancement		
Lorazepam			Suppression
Azapirone			
Buspirone	Enhancement	Enhancement	Enhancement
Antidepressants			
Tricyclic antidepressants			
Amitriptyline	Suppression	Suppression	Suppression
Amoxapine	Suppression	Suppression	Suppression
Clomipramine	Suppression	Suppression	Suppression
Desipramine			
Imipramine	Suppression	Suppression	Suppression
Maprotiline	Suppression	Suppression	Suppression
Nortriptyline	Suppression	Suppression	Suppression
Protriptyline	Suppression	Suppression	Suppression
MAO-inhibitors			
Iproniazid		Suppression	Suppression
Isocarboxazid		Suppression	
Mebanazine			Suppression
Pargyline		Suppression	Suppression
Phenelzine	Enhancement	Suppression	Suppression
Transcypromine	Enhancement		
Trazodone	Enhancement	Enhancement	Enhancement
5HT uptake inhibitors			
Fluoxetine	Suppression	Suppression	Suppression
Paroxetine	Suppression	Suppression	Suppression
Sertraline	Suppression	Suppression	Suppression
NE uptake inhibitors			
Viloxazine	Enhancement		
DA uptake inhibitors			
Bupropion	Enhancement		
Nomifensine	Enhancement		
Lithium	Suppression	Suppression	

Table 15.1. (cont'd)

Drug type	Sexual side-effects reported*		
	On libido	On erection	On ejaculation
Opioid agonist			
Methadone	Suppression	Suppression	Suppression
Opioid antagonists			
Naloxone		Enhancement	
Naltrexone		Enhancement	
Endocrine therapies			
Oestrogen			
Ethinyl oestradiol	Suppression		
Androgen			
Methandrostenenolone	Suppression		
Norethandrolone	Suppression		
Progestin			
Hydroxyprogesterone	Suppression	Suppression	
Medrogesterone	Suppression		
Medroxyprogesterone	Suppression		
Progesterone	Suppression	Suppression	
Anti-androgen			
Cyproterone acetate	Suppression		
Miscellaneous			
Amphetamine		Suppression	Suppression
Baclofen		Suppression	Suppression
Barbiturates	Suppression/?	Suppression	
Cimetidine	Suppression	Suppression	
Clofibrate	Suppression	Suppression	
Digoxin	Suppression	Suppression	
Disopyramide	Suppression	Suppression	
Disulfiram		Suppression	
Ethosuximide	Suppression		
Fenfluramine	Suppression	Suppression	
Heparin		(Priapism)[†]	
Hydralazine		Suppression?	
Metoclopramide	Suppression	Suppression	
Naproxen			Suppression
Nifedipine		Mixed	
Phenytoin	Suppression	Suppression	
Primadone	Suppression	Suppression	
Verapamil		Mixed	

*Suppression, mixed and enhancement, indicate the types of disorders reported. [†](Priapism) denotes an infrequent observation of sustained erection. (Data from refs. 4–8, 10–12 and 15.)

There are several classification schemes for grouping drugs with sexual side effects. The most common has been categorization by therapeutic indication, for example antihypertensives, antidepressants and anti-androgens.[4–7] However, therapeutic indications do not necessarily describe the mechanism or site of action of the iatrogenic effects, with the exception of androgen blockers. An alternative scheme is to segregate drugs by their mechanisms of action on the sexual response cascade: interest → performance → satisfaction.[8] Since this classification is the same as that used for designing new drugs to alleviate sexual disorders, it provides a link between preclinical studies that explore the origins of male sexual function and clinical studies that exploit novel or existing pharmacological preparations for the treatment of sexual interest, performance and satisfaction.[9,10] The subdivisions of this classification scheme include: a central behavioural component, a central–spinal reflex component and an end-organ component. Drugs are also segregated by effect, as psychopharmacological, neuropharmacological and smooth muscle or vascular drugs.[9]

DRUG-INDUCED EFFECTS ON THE BEHAVIOURAL COMPONENT OF SEXUAL RESPONSE

The behavioural component of sexual response encompasses the integration of sensory inputs with cognitive, emotional and desire components for the initiation and maintenance of sexual drive.[10–12] These agents are often separated into psychopharmacological drugs and neuropharmacological drugs; however, the distinction between psychopharmacological and neuropharmacological is ambiguous, because specific neural pathways of human male sexual function have not been completely identified and psychotropic effects could influence any aspect of the neural integration. The most obvious effects noted by the patient and the clinician are those on general behavioural or specific sexual behaviour. Drugs with general sedative effects that can alter sexual behaviour include antihypertensives, anticonvulsants, hypnotics, anorexics, antidepressants, antipsychotics and anxiolytics.[8,11]

Direct effects on sexual behaviour occur through effects on the brain areas responsible for regulating sexual drive. These areas include the medial pre-optic area (MPOA) of the ventral diencephalon, the mesencephalic central grey nucleus, the amygdala and the hippocampus.[1,10,13] These areas, particularly the MPOA, are thought to be responsible for sexual drive and emotional control of peripheral sexual reflexes. Pharmacological and histochemical studies have identified a variety of receptor subtypes in the MPOA, including peptidergic, cholinergic, dopaminergic, adrenergic and serotonergic receptors, and receptors for reproductive hormones.[10,13–16] Among these receptors, monoaminergic and hormonal receptors have been the most extensively studied.

Sexual dimorphism of the central nervous system (CNS) is regulated by foetal and neonatal levels of circulating androgens and oestrogens: sexual behaviour can be altered by changes in the MPOA induced by supplementation or denial of sex steroids. Yet, in adults, there is poor correlation between circulating testosterone levels and measures of sexual interest, activity or erectile function. Among geriatric patients, the complaint of impotence and the incidence of hypogonadism are statistically independent.[17,17a] Not surprisingly, endocrinopathy as the cause of impotence is variable, from 1 to 35%.[18] Despite routine endocrine screening in the evaluation of male sexual dysfunction, the exact role of androgen levels in erectile dysfunction has remained elusive: for example, prepubertal boys have reflexogenic and castrate men can have psycho-erotic erections.[19]

With castration, sexual function may range from a complete loss of libido to continued normal sexual activity. Spontaneous nocturnal erections are androgen dependent. Erections in response to visual erotic stimuli, on the other hand, appear independent of androgens. Rousseau followed prostate cancer patients treated with either bilateral orchiectomy or flutamide/leuprolide and reported preservation of erection in 20%.[20] Drugs with anti-androgenic activity — such as cyproterone acetate, flutamide, finasteride and cimetidine — will decrease libido and erectile dysfunction.[1,7] The luteinizing-hormone-releasing hormone (LHRH) agonists leuprolide acetate and goserelin rapidly induce hypogonadal levels of testosterone. Each of these will yield variable rates of decreased libido and erectile dysfunction.[7] Sexual dysfunction is also associated with the antihypertensive agent spironolactone, which has anti-androgenic activity and also suppresses the synthesis of androgens.

Another consequence of pharmacological or surgical castration is hot flushes, which occur in the majority of patients (77 and 58%, respectively). The physiology is poorly understood, but is believed to be related to changes in the hypothalamus which is in proximity to the thermoregulatory system. A decrease in intrahypothalamic endogenous opioids and an increase in the concentration of catecholamines has been associated with menopausal hot flushes.[21,22] In men, the vasomotor instability is marked by a reddening of the skin, sweating, an increased sensation of temperature and sometimes a sense of foreboding or doom; episodes may occur from seven to 50 times per week. Therapies have included 1 mg stilboestrol (diethylstilbestrol; DES) daily; phenobarbitone (phenobarbital) and ergotamine (one tablet each); clonidine 1 mg daily, megestrol acetate 20 mg twice a day. In a review of side effects following hormonal ablation for prostate cancer, Kirschenbaum concluded that megestrol acetate was the optimal therapy.[23] Furthermore, drugs that decrease dopaminergic receptor activity (antipsychotics or catecholamine-depleting agents) may suppress sexual function through the induction of hyperprolactinaemia.

Dopaminergic mechanisms

One of the milestone observations on the psycho-pharmacological control of sexual response was the finding of increased libido in parkinsonian, psychiatric and impotent patients receiving the catecholamine precursor L-dopa.[24–28] In laboratory animals and patient populations, similar effects were also observed with deprenyl (a monoamine oxidase B inhibitor), cocaine (a catecholamine re-uptake inhibitor) and amphetamine (a catecholamine-releasing agent).[7,11,12,14,29,30] In contrast to these stimulatory effects, suppression of sexual behaviour in animals and libido in patients has been reported with reserpine and alpha-methyldopa, which deplete functional pools of catecholamines in neurons.[13,12] These results suggest the involvement of dopaminergic and/or adrenergic receptors in the central regulation of sexual drive.

The theory of dopaminergic receptor involvement is further supported by the observations of increased libido in patients treated with dopamine agonists (apomorphine and pergolide) and dopamine re-uptake inhibitors (nomifensine and bupropion).[31–35] In animal studies, activation of D2 or D3 dopaminergic receptors by systemic administration of the agonists apomorphine or quinelorane increases sexual behaviour in rats at doses that do not affect prolactin secretion or elicit other responses.[36] In contrast to dopaminergic agonists, dopaminergic antagonists (antipsychotics) suppress sexual drive in both patients and animals.[1,7,11] In addition to the effects on central and peripheral neuronal function, dopaminergic antagonists can also suppress sexual responses through the induction of hyperprolactinaemia and secondary hypogonadism. Currently, bromocriptine is the only dopaminergic agonist approved for treating erectile disorders, but only for hyperprolactinaemia-induced dysfunction.

Adrenergic mechanisms

Adrenergic receptors have important roles in the central control of sexual response. Amplification of noradrenergic transmission with a selective noradrenaline re-uptake inhibitor, viloxazine, markedly increased libido in depressed patients.[11,37] These effects did not correlate with the antidepressant activity of this compound. There have been a few clinical reports of decreased libido with alpha-1-adrenergic antagonists (prazosin and phenoxybenzamine), alpha-2-adrenergic agonists (clonidine) or beta-adrenergic antagonists (propranolol).[11] The reports match animal investigations in males with either prazosin or clonidine suppressing mating behaviour and yohimbine, an alpha-2-adrenergic antagonist, increasing sexual behaviour.[38–40] The psycho-pharmacological effects of yohimbine may, in part, be responsible for its reported efficacy in the treatment of subgroups of patients with erectile dysfunction.[41–43] The stimulatory effect of yohimbine has recently been used to counteract the sexual disorders induced by serotonin re-uptake inhibitors (SRIs, see below).[44] From these discoveries, other preclinical candidates that alter central adrenergic activity are being evaluated.[45,46]

Serotonergic mechanisms

With the recent success of SRIs and other newly developed serotonergic drugs, knowledge both of the sexual side effects and of new uses of these agents has rapidly expanded. In preclinical studies, suppression of sexual behaviour and subsequently of erectile and ejaculatory response has been demonstrated, with direct or indirect augmentation of central serotonin activity with 5HT (5-hydroxytryptamine, serotonin) loading, uptake inhibitors (SRIs), releasing agents or postsynaptic agonists.[14,47] These effects correlated with reports of suppressed libido and anorgasmia in patients treated with the 5HT-releasing agent fenfluramine and various other SRIs.[48–50] The effects of SRIs in prolonging the latency of the ejaculatory reflex in animals and men has been sufficiently reproduced to be proposed as a therapy for premature ejaculation.

Serotonin may have both facilitating and inhibiting effects on sexual behaviour, depending on the receptor subtype, location of receptors and species examined. 5HT1A agonists can inhibit erection and promote ejaculation; 5HT1C agonists promote erection; 5HT2 agonists both inhibit and facilitate various aspects of sexual behaviour. 5HT1A autoreceptor agonists, such as buspirone, increase sexual behaviour in male rats and rhesus monkeys.[51–54] These studies correlate with the clinical findings on buspirone. In one human trial, buspirone increased libido and other sexual responses in male and female patients with generalized anxiety disorders.[55] Several more selective and potent 5HT1A agonists have been reported to have robust effects on sexual performance and may become clinical candidates.[52,56–58] In addition to 5HT1A autoreceptor agonists, postsynaptic 5HT2 receptor antagonists augment sexual behaviour and indirectly enhance peripheral sexual reflexes.[16,47,59] These laboratory studies suggest that 5HT2 receptor antagonism can contribute to the enhanced libido and erectile response noted in clinical studies with trazodone.[60,61]

■ DRUG-INDUCED EFFECTS ON ERECTILE REFLEXES

In addition to their effects on the diencephalic areas involved in sexual regulation, drugs can also suppress or induce the erectile reflex through actions on sites in the brain stem and spinal cord that regulate the autonomic control of erection.[10] These drug-induced disorders of the erectile reflex include failure to initiate, failure to maintain, spontaneous erections unaccompanied by interest, and priapism.

Dopaminergic mechanisms

Dopaminergic agents also affect erectile responses in men and laboratory animals without changing sexual behaviour, presumably by altering reflex pathways. Spontaneous erections were first noted as side effects in patients treated with L-dopa or dopaminergic agonists.[24,34] Recently, subcutaneously administered apomorphine has been shown to induce penile erections in normal volunteers and patients. Apomorphine induces yawning,

stereotypical sexual behaviour and erections in rodents. Erections have been induced in 67% of psychogenically impotent patients in one series; dosage-related nausea and vomiting have been a problem with both subcutaneous and oral formulations. Presumably, patients must have an intact end organ (non-vasculogenic erectile dysfunction) to respond to apomorphine.[32,62–65] The response to dopaminergic receptor stimulation with apomorphine is not accompanied by increases in libido.[62] Although erections have been noted as side effects of oral dopaminergic agonist therapy, the incidence of this response appears to be far greater with subcutaneous administration. In parallel to these clinical studies, dopaminergic agonist-induced erections have also been observed in rats and rhesus monkeys.[52,66–68] In contrast to agonists, erectile dysfunction is a reported side effect of drugs with dopaminergic antagonist activity.[7,12]

Serotonergic mechanisms

Unlike dopamine, serotonin appears to have different effects on the central and peripheral components of the sexual response. Amplification of serotonergic activity through the administration of serotonin-releasing agents or agonists also induces spontaneous erections in rats and rhesus monkeys.[69,70] In contrast, in humans SRIs result in sexual effects that are primarily suppressive, although case reports of improvements in erectile function have been published.[71,72] The erectogenic effects of serotonin have been proposed to be mediated by the 5HTC receptor subtype.[10,69] These effects may contribute to the induction of priapism in patients treated with the antidepressant trazodone and to the increase in erectile activity during rapid eye movement (REM) sleep.[64,73,73a,40] The primary trazodone metabolite *meta*-chlorophenyl piperazine (mCPP) is a serotonergic agonist that induces erections in rats and rhesus monkeys and selectively increases the firing rate of the penile nerve and cavernosal blood pressure in rats.[69,70,74] These studies indicate that a serotonergic agonist could be useful for erectile dysfunction, particularly if drugs with appropriate receptor specificity can be developed. Again, it must be emphasized that serotonin has both facilitating and inhibiting effects on sexual behaviour, depending on the receptor subtype, location of receptors and species being tested.

Major roles for opioid receptors have been proposed, based on a variety of laboratory and clinical studies.[15,75,75a] The loss of the ability to achieve or maintain erection has been a noted side effect in heroin- and methadone-addicted patients.[7,12,15] Decreased sexual desire was also noted in many of these patients, suggesting a CNS-depressant effect. Spontaneous erections are reported side effects during treatment with the opiate antagonists naloxone and naltrexone in heroin- or methadone-addicted patients. In a single-blind study with impotent patients, naltrexone produced significant increases compared with placebo in both sexual performance and the number of morning and spontaneous erections; improved sexual performance was reported in 11 of 15 patients with psychogenic impotence.[76] In an uncontrolled study, six of seven idiopathic impotent patients were restored to full erectile function with naltrexone therapy.[77] Naloxone has also been reported to induce full erections lasting an hour in normal volunteers when combined with yohimbine, presumably through the additive effects of these agents on sexual response.[78]

Until recently, iatrogenic erectile dysfunction associated with anticholinergic drugs was thought to be mediated exclusively through a vascular pharmacological mechanism. In this mechanism, anticholinergic drugs block the effects of parasympathetic-induced release of endothelial cell-derived relaxation factors (nitric oxide) that relax the cavernosal smooth muscle.[79,80] However, Maeda and co-workers (1994) recently discovered that muscarinic agonists induce erections in rats through effects on a hippocampal–spinal pathway.[81] According to this novel theory, cholinergic, serotonergic and dopaminergic pathways are linked in a central neuropharmacological control of the erectile reflex response. Regardless of the mechanism, blockade of muscarinic receptors appears to be responsible for the reported erectile failures associated with drugs such as imipramine and other tricyclic antidepressants.[1,6,7,12] The best evidence for this was the discovery that bethanechol could reverse erectile failure due to these drugs.[82]

Drug therapies that alter sympathetic neural activity also are associated with erectile disorders. The maintenance of the penis in a flaccid condition is dependent upon a continuous stimulation of alpha-1-adrenergic receptors on the smooth muscle of the corpora cavernosa through the tonic release of noradrenaline from sympathetic terminals. It has been proposed that the sinusoidal endothelium also contributes to the maintenance of tone (flaccidity) by synthesis and release of endothelins. Drug regimens that increase peripheral adrenergic tone have been reported to cause erectile failure, whereas those that decrease postsynaptic alpha-1-adrenergic receptor activity are associated with reports of priapism.[6] Chronic treatments with amphetamine and cocaine, which indirectly increase alpha-1-adrenergic receptor activity, have been associated with the side effect of erectile failure. In contrast, a variety of drugs with alpha-1-adrenergic antagonist activity, as is the case with some antihypertensives and antipsychotics, have been reported to cause priapism. The priapism associated with trazodone has also been theorized to be mediated through its alpha-1-adrenergic antagonist activity.[73] This mechanism may explain the sporadic observation of priapism with drugs possessing alpha-1-adrenergic antagonist activity.[6] These effects also justify the current evaluations of oral alpha-1-adrenergic antagonists for erectile disorders.

Pharmacological studies in vitro on corporal smooth muscle have provided evidence that many new vascular therapies have erectogenic effects.[83–85] Since the inadvertent discovery that hypogastric arterial infusion of papaverine induces erection, these agents have been clinically exploited in pharmacological erection programmes.[86] The erectile reflex has been modulated at the level of the end organ by intracavernous injection, and by topical or urethral agents. The most efficacious corporal relaxants act by increasing corporal smooth muscle levels of cyclic adenosine monophosphate (cAMP) (e.g. prostaglandin E1; PGE1), cyclic guanosine monophosphate (cGMP) (e.g. nitric oxide releasers), or cAMP and cGMP (papaverine and other phosphodiesterase inhibitors).[80,84]

▉ DRUG-INDUCED EFFECTS ON EJACULATORY REFLEX CONTROL

The ejaculatory-phase events include the induction of seminal emission, ejaculation and perceptual changes associated with orgasm.[1] Agents that alter the ejaculatory phase may do so directly by affecting performance, or indirectly by affecting sexual satisfaction. The predominant drug-induced disorders of this phase include delayed or absent ejaculation, retrograde ejaculation and suppressed seminal emission.[75] These side effects are associated with agents that alter the central or peripheral components of the seminal emission–ejaculation reflex. As in the case of the behavioural and erectile phases, drugs that affect dopaminergic or serotonergic receptor activity are thought to modulate the central component of the ejaculatory reflex.[12]

In laboratory animals, pharmacological agents that increase dopaminergic receptor activity shorten ejaculatory latency and induce seminal emission in normal animals and restore ejaculatory capacity to dysfunctional animals.[14,36] Examples of such agents include L-dopa, deprenyl and dopaminergic agonists.[4,14,29,30] Conversely, agents that decrease dopaminergic activity (antagonists) increase ejaculatory latency and reduce ejaculatory capacity.[14,87] The clinical correlates include premature seminal emission or ejaculation in parkinsonian patients treated with L-dopa or pergolide, and delayed or absent ejaculation in patients treated with antipsychotics.[12,24,34] A practical application of this latter side effect has been the use of low-dose therapies of thioridazine or metoclopramide to treat premature ejaculation.[12,87]

The effects of serotonergic agents on ejaculatory reflexes in laboratory animals have been more controversial. In experiments with mating animals, pharmacological agents that increase release or inhibit synaptic uptake of 5HT or directly stimulate postsynaptic 5HT receptors have been shown to delay or suppress ejaculatory responses.[10] Agents that decrease serotonergic activity, such as serotonergic neurotoxins or antagonists, have the opposite effects. However, serotonergic agonists and releasing agents can also induce spontaneous ejaculation in animals.[88,89] In clinical studies with SRIs, protracted ejaculatory latencies in patients were so reproducible that these agents were employed as treatments for premature ejaculation.[49,90] Other antidepressants that inhibit 5HT uptake, e.g. tricyclic antidepressants, also produce these side effects.[12,91] These clinical effects appear to correlate to the effects observed in animals during mating conditions. Further, anorgasmia induced by tricyclic antidepressants and monoamine oxidase inhibitors (which suppress metabolism of 5HT) can be reversed by the administration of a serotonergic antagonist, cyproheptadine.[12]

As seminal emission and antegrade ejaculation are processes that are primarily controlled by sympathetic activity, pharmacological agents that deplete functional pools of catecholamines or have alpha-1-adrenergic antagonist activity are known to suppress ejaculatory capacity and induce retrograde ejaculation.[6,11,75] The agents that diminish presynaptic noradrenaline release include reserpine, alpha-methyldopa, guanethidine, guanadrel, bethanidine and derisoquine. Other drugs associated with this side effect have significant alpha-1-adrenergic antagonist activity: these include the antihypertensives phenoxybenzamine, phentolamine, prazosin and tamsulosin, and the antipsychotics thioridazine, chlorpromazine, triflupromazine and mesoridazine. In contrast to the effects of alpha-1-adrenergic antagonists, sympathomimetic agents such as pseudoephedrine, ephedrine and phenylpropanolamine have been used to treat retrograde ejaculation.[75]

■ SURGICAL MORBIDITY

Contemporary appreciation of the anatomy, ultrastructure and haemodynamics of erection have resulted in refinements of urosurgical technique that have decreased sexual morbidity following procedures for both benign and malignant disease. The majority of studies examine sexual morbidity following surgical therapy for pelvic malignancies; few have examined the impact of radiation or chemotherapy. These surgical series have been criticized for lack of comparative testing before and after operation, for significant disparity between objective reports of potency and subjective reports of coital frequency, and for failure to account for the impact of preoperative medical risk factors for impotence (age, hypertension, diabetes mellitus, vascular disease, hyperlipidaemia, alcohol/nicotine consumption). As preoperative levels of sexual activity are important predictors of sexual adjustment to surgery, normative data on the patient population undergoing operation are essential.

The current estimate of the number of men in the United States with complete erectile dysfunction is 10–20 million; when partial erectile dysfunction is included, the estimate jumps to a total of 30 million. The majority of these men are 65 years of age or older. The age-specific prevalence of male sexual dysfunction is 5% at the age of 40, increasing to 15–25% by the age of 65.[92] Weekly coitus is reported among 37% of patients aged 61–65 years and 28% of patients aged 66–71 years; 75% of men in their seventh decade report coital activity once monthly. The National Institutes of Health Consensus Statement on Impotence acknowledges the likelihood of erectile dysfunction increasing with age, but emphasizes that progression is not inevitable. Erectile dysfunction may be influenced more by the concurrence or progression of medical illnesses and by the specific pharmacotherapies employed to control diabetes, atherosclerotic, peripheral and coronary vascular disease, hypertension, renal insufficiency and depression.[92]

Radical prostatectomy

The preservation of sexual quality of life is an important issue as cancer survival following treatment improves; it is an especially important issue in prostate cancer and, for some patients, may actually dominate selection of therapy. In a study examining decision-making in patients with localized prostate cancer, Singer found that some patients were willing to choose an intervention with lower long-term survival in order to preserve sexual potency.[93]

Enthusiasm for the surgical management of prostate cancer followed the elegant anatomical dissections by Donker and Walsh[94] and by Lepor and Walsh.[95] Injury to the neural pathways of erection during radical pelvic surgery typically occur at or below the pelvic plexus. The sympathetic preganglionic nerve fibres to the penis arise from neurons in intermediolateral grey matter of the lower thoracic spine; the segmental origin is from T10 to T12. Preganglionic fibres leave the cord via the ventral roots of the corresponding spinal nerves and pass via the white rami communicantes to the paravertebral sympathetic chain ganglia. The chain ganglion cells projecting to the penis are located in the sacral and caudal lumbar ganglia. By way of the grey rami, the postganglionic axons reach the urogenital tract through the pelvic plexus. The parasympathetic efferent activity of the penis is located in the intermediate grey matter of spinal cord segments S2–S4. The sacral preganglionic nerves travel to the pelvic plexus in the pelvic nerves. The pelvic nerves also receive input from the sacral sympathetic chain ganglia, via the grey rami. Fibres from the inferior hypogastric nerves join the pelvic nerves to form the pelvic plexus. The autonomic nerve fibres projecting to the penis from the pelvic plexus are known as the cavernous nerves.

Donker and Walsh[94] demonstrated the anatomical relationships of the cavernous nerves to the pelvic plexus, lateral pelvic fascia, Denonvilliers' fascia, prostatovesicular vessels, prostate, urethra and rectum. Fibres of the pelvic plexus are microscopic, travelling laterally and posteriorly to the seminal vesicles; they coalesce along the posterolateral surface of the prostate from a group of fibres 11 mm wide to a group 5 mm wide at the apex of the prostate, where they are only 1–3 mm from the urethral lumen. Distal to the membranous urethra, fibres penetrate the tunica albuginea of the corpus spongiosum; the remaining fibres, lying at the 1 and 11 o'clock positions, enter the penile crura along with terminal branches of the pudendal artery and cavernous veins. Operatively, these nerves are only identifiable by their relationship to the capsular vessels of the prostate.[96,97] Injury and consequent impotence commonly occurs during apical dissection and transection of the urethra from the prostate, or separation of prostate from rectum, or dividing lateral pelvic fascial attachments. Refinements in surgical technique not only have improved postoperative potency rates, but also have lowered morbidity secondary to intra-operative bleeding from the dorsal venous complex.

Potency after radical retropubic prostatectomy (RRP) is a function of patient age, volume of prostatic disease, and preservation of neurovascular bundles. Patients with cancer pathologically confined to one lobe of the prostate in their fifth decade of life have a 83% recovery of sexual function by 12 months; similarly, for men aged 60–69 the rate of recovery is 60%, but it is less than 50% for men aged 70–79. More extensive disease, pathologically involving both lobes of the prostate, is often associated with a desmoplastic–fibrotic response surrounding the neurovascular bundles, and postoperative potency for men in their sixth decade falls dramatically to 38%.[98] Experience at other academic centres corroborates the importance of age at operation, tumour volume and the role of neurovascular preservation. Catalona reported on 295 men with a mean age of 64 years: bilateral nerve sparing was performed in 236 cases with 63% potency rate and unilateral nerve sparing in 59 cases with a potency rate of 41%.[99] Stamey correlated surgical technique with outcomes recorded by health professionals other than the operating surgeon. Potency was defined for the patient as unassisted intercourse with vaginal penetration. In 69 men who received bilateral nerve-sparing surgery, 31.2% reported potency; of 203 receiving unilateral nerve-sparing, only 13.3% reported potency.[100] Unilateral wide resection of the neurovascular bundle has been advocated by surgeons concerned with establishing an adequate cancer margin, in recognition of the fact that local tumour spread through the prostate capsule may be in or along perforating neural sheaths. In a community series detailing complications of radical prostatectomy in Medicare patients, postoperative potency was notably meagre, at 11%; all patients were 65 years or older, with no data correlating surgical technique, pathological stage or tumour volume.[101]

There are a few prospective studies before and after RRP.[102,103] These studies suggest that a patient's perceptions of potency do not always correspond with those of his spouse, or correlate with frequency of

159

postoperative coital activity. Most significantly, when diagnostic testing (response to intracavernous vasoactive agents or nocturnal penile tumescence (NPT) and rigidity testing) is applied, preoperative erectile dysfunction is revealed at significant rates. One such study serially re-examined as well as re-interviewed patients for adequacy of erections, finding a 50% potency rate at 24 months following nerve-sparing radical prostatectomy, with only 7% of patients showing further improvement beyond 12 months.[102]

Erectile dysfunction following RRP is presumably neurogenic. Today, when postoperative potency rates are less than optimal, speculation arises about technique, candidate selection and volume of disease; adding to this controversy is the recent supposition that erectile dysfunction after RRP may be a consequence of vascular injury.[104] Cadaver dissections by Breza and Lue revealed that, in addition to primary inflow from the internal pudendal artery, corporal blood supply was provided by an accessory pudendal artery in seven of ten specimens. The accessory pudendal artery was noted to take origin from the obturator, inferior vesical or superior vesical arteries.[105] The same group examined 20 patients before and after nerve-sparing radical prostatectomy with vasoactive intracavernous injection. The mean age of patients was 65 years; each received the same pre- and postoperative dosage and all were evaluated with duplex Doppler ultrasonography. A decreased response to vasoactive agent was noted in 40%.[106] Unfortunately, the accessory pudendal vessel pierces the endopelvic fascia through the middle of the dorsal venous complex; its preservation may engender significant haemorrhage, compromising the subsequent nerve-sparing dissection. Polascik and Walsh[107] identified an accessory pudendal artery in only 4% of 835 patients; postoperatively, 67% of patients who had the accessory pudendal artery spared reported unassisted intromission, but so did 50% of patients in whom the vessel was sacrificed. Polascik and Walsh concluded that the occurrence of an accessory pudendal vessel was less frequent than originally proposed, and that its preservation during prostatectomy may not be productive.[107]

Cystoprostatectomy

Walsh's anatomical nerve-sparing modifications have been applied to radical cystectomy, with consequent improvement in postoperative potency, albeit less dramatic improvements than those noted for radical prostatectomy. Removal of the bladder, prostate and urethra en masse requires wider mobilization and dissection. Injury to the cavernous nerves probably occurs during mobilization and excision of the membranous urethra: the cavernous nerves pierce the genitourinary diaphragm at 3 and 9 o'clock, 1–3 mm from the urethra. Brendler has described the technique of potency-preserving urethrectomy based on earlier modifications of radical prostatectomy.[108]

Despite improved surgical extirpation, creation of a stoma for benign or malignant disease produces postoperative anxieties associated with hygiene, and alters the patient's body image. Altered body image, depression, anger and fear of repugnance contribute to patterns of sexual avoidance following urinary and faecal diversions.[109] Just as there is a cohort of patients who will avoid prostatectomy for fear of impotence, there are patients who will accept a higher incidence of complications from operations that accomplish continent diversion.[110]

Radiotherapy for prostate cancer

Assessments of post-radiation impotence share the same flaw as most surgical series, in a lack of pre-therapy diagnostic testing. The incidence of post-radiation impotence has been reported to range from 30 to 65% for external beam therapy and to be 25% for interstitial therapy.[111] Bagshaw subsequently reported on 434 potent patients who received external beam radiotherapy (XRT) and found a 2-year actuarial potency rate of 80% with median follow-up of 2 years.[112] In two retrospective series utilizing the same survey instrument to assess sequelae of radical prostatectomy and definitive radiation therapy for prostate cancer, 84% of patients reported potency before surgery, with 9% able to have full erections and 38% partial erections after nerve-sparing RRP; 77% of men claimed potency before radiation and 22% were able to have full erections and 41% partial erections after XRT.[113,114]

Potency rates seem to decline with time following XRT: Goldstein noted that 79% of men had progressive deterioration of sexual function following XRT, hypothesizing that vascular damage may be the aetiology.[115] Radiation for the management of Peyronie's disease had been utilized as an alternative to surgery. Recently, extensive corporal fibrosis has been noted following irradiation of the penis for Peyronie's disease: corporal biopsy obtained during subsequent prosthetic surgery demonstrated extensive fibrosis and arterial vasculopathy with diminished trabecular smooth muscle content (26% compared with the normal 40–52%).[116] Ionizing radiation damages vascular endothelium: in an animal model, 2000 rad (= 20 Gy) to the myocardium induced progressive capillary injury leading to myocardial fibrosis.[117,118] A retrospective series compared patients complaining of persistent erectile dysfunction 12–18 months following RRP or definitive XRT for localized prostate cancer: XRT patients were notably older than RRP patients, with mean ages of 70 years for XRT and 63 years for RRP patients. When duplex Doppler data following intracavernous PGE1 were age matched, comparison revealed significantly lower peak systolic velocities and resistive indices for XRT patients than for RRP patients. Erectile failure among XRT patients was predominantly arterial (91%), suggesting that XRT patients would require higher dosages or combination therapy of intracavernous agents for sexual rehabilitation.[119]

Colorectal operation

Colorectal operation, especially abdominoperineal resection (APR) and protocolectomy for cancer, can result in damage or ligation of the nerves and vessels necessary for erection. Early reports documented high (95%) impotence rates following APR for malignancy and following proctocolectomy for benign disease.[120] Contemporary reviews cite significant reductions (0–20%) in the incidence of erectile failure following rectal excision for benign disease, but no improvement following APR for malignancy, with iatrogenic impotence occurring in 33–100% of patients.[121,122]

Sympathetic preganglionic fibres exit the ventral roots as the white rami to the paravertebral chain ganglia, making synaptic connection with the postganglionic fibres of the preaortic plexus. These postganglionic fibres enter the pelvic plexus where they intermingle with sacral parasympathetic fibres. Autonomic nerves leaving the pelvic plexus are protected by the parietal pelvic fascia and run on the surface of the pyriformis muscles, where they join the hypogastric nerves. Half of the pelvic plexus lies close to the anterolateral wall of the lower rectum; the other half rests on the posterior and lateral aspect of the bladder and prostate.

Havenga and Welvaart[123] reported on 26 men with rectosigmoid carcinoma: only 22% of patients undergoing APR returned to sexual functioning, the remainder experiencing erectile dysfunction and/or anorgasmia; in contrast, 70% of patients who underwent low anterior resection retained sexual function.[123] Koukouras[124] reported on a larger series of sexually active males with colorectal cancer, who underwent anterior resection, low anterior resection or APR: APR patients had the highest level of sexual dysfunction, with 65% experiencing sexual dysfunction.[124] The pelvic autonomic plexus runs anterolateral to the rectal ampulla below the lateral pelvic fascia; if dissection is extended to the walls of the pelvis for removal of lymph nodes in the case of operation for malignancy, parasympathetic nerve damage and neurogenic erectile compromise invariably ensues. Hojo and colleagues[125] performed extended pelvic lymphadenectomy and selective pelvic autonomic nerve preservation in 134 patients; they classified pelvic autonomic nerve preservation into five degrees, the first degree being complete preservation and the fifth degree no preservation. There was a progressive decline in bladder sensation, voiding function and sexual function with increasing degrees of pelvic dissection. Most patients who underwent first-degree preservation spontaneously voided by 7–10 days, whereas 78% of fifth-degree patients remained in retention at postoperative day 60. Only 31% of men (all under 60 years) recovered erectile function and 19% recovered ejaculatory function, following first-degree preservation. Hojo and colleagues conclude that preservation of male sexual function is more difficult than preservation of voiding function during rectal resection for cancer; dissection of lymph nodes around the middle rectal artery is impossible if the pelvic nerve plexus is to be preserved and attempts should be restricted to patients with Dukes' A and B carcinomas.[125]

Isolated sympathetic nerve damage, sparing erectile function but altering fertility status through failure of emission or retrograde ejaculation, is possible. During emission, the secretions from the periurethral glands, seminal vesicles and prostate, and sperm from the vas deferens and ampulla of the vas, enter the posterior urethra, all under sympathetic stimulation. Ejaculation involves both sympathetic and somatic nerve control, with closure of the bladder neck under autonomic regulation and opening of the external sphincter and contraction of bulbospongiosal muscles under somatic control. The postganglionic sympathetic nerves may be damaged during separation of the rectum from the sacrum, in the pre-aortic tissues below the inferior mesenteric artery near the aorto-iliac bifurcation and where they enter the seminal vesicles. Fertility following colorectal surgery is similarly a function of patient age at the time of operation, of how low the resection is performed and of how wide the dissection is carried — all of which preselect for sexual dysfunction in nearly 100% of elderly patients following APR for cancer.

Another important and rarely addressed factor of co-morbidity is alteration of sexual self-image following cancer procedures creating abdominal stomas for the collection of faeces. A psychosexual profile of the male cancer patient with an abdominal stoma suggests that, even in the face of maintained erectile ability, sexual self-esteem is reduced.[126] Furthermore, patients with urinary ileostomies who undergo reoperation for continent urinary diversion show improved sexual self-image and levels of sexual activity.[110,127,128]

Transurethral operations

As described above, the neurovascular bundles of the prostate run posterolateral and contain the postganglionic autonomic nerves of erection; during transurethral resection of the prostate (TURP), therefore, potential nerve trauma could result from capsular penetration or current spread during electrocautery of bleeding vessels within the posterior urethra from the 3–5 o'clock or 7–9 o'clock positions. Urologists have traditionally asserted that there is no causal relationship between TURP and impotence, citing patient age, patient anxiety at the occurrence of retrograde ejaculation and concurrent medical risk factors predisposing erectile dysfunction as primary culprits. Clearly, the incidence of retrograde ejaculation is 50–60% and often will be the basis for the patient's complaint.[121,129–132] Older series reported erectile dysfunction following TURP in 4–40% of patients. A cooperative retrospective study of 13 institutions found the incidence of impotence following transurethral resection to be 4% among 3885 patients.[130] One recent prospective study used Snap-Gauge testing (Dacomed, Minneapolis, MN, USA) both to recruit potent patients prior to TURP and to test them postoperatively. Tscholl and colleagues[133] followed 98 men who broke all three bands (force constants of 226, 340 and 453 g) the night before surgery: on the fourth night following Foley catheter removal, 64/98 broke all bands; 3 months later an additional 26/98 broke three bands, with post-TURP impotence defined by Snap-Gauge testing at 3 months being 8.3%.[133] According to the meta-analysis by the Benign Prostatic Hyperplasia

(BPH) Guideline Panel,[134] the incidence of retrograde ejaculation following TURP is 73%; that of erectile dysfunction following transurethral incision of the prostate (TUIP) is 4–24% and following TURP is 3–32%.[134] In a prospective study based on interviews, Hanbury and Sethia[135] noted that the overall risk of impotence was 28.1% if the prostate capsule was breached during TURP, and 10% if it was not. Preoperatively, only 55.7% of patients described themselves as fully potent; 17% were capable of partial erections. Of the fully potent, 14.6% described themselves as partially potent, 3 months following TURP, and 2.9% as impotent.[135]

Visual laser ablation of the prostate

Visual laser ablation of the prostate (VLAP) and medical management of BPH are replacing TURP, which was once the most commonly performed urological procedure requiring anaesthetic. It is anticipated that the incidence of sexual dysfunction (retrograde ejaculation or erectile dysfunction) will be less than that reported for TURP. There are two modes of ablating prostate tissue — coagulation and vaporization. Coagulation necrosis is accomplished at lower powers, with tissue temperatures reaching 60–70°C; vaporization requires higher power, with surface temperatures in excess of 100°C but considerably less tissue penetration than occurs with coagulation. Excessive photocoagulation could potentially cause tissue damage beyond the prostatic urethra, including nerve and bowel injury.[136] In the only prospective, randomized series comparing VLAP with TURP, coagulation necrosis at 40 W of neodymium: yttrium aluminium garnet (Nd:YAG) laser energy resulted in no retrograde ejaculation, but in complaints of erectile dysfunction in 5.4% of patients.[137]

Optical urethrotomy

Optical internal urethrotomy (OIU) permits direct and precise incision of urethral strictures, usually without electrocautery. In 1981, McDermott and colleagues reported four cases of temporary or permanent erectile dysfunction among 179 patients receiving OIU.[138] In 1990, Graversen and colleagues[139] reported a 10% incidence of partial or total erectile dysfunction following OIU; assessment was made by interviews and dynamic testing using Doppler ultrasonography and cavernosography.[139] Graversen and colleagues postulated that shunting of the normally sequestered corpus cavernosum blood during erection was occurring via communication with the corpus spongiosum — a communication established by the urethrotomy. Incision for OIU is typically performed at the 12 o'clock position where this section of urethra is surrounded by the least amount of spongiosum. Cross-sectional anatomy of the urethra reveals that it resides within the corpus spongiosum in an eccentric position, superiorly. If impotence after direct-vision internal urethrotomy (DVIU) were actually due to inadvertent surgical communication between the spongiosum and corporal bodies, this long-term complication would be associated with the immediate postoperative complication of excessive bleeding per urethram; however, no such association has been described. As the level of the prostate, cavernous nerves run in the 5 and 7 o'clock positions; at the external sphincter they approximate the 3 and 6 o'clock positions; thereafter ascending to 11 and 1 o'clock in the proximal bulbar urethra to enter the cavernous bodies.[120] The majority of OIUs are performed for stricture in the bulbar or pendulous urethra, sites well distal to the entry of the cavernous nerves into the corpora cavernosa. Confounding this complex issue of post-OIU potency is the recognition that a predominant aetiology of urethral stricture is scar formation after transurethral resection.

Haemodialysis
Chronic uraemia and haemodialysis result in progressive impotence in 90% of men.[140,141] The pathogenesis of male sexual dysfunction in uraemic patients on haemodialysis is multifactorial and is compounded by the medical conditions that promoted the chronic renal failure (CRF): these include uraemic toxins, zinc deficiency, hyperparathyroidism, decreased levels of free testosterone and dihydrotestosterone, hyperprolactinaemia, autonomic neuropathy, diabetes mellitus, and hypertensive and atherosclerotic vascular disease. Chronic haemodialysis patients have accelerated atherosclerosis associated with small-vessel occlusive disease and penile vascular calcifications.[142] Autonomic and peripheral neuropathies have been described in CRF patients: abnormal heart rate responses to the Valsalva manoeuvre have been correlated with abnormal NPT and rigidity testing; bulbocavernosus reflex latency abnormalities have, similarly, been found among men with CRF.[143–145] Testicular morphology in haemodialysis is altered, showing maturational arrest, germ cell aplasia and interstitial cell abnormalities. Most patients on

haemodialysis have low or low normal testosterone levels secondary to both decreased production and increased clearance. Sex-hormone-binding globulin is elevated in some haemodialysis patients, which further reduces the level of free serum testosterone.[146,147] Correspondingly, luteinizing hormone (LH) levels may be mildly elevated in uraemic men ($\geq$ 20% of normal). Pituitary response to stimulation (gonadotrophin-releasing hormone) is usually normal, but there may be loss of diurnal variation/pulsatile release of LHRH.[148]

Hyperprolactinaemia is evident in 50% of dialysis patients and is a well-known central inhibitor of gonadotrophin secretion; however, it is typically associated with low T and low LH rather than low T and high LH as seen in non-uraemic patients with prolactin-secreting pituitary adenomas. The increased prolactin levels found in CRF patients on dialysis is a function of increased secretion and decreased degradation. Prolactin release is further stimulated by medications such as methyldopa, cimetidine, metoclopramide and digoxin.[144] Treatment of chronic anaemia in CRF men with erythropoietin has reportedly improved erectile function/libido.

Renal transplantation
Men with long-term renal allografts may regain their potency (50–80%). Similarly, improvements in fertility secondary to increased testosterone and sperm density are reported. Revascularization of the transplant is typically accomplished either end-to-end to the internal iliac artery or end-to-side to the external iliac artery.[149,150] If erectile dysfunction following renal transplantation were due solely to a vascular steal phenomenon, then modification of the technique — end-to-side (external iliac artery) rather than end-to-end internal iliac arterial anastomosis — should improve postoperative potency. The risk of vasculogenic erectile failure following anastomosis of renal graft to the internal iliac artery is 10% but, following a second transplant to the left pelvis and internal iliac artery, the incidence climbs to 65%.[151] Salvatierra[152] recommends that, if there is moderate atherosclerosis extending into the bifurcation of the iliacs, then an end-to-side anastomosis with the external iliac artery is preferable; similarly, in the case of cadaver donor with multiple renal arteries, a patch of aorta with renal arteries intact is taken (Carrel patch) for end-to-side external iliac anastomosis. In the case of a living related donor transplantation, the graft is obtained from

the donor simultaneously in parallel operating rooms. In this situation, if there are multiple renal arteries a Carrel patch is not possible but a variety of vascular anastomotic options remain: these include double end-to-side renal arteries to the common or external iliac artery, or end-to-end superior renal artery to internal iliac artery with end-to-side inferior renal artery to external iliac artery; alternatively, it may be necessary to mobilize the internal iliac artery of the recipient and to use its branches to perform multiple end-to-end anastomoses.[152] Interestingly, in the primate model, a reduction of internal iliac flow of 85% or more is necessary before the erectile response initiated by direct neurostimulation can be suppressed.[153]

Aorto-iliac operation

The incidence of iatrogenic erectile dysfunction following aorto-iliac revascularization ranges from 21 to 88%. Preoperative sexual dysfunction is equally high in this group of patients, ranging from 25 to 60%. Leriche's syndrome, described in 1923, is characterized by fatigue and claudication in the buttocks and legs with exercise, absence of pulsations in the femoral arteries and the complaint of impotence.[154] In 1969, a 21% incidence of impotence following aortic aneurysmectomy and a 34% incidence following revascularization for thrombo-occlusive disease were reported; the associated incidence of ejaculatory dysfunction was 63% and 49%, respectively.[155,156]

Technical modifications sparing sexual function include the following: omitting lumbar sympathectomy; opening the aorta on its right lateral surface, reflecting the overlying tissue to the left but not incising the pre-aortic tissue; tunnelling aortofemoral bypass grafts directly anterior to the native common and external iliac vessels deep to the ureters and pelvic plexus; dissection in the longitudinal plane over the proximal external iliac arteries; preserving or restoring hypogastric flow during aortofemoral reconstruction; not resecting aortic aneurysm sacs but controlling back-bleeding from the inferior mesenteric artery from within the sac.[157–159] In a series of 148 men with preoperative impotence undergoing aorto-iliac/femoral reconstruction, Gorssetti and colleagues noted that 80% had unilateral or bilateral hypogastric occlusions; only 20% regained erections when standard aortofemoral bypass was performed; when distal anastomosis to the common iliac artery was performed, 75% regained function.[160]

There are, clearly, morphological changes in the arterioles, capillaries and smooth muscle cells of the corpus cavernosum of patients undergoing penile implants.[161] These changes parallel the extent of occlusive disease in the aorto-iliac system, with significant decreases in smooth muscle content noted in men with cavernous arterial insufficiency. There is at this time no clinical role for corporal biopsy for diagnosis or for amelioration of potency, but this line of research does suggest that, despite technical refinements in the management of aorto-occlusive disease — including thrombo-endarterectomy and angioplasty — high rates of preoperative impotence are to be expected and postoperative improvement does not rest entirely in the hands of the surgeon.

■ REFERENCES

1. Bancroft J. Human sexuality and its problems. Edinburgh: Churchill Livingstone, 1989
2. Bracket N L, Bloch W E, Abae M. Neurological anatomy and physiology of sexual function. In: Singer C, Weiner W J (eds) Sexual dysfunction: a neuromedical approach. Armonk: Futura, 1994: 1–45
3. Kaplan H S. The evaluation of sexual disorders: psychological and medical aspects. New York: Brunner Mazel
4. Buffum J. Pharmacosexology: the effects of drugs on sexual function. J Psychoactive Drugs 1982; 14: 5–44
5. Abramowicz M. Drugs that cause sexual dysfunction. Med Lett 1987; 29: 65–70
6. Wein A J, Van Arsdalen K N. Drug-induced male sexual dysfunction. Urol Clin North Am 1988; 15: 23–31
7. Rosen R C. Alcohol and drug effects on sexual response: human experimental and clinical studies. Ann Rev Sex Res 1991; 2: 119–179
8. Broderick G, Foreman M. Iatrogenic sexual dysfunction. In: Singer C, Weiner W J (eds) Sexual dysfunction: a neuromedical approach. Armonk: Futura, 1994: 299–331
9. Foreman M M, Wernicke J F. Approaches for the development of oral drug therapies for erectile dysfunction. Semin Urol 1990; 8: 107–112
10. Foreman M M. Disorders of sexual response: pioneering new pharmaceutical and therapeutic opportunities. Expert Opin Invest Drugs 1995; 7: 621–636
11. Segraves R T. Drugs and desire. In: Leiblum S R, Rosen R C (eds) Sexual desire disorders. New York: Guilford Press, 1988: 313–347
12. Segraves R T. Effects of psychotropic drugs on human erection and ejaculation. Arch Gen Psychiatry 1989; 46: 275–284
13. Sachs B D, Meisel R L. The physiology of male sexual behavior. In: Knobil E, Neil J D, Ewing E E (eds) The physiology of reproduction, Vol 2. New York: Karger, 1988: 1393–1423

14. Bitran D, Hull E M. Pharmacological analysis of male rat sexual behavior. Neurosci Biobehav Rev 1987; 11: 365–389

15. Pfaus J G, Gorzalka B. Opioids and sexual behavior. Neurosci Biobehav Rev 1987; 11: 1–34

16. Wilson C. Pharmacological targets for the control of male and female sexual behavior. In: Riley A J, Peet M, Willson C (eds) Sexual pharmacology. Oxford: Clarendon, 1993: 1–59

17. Korenman S G, Morley J E, Mooradian A D et al. Secondary hypogonadism in older men: its relationship to impotence. J Clin Endocrinol Metab 1990; 71(4): 963–969

17a Krane R, Goldstein I, Saenz de Tejada I. Impotence: secondary hypogonadism. N Engl J Med 1989; 8: 1659

18. Johnson A R, Jarow J P. Is routine endocrine testing of impotent men necessary? J Urol 1992; 147: 1542

19. Heim N. Sexual behavior of castrated sex offenders. Arch Sex Behav 1981; 10: 11

20. Rousseau R, Dupont A, Labrie F et al. Sexuality changes in prostate cancer patients receiving anti-hormonal therapy combining the antiandrogen flutamide with medical (LHRH agonist) or surgical castration. Arch Sex Behav 1988; 32: 128–133

21. Casper R F, Yen S S C. Neuroendocrinology of menopausal flushes: an hypothesis of the flush mechanism. Clin Endocrinol 1985; 22: 293–312

22. Radlmaier A, Barmacher K, Neumann F. Hot flushes: mechanism and prevention. Prof Clin Biol Res 1990; 359: 131

23. Kirschenbaum A. Management of hormonal treatment effects. Cancer 1995; 75(7): 1983–1986

24. Barbeau A. L-Dopa therapy in Parkinson's disease: a critical review of nine years' experience. Can Med Assoc J 1969; 101: 59–69

25. Yaryura-Tobias J, Diamond B, Merlis S. The action of L-dopa on schizophrenic patients (a preliminary report). Curr Ther Res 1970; 12: 528–531

26. Benkert O, Crombach G, Kockott G. Effect of L-dopa on sexually impotent patients. Psychopharmacologia 1972; 23: 91–95

27. Angrist B, Gershon S. Clinical effects of amphetamine and L-dopa on sexuality and aggression. Compr Psychiatry 1976; 17: 715–722

28. Brown E, Brown G M, Kofman O, Quarrington B. Sexual function and affect in Parkinsonian men treated with L-dopa. Am J Psychiatry 1978; 135: 1552–1555

29. Dallo J, Lekka N, Knoll J. The ejaculatory behavior of sexually sluggish male rats treated with (−)deprenyl, apomorphine, bromocriptine and amphetamine. Pol J Pharmacol Pharm 1986; 38: 251–255

30. Malmnas C O. The significance of dopamine, versus other catecholamines, for the L-dopa induced facilitation of sexual behavior in the castrated male rat. Pharmacol Biochem Behav 1976; 4: 521–526

31. Crenshaw T, Goldberg J, Stern W. Pharmacologic modification of psychosexual dysfunction. J Sex Marital Ther 1987; 13: 239–250

32. Del Bene E, Fanciullacci M, Poggioni M et al. Apomorphine and other dopamine modifiers of human sexual and nocioceptive tonus. In: Segal M (ed) Psychopharmacology of sexual disorders. London: Libbey, 1985: 145–153

33. Freed E. Increased sexual function with nomifensine. Med J Aust 1983; 1: 551

34. Jeanty P, Van den Kerchove M, Lowenthal A, DeBruyne H. Pergolide therapy in Parkinson's disease. J Neurol 1984; 231: 148–152

35. Uitti R J, Tanner C M, Rajput A H. Hypersexuality with antiparkinsonian therapy. Clin Neuropharmacol 1989; 5: 375–383

36. Foreman M M, Gehlert D R, Schaus J M. Quinelorane, a potent and selective dopamine agonist for the "D2-like" receptor family. Neurotransmissions 1995; 11: 1–5

37. DeLeo D, Magni G. Does viloxazine really improve sex drive? A double blind controlled study. Br J Psychiatry 1986; 148: 597–599

38. Clark J T, Smith E R, Davidson J. Evidence for modulation of sexual behavior by alpha adrenoceptors in male rats. Neuroendocrinology 1985; 41: 36–43

39. Sala M, Braida D, Leone M et al. Central effect of yohimbine on sexual behavior in the rat. Physiol Behav 1990; 47: 165–173

40. Smith E, Lee R, Schnur S, Davidson J. Alpha2-adrenoceptor antagonists and male sexual behavior. Physiol Behav 1987; 41: 7–14

41. Morales A, Condra M, Owen J et al. Is yohimbine effective in the treatment of impotence? Results of a controlled trial. J Urol 1987; 137: 1168–1172

42. Riley A J, Goodman R, Kellett J M, Orr R. Double blind trial of yohimbine hydrochloride in the treatment of erection inadequacy. Sex Marital Ther 1989; 4: 17–26

43. Susset J, Tessier C, Wincze J et al. Effect of yohimbine hydrochloride on erectile impotence: a double-blind study. J Urol 1989; 141: 1360–1363

44. Jacobsen F M. Fluoxetine-induced sexual dysfunction and an open trial of yohimbine. J Clin Psychiatry 1992; 53: 119–122

45. Brown C, Mackinnon A, Redfern W et al. The pharmacology of RS-15385-197, a potent and selective α2-adrenoceptor antagonist. Br J Pharmacol 1993; 108: 516–525

46. Linnankoski I, Gronosoos M, Carlson S, Pertovaara A. Atizepamezole, an alpha-2-adrenoreceptor increases sexual behavior in male monkeys. Proc Soc Neurosci 1991; 17: 282

47. Foreman M, Fuller R, Nelson D et al. Preclinical studies on LY237733, a potent and selective serotonergic antagonist. J Pharmacol Exp Ther 1992; 260: 51–57

48. Forster P, King J. Fluoxetine for premature ejaculation. Am J Psychiatry 1994; 151: 1523

49. Mendels J, Camera A, Sikes C. Seratraline treatment for premature ejaculation. J Clin Psychopharmacol 1995; 15: 341–346

50. Pinder R M, Brogen R N, Sawyer P R. Fenfluramine: a review of its pharmacological properties and efficacy in obesity. Drugs 1975; 10: 241–323

51. Ahlenius S, Larsson K, Svensson D et al. Effects of a new type of 5-HT receptor agonist on male rat sexual behavior. Pharmacol Biochem Behav 1981; 15: 785–792

52. Glaser T, Dompert W, Schuurman T et al. Differential pharmacology of the novel 5-HT1A receptor ligands 8-OH-

DPAT, BAY R 1531 and ipsapirone. In: Dourish C T, Ahlenius S, Hutson P T (eds) Brain 5-HT1A receptors. New York: Ellis Horwood, 1987: 106–119

53. Pomerantz S D. Quinelorane (LY163502), a D2 dopaminergic receptor agonist, acts centrally to facilitate sexual behavior of rhesus monkeys. Pharmacol Biochem Behav 1991; 39: 123–128

54. Pomerantz S D, Hepner B, Wertz J M. Serotonergic influences on male sexual behavior of rhesus monkeys: effects of serotonin agonists. Psychopharmacology 1993; 111: 47–54

55. Othmer E, Othmer S. Effect of buspirone on sexual dysfunction in patients with generalized anxiety disorder. J Clin Psychiatry 1987; 48: 201–203

56. Armone M, Baroni M, Gai J et al. Effect of SR59026A, a new 5-HT1A receptor agonist, on sexual activity in male rats. Behav Pharmacol 1995; 6: 276–282

57. Foreman M, Fuller R, Benvenga M et al. Pharmacological characterization of LY293284: an extremely potent and selective 5-HT1A agonist. J Pharmacol Exp Ther 1994; 270: 1270–1281

58. Foreman M, Fuller R, Zhang L et al. Preclinical studies on LY228729: a potent and selective 5-HT1A agonist. J Pharmacol Exp Ther 1993; 268: 58–71

59. Klint T, Dahlgren I L, Larsson K. The selective 5-HT2 receptor antagonist amperozide attenuates 1-(2,5-dimethoxy-4-iodophenyl)-2-aminopropane-induced inhibition of male rat sexual behavior. Eur J Pharmacol 1992; 212: 241–246

60. Kurt U, Ozkardes H, Altug U et al. The efficacy of antiserotonergic agents in the treatment of erectile dysfunction. J Urol 1994; 152: 407–409

61. Sullivan G. Increased libido in three men treated with trazodone. J Clin Psychiatry 1988; 49: 202–203

62. Danjou P, Alexandre L, Warot D et al. Assessment of erectogenic properties of apomorphine and yohimbine. Br J Clin Pharmacol 1986; 26: 733–739

63. Heaton J P W, Morales A, Adams M A et al. Recovery of erectile function by the oral administration of apomorphine. Urology 1995; 45(2): 200–206

64. Lal S, Tesfaye Y, Thavundayil J et al. Apomorphine: clinical studies on erectile impotence and yawning. Prog Neuropsychopharmacol Biol Psychiatry 1989; 13: 329–339

65. Segraves R T, Bari M, Segraves K, Spirnak P. Effect of apomorphine on penile tumescence in men with psychogenic impotence. J Urol 1991; 145: 1174–1175

66. Doherty P C, Wisler P, Foreman M M. Effects of quinelorane on yawning, penile erection and sexual behavior in the male rat. Proc Soc Neurosci 1991; 17: 328

67. Ferrari F, Pelloni F, Giuliani D. Behavioral evidence that different neurochemical mechanisms underly stretching–yawning and penile erection induced in male rats by SND 919, a selective D2 dopaminergic receptor agonist. Psychopharmacology 1993; 113: 172–176

68. Gower A, Berendsen H, Princen M, Broekkamp C L E. The yawing–penile erection syndrome as a model for putative dopamine autoreceptor activity. Eur J Pharmacol 1984; 103: 81–89

69. Berendsen H, Jenck F, Broekkamp C. Involvement of 5-HT1c receptors in drug induced penile erections in rats. Psychopharmacology (Berlin) 1990; 101: 57–61

70. Szele F G, Murphy D L, Garrick N A. Fenfluramine, m-chlorophenylpiperazine and other serotonin reuptake agonists and antagonists on penile erections in non-human primates. Life Sci 1988; 43: 1297–1303

71. Power-Smith P. Beneficial sexual side-effects from fluoxetine. Br J Psychiatry 1993; 164: 249–250

72. Smith D M, Levitte S S. Association of fluoxetine and return of sexual potency in three elderly men. J Clin Psychiatry 1993; 54: 317–319

73. Saenz de Tejada I, Ware C J, Blanco R. Pathophysiology of prolonged penile erection associated with trazadone use. J Urol 1991; 145: 60–64

73a Scher M, Krieger J, Juergens S. Trazodone and priapism. Am J Psychiatry 1983; 140: 1362–1363

74. Steers W D, de Groat W C. Effects of m-chlorophenylpiperazine on penile and bladder function in rats. Am J Physiol 1989; 257: R1441–1449

75. Murphy J B, Lipshultz L I. Abnormalities of ejaculation. Urol Clin North Am 1987; 14: 583–596

75a Murphy M R. Endogenous opiates and the mechanisms of male sexual behavior. In: Segal M (ed) Psychopharmacology of sexual disorders. London: Libbey, 1988: 51–62

76. Fabbri A, Jannini A, Gnessi L. Endorphins in male impotence: evidence for naltrexone stimulation of erectile activity in patient therapy. Psychoneuroendocrinology 1989; 14: 103–111

77. Goldstein J A. Erectile function and naltrexone. Ann Intern Med 1986; 105: 799

78. Charney D S, Heninger G R. Alpha2-adrenergic and opiate receptor blockade. Synergistic effects on anxiety in healthy subjects. Arch Gen Psychiatry 1986; 43: 1037–1041

79. Adaikan P G, Lan L C, Nag S C, Ratnam S S. Physiopharmacology of human penile erection — autonomic/nitrergic neurotransmission and receptors of the human corpus cavernosum. Asia Pac J Pharmacol 1991; 6: 213–227

80. Saenz de Tejada I. Commentary on mechanisms for the regulation of penile smooth muscle contractility. J Urol 1995; 153: 1762–1763

81. Maeda N, Matsuoka N, Yamaguchi I. Role of the dopaminergic, serotonergic and cholinergic link in the expression of penile erection in rats. Jpn J Pharmacol 1994; 66: 59–66

82. Gross M D. Reversal by bethanechol of sexual dysfunction caused by anticholinergic antidepressants. Am J Psychiatry 1982; 139: 1193–1194

83. Andersson K-E. Pharmacology of lower urinary tract smooth muscle and penile erection. Pharmacol Rev 1993; 45: 253–308

84. Andersson K E, Wagner G. Physiology of penile erection. Physiol Rev 1995; 75(1): 191–236

85. Rayner H C, May S, Walls J. Penile erection due to nifedipine. Br Med J 1988; 296: 137

86. Virag R. Intracavernous injection of papaverine for erectile failure. Lancet 1982; 2: 398

87. Falaschi P, Rocco A, De Giorgio G et al. Brain dopamine and premature ejaculation: results of treatment with dopamine antagonists. In: Gessa G L, Corsini G U (eds) Apomorphine and other dopaminomimetics. New York: Raven Press, 1981: 117–121

88. Renyi L. Ejaculations induced by p-chloroamphetamine in the rat. Neuropharmacology 1985; 24: 697–704

89. Renyi L. The effect of selective 5-hydroxytryptamine uptake inhibitors on 5-methoxy-N,N-dimethyltryptamine-induced ejaculation in the rat. Br J Pharmacol 1986; 87: 639–648

90. Herman J B, Brotman A W, Pollack M H et al. Fluoxetine-induced sexual dysfunction. J Clin Psychiatry 1990; 51: 25–27

91. Girgis S, El-Haggar S, El-Hermouzy S. A double-blind trial of chlomipramine in premature ejaculation. Andrologia 1982; 14: 364–368

92. Consensus Development Conference Statement. Impotence. National Institutes of Health. JAMA 1993; 270: 83–90

93. Singer P A, Tasch E S, Stocking C et al. Sex or survival trade-offs between quality and quantity of life. J Clin Oncol 1991; 9: 328–334

94. Donker P J, Walsh P C. Impotence following radical retropubic prostatectomy: insight in etiology and prevention. J Urol 1982; 128: 492–497

95. Lepor H, Gregerman J, Crosby R et al. Precise localization of the autonomic nerves from the pelvic plexus to the corpora cavernosa: a detailed anatomical study of the adult male pelvis. J Urol 1985; 133: 207–212

96. Walsh P C, Lepor H, Eggleston J C. Radical prostatectomy with preservation of sexual function: anatomical and pathological considerations. Prostate 1983; 4: 474

97. Walsh P C. Radical prostatectomy with preservation of sexual function: evolution of a surgical procedure. AUA Update Ser 1985; 5(5): 2–9

98. Quinlan D M, Epstein J I, Carter B S, Walsh P C. Sexual function following radical prostatectomy: influence of preservation of neurovascular bundles. J Urol 1991; 145: 998

99. Catalona W J, Basler J W. Return of erections and urinary continence following nerve sparing radical retropubic prostatectomy. J Urol 1993; 150: 905

100. Geary E S, Dendinger T E, Freiha F S, Stamey T A. Nerve sparing radical prostatectomy: a different view. J Urol 1995; 154: 145–149

101. Fowler J E, Barry M J, Lu-Yao G et al. Patient reported complications and follow-up treatment after radical prostatectomy. The national Medicare experience: 1988–1990 (updated June 1993). Urology 1993; 42: 622

102. Leach G, Zimmern P E, Roskamp D, Faswick J. Prospective evaluation of potency following nerve sparing radical retropubic prostatectomy. J Urol 1992; 147(4): 358A

103. Padma-Nathan H, Kanellos A, Lieskovsky G. Prospective erectile function testing prior to nerve sparing prostatectomy will predict successful potency preservation. J Urol 1992; 147(4): 359A

104. Bergman B, Silvertsson R, Suurkula M. Penile blood pressure in erectile impotence following cystectomy. Scand J Urol Nephrol 1982; 16: 81–84

105. Breza J, Aboseif S R, Orivs B R et al. Detailed anatomy of penile neurovascular structures: surgical significance. J Urol 1989; 141: 437–443

106. Aboseif S, Shinohara K, Breza J et al. Role of penile vascular injury in erectile dysfunction after radical prostatectomy. Br J Urol 1994; 73: 75–82

107. Polascik T J, Walsh P C. Radical retropubic prostatectomy: the influence of accessory pudendal arteries on the recovery of sexual function. J Urol 1995; 153: 150–152

108. Brendler C B, Schlegel P N, Walsh P C. Urethrectomy with preservation of potency. J Urol 1990; 144: 270–273

109. Hurny C, Holland J C. Psychosocial sequelae of ostomies in cancer patients. Cancer 1985; 36: 170–183

110. Broderick G A, Stone A R, deVere-White R W. Neobladders: clinical management and considerations for patients receiving chemotherapy. Semin Oncol 1990; 17(5): 598–605

111. Bagshaw M A, Cox R S, Ray G R. Status of radiation treatment of prostate cancer at Stanford University. NCI Monogr 1988; 7: 47–60

112. Bagshaw M A, Cox R S, Hancock S L. Control of prostate cancer with radiotherapy: long-term results. J Urol 1994; 152: 1781–1785

113. Jonler M, Messing E M, Rhodes P R, Bruskewitz R C. Sequelae of radical prostatectomy. Br J Urol 1994; 74: 352–358

114. Jonler M, Ritter M A, Brinkmann R et al. Sequelae of definitive radiation therapy for prostate cancer localized to the pelvis. Urology 1994; 44: 876–882

115. Goldstein I, Feldman M, Deckers P et al. Radiation-associated impotence, a clinical study of its mechanism. JAMA 1984; 251: 903

116. Hall S J, Basile G, Bertero E B et al. Extensive corporeal fibrosis after penile irradiation. J Urol 1995; 153: 372–377

117. Fajardo L F, Berthong M. Vascular lesions following radiation. Pathol Annu 1988; 23: 297

118. Fajardo L F, Berthong M. Pathogenesis of radiation-induced myocardial fibrosis. Lab Invest 1973; 29: 244

119. Broderick G A, Malkowicz S B, VanArsdalen K, Wein A J. Erectile dysfunction following therapy for localized prostate cancer; the role of the penile blood flow study. J Urol 1995; 153(4): A405

120. Lue T F, Zeineh S J, Schmidt R A et al. Neuroanatomy of penile erection: its relevance to iatrogenic impotence. J Urol 1984; 131: 273–280

121. Melman A. Iatrogenic causes of erectile dysfunction. Urol Clin North Am 1988; 15(1): 33–40

122. Weinstein M, Roberts M. Sexual potency following surgery for rectal carcinoma. Ann Surg 1985; 185: 295–300

123. Havenga D, Welvaart K. Sexual dysfunction in men following surgical treatment for rectosigmoid carcinoma. Ned Tijdschr Geneesk 1991; 135: 710–713

124. Koukouras D, Spiliotis J, Scopa C D et al. Radical consequence in sexuality of male patients operated for colorectal carcinoma. Eur J Surg Oncol 1991; 17: 285–288

125. Hojo K, Vernava A M, Sugihara K, Katumata K. Preservation of urine voiding and sexual function after rectal cancer surgery. Dis Colon Rectum 1991; 34(7): 532–539

126. Santangelo M L, Romano G, Sassaroli C. Sexual function after resection for rectal cancer. Am J Surg 1987; 154: 502–504

127. Boyd S D, Feinberg S M, Skinner D G et al. Quality of life survey of urinary diversion patients: comparison of ileal conduits versus continent Kock ileal reservoirs. J Urol 1987; 138: 1386

128. Goldwasser B, Webster G D. Continent urinary diversion. J Urol 1985; 134: 227–236

129. Finkle A L, Prien D V. Sexual potency in elderly men before and after prostatectomy. JAMA 1966; 196: 139–143

130. Mebust W K. A review of TURP complications and the AUA national cooperative study. AUA Update Ser 1989; 8(24): 186–191

131. So E P, Ho P C, Bodestab W et al. Erectile impotence associated with transurethral prostatectomy. Urology 1982; 19(3): 259–262

132. Zohar J, Meiraz D, Maoz B et al. Factors influencing sexual activity after prostatectomy. J Urol 1976; 116: 332–334

133. Tscholl R, Largo M, Poppinghaus E et al. Incidence of erectile impotence secondary to transurethral resection of benign prostatic hyperplasia, assessed by preoperative and postoperative snap gauge tests. J Urol 1995; 153: 1491–1493

134. McConnell J D, Barry M J, Bruskewitz R C et al. Benign prostatic hyperplasia: diagnosis and treatment. Clinical practice guideline 8, AHCPR publication 94–0582. Rockville, MD: Agency for Health Care Policy and Research, Public Health Service, US Department of Health and Human Services, 1994

135. Hanbury D C, Sethia K K. Erectile function following transurethral prostatectomy. Br J Urol 1995; 75(1): 12–13

136. Stein B S. Laser prostatectomy. AUA Update Ser 1996; 14(6): 41–48

137. Cowles R S, Kabalin J N, Childs S et al. A prospective randomized comparison of transurethral resection to visual laser ablation of the prostate for the treatment of benign prostatic hyperplasia. Urology: in press

138. McDermott D W, Bates R J, Heney N M, Althausen A. Erectile impotence as complication of direct vision cold knife urethrotomy. Urology 1981; 18: 467–469

139. Graversen P H, Rosenkilde P, Colstrup H. Erectile dysfunction following direct vision internal urethrotomy. Scand J Urol Nephrol 1991; 25: 175–178

140. David R D, Koyle M A. Impotence in chronic renal failure. In: Rajfer J (ed) Common problems in infertility and impotence. Chicago: Year Book Medical, 1990: 368–375

141. Salvatierra O Jr, Fortmann J L, Belzer F O. Sexual function in males before and after renal transplantation. Urology 1975; 5: 64–66

142. Dalal S, Gandhi V C, Yu A W et al. Penile calcification in maintenance hemodialysis patients. Urology 1992; 40: 442

143. Campese V M, Procci W R, Levitan D et al. Autonomic nervous system dysfunction and impotence in uremia. Am J Nephrol 1982; 2: 140

144. Carson C C. Impotence and chronic renal failure. In: Bennett A H (ed) Impotence: diagnosis and management of erectile dysfunction. Philadelphia: Saunders, 1994: 124–134

145. Kersh E S, Kronfield S J, Unger A et al. Autonomic insufficiency in uremia as a cause of hemodialysis-induced hypotension. N Engl J Med 1974; 290: 650

146. Altman J J. Sex hormones and chronic renal failure of the diabetic. Ann Endocrinol 1988; 49: 412

147. Ramirez G, Butcher D, Bruggenmyer C D, Gungangly A. Testicular defect: the primary abnormality in gonadal dysfunction of uremia. South Med J 1987; 80: 698

148. Rodger R S C, Dewar J H, Turner S J et al. Anterior pituitary dysfunction in patients with chronic renal failure treated by hemodialysis or continuous peritoneal ambulatory dialysis. Nephrology 1986; 43: 169

149. Hefty T R. Complications of renal transplantation: the practising urologist's role. AUA Update Ser 1991; 10(8): 64

150. Hodge E E, Banowsky E H. Renal transplantation, parts I–II. AUA Update Ser 1990; 9(13,14): 98–111

151. Gittes R F, Waters W B. Sexual impotence: the overlooked complication of a second renal transplant. J Urol 1979; 121: 719–720

152. Salvatierra O Jr. Renal transplantation. In: Walsh P C, Gittes R F, Perlmutter A D, Stamey T A (eds) Campbell's Urology, 5th edn. Philadelphia: Saunders, 1986: 2534–2555

153. Junemann K P, Personn-Junemann C, Alken P. Pathophysiology of erectile dysfunction. Semin Urol 1990; 8(2): 80–93

154. Leriche R. Des oblitérations arterielles hautes (oblitération de la terminasion de l'aorte) comme causes des insuffisances circulatoires des membres inférieurs. Bull Mem Soc Chir 1923; 49: 1404

155. May A G, DeWeese J A, Rob C G. Changes in sexual function following operation on the abdominal aorta. Surgery 1969; 65: 41–47

156. Weinstein M H, Machleder H I. Sexual function after aorto-iliac surgery. Ann Surg 1975; 181: 787–790

157. DePalma R G, Levine S B, Feldman S. Preservation of erectile function after aortoiliac reconstruction. Arch Surg 1978; 113: 985

158. Flanigan P D, Schuler J J, Keifer T et al. Elimination of iatrogenic impotence and improvement of sexual function after aortoiliac revascularization. Arch Surg 1982; 117: 544–550

159. Oshiro T, Kosaki G. Sexual function after aorto-iliac vascular reconstruction. J Cardiovasc Surg 1984; 25: 47–50

160. Gorssetti B, Gattuso R, Irace L et al. Aorto-iliac femoral reconstructions in patients with vasculogenic impotence. Eur J Vasc Surg 1991; 5: 425

161. Persson-Junemann C, Diedrichs W, Lue T F. Alteration of penile ultrastructure in impotence: morphology and clinical correlation. In: Rubben H, Jocham D, Joacobi G H (eds) Investigative urology 3. Berlin: Springer-Verlag, 1989: 53–59

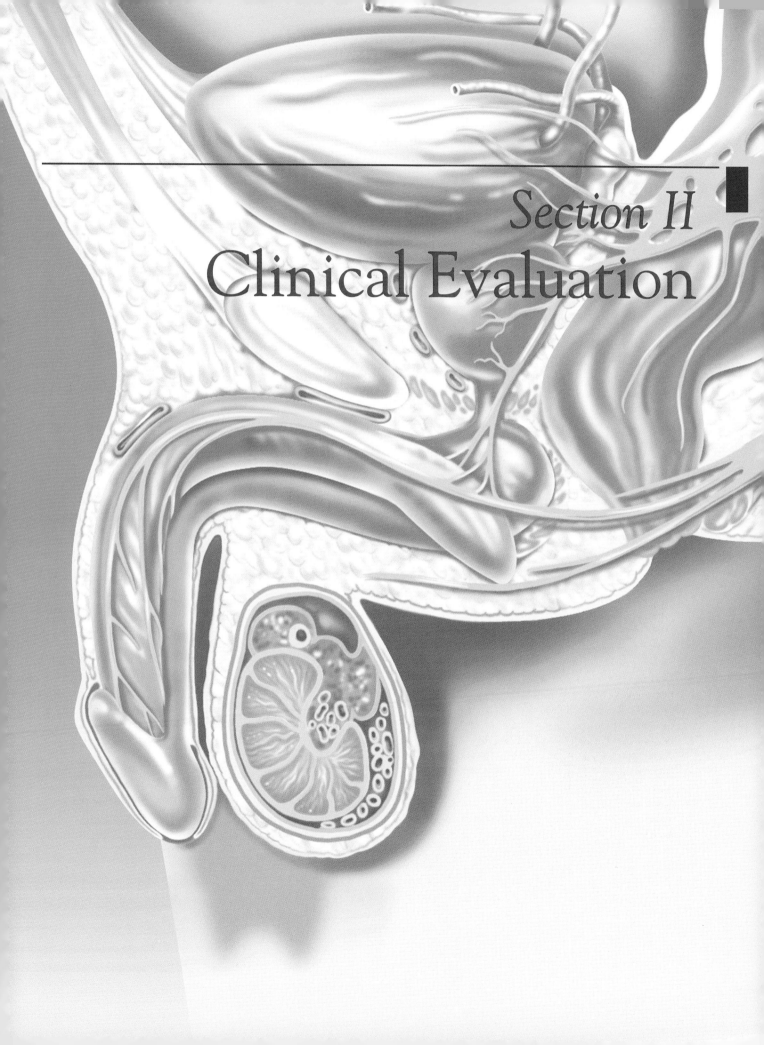

Section II
Clinical Evaluation

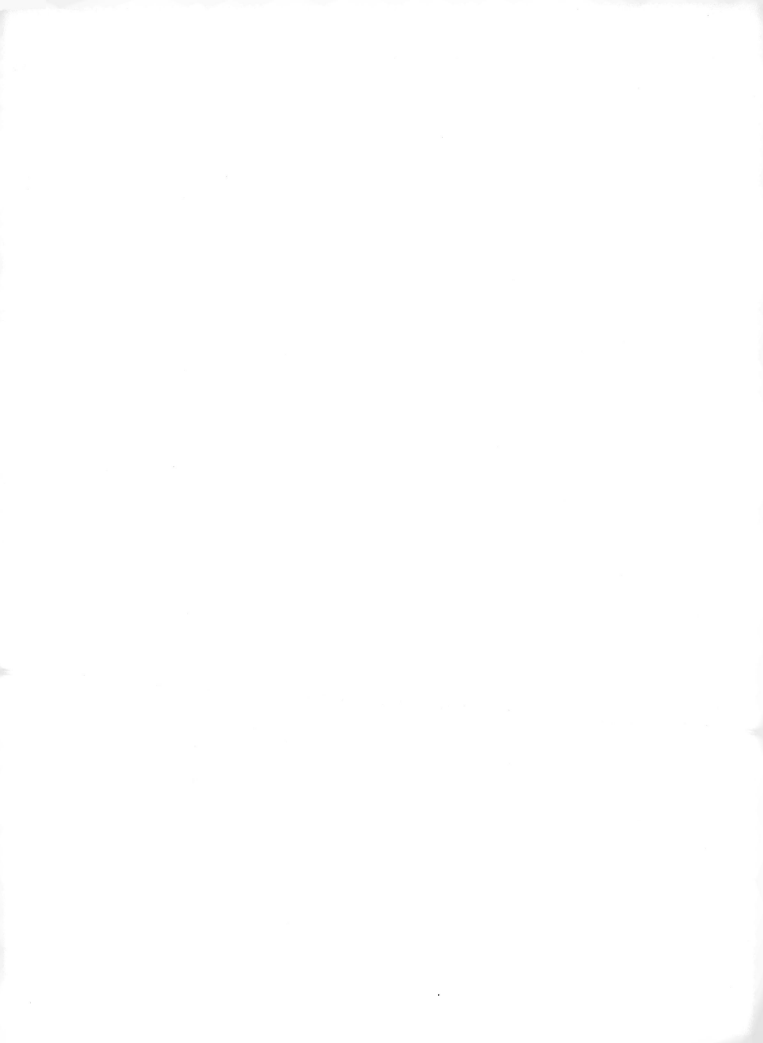

Chapter 16

Design and methodology of clinical trials of erectile dysfunction

R. C. Rosen

■ INTRODUCTION

Clinical trials of erectile dysfunction (ED) have proliferated in the past decade, as a wide range of injectable, transurethral and oral agents have become available.[1–9] Crucial to the development of these new treatments has been the design, conduct and interpretation of clinical trials in selected patient groups. Conversely, the advent of novel pharmacological agents has served as a major impetus for innovations in research design and methodology. This is especially evident in the area of sexual function assessment, where advances have taken place in the measurement of objective (physiological) and subjective (self-report) indices of male sexual function.[10–15] Changes are also evident in the types of research design employed, the criteria used for patient selection, and the evaluation of treatment efficacy and outcome. Quality-of-life (QL) measures are an essential component of outcome assessment, and two disease-specific QL instruments have been proposed recently.[16,17] Despite these advances, significant limitations and weaknesses are apparent in some areas, and these are addressed below. Specific goals of this chapter are (a) to provide a conceptual overview for evaluating clinical trials of ED, (b) to review and evaluate current trial methodologies, and (c) to identify critical gaps and needs for future research.

■ CLINICAL TRIALS: BASIC ISSUES IN RESEARCH DESIGN

The concept of a clinical trial originated in the 18th century with Lind's classic study of dietary control of scurvy.[18,19] However, the key principles of blinding and random assignment of subjects to study groups were first reported in 1931 by Amberson and colleagues,[20] in a study of sanocrysin treatment of tuberculosis. Similarly, the term 'placebo' can be traced to a study by Diehl and colleagues[21] in 1938, in which the effectiveness of a cold vaccine was compared with that of a neutral (saline) solution. Since that time, the clinical trial has assumed a dominant role as the preferred method of evaluating new and existing treatments in almost all areas of medical practice. Despite the numerous refinements in study design and analysis that have taken place in the subsequent half-century,[22–25] the basic principles of blinding, random assignment to treatment conditions, and use of placebo controls remain at the core of most clinical trial designs. With few exceptions, all of the major clinical trials in the past decade have been based on these core principles.

A clinical trial may be defined as 'a prospective study comparing the effect and value of intervention(s) against a control in human beings'.[26] Several elements of this definition are worth emphasizing. First, patients must be followed prospectively from a clearly specified point in time (i.e. study baseline). Second, a clinical trial must employ one or more defined treatments or interventions, each of which is capable of being evaluated objectively. Current treatment options for ED include surgical, medical, or psychological interventions, or combinations thereof. Third, a control group must be included, against which the effectiveness and value of each intervention is compared. Several types of control group are available, including a standard treatment or usual care group, a placebo condition, or a waiting-list (i.e. no-treatment) control. Clinical trials of ED have typically made use of placebo controls, in preference to either standard treatment or usual care controls. This may reflect a lack of agreement among investigators regarding the definition of standard treatment or usual care for ED, as well as a reluctance by patients to be assigned to these conditions. Owing to the obvious significance of psychological factors in ED, placebo controls are an essential consideration in the design of clinical trials of ED. Various types of placebo control are available, as discussed below. Finally, although animal studies have contributed significantly to the understanding of pathophysiology and mechanisms of action, only studies on humans are properly considered as clinical trials.[26]

Design of clinical trials

Two key elements in the design of any clinical trial are (1) definition of the study population, and (2) selection of response variables or study endpoints to be monitored. Definition of the study population will determine which patients are recruited for the study, the eligibility requirements (inclusion and exclusion criteria), and the generalizability of the findings. Given the heterogeneity of most ED samples and the lack of a standardized approach to diagnosis,[27-29] patient selection criteria may vary widely from one trial to another. Disease severity and duration of illness are two fundamental dimensions along which patient populations differ, in addition to age, marital status and presence of concomitant illnesses. Clinical trials of ED also differ markedly in the proportion of patients with organic versus psychogenically based dysfunction,[2,4,7,8] as well as the means for assessing these factors.

The selection of response variables or study endpoints is highly variable from one ED trial to another. Physiological measures of penile engorgement or rigidity, self-administered questionnaires, patient diaries or event logs, and partner reports have all been used to varying degrees.[30-33] Standardized definitions of a treatment responder are lacking, as are well-established criteria for clinical improvement or change. An important implication of the inconsistency in patient selection criteria and choice of study endpoints is that caution needs to be exercised in drawing comparisons of treatment outcome from one trial to another. Regrettably, no prospective studies to date have included direct (i.e. head-to-head) comparisons of different treatment interventions in the same trial.

A number of study designs have been used in clinical ED trials, all of which incorporate the basic principles of randomization and placebo control. In the simplest type of design, patients are randomly assigned to one of two or more parallel treatment conditions for a specified period (usually 1–3 months). Each patient is exposed to one treatment condition only, and comparisons are made between groups at various points in time. Baseline evaluation is necessary to demonstrate that treatment groups are equivalent prior to randomization. Treatment efficacy is assessed by analysis of between-group differences during or following treatment. Parallel designs are typically employed in large-scale, multicentre, phase III or IV ED trials with relatively large patient samples (e.g. >100 patients). In contrast, crossover or within-subject designs, in which each patient serves as his own control, are used in phase I or II trials. Crossover designs may include as few as two periods — intervention and control — which patients receive in randomized or counterbalanced order. Three- or four-period crossover designs are used infrequently in clinical trials. The major advantage of a crossover design is the reduction in variability due to individual patient differences, although use of the design should be restricted to situations in which carryover effects are absent or unlikely.[34,35] Given the strong potential for psychological carryover effects, crossover designs may have limited applicability in phase III clinical trials of ED.

Withdrawal designs are used to assess the effects of treatment discontinuation or dosage reduction. This type of study design is useful in evaluating the need for continued therapy in patients with various chronic diseases. For example, withdrawal designs have been used to evaluate the need for chronic antihypertensive or anticoagulant therapy in several large-scale clinical trials.[36,37] Few withdrawal studies have been performed on the treatment of ED, although the chronic nature of the condition and need for long-term therapy are strong arguments in favour of conducting more of these trials in the future. A withdrawal design can also be valuable in assessing the effectiveness of a treatment with uncertain benefits, such as yohimbine.[38,39] This type of study has not been conducted to date.

Blinding procedures

Blinding procedures are a key element in the design of all clinical trials. Blinding is necessary to prevent response bias associated with treatment-related expectations on the part of either investigators or participants. These biases may influence the outcome of the trial in either a positive or negative direction. In addition to the usual double-blind treatment phase, clinical trials of ED frequently include a single-blind, lead-in phase, which is used to screen out patients who are most susceptible to placebo effects. Although this design has potential benefits in limiting the magnitude of subsequent placebo effects, it may lead to exclusion of a potentially important group of study subjects — namely, those who respond positively to both psychological and pharmacological interventions. In this sense, the design may introduce a form of type II error. There is also a tendency, in some instances, for patients or staff to 'bend the rules' in order to have patients admitted to a study. Patients may be encouraged to fake good or bad if the single-blind contingencies are inadvertently revealed.

Following the single-blind lead-in or no-treatment baseline phase, patients are typically assigned to the double-blind, randomized phase of the study. This phase may last from several weeks to several months, and is the core feature of most clinical trials. All major clinical trials of ED to date have included designs of this type, with minor variations. The obvious advantages are in controlling for patient or experimenter bias, although these sources of bias are never entirely eliminated. For example, when a drug is associated with characteristic side effects (e.g. facial flushing, tachycardia), patients or investigators may infer that the active drug is being taken, thus effectively 'breaking the blind'. To assess the potential degree of unblinding that may have occurred, participants and clinical staff can be asked, following the termination of the trial, to guess to which condition (drug or placebo) the patient was assigned. Assuming equal probability of the patient being assigned to drug or placebo, estimates by staff and patients should be correct approximately 50% of the time; marked deviations in either direction are an indication of blinding failure. Post-treatment assessment of blinding has provided useful data in some large-scale trials of cardiovascular disease,[40–42] but has yet to be applied in clinical trials of ED. This would make a useful addition to the design of future clinical trials in this area.

Blinding may also be compromised by the need for safety or interim data-monitoring procedures. In large-scale trials, safety and data monitoring will usually be assumed by a separate entity, typically a data-monitoring committee or agency. To guard against possible biases in this monitoring agency, some studies are conducted in a 'triple-blind' fashion — i.e. the patient, investigator, and monitoring agency are all blind as to the study conditions. This type of design is not commonly used in clinical trials of ED, perhaps owing to the lack of major safety issues or perceived need for potential early termination of the trial,

as is more likely to occur in trials of cardiovascular disease, cancer or other life-threatening conditions. Triple-blind study designs have yet to be reported in the clinical trial literature for ED.

Open-label extension trials

Following the double-blind phase, it is common practice in ED trials for patients to be offered entry into an open-label extension trial with the study drug. Patients are usually titrated to an optimal dosage level in this phase. This open-label phase serves two important functions: (1) it serves as an incentive for patients to participate in the trial, and (2) it provides additional long-term safety and efficacy data. Open-label treatment typically lasts from 6 to 12 months, or up to 2 years in some instances. Patients are required to return for follow-up visits at regular intervals, at which time safety and efficacy variables are monitored. Despite the lack of patient or investigator blinding, open-label studies provide useful data concerning long-term safety and potential discontinuation rates over time. Investigators also acquire first-hand experience in the clinical use of the drug, including potential benefits or risks associated with long-term use.

Historical or concurrent controls

Finally, non-randomized control studies may provide limited information concerning the effects of a new intervention in comparison with either historical or concurrent control conditions. For example, the author and colleagues have recently reported on the use of a concurrent control design for evaluating the effects of several pharmacological antidotes for treatment of serotonin re-uptake inhibitor (SRI)-related sexual dysfunctions in a large sample of psychiatric patients.[43] Patients were treated with either yohimbine, amantadine or cyproheptadine, based upon patients' preferences and/or prior experience with one or another of these drugs. Retrospective comparison of the effects of these agents, compared with SRI treatment alone, provided information concerning the effectiveness of each drug in alleviating SRI-related dysfunction. Other studies have made use of historical controls, in which the use of a new intervention is compared with outcomes in previous patient groups or clinical trials. Several authors have argued that historical control data can contribute substantially to clinical decision-making.[44,45] Despite the potential advantages of non-randomized designs in more highly developed areas of clinical research, such as cancer or heart disease, use of these designs has been extremely limited in clinical trials of ED.

DEFINING THE STUDY POPULATION

It is axiomatic in any clinical trial that the study population should be defined as clearly as possible in advance, using unambiguous inclusion and exclusion criteria. In describing the study, investigators should state specifically how participants were recruited for the study, which eligibility requirements were used for inclusion, and the baseline characteristics of the population. The age range of participants should be specified, in addition to overall health status, use of concurrent medications, and the criteria used for determining the level and duration of dysfunction. Study populations in clinical trials of ED have varied along three important dimensions: (1) the degree of severity or duration of ED; (2) the diagnosis of organic versus psychogenic aetiology; and (3) the presence of concomitant illnesses or medications. Additionally, some studies have required all participants to be in a committed heterosexual relationship, and the involvement of participants' wives or partners has been a requirement for participation in some studies. Eligibility criteria such as these have a significant effect on the degree of efficacy observed, as well as determining the generalizability of the findings.

Homogeneity

The degree of homogeneity of the study population is an important design element in any clinical trial. Arguments in favour of a more homogeneous study group (e.g. psychogenic or diabetic patients) are the potential reduction of patient-related variability and the increased likelihood of observing a significant treatment effect. Results may also be easier to interpret and the applicability to clinical practice may be clearer. For example, if only those patients with mild or psychogenic ED are included in the trial, practitioners may be less likely to make use of the treatment in more severe cases. On the other hand, restriction of the entry criteria may limit the trial's potential for showing positive treatment effects in other patient groups. Heterogeneous patient groups are also easier to recruit in large numbers. Additionally, highly selected patient groups may not be representative of actual clinical practice, where a more heterogeneous group of patients is likely to be encountered. Recently, the trend in

randomized clinical trials is towards simplification of entry criteria and admission of less-selected patient groups to the trial. This is especially evident in large-scale trials of cardiovascular disease.[46,47] Similarly, recent trials of the new phosphodiesterase type-5 inhibitor (sildenafil) have included large numbers of relatively unselected ED patients.[8] The high level of safety and efficacy shown in this heterogeneous population suggests that the drug may be well suited as a first-line therapy for ED in general office practice.

Subgroup analyses

In large-scale trials with heterogeneous patient populations, subgroup analyses are frequently used to evaluate treatment efficacy and safety in selected patient groups. Although useful findings may be generated in some instances by this approach, there is also a danger of spurious findings being reported. The potential risks and limitations of subgroup analyses have been described by Collins and colleagues.[48] These authors note that most subgroup analyses lack sufficient power to demonstrate significant interaction effects, even where these may exist. Conversely, subgroup analyses may occasionally demonstrate a significant interaction effect (i.e. greater or lesser therapeutic efficacy or safety in specific subgroups) due to the effects of chance or uncontrolled variables in the study. To limit the potential for false positives, a limited number of subgroup analyses should be specified in advance. Moreover, these should be justified on the basis of a priori predictions about the probable interaction effects to be evaluated.

STUDY OUTCOMES AND RESPONSE VARIABLES

Response variables are the endpoints or outcomes to be measured during the course of a clinical trial. In principle, one or two response variables should be selected in advance as the primary endpoints of the trial, although in practice several response variables are usually reported. In these situations, special care needs to be taken to correct statistically for the number of comparisons made, and possible interrelationships between the response variables. Whereas measures of morbidity or mortality are relatively standardized and well accepted in some areas of medicine, this is less true in clinical trials of ED. The choice of primary endpoints in a clinical trial is clearly essential, and response variables should be clearly defined and justified prior to initiation of the trial. In the absence of standardized outcome measures, comparison of results from one ED trial to another should be viewed with considerable caution.

Among the response variables most frequently used in trials of ED are objective measures of penile rigidity or tumescence (e.g. RigiScan), patient-based questionnaires or diary reports of sexual function, partner assessments, and global ratings of clinical improvement. Each of these measures has certain advantages and limitations.

Objective measures

Several methods for objective measurement of penile rigidity and engorgement have been described,[10–12] the most widely used of which is the RigiScan system (Urohealth Corporation, Atlanta, Georgia). This method was first described by Bradley and colleagues,[49] who recommended use of the device in the home setting for monitoring of nocturnal penile tumescence and rigidity (NPTR). The device is attached to the patient's inner thigh, with two loops placed around the base and tip of the penis proximal to the coronal sulcus. Measures of radial rigidity are obtained by application of a predetermined force to each loop every 3 minutes initially, and at 30-second intervals when an increase of more than 10 mm at the base is detected. Penile rigidity is expressed as a function of displacement when the loop is tightened around the penis, and rigidity is defined in terms of penile stiffness as determined by cross-sectional response to radial compression.[10] Although the technique was developed originally for home monitoring of NPT, it has been used for real-time assessment of penile tumescence and rigidity in response to pharmacological or visual sexual stimulation (VSS). For example, in-office RigiScan measures of penile rigidity were reported as a primary endpoint in a pivotal dose-finding study of intracavernosal alprostadil for ED.[1] RigiScan changes in response to VSS have similarly been reported in recent trials of oral apomorphine[6] and sildenafil.[50]

Several potential limitations have been identified, the most serious of which is the assumption of equivalence between radial and axial rigidity. Although there is limited evidence for this assumption, at least one study compared measurements of axial and radial rigidity at constant corporal pressures.[51] Axial and radial rigidity were found to be functionally related, and both measures were moderately correlated with intracavernous pressure. In a comparison of RigiScan with sleep laboratory measures of tumescence and rigidity, Licht and

colleagues[52] reported that a base rigidity of 55% or more predicted functional erection with a sensitivity of 85% and specificity of 91%. Other investigators have reported that tip rigidity of 70% for more than 5 minutes provides the best cutoff for diagnostic classification.[53] Additional limitations of the device include lack of adequate standardization of normal values, limited time sampling of tumescence and rigidity, inflexibility of the accompanying software, and potential intrusiveness of the device for some patients. Despite these limitations, RigiScan recording continues to have an important role as an objective and quantifiable measure of erectile response.

Other physiological measures of penile tumescence and rigidity include volumetric and strain-gauge plethysmography,[54,55] and the erectiometer.[56] Volumetric plethysmography provides a highly sensitive measure of penile engorgement, which has been used extensively in studies of sexual preference or paraphilias.[57–59] However, the measurement apparatus is obtrusive and inconvenient to use, and provides no information on penile rigidity. Similarly, mercury-in-rubber and electromechanical strain-gauges provide sensitive measures of changes in penile circumference and have been widely used in laboratory studies of sexual arousal.[60–62] Again, the lack of rigidity assessment is a major disadvantage of these approaches in clinical trials of ED.

Lastly, the erectiometer provides a crude measure of both rigidity and tumescence (circumference change). This device consists of a felt band 2 cm wide with a sliding collar fastened to one end. The felt band expands with tumescence, but requires a force of about 250 g to initiate expansion. In this way, the device provides a combined assessment of changes in both circumference and rigidity.[56] It has been used to differentiate response patterns in clinical studies with normal and sexually dysfunctional men,[63,64] although the erectiometer provides less sensitivity and reliability than either the RigiScan or mercury strain-gauge devices.[65]

Self-report measures

Self-report measures of sexual function are divided into three major categories — self-administered questionnaires, daily diaries or event logs, and structured interviews. Each of these approaches has been used in recent clinical trials, although the primary emphasis in most validation studies has been on self-administered questionnaires (SAQs). These measures have the potential advantage of providing standardized and relatively cost-efficient assessment of current and past sexual functioning. Patient burden is generally low, and some measures have been designed specifically for use in multicentre, clinical trials.[14,15] Only one structured interview method has been evaluated to date.[66] At present, the most widely used measures are those described below.

The Derogatis Sexual Function Inventory (DSFI)

The DSFI is a comprehensive measure of male and female sexual function.[67] The complete DSFI scale consists of 245 items, requiring 40–60 minutes to complete. Ten different domains of sexual function are assessed, including information, experience, drive, attitudes, psychological symptoms, effects, gender role definition, fantasy, body image and sexual satisfaction, in addition to a global sexual satisfaction index. The test has been psychometrically validated, and has been widely used in studies of normal and dysfunctional individuals. Its major drawbacks are the length and complexity of the instrument, which render it generally unsuitable for use in clinical trials.

The Center for Marital and Sexual Health Questionnaire (CMSH-SFQ)

This brief 18-item, self-report questionnaire assesses current sexual function in the areas of erection, orgasm, desire and satisfaction.[68] Initial psychometric assessment of the instrument has been performed, although data regarding sensitivity and specificity are lacking. In this study, the measure showed adequate reliability and construct validity. It has had limited use to date in clinical trials of ED.

The Brief Male Sexual Function Inventory (BMSFI)

This is an 11-item questionnaire scale that assesses several components of male sexual function, including sexual drive, erection, ejaculation, sexual problems, and overall satisfaction.[14] Major advantages of this scale are (a) a relatively high degree of internal consistency and test–retest reliability, (b) adequate discriminant validity for three of the domains (erectile function, problems, overall satisfaction), and (c) ease of use. Potential limitations are the restricted evaluation of erectile and orgasmic function, and lack of evidence concerning sensitivity or treatment responsiveness.

The International Index of Erectile Function (IIEF)

A recent measure designed specifically for assessment of sexual function in clinical trials is the IIEF.[15] This instrument consists of 15 items and assesses sexual functioning in five domains — erectile function, orgasmic function, sexual desire, intercourse satisfaction, and overall satisfaction. Average scores are calculated in each of the major domains, and a severity algorithm is available for clinical interpretation of scores. Psychometric validation has demonstrated a high degree of reliability (internal consistency and test–retest reliability) in both clinical and non-clinical samples. Sensitivity and specificity (treatment responsiveness) are excellent, as has been shown in recent clinical trials.[69] The IIEF is available in 23 languages, and is currently in use in several large-scale multinational trials.

Major advantages of this measure are its relative brevity and ease of use, inclusion of multiple domains of sexual function and strong psychometric profile. Potential disadvantages are the limited assessment of certain domains (e.g. sexual desire, orgasmic function), restricted time-frame (4 weeks), and uncertain validity in selected populations (e.g. spinal cord injured, psychiatric patients).

Structured interview of sexual function

Despite potential advantages in sensitivity and reliability, as previously stated, only one structured interview method for assessment of sexual function has been reported to date.[66] The Derogatis Interview for Sexual Functioning (DISF-SR), is a set of brief, gender-specific, interview questions designed to assess an individual's quality of sexual functioning in several domains. The major disadvantages of this method are the increased time of administration and the need for interviewer training. Additionally, the DISF-SR may not be suitable for use in multicentre or multinational trials, given the need for standardization of interviewer ratings across sites. Cross-cultural validation data are also lacking.

Daily diary and event logs

Daily diary forms or sexual event logs are frequently used measures of sexual function in clinical trials. These typically include assessment of variables such as intercourse frequency and satisfaction, quality of erection, and medication use. Despite their widespread use, validation studies of these measures are notably lacking. The author and colleagues have recently conducted a validation study of the Sexual Encounter Profile (SEP), an event log used in clinical trials of oral phentolamine and other agents.[70] Data from this preliminary study indicates a high degree of correlation between erection and intercourse satisfaction ratings between SEP and IIEF measures in patients with mild to moderate degrees of ED.

QUALITY-OF-LIFE ASSESSMENT IN TRIALS

QL measures, such as physical functioning, mood state and overall life satisfaction, are routinely used in large-scale clinical trials. Although measurement of these domains remains controversial, marked progress has been made towards development of a range of instruments for QL assessment.[71–73] These measures are usually employed as either baseline covariates or secondary outcome variables in clinical trials, particularly in the areas of cardiovascular disease and cancer. In the treatment of hypertension, for example, QL outcomes have been used to differentiate between drugs with approximately similar effects on morbidity and mortality.[74,75] Recent clinical trials of ED have included QL measures as secondary endpoints. Although these measures provide a potentially broader understanding of treatment effects, several limitations and problems are evident.

First, most QL scales are designed for use in medically ill patients, whose disease or treatment has a noticeable impact on physical or psychological functioning. Although ED patients in the general population may have deficits in some areas,[76] clinical trials of ED typically exclude patients with major medical or psychiatric disease. As a result, baseline differences between these patients and age-matched controls tend to be minimal. Additionally, most domains of QL assessment, such as physical functioning, cognitive functioning and global health perceptions, are unlikely to be affected by the symptoms of ED or its treatment. Patients may also be unwilling to acknowledge emotional concomitants of the disorder, for fear of their condition being labelled 'psychogenic'.

In response to the need for a more 'disease-specific' approach, two new instruments for QL assessment in ED trials have been developed. Wagner and colleagues[16] have reported the development of a 19-item scale (QOL-MED), based on semi-structured interviews with a representative sample of ED patients. This measure has a high degree of reproducibility and internal consistency, but has received little validation in ED patients or controls. More recently, Fugl-Meyer and colleagues[76] have described the use of a brief, eight-item life satisfaction checklist for specific QL assessment in ED

trials. This measure was found to differentiate between ED patients and controls on several dimensions, although few differences were found between patients diagnosed with organic ED and non-dysfunctional controls. As predicted, significant improvements on two scale dimensions (sexual life and overall life satisfaction) were found, following successful treatment with prostaglandin injections. This measure provides a simple, crude assessment of QL dimensions of potential interest in ED patients, and may be of value in future clinical trials. However, there is a clear need for more sophisticated and sensitive measures of ED-related QL assessment.

ADVERSE-EVENT MONITORING

An important component of all clinical trials is the monitoring and reporting of adverse events. Evaluation of adverse events is typically conducted over several stages, ranging from phase I safety and toxicology studies in humans and animals, to large-scale, phase III trials during which multiple adverse events are monitored and evaluated. Post-marketing surveillance studies provide additional data on side effects associated with long-term use of the drug. Although most pharmacological agents are extensively evaluated prior to and following regulatory approval, several issues and concerns in adverse-event monitoring in clinical ED trials are worth noting.

First, the means by which adverse events are ascertained can influence the frequency and type of reports obtained. Checklist or interview approaches each have certain advantages and disadvantages. Symptom checklists have the major advantage of allowing standardization of reporting between and within trials, whereas interview approaches encourage more in-depth assessment and recording of unanticipated adverse events. Some trials use a combination of these approaches. The number of patients and duration of the trial can have a significant impact on the frequency of adverse events reported. Since sample size is invariably calculated on the basis of estimated changes in the primary response variables, most trials lack adequate power for reliably assessing adverse-event frequency, particularly in the area of low-frequency but potentially serious adverse events. A related problem is the relatively high rate of adverse events often observed in the control group, which could be related to the age and health status of the patients or to the influence of placebo effects. Long-term follow-up studies of

ED treatment are relatively rare, although such trials are obviously necessary for adequate safety assessment.

With the advent of a wide range of treatment options for ED, it might be anticipated that safety issues and reporting of adverse events will assume even greater significance in the years to come. Regulatory agencies, in particular, are likely to place increasing emphasis on adverse-event reporting, since ED is regarded as neither life threatening nor a serious medical condition. Manufacturers are tending to pay greater attention also to safety issues, in an attempt to differentiate their product from those of competitors. A positive effect of these trends is that clinical trials of ED are including increasingly larger numbers of patients for longer periods.

■ DATA ANALYSIS AND REPORTING OF RESULTS

A variety of data-analytic methods have been employed in recent clinical ED trials. Although a detailed discussion of these methods is beyond the scope of this chapter, some general comments and recommendations are as follows. To a large degree, the type of statistical model employed depends upon the nature of the research design (e.g. parallel, between-group versus counterbalanced, crossover design) and the response variables being analysed (e.g. continuous versus dichotomous variables). Sample power should be calculated in advance, using best available estimates of the means and variances of the primary response variables, and anticipated changes associated with treatment. All subjects randomized to treatment or control conditions should be included in an 'intention-to-treat' analysis, in which data from drop-outs or withdrawals are included in the final analysis of treatment outcome. This general rule should not be applied to the assessment of adverse events, however, where it may be preferable to report the frequency of side effects only among those who actually received the treatment.[48] Covariate adjustments are often used to control for differences between the study groups in baseline or prognostic factors (e.g. age, duration of illness), although covariance analysis should be performed only when specific statistical assumptions are met.[77,78] As noted above, a limited number of subgroup analyses may be conducted, paying careful attention to the potential lack

of power and possibility of type I errors associated with these analyses.[48]

Assessing the magnitude of treatment effects is a potentially thorny issue, which involves both statistical and clinical considerations. Effect-size calculations can be used to provide a statistical estimate of the magnitude of treatment effects, although this approach has not been widely used in clinical trials of ED. Rather, most investigators report the magnitude of treatment effects in terms of percentages of responders in the active compared with control groups.[1,2] Such comparisons involve prior definition of a response threshold or cutoff, which may be subject to criticism. For example, in the recent multicentre trial of transurethral alprostadil,[2] a treatment responder was defined as any individual who completed sexual intercourse at least once during the study period. It could be argued that this definition is overly liberal and not in keeping with the usual clinical criteria for successful treatment. Unfortunately, normative population data are lacking to establish response criteria for adequate sexual performance at each age-group; in the absence of such data, continued disagreement on this issue is likely. One approach to the problem is to report several measures of treatment efficacy, including both quantitative (e.g. number of successful intercourse attempts) and non-quantitative (e.g. global satisfaction) indices. This allows for a broader assessment of the magnitude and consistency of treatment effects.

Finally, meta-analysis is a potentially powerful statistical technique for assessing the direction and magnitude of treatment effects over several independent trials.[79,80] First, the method requires careful selection of trials for inclusion in the analysis, based upon predetermined criteria for assessing methodological adequacy (i.e. randomization, double-blinding). Results from all eligible trials are then standardized and combined according to strict statistical rules. An odds ratio or relative risk analysis is then performed on the resulting data. To date, only one meta-analysis has been reported for clinical trials of yohimbine hydrochloride in the treatment of ED;[81] this analysis showed a moderate, although inconsistent, effect for yohimbine across clinical trials. The author and colleagues have recently proposed that this inconsistency in outcome may be related to unpredictable patterns of absorption and bioavailability observed with the drug.[82,83] As the number of clinical trials of ED increases, it is anticipated that meta-analytical techniques will play an increasingly important role.

■ SUMMARY AND CONCLUSIONS

Major advances have taken place in the diagnosis and treatment of ED in the past decade. The advent of new pharmacological treatment agents, in particular, has raised a number of important issues regarding the design and conduct of clinical trials for ED. Randomized clinical trials are a relatively recent innovation in this area, and methodological issues and concerns have been identified in several areas: these have included problems in study design, selection of patients, blinding procedures, response measures and outcome variables, and types of statistical analysis employed. Of particular concern are the lack of standardization in response measures across trials, use of single-blind lead-in procedures, lack of assessment of blinding efficacy, and limited range of interventions and controls in most trials. Despite these limitations, an impressive body of data has accumulated in recent years, owing, in part, to significant advances in the design and conduct of ED trials.

A major focus of this chapter is the choice of response variables for outcome assessment. These include objective (e.g. RigiScan) and self-report (e.g. IIEF, BMSFI) measures of response, each of which has certain strengths and weaknesses.

One measure in particular, the IIEF, has demonstrated a high degree of sensitivity and specificity to treatment effects.[15] Self-report questionnaires have important advantages in cost efficiency and inclusion of other dimensions of sexual function (e.g. sexual desire, orgasmic capacity). Additional studies are needed to determine the ideal measure, or combination of measures, for outcome evaluation in clinical trials of ED. QL assessment is increasingly important as an additional study endpoint, and two disease-specific QL measures have recently been proposed.[75,76] The ultimate value of these measures in large-scale clinical trials has yet to be determined.

Final issues considered in this chapter are the assessment of magnitude of treatment effects and the definition of a treatment responder. Currently, these are highly controversial issues, as response criteria have varied widely from study to study. Additional normative data are urgently needed to address this issue, as are comparative studies of outcome assessment across trials. Meta-analytic techniques provide useful information on the direction and magnitude of effects over multiple independent trials, although this approach has rarely been used to date in trials of ED. As the number and variety of new pharmacological agents increases, and increasing numbers of clinical trials are undertaken, meta-analytic studies are likely to assume an increasingly important role in the future.

■ REFERENCES

1. Linet O I, Ogrinc F G, for the Alprostadil Study Group. Efficacy and safety of intracavernosal alprostadil in men with erectile dysfunction. N Engl J Med 1996; 334: 873–877

2. Padma-Nathan H, Hellstrom W J G, Kaiser F E et al. Treatment of men with erectile dysfunction with transurethral alprostadil. N Engl J Med 1997; 336: 1–7

3. Roy J B, Petrone R L, Said S I. A clinical trial of intracavernous vasoactive intestinal peptide to induce penile erection. J Urol 1989; 143: 302–304

4. Cavallini G. Minoxidil versus nitroglycerin: a prospective double-blind controlled trial in transcutaneous erection facilitation for organic impotence. J Urol 1991; 146: 50–53

5. Korenman S G, Viosca S P. Treatment of vasculogenic sexual dysfunction with pentoxifylline. J Am Geriatr Soc 1993; 41: 363–366

6. Heaton J P W, Morales A, Adams M A et al. Recovery of erectile function by the oral administration of apomorphine. Urology 1995; 45: 200–206

7. Morales A, Heaton J P, Johnson B, Adams M. Oral and topical treatment of erectile dysfunction: present and future. Urol Clin North Am 1995; 22: 879–886

8. Boolel M, Gepi-Attee S, Gingell J C, Allen M J. Sildenafil, a novel effective oral therapy for male erectile dysfunction. Br J Urol 1996; 78: 257–261

10. Levine L A, Lenting E L. Use of nocturnal penile tumescence and rigidity in the evaluation of male erectile dysfunction. Urol Clin North Am 1995; 22: 775–788

11. Burris A S, Banks S M, Sherins R J. Quantitative assessment of nocturnal penile tumescence and rigidity in normal men using a home monitor. J Androl 1989; 10: 492–498

12. Slob A K, Blom J H, van der Bosch J J. Erection problems in medical practice: differential diagnosis with a relatively simple method. J Urol 1990; 143: 46–50

13. Corty E W, Althof S E, Kurit D M. The reliability and validity of a sexual functioning questionnaire. J Sex Marital Ther 1996; 22: 27–34

14. O'Leary M P, Fowler F J, Lenderking W R et al. A brief male sexual function inventory for urology. Urology 1995; 46: 697–706

15. Rosen R C, Riley A, Wagner G et al. The International Index of Erectile Function (IIEF): a multidimensional scale for assessment of erectile dysfunction. Urology 1997; 49: 822–830

16. Wagner T H, Patrick D L, McKenna P, Froese P S. Cross-cultural development of a quality of life measure for men with erection difficulties. Qual Life Res 1996; 5: 443–449

17. Fugl-Meyer A R, Lodnert G, Branholm I-B, Fugl-Meyer K S. On life satisfaction in male erectile dysfunction. Int J Impot Res 1997; 9: 141–148

18. Bull J P. The historical development of clinical therapeutic trials. J Chronic Dis 1959; 10: 218–248

19. Lilienfeld A M. Ceteris paribus: the evolution of the clinical trial. Bull Hist Med 1982; 56: 1–18

20. Amberson J B, McMahon B T, Pinner M. A clinical trial of sancrosyn in pulmonary tuberculosis. Am Rev Tuberc 1931; 24: 401–435

21. Diehl H S, Baker A B, Cowan D W. Cold vaccines: an evaluation based on a controlled study. JAMA 1938; 111: 1168–1173

22. Hill A B. The clinical trial. N Engl J Med 1952; 247: 113–119

23. Doll R. Clinical trials: retrospect and prospect. Stat Med 1982; 1: 337–344

24. Schaefer A. The ethics of the randomized clinical trial. N Engl J Med 1982; 301: 719–724

25. Bulpitt C J. Randomized controlled clinical trials. The Hague: Martinus Nijhoff, 1983

26. Friedman L M, Furberg C D, DeMets D L. Fundamentals of clinical trials, 3rd edn. St Louis: Mosby, 1996

27. Meuleman E J, Diemont W L. Investigation of erectile dysfunction: diagnostic testing for vascular factors in erectile dysfunction. Urol Clin North Am 1995; 22: 803–819

28. Hatzichristou D G, Bertero E B, Goldstein I. Decision making in the evaluation of impotence: the patient profile-oriented algorithm. Sex Disabil 1994; 12: 29–37

29. Davis-Joseph B, Tiefer L, Melman A. Accuracy of the initial history and physical examination to establish the etiology of erectile dysfunction. Urology 1995; 45: 498–502

30. Althof S E, Turner L A, Levine S B et al. Through the eyes of women: the sexual and psychological responses of women to their partner's treatment with self-injection or external vacuum pump therapy. J Urol 1992; 147: 1024–1027

31. Derogatis L R, Melisaratos N. The DSFI: a multidimensional measure of sexual functioning. J Sex Marital Ther 1979; 5: 244–281

32. Reynolds C F, Frank E, Thase M E et al. Assessment of sexual function in depressed, impotent and healthy men: factor analysis of a brief sexual function questionnaire for men. Psych Res 1988; 24: 231–250

33. Rosen R C. Physiological and self-report measures in the male. Int J Impot Res (in press)

34. Brown B W. The crossover experiment for clinical trials. Biometrics 1980; 35: 69–80

35. Fleiss J L. A critique of recent research on the two treatment crossover design. Controlled Clin Trials 1989; 10: 237–243

36. Stamler R, Stamler J, Grimm R et al. Nutritional therapy for high blood pressure — final report of a four-year randomized controlled trial — the Hypertension Control Program. JAMA 1987; 257: 1484–1491

37. Report of the Sixty Plus Reinfarction Study Research Group: A double blind trial to assess long-term oral anticoagulant therapy in elderly patients after myocardial infarction. Lancet 1980; ii: 989–994

38. Reid K, Morales A, Harris C et al. Double blind trial of yohimbine in treatment of psychogenic impotence. Lancet 1987; i: 421–423

39. Riley A J, Goodman R E, Kellett J M, Orr R. Double blind trial of yohimbine hydrochloride in the treatment of erection inadequacy. Sex Marital Ther 1989; 4: 17–26

40. Howard J, Whittemore A S, Hoover J J et al. How blind was the patient blind in AMIS? Clin Pharmacol Ther 1982; 32: 543–555

41. Byington R P, Curb J D, Mattson M E. Assessment of double-blindness at the conclusion of the Beta-Blocker Heart Attack Trial. JAMA 1985; 253: 1733–1736

42. Jespersen C M and the Danish Study on Verapamil in Myocardial Infarction. Assessment of blindness in the Danish Verapamil Infarction Trial II (DAVIT II). Eur J Clin Pharmacol 1990; 39: 75–76

43. Ashton A K, Hamer R, Rosen R C. Serotonin reuptake inhibitor-induced sexual dysfunction and its treatment: a large-scale retrospective study of 596 psychiatric outpatients. J Sex Marital Ther 1997; 23: 165–175

44. Lasagna L. Historical controls: the practitioner's clinical trials. N Engl J Med 1982; 307: 1339–1340

45. Gehan E A. The evaluation of therapies: historical control studies. Stat Med 1984; 3: 315–324

46. Hypertension Detection and Follow-up Program Cooperative Group. Five-year findings of the Hypertension Detection and Follow-up Program. 1. Reduction in mortality of persons with high blood pressure, including mild hypertension. JAMA 1979; 242: 2562–2571

47. ISIS-3 (Third International Study of Infarct Survival) Collaborative Group. ISIS-3: a randomised comparison of streptokinase vs tissue plasminogen activator vs anistreplase and of aspirin plus heparin vs aspirin alone among 41,299 cases of suspected acute myocardial infarction. Lancet 1992; iii: 753–770

48. Collins R, Peto R, Gray R, Parish S. Large-scale randomized evidence: trials and overviews. In: Weatherall D J, Ledingham J G G, Warrell D A (eds) Oxford textbook of medicine, 3rd edn. Oxford: Oxford University Press, 1996: 21–32

49. Bradley W E, Timm G W, Gallagher J M et al. New method for continuous measurement of nocturnal penile tumescence and rigidity. Urology 1985; 26: 4–9

50. Levine L A, Lenting L. Use of nocturnal penile tumescence and rigidity in the evaluation of male erectile dysfunction. Urol Clin North Am 1995; 22: 775–788

51. Frohib D A, Goldstein I, Payton T R et al. Characterization of penile erectile states using external computer-based monitoring. J Biomech Eng 1987; 109: 110

52. Licht M R, Lewis R W, Wollan P C, Harris C D. Comparison of Rigiscan and sleep laboratory nocturnal penile tumescence

in the diagnosis of organic impotence. J Urol 1995; 154: 1740–1743

53. Benet A E, Rehman J, Holcomb R G, Melman A. The correlation between the Rigiscan plus software and the final diagnosis in the evaluation of erectile dysfunction. J Urol 1996; 156: 1947–1950

54. Rosen R C, Keefe F J. The measurement of human penile tumescence. Psychophysiology 1978; 15: 366–376

55. Freund K, Langevin R, Barlow D H. A comparison of two penile measures of erotic arousal. Behav Res Ther 1974; 12: 355–359

56. Slob A K, Blom J H, van der Werff J J. Erection problems in medical practice: differential diagnosis with a relatively simple method. J Urol 1990; 143: 46–50

57. Freund K, Scher H, Chan S, Ben-Aron M. Experimental analysis of paedophilia. Behav Res Ther 1982; 20: 105–112

58. Freund K, Langevin R. Bisexuality in homosexual pedophilia. Arch Sex Behav 1976; 5: 415–423

59. Freund K, Chan S, Coulthard R. Phallometric diagnosis with 'nonadmitters'. Behav Res Ther 1979; 17: 451–457

60. Barlow D H, Becker R, Leitenberg H, Agras S. A mechanical strain gauge for recording penile circumference change. J Appl Behav Anal 1970; 6: 355–367

61. Rosen R C, Kopel S A. Penile plethysmography and biofeedback in the treatment of a transvestite-exhibitionist. J Consult Clin Psychol 1977; 45: 908–916

62. Julien E, Over R. Male sexual arousal across five modes of erotic stimulation. Arch Sex Behav 1988; 17: 131–143

63. Rowland D L, Slob A K. Vibrotactile stimulation enhances sexual response in sexually functional men: a study using concomitant measures of erection. Arch Sex Behav 1992; 21: 387–400

64. Rowland D L, den Ouden A H, Slob A K. The use of vibrotactile stimulation for determining sexual potency in the laboratory in men with erectile problems: methodological considerations. Int J Impot Res 1994; 6: 153–161

65. Rosen R C, Weiner D N, Gendrano N. Objective and subjective measures of sexual arousal in sexually dysfunctional and non-dysfunctional men. Int J Impot Res 1996; 8: 118

66. Derogatis L R. The Derogatis Interview for Sexual Functioning (DISF/DISF-R): an introductory report. Arch Sexual Behaviour: in press

67. Derogatis L R, Melisaratos N. The DSFI: a multidimensional measure of sexual functioning. J Sex Marital Ther 1979; 5: 244–281

68. Corty E W, Althof S E, Kurit D M. The reliability and validity of a sexual functioning questionnaire. J Sex Marital Ther 1996; 22: 27–34

69. Cappelleri J C, Rosen R C, Smith M D et al. Evaluating the erectile function domain of the International Index of Erectile Function (IIEF) as a diagnostic tool. Unpublished

70. Rosen R C, Ferguson D. The Sexual Encounter Profile (SEP): validation of a simple event log for sexual function assessment. Unpublished

71. Aaronson N K. Quality of life: what is it? How should it be measured? Oncology 1988; 2: 69–74

72. Gill T M, Feinstein A R. A critical appraisal of the quality of quality-of-life measurements. JAMA 1994; 272: 619–626

73. Guyatt G H, Feeny D H, Patrick D L. Measuring health-related quality of life. Ann Intern Med 1993; 118: 622–629

74. Applegate W B, Phillips H L, Schnaper H et al. A randomized, controlled trial of the effects of three antihypertensive agents on blood pressure control and quality of life in older women. Arch Intern Med 1991; 151: 1817–1823

75. Wassertheil-Smoller S, Blaufox D, Oberman A et al. Effects of antihypertensives on sexual function and quality of life: the TAIM study. Ann Intern Med 1991; 114: 613–620

76. Fugl-Meyer A R, Lodnert G, Branholm I-B, Fugl-Meyer K S. On life satisfaction in male erectile dysfunction. Int J Impot Res 1997; 9: 141–148

77. Beach M L, Meier P. Choosing covariates in the analysis of clinical trials. Controlled Clin Trials 1989; 10: 161S–175S

78. Canner P L. Covariate adjustment of treatment effects in clinical trials. Controlled Clin Trials 1991; 12: 359–366

79. Chalmers T C, Levin H, Sacks H S et al. Meta-analysis of clinical trials as a scientific discipline. Stat Med 1987; 6: 315–326

80. DeMets D L. Methods for combining randomized clinical trials: strengths and limitations. Stat Med 1987; 6: 341–348

81. Carey M P, Johnson B T. Effectiveness of yohimbine in the treatment of erectile disorders: four meta-analytic integrations. Arch Sex Behav 1996; 25: 341–360

82. Grasing K, Sturgill M G, Rosen R C et al. Effects of yohimbine on autonomic measures are determined by individual values for area under the concentration–time curve. J Clin Pharmacol 1996; 36: 814–822

83. Sturgill M G, Grasing K, Rosen R C et al. Yohimbine elimination in normal volunteers is characterized by both one- and two-compartment behavior. J Cardiovasc Pharmacol 1997; 29: 697–703

Chapter 17
Psychological assessment of erectile dysfunction

J. LoPiccolo

■ INTRODUCTION

This chapter presents a model for psychological assessment of erectile failure, in the context of a 'post-modern' view that most cases of erectile failure involve both psychological *and* physiological aetiology.[1] A functional analysis-based model for psychological assessment is offered, with emphasis on identification of issues that need to be considered in treatment planning for either medical or psychotherapeutic treatment.

■ MODERN SEX THERAPY: MASTERS AND JOHNSON

The book by Masters and Johnson,[2] entitled *Human Sexual Inadequacy* and published in 1970, revolutionized thinking about erectile failure. Their assessment featured a detailed sex-history interview on childhood, adolescent and adult events resulting in erectile failure. Masters and Johnson basically proposed that, although a variety of life experiences might result in the first occasion of erectile dysfunction, the performance anxiety resulting from this failure and the development of an anxious, self-evaluative, spectator role maintained the occurrence of erectile failure.

In the Masters and Johnson schema for sexual dysfunction, assessment focuses on two issues. First, an extensive and detailed sex history is taken to identify the original pathogenic life experiences. Secondly, a careful assessment is made of the patient's actual sexual behaviour, so that new sexual techniques (e.g. non-demand sensual massage) that disrupt the vicious cycle of performance anxiety–spectator role–erectile failure can be implemented.

■ THE BEGINNINGS OF POST-MODERNISM IN COGNITIVE/BEHAVIOURAL THERAPY

The next major change in the thinking about erectile failure occurred with the development of cognitive–behavioural therapy. Within the field of sex therapy, the cognitive–behavioural approach led to an emphasis on the patient's *thinking* about sex. Assessment of erectile failure came to include evaluation of the patient's cognitions regarding sexual issues. Unrealistic expectations, negative self-images, distorted views of the opposite sex's needs and requirements, and tendencies to catastrophic thinking became a major focus of assessment. While these changes developed as part of the cognitive revolution in psychotherapy, they were also a response to treatment failures when using the Masters and Johnson[2] model. The Masters and Johnson approach of anxiety reduction plus skill training may not work well if the patient's distorted cognitions about sexual functioning are paramount factors. In such cases, instructions to relax and enjoy sensual massage are as ineffective as advising a depressed patient to 'just cheer up'.

■ THE POST-MODERN VIEW OF ERECTILE FAILURE

While acknowledging the importance of life history events and the central role of performance anxiety and attitude factors, the post-modern view of erectile failure[1] emphasizes four other elements as perhaps even more important for assessment. These are: (i) the impact of couple systemic issues on the erectile failure, (ii) the male's individual psychological issues, (iii) physiological impairment, and (iv) the couple's sexual behaviour pattern.

Systemic therapy for marital distress traditionally posited that sexual dysfunctions were just symptoms of underlying marital dynamics, and the dysfunction was not directly addressed in assessment or therapy. In a similar fashion, sex therapy until recently would not focus on marital issues that coexisted with erectile failure, attributing these problems to the corrosive effects of erectile failure on the relationship.

In more recent years, there has come to be a realization that erectile failure and marital systemic issues are mutually and reciprocally causative and resultant of each other.[3] In cases of erectile failure, systemic issues often maintain this failure. For example, a wife who is dominated by her husband may gain power if he develops erectile failure. In a similar manner, erectile failure may have systemic value for a man, in that it creates the degree of distance in the relationship that he needs, in contrast to his wife's pushing for more closeness. In cases where there is major systemic value associated with erectile failure, patients often 'resist' standard sex therapy procedures, by not performing the sensate focus exercises, breaking the initial prohibition on further attempts at intercourse, and so forth. These so-called resistant cases often fail in modern sex therapy. Kaplan[4] suggested that, when patients resist standard techniques, sex therapy must be discontinued and individual analytic therapy conducted to attain insight into underlying individual psychoanalytic issues that are blocking progress. Heiman and colleagues[5] first offered the alternative view that a more broadly focused assessment that includes the systemic value of the erectile dysfunction for the patient couple must be undertaken, so that treatment planning can address the search for ways to meet the systemic needs currently being met in a maladaptive way by the sexual dysfunction. Rather than beginning with standard sex therapy and considering cognitive/dynamic/systemic factors only when resistance occurs, a post-modern view suggests that these issues be assessed initially, and resistance prevented by dealing with such factors in a proactive fashion. In post-modern sex therapy, then, patient 'resistance' is viewed as actually caused by the therapist's conceptual error in failing to make an adequate assessment of all the factors involved in the dysfunction.

In the post-modern view, then, six factors involved in erectile failure need to be carefully assessed, and a treatment plan developed to address each of the factors.

The first factor to be considered, as noted above, is the value that erectile failure may have in maintenance of emotional homoeostasis in the patient couple's relationship. Erectile failure may have an impact on issues such as intimacy, closeness, trust, power sharing, conflict resolution, time spent together, and so forth. Sometimes the erectile failure develops as a result of problems in these areas, but an erectile problem that develops for entirely other reasons can come to have systemic adaptive value in these areas, as a sort of positive side effect of the erectile failure.

In broaching the systems theory notions, the therapist must be very careful. Stated improperly, a systems theory interpretation can sound as if the therapist is accusing the patient of having the problem 'on purpose', to punish their partner, or gain something from their partner. Similarly, a systemic assessment question can sound as if the therapist is accusing the wife of *causing* the husband's erectile problem, because the problem does benefit her, in some way. It must always be stressed that systems function to maintain homoeostasis, and do not develop unless there is a positive value for both partners in the system.

One way to avoid a systems theory assessment question sounding accusatory is to present the notion of *secondary gain*. The clinician should explain to the patients that it is very apparent that they are each suffering greatly from their sexual dysfunction and it is causing each of them great pain. I tell them that there are two victims, and no villains, involved in their difficulties. I then go on to explain, however, that as we humans are adaptable, people do adjust to having the problem with erection. The dysfunction therefore comes to have some effect on how their relationship is structured. I ask the couple what effect the sexual dysfunction has had on their relationship.

As might be expected, virtually all couples indicate some negative effects on their emotional relationship. I then ask if they have seen any positive effects on their relationship. That is, I ask if the erection problem has any positive 'side effects' for each of them. Not too surprisingly, most patients say 'no'. The clinician should ask this 'side effect' question late in the assessment interview, by which time the clinician should have a very good idea of just what the functional value of the erectile failure may be for the couple.

I first offer the patients an example of the adaptive value of sexual dysfunction, focusing on a presenting complaint other than their erectile failure. By doing this, the patients' defences are not activated, and they can more easily hear the notion of functional value of a sexual dysfunction. Therefore, in cases of erectile failure, I will give a female-dysfunction example. This might be an explanation that in cases of female lack of arousal, while the husband is frustrated and upset, he also has the positive gain of not worrying about his wife having sex with other men, or of worrying whether he will be able to satisfy a high level of her sexual needs.

Following explanation of an opposite-sex example, I may then give one or two examples of positive side effects of erectile failure, carefully emphasizing that I do not mean that I think these examples necessarily apply to them. These focused examples are offered only to those couples who seem at a loss following my explanation and 'opposite sexed problem' example.

I then ask the couple if they are now aware of any positive effects of their sexual problem. At this point, many couples will be able to offer a systemic value. For those who cannot as yet see such an issue, an alternative approach is to ask the client to speculate about any possible negative effects, on their marital stability, of recovering erectile functioning, to raise awareness of systemic value of erectile failure.[6] For example, might the husband feel more powerful and revert to a more authoritarian role with the wife, if he became 'potent' again? Might the wife find his sexual needs burdensome, if he regained erectile function?

It is often difficult for the patient couple to identify these issues of current positive side effects of the dysfunction, and risks or losses that might be involved in the male regaining erectile function. Rather than pressing them to accomplish this task during an initial interview, I often ask them to do a bit of 'homework', to assist me in being able to assist them. I ask them to each, separately, write me two lists. One list will be of possible positive side effects now occurring, and the other list will be of risks or possible losses with the restoration of functioning. I ask that each list contain at least five — and preferably ten — items. I encourage them to list even those items that they doubt are operative or true, in order that some ideas may be forthcoming. I stress that many items on the risks list, for example, may be things that logically they know are not valid, but that at an emotional level, there may be some impact. An example I may give is that many, if not

most, wives have a logical fear that their husband's erectile problem may mean that he no longer finds them sexually arousing, or he is having an affair. Additionally, however, there may be an emotional fear that if he were to regain erectile functioning, *then* he would have an affair.

It is to be hoped that the patients will attain insight into the systemic value of their problem during initial assessment, so that therapy can begin immediately to address the needs that are now being served by the erectile failure. However, if the patients cannot see a systemic value to the problem that is identified by the assessing clinician, there should not be an attempt to convince them. If the therapist is incorrect, and there is no homoeostatic value attached to the dysfunction, the issue will not disrupt therapy. If the assessment is correct and there is systemic value, at some point the patients will begin to show 'resistance' to therapeutic manipulations. At this point, the therapist can remind the patients of the notion that was raised at assessment about the value of the problem, and fears about the effect of losing the problem. With this explanation, patients often are now more receptive to working directly on the systemic issues identified during the assessment. Although it is preferable to avoid 'resistance' by assessing and then addressing systemic issues at the beginning of therapy, if the patients are amenable to this approach, a good systemic assessment also sets the stage for doing this work later, when problems do arise.

A wide variety of couple-relationship issues may be involved in the systemic aetiology of erectile failure. These issues include the following as commonly occurring systemic factors: lack of attraction to partner; poor sexual skills of the partner; general marital unhappiness; fear of closeness; differences between the couple in degree of 'personal space' desired in the relationship; passive–aggressive solutions to a power imbalance; poor conflict resolution skills; inability to blend feelings of love and sexual desire, and reaction to the problems caused by lack of knowledge about normal age-related changes in male erectile functioning.

Consistent with the approach taken to systemic issues, assessment should also address the role, in the aetiology of erectile failure, of the patient's individual cognitive processes or 'psychodynamics'. For example, erectile failure may be valuable to a patient in avoiding anxiety about what it would mean to be a sexually functional man. For some such men, erectile failure is a way of resolving negative feelings about their sexuality. These negative feelings may be moralistically based, or result from cultural negative messages about sexuality. Similarly, erectile failure may ward off depression about some highly distressing life situation, by simply giving the man another problem upon which to focus. A man who is very unhappy in his marriage, but who finds divorce too threatening an idea to process, exemplifies this issue. Erectile failure may also be an adaptive dynamic mechanism for avoiding repressed homosexual urges. Some men with ego dystonic homosexual impulses experience a breakdown of repression during intercourse with their wife, and have intrusive mental images or fantasies of sex with a man. Other men may find that, during erection and intercourse, deviant fantasies such as sex with a child occur. In such cases, erectile failure fosters repression of unacceptable sexual impulses and allows maintenance of one's self-image as a decent, moral person. Additionally, there are some cases seen for assessment that do not have erectile failure except with their wife, who is responsible for them appearing for assessment. That is, some men have good erections with a lover, but not with their wife. These men agree to come for evaluation/therapy because, as one patient explained, 'I was afraid that if I didn't seem to care about not having erections, she would figure out I was doing it with someone else'. Other men have admitted to sexually deviant behaviours, including voyeurism, exhibitionism, and a variety of fetishistic paraphilia, during which they have good erections and of which the wife is unaware.

Very few men will admit to such taboo issues as factors in their erectile failure if only interviewed with the wife present. The clinician should see each member of the couple alone briefly, explaining that all people in a couple relationship each have some issues that are not comfortably spoken about with the partner present. I explain that I do need to obtain a complete picture, to assess their problem accurately. The ground rule for these individual interview sessions is that, unless the patient informs me that they do not want their partner to know about a particular item they mention to me, I will assume that we can, if needed, discuss such items with the partner when we rejoin. I tell them that, if one of them asks for confidentiality on some item, I may agree that there is no need for the partner to hear about it. However, I also tell them that there may be some item that I feel the partner needs to know so that therapy can

succeed. In such a case, I will not simply tell the partner the 'secret'. Nevertheless, I also will not waste the patients' time and money (and my time) by working with them in a context that is doomed to failure. I will suggest instead that either we tell the partner and deal with the consequences of this disclosure, or we simply do not begin therapy.

The most common secret is the ongoing affair. When a man tells me that he does have good erections with his lover, but not with his wife, I ask if he wants to end the marriage, or to stop the affair and work on regaining erections with his wife. Many men do not want either — they want simply to continue the affair and to regain (or not regain) erections with the wife, but chiefly to allay her suspicion about his lack of erection by coming to assessment and therapy. If the man will not agree to stop the affair at least for the duration of therapy (so that the therapist is not also deceiving the wife), I suggest that, when we rejoin the wife, I should explain that the erection problem is not really the problem. That is, it seems to me that the marriage has become rather emotionally distant and that the couple should think of marital therapy, either to regain emotional closeness or to consider whether a divorce should be explored. Men usually do not like this alternative, and I then ask for some other way to explain to the wife why we are not going to do therapy for erectile failure, which does not tell his secret and does not require me to lie to his wife. That is, the reason I give for not starting therapy is, indeed, the truth, as far as it goes. Of course, the patient can lie to the clinician and not stop the affair, but this is preferable to the clinician doing therapy with the couple under a set of conditions that is a betrayal of the wife's trust in the clinician.

A past affair is a different matter. If the affair is genuinely over, and the patient is committed to the marriage, assessment need focus only on what made sex work in the affair and how that can be applied to the marriage. Some patients (not many) do express, during the solo assessment interview, a wish to tell the wife about the affair. The clinician should carefully enquire about the motivation to disclose: that is, often one hears about wishes to be honest, to be forgiven, and so forth. Although these may be sincere, there are often also less benign motivations as well, such as reminding the wife that the patient is attractive to other women, that he could end the marriage, that she should make more efforts to please him, and so forth. All of these issues can be addressed during therapy, but revealing the affair may, indeed, simply end the marriage. For some women, learning of the husband's affair puts a fracture in the foundation of the marriage that cannot be repaired.

Another, and related, secret topic is whether the patient still loves his wife, or is he remaining in the marriage for reasons such as social conformity, parenthood, or even to avoid the financial consequences of divorce? Similarly, the patient should be asked if he finds his wife physically attractive. Sometimes, when the answer is 'no', this reflects issues in the man's thinking that will need to be addressed in therapy. For example, one patient answered 'No. After all, she's an old lady — a grandmother, in fact. Who wants to have sex with an old lady?' In point of fact, the wife was quite an attractive woman, and the fact that the patient was himself an 'old gentleman and grandfather' somehow did not enter into his view of his wife. However, sometimes the lack of attraction is more based in reality than in our ageist–sexist views of women's attractiveness. One patient explained that he couldn't be aroused by his wife, owing to her weight. She had weighed 127 pounds (≈ 57 kg) when they married, 9 years previously; at assessment, she did not know her weight, as their home scale only went to 300 pounds (135 kg), and she was over this amount. In assessment in such cases, the clinician needs to consider not just the male's erectile problem, but also the issue of whether the weight gain helps the wife to avoid having sexual intercourse with her husband. Of course, in this case, the issue of the health risk, for the wife, of this weight gain was also raised during assessment.

In addition to the topics of affairs, love, and physical attraction, the clinician should, during individual interviews, enquire about the following commonly revealed 'secrets' in cases of erectile failure: religious issues; gender identity conflicts; homosexual orientation or conflict; anhedonic or obsessive–compulsive personality; sexual phobias or aversions; fear of loss of control over sexual urges; masked sexual deviation; fears of having children; the 'widower's syndrome' (unresolved feelings about death of the first wife); underlying depression; ageing concerns, and attempting sex in a context or situation that is not psychologically comfortable for the patient.

The third component element for assessment is the impact of unresolved family-of-origin issues on erectile functioning. A patient raised in a family in which the mother was emotionally erratic or abusive may have difficulty in letting himself feel sexual pleasure and desire for his partner. Of course, men who were sexually abused by parents or other adults are very vulnerable to sexual dysfunction in adulthood.

Although the time constraints of most therapy settings preclude detailed sex-history interviews (which may take up to 8 or 10 hours in classical 'sex therapy'), some assessment of life history is indicated. Patients can be directly asked about their thoughts on any life history events that may be contributing to their erectile problem. Similarly, patients can be asked what they learned, directly or indirectly, from their family, their religion, their school and their friends, over the course of their lives, that may have made them more vulnerable to the development of erectile problems.

Another area to be considered in assessing the cause of erectile failure concerns the possible operant value the dysfunction may have for either partner. 'Operant value' here refers to reinforcing consequences of the erectile failure that come, not from the relationship with the partner or from the patient's own psyche, but from the external world. For example, the patient's erectile failure may lead him to devote long hours to his business or profession, resulting in great financial reward. Similarly, in one recent case, the wife informed all her friends and relatives of her husband's history of erectile failure in their 20-year marriage, and received admiration and praise for her loyalty, self-sacrifice and fidelity.

In summary, post-modernism holds that erectile failure is not just a function of performance anxiety and lack of sexual skills, as was proposed in modern sex therapy.[2,4] While acknowledging that erectile failure is a painfully distressing condition, post-modernism stresses that erectile failure has positive value for the patient and his partner in terms of couple-systemic issues, individual intrapsychic conflicts, unresolved family-of-origin issues, and reinforcing consequences in the external environment.

Post-modern sex therapy arose partly out of the move to an integrated cognitive/behavioural/systemic approach as the mainstream of current thinking. However, post-modern sex therapy also arose in response to treatment failures. That is, the basic anxiety-reduction/skill-training approach called sensate focus by Masters and Johnson[2] has been widely publicized in the popular media, and effective self-help books[7] using this approach are widely available. Many of the cases seen by professionals today are failures of such 'bibliotherapy' or guided self-treatment. Often, the reason that the patient has not been able to follow a self-help programme, or to succeed if the programme was followed, involves the functionally useful nature of erectile failure. Assessment now includes making a functional analysis of the positive value of the problem, and helping the patient to find more adaptive mechanisms for dealing with systemic, psychodynamic, family of origin, and environmentally reinforcing issues related to the maintenance of erectile failure. However, there is now another issue that needs to be assessed in cases of erectile problems: this issue involves the fact that erectile failure very commonly involves both complex psychological factors *and* coexisting physiological impairment of erectile capability.

In 1970, Masters and Johnson[2] stated that almost all cases of erectile failure were purely psychogenic. More recently, new diagnostic procedures have revealed that neurological, vascular and hormonal abnormalities are involved, to some degree, in a considerable percentage of cases of erectile failure.[8] The assessment of physical factors is covered elsewhere in this volume; however, it is important to realize that psychological factors do interact with physical factors, and to assess this interaction.

The high incidence of physical pathology has led to the argument that sex therapy is no longer a viable treatment for erectile failure. One has only to look in the sports pages of any major newspaper to see advertisements typically headed something like 'Impotence is a Medical Problem — Effective Medical Treatment Available'. These advertisements are usually from centres that offer a treatment array of penile prostheses, vasoactive injections, revascularization surgery, vacuum erection devices and recently, oral medication. Although such centres usually offer some assessment prior to intervention, this assessment is typically aimed at making a differential diagnosis into organic or psychogenic categories, with the latter presumably a rare phenomenon. However, in many cases, both organic *and* psychogenic factors are involved. A recognition of this combined causality[9] diagnosed patients with erectile failure along a bipolar scale, from exclusively psychogenic, through mixed aetiology, to exclusively organic in origin. Although this bipolar scale is an advance over a simplistic two-category typology, there is a logical problem: the factors of organic and psychogenic causes of erectile problems logically are not the opposite ends of a unidimensional bipolar scale but, rather,

represent two separate and independently varying dimensions. That is, a man may have a high degree of *both* organic and psychogenic causes of erectile failure, or a low degree of both factors, or any combination of high and low degrees of impairment on each separate dimension. While this fact may seem obvious, there are statements in the clinical literature that, if one finds a clear psychological cause of the erection problem, one need not conduct any physiological evaluation. This point of view suggests, for example, that having a serious problem in a marital relationship prevents one from developing atherosclerotic disease processes in the arteries leading to the penis.

Similarly, many physicians currently will perform surgery to implant a penile prosthesis if *any* degree of organic abnormality is found at assessment. In many such cases the patient has only a mild organic impairment, which then makes his erection extremely vulnerable to being disrupted by psychological, behavioural and sexual-technique factors. In many cases, such partial organic impairment can be treated successfully by sex therapy. If psychological and behavioural difficulties are assessed and then focused upon in sex therapy, the patient's mildly impaired physiological capacity may be sufficient to easily produce good erection.

In one study of aetiology of erectile failure,[1] 63 men were independently rated for degree of psychological impairment (scored 0–4) and degree of organic impairment (also scored 0–4), following complete psychological, vascular, hormonal, neurological and nocturnal penile tumescence (NPT) evaluations. These ratings were determined by having three separate clinicians review the patient's evaluation report, which contained all the raw data from the vascular, neurological, hormonal and NPT laboratories. The three raters also reviewed the written psychological evaluation report, which was based on questionnaire assessment and interviews with both patient and spouse. These ratings were not completely subjective judgements as, whenever possible, scores were anchored to objective criteria. For example, a score of 4 on organic impairment required either a complete absence of NPT, or markedly impaired NPT *plus* abnormality in at least one of the other systems assessed. Although initial inter-rater reliability scores were good (ranging from .74 to .92 between individual raters on each dimension), in cases where there were disagreements the raters jointly reviewed the evaluation data and arrived at a consensus score.

The results of these evaluations are shown in Figure 17.1, with each circle representing one patient. The distribution in Figure 17.1 indicates that there is only a moderate negative correlation (–.58) between degrees of organic and psychological impairment, so a unidimensional, bipolar scale is not an accurate representation of clinical reality. Furthermore, Figure 17.1 indicates that, of these 63 patients, only ten men were found to have erectile dysfunction that was purely psychogenic, and only three men to have dysfunction that was purely organic in aetiology, so an 'either/or' two-category typology is even more inappropriate. Figure 17.1 also indicates that there are a considerable number of men (19/63 or 30%) with mild organic impairment (0.5–1.0 on this scale), but significant psychological problems (2.0 or more on this scale). These men might, in a two-part typology, be considered to be 'organic' cases of erectile failure, as there is some demonstrated physiological impairment. However, the greater degree of psychological aetiology seen in these cases argues against this categorization, and suggests that a physical intervention is probably not necessary to restore normal erectile functioning for these men.

Diagnostic classification into a two-dimensional schema also offers a caution on the need for prospectively assessing for possible patient and spouse adjustment to purely medical interventions such as vasoactive injection. Consider, in Figure 17.1, the 16 men who scored at least 2.5 on the organic impairment scale, and for whom a medical intervention might therefore be an appropriate treatment. Of these 16 men, 5 (31%) received a rating of 2.0, 2.5, or 3.0 for presence of concurrent psychological problems. It might be anticipated that, with this degree of psychological disturbance, long-term adjustment to the

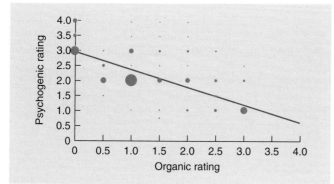

Figure 17.1. Relationship between psychogenic and organic rates of impairment in cases of erectile dysfunction. (Each circle represents one patient.)

restoration of erection would be poor. Although patients are often very eager to have a medical intervention, and report being very happy with it initially, longer-term follow-up indicates poor sexual adjustment in a significant percentage of cases.[10] If a man and his wife have a number of psychological/sexual behaviour problems involved in his erectile failure, the medical intervention will result only in their now having these same difficulties, but with an artificially rigid penis. Although erection is now present, one would not expect the frequency or quality of sexual activity to be high in such cases and this result is what, in fact, was found.[10] A thorough psychological evaluation is therefore indicated for all cases of erectile failure, even when an organic aetiology is clearly established and a medical treatment is planned. A post-modern view of erectile failure argues that brief concurrent psychotherapy will often be needed when a medical intervention is used, because of the functional adaptive value of erectile failure, even when there is an organic impairment involved in causality.

The focus in much of the clinical literature, on making a differential diagnosis into mutually exclusive categories of organic or psychogenic aetiology, is often at the expense of formulating the best treatment plan, which is ultimately the purpose of diagnostic assessment. The focus of assessment should be not only to quantify the degrees of psychological/physiological causality of the erection problem, but to identify, through the four-element functional analysis discussed previously, issues to be focused upon in treatment, and to assess prognosis for response to physical interventions such as oral medication, vasoactive injections, vacuum erection devices or prostheses. As it seems to be true that most cases of erectile failure involve major psychological aetiology (regardless of degree of organic impairment present), assessment should focus on which psychological and/or somatic interventions are most likely to help each particular patient. As Mohr and Beutler[11] have noted, prognosis, not diagnosis, must be the deciding factor in choice of treatment, and psychological evaluation is critical in making prognostic evaluations for physical interventions.

Assessment of prognosis is made with information gathered by semi-structured interviews and symptom-focused questionnaires.[6] Given the restrictions on contact hours typical of virtually all 'managed care' arrangements, the use of written questionnaires to gather information and guide interview content is very useful. Specifically, a sexual-functioning questionnaire[12] and a marital adjustment test[13] guide the initial assessment. For couples who will then be seen for sex therapy, a detailed analysis of the nature of the couple's actual sexual behaviour with the Sexual Interaction Inventory[14] is very useful in treatment planning.

■ PROGNOSTIC INDICATORS AND CHOICE OF TREATMENT

Based on the information gathered from the interview and questionnaire materials discussed above, the clinician can now make a prognostic decision about which type of treatment will best suit the individual patient couple. What follows is a brief review of prognostic indicators for psychotherapeutic treatment and for medical interventions such as implantation of a prosthesis, use of a vacuum erection device, vasoactive injections or oral medication.

Good prognostic indicators for psychotherapy

The best prognosis for successful psychotherapy occurs in cases in which clear behavioural deficits or maladaptive thinking patterns that contribute to lack of erection can be identified. The most common behavioural, cognitive, dynamic and systemic problems that respond well to post-modern sex therapy are listed below:

1. *Lack of adequate sexual stimulation.* If the wife does not engage in any manual or oral stimulation of her husband's penis, but expects him to have an erection because he is kissing and caressing her, relatively simple behavioural directions for increasing physical stimulation have a good chance of success. These behavioural deficits can be identified clearly with the Sexual Interaction Inventory.[14] This intervention is indicated in cases of partial organic impairment or in ageing males, where the erection response requires a high degree of intensity of physical stimulation of the penis.[1]

2. *The wife's sexual gratification is currently dependent upon the male obtaining an erection.* If the wife has orgasm only during coitus, and does not consider an orgasm produced by her husband's manual, oral, or electric-vibrator stimulation to be normal, there is a good prognosis for sex therapy. If the husband can be reassured that he is providing full sexual satisfaction for his wife through manual, oral, or electric-vibrator stimulation of her genitals, the pressure on him to perform for her by getting an erection will be greatly reduced.

3. *Lack of knowledge about age-related changes in sexual functioning.* Erectile failure is most commonly seen in men aged 50 or older. In ageing men, the slowing down of the erection response, the greater dependence upon physical as opposed to psychological stimulation to produce an erection, the longer duration of the refractory period, and the inability to ejaculate on every occasion of intercourse, are normal ageing changes.[15] However, many couples overreact to these changes with anxiety and distress, which leads to erectile failure in the male.[1] Simple education about normal ageing changes in sexuality, and behavioural techniques for dealing with these changes, can resolve the erectile failure.

4. *Cognitive distortions regarding the male sex role stereotype,* leading to unrealistic demands upon the male for sexual performance. Many men and women labour under a 'macho' set of unrealistic role demands for male sexual performance.[12] Education to promote a realistic view of male sex roles and sexual performance can be very helpful.

5. As noted above, *individual dynamic, relationship-system, unresolved family-of-origin, or operant reinforcement issues that make it functionally adaptive for the erectile failure to continue to occur.* Although long-term therapy in such cases is often indicated, the prognosis is good if such functional issues can be identified.

Negative prognostic indicators for psychotherapy

The following factors suggest a poor prognosis for psychotherapeutic intervention in erectile dysfunction:

1. An *unwillingness* on the part of either the patient or his wife *to reconsider* male sex-role demands, the role of the female in providing adequate stimulation for the male, or the means of stimulation by which the female reaches her orgasm.

2. *Sexual deviation.* If the male is, for example, a paedophile or a transvestite, therapy becomes much more difficult.

3. *Extreme religiosity,* with religious beliefs about sex interfering with sexual performance. These cases are best referred to a pastoral counsellor, who may have some credibility in changing (or at least helping the patient to re-examine) these beliefs.

4. *Clinical depression.* Sex therapy is routinely unsuccessful in cases of actual clinical depression. However, subclinical depression, which may be a reaction to erectile and marital distress, may respond well to sex therapy.

Good prognostic indicators for medical treatments

Positive prognostic indicators for a prosthesis, use of a vacuum-aided device, or vasoactive injections include the following:

1. A *currently adequate range of sexual stimulation* is provided for the male by the female, in terms of manual and oral stimulation of the penis during foreplay; however, this stimulation is ineffective in producing an erection.
2. *There is a clear understanding of exactly what sexual behaviour can be expected* following the medical treatment, *and a willingness to adapt* to the marked changes in sexual behaviour patterns that are necessitated by any of these medical procedures.[10]
3. The female does enjoy penile–vaginal intercourse, but reports that *size of the penis is not important to her*. As a prosthesis does not increase the size of the penis, as occurs when a man gets a physiological erection, some women do report dissatisfaction with the prosthesis, if they previously enjoyed the sensation of containment of the larger normally erect penis. These cases are routinely dissatisfied with the prosthetic implant.[14] Very recently, a new version of the inflatable prosthesis has been developed that does increase both diameter and length of the penis. It is possible that the spouse's satisfaction will be increased with this device.

Poor prognostic indicators for medical treatments

There are also some indicators of poor prognosis for long-term adjustment to a medical intervention. The more commonly seen factors include the following:

1. *Strong positive functional value*, for either the wife or husband, *in the continuance of the erectile failure*. If either a husband or wife is invested in maintenance of the erectile failure because it helps them deal with issues in the relationship or has other functional value, adjustment to a prosthesis or medical procedure will

be poor, unless psychotherapy is also provided, preferably prior to surgery.
2. *The wife is essentially uninterested in resuming an active sex life*. In a recent case, the wife stated, 'I've always done my wifely duty, but it's been a great relief not to have to do it these last five years, since he's been impotent'. The husband in this case was given a penile prosthesis: as might be expected, the results were psychologically disastrous, with severe marital distress and ultimately, divorce occurring.
3. *Unrealistic expectations that an artificial erection will resolve conflicts* about desired frequency of intercourse, willingness to engage in other forms of sexual activity, such as manual or oral stimulation, and general dissatisfaction with the partner's sexual techniques.

Sexual behaviour pattern

Thus far, it has been stressed that a post-modern view of erectile failure leads to the assessment of a complex interaction of psychological and physiological factors. There is another, less complex but no less important, element for assessment in erectile failure cases: this element is the actual sexual behaviour pattern of the couple, alluded to briefly in the preceding section on prognosis.

Modern sex therapy, as developed by Masters and Johnson,[2] suggests that, if performance anxiety and the spectator role are eliminated by substituting sensate focus (non-genital body massage) for further attempts at intercourse, erections will occur spontaneously. Assessment should look for the presence of two factors that reduce the effectiveness of sensate focus.

First, sensate focus is, in some fashion, a form of paradoxical treatment. The therapist instructs the patient to relax, not to be sexual, not to expect an erection, and only to enjoy the sensual body massage. Of course, a nude massage by a nude partner, even without direct genital caressing, is a highly sexual—not just sensual—situation and, with performance anxiety eliminated, erection should therefore occur. The paradox is in labelling, for the patient, a sexual situation as non-sexual, so that he is not expecting an erection, and neither he nor his partner are placing any performance demands on him. Like most paradoxical procedures, sensate focus works only if the patient is unaware of the underlying paradox (for example, telling a negativistic adolescent to do the opposite of what you actually want him to do will not work if he is aware that you are using 'reverse psychology'). Of course, with modern sex therapy procedures widely explained in books, magazines, newspaper columns and television talk-shows, it is a rare patient today who is unaware that the therapeutic effect of sensate focus lies in reduction of performance pressure. In fact, many have already tried the sensate focus procedure, often using a self-help guidebook. These patients who now appear for assessment have 'meta-performance anxiety'. Meta-performance anxiety refers to a type of higher-order anxiety, nicely explained by a patient as follows:

> I found myself lying there, thinking — I'm now free of pressure to perform. I'm not supposed to get an erection, and we're not allowed to have intercourse even if I do get one. So now that all the pressure is off, why am I not getting an erection? I'm relaxed, I'm enjoying this, so where's the erection?

What this patient described is something that does need to be explored at assessment — knowledge of, and attempts to use, the basic procedures of sex therapy for erectile problems.

Assessment is also needed of how actual sexual behaviour patterns can defeat sensate focus procedures. This failure involves the one-third to two-thirds of men who have some degree of organic impairment of their erectile capability. For these men, it is unrealistic to expect that physiological arousal (erection) will occur without direct, intense genital stimulation, regardless of the degree of sensual pleasure and subjective arousal experienced in sensate focus. Furthermore, erectile failure is much more common in ageing men, and even healthy ageing men require direct, and intense, physical stimulation of the penis for erection to occur.[15]

Because sensate focus is often ineffective in reducing performance anxiety in today's sophisticated patients, and because the typical patient with erectile failure needs intense stimulation for erection, the actual behaviour pattern of the patient couple has become crucial in a post-modern therapeutic approach and therefore does need to be assessed.

Far more effective than sensate focus in reducing performance anxiety is the patient's knowledge that his partner's sexual gratification does not depend on his achieving an erection. If the patient can be reassured that his partner finds their lovemaking highly pleasurable, and that she is sexually fulfilled by the orgasms he gives her through manual and oral stimulation, his performance anxiety will be greatly reduced. If these options have never been discussed or tried, therapy may be relatively simple. However, if assessment reveals that the sexual partner finds alternative routes to orgasm unacceptable, the therapist may find it more difficult to introduce these activities as a vehicle for therapeutic progress. A recent patient's partner, in response to assessment questions regarding him bringing her to orgasm by manual or oral stimulation, replied, 'If he can't give me the real thing, I don't want him to get me all hot and bothered'. In such cases, assessment may reveal nothing more than the fact that the wife of the typical elderly patient with erectile failure was raised in a culture that was very sex-negative for women, indicating a need for therapeutic support to enable her to re-examine her sexual attitudes.[15,16] However, as noted above, couple systemic issues should also be explored when strong statements regarding 'taboo' sexual behaviours are encountered at assessment.

The couple's acceptance of manual and oral stimulation of the female's genitals as a route to sexual satisfaction for her is important in most cases of erectile failure. However, at least as important is the wife's direct manual and oral stimulation of the patient's penis. While the importance of adequate direct penile stimulation is obvious in cases of major organic pathology, it is also important because of normal ageing changes in sexual response in healthy men.[15]

One especially important normal change that can cause problems is that the erection response slows down, and it takes longer for men to get an erection as they age. Similarly, with ageing, the erection response becomes more dependent on direct physical stimulation of the penis and less responsive to visual, psychological or non-genital physical stimulation. Rigidity of the penis and angle of erection both decline somewhat, but typically not enough to interfere with intercourse. All these changes are minor and need not interfere with a full sexual life; however, for patients who are unaware of the normality of these changes, there may be great anxiety and distress about them. The couple begins to make love, and they notice that the man does not immediately obtain an erection, so they cease all sexual activity, assuming that he is 'impotent', perhaps because of his age. If the couple simply continued with direct physical stimulation of the man's penis for a while longer, he would probably obtain an erection. Such a couple typically does not profit from sensate focus-based therapy, so assessment needs to focus directly upon the degree of direct physical stimulation that the partner has been providing to the patient's penis.

The need for more direct physical stimulation of the penis is especially problematic in the older couple, for whom direct physical stimulation of the penis has not previously been a major component of their sexual activity. A couple who are in their sixties or seventies grew up in a culture in which 'decent' women were not encouraged to be sexually active, and did not necessarily engage in touching the man's penis.[16] Their sexual repertoire may have consisted of hugging and kissing, some breast caressing, and intercourse. As the male ages, this repertoire will often not be sufficient to produce erection for the male, even though he feels psychologically aroused. When the assessing clinician encounters this situation, a brief explanation should be given, explaining that erection is not subject to voluntary control and is neither spontaneous nor instantaneous (especially in older men) but it will occur automatically, given sufficient stimulation. The clinician should then ask if the wife is willing to consider providing more direct manual, oral or electric-vibrator stimulation of his penis. Whereas some women are very open to this idea, others are not: for example, one patient's wife stated, 'Real men don't need that stuff—that's what homosexuals do'. If the wife makes demanding or derogatory statements about her husband's sexual abilities, the assessing clinician should note this for a focus in therapy but should also attempt to support both members of the couple. The clinician should not simplistically assume that all such women are hostile, demanding or deriving secondary benefits from the man's dysfunction. It should be remembered that it is personally very threatening, to all but the most secure women, for their husbands to have erectile failure. A wife commonly interprets her husband's erectile failure as an indication that he does not love her, is having an affair, is no longer sexually attracted to her, and so forth. The critical statements one hears at assessment may be a reflection of inner anxiety, despair and depression, rather than of hostility. In such cases, reassurance on these issues by the clinician — and, more importantly, by the husband — during the assessment interview is needed, or the assessment may, indeed, be quite upsetting to the couple.

CONCLUSIONS

A post-modern view argues that erectile failure represents a complex, over-determined psycho-physiological problem. In a sense, erectile failure is a sexual representation of the old mind–body problem that first philosophers, and now neuroscientists and psychologists, have debated with great passion. Like many 'either–or' debates, this one ignores the reality of complex, multiple causality in seeking a single unifying principle.[17] Perhaps we should cease speaking of erectile failure in the singular and, instead, refer to a plurality of erectile failures. Erectile failure is a form of 'final common pathway', to which many tributary factors contribute. Although unitary approaches may make for elegantly simple theory, they are also likely to result in ineffective clinical practice with many of our patients who struggle with erectile failure. We owe each patient a thorough assessment of the factors involved in his unique case, and a treatment plan individualized for maximum possibility of therapeutic success.

REFERENCES

1. LoPiccolo J. Post modern sex therapy for erectile failure. In: Rosen R C, Leiblum S R (eds) Erectile disorder: assessment and treatment. New York: Guilford Press, 1992: 171–197

2. Masters W H, Johnson V E. Human sexual inadequacy. Boston: Little, Brown, 1970

3. LoPiccolo J, Friedman J. Sex therapy: an integrative model. In: Lynn S, Garske J (eds) Contemporary psychotherapies: models and methods. New York: Merrill, 1985

4. Kaplan H S. The new sex therapy. New York: Brunner/Mazel, 1974

5. Heiman J, LoPiccolo L, LoPiccolo J. Treatment of sexual dysfunction. In: Gurman A S, Kniskern D P (eds) Handbook of family therapy. New York: Brunner/Mazel, 1981

6. LoPiccolo J, Daiss S. The assessment of sexual dysfunction. In: O'Leary K D (ed) Assessment of marital discord. New Jersey: Lawrence Erlbaum Associates, 1987

7. Zilbergeld B. Male sexuality. New York: Bantam Books, 1978

8. Rosen R C, Leiblum S R (eds) Erectile disorders: assessment and treatment. New York: Guilford Press, 1992

9. Melman A, Tiefer L, Pedersen R. Evaluation of the first 406 patients in urology department based center for male sexual dysfunction. Urology 1988; 32: 6–10

10. Tiefer L, Pedersen B, Melman A. Psychosocial follow-up of penile prosthesis implant patients and partners. J Sex Marital Ther 1988; 14: 184–201

11. Mohr D C, Beutler L E. Erectile dysfunction: a review of diagnostic and treatment procedures. Clin Psychol Rev 1990; 10(1): 123–150

12. Schover L R, Friedman J, Weiler S et al. A multi-axial diagnostic system for sexual dysfunctions: an alternative to DSM-III. Arch Gen Psychiatry 1982; 39: 614–619

13. Kimmel D, VanderVeen F. Factors of marital adjustment in Locke's Adjustment Test. J Marriage Fam 1974; 29: 57–63

14. LoPiccolo J, Steger J. The sexual interaction inventory: a new instrument for assessment of sexual dysfunction. Arch Sex Behav 1974; 3: 585–595

15. Schover L. Prime time: sexual health for men over fifty. New York: Holt, 1984

16. LoPiccolo J, Heiman J R. The role of cultural values in the prevention of sexual problems. In: Qualls C B, Wincz J P, Barlow D H (eds) The prevention of sexual disorders. New York: Plenum Press, 1978: 43–74

17. Ackerman M D, Carey M P. Psychology's role in the assessment of erectile dysfunction: historic precedents, current knowledge, and methods. J Consult Clin Psychol 1995; 63(6): 862–876

Chapter 18

Basic assessment of the patient with erectile dysfunction

R. S. Kirby

■ INTRODUCTION

Recently, knowledge of the pathogenesis of erectile dysfunction (ED) has expanded considerably and, with this, there has been a parallel increase in the variety and complexity of investigations employed to establish the cause of the disorder in the individual patient. However, despite the highly technological diagnostic modalities now available, the basic principle taught to every medical student — and one that is especially important in the evaluation of the man with erectile dysfunction — must not be forgotten: that accurate diagnosis depends on a careful history and physical examination, the results of which are supplemented by special investigations. Subsequent chapters dwell in some depth on the still-evolving and increasingly sophisticated modalities of diagnosis used in ED, but in this chapter the question of how the patient should be assessed initially is addressed.

■ HISTORY

Because of the sensitive nature of the complaint of ED, it is of paramount importance to establish a relationship of trust between patient and clinician at an early stage. Building this rapport requires more time and patience than is usually required in, for example, the assessment of a patient with benign prostatic enlargement, and appointment schedules need to be adjusted accordingly. Recently, several formal symptom scores have been developed and validated, which aim to quantify the extent of ED. The two with the greatest facility are those developed by O'Leary et al.[1] and Rosen et al.,[2] which are reproduced as Tables 18.1 and 18.2. Although such questionnaires are undoubtedly valuable,

they do focus exclusively on the functional element of ED. A more complex question is the extent to which sexual dysfunction affects the quality of life; recently, Wagner et al.[3] have addressed this important issue. Their questionnaire, developed following interviews with patients presenting with ED both in the UK and the USA, is set out in Table 18.3.

Notwithstanding the value of these questionnaires, it is often helpful to start a face-to-face interview with a brief explanation of the distinction between loss of libido, ED and ejaculatory disturbance. By far the most common presenting complaint is that of reduced rigidity of erections; less commonly, the patient complains of a total absence of erectile activity. Enquiry should concentrate initially on this element of the symptoms and their duration, as well as the rapidity and particular circumstances of onset. A key question is obviously whether the impairment of erections is consistent, rather than 'situational' with preservation of nocturnal and early morning erections. Although the majority of physicians are now acquainted with the loose association between preservation of the latter and psychogenic impotence, most patients do not make this connection. A useful guide to the severity of the problem is to enquire when penetrative intercourse was last possible — not uncommonly, the surprising reply is received, that this was accomplished only a few days ago!

Discreet enquiry should also be made as to whether the problem is confined to sexual encounters with one partner or whether it is also present with other partners. The partner's attitude to the potency problem should also be established. Questions about deviant sexual behaviour or taboo practices at this early stage, although relevant, risk compromising the developing relationship between

Table 18.1. A brief sexual function inventory. (From ref. 1, with permission)

SEXUAL DRIVE — Let's define sexual drive as a feeling that may include wanting to have a sexual experience (masturbation or intercourse), thinking about having sex or feeling frustrated due to lack of sex.

1. During the past 30 days, on how many days have you felt sexual drive?	No days 0	Only a few days 1	Some days 2	Most days 3	Almost every day 4
2. During the past 30 days, how would you rate your level of sexual drive?	None at all 0	Low 1	Medium 2	Medium High 3	High 4
ERECTIONS 3. Over the past 30 days, how often have you had partial or full sexual erections when you were sexually stimulated in any way?	Not at all 0	A few times 1	Fairly often 2	Usually 3	Always 4
4. Over the past 30 days, how often have you had erections; how often were they firm enough to have sexual intercourse?	0	1	2	3	4
5. How much difficulty did you have getting an erection during the last 30 days?	Did not get erections at all 0	A lot of difficulty 1	Some difficulty 2	Little difficulty 3	No difficulty 4
EJACULATION 6. Over the past 30 days, how much difficulty have you had in ejaculating when you have been sexually stimulated?	Have had no sexual stimulation in past month 0	A lot of difficulty 1	Some difficulty 2	Little difficulty 3	No difficulty 4
7. In the past 30 days, how much did you consider the amount of semen you ejaculate?	Did not climax 0	Big problem 1	Medium problem 2	Small problem 3	No problem 4
PROBLEM ASSESSMENT 8. In the past 30 days, to what extent have you considered a lack of sex drive to be a problem?	Big problem 0	Medium problem 1	Small problem 2	Very small problem 3	No problem 4
9. In the past 30 days, to what extent have you considered your ability to get and keep an erection a problem?	0	1	2	3	4
10. In the past 30 days, to what extent have you considered your ejaculation to be a problem?	0	1	2	3	4
OVERALL SATISFACTION 11. Overall, during the past 30 days, how satisfied have you been with your sex life?	Very dissatisfied 0	Mostly dissatisfied 1	Neutral or mixed 2	Mostly satisfied 3	Very satisfied 4

Table 18.2. Individual items of International Index of Erectile Function (IIEF) Questionnaire and response options (US version). (From ref. 2, with permission)

Question*	Response options
Q1: How often were you able to get an erection during sexual activity? Q2: When you had erections with sexual stimulation, how often were your erections hard enough for penetration?	0 = No sexual activity 1 = Almost never/never 2 = A few times (much less than half the time) 3 = Sometimes (about half the time) 4 = Most times (much more than half the time) 5 = Almost always/always
Q3: When you attempted sexual intercourse, how often were you able to penetrate (enter) your partner? Q4: During sexual intercourse, *how often* were you able to maintain your erection after you had penetrated (entered) your partner?	0 = Did not attempt intercourse 1 = Almost never/never 2 = A few times (much less than half the time) 3 = Sometimes (about half the time) 4 = Most times (much more than half the time) 5 = Almost always/always
Q5: During sexual intercourse, *how difficult* was it to maintain your erection to completion of intercourse?	0 = Did not attempt intercourse 1 = Extremely difficult 2 = Very difficult 3 = Difficult 4 = Slightly difficult 5 = Not difficult
Q6: How many times have you attempted sexual intercourse?	0 = No attempts 1 = One to two attempts 2 = Three to four attempts 3 = Five to six attempts 4 = Seven to ten attempts 5 = Eleven+ attempts
Q7: When you attempted sexual intercourse, how often was it satisfactory for you?	0 = Did not attempt intercourse 1 = Almost never/never 2 = A few times (much less than half the time) 3 = Sometimes (about half the time) 4 = Most times (much more than half the time) 5 = Almost always/always
Q8: How much have you enjoyed sexual intercourse?	0 = No intercourse 1 = No enjoyment 2 = Not very enjoyable 3 = Fairly enjoyable 4 = Highly enjoyable 5 = Very highly enjoyable

*All questions are preceded by the phrase "Over the past 4 weeks".

Table 18.2. (Cont'd)

Question*	Response options
Q9: When you had sexual stimulation *or* intercourse, how often did you ejaculate? Q10: When you had sexual stimulation *or* intercourse, how often did you have the feeling of orgasm or climax?	0 = No sexual stimulation/intercourse 1 = Almost never/never 2 = A few times (much less than half the time) 3 = Sometimes (about half the time) 4 = Most times (much more than half the time) 5 = Almost always/always
Q11: How often have you felt sexual desire?	1 = Almost never/never 2 = A few times (much less than half the time) 3 = Sometimes (about half the time) 4 = Most times (much more than half the time) 5 = Almost always/always
Q12: How would you rate your level of sexual desire?	1 = Very low/none at all 2 = Low 3 = Moderate 4 = High 5 = Very high
Q13: How satisfied have you been with your overall *sex life*? Q14: How satisfied have you been with your *sexual relationship* with your partner?	1 = Very dissatisfied 2 = Moderately dissatisfied 3 = About equally satisfied and dissatisfied 4 = Moderately satisfied 5 = Very satisfied
Q15: How do you rate your *confidence* that you could get and keep an erection?	1 = Very low 2 = Low 3 = Moderate 4 = High 5 = Very high

*All questions are preceded by the phrase "Over the past 4 weeks".

interviewer and patient. Although libido is usually preserved in men presenting with ED, inevitably increasing the psychological frustrations of the patient, a decline of sexual drive may suggest an endocrinological cause of the problem and this should be carefully documented. Ejaculation is much less commonly affected than erection itself, but enquiry should be made as to whether ejaculation is premature, delayed or dry (as commonly occurs following transurethral resection of the prostate).

The previous medical history should include a brief survey of sexual history, which may provide a clue to a congenital problem due, perhaps, to a veno-occlusive disorder or congenital chordee. Previous surgery, especially pelvic surgery for bowel, bladder or prostatic malignancy, reconstructive vascular surgery or renal transplantation, may obviously be relevant. Multisystem disorders may result in impotence and can sometimes present with this symptom. Hypertension

Table 18.3. QOL-MED questionnaire: item list

1. I feel frustrated because of my erection problem
2. My erection problem makes me feel depressed
3. I feel like less of a man because of my erection problem
4. I have lost confidence in my sexual ability
5. I worry that I won't be able to get or keep an erection
6. My erection problem is always on my mind
7. I feel that I have lost control over my erections
8. I blame myself for my erection problem
9. I feel angry because of my erection problem
10. I worry about the future of my sex life
11. I have lost pleasure in sex because of my erection problem
12. I am embarrassed about my problem
13. I worry about being humiliated because of my problem
14. I try to avoid having sex
15. I feel different from other men because of my erection problem
16. I get less enjoyment out of life because of my erection problem
17. I feel guilty about my erection problem
18. I am afraid to 'make the first move' towards sex
19. I worry that my partner blames herself for my erection problem
20. I worry about letting her down because of my erection problem
21. I worry that I'm not satisfying her because of my erection problem
22. I worry that we are growing apart because of my erection problem
23. I worry that she is looking for someone else because of my problem
24. I feel that she blames me for my erection problem
25. I worry that she thinks I don't want her because of my erection problem
26. I have trouble talking to her about my problem
27. My erection problem interferes with my daily activities

(Reproduced from ref. 3 with permission.)

and diabetes mellitus are by far the most common of these (and the family history may provide a clue), but alcoholism, thyroid dysfunction, haemochromatosis and other systemic disorders should be borne in mind (Table 18.4).

Of the neurological disorders that may cause impotence, multiple sclerosis is the most frequently encountered, but this is seldom a presenting feature of the disease. Another diffuse disease affecting the central nervous system, however, may produce ED as its earliest presenting manifestation: this disease, originally known as the Shy–Drager syndrome, but now more commonly termed multiple system atrophy (MSA) is characterized by selective degeneration of autonomic neurons in the central nervous system (CNS). In this disorder there is progressive selective cell loss from the pons, medulla and cerebellum, as well as degeneration of the neurons of the intermediolateral cell column of the thoracolumbar sympathetic outflow and sacral parasympathetic outflow (Fig. 18.1). The condition affects patients in their middle age, with a male:female ratio of 2:1. In the male, erectile dysfunction is accompanied by frequency and urgency of micturition, which may be confused with bladder outflow obstruction due to benign prostatic enlargement. An important sign that may provide a clue to this sometimes elusive diagnosis is postural (orthostatic) hypotension due to impaired sympathetic vasoconstrictor tone, and this can usually be demonstrated on measuring blood pressure in the standing and lying positions.[4]

DRUG HISTORY

A detailed history of all concomitant medications is important in the evaluation of patients with ED, since many pharmacological agents may be associated with problems of potency (Table 18.5). Often, it is difficult to decide whether it is the drug itself, or the condition for which it is being administered (e.g. hypertension), that has caused the symptom.

Antihypertensive agents have often been cited as the most common medication-related cause of ED.[5] Clonidine, methyldopa and reserpine, all of which share a centrally acting sympatholytic effect, are associated with an incidence of erectile dysfunction in about one-third to one-quarter of patients treated, but these agents are now seldom used therapeutically. The

Table 18.4. Organic causes of erectile dysfunction

Congenital deformities
  Epispadias
  Hypospadias
  Congenital chordee
  Microphallus

Mechanical
  Morbid obesity
  Peyronie's disease
  Bilateral hydrocoele
  Phimosis
  Tethered frenulum
  Carcinoma of penis

Postsurgical
  Cystectomy, urethrectomy
  Radical prostatectomy
  Abdominoperineal resection of rectum
  Low anterior resection of rectum
  Rectal pull-through procedures
  Transurethral resection of prostate
  External sphincterotomy

Vascular insufficiency
  Aorto-iliac disease (Leriche syndrome)
  Internal iliac atheroma
  Atheroma of pudendal vessels
  Distal vessel disease
  Post-priapism
  Smoking
  Anaemia
  Veno-occlusive dysfunction
  Post-pelvic fracture

Metabolic disorders
  Diabetes mellitus
  Haemochromatosis
  Alcoholism
  Sickle-cell disease
  Hepatic/renal failure
  Scleroderma
  Thyroid disease
  Adrenal disease

Neurogenic disorders
  Multiple system atrophy
  Spinal cord lesions
  Multiple sclerosis
  Tabes dorsalis
  Peripheral neuropathies
  Spina bifida
  Amyotrophic lateral sclerosis

Abnormalities of hypothalamopituitary function
Congenital
  LH-FSH deficiency (Kallmann's syndrome)
  Congenital hypogonadotrophic hypogonadism
  Panhypopituitarism
Acquired
  Trauma, infiltrative disease, tumours of
    pituitary, etc.
  Exogenous hormones
  Hyperprolactinaemia

Primary gonadal abnormalities
  Chromosomal abnormalities
    (e.g. Klinefelter's syndrome)
  Bilateral anorchia
  Gonadal toxins
  Drug-induced gonadal damage
    (chemotherapeutic agents)
  Gonadal injury (trauma/mumps/torsion)

precise mechanism by which they impair potency is unclear, but probably they directly reduce libido by a central effect and they may also elevate serum prolactin levels. Peripherally acting alpha-adrenoceptor blockers, such as phenoxybenzamine (mixed alpha-1 and alpha-2 blockade) and the newer alpha-1-selective adrenoceptor blockers prazosin, doxazosin and terazosin, are less commonly associated with ED. In fact, from their vasodilator action on cavernosal vessels, one might expect their effect to be mildly beneficial but, by blocking the sympathetically mediated closure of the bladder neck at the time of ejaculation, they may

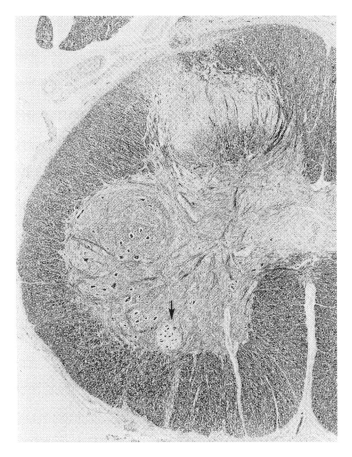

Figure 18.1. A section through the spinal cord of a man who suffered from MSA. There is selective loss of cell bodies from Onuf's nucleus.

occasionally produce retrograde ejaculation. Indeed, the alpha-1A-selective adrenoceptor-blocker tamsulosin seems to be particularly potent in this respect.[6] In the recently conducted Treatment of Mild Hypertension Study (TOMHS), most classes of antihypertensive agent (diuretic, beta blocker, angiotensin-converting enzyme [ACE] inhibitor and calcium-channel blocker) were associated with a higher incidence of sexual dysfunction than placebo.[7] By contrast, the alpha-1-adrenoceptor blocker doxazosin appeared less likely than placebo to produce this effect, suggesting a beneficial action of reduced alpha-1-adrenoceptor tone (Fig. 18.2).

In other studies, beta-adrenoceptor blockers have often been reported to cause ED (especially at higher doses), directly by a peripheral action on the corporal tissue and also perhaps by a central effect on libido.[8] Their ability to penetrate the CNS and induce a sympatholytic effect depends on their lipid solubility. Newer beta blockers, such as atenolol, are less lipid soluble and seem to cause less impairment of sexual

function. Diuretics have also been linked with ED: in particular, spironolactone has been reported to induce gynaecomastia, erectile dysfunction and reduced libido in some patients,[9] and vasodilators such as hydralazine also seem to produce ED.[10]

It must be remembered that, in some patients with partial vasculogenic ED, high systolic arterial pressures may be required to achieve sufficient cavernosal artery flow for erection. Lowering blood pressure into the normal range, in itself may, therefore, to some extent compromise penile blood flow and induce or exacerbate erectile dysfunction.[11]

Many major and minor tranquillizers and hypnotics have been reported to cause both diminished libido and erectile dysfunction.[12] Antidepressants such as monoamine oxidase (MAO) inhibitors and tricyclic compounds may cause ED, probably by decreasing libido. The minor tranquillizers or anxiolytic agents, particularly the benzodiazepines, exert a depressive effect on the brain stem, limbic system and septal region; libido can also be reduced and ED may follow. Meprobamate, barbiturates and other sedative hypnotics all exert a central effect similar to that of the benzodiazepines, with consequent effects on erectile function and libido.

Drugs with anti-androgenic activity, such as ketoconazole, cyproterone acetate and the histamine-receptor blocker cimetidine,[13] are known to cause diminished potency; however, interestingly, Casodex and flutamide, which are pure anti-androgens, seem to spare both potency and libido, while still effectively blocking androgen receptors. This effect has been suggested to be the result of elevated serum testosterone levels. The luteinizing-hormone-releasing hormone (LHRH) analogues, such as goserelin and leuprolide, induce medical castration and are almost always associated with ED, as well as with profound suppression of libido. By contrast, 5-alpha-reductase inhibitors produce ED and loss of libido in only 3–5% of patients.[14] This suggests that testosterone, rather than its 5-alpha-reduced form dihydrotestosterone, is mainly responsible for the maintenance of erectile function and libido.

Recreational drugs such as marijuana, and especially cocaine and heroin,[15] may also cause impotence and reduce libido, and are associated with a reduction of testosterone levels. Cigarette smoking, probably by virtue of its vasoconstricting effect or by the induction of

Table 18.5. Pharmacological agents associated with erectile dysfunction

Major tranquillizers
    Phenothiazines, e.g. fluphenazine, chlorpromazine, promazine, mesoridazine
    Butyrophenones, e.g. haloperidol
    Thioxanthines, e.g. thiothixene, chorprothixene

Antidepressants
    Tricyclics, e.g. nortriptyline, amitriptyline, desipramine, doxepin
    MAO inhibitors, e.g. isocarboxazide, phenelzine, tranylcypromine, pargylene, procarbazine
    Lithium

Anxiolytics
    Benzodiazepines, e.g. chlordiazepoxide, diazepam, chlorazepate

Anticholinergics
    Atropine
    Propantheline
    Benztropine
    Dimenhydrinate
    Diphenhydramine

Cardiac
    Digoxin
    Lipid-lowering agents

Antihypertensives
    Diuretics, e.g. thiazides, spironolactone
    Vasodilators, e.g. hydralazine
    Central sympatholytics, e.g. methyldopa, clonidine, reserpine
    Ganglion blockers, e.g. guanethidine, bethanidine
    Beta blockers, e.g. propranolol, metoprolol, atenolol
    Calcium-channel blockers
    ACE inhibitors

Recreational drugs
    Alcohol
    Marijuana
    Amphetamines
    Barbiturates
    Nicotine
    Opiates

Anti-androgenic
    Cyproterone acetate
    Flutamide
    Casodex
    LHRH analogues
    Oestrogens
    5-alpha-reductase inhibitors

Miscellaneous
    Cimetidine
    Clofibrate
    Metoclopramide
    Baclofen
    Indomethacin
    (+ many others)

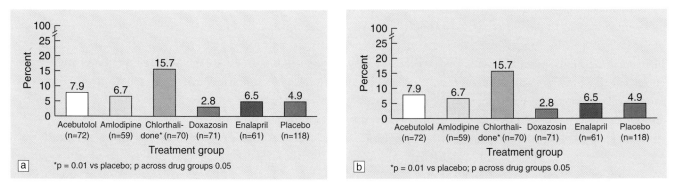

Figure 18.2. Impact of various classes of antihypertensive therapy on erectile function as reported in the TOMHS study by Grimm et al. Incidence of men reporting (a) an inability to obtain erection, (b) an inability to maintain erection, by treatment group (24 months).

atheroma, has also been reported to cause impaired potency.[16] Alcoholism may induce ED by several mechanisms: these include peripheral neuropathy, testicular dysfunction and an effect on the hypothalamopituitary axis, as well as impaired hepatic function resulting in increased serum oestrogen levels.[17] Even moderate doses of alcohol may impair erectile function (although, frustratingly, they also increase libido). As a consequence, patients with potency problems should usually be advised to reduce their alcohol consumption, as well as to refrain from cigarette, cigar and pipe smoking.

PHYSICAL EXAMINATION

A thorough physical examination is an important part of the basic assessment of the man with ED; care should be taken to look for clinical signs of thyroid underactivity or overactivity, as well as stigmata of liver failure or anaemia. Hypertension and other serious cardiovascular pathology must also be excluded. All peripheral pulses should be palpated and any cardiac murmurs or arrhythmias identified. A focused neurological examination is valuable, with special attention being paid to the sacral spinal outflow. Saddle anaesthesia, with loss of bulbocavernosus reflex in combination with a lax anal sphincter, may suggest the presence of an occult cauda equina lesion. This disorder may occasionally present with ED due to a central prolapse of an intervertebral disc or a slow-growing lumbar or sacral intraspinal tumour.

Examination of the external genitalia should be performed with a view to excluding congenital or acquired abnormalities of the penis itself. Peyronie's plaques should be sought along the palpable length of the corpora and the patient questioned about the presence of pain on intercourse, or erectile deformity. Preputial abnormalities, such as tethering of the frenulum or phimosis, may occasionally present with ED, as may a spectrum of other genital abnormalities including microphallus, epispadias and squamous cell carcinoma of the penis. The presence of small testes and reduced or absent secondary sexual characteristics may suggest hypogonadism, and it is worth enquiring about the frequency of necessity for facial shaving, as this may decline with androgen insufficiency. The anterior chest wall should be examined to exclude gynaecomastia, and enquiry made concerning galactorrhoea. Causes of primary hypogonadism and testicular failure are listed in Table 18.4; when any of these are present they are usually an indication for referral for specialist endocrine opinion.

Digital rectal examination should be performed in men with erectile dysfunction to assess prostatic size and consistency. If the presence of benign prostatic enlargement is detected, a urinary flow rate should be determined and the patient warned that androgen therapy may risk exacerbation of bladder outflow obstruction. The presence of prostatic nodules should raise the possibility of early prostatic cancer and a prostate-specific antigen (PSA) value should usually be measured, at least in men over the age of 45. If the level of this marker is raised, a prostatic biopsy under transrectal ultrasound control may be necessary; in these circumstances, androgen replacement therapy is contraindicated, at least until adenocarcinoma of the prostate is excluded.

SPECIAL INVESTIGATIONS

Investigation of the male patient with ED must, obviously, be tailored specifically to the individual concerned and any leads given by the history or examination. Baseline haematological and biochemical screens are necessary, which should exclude diabetes mellitus. Also included are liver function tests to exclude hepatic impairment, which may be associated with increased serum oestrogen levels and a reduced plasma testosterone. The baseline values are also useful if papaverine or hormone-replacement therapy is subsequently employed, because of the occasional hepatoxicity associated with these treatments.

Estimation of serum hormone levels is expensive, and some investigators suggest that a single measurement of serum testosterone is all that is required.[18] In occasional cases of hyperprolactinaemia, however, serum testosterone may be just within normal limits and a space-occupying lesion of the pituitary fossa (Fig. 18.3) is obviously something that must not remain undetected.[19,20] Many clinicians dealing with ED routinely measure testosterone, prolactin and sex-hormone-binding globulin. Patients with significant abnormalities of serum testosterone and/or prolactin levels often respond well to treatment.[21] As discussed previously, a prostate-specific antigen (PSA) value should

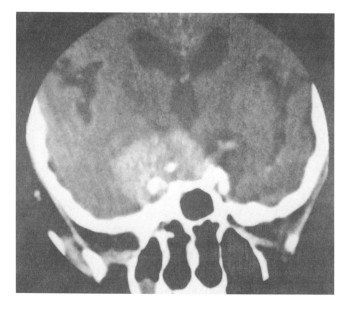

Figure 18.3. A CT scan demonstrating a craniopharyngioma in a man presenting with hyperprolactinaemia resulting in ED. The patient also complained of headaches and visual disturbances.

be obtained to assess the probability of the patient harbouring an incidental prostate carcinoma.

While sophisticated neurological testing is not possible in the office setting and there are currently no accurate methods for testing the autonomic nerve supply to the genitalia, biothesiometry is an accurate measure of peripheral sensation and can be applied to the penis (Fig. 18.4). The device tests vibratory sensation and can be

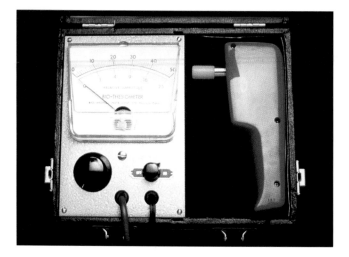

Figure 18.4. The biothesiometer consists of a hand-held vibratory wand, a rheostat for control and a measurement guage.

compared with a normal age-adjusted nomogram for standardization (Fig. 18.5). The sensation is first tested on the index fingers by applying the vibrating wand lightly and increasing vibration frequency with the rheostat until first sensation. The procedure is repeated on the inner thighs, penile shaft and finally the glans penis. Patients with peripheral neuropathy, penile nerve damage and Peyronie's disease will exhibit reduced sensation for age.

Often, the most valuable information obtained in an outpatient or office setting is the assessment of response to intercavernosal prostaglandin E1 (PGE1).[22] Although some clinicians withhold this diagnostic test until the second visit, it is often convenient to employ a small test dose (5–10 µg) on the first attendance. Prior to administration of this compound, the patient must be warned about the possibilities of bruising (which is of little significance) and of a prolonged response (>6 h), which must be treated by corporal aspiration or intracorporal phenylephrine or other alpha-adrenergic injection within 6–8 h. A signed consent form is useful, as well as a detailed description of who to contact and what to do should the erection fail to disappear spontaneously. An absent or impaired response may be an indication for colour Doppler scanning of the cavernosal and dorsal penile arteries, with higher dosage of PGE1 to exclude arterial insufficiency or venous leakage. This investigation is indicated in patients in whom reconstruction would be considered, and this test can be arranged before the second consultation.

Further details of this and other special investigations for elucidating the cause of impaired erectile potency are discussed in greater detail in subsequent chapters.

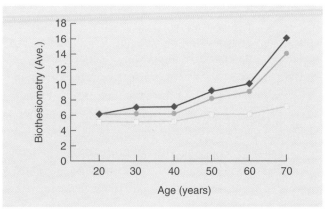

Figure 18.5. A standard nomogram for vibratory sensation and age was compiled by measurement of biothesiometry on 350 normal patients. (Courtesy of C. Carson, MD.)

■ CONCLUSIONS

The initial basic assessment of ED is of some importance, because it is the main opportunity for the clinician to establish a rapport with the patient. This first meeting, if effectively and sympathetically handled, can set this relationship on the course towards a successful outcome for both parties.

With the advent of new, effective non-invasive therapies, such as intra-urethral prostaglandin E1 and the phosphodiesterase type 5 inhibitor, sildenafil, the history and examination have assumed an even more important role in ED, since many patients will wish to start therapy without proceeding with invasive investigations. The importance of excluding other important pathologies, such as diabetes mellitus, hypertension, or pituitary tumour, should not be underestimated.

Many of the issues raised in this chapter are addressed more extensively in subsequent chapters; however, as in most other areas of life, the need for especial care and attention to detail at the outset of the process of diagnosis and treatment remain paramount.

■ REFERENCES

1. O'Leary M P, Fowler F J, Lenderking W R et al. A brief male sexual function inventory for urology. Urology 1993; 46: 697–706

2. Rosen R C, Riley A, Wagner G et al. An international index of erectile function (IIEF): a multidimensional scale for assessment of erectile dysfunction. Urology 1997; 49: 822–830

3. Wagner T H, Patrick D L, McKenna S P, Froese P S. Cross-cultural development of a quality of life measure for men with erection difficulties. Qual Life Res 1996; 5: 443–449

4. Bannister R. Clinical features of progressive autonomic failure. In: Bannister R (ed) Autonomic failure. a textbook of clinical disorders of the autonomic nervous system, 2nd edn. Oxford: Oxford University Press, 1988: 267–288

5. Forsberg L, Gustavii B, Hojerback T, Olsson A M. Impotence, smoking and orgasmic-ejaculatory response in human males. Fertil Steril 1979; 31: 589

6. Abrams P, Schulman C C, Vaage S. Tamsulosin, a selective alpha 1c adrenoceptor antagonist: a randomized controlled trial in patients with benign prostatic obstruction. Br J Urol 1995; 76: 325–336

7. Grimm R H, Gregory A, Prineas R J et al. Long-term effects on sexual function of five antihypertensive drugs and nutritional hygienic treatment in hypertensive men and women. Hypertension 1997; 29: 8–14

8. Horowitz J D, Gobel A J. Drugs and impaired male sexual function. Drugs 1979; 18: 206

9. Greenblatt D J, Kochweser J. Gynaecomastia and impotence: complication of spironolactone. JAMA 1983; 223: 83–87

10. Papadopoulos C. Cardiovascular drugs and sexuality. Arch Intern Med 1980; 140: 1341

11. Wein A J, Van Arsdalen K. Drug-induced male sexual dysfunction. Urol Clin North Am 1988; 15: 23–31

12. Mitchell J E, Popkin M K. Antidepressant drug therapy and sexual dysfunction in men: a review. J Clin Psychopharmacol 1983; 3: 76–84

13. Pedan N R, Cargill J M, Browning M C K et al. Male sexual dysfunction during treatment with cimetidine. Br Med J 1979; i: 659

14. Gormley G, Stoner E, Bruskewitz R C et al. The effect of finasteride in men with benign prostatic hyperplasia. N Engl J Med 1992; 327: 1185–1191

15. Mirin S M, Meyer R E, Mendelsohn J H, Ellinghoe J. Opiate use and sexual function. Am J Psychiatry 1980; 137: 909

16. Shabsigh R, Fishman I, Schum C, Dunn J K. Cigarette smoking and other vascular risk factors in vasculogenic impotence. Urology 1991; 38: 227–232

17. Whalley L J. Sexual adjustment of male alcoholics. Acta Psychiatr Scand 1978; 56: 281–287

18. Pryor J L, Johnson A R, Jarrow J P. Editorial comment. Is routine endocrine testing of impotent men necessary? J Urol 1992; 147: 1542–1544

19. McClure R D. Endocrine investigation and therapy. Urol Clin North Am 1987; 14: 471–488

20. Leonard M P, Nickel C J, Morales A. Hyperprolactinaemia and impotence: why, when and how to investigate. J Urol 1989; 142: 992–994

21. Carini C, Zini D, Balini A et al. Effects of androgen treatment in impotent men with normal and low levels of free testosterone. Arch Sex Behav 1990; 19: 223–234

22. Stackl W, Hasun R, Marberger M. Intracavernous injection of prostaglandin E1 in impotent men. J Urol 1988; 140: 66–71

Chapter 19

Pharmacological testing: Doppler

U. Patel and W. R. Lees

■ INTRODUCTION

This chapter presents the application of Doppler ultrasound in the evaluation of penile haemodynamics. The penile Doppler study (PDS) has undergone the course typical of modern medical innovations: after initial enthusiasm and wide application,[1–7] more recent publications have been cautionary,[8–11] veering at times to full scepticism. In the opinion of the present authors, based on their own experience and studies, this last view is an overreaction. As well as technical aspects, a review of the theoretical soundness of the test is presented in this chapter; areas of controversy are explored, and the limitations and validity of the test are discussed.

■ PHARMACOLOGICAL TESTING: DOPPLER

Thorough understanding of penile anatomy and of the physiology of erection are both essential to the successful use of Doppler ultrasound in erectile dysfunction. These aspects are covered more fully elsewhere in this book, but a brief review of the immediately relevant points is given here.

Anatomy

The erectile bodies of the penis are the paired, dorsolateral spongy corpora cavernosa encased by the stiff multilayered fibroelastic tunica albuginea. Each cavernosum is supplied by a single end artery — the cavernosum artery, a branch of the penile artery, which is itself a branch of the internal pudendal artery (Fig. 19.1). Variations of this arterial anatomy are not uncommon (e.g. accessory pudendal artery, distal dorsal to cavernosal artery collaterals and unilateral absence of dorsal artery).[12] Whether such variations affect erectile

dysfunction is still disputed, but they do greatly influence diagnostic imaging — both Doppler ultrasound and (especially) arteriography. The cavernosal artery further branches into helicine arteries and finally into arterioles terminating in cavernosal sinusoids lined by smooth muscle. The sinusoid is capable of considerable expansion in volume and this is the fundamental basis of penile enlargement and rigidity. Sinusoids drain into subtunical venules which merge into the emissary veins; these pierce obliquely through the tunica albuginea and further empty into the midline dorsal penile vein (Fig. 19.2). With sinusoidal distension, the subtunical venules and the obliquely aligned emissary veins are compressed against the tunica albuginea, and this is the postulated anatomical/ mechanical mechanism of venous occlusion (Fig. 19.2). Alternative pathways of cavernosal drainage (such as the cavernosal and crural veins at the root of the cavernosa) are minor routes in the normal man.

Physiology

At baseline, the tone of the smooth muscle of the cavernosal arterioles and sinusoids is high, restricting cavernosal artery flow; and inflow and outflow are in equilibrium at low volume flow. The haemodynamic changes of erection are initiated by neurophysiologically driven relaxation of smooth muscle of the sinusoids and arterioles. This acutely reduces the peripheral resistance, stimulating an up to tenfold rise in cavernosal artery volume flow. Increased inflow is accommodated by engorgement of the relaxed cavernosal sinusoids, and penile lengthening and tumescence commences. Sinusoidal distension progressively compresses the subtunical venules and the obliquely aligned emissary veins. Thus, active relaxation and congestion of sinusoids leads to passive restriction of venous outflow (Fig. 19.2). This state of high inflow and restricted outflow will continue until full erection, when cavernosal pressure will

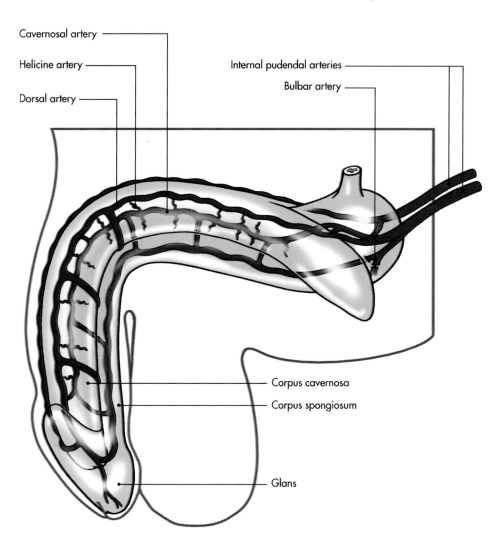

Cavernosal artery

Helicine artery

Dorsal artery

Internal pudendal arteries

Bulbar artery

Corpus cavernosa

Corpus spongiosum

Glans

Figure 19.1. Normal arterial anatomy of the penis; note that variations are common and easily recognizable on ultrasound.

reach systolic pressure and inflow will also diminish, or even cease. The cavernosal pressure may further rise above systolic levels with contraction of the bulbocavernosus muscles during pelvic thrusting.[13]

Smooth muscle relaxation, marked augmentation of arterial inflow and passive venous occlusion are the key steps of the haemodynamic model. The mechanism may malfunction at any of these three points. This simplified view of erectile dysfunction is useful when considering the PDS, as this test can only provide this broad mechanistic subdivision. It should, however, be remembered that there are areas of as yet incomplete understanding with this model, and future advances may modify the application of the PDS. A recent theory proposes finely balanced smooth muscle tone as the chief controller of penile erection, with either deficient relaxation or augmented contraction causing erectile dysfunction; mechanical factors, such as arteriopathy or tunical rigidity (or a mechanical cause of venous leak),

are secondary or even unimportant factors.[14] Although this model has attractions, it fails to explain the most striking finding of the PDS — that a man with a high-velocity normal inflow can still be impotent, unless relaxation of arterioles and centrally placed sinusoids, permitting high cavernosal artery inflow, can coexist with continued contraction of peripheral and subtunical sinusoidal smooth muscle preventing venous occlusion.

■ THEORETICAL FOUNDATIONS OF THE PENILE DOPPLER STUDY: DOPPLER PHYSICS AND ITS APPLICATION IN ERECTILE PHYSIOLOGY

Doppler ultrasound exploits the frequency change (the so-called Doppler shift) that occurs when a sound wave is reflected by a moving interface. The principal interface in

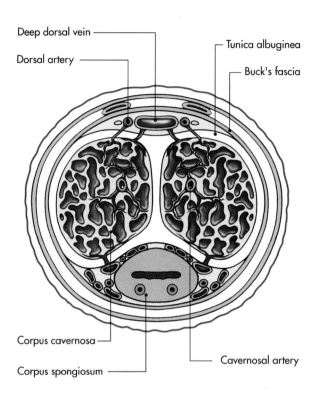

Deep dorsal vein

Dorsal artery

Tunica albuginea

Buck's fascia

Corpus cavernosa

Corpus spongiosum

Cavernosal artery

a

Figure 19.2. (a) Cross-sectional diagram of the penis demonstrating the location of the arteries and veins in relationship to the corporal bodies and the fascial coverings. Further cross-sectional diagrams (b, flaccid; c, erect) illustrate the mechanism of venous occlusion which is activated by distension of the venous sinusoids. Note compression of subtunical venules and emissary veins secondary to sinusoid distension.

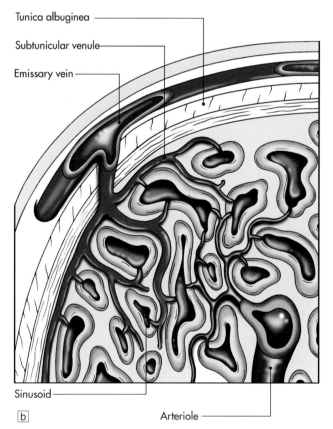

Tunica albuginea

Subtunicular venule

Emissary vein

Sinusoid

Arteriole

b

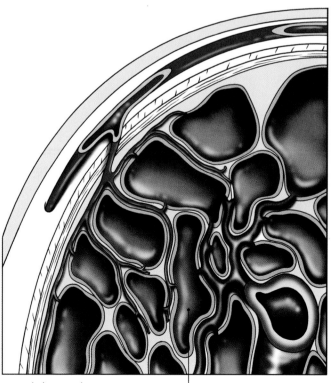

Distended sinusoid

c

209

vascular ultrasound is the surface of red blood cells. The frequency change, detected by the ultrasound probe, and the velocity of red blood cells are related by the formula: $\Delta D = 2fV_2.\text{cosine } \theta/V_1$ (where ΔD is frequency change, f and V_1 are the frequency and velocity of the ultrasound beam emitted by the probe, and θ is the angle between the beam and the direction of blood. All these factors are known; thus, the velocity of the moving interface of the red blood cells (V_2) can be calculated by the software of the ultrasound machine).[15]

Calculated velocities can be displayed in real time either as a semi-quantitative colour map (colour Doppler) or quantitatively as the Doppler waveform (spectral Doppler, duplex Doppler or continuous-wave Doppler). Such a waveform represents the full spectrum of measured velocities within the volume of artery being insonated. However, the shape of the Doppler waveform is not merely a velocity record but also encodes further useful information.

The shape of the waveform is governed by two cardinal factors: these are, first, the characteristics of the tissue bed supplied and, secondly, the elasticity of the vessel wall both upstream and at the point of measurement.[16] Briefly, a low-resistance tissue bed (such as most organs, exercising muscle or cavernosal sinusoids relaxed as in early erection) will allow forward flow throughout the cardiac cycle with high diastolic velocity, whereas the high-resistance bed (tonic cavernosal sinusoids in the flaccid penis or the engorged sinusoids of the erect penis) will allow flow only during the high-pressure systolic portion of the cycle. During diastole the pressure will be insufficient to overcome the peripheral vascular resistance and the diastolic flow (and velocity) will be low, or reversed. Further, more subtle, waveform shapes are also recognizable, e.g. impedance to flow upstream as in, say, iliac stenosis will lengthen the time of the initial systolic upstroke (the so-called 'damped waveform') and increasing peripheral resistance will herald the onset of the dicrotic notch. All these waveform characteristics can be quantified and the various waveform measurements used and of value in the PDS are illustrated in Figure 19.3.

Uniquely, the penile erectile cycle encompasses every possible combination of the interplay between tissue pressure, peripheral resistance and arterial flow. Figure 19.4 schematically summarizes the six phases of erection (as defined by Aboseif and Lue),[13] in terms of pudendal artery flow and intracavernosal pressure, as well as the corresponding changes in peripheral resistance. From

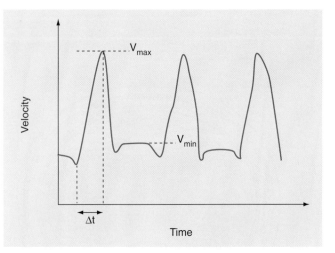

Figure 19.3. Diagrammatic representation of a Doppler waveform and those measurements useful in the evaluation of penile haemodynamics. For the cavernosal artery, flow is conventionally recorded in cm/s. V_{max}, peak systolic velocity (PSV); V_{min}, end-diastolic velocity (EDV); Δt, systolic rise time or acceleration time; resistive index (RI), $(V_{max}-V_{min})/V_{max}$; pulsatility index (PI), $(V_{max}-V_{min})/V_{mean}$.

these three interrelated trends a Doppler waveform pattern can be extrapolated. The soundness of this pressure–flow Doppler waveform model can be experimentally confirmed by the direct correlation of cavernosal artery waveforms with intracavernosal pressure during pharmacocavernosometry, and an example is shown in Figure 19.5. This intimate relationship between cavernosal pressure–flow and Doppler waveforms illustrates why Doppler ultrasound should be especially suited to the study of erectile haemodynamics.

It is more useful to consider the PDS in these terms (i.e. as a means of dynamic evaluation of the changing patterns of flow, velocity and intracavernosal pressure) than merely as involving single, isolated, velocity or waveform measurements. The diagnostic value of this test is fully expressed only when it is used for frequent sampling (every 2 minutes) until the entire normal or abnormal erectile cycle has been adequately evaluated, and this may take up to 30 minutes in some men. Furthermore, using the prevailing haemodynamic model for erectile dysfunction — i.e. failure of initiation (inadequate cavernosal smooth muscle relaxation as in psychogenic impotence, anxiety or sinusoidal parenchymal rigidity), failure of inflow augmentation (arteriogenic impotence) or ineffective veno-occlusion (venous leakage) — it can be predicted that each of these three diagnostic subgroupings will

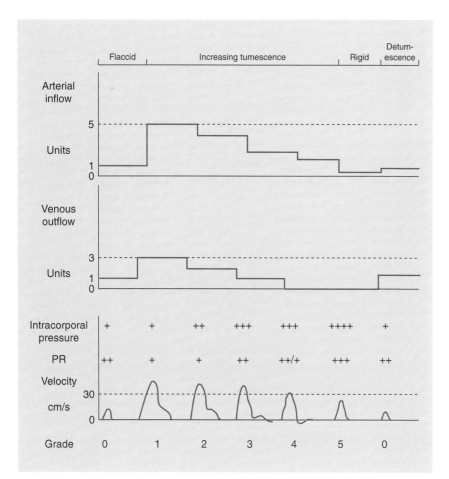

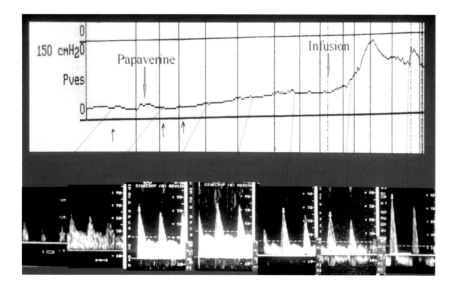

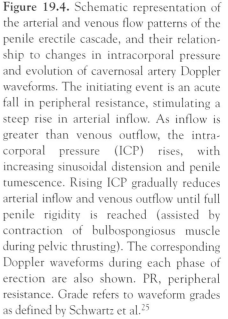

Figure 19.4. Schematic representation of the arterial and venous flow patterns of the penile erectile cascade, and their relationship to changes in intracorporal pressure and evolution of cavernosal artery Doppler waveforms. The initiating event is an acute fall in peripheral resistance, stimulating a steep rise in arterial inflow. As inflow is greater than venous outflow, the intracorporal pressure (ICP) rises, with increasing sinusoidal distension and penile tumescence. Rising ICP gradually reduces arterial inflow and venous outflow until full penile rigidity is reached (assisted by contraction of bulbospongiosus muscle during pelvic thrusting). The corresponding Doppler waveforms during each phase of erection are also shown. PR, peripheral resistance. Grade refers to waveform grades as defined by Schwartz et al.[25]

Figure 19.5. Cavernosal artery waveforms recorded during dynamic pharmacocavernosometry (please note that the vertical axis is incorrectly labelled, it should read mmHg). Intracavernosal injection of pharmacostimulant (papaverine) induces increased systolic and diastolic arterial inflow, secondary to smooth muscle relaxation and reduced peripheral resistance. Increased inflow causes only a small rise in intracorporal pressure in this case (from baseline of 20 mmHg up to <50 mmHg), and the Doppler waveforms continue to be of a low peripheral resistance pattern. On infusion of saline (at 100 ml/min) the intracorporal pressure rises rapidly up to systolic occlusion level (>100 mmHg), and the cavernosal artery waveforms evolve into high peripheral resistance forms with reduced diastolic flow. These recordings demonstrate how closely Doppler waveforms reflect intracorporal pressure and how they can be used to evaluate penile haemodynamics.

211

undergo characteristic patterns of waveform evolution. Thus, with failure of sinusoidal relaxation secondary to anxiety or receptor antagonism/failure, there will be no velocity increase and waveforms will not progress beyond grade 0 (Fig. 19.4). With arteriogenic impotence, cavernosal artery flow will be insufficient to engorge sinusoids and activate the venous occlusion mechanism, so waveforms will show low systolic velocity and elevated diastolic velocity with no evidence of rising cavernosal pressures. In comparison, with defective venous occlusion both systolic and diastolic velocities will remain high (particularly end-diastolic velocity, or EDV) with no evidence of rising intracavernosal pressure. Finally with psychogenic or neurogenic impotence the full waveform cascade will be seen, as pharmacostimulation will bypass the pathophysiological defect. These various patterns are schematically presented in Figure 19.6.

■ THE PENILE DOPPLER STUDY: PRACTICAL DETAILS

Only some patients benefit from the investigation of penile haemodynamics. Selection of suitable patients

and the place of the PDS in the diagnostic algorithm is covered elsewhere in this book. The essential test requirements are cavernosal pharmacostimulation, a colour Doppler ultrasound machine with a 7.5–10 MHz linear array probe, and facilities for making multiple hard copies.[17] The test should be conducted in comfortable, calm and private surroundings to alleviate anxiety and adrenergic smooth muscle tonicity. The penis can be scanned by a dorsal or ventral approach at the base of the penis, with the probe held transversally or in an oblique–longitudinal position (Fig. 19.7). The authors prefer dorsal scanning, transversely in the early phases and oblique–longitudinal once tumescence starts. Their choice of probe position has evolved empirically over time and is the one that they find most comfortable, but it also ensures good reproducibility of velocity records. The transverse position is ideal for consistency of technique. By angling the probe 20–30 degrees cephalad, the artery can be visualized in the root of the cavernosa where it has a vertical course for 1–2 cm, and blood flow is directed towards the probe. Thus, the cavernosal artery can be insonated at a Doppler angle of 0 degrees.

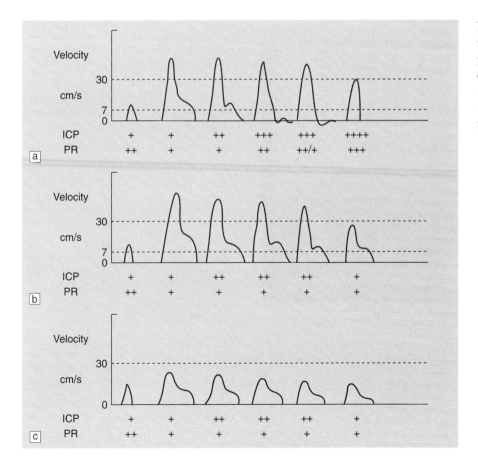

Figure 19.6. Illustration of the waveform cascades as seen with (a) an intact penile haemodynamic mechanism, (b) defective venous occlusion and (c) inadequate arterial inflow. ICP, intracorporal pressure; PR, peripheral resistance.

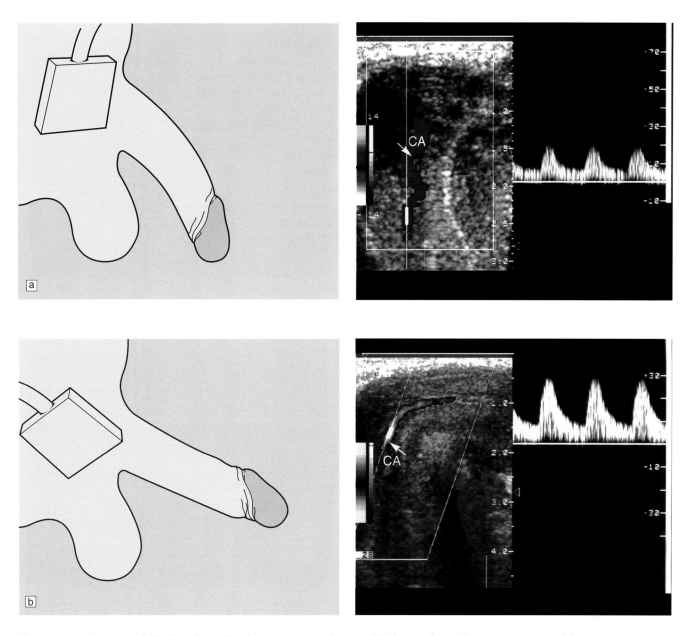

Figure 19.7. Position of the Doppler probe during cavernosal artery (CA) recordings. Transverse position (a) ensures consistent Doppler angle correction and velocity recordings close to the origin of the artery and consistently in the same portion of the artery. The technique is most reproducible in this position. An alternative is the oblique–longitudinal position (b) which is easier in the semi-erect penis; however, reproducibility is slightly difficult in this position, and angle correction has a wider margin of error.

Angle correction is crucial: the angle should always be less than 60 degrees (otherwise the cosine θ in the equation above is too large) and always corrected to match the direction of the artery. In the oblique– longitudinal position the curving course of the artery can make angle correction difficult, and a discrepancy of as little as 20 degrees can introduce substantial computational error (Fig. 19.8). Velocity recordings are also most accurate and reproducible if measured near the origin of the artery and consistently at the same point, since there is a velocity gradient between the base and the tip of the penis. Waveform indices such as resistive index and pulsatility index (Fig. 19.3) are angle-independent measurements, which places them at an advantage over angle-dependent velocity values. However, they are less informative overall, as patients with venous leak cannot be distinguished from those with deficient inflow; the authors, therefore, do not use them routinely.

The choice of pharmacostimulant is important. A variety of intracavernosal drugs can induce erection, but

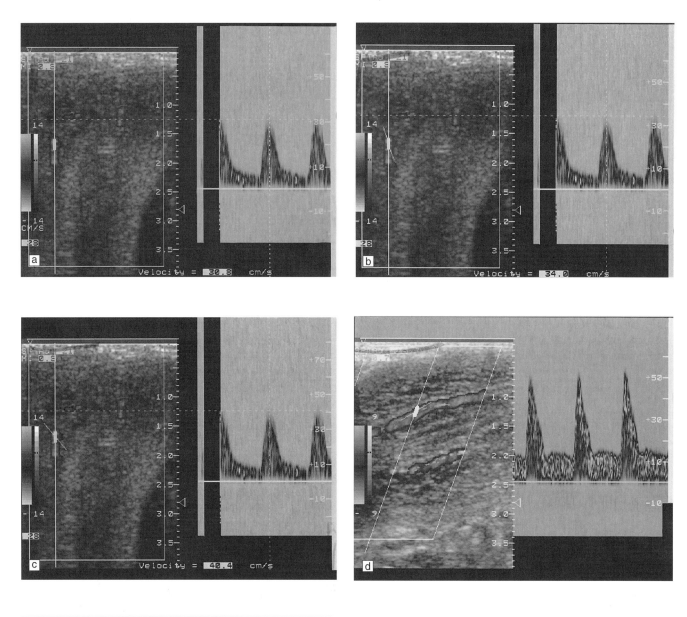

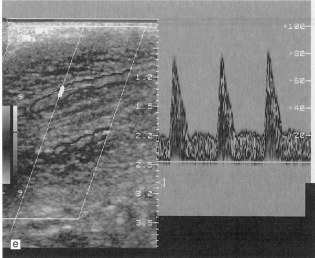

Figure 19.8. This montage of five images demonstrates the measurement errors possible unless the Doppler angle is accurately aligned along the direction of blood flow. (a–c) illustrate the errors introduced by lack of angle correction in the transverse position, in this case the difference between a normal and abnormal study. (d) and (e) illustrate errors in the oblique–longitudinal position. Angle correction is easier in the transverse scanhead position when insonating close to the base of the penis along the vertical portion of the artery.

the two favoured agents are prostaglandin E1 (PGE1) or papaverine,[18,19] with or without the addition of phentolamine (the addition of phentolamine allows a reduction in the dose of pharmacostimulant and so causes less penile ache, which is sometimes a feature with the use of PGE1). There is no published experience regarding the use of the newer oral and intra-urethral formulations.

The authors favour intracavernosal PGE1, as it has a superior side-effect profile;[20] in particular, the incidence of priapism is lower. Because maximal stimulation is crucial, 20 µg of PGE1 is used initially, unless there is a suspicion of neurogenic impotence when 5–10 µg is used, with repeat dosing if there is poor evidence of sinusoidal relaxation by 5 minutes after injection. Adjunctive measures, such as self-stimulation, massaging of the injectate and visual stimulation have all been advocated,[21–23] but the authors prefer repeat pharmacostimulation. Adequate sinusoidal relaxation is best heralded by a significant rise in diastolic velocity. Anxiety may attenuate the effect of the drug;[25] indeed, it is the single dominant confounding factor with the PDS. A feature that helps to identify anxiety is improvement in flows (particularly diastolic forward flow) if the patient is left in private. Improved diastolic flow indicates improved sinusoidal relaxation, which disappears rapidly once privacy is interrupted.

Waveform recording should begin within a minute of injection and be repeated frequently (the authors' protocol is shown in Table 19.1) until a stepwise evaluation of the entire erectile cycle has been accomplished. Infrequent recordings or, worse still, single recordings (often at 5 minutes alone) are inadequate in the evaluation of a dynamic physiology such as the penile erection, and are a predictable source of diagnostic inaccuracy. Guidelines for a technically

Table 19.1. Protocol of a technically adequate study

1. Maximal pharmacostimulation ensured and anxiety minimized.

2. Waveforms recorded from the cavernosal artery, close to the base of the penis and consistently at the same point. Ideally, this should be with a transversely held probe.

3. Doppler parameters optimized for velocity measurements. The important factors are a Doppler angle of less than 60 degrees and corrected for the direction of flow using a narrow sampling gate, aligned along a straight part of the cavernosal artery. Machine settings should also be optimized for flow in small vessels (i.e. the lowest pulse repetition frequency, highest Doppler gain and lowest wall filter without increasing background 'noise'). The interested reader is advised to refer to a standard book of Doppler physics, for further details of these and other minor sources of error in Doppler ultrasound.[15,16]

4. Baseline velocity recordings have no diagnostic value and measurements should start 1 min after injection and be repeated until maximal peak systolic velocity (PSV) and minimal diastolic velocity have been reached. Diastolic velocity will reach its nadir after maximal systolic velocity and can be delayed up to 25 min after injection (see below).

5. Waveform progression should be evaluated in a step-like fashion. Thus, the first few waveforms should demonstrate the effects of smooth muscle relaxation with elevating velocities (particularly diastolic velocity); if this does not occur, further PGE1 should be given. Once adequate smooth muscle relaxation has been ensured, the PSV should be followed. After PSV has reached its maximum, and if it is within the normal range for a sustained period (>5 min), the waveforms should be studied for evidence of rising intracavernosal pressure (narrowing of the upstroke of the waveform, development of a dicrotic notch and gradual reduction of the end-diastolic velocity). After the minimal diastolic velocity has been reached, the examination can be considered complete.

adequate study (i.e. one where the operator can be confident of having recorded all phases of the erectile cascade) are given in Table 19.1. Diagnostic details of temporal systolic and diastolic velocity profiles, with waveform changes, are also given, as well as what constitutes a normal study.

THE NORMAL AND ABNORMAL PENILE DOPPLER STUDY

There are no published large studies of true normals (i.e. potent volunteers) encompassing the entire adult age range to allow the incontestable definition of the normal cavernosal artery velocity range, and this type of study is unlikely to be conducted with injectable pharmacostimulants. Those small studies available (the most thorough studied only seven subjects)[25] report a wide range of peak systolic velocities (PSVs)[2,5,25] from 19 cm/s upwards. The largest study (of 44 volunteers) used a low dose of pharmacostimulation; the age of volunteers, who had been selected from a hospital urology clinic, was relatively high; and a fixed 15 min study protocol was used; however, a mean PSV of 44 cm/s (range 19–120 cm/s) was reported.[26] Incidentally, this paucity of true normal data also applies to some other aspects of evaluation of impotence, such as angiography (see below).

To determine the normal velocity range, data must be inspected on patients with psychogenic or neurogenic impotence who developed a full erection after pharmacostimulation,[4,6] as it is a reasonable assumption that full erection can occur only with a competent haemodynamic circuit. Figure 19.9 documents the range of normality defined in the authors' practice, after papaverine or PGE1. These curves demonstrate the striking temporal variation in both systolic and diastolic velocities and underline the importance of prolonged sampling and waveform correlation.

Two further points are worthy of discussion on the subject of normal ranges. First, like other aspects of human physiology (e.g. systemic blood pressure), a sharp cutoff point between the normal and abnormal cavernosal velocity cannot be expected; rather, there will always be an intermediate zone or an overlap between the two groups. Similarly, the choice of cutoff or threshold values for any test also has a grey area and the operator has to trade off sensitivity against the specificity demanded from the test. These two points may explain some of the variation in reported literature over threshold values. A

further source of conflict in the published literature is discrepancy in technique, particularly sampling frequency and different machines and probes. It is, perhaps, advisable for each interested group to develop their own normal values and range, according to local circumstances and equipment.

The authors' results from normal responders to pharmacostimulation have led them to a definition of normal velocities as being more than 35 cm/s for PSV and less than 5 cm/s for EDV, sustained over a period of more than 5 minutes. Transient values within the normal range should be ignored. Abnormal values are PSV less than 25 cm/s and EDV more than 7 cm/s. Values in between (PSV 25–35 cm/s and EDV 5–7 cm/s) are considered by the authors to be an intermediate zone (Fig. 19.9). This formulation is a recognition of the limitations of the test outlined above and the dangers that lie in rigid diagnostic categorization. In the authors' experience, up to 20% of all patients studied will fall within the intermediate zone with papaverine as stimulant; this figure, in the authors' opinion, is lower with PGE1. Patients in this intermediate group require further evaluation. It is difficult at the moment to say what form further diagnostic workup should follow. One policy is to try repeat stimulation in privacy at home, perhaps at a higher dose. This will help to separate those with anxiety-induced pharmaco-antagonism from those with mild venous leakage or mild arteriogenic impotence. This is to be preferred to subjecting all these patients to cavernosometry, or arteriography. The authors have insufficient personal experience with repeating Doppler studies in this group and, indeed, at the moment there are very few published data on the reproducibility of the penile Doppler study. Other waveform measurements have also been used in diagnosis, especially resistivity index. As stated earlier, the authors do not use any routinely but their relative values are given in Figure 19.9 for completeness.

VALIDITY OF THE PENILE DOPPLER STUDY

As argued above, the PDS is based on existing, well-grounded understanding of Doppler physics and the prevailing haemodynamic model of penile erection. In practice, however, the test does not perform as well as the model would predict. This is partly accountable by the

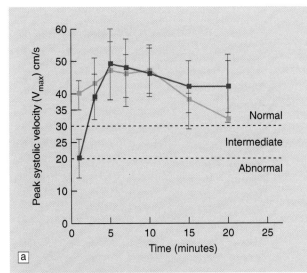

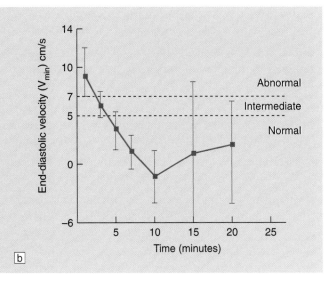

Waveform assessment	Normal range
Pulsatility index	>300
Resistivity index	>0.80
Systolic rise time (ΔT)	<0.1s
Cavernosal artery diameter	0.2–1.0 mm, with >50% diameter increase post stimulation
Acceleration index	>400

Figure 19.9. Normal systolic (a) and diastolic (b) time–velocity curves using papaverine (▨) or prostaglandin E1 (■) as sinusoidal muscle relaxant (diastolic curves shown post-papaverine alone). Values are means with 95% confidence intervals from men who developed a full erection after an appropriate dose of either drug. The dose varied between patients (40–80 mg papaverine or 10–20 μg prostaglandin E1). The graphs also incorporate the normal and abnormal range as used in the authors' practice; note the intermediate range where firm diagnostic characterization is unreliable. (c) tabulates the normal ranges reported for a variety of waveform and morphological measurements. The authors do not use these measurements routinely.

expected centre-to-centre and person-to-person variability in any test performance. Put another way, the enthusiast and the specialist centre will always perform better. A separate factor, as emphasized above, is the natural variability of human physiology. The haemodynamic model may also be incomplete. But once these factors are accounted for, how firmly validated is the PDS?

This is difficult to answer categorically, as ideally, validity can be established only by careful patient follow-up and the response to specific treatment, or, in its absence, by correlation with other investigations: this highlights some core difficulties, e.g. the lack of predictably successful treatments for arterial or venous disease (except for intracavernosal agents) and the absence of solid standard reference investigations for comparison. Venous ligation and ablation has had poor long-term results and arterial reconstruction is not yet feasible. The comparative tests that are available are unsatisfactory for a variety of reasons.

Patients with full response to pharmacostimulation are presumed to have a psychogenic or neurogenic impotence with a competent sinusoidal, arterial and venous system, but external confirmation of psychogenic or neurogenic defects is not easy.[24] Psychogenic impotence is a subjective diagnosis based on clinical assessment and psychometric questionnaire analysis. It is usually backed up by nocturnal penile tumescence and rigidity testing, which can be cumbersome;[27] furthermore, it has been suggested that the nocturnal erection may differ from the sexual erection, while tests for neurogenic impotence have not yet been standardized.[24,28] With venous leakage, diagnostic characterization is more secure, in that there is a relatively robust reference standard investigation in use (pharmacocavernosometry). Experimental results of pharmacocavernosometry concur with the haemo-dynamics predicted by the penile erection model. Although there are still some unresolved technical disagreements about its method and interpretation, pharmacocavernosometry can be used to validate the diagnostic accuracy of venous leakage on PDS.[29] However, it is with arteriogenic impotence that relative comparisons are most difficult: there is, at the time of writing, no satisfactory, readily available reference investigation. Searching for risk factors for arteriopathy, although of clinical value, cannot be sufficiently thorough to be reliable in the individual patient. Arteriography has been widely advocated and accepted as a reference diagnostic test for arteriogenic impotence; this is unsatisfactory, for several reasons, as follows.

Penile arteriography continues to be one of the most technically demanding aspects of peripheral vascular radiology; indeed, one of its chief exponents termed it the 'last frontier of arteriography'.[30] 'Normal' variations in penile arterial anatomy are so common that they defy definition of normality.[31] Super-selective catheterization of the internal pudendal artery can be time consuming and difficult, particularly in the presence of catheter-related spasm. When selective catheterization is achieved, the study represents (even with maximal pharmacological stimulation, given as an intracavernosal injection) only a snapshot image in time of a rapidly evolving haemodynamic cascade. Because this is a static investigation, information about physiological status has to be extrapolated from the arterial morphology, chiefly the cavernosal artery diameter. The angiogram should, therefore, be timed to coincide with the phase of maximal cavernosal artery distension; unfortunately, in a given patient it is impossible to be certain that the study was recorded at the moment of maximal response. This is important, as the 'normal' cavernosal arteriogram is defined as showing a smooth cavernosal artery in its entirety, with sufficient helicine branches. As for direct size measurements, it has to be remembered that the cavernosal artery is between 0.2 and 1 mm in diameter at rest, and undergoes only up to an 80% increase in diameter size with maximum distension. At this level (1–1.5 mm), the most modern digital subtraction vascular imaging equipment, indispensable for the contrast resolution and magnification necessary for cavernosal arteriography, will have an error margin of 20–30% in spatial resolution as well as the inevitable human errors in the placement of the computer-generated measurement callipers. These uncontrollable sources of technical error should be remembered when reviewing articles claiming to categorize 50% or even 80% cavernosal artery stenosis accurately.[32] Some of the other described signs of cavernosal arterial disease are also disputable: for instance, does the non-visualization of helicine branches necessarily mean that the artery is functionally incompetent?

That is not to say that arteriography does not have a role. In the diagnosis of proximal arterial disease, for instance in the young man after pelvic trauma or with the pelvic steal syndrome, it has a secure diagnostic role. However, with the more common distal or small artery disease, as the above arguments show, it cannot serve as a firm diagnostic or reference investigation to compare against the PDS.

■ CONCLUSIONS

To summarize, the achievement of a full erection with PGE1 and dynamic pharmacocavernosometry are the only two readily available comparative tests to validate the PDS. Using the former, a receiver–operating-characteristic (ROC) curve can be generated for various 'normal' PSVs for identification of an intact haemodynamic circuit (Fig. 19.10a). The validity of the PDS in diagnosis of venous leakage can be established by reference to cavernosometry findings; Figure 19.10b is a similar ROC curve for the sensitivity and specificity values at various threshold values of diastolic velocity. Note that this exercise serves to diagnose positively those men with an intact haemodynamic circuit and those men with normal inflow but defective venous occlusion, leaving a third group who are best considered as showing deficient arterial inflow for whatever reason: they may have true organic or structural arterial disease, pharmacological resistance, receptor defects or subtle undefined defects of sinusoidal relaxation, without any inference possible about the state of their venous occlusion mechanism. This diagnostic flow path is summarized in Figure 19.11. This approach is not flawless, but in the authors' view it is the one most congruous with the current state of knowledge about penile haemodynamics. Future information will, of course, lead to modifications, particularly as understanding of the venous occlusion mechanism, cavernosal smooth muscle control and the role of the tunica albuginea advances. The current haemodynamic model may even be rendered obsolete, but it is more likely that there will be improvements in subcharacterization.

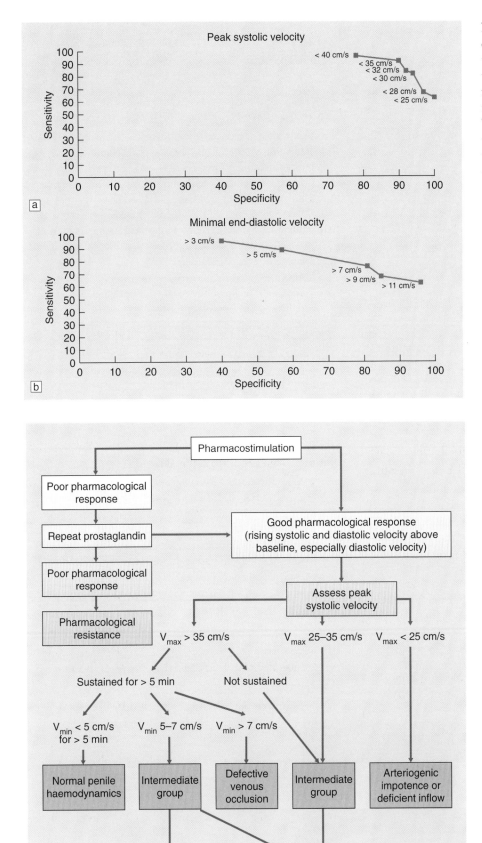

Figure 19.10. Receiver–operating characteristic (ROC) curves plotting the specificity and sensitivity values of various threshold levels for identification of normal arterial inflow and normal venous occlusion mechanism. To generate these curves, 'truth' data were established using full erection with pharmacostimulation or normal cavernosometric findings as the reference standards (see text).

Figure 19.11. A suggested practical diagnostic pathway for the penile Doppler study. For accuracy and reproducibility test conditions must be optimized (see text).

219

■ REFERENCES

1. Mueller S C, Lue T F. Evaluation of vasculogenic impotence. Urol Clin North Am 1988; 15: 65–76

2. Shabsigh R, Fishman I J, Quesada E T et al. Evaluation of vasculogenic erectile impotence with penile duplex ultrasonography. J Urol 1989; 142: 1469–1474

3. Paushter D M. Role of duplex sonography in the evaluation of sexual impotence. AJR 1989; 153: 1161–1163

4. Benson C B, Vickers M A. Sexual impotence caused by vascular disease: diagnosis with duplex sonography. AJR 1989; 153: 1149–1153

5. Merckx L A, De Bruyne R M G, Goes E et al. The value of duplex scanning in the diagnosis of venogenic impotence. J Urol 1992; 148: 318–320

6. Patel U, Amin Z, Friedman E et al. Colour flow and spectral Doppler imaging after papaverine induced erection in 220 impotent men: study of temporal patterns and the importance of repeated sampling, velocity asymmetry and vascular anomalies. Clin Radiol 1993; 48: 18–24

7. Patel U, Kirby R S, Rickards D. Impotence: the radiologist's role. Clin Radiol 1994; 49: 75–76

8. Valji K, Bookstein J J. Diagnosis of arteriogenic impotence: efficacy of duplex sonography as a screening tool. AJR 1993; 160: 65–69

9. Valji K. What is the radiologist's current role in the diagnosis and treatment of sexual impotence in men? AJR 1994; 163: 217

10. Kropman R F, Schipper J, van Oostayen J A et al. The value of increased end diastolic velocity during penile duplex sonography in relation to pathological venous leakage in erectile dysfunction. J Urol 1992; 148: 314–317

11. Allen R P, Engel R M, Smolev J K, Brendler C B. Comparison of duplex ultrasonography and nocturnal penile tumescence in evaluation of impotence. J Urol 1994; 151: 1525–1529

12. Bahren W, Gall H, Scherb W et al. Pharmacoarteriography in chronic erectile dysfunction. In: Jonas W, Thon W F, Stief C G (eds) Erectile dysfunction. Berlin: Springer-Verlag, 1991: 137–161

13. Aboseif S R, Lue T F. Haemodynamics of penile erection. Urol Clin North Am 1988; 15: 1–7

14. Lerner S E, Melman A, Christ G J. A review of erectile dysfunction: new insights and more questions. J Urol 1993; 149: 1246–1255

15. Zagzebski J A. Physics and instrumentation in Doppler and B mode ultrasonography. In: Zweibel W J (ed) Introduction to vascular ultrasonography. Philadelphia: Saunders, 1992: 19–44

16. Zweibel W J. Spectrum analysis in vascular diagnosis. In: Zweibel W J (ed) Introduction to vascular ultrasonography. Philadelphia: Saunders, 1992: 45–65

17. Patel U, Lees W R. Penile sonography. In: Solbiati L, Rizzato G (eds) Ultrasound of superficial structures. Edinburgh: Churchill Livingstone, 1995: 229–242

18. Liu L C, Wu C C, Chiang C P et al. Comparison of the effects of papaverine versus prostaglandin E_1 on penile blood flow by colour duplex sonography. Eur Urol 1991; 19: 49–53

19. Meuleman E J, Bemelmans B L, Doesberg W H et al. Penile pharmacological duplex ultrasonography : a dose–effect study comparing papaverine, papaverine/phentolamine and prostaglandin E_1. J Urol 1992; 148: 63–66

20. Gerber G S, Levine L A. Pharmacological erection program using prostaglandin E_1. J Urol 1991; 146: 786

21. Montorsi F, Guazzoni G, Barbieri L et al. The effect of intracorporeal injection plus genital and audiovisual sexual stimulation versus second injection on penile color Doppler sonography parameters. J Urol 1996; 155: 536–540

22. Katlowitz N M, Albano G J, Morales P, Golimbu M. Potentiation of drug-induced erection with audiovisual sexual stimulation. Urology 1993; 41: 431–434

23. Donatucci C F, Lue T F. The combined intracavernous injection and stimulation test: diagnostic accuracy. J Urol 1992; 148: 61–62

24. Steers W D. Editorial: Impotence evaluation. J Urol 1993; 149: 1284

25. Schwartz A N, Wang K Y, Mack L A. Evaluation of normal erectile function with color Doppler sonography. AJR 1989; 153: 1155

26. Meuleman E J H, Bemelmans B L, van Austen W N J L et al. Assessment of penile blood flow by duplex ultrasonography in 44 men with normal erectile potency in different phases of erection. J Urol 1992; 147: 51–56

27. Karachan I. Sleep environment crucial in NPT assessment. Urology 1988; 30: 416–419

28. Merckx L A, de Bruyne R M, Keuppers F I. Electromyography of cavernous smooth muscle during flaccidity: evaluation of technique and normal values. Br J Urol 1993; 72: 353–358

29. Wespes E, Schulman C. Venous impotence: pathophysiology, diagnosis and treatment. J Urol 1993; 149: 1238–1245

30. Bookstein J J. Penile angiography: the last angiographic frontier. AJR 1988; 150: 47–54

31. Bookstein J J, Lang E V. Penile magnification arteriography: details of intrapenile arterial anatomy. AJR 1987; 148: 883–888

32. Rosen M P, Greenfield A J, Walker T G et al. Arteriographic impotence: findings in 195 impotent men examined with selective internal pudendal angiography. Radiology 1990; 174: 1043–1048

Chapter 20

Radionuclide imaging in the diagnosis of vasculogenic impotence

J. A. Vale

■ INTRODUCTION

With the realization that as many as 50% of cases of erectile dysfunction may have a vasculogenic basis,[1] a number of tests have been introduced to try to measure penile blood flow. Some (such as the penile brachial index) have already fallen into disrepute, whereas others have become increasingly widely accepted without much prior validation. Colour Doppler imaging (CDI) is in common use, yet is highly observer dependent and does not correlate well with arteriography;[2] in addition, recently there have been questions about its interpretation.[3] Of course, one of the problems is that the so-called 'gold standard' arteriography is itself flawed in that it is anatomical and gives no information about perfusion.

Isotope techniques for assessing tissue perfusion were first introduced in the 1960s, and would seem to provide an ideal method for assessing penile blood flow. They are relatively non-invasive, involve less radiation dose than arteriography or cavernosography and do not require a great deal of operator skill; however they have not received wide acceptance. This chapter reviews the reasons for this, the current state-of-the-art techniques, and the reasons why we should perhaps consider using these techniques more.

■ HISTORICAL PERSPECTIVE

Radionuclide techniques for the assessment of the penile circulation have been adapted from limb-perfusion studies. The first of these was the Xenon washout technique developed in the 1960s. This involved the injection of Xenon-133 into a muscle, and subsequent scintigraphy.[4] Xenon is so lipid soluble that it rapidly equilibrated between the extravascular and intravascular compartments and its clearance from the limb reflected blood flow. It relied on the fact that the limb has a constant volume and arterial inflow equals venous outflow. Although this technique has been applied to the penis using Xenon injected into the corpora cavernosa or subcutaneously,[5,6] these basic assumptions do not apply to the penis: it does not have a fixed volume, and arterial inflow does not equal venous outflow during tumescence or detumescence. Xenon washout techniques will actually reflect venous outflow, not arterial blood supply; indeed, they have been used for this purpose.[7,8] However, these studies were limited by lack of effective pharmacostimulation, and although one study[7] suggested that flaccid state washout is diagnostically helpful, this has not been corroborated by other workers[8] and certainly is inconsistent with our basic understanding of penile vascular physiology.

The second isotopic approach that has been used to measure limb blood flow is the technique of blood-pool labelling. The original description relied upon intravenous ^{99m}Tc-labelled human serum albumin, and the shape of the time–activity curve was recorded as tracer reached the limb extremity — the so-called first-pass effect.[9] However, this did not produce an absolute measure of blood flow, and various modifications were made subsequently to facilitate this goal, the most important of which was isolation of the limb circulation until the tracer had equilibrated throughout the intravascular compartment.[10] In this situation, when the tourniquet is released and the limb is scanned using a scintigraph there are three phases of perfusion (Fig. 20.1). Initially, there is a linear increase in radioactivity as labelled blood flows rapidly into the limb; this is phase 1

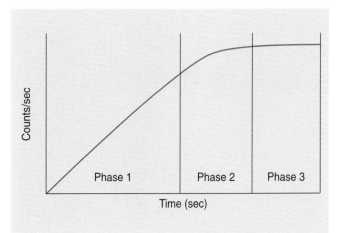

Figure 20.1. Blood-pool labelling technique with isolation of the circulation: phases of scintigraphic activity following tourniquet release. Phase 1 (initial) corresponds to initial uptake and reflects blood flow. Phase 2 (exponential) occurs as labelled blood mixes with unlabelled blood and starts to drain away from the limb in venous channels. Phase 3 (equilibrium) develops when inflow of isotope equals outflow. Any further change will be a decline according to the half-life of the isotope.

and is independent of venous drainage. After a short time, the labelled blood entering the limb mixes with unlabelled blood and starts to reach the veins. There is a progressive decline in the rate of isotope uptake as some activity starts to 'leak' back into the general circulation; this is phase 2 or the exponential phase of the curve. Phase 3 (equilibrium) occurs when there has been complete mixing of the labelled and unlabelled blood, and thus isotopic activity flowing in is the same as that flowing out and any subsequent decline will reflect the half-life of the isotope. The product of the gradient of the initial phase of the curve and blood-pool activity provides an absolute measure of limb blood flow.

Blood-pool labelling techniques have been applied to the penis, but once again the earlier studies were hampered by the complicating factor of volume change during an erection. These early studies did not use a cuff to isolate the penile circulation at the time of isotope injection, and peak scintigraphic activity after stimulation was measured and compared with activity before stimulation.[11,12] Peak activity will reflect the volume of the penis rather than perfusion, assuming that the isotope is fully equilibrated in the bloodstream, and studies using this endpoint actually measured change in penile volume rather than blood flow. These early studies were also hampered by the absence of a reliable

vasodilator to stimulate blood flow changes normally associated with an erection, and relied on visual sexual stimulation[11,13] or intravenous isoxsuprine.[12]

Blood-pool techniques using the isolated circulation[10] and maximal stimulation with prostaglandin E1 or papaverine should be the ideal means of measuring penile blood flow. The cuff ensures that labelled blood only enters the penis as a bolus, displacing unlabelled blood. The influences of changes in venous flow and change in volume are therefore removed, and the rate of uptake of isotope (phase 1) should reflect penile perfusion. There have been relatively few results described using this technique, but it is now in routine clinical usage in the author's institution.

METHOD OF PENILE BLOOD FLOW ESTIMATION USING BLOOD-POOL LABELLING AND ISOLATION OF THE PENILE CIRCULATION

At the outset, the flaccid penile volume is estimated by measuring length and girth, and calculating volume on the basis that the penis is a cylinder; this information is necessary only to allow a blood-flow value to be derived per unit volume of tissue. In the original description by Grech and colleagues,[14] blood-pool labelling was performed with initial pretreatment in vivo with stannous medronate to sensitize the red blood cells. The isotope ^{99m}Tc (925 MBq) was administered intravenously 30 minutes later, after inflation of a 19 mm cuff around the base of the penis to a pressure above systolic. Intracavernosal vasodilator was injected at this stage (papaverine 60 mg or papaverine 40 mg with 1 mg phentolamine or prostaglandin E1) and the cuff was kept inflated for a further 10 minutes to allow maximal cavernosal smooth muscle relaxation/arteriolar dilatation to develop. The cuff was then released and a venous blood sample was taken to assess blood-pool activity.

The whole event can be recorded on a gamma camera, and scintigraphy continued until 3 minutes after release of the cuff (Fig. 20.2). Count rates are plotted against time and the computer applies a 'best fit' line through the initial uptake phase (phase 1) — this should approximate to a straight line. Penile blood flow (F) is calculated using the formula: F (ml/s/100 ml tissue) = G/C x 100/V, where G is the initial portion of the curve in counts/s/s, C is blood-pool activity in counts/s/ml, and V is penile volume in ml.

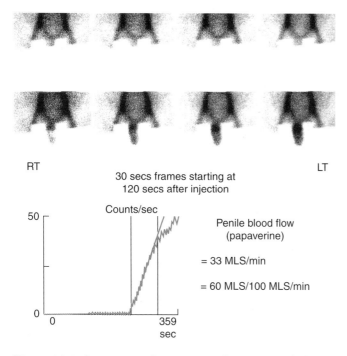

RT   LT

30 secs frames starting at
120 secs after injection

Counts/sec

Penile blood flow
(papaverine)

= 33 MLS/min

= 60 MLS/100 MLS/min

Figure 20.2. Scintigram of a patient undergoing penile blood flow estimation after injection of papaverine (60 mg), using an isolated penile circulation/labelled blood-pool method. The first of the two vertical lines corresponds to tourniquet release; the second to the end of phase 1. The gradient G is computed from the segment of curve between these lines.

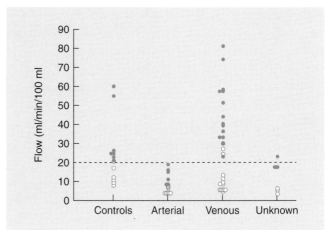

Figure 20.3. Correlation of penile blood flow as determined by the blood-pool technique with presumed diagnosis. This shows a good correlation using a cutoff value of 20 ml/min/100 ml tissue in the stimulated state (○, without papaverine; ●, with papaverine). Flaccid blood flow was of no diagnostic value. (From ref. 14 with permission.)

Using this type of technique, Grech and colleagues[14] were able to separate those patients with presumed arteriogenic impotence from those without, using a cutoff of 20 ml/min/100 ml (Fig. 20.3). Unfortunately, no attempt was made to correlate this technique with arteriographic findings, as it is hard to justify selective pudendal arteriography if reconstructive surgery is not contemplated. The group of patients with a poor papaverine response but normal arterial flow were presumed to have venous insufficiency, and there was an excellent correlation with cavernosography. This suggests that dual isotope techniques[15] (labelled red cells to measure arterial inflow and Xenon washout to assess venous outflow) are probably unnecessary.

One of the problems, when introducing any new technique for the evaluation of penile blood flow, remains the need to correlate it with the 'gold standard', yet the latter is really a Holy Grail. Selective arteriography is not indicated unless surgery is under consideration — seldom the case — and in addition it is an anatomical, not a functional, means of assessment. CDI has been widely adopted as a means of diagnosing arteriogenic impotence yet, once again, there has been little attempt at

validation. In view of this, the author and colleagues compared the results of isotope penile blood flow determination and CDI in a group of patients presenting with erectile failure.[16] Each patient underwent both investigations at least 1 week apart, using the same intracavernosal stimulation, and thus each served as his own control. Colour Doppler scanning was performed by a single operator using a 7.5 MHz linear-array probe (Hewlett-Packard Sonos, USA), and flow velocity measurements were taken from both right and left cavernosal arteries 5–10 minutes and 20–30 minutes after intracavernosal injection. Penile blood flow was determined isotopically using a technique similar to that described by Grech and colleagues,[14] except that ^{99m}Tc-labelled human serum albumin (800 MBq) was used instead of labelled red blood cells; labelled albumin is simpler to use and equally good as it remains in the intravascular compartment. There was no correlation between blood flow velocity determined on CDI (cutoff V_{max} 30cm/s) and blood flow as measured by the isotopic technique, and the latter correlated better with response to papaverine, taking a cutoff of 20 ml/min/100 ml tissue.

■ WHY HAVE RADIONUCLIDE TECHNIQUES BEEN FORGOTTEN?

Despite encouraging results from recent studies,[14,16] isotope techniques for estimating penile blood flow have assumed little general acceptance. The reasons for this are multiple and include the fact that many of the early approaches — such as the xenon washout study — were fundamentally flawed and claims made about them were clearly incorrect. Secondly, CDI has been developed over the same time-scale and rapidly adopted in many units, as it is easy to perform and its ability to generate numbers has fostered a belief that it is in some way objective. However, there has been little effort to compare CDI with the results of arteriography and, when this has been achieved, the results have often been disappointing.[2] CDI has also come under scrutiny for other reasons. Thus, V_{max} is a measure of the speed with which blood flows within a vessel. It is not a measure of blood flow or perfusion and, alone, is an inadequate discriminant of arterial disease;[3] it may be artefactually high in calcified vessels which fail to dilate in response to demand and are poor sources of perfusion. It is highly variable when measured in men with normal erectile function,[17] and correlates poorly with the results of nocturnal penile tumescence monitoring.[18] Finally, it looks only at small distal vessels, which is inconsistent with vascular assessment elsewhere in the arterial tree: to assess claudicants it is normal practice to look at the proximal arterial tree, not to measure flow velocity in the digital arteries. In this regard, radionuclide studies are anatomy independent.

■ CONCLUSIONS

Modern isotope techniques using blood-pool labelling and isolation of the penile circulation are an objective means of measuring penile blood flow in the excited state after injection of an intracavernosal vasodilator. Although the methods require some initial calibration and effort to establish, they are quick and simple to carry out and there is no opportunity for observer bias. This represents a significant advantage over some of the other available techniques, and perhaps the most logical investigative algorithm for vasculogenic impotence would be isotope assessment of perfusion, followed by selective arteriography to evaluate the anatomy if surgical revascularization is under consideration.

■ REFERENCES

1. Virag R, Bouilly P, Frydman D. Is impotence an arterial disorder? Lancet 1985; i: 181–184
2. Rajfer J, Canan V, Dorey F J, Mehringer C M. Correlation between penile angiography and duplex scanning of cavernous arteries in impotent men. J Urol 1990; 143: 1128–1130
3. Oates C P, Pickard R S, Powell P H et al. The use of ultrasound in the assessment of arterial supply to the penis in vasculogenic impotence. J Urol 1995; 153: 354–357
4. Lassen N A, Lindbjerg J, Munck O. Measurement of blood flow through skeletal muscle by intramuscular injection of xenon-133. Lancet 1964; i: 686–688
5. Nseyo U O, Wilbur H J, Kang S A et al. Penile xenon (^{133}Xe) washout: a rapid method of screening for vasculogenic impotence. Urology 1984; 23: 31–34
6. Lin S N, Liu R S, Yu P C et al. Diagnosis of vasculogenic impotence: combination of penile xenon-133 washout and papaverine tests. Urology 1989; 34: 28–32
7. Yeh S H, Liu R S, Lin S N et al. Corporeal Xe-133 washout for detecting venous leakage. J Nucl Med 1987; 28: 650 (abstr 388)
8. Haden H T, Katz P G, Mulligan T, Zasler N D. Penile blood flow by xenon-133 washout. J Nucl Med 1989; 30: 1032–1035
9. Oshima M, Ijima H, Kohda Y et al. Peripheral arterial disease diagnosed with high-count-rate radionuclide arteriography. Radiology 1984; 152: 161–166
10. Parkin A, Robinson P J, Wiggins P A et al. The measurement of limb blood flow using technetium-labelled red blood cells. Br J Radiol 1986; 59: 493–497
11. Shirai M, Nakamura M, Ishii N et al. Determination of intrapenile blood volume using ^{99m}Tc-labelled autologous red blood cells. Tohoku J Exp Med 1976; 120: 377–383
12. Fanous H N, Jevtich M J, Chen D C P, Edson M. Radioisotope penogram in diagnosis of vasculogenic impotence. Urology 1982; 20: 499–502
13. Shirai M, Nakamura M. Diagnostic discrimination between organic and functional impotence by radioisotope penogram with ^{99m}TcO$_4^-$. Tohoku J Exp Med 1975; 116: 9–15
14. Grech P, Dave S, Cunningham D A, Witherow R O'N. Combined papaverine test and radionuclide penile blood flow in impotence: method and preliminary results. Br J Urol 1992; 69: 408–417
15. Kursh E D, Jones W T, Thompson S et al. A dynamic dual isotope radionuclide method of quantifying penile blood flow. J Urol 1992; 147: 1524–1529
16. Glass J M, Vale J A, Belcaro G et al. A comparison of isotope penile blood flow and colour Doppler ultrasonography in the assessment of erectile dysfunction. Br J Urol 1996; 77: 566–570
17. Meuelman E J H, Bemelmans B H L, van Asten W N J C et al. Assessment of penile blood flow by duplex ultrasonography in 44 men with normal erectile potency in different phases of erection. J Urol 1992; 147: 51–56
18. Allen R P, Engel R M E, Smolev J K, Brendler C B. Comparison of duplex ultrasonography and nocturnal penile tumescence in evaluation of impotence. J Urol 1994; 151: 1525–1529

Chapter 21
Radiological diagnosis of venous leakage

J. Richenberg and D. Rickards

■ INTRODUCTION

Erectile dysfunction is a complex pathophysiological process, consequent upon several interrelated causes. Incompetence of the penile venous system is a cause that can be rectified by surgery.[1]

Penile tumescence relies on venous occlusion, a keystone in the initiation and maintenance of erection. The venous occlusion is brought about passively, the emissary veins being compressed between the fibrous tunica albuginea and the engorging corpus cavernosum. The pressure in the corpora cavernosa increases when neuroendocrine-mediated arteriolar smooth muscle relaxation leads to a dramatic rise in cavernosal artery inflow. A positive feedback loop ensues, with rising cavernosal pressure causing further venous compression leading, in turn, to progressive cavernosal engorgement and the storage phase of penile erection is achieved (Fig. 21.1).[2,3]

The veno-occlusive mechanism may fail[4] for the following reasons:

1. Inability to initiate a rise in cavernosal pressure — arterial or neurogenic factors.
2. Structural abnormalities (in the tunica albuginea) e.g. Peyronie's disease or trauma.[5–7]
3. Venous incompetence: non-occluded veins or fistulae.
4. A combination of factors, often arterial and venous abnormalities, for instance, coexisting.

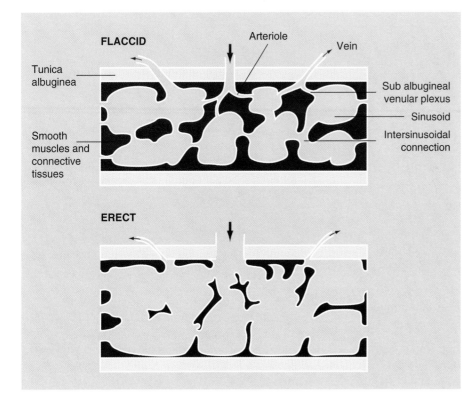

Figure 21.1. Schematic drawing of the corpora in the flaccid and erect states, demonstrating how the veins are obstructed in the erect state by the tunica albuginea.

The incidence of pure veno-occlusive disease amongst patients with organic erectile dysfunction is quoted as between 20 and 30%, and combined arterial and venous abnormalities may be seen in up to 60% of cases.[4,7]

■ INDICATIONS

The history may well suggest veno-occlusive disease as the cause of impotence, especially in younger patients, in whom arterial disease is rare. The most common presentation is with secondary impotence, progressing over several years, with inability to sustain an erection, and rapid detumescence prior to ejaculation. 'Spike' erections recorded during nocturnal tumescence studies point to a venous abnormality. Before radiological investigation, patients should be screened:[8] only those who fail to achieve a satisfactory erection after intracavernosal injection of a suitable pharmacological agent on two occasions should be investigated. Failure to induce any tumescence after intracavernosal smooth muscle relaxants is highly suggestive of veno-occlusive dysfunction.[1,9] Those patients who have previously undergone venous ligation surgery, but in whom impotence persists, also warrant investigation.

■ COLOUR/POWER DOPPLER ULTRASOUND

In all patients being considered for venous leak studies, documentary proof that the arterial aspect is normal should be obtained. This is achieved radiologically by ultrasound: 20 μg prostaglandin E1 is injected into the proximal corpus cavernosum using a 23 gauge needle, and the Doppler probe (linear array 7–10 MHz) is placed on the ventral surface at the base of the penis; this permits interrogation of both the arterial and venous systems.[10,11] Assuming a normal arterial peak systolic velocity (> 30 cm/s), veno-occlusive disease can be inferred if there is persistent forward diastolic flow in the presence of normal arterial inflow (Fig. 21.2). The exact threshold for peak diastolic flow, above which venous leak is diagnosed, is not universally accepted. Studies on patients who have received pharmacological stimulation and then have undergone penile Doppler and cavernosometry have generated receiver–operating-characteristic (ROC) curves for the sensitivity and specificity for various peak diastolic thresholds (Fig.

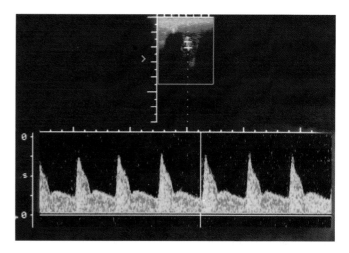

Figure 21.2. Power Doppler study in a patient with impotence, showing that, at maximum tumescence for this particular patient, systolic flow was measured at 0.64 m/s (equivalent to 64 cm/s) whereas diastolic flow was 0.15 m/s (equivalent to 15 cm/s). Such criteria conform to normal arterial inflow and increased forward flow in diastole, and are strongly suggestive of a venous leak.

21.3). The data suggest that there is a significant venous leak if the peak diastolic flow is 5 cm or more.[12]

Penile Doppler studies are not 100% sensitive in the detection of significant and potentially correctable venous leak. Once arterial disease has been excluded by pharmacologically stimulated penile Doppler, cavernosometry and cavernosography are indicated to define veno-occlusive abnormalities more fully,[13] as

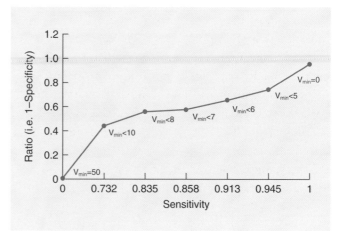

Figure 21.3. ROC curve plotted for different values of V_{min} (cm/s) derived from patients who have undergone combined penile Doppler and dynamic pharmacocavernosography after prostaglandin E1. The varying sensitivities at increasing forward flow rates in diastole in those with venous leakage can be identified.

ultrasound gives no information regarding the anatomy of the leak or which veins are involved.

DYNAMIC PHARMACO-CAVERNOSOGRAPHY (PCMG)

The early enthusiasm for cavernosometry,[14,15] and the advocacy of the use of intracavernosal vasoactive compounds,[16–18] have been justified: pharmaco-cavernosography remains the 'gold standard' in investigating penile venous leak and always involves the use of a smooth muscle relaxant.[19,20] Not only does drug-induced penile arteriolar relaxation supersede any psychological inhibition, but the drug's action mimics the physiological trigger for erection (unlike dynamic cavernosometry which induces veno-occlusion merely by passive cavernosal engorgement with infusant). In the authors' practice, any patient with normal arterial studies (by ultrasound Doppler criteria) proceeds directly to cavernosography, under the same intracavernosal pharmacological stimulant.

Technique

On the screening table, the proximal third of the penis is disinfected and two 21 gauge needles are inserted into both distal corpora cavernosa (Fig. 21.4); they are angled along the shaft so that the risk of dislodgement with erection is minimized. Confirmation that the needles are correctly sited is achieved by the injection of a small amount of contrast (Fig. 21.5). One needle is then connected to a pressure monitor (Medical Measurement Systems, Sensor Noras™ transducer pressure domes); the transducer is levelled to the height of the needle tip, allowing initial intracavernosal pressure measurement. The other is connected, via a variable-rate pump, to radiographic contrast medium (Omnipaque 140™) (Fig. 21.6). Modern urodynamic systems usually have a programme within them for PCMG studies. The initial rate of infusion is 10 ml/min and this is gradually increased to 100 ml/min until a steady-state intracavernosal pressure of 100 mmHg is achieved ($\approx$ 136 cmH$_2$O). The infusion is slowed automatically until the rate required to maintain an intracavernosal pressure of 100 mmHg is found; this is the maintenance flow rate. Once this has been measured, the pump stops, the rate of intracavernosal pressure decline is measured and the pressure 30 s later is recorded. During this process, visual inspection and

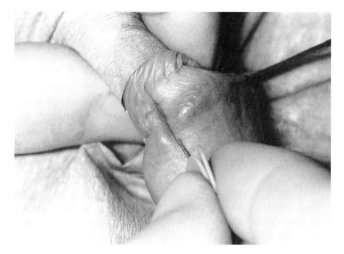

Figure 21.4. For PCMG, the foreskin (if present) is retracted and two 21 gauge butterfly needles are inserted into the distal corpora and angled along the shaft of the corpora.

subjective assessment of the erection are noted. Intermittent screening confirms free communication between the two corpora. Spot films are exposed to demonstrate the anatomy of the corpora and of the draining veins, if appropriate.

The diagnostic accuracy of PCMG relies on measurement of several parameters during cavernosography. These are the flow rate required to induce erection, the flow rate to maintain erection, the rate of intracavernosal pressure drop (on cessation of infusion) and the intracavernosal pressure 30 s after cessation.[21] Reliance on a single parameter can lead to misdiagnosis.[22]

Once the procedure has been completed, the needles are disconnected from the contrast medium and pressure transducer and, where the patient did achieve tumescence, drainage from the needles is allowed until near-full detumescence has been achieved. Aspiration with a 50 ml syringe will accelerate the process. The needles are then removed, a pressure bandage is applied to the distal penis and the patient is warned that bruising is likely to occur. The complication of priapism is explained to the patient.

Interpretation

A representative range of maintenance rates after papaverine injection have been recorded as 59 ml/min in patients with venous leakage, 14.6 ml/min in impotent patients without venous leakage and 14.1 ml/min in a control group.[23] Maintenance flow rates of 30 ml/min or more, and a fall in intracavernosal pressure of more than 40 mmHg (after achieving full erection) within 30 s of the infusion being stopped, are taken as signs of veno-

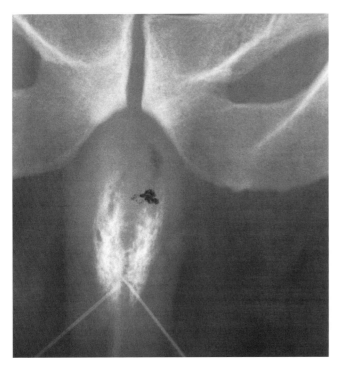

Figure 21.5. To confirm that the needles are correctly sited, a small test injection of contrast is given. Both corpora can be seen to be partially filled with contrast. This injection should be painless; any discomfort experienced by the patient should arouse suspicion of incorrect placement.

Table 21.1. Diagnostic criteria (maintenance flow rates in ml/s following prostaglandin E1) for a venous leak

Effect on erection	Diagnosis		
	Psychogenic	Organic	Venous leak
Induce	30–40	20–65	50–120
Maintain	0–5	5–10	25–40

occlusive disease.[24] The diagnostic criteria for venous leakage are summarized in Table 21.1.

The concept of dysfunction rather than frank veno-occlusive disease has been raised by Vickers and colleagues.[25] They propose that the widely accepted thresholds are too stringent, having studied men with non-organic erectile dysfunction which spontaneously resolved (without any therapeutic intervention). All six patients had maintenance rates of more than 5 ml/min; five had initial decompression rates of more than 48 mmHg within 30 seconds, and four had 5 minute postinfusion steady-state values of less than 50 mmHg — criteria that have been used to define corporovenous dysfunction.

Radiological findings

Filling of the superficial and deep veins may occur during the flaccid phase in normal controls (Fig. 21.7); this disappears with induced erection, underpinning the need for intracavernous prostaglandin injection (Fig. 21.8). However, even after intracavernosal injection, the finding of a venous leak by cavernosography must not be considered a sine qua non diagnosis of venogenic impotence, since a certain percentage of potent men will demonstrate this radiographic finding.[26] Opacification of the glands during cavernosography (Fig. 21.9) may be a normal variant rather than a sign of pathological shunts between the glans and the corpora cavernosa.[27] In the group studied by Vickers and colleagues with veno-occlusive dysfunction, the cavernous, external pudendal and deep dorsal veins were identified during pharmaco-cavernosography, performed at pressures of 100 mmHg.[25]

The venous channels abnormally opacified in impotent males during PCMG include the deep dorsal vein in 55–100% (Fig. 21.10), proximal cavernosal and

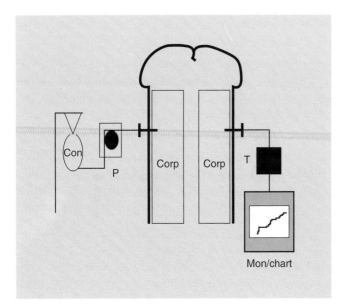

Figure 21.6. Schematic drawing of PCMG. One needle is connected via a variable-speed roller pump (P) to non-ionic contrast medium; the other is connected via a pressure transducer (T) to a pressure-recording device. Con, contrast medium; Corp, corpus cavernosum; Mon/chart, monitor and print-out.

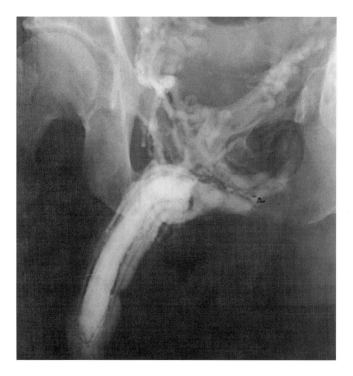

Figure 21.7. An injection of contrast has been given by a single needle in this patient in whom there is suspicion of cavernosal trauma; no prostaglandin has been given. Both corpora are outlined and a plethora of normal veins draining the corpora can be seen.

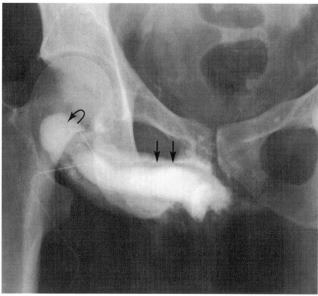

Figure 21.9. Spot film exposed in this patient with a proven venous leak. The glans penis (curved arrow) is opacified as well as the dorsal vein (straight arrows).

crural veins in 55–70% (Fig. 21.11), and corpus spongiosum in 25–30% (Fig. 21.12). Approximately 15% of studies reveal aberrant veins, which may communicate with the saphenous vein, scrotal veins or femoral vein (Fig. 21.13). Almost one-third of men with pathological cavernosal leak drain via a single

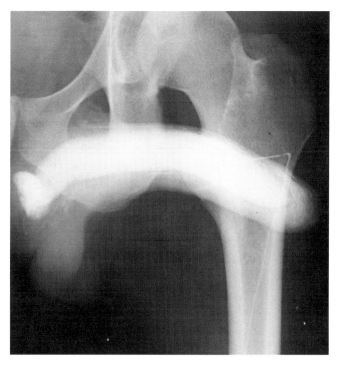

Figure 21.8. Spot film exposed in this patient who achieved full erection during PCMG. The corpora are outlined, but no draining veins can be identified.

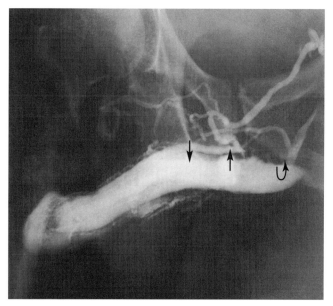

Figure 21.10. Spot film exposed in a patient with a venous leak. The deep crural veins (curved arrow), dorsal vein (straight arrows) and glans penis are opacified.

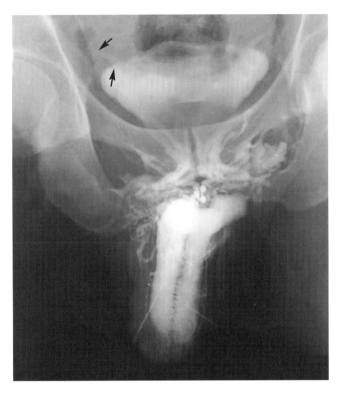

Figure 21.11. Spot film exposed in a patient with a venous leak. Numerous veins are seen at the base of the corpora. There is leak from dorsal vein, superficial and deep crural veins.

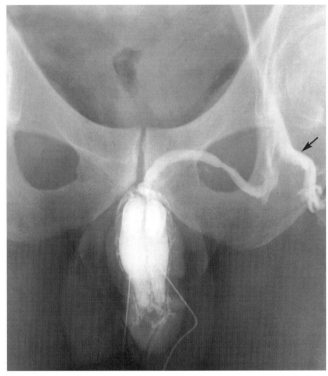

Figure 21.13. Spot film in a patient with venous leakage. The left femoral vein (arrow) is opacified.

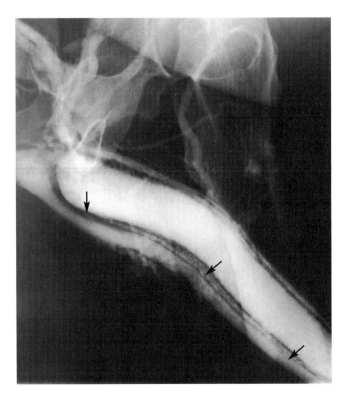

Figure 21.12. Spot film in a patient with venous leakage. There is opacification of the corpus spongiosum (arrows) and the dorsal vein.

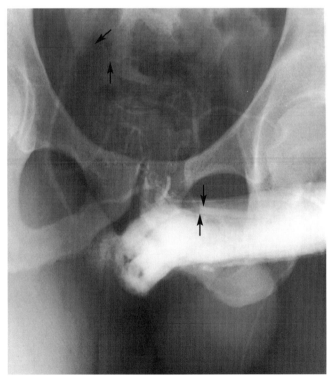

Figure 21.14. Spot film in a patient who has undergone venous leak surgery and who has recurrent symptoms. The ligated dorsal vein can be identified (arrows).

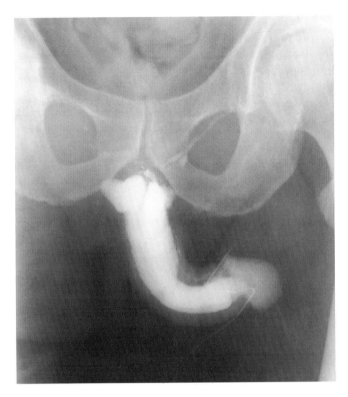

Figure 21.15. Spot film during PCMG showing chordee.

venous system; the remainder demonstrate combined venous leakage. Following venous leak surgery, the tied-off dorsal vein is usually seen, but not any of the other veins that might have been ligated (Fig. 21.14). The type of leakage does not seem to be related to either the maintenance flow or the response to intracavernosal injections.[28,29] Digital subtraction (when available) provides better definition of abnormal veins. In particular, deep crural veins are more clearly seen than in conventional studies and these may be of more importance than was previously thought.[30] Moreover, digital subtraction permits the use of shorter examination times and lower doses of contrast medium.[31]

Other radiological findings
In addition to venous leakage, chordee (Fig. 21.15), and filling defects within the corpora representing Peyronie's disease, may be seen.

■ COMPLICATIONS

Penile bruising is minimized by tight bandaging on removal of the needles. Contrast reactions are rare when non-ionic media are used, and may be anticipated by pretreatment with oral steroids in those deemed at high risk. Priapism can be expected in 10–15% of those undergoing PCMG.[31] Conventional treatment by aspiration puncture of the cavernous body is often successful, and can be safely combined with intracavernosal injection of an alpha-adrenergic agent (pharmacological reversal).[32,33]

The combined ultrasound and cavernosographic protocol outlined provides ample data to stratify patients with erectile dysfunction into those with arterial disease, those with veno-occlusive disease and those with non-vasculogenic impotence. This protocol is more tolerable and rapid than some others that have been advocated,[34,35] without loss of diagnostic accuracy.

■ REFERENCES

1. Williams G, Mulcahy M J, Hartnell G, Kiely E. Diagnosis and treatment of venous leakage: a curable cause of impotence. Br J Urol 1988; 61(2): 151–155
2. Porst H, Altwein J E, Bach D, Thon W. Dynamic cavernosography: venous outflow studies of cavernous bodies. J Urol 1985; 134(2): 276–279
3. Krysiewicz S, Mellinger B C. The role of imaging in the diagnostic evaluation of impotence. AJR 1989; 153(6): 1133–1139
4. Kaufman J M, Borges F D, Fitch W P et al. Evaluation of erectile dysfunction by dynamic infusion cavernosometry and cavernosography (DICC). Multi-institutional study. Urology 1993; 41(5): 445–451
5. Jordan G H, Angermeier K W. Preoperative evaluation of erectile function with dynamic infusion cavernosometry/cavernosography in patients undergoing surgery for Peyronie's disease: correlation with postoperative results. J Urol 1993; 150(4): 1138–1142
6. Abrahamy R, Leiter E. Post-traumatic segmental corpus cavernosum fibrosis: the diagnostic value of cavernosography and the surgical correction by cavernosum–cavernosum shunt. J Urol 1980; 123(2): 289–290
7. Jantos C, Weidner W. Pharmacocavernosography in the evaluation of erectile failure. Urol Int 1988; 43(4): 225–230
8. DePalma R G, Schwab F J, Emsellem H A et al. Noninvasive assessment of impotence. Surg Clin North Am 1990; 70(1): 119–132
9. Pescatori E S, Hatzichristou D G, Namburi S, Soldstein I. A positive intracavernosal injection test implied normal veno-occlusion but not necessarily normal arterial function: a hemodynamic study. J Urol 1994; 151: 1209–1216
10. Gall H, Sparwasser C H, Stief C G et al. Diagnosis of venous incompetence in erectile dysfunction. Comparative study of cavernosography and Doppler ultrasound. Urology 1990; 35(3): 235–238

11. Hampson S J, Cowie A G, Richard D, Lees W R. Independent evaluation of impotence by colour Doppler imaging and cavernosometry. Eur Urol 1992; 21(1): 27–31

12. Quam J P, King B F, James E M et al. Duplex and colour doppler sonographic evaluation of vasculogenic impotence. AJR 1989; 153: 1141

13. Vickers M A J, Benson C B, Richie J P. High resolution ultrasonography and pulsed wave Doppler for detection of corporovenous incompetence in erectile dysfunction. J Urol 1990; 143(6): 1125–1127

14. Velcek D, Evans J A. Cavernosography. Radiology 1982; 144(4): 781–785

15. Lue T F, Hricak H, Schmidt R A, Tanagho E A. Functional evaluation of penile veins by cavernosography in papaverine-induced erection. J Urol 1986; 135(3): 479–482

16. Stief C G, Benard F, Diederichs W et al. The rationale for pharmacologic cavernosography. J Urol 1988; 140(6): 1564–1566

17. Bookstein J J, Fellmeth B, Moreland S, Lurie A L. Pharmacoangiographic assessment of the corpora cavernosa. Cardiovasc Intervent Radiol 1988; 11(4): 218–224

18. Porst H, van Ahlen H, Vahlensieck W. Relevance of dynamic cavernosography to the diagnosis of venous incompetence in erectile dysfunction. J Urol 1987; 137(6): 1163–1167

19. Stief C G, Wetterauer U, Sommerkamp M. Intraindividual comparative study of dynamic and pharmacocavernosography. Br J Urol 1989; 64: 93–97

20. Delcour C, Wespes E, Vandenbosch G et al. Impotence: evaluation with cavernosography. Radiology 1986; 161(3): 803–806

21. Rudnick J, Bödecker R, Weidner W. Significance of the intracavernosal pharmacological injection test, pharmacocavernosography, artificial erection and cavernosometry in the diagnosis of venous leakage. Urol Int 1991; 46(4): 338–343

22. Martins F E, Padma-Nathan H. Diffuse veno-occlusive dysfunction: the underlying hemodynamic abnormality resulting in failure to respond to intracavernous pharmacotherapy. J Urol 1996; 156(6): 1942–1946

23. Sargin S, Esen A, Ergen A et al. Dynamic cavernosography in the evaluation of impotence. Int Urol Nephrol 1991; 23(6): 599–604

24. Motiwala H G. Dynamic pharmacocavernosometry: a search for an ideal approach. Urol Int 1993; 51(1):1–8

25. Vickers M A J, Benson C, Dluhy R, Ball R A. The current cavernosometric criteria for corporovenous dysfunction are too strict. J Urol 1992; 147(3): 614–617

26. Fuchs A M, Mehringer C M, Raifer J. Anatomy of penile venous drainage in potent and impotent men during cavernosography. J Urol 1989; 141(6): 1353–1356

27. Delcour C, Wespes E, Vandenbosch G et al. Opacification of the glans penis during cavernosography. J Urol 1988; 139(4): 732–733

28. Shabsigh R, Fishman I J, Toombs B D, Skolkin M. Venous leaks: anatomical and physiological observations. J Urol 1991; 146(5): 1260–1265

29. Stief C G, Wetterauer U. Quantitative and qualitative analysis of dynamic cavernosographies in erectile dysfunction due to venous leakage. Urology 1989; 34(5): 252–257

30. Hassouna M, Elgammal M, Gafir S et al. Digital subtraction cavernosography: method to detect venous leakage. Urology 1991; 38(6): 577–581

31. Hartnell C G, Mulcahy M J, Kiely E A et al. Digital subtraction dynamic cavernosography. Br J Radiol 1988; 61(728): 679–682

32. Fuselier H A J, Allen J M, Annaloro A, Morgan J O. Incidence and simple management of priapism following dynamic infusion cavernosometry–cavernosography. South Med J 1993; 86(11): 1261–1263

33. Block T, Sturm W, Ernst G, Schmiedt E. The intravenous applications of alpha drugs in the treatment of priapism. World J Urol 1987; 5: 178–181.

34. Rosen M P, Schwartz A N, Levine F J, Greenfield A J. Radiologic assessment of impotence: angiography, sonography, cavernosography, and scintigraphy. AJR 1991; 157(5): 923–931

35. Chen K K, Chen M T, Lo K Y, Chang L S. Dynamic infusion cavernosometry and cavernosography (DICC) in the evaluation of vasculogenic impotence. Chung Hua I Hsueh Tsa Chih 1996; 57(4): 266–273.

Chapter 22

Non-invasive vascular imaging for erectile dysfunction

G. A. Broderick

■ INTRODUCTION: DO WE NEED IMPOTENCE TESTING?

If, when conducted by an expert, a good sexual history and physical examination have a 95% sensitivity and 50% specificity for making a diagnosis of organic erectile dysfunction, is impotence testing necessary? In the author's opinion, it is the obligation of the urologist to establish the aetiology of erectile dysfunction (end-organ vascular failure versus neurological dysfunction versus psychosexual dysfunction), to grade the severity of that dysfunction, and to select a therapy that both is acceptable to the patient and addresses his pathology.

In a prospective review, Melman compared the accuracy of making a diagnosis of organic impotence versus psychogenic impotence through initial, careful history and physical examination with diagnostic testing.[1] He concluded that history and physical examination (PE) had a 95% sensitivity but only a 50% specificity for diagnosing organic erectile dysfunction (ED); in Melman's hands the accuracy of history alone was 80%, and PE alone 60%. This level of accuracy presupposes expertise: it requires full knowledge of the medical risk factors for ED and skill in sexual history taking. Clinicians specializing in male sexual dysfunction have gone as far as to formalize this strategy for managing ED: it is known as the patient's goal directed approach.[2] From a managed care perspective, establishing a diagnosis with 95% sensitivity without testing is clearly preferable when compared with the costs of a comprehensive evaluation for ED. However, from the patient's perspective, is a successful outcome only defined as receipt of a method of enhancing rigidity? Similarly, what will be the sensitivity and specificity of a male sexual history and physical

examination in the hands of a general practitioner who may rely solely on the responses to a sexual questionnaire? It must be acknowledged that significant numbers of men present themselves as patients with ED because they are interested in information (establishing why their erectile quality is diminishing), and not necessarily because they are motivated to pursue therapy. Furthermore, as available treatments for ED grow into a 'laundry list' of options, the role of impotence testing will assume a twofold import: establishing an aetiology-specific diagnosis and formulating an effective treatment plan.

■ PREVALENCE OF VASCULAR ERECTILE DYSFUNCTION: WHO ARE THESE PATIENTS?

A recent estimate of the number of men in the United States suffering from 'complete impotence' is 10–20 million; when 'partial impotence' is included, the estimate jumps to 30 million.[3] Epidemiological studies suggest that the age-specific prevalence of impotence is 5% at 40 years increasing to 15–25% by 65 years. In clinical series, the ratio of organic to psychological male sexual dysfunction also varies with age, 70% of patients under 35 years of age having a psychogenic aetiology, and 85% of men over 50 years of age having organic impotence. Patient accounts of coital frequency likewise vary with age, 75% of men in their seventh decade reporting coitus once monthly and 37% of patients 61–65 years old claiming weekly coitus.

Reliable normative data on the prevalence of impotence in the community have only recently become available.[4] The Massachusetts Male Ageing Study

(MMAS) assessed the prevalence of 'impotence' among 1290 community-dwelling men ranging in ages from 40 to 70 years. Men rated their potency on a four-point scale — not impotent, minimally impotent, moderately impotent and completely impotent. A complaint of impotence was offered by 51% of men surveyed — 16% minimally, 25% moderately and 10% completely impotent. Diabetes, hypertension and coronary artery disease were each associated with increased probability of impotence complaints; these risks were amplified by concurrent smoking. Complete impotence was more prevalent among men taking medications, such as hypoglycaemics, antihypertensives, vasodilators and cardiac drugs. Normative data confirm a relationship between ageing and male sexual dysfunction and, more importantly, the data demonstrate the importance of vascular risk factors. In 1992, the National Institutes of Health sponsored a Consensus Conference on Impotence; participants recommended adoption of precise terminology when referring to male sexual dysfunction, specifically defining erectile dysfunction as the inability to achieve or maintain erection of sufficient rigidity and duration to permit satisfactory sexual performance. The consensus statement acknowledged not only the role of ageing in ED but also its relationship to para-ageing phenomena — precisely, the vascular risk factors: diabetes mellitus, atherosclerosis, hypertension, smoking and chronic renal insufficiency.[5]

This chapter reviews arterial vascular testing for ED, which is based on the simple but well-substantiated observation that organic ED is due to deficiencies of penile blood flow — either failure to fill the penis because of too little inflow (arterial insufficiency), or failure to trap blood within the penis because of too much outflow (venous insufficiency).

■ HISTORY OF PENILE ARTERIAL TESTING

Numerous diagnostic tests have been employed to evaluate penile blood flow: these include penile plethysmography, penile blood pressures, penile/brachial pressure index, penile pharmaco-angiography, duplex Doppler sonography, dynamic infusion cavernosometry/cavernosography (DICC), nuclear washout radiography, colour duplex Doppler ultrasonography, penile near-infrared spectro-photometry and magnetic resonance angiography.

In 1971, Gaskell[6] described a non-invasive test of penile arterial inflow: he used a photometer to quantify the absorption of light by the pigment oxyhaemoglobin in the glans penis. An occlusive cuff at the base of the penis was slowly loosened, and the pressure at which oxyhaemoglobin became measurable in the glans indicated the penile systolic blood pressure. A contemporary version of this tool is under development: it employs near-infrared spectrophotometry to measure change and rate of change of blood volume in the penis by monitoring oxyhaemoglobin and deoxyhaemoglobin.[7]

In 1975, Abelson[8] described the use of a Doppler stethoscope to measure penile blood pressure in flaccidity, comparing it with systolic brachial pressure and thus yielding the penile/brachial index (PBI; maximal systolic penile pressure divided by systolic brachial artery pressure). Michal and colleagues[9] and Goldstein and colleagues[10] modified the PBI test with a dynamic component by adding lower extremity and pelvic musculature exercises, with Doppler stethoscope auscultation before and after exercise. A decrease in the ratio of penile systolic pressure (< 0.15) was indicative of pelvic steal, or significant penile inflow disease. Subsequent reviews comparing the PBI with pharmacopenile angiography found that PBI values from normal patients overlapped with those from impotent patients. Although auscultation of penile pressures was easily performed in the office with affordable equipment, results were confounded by the tendency to measure dorsal and not central cavernous arterial flows.[11] In 1985, Lue and colleagues[12] introduced the technique of high-resolution sonography and quantitative Doppler spectrum analysis. Duplex Doppler allows real-time imaging of the central cavernous arteries with measurement of dynamic changes in cavernous arterial diameter and flow following intracorporal injection of papaverine.

Vascular testing: contemporary practice patterns

There are few objective data on US nationwide practice patterns in impotence testing, but a survey of urologists in six European countries has recently been conducted and the findings are quite revealing.[13] A total of 3000 urologists practising in France, Germany, Italy, Spain, Sweden and the United Kingdom were surveyed as to how they managed ED. The questionnaire (sponsored by Pharmacia Upjohn) was designed to provide an overview of evaluation and treatment strategies; the response rate was 60%. The data reflect differences in diagnostic and treatment strategies, highlighting the influences of healthcare structure, medical economics and cultural diversity. Perhaps more importantly, the data paint a picture revealing the state of the art in ED testing and treatments (in 1996), immediately prior to the introduction of oral pharmacotherapy designed specifically to improve penile haemodynamics.

In Germany, Spain, Sweden and the UK, most urologists work alone when it comes to the evaluation of ED. Both France and Italy report high proportions of multidisciplinary teams, 72 and 78% respectively. In Germany, most patients are self-referred (60%), whereas in the UK and Sweden most are referred by general practitioners (60–73%). In each country more than 90% of men complete a sexual questionnaire and have a physical examination during the initial visit. With the exception of Sweden (40%), urologists in European countries routinely investigate the aetiology of ED before initiating therapy (Fig. 22.1). The most commonly performed evaluation is hormonal screening (62–68%); the second most commonly performed test is in-office intracavernous injection (ICI; 53–81%). The preferred radiological investigation is duplex Doppler combined with ICI, which is performed by 30–65% of urologists, with the exception of the UK (5%) (Fig. 22.2). The remaining investigations are performed with much less frequency: these are nocturnal penile tumescence and rigidity testing (12%), visual erotic stimulation (6%), DICC (6%), electromyography (6%), and psychological assessments (16%). The average number of visits following the first consultation is 2.9. Surprisingly few physicians (< 40%) involve the partner during the initial visits.

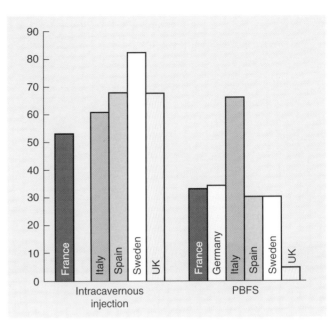

Figure 22.2. Survey of 3000 European urologists, percentage by country who utilize intracavernous injection pharmacotesting and penile blood flow studies (PBFS).

Investigating penile inflow

Penile angiography set the initial standards for diagnosis of vascular ED. Accurate penile angiography requires pharmacologically induced erection, as the vessels of the flaccid shaft are contracted and tortuous; this was not appreciated in the earliest investigations. High-osmolality contrast agents are painful, may induce anaphylaxis, and require intravenous sedative-anaesthesia. Some centres use epidural or spinal anaesthesia because of the additional benefit of reducing vasospasm.[14,15] Low-osmolality contrast agents reduce angiographic morbidity but are more expensive. State-of-the-art examinations are performed with intracavernous injection of vasodilator (prostaglandin E1 [PGE1], papaverine and phentolamine), intra-arterial dilators (nitroglycerine), digital subtraction techniques and superselective catheterization of pelvic vessels bilaterally, with visualization of internal pudendal, accessory pudendal and inferior epigastic arteries (Fig. 22.3). The inferior epigastrics are the vessels most commonly harvested in penile revascularization.

Indisputably, arteriography provides the best anatomical information about the origin of the common penile arteries, but these data have been difficult to correlate with patient complaints and with erection dynamics.[16] The common penile artery typically arises from the third segment of the internal pudendal artery (IPA) as it passes through the urogenital diaphragm. The

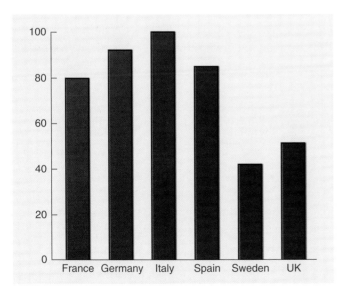

Figure 22.1. Survey of 3000 European urologists, percentage by country who routinely investigate the cause of erectile dysfunction.

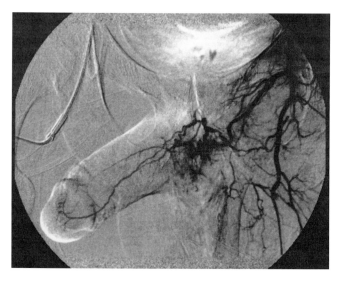

Figure 22.3. Selective internal pudendal pharmacopenile angiography with digital subtraction.

IPA arises from the inferior gluteal artery, which originates as a posterior branch of the internal iliac. The first branch of the IPA is the superficial perineal artery to the scrotum; the IPA continues as the common penile artery, with the artery to the bulbar urethra as its first branch. The paired common penile arteries may originate from one internal pudendal artery, or from an accessory internal pudendal artery. The accessory IPA may take origin from the hypogastric, remnant of the umbilical, ischial, or obturator arteries; an accessory IPA should be suspected if the IPA ends in the perineal artery. An accessory IPA is more common on the right, and prevalence has been variably described as from 4 to 70%. Therefore, performing selective internal pudendal arteriography (and missing an accessory IPA) has an inherent false-positive rate for diagnosing penile inflow disease.[15–19] In post-traumatic impotence secondary to pelvic fracture, penile inflow may originate in collaterals from the obturator arteries (in 20% of patients the IPA arises from the obturator).

As far as intrapenile anatomy is concerned, deviation from paired common penile arteries has been documented in 50% of normally potent volunteers; unilateral absence or hypoplasia of a dorsal artery has been shown in up to 30% of volunteers.[14] Anatomical variation of intrapenile arterial anatomy appears to be the rule rather than the exception, with unilateral or bilateral origin of the cavernous arteries, distal shaft communications between the dorsal and central cavernous arteries and collaterals to the corpus spongiosum.[20] The problem for the arteriographer is twofold — how to distinguish congenital variations in penile arterial anatomy from acquired abnormalities and how to correlate anatomical alterations in the pattern of vascular inflow with the complaints of impotence.

For the patient there remains the discomfort of the intra-arterial contrast, exposure to ionizing radiation, risk of minor or severe dye reaction and potential for endothelial cell and smooth muscle damage following corporal exposure to ionic contrast agents. As a screening test, pharmacopenile arteriography is overly invasive and non-specific of penile haemodynamics. Current penile arteriography studies have been compared with non-invasive imaging, specifically duplex Doppler. One such study utilized intra-arterial dilator (tolazoline) and intracavernous papaverine, finding severe or moderate arterial insufficiency in 11/11 patients with peak systolic velocity (PSV) values in the cavernous arteries of less than 25 cm/s, and in 13/17 patients with PSV values of 25–34 cm/s, and arteriographic inflow disease in only 1/12 patients with PSV of more than 35 cm/s.[21] There is consensus in the literature that the duplex Doppler parameter of PSV greater than 35 cm/s indicates normal arterial supply to the penis, and that arteriography is unwarranted in these men. Pharmacopenile angiography provides a 'road map' of pre-penile vessels and is reserved for men who are candidates for revascularization.[17,22]

Pharmacotesting: intracavernous injection (ICI)

In 1982, during the course of vascular reconstructive surgery, Ronald Virag noted that infusion of papaverine into the hypogastric artery produced an erection.[23] In 1983, a dramatic demonstration of the efficacy of penile self-injection was offered by Charles Brindley, who injected himself in front of an audience at a national meeting; he subsequently popularized the use of alpha blockers (phenoxybenzamine and phentolamine) for intracorporal injection in the management of erectile dysfunction.[24,25] Zorgniotti and Lefleur promoted injection therapy with the drug combination papaverine/phentolamine.[26] In 1986, Ishii and colleagues published the first clinical series of the use of PGE1 for investigation and treatment of ED.[27,28] Clinicians have subsequently turned to the benefits of combination therapy, exploiting the specific pharmaco-relaxing properties of different intracavernous agents to reduce the pain associated with PGE1, to reduce the risk of corporal fibrosis and hepatic dysfunction associated with papaverine, and to minimize the cost and volume of penile injections. In 1991, Bennett and colleagues[29] first described the clinical efficacy of the 'trimix' — papaverine, phentolamine and PGE1. In July 1995, Upjohn Company (Kalamazoo, MI, USA) received Food and Drug Administration (FDA) approval to market injectable PGE1 (Caverject®) specifically for the diagnosis and treatment of 'male impotence'. The demonstration that vasoactive injections could produce penile erection without benefit of psychic or tactile stimuli revolutionized the diagnosis and treatment of erectile dysfunction by providing a direct test of end-organ integrity and therapy specifically for vascular deficiency.

Pharmacotesting (ICI) consists of an intracavernous injection and visual rating of the subsequent erection; the test is the most commonly used in-office diagnostic procedure for impotence. It is simple, minimally invasive, and performed without monitoring equipment. A positive response in a neurologically normal patient implies psychogenic impotence, presumably excluding significant venous or arterial pathology.[30,31] Unfortunately, a standard intracavernous test dosage has never been established for any agent. Furthermore, a contemporary haemodynamic investigation suggests that a positive injection test is associated with normal veno-occlusion (low flow to maintain erection values of 0.5–3ml/min and minimal (or no) contrast medium leakage during DICC), but not necessarily with normal arterial function. In as many as 19% of patients the test may be a false negative. Despite the presence of an erection, there may be a significant disparity between the systemic and cavernous systolic arterial pressures, which can be correlated with abnormalities on pharmacopenile angiography. A normal ICI test then indicates meeting or exceeding a threshold response for intracavernous pressure ($\geq$ 80 mmHg), but this may occur in the presence of a significant gradient between systemic systolic pressure and cavernous systolic pressure. A positive injection test helps select patients for home injection therapy; it does not rule out mild arterial insufficiency.[32]

McMahon[33] has proposed standards for ICI and investigated three dosages of PGE1 (10, 20 and 30 µg). In his series a correct diagnosis of arterial insufficiency was made in 71, 89 and 90% of patients at the respective dosages of PGE1. A correct diagnosis of psychogenic ED was made in 72, 95 and 98% of patients at the corresponding dosages. Although specification of the aetiology of ED required additional testing beyond ICI, this series supports optimal pharmacological dosing

(without visual or tactile stimulation) at 20 µg of PGE1.[33] When visually assessing the erectile response to ICI it is helpful to have a consistent rating system; again, there is no consensus. The author has found that, for clinical purposes, rating the erectile response as (a) inadequate, (b) adequate for penetration or (c) excellent unbending rigidity of at least 20 minutes is most helpful.[34]

■ COLOUR DUPLEX DOPPLER ULTRASOUND

Introduction

All too often the penile response is suboptimal, leaving the clinician wondering whether the patient has severe arterial insufficiency, venous leakage or a high degree of anxiety. When diagnostic testing is indicated or desired, the penile blood flow study (PBFS), which consists of an intracavernous challenge of a vasoactive agent (ICI) and assessment by colour duplex Doppler ultrasound (CDDU), is the most reliable and least invasive means of screening for vasculogenic ED. Duplex sonography is more accurate than continuous-wave sonography because the examiner can see in real-time grey scale the central cavernous arteries, avoiding the pitfall of erroneously measuring the dorsal vessels. Colour duplex Doppler is a further advance in sonography: it aids in visualizing vessels, with the Doppler computer assigning colour to flowing blood, highlighting the arteries against the grey-scale background of corporal tissue. PBFS efficiently selects patients who are candidates for invasive testing.[34–37] The principles and techniques of PBFS with CDDU have been reviewed, as have the most recent criteria for distinguishing arterial insufficiency from cavernous venous occlusive disease, and high-flow from low-flow priapism, and for preoperative staging of Peyronie's disease.

Anatomy

The human penis consists of three corpora: these are the paired corpora cavernosa and the ventral corpus spongiosum, which forms the glans penis distally. The cavernous bodies share a fenestrated septum, which allows them to function neurophysiologically and to respond pharmacologically as a single unit. The tunica albuginea of the corpora cavernosa has a thickness of 2–3 mm in the flaccid state. The tunica albuginea of the corpus spongiosum is much thinner than that of the corpora cavernosa. Each of the corporal bodies is surrounded by a dense fascial structure, Buck's fascia. Additionally, Buck's fascia forms a thin non-fenestrated septum between the corpora cavernosa and the corpus spongiosum (there are connections through perforating arteries and emissary veins). With real-time ultrasound the corpus cavernosum and spongiosum have a homogeneous medium echogenicity which is distinguished from the hyperechoic tunica albuginea and septum. The tunica albuginea should have uniform thickness and echogenicity; the subcutaneous tissues and Buck's fascia are not identifiable sonographically except by the location of the dorsal vascular bundle comprising the paired dorsal arteries (DAs) and deep dorsal vein complex (DDV) (Fig. 22.4). The proximal penis (crural bodies) is anchored to the inferior pubis. The penile bulb is surrounded by the bulbocavernosus (or bulbospongiosus) muscle. The crura and proximal part of the shaft are covered by the ischiocavernosus muscles. Whereas the pendulous penis is easily imaged from either the dorsal (Fig. 22.5) or ventral projection, the proximal third of the penis may be imaged in transverse or sagittal view only by scanning from the ventral penis or below the scrotum. The urethral lumen will be compressed, but can be imaged by retrograde filling with sterile gel or water (Fig. 22.6).[38,39] The glans penis is covered with very thin and firmly adherent skin, has no fibrous sheath and contains much connective tissue.

Penile inflow

CDDU both provides a detailed examination of the vascular anatomy of the penis and records the dynamics of erection. The penis is supplied mainly by the IPA: pre-penile inflow vessels are not seen during penile sonography. Branches of the common penile artery consist of the bulbar, urethral (spongiosal), dorsal and cavernous arteries, each of which can be identified by CDDU. The cavernous artery penetrates the tunica albuginea and enters the crura of the corpora cavernosa along with the cavernous veins and cavernous nerves. The cavernous arteries are easily identified by their echogenic walls: in the flaccid state the arteries are tortuous and 0.5 mm or less in diameter. With CDDU, low blood flows are visible, but detection of flow prior to injection of vasodilator depends on the patient's level of sympathetic tone (affected by anxiety and room temperature) and is of no predictive value.[34,40] Cavernosal tissue is sponge-like and composed of a meshwork of interconnected cavernosal spaces, which are lined by vascular endothelium and separated by trabeculae, containing bundles of smooth muscle in a framework of

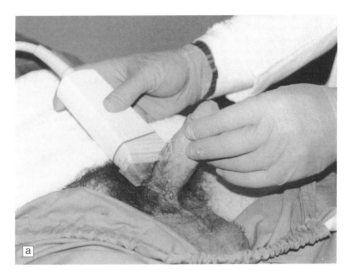

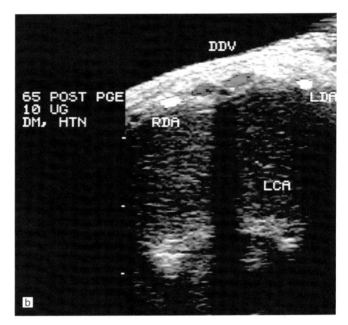

Figure 22.4. (a) The penis is held in the position of erection to straighten the cavernous vessels; imaging is begun in the transverse plane to assess anatomy. (b) Corresponding transverse colour duplex Doppler ultrasound (CDDU) image showing right dorsal artery (RDA), deep dorsal vein complex (DDV), left dorsal artery (LDA) and left cavernous artery (LCA).

collagen, elastin and fibroblasts. The terminal helicine arteries are multiple muscular and corkscrew-shaped arteries (150–350 µm) that open directly into the cavernous spaces and act like resistance arteries. The corporal tissue becomes more hypo-echoic (darker) as the sinusoids distend with blood, making the echogenic walls of the cavernous arteries more distinct sonographically (Fig. 22.7). The dorsal artery enters the penis and continues distally beneath Buck's

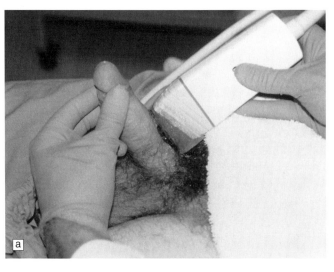

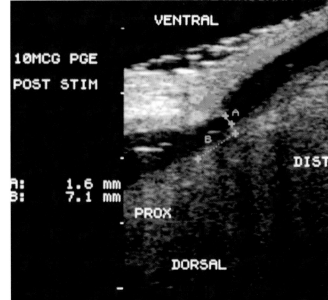

Figure 22.6. Sono-urethrogram performed during PBFS in 55-year-old patient complaining of impotence following optical internal urethrotomy. Scanning is performed in the sagittal plane from the ventral aspect of the penis, with lignocaine jelly filling the urethra; a persistent 7 mm stricture is seen.

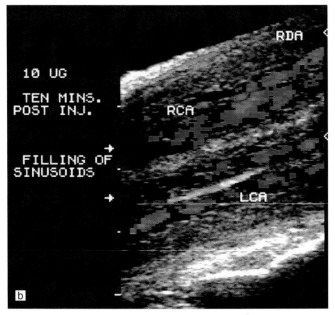

Figure 22.5. (a) The penis is held in the position of erection to straighten the cavernous vessels; imaging in the sagittal plane from the dorsum. (b) Sagittal image of the penis 10 minutes following injection of PGE1 (10 μg). The right dorsal artery (RDA), right cavernous artery (RCA), and left cavernous artery are imaged (LCA).

fascia. Between the dorsal arteries are one or more deep dorsal vein(s) and flanking each dorsal artery is a dorsal nerve (Fig. 22.4b). The urethral artery runs longitudinally through the corpus spongiosum lateral to the urethra. This supplies the corpus spongiosum, urethral tissue and glans penis. The bulbar artery enters the bulb of the penis shortly after its origin. It supplies blood to Cowper's gland and the proximal urethral bulb. Anatomical variations of the penile arterial supply include dorsal-to-cavernous, cavernous-to-cavernous and cavernous-to-urethral collaterals, duplication of the cavernous artery, and unilateral absence of a dorsal artery.[14,34]

Penile outflow

On the basis of scanning electronic microscopy of vascular corrosion casts, Banya and colleagues[41] suggested two circulatory routes in the human corpora. One route goes from the cavernous artery to capillary networks collected into the venular plexus just beneath the tunica albuginea; this is suggested to serve as a main circulatory pathway during the flaccid state. The other route is through anastomoses from the cavernous artery, via the helicine arteries to the cavernae (sinusoids), which are then emptied into the post-cavernous venules. This ultrastructural detail is not visualized sonographically.

There are three sets of veins draining the penis — the superficial, intermediate and deep. The deep venous system drains both the corpora cavernosa and the corpus spongiosum. The post-cavernous venules coalesce to form larger emissary veins, which pierce the tunica albuginea. The emissary veins of the middle and distal penis join to form the circumflex veins, which empty into the deep dorsal vein (Fig. 22.8). Both the emissary and circumflex veins have valves. The emissary veins of the proximal

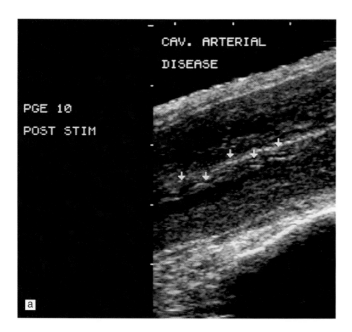

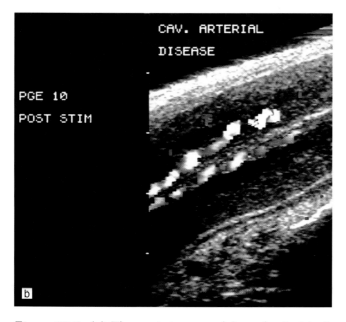

Figure 22.7. (a) The penis is scanned from the 3 o'clock position with grey-scale imaging: the sinusoids are hypo-echoic compared with the septum; the left cavernous artery walls are relatively hyperechoic in comparison to sinusoidal tissues. (b) Colour duplex Doppler image of the same patient as in (a); note how close the cavernous arteries are to the septum.

penis form the cavernous vein, which empties into the internal pudendal vein.

The intermediate set of veins is deep to Buck's fascia. Veins from the glans penis form a retrocoronal plexus that drains into the deep dorsal vein. The deep dorsal vein courses proximal in the midline and empties into the periprostatic plexus. The superficial dorsal vein drains the skin and the subcutaneous tissue superficial to Buck's fascia. It drains into the superficial external pudendal vein.

Erection haemodynamics

Erection is a complex event regulated by the tone of smooth muscle composing the cavernous arterioles, venules and sinusoids. Tumescence follows a decrease in corporal smooth muscle tension, decreasing arterial, arteriolar and sinusoidal resistance. Decreasing resistance to arterial inflow bathes the cavernous tissues in highly oxygenated arterial blood. Venous outflow during erection is dynamically limited by distension of the sinusoids compressing the subtunical venular plexus against the inner layer of the tunica albuginea. The differential stretching of the two primary layers of the tunica albuginea, during erection, scissors closed the exiting emissary veins (Fig. 22.8). The rigid penis is veno-occluded, in a low-outflow state, with distended sinusoids and elevated intracorporal pressure. During rigid erection, arterial inflows are paradoxically very low (by Doppler estimation 1.5–5.6 ml/min, by phalloarteriography 4.7 ml/min, by radioisotope study < 5 ml/min). Dynamic cavernosometry similarly reveals that rigid erection is associated with low flow to maintain values of 0.5–3 ml/min.[12,32,42] Detumescence and flaccidity are initiated and maintained by corporal smooth muscle contraction.

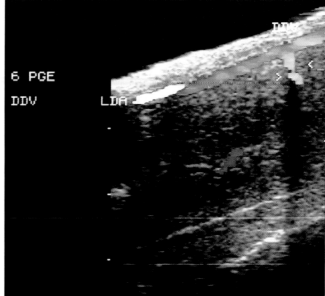

Figure 22.8. The deep dorsal vein (DDV) and part of the left dorsal artery (LDA) are imaged from the dorsum; the open arrowheads outline a perforating emissary vein.

Lue and Wagner and their associates have studied the dynamics of erection in several species and have divided the progress from flaccidity to erection into distinct phases (Fig. 22.9).[43,44] In the flaccid phase there is a dominant sympathetic influence, and the terminal arterioles and cavernous smooth muscles are contracted. In the filling phase, parasympathetic nervous activity dominates and there is an increased blood flow through the internal pudendal and cavernous arteries; penile resistance decreases, owing to dilatation of the cavernosal and helicine arteries; the penis elongates. During the tumescence phase the intracavernous pressure increases rapidly; the compliance of the sinusoidal muscle increases, causing penile engorgement. In full erection the relaxed trabecular muscle expands and, together with the increased blood volume, compresses the plexus of subtunical venules, reducing venous outflow, and increasing intracavernous pressure to 10–20 mmHg below the systolic blood pressure (minimum of 80 mmHg). In the rigid erection phase, cavernous pressure may transiently increase above the systolic pressure. As a consequence of voluntary or reflexogenic contraction of the ischiocavernosus and bulbocavernosus muscles, suprasystolic pressures may be achieved during pelvic thrusting; maximal penile rigidity is compromised when bulbocavernous reflex is absent.

The separate phases of erection documented in laboratory animals do have correlates with human erectile responses during PBFS. There are many variables in clinical testing that may alter the normal progression of erection phases. The threshold dosage for a single agent or multiple agents to promote complete smooth muscle relaxation reliably has not been established, and quite probably varies with levels of patient sympathetic tone (anxiety). Available data on the minimal effective dosage of PGE1 suggest that 2 µg will produce erection in 38% of men with psychogenic impotence and 20% of men with vasculogenic ED.[45] A pattern of spectral waveform progression on CDDU has been correlated with a normal rigid response during PBFS.[46] In the filling phase, when sinusoidal resistance is low (5 minutes) following injection, the waveform is characterized by high forward flow during diastole (Fig. 22.9). As intrapenile pressure increases, diastolic velocities decrease; with full erection the systolic waveforms will peak sharply and may be slightly less than during full tumescence; diastolic flow will be zero. In rigid erection, cavernous pressure will exceed systemic diastolic blood pressure and reversal of diastolic flow occurs. Similarly, in the rigid erection phase the systolic waveform may be dampened. The bulbocavernous reflex may be stimulated by intermittent glans compression during examination, which will alter the Doppler waveform, transiently reducing diastolic flows (Fig. 22.10).[34]

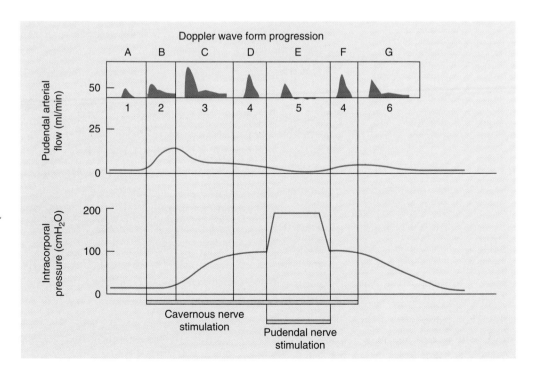

Figure 22.9. Phases of the erectile response in the animal model, first stimulated by the cavernous nerve then additionally stimulated by the pudendal nerve. Pudendal arterial flow and intracavernous pressures are graphically compared with the Doppler waveform progression of a normal erection: (A) flaccid phase; (B) latent phase; (C) tumescence; (D) full erection; (E) rigid erection with reversal of diastolic flow; (F) rigid erection with suppression of diastolic flow; (G) detumescence.

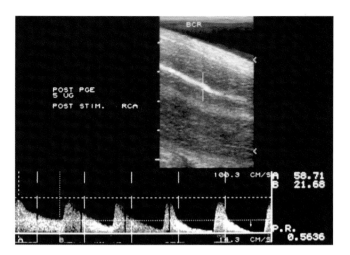

Figure 22.10. Right cavernous arterial flow (RCA) following 5 μg of PGE1; the PSV is 58 cm/s and EDV 21 cm/s. Squeezing the glans stimulates a bulbocavernous reflex; contraction of these muscles transiently alters diastolic flows (large, medium and small arrows).

■ TECHNIQUE

Instruments

Since its introduction by Lue in 1985, duplex Doppler penile sonography has proved to be an accurate and reproducible technique for evaluating erectile dysfunction. With the initial grey-scale imaging of duplex sonography, study quality was highly dependent on the skill of the examiner. Vessel localization within the corporal tissue was difficult and dorsal vessel imaging all but impossible. The addition of colour has facilitated consistent detection of dorsal, cavernous and urethral vessels. CDDU permits the rapid acquisition and measurement of small vessels in low-flow states.[47–49] High-frequency linear array transducers (5–10 MHz) provide the best images of the penis: the higher the frequency the better the near-field resolution. For this chapter all images were retrieved from 7.0–10.0 MHz linear array transducers with a standoff wedge; these permit continuous colour encoded grey-scale images during Doppler sampling. Others have reported adequate high-resolution penile imaging with (non-colour) grey scale 13.5 MHz probes.[50]

Colour flow uses the imaging principles of pulsed Doppler: a pulse of ultrasound is emitted from the transducer, is reflected back and received. When the returning echo has a frequency that differs from the emitted frequency, a Doppler shift has occurred (ultrasound reflecting back off a moving object [e.g. penile blood] causes a Doppler shift). Doppler frequency shift depends on several factors: these include frequency of the transducer, velocity of the moving object (penile blood), speed of sound through the medium (penile tissue) and angle between the Doppler beam and direction of blood flow. The blood flowing in a vessel approaching the transducer will produce echoes with a higher frequency than was emitted; blood flowing away produces a lower frequency. As blood-flow velocities increase, Doppler shift increases. The Doppler shift is displayed on a grey scale as a spectrum (waveform) or in CDDU as a two-dimensional colour image. In CDDU the colour display has an angle dependence just like the grey-scale spectrum of the Doppler shift. If the vessel runs parallel to the skin surface, ultrasound scanning lines are perpendicular (90-degree Doppler angle); this will yield no Doppler shift and no colour within the vessel. To correct this problem of physics, linear array transducers use phasing to steer the scan lines at a more appropriate angle, or an angled standoff wedge on the end of the transducer to provide a non-perpendicular Doppler angle. The angled standoff wedge is acoustically neutral and is ideal for imaging penile vessels that are parallel to, and near the surface of, the penile skin. Arterial flow velocity determinations depend on the ultrasound beam–vessel angle; the optimal angle is 60 degrees; the angle correction is set by the examiner. Since arterial flow velocity measurements will be repeated several times after injecting vasodilator, particular attention should be paid to maintaining the same angle of insonation: for example, arterial velocities in the same vessel will be recorded at 20, 25, 31 or 203 cm/s if the probe–vessel angle is altered from 30 to 45 to 55 to 85 degrees respectively.[51–55]

Examination protocol

The examination should be performed in a warm, darkened room. A warm, secure setting is essential to reduce anxiety and thus sympathetic cavernous smooth muscle tone. The patient should be assured that no one will come walking in during his testing. The patient should be supine; he need disrobe only from the waist down. His attention should be directed at the video monitor with a periodic explanation of images displayed, for example: 'you are going to see ultrasound views of your penile vessels; some of these run on the surface of the penis and two are central arteries providing the pressure to your erection. When the Doppler is activated the sound you hear will be blood flowing into your penis with each heartbeat.'

The corporal bodies should be scanned in the transverse plane from base to tip, to demonstrate normal anatomy (paired cavernous and dorsal arteries); the echotexture should be homogeneous; fibrotic processes are relatively hyperechoic in comparison (Fig. 22.11). Peyronie's plaques will be denser than normal tunica; they may be visible as linear echogenic thickenings. If they cast an acoustic shadow like a renal stone, then calcification should be suspected and plain radiographs taken following PBFS/CDDU. The penile vessels and flow velocities are assessed in the sagittal plane (parallel to the long axis of the penis). Vessels may be scanned from a dorsal or ventral approach. Lateral scanning will demonstrate both cavernous vessels in the same image, with the hyperechoic septum between both arteries. (Fig. 22.12). Cavernous-to-cavernous collaterals are best imaged in the sagittal projection from the lateral penis (3 or 9 o'clock). The author has noted these vessels perforating the septum in 50% of men examined. They are seen in patients with neurogenic and psychogenic impotence suggesting congenital origin. The dynamics of collateral flow are important: high-flow collaterals may supplement unilateral cavernous arterial insufficiency. A dorsal projection is required to image the dorsal artery and ipsilateral cavernous artery simultaneously (Fig. 22.13). Following the injection of vasodilator, dorsal-to-cavernous collaterals

were demonstrated recently in 59% of men; these were haemodynamically significant in only 15% of patients (≥ 25 cm/s).[56] The dorsal arteries are not subjected to intracorporal pressure changes at each progressive erection phase; therefore, even in well-sustained rigidity, antegrade diastolic flow persists. During peak erection, dorsal systolic flow is maximal; copious acoustic gel on the surface of the penis and a light touch are needed to prevent alteration of the flow dynamics of dorsal vessels.

All four penile arteries should be scanned at least from the level of the penoscrotal junction to the glans. When

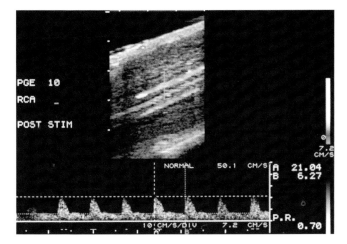

Figure 22.12. Lateral scanning images both cavernous arteries; the right cavernous artery is measured and has a PSV of 21 cm/s, EDV of 6 cm/s and RI of 0.7.

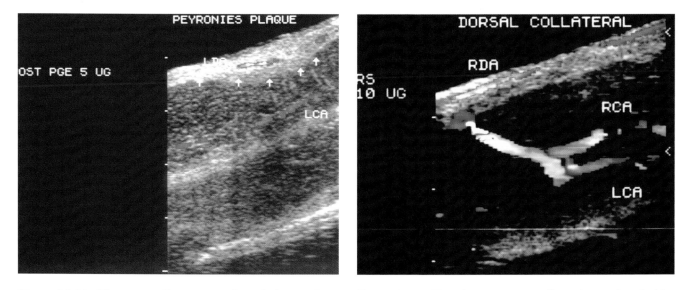

Figure 22.11. The tunica albuginea is relatively hyperechoic compared with the corporal tissues; a Peyronie's plaque is seen as a relative thickening beneath the left dorsal artery (LDA).

Figure 22.13. Dorsal-to-cavernous collaterals are identified by scanning in the sagittal plane; here the right dorsal artery (RDA) supplies collateral flow to both right and left cavernous arteries (RCA, LCA).

there is asymmetry of cavernous flows (≥ 10 cm/s), or when collaterals are seen, the crura should be examined to determine whether proximal inflow disease exists (prepenile) or if intracorporal stenosis has resulted in a decreased unilateral CDDU signal. Reversal of arterial flow in systole signals severe unilateral inflow disease: blood should be flowing in an antegrade direction in both cavernous arteries during each phase of erection. If the patient's legs are abducted in a frog-leg position, the perineum can be scanned, revealing the entry of the cavernous arteries into the penis. This view is especially helpful when searching for arterial sinusoidal malformations, which may develop as a result of straddle injury causing high-flow priapism. As distal flows will rapidly drop off in a normal erection if the examiner waits too long and the erection is rigid, cavernous inflow should be measured at the perineum; otherwise, Doppler data will be inconsistent with observed rigidity (Fig. 22.14). Cavernous flow velocities will be highest at the perineum and will segmentally diminish, distally. Several investigators have confirmed that systolic velocities of the cavernous arteries vary significantly as a function of sampling location.[57,58] Traditionally, arterial velocities are measured at the penoscrotal junction (proximal pendulous shaft), from either the ventral or lateral–sagittal projections. If the penis has not assumed an erect posture, it should be held upright by the glans; this is the anatomical position of erection and serves to straighten the course of the cavernous and dorsal arteries. The principal source of error in flow-velocity determinations is an incorrectly assigned Doppler angle. Holding the shaft upright stretches the normally tortuous cavernous vessels and permits consistent measurements, with the probe–vessel Doppler angle remaining set.

Timing is important: arterial diameter and cavernous PSV values will maximize before rigid erection (maximal intracavernous pressure). Some investigators advocate continuous penile sampling for up to 30 minutes following penile injection;[59] Meuleman and colleagues[60] found peak velocities to be highest 5–10 minutes following vasodilator; Fitzgerald and colleagues[61] found that 24% of patients tested did not reach maximum cavernous flow until 10–15 minutes after injection. Patel and colleagues[62] noted that PSV values maximized between 5 and 6.5 minutes following injection; 22% of patients had a delayed response (1–18 minutes). If initial measurements are made 5–10 minutes after injection, and full or rigid erection waveforms are not seen, a period of

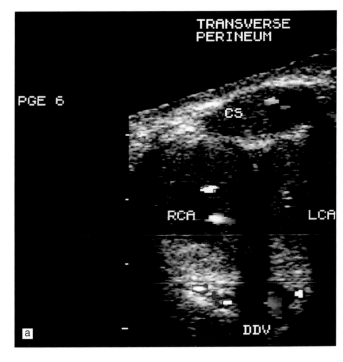

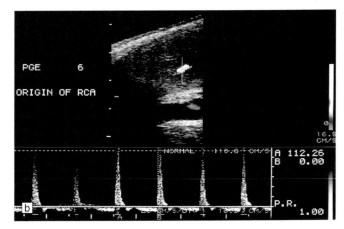

Figure 22.14. (a) Scanning from through the perineum in the transverse plane reveals the corpus spongiosum (CS), paired cavernous bodies, and dorsal vessels. (b) Scanning from through the perineum in the sagittal plane for measurement of cavernous artery flow (RCA) at site of entry in the crura. Crural flows are normally several orders of magnitude higher than pendulous penis flows, here 112 cm/s.

privacy and self-stimulation will enhance the penile response in 70% or more of patients. CDDU assessment is repeated immediately following self-stimulation, and note is made of whether the response weakens or is sustained. Lue and Donatucci[63] found that, among 90 patients performing self-stimulation after PGE1 challenge, 74% improved; among those whose responses weakened within 5 minutes of stimulation, 84% were noted to have moderate venous leakage on follow-up cavernosography. Montorsi and colleagues[64] evaluated initial dosing with PGE1 10 μg and redosing with 10 μg versus the effects of a single dosage followed by genital plus audiovisual sexual stimulation. Erectile responses after the genital stimulation session were significantly greater than after redosing, and patients more frequently achieved erections equal to (or greater than) those achieved at home.

Again, it is very useful to rate the erectile quality visually during Doppler assessment, e.g. (a) inadequate versus (b) adequate versus (c) unbending rigidity sustained for 20 minutes. Correlation of visual erection rating and Doppler parameters is an essential element in the diagnostic process: although the Doppler parameters are distinctly different, tumescence without rigidity is characteristic of both severe veno-occlusive disease and arterial insufficiency. According to Goldstein,[50] the aim of penile vascular testing is to obtain haemodynamic data on the same quality of erection that the patient gets in the privacy of his own bedroom, i.e. the best quality erection. If this is not the case then the patient can be redosed to achieve maximal smooth muscle relaxation.[65]

The choice of intracavernous vasoactive agent for CDDU has never been standardized. The initial duplex Doppler studies were performed following injection of 60 mg papaverine.[16,66,67] 'Trimix' has been used recently in efforts to achieve maximal smooth muscle relaxation (0.2 ml papaverine [6 mg], phentolamine [0.2 mg] and PGE1 [2 μg]).[29] Of the currently used agents, PGE1 is thought to have the greatest biocompatibility. PGE1 is a corporal smooth muscle relaxant and has anti-adrenergic activity that may explain its efficacy in patients suffering from high-anxiety psychogenic ED.[28,68–70] PGE1 (Caverject®, Upjohn Co.) is the only FDA-approved injectable for the treatment of ED. In a recent dose-finding study, the median effective dosage was 5.0 μg in patients with vasculogenic dysfunction, producing a mean duration of erection of 37 minutes; penile discomfort was noted in 34%, and prolonged erection (4–6 hours) in 5%.[45] In the author's experience with initial diagnostic intracavernous challenges, PGE1 is highly effective in neurologically intact males with vascular risk factors, at a dose of 10 μg when coupled with privacy and self-stimulation. With this regimen only 4% of patients develop persistent rigidity of 2 hours. Patients are successfully managed with simple aspiration and/or direct corporal injection of the alpha-adrenergic phenylephrine (100 μg/ml, using 1–3 ml).

Treatment is uniformly successful if given within 2–4 hours of ICI challenge.

CDDU and penile inflow: arterial adequacy

The original parameter used to deduce the adequacy of penile circulation was cavernous PSV. In efforts to refine further the diagnosis of cavernous inflow disease, Doppler parameters have been expanded: these include end-diastolic arterial velocity (EDV), which is the flow velocity measured during diastole immediately prior to take-off of the systolic waveform, systolic rise time (measured in ms) from the start of systolic velocity to the maximum value, and cavernous artery acceleration, which is calculated by dividing peak flow velocity by systolic rise time.[40,71,72] Flow velocities should be measured 5–10 minutes after injection; a delay in response is typical in both the hypertensive and the anxious patient. A visual rating of erectile quality should be recorded each time a set of Doppler parameters is recorded.

Penile inflow is a function of both velocity and vessel diameter. Lue and Tanagho[73] originally proposed that an adequate response in the cavernous arteries should produce a postinjection arterial diameter of more than 0.7 mm and a PSV of 25 cm/s or more. They found that, if the cavernous arteries did not dilate by 75%, there was a high likelihood of arterial disease. Other investigators suggested increases of more than 100%, or could not confirm significant changes in pre- and post-injection cavernous arterial diameters.[49,74–76] Subsequent investigations have shown that cavernous arterial diameters normally decrease from proximal to distal and that measurement of cavernous arterial lumens actually exceeds ultrasound resolution of 7–10 MHz probes (Fig. 22.15). In the University of California at San Francisco (UCSF) series, normal subjects had a mean PSV of 34.8 cm/s and a mean arterial diameter of 0.89 mm.[55] In a study from Baylor University, normal volunteers had a mean PSV of 40 cm/s and mean arterial diameter of 1.0 mm.[75,77] Normal volunteers at the Harvard Medical School study had a mean PSV of 47 cm/s.[74] Each of these groups concurs that a PSV of less than 25 cm/s suggests arterial disease. When penile angiography is compared with duplex Doppler examinations of the same patients, a PSV of less than 25 cm/s is consistently associated with severe arterial disease; in the Mayo Clinic series, a PSV of less than 25 cm/s had a sensitivity of 100% and specificity of 95% in selection of patients with abnormal pudendal

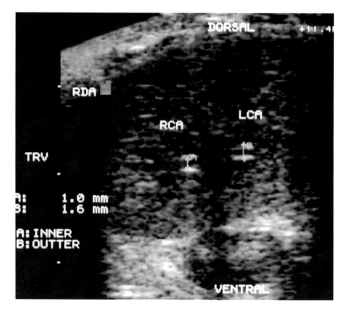

Figure 22.15. Transverse image of the paired cavernous arteries; variance in arterial diameters is a function of measuring lumen versus vessel wall (1.0 vs 1.6 mm).

arteriography (Fig. 22.16).[78] A PSV of 35 cm/s or more is generally associated with a normal penile arteriogram.[76] The Mayo Clinic group has recommended that, if a patient has a good clinical response to a vasodilating injection and bilateral PSV values are more than 30 cm/s with arterial dilatation to 0.7 mm, arteriography should not be performed. When PSV is compared with cavernous arterial systolic occlusion pressures (CASOPs) generated during dynamic infusion cavernosometry, a PSV of 25 cm/s or more predicts a normal CASOP with a sensitivity of 95% and specificity of 95%.[79] If cavernous inflows are asymmetric or absent at the perineum, pre-penile (pudendal) arterial disease should be suspected (Fig. 22.17). Intrapenile arterial disease is confirmed when crural inflows are adequate and symmetric, but asymmetry of R/L PSVs is noted in the pendulous shaft. On CDDU, severe unilateral cavernous arterial insufficiency may be associated with reversal of systolic flow proximal to the entry of a collateral (Fig. 22.18).

Schwartz and colleagues[80] correlated progressive changes in Doppler spectral waveform pattern with increasing intracorporal pressure in potent volunteers stimulated with papaverine/phentolamine. Rigid erection was associated with intracorporal pressures ranging from 83 to 106 mmHg. During tumescence both PSV and EDV increased, with corporal pressure ranging from 11 to 25 mmHg. With rigidity, EDV approached 0, and diastolic

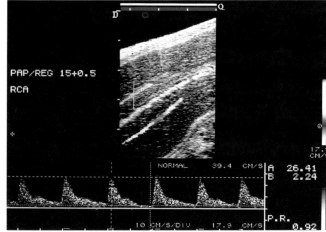

Figure 22.16. Suboptimal arterial response in a 49-year-old diabetic patient, PSV 26 cm/s. The erection was rated as adequate for penetration; note RI 0.92.

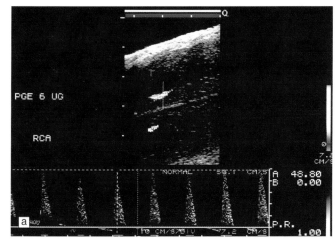

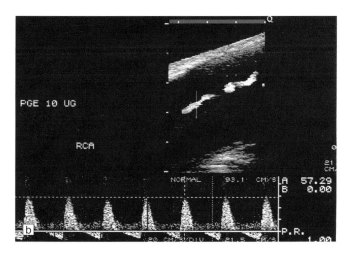

Figure 22.17. (a) Excellent erectile response following 6 μg of PGE1 in 49-year-old associated with PSV 49 cm/s and suppression of diastolic flow. (b) Excellent erectile response following 10 μg of PGE1 in 72-year-old associated with PSV 57 cm/s and reversal of diastolic flow.

flow reversed when intracorporal pressures reached 63–83 mmHg.

In 1974, Planiol and Pourcelot[81] derived the index of vascular resistance from the Doppler spectrum. The formula for resistive index is RI = (PSV – EDV)/PSV. RI calculation is not directly dependent on the probe vessel angle:[81] the value of RI depends on the resistance to arterial inflow and, in the context of corporal physiology, this is a function of sympathetic tone in the flaccid state and of changing intracorporal pressure during the various phases of erection. As penile pressure equals or exceeds diastolic pressure, diastolic flow in the corpora will approach zero and the value for RI approaches 1. During tumescence and until full rigidity, diastolic flow is antegrade and the value for RI remains less than 1.0. The RI correlates very well with visual rating of erectile responses, as both are descriptions of penile rigidity and pressure. Both EDV and RI are useful parameters in predicting the adequacy of veno-occlusion (see below).

CDDU and penile outflow: documenting veno-occlusive adequacy

Failure of the veno-occlusive mechanism is reflected in the Doppler spectral waveform of the cavernous artery.

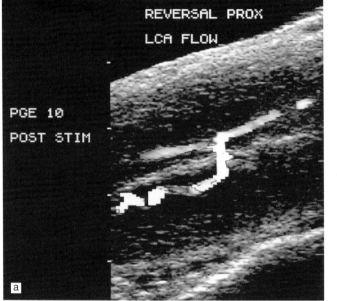

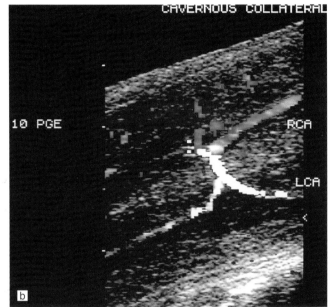

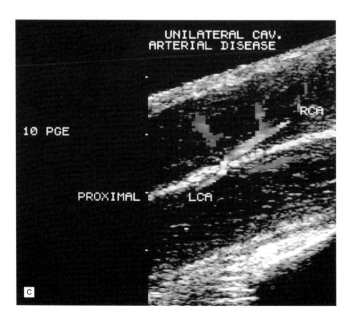

Figure 22.18. (a) Cavernous collateral with reversal of systolic flow in the left cavernous artery (LCA), consistent with severe unilateral cavernous insufficiency. (b) Cavernous collateral with antegrade flows in both cavernous arteries. (c) Cavernous collateral from the left to right cavernous artery; no flow seen in proximal right cavernous artery (RCA).

The suspicion of venous leakage is raised when the patient has an excellent arterial response to injected vasodilator (≥ 30 cm/s PSV), with well-maintained EDV (> 3–5 cm/s), accompanied by transient rigidity after self-stimulation.

Quam and colleagues[47] found EDVs ranging between 0 and 24 cm/s after intracavernous papaverine (60 mg). Among patients with PSVs above 25 cm/s, venous leakage on cavernosometry was predicted with a sensitivity of 90% and specificity of 56% when end-diastolic flow was more than 5 cm/s.[47,78] Fitzgerald and colleagues,[61] using criteria of cavernous arterial adequacy (>25 cm/s PSV) and venous leakage (>5 cm/s EDV), noted that only three-quarters of patients achieved maximal responses to papaverine (60 mg) at 5 minutes; data acquisition for a total of 30 minutes yielded a sensitivity of 95% and specificity of 83% for prediction of venous leakage. Merckx and colleagues[82] injected patients with PGE1 (20 μg) followed by Doppler analysis at intervals of 5 minutes. Doppler parameters among 26 psychogenically impotent men were statistically identical to those of eight potent volunteers: (at 5 minutes) maximum PSV 49 cm/s, maximum EDV 11 cm/s, RI 0.78; (at 10 minutes) PSV 38.8 cm/s, EDV 3.7 cm/s, RI 0.91. The RI was the only parameter that statistically differentiated the venous incompetence. Using this 5 and 10 min scanning protocol, Merckx and colleagues noted a 93% correlation between CDDU and cavernosometry. In the Mayo Clinic series of 1994, Lewis and King[78] noted an EDV of more than 3 cm/s measured 15–20 minutes after injection yielded a specificity of 94% and sensitivity of 69% for detection of venous leakage when compared with dynamic cavernosometry. McMahon and Daley[83] found that RI calculations 15 minutes after injection correlated well with maintenance flow rates (from dynamic infusion cavernosometry) and cavernosal decay rates. In a study from Japan, Naroda and colleagues[84] found that an RI of more than 0.9 was associated with normal dynamic infusion cavernosometry in 90%, whereas one of less than 0.75 was associated with venous leakage in 95% of patients. The conclusion reached from these investigations is that measurement of RI 20 minutes after injection and stimulation (or redosing) is a reliable, non-invasive method by which to diagnose cavernous venous leakage (Fig. 22.19).

Although the definitive criteria for CDDU-diagnosed venous leakage have not been agreed upon, the examiner will reliably be able to select patients for DICC. When the Doppler spectral waveform continues to exhibit forward diastolic flow despite peak systolic flow (> 35 cm/s) a low-resistance state persists in the sinusoids and the patient may have venogenic impotence (Fig. 22.20). The dorsal arteries are not subjected to the intracorporal pressure changes with each phase of erection and well-sustained rigidity is associated with antegrade diastolic flow. Deep dorsal vein (DDV) flow persists during rigid erection; DDV flows are a function of dorsal arterial flow to the glans and should not be interpreted as evidence of corporal venous leakage. When DDV flows are high, a pattern of respiratory venous variation often may be seen (Fig. 22.21): the primary veno-occlusive mechanism

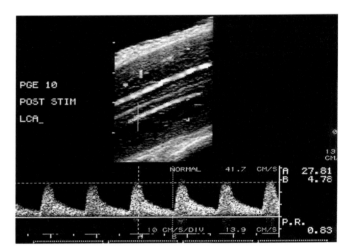

Figure 22.19. Mixed vascular insufficiency with PSV 27 cm/s and RI 0.83.

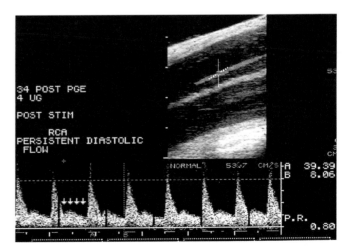

Figure 22.20. Cavernous venous occlusive disease is properly diagnosed when PSV exceeds 35 cm/s and diastolic flows persist, RI < 0.9.

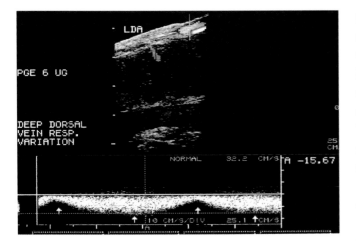

Figure 22.21. Respiratory variation in the deep dorsal vein (DDV); high DDV flow does not indicate veno-occlusive disease.

consists of passive compression of the subtunical venular plexus by the distended sinusoids; the secondary mechanism is the scissoring-off of the emissary veins as they exit through the two layers of the tunica albuginea. Emissary veins, unlike dorsal artery to cavernous artery collaterals, are difficult to localize with CDDU, presumably because of their low-flow state and easy compressibility (Fig. 22.8).

Priapism: CDDU characteristics of low flow and high flow

Priapism is a persistent erection that fails to subside after climax and is accompanied by penile pain and tenderness; it is an overfunction of a normal mechanism.[85] Traditionally, priapism has been categorized as primary (spontaneous–idiopathic) or secondary to specific pathologies such as sickle-cell disease, leukaemia, fat emboli, malignant infiltration, neurological injury, alcohol and psychotropic drugs. Aetiology-specific classification has now been abandoned, and priapism is currently described as low-flow/ischaemic versus high-flow/arterial, based on erection haemodynamics. With the increasing popularity of pharmacological erection programmes iatrogenic or therapeutically induced prolonged erection has become the most common cause of low-flow priapism.[86]

Ischaemic priapism is an obvious failure of the detumescence mechanism, which may result from direct dysregulation of the cavernous–arterial–sinusoidal system through persistent stimulation of corporal relaxing factors, inhibition of the neurotransmission that normally terminates erection, or inactivation of the smooth muscle cellular cofactors that regulate corporal smooth muscle tone, such as an altered metabolic environment (hypoxia, hypercarbia, acidity or sickling of red cells).[87] It is known that, beyond a certain (and, as yet, undefined) time, the cavernous smooth muscle becomes refractory to recoiling. This condition is clinically well recognized in emergency rooms and remains one of the few true urological emergencies.

Histological investigations reveal that after 24 hours of ischaemic priapism, the corporal tissues become thickened and oedematous. The natural history of untreated priapism is impotence with perhaps some erectile activity maintained in the proximal crura. More recent electron microscopic work by Spycher and Hauri has demonstrated trabecular interstitial oedema after 12 hours, followed by the destruction of sinusoidal endothelium, exposure of the basement membrane and thrombocyte adherence by 24 hours. By 48 hours, actual thrombus formation occurs in the sinusoidal spaces and the smooth muscle undergoes fibroblast-like cell transformation. The diagnosis is established by history and measurement of penile blood gas. CDDU may be useful in the follow-up of ischaemic priapism, to determine the extent of corporal fibrosis and the patency of the cavernous arteries or in localizing the sinusoidal arterial fistula producing a high-flow state (Fig. 22.22).

Understanding normal penile haemodynamics has led to classification of the prolonged erection as either

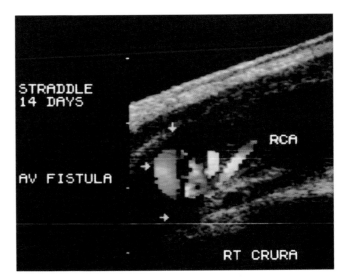

Figure 22.22. Sagittal perineal imaging in a 12-year-old boy with persistent erection following straddle injury reveals a sinusoidal fistula and high-flow priapism.

ischaemic–veno-occlusive or high-flow–arterial. Of the various aetiologies for priapism, only one — trauma — has been attributed to 'dysregulation' of inflow and production of high-flow priapism.[88,89] Hakim and colleagues[90] have demonstrated the utility and accuracy of duplex Doppler in the diagnosis and management of high-flow priapism when compared with selective internal pudendal arteriography. The investigators followed ten men with selective internal pudendal arteriography, duplex Doppler ultrasonography and physical examinations. The duration of priapism was startling — from 21 days to 36 years; at the time of initial evaluation all patients gave a history of blunt perineal or shaft trauma, and had bright red corporal aspirates. Six patients who had emboli had retrograde unilateral cavernous flows on CDDU follow-up, suggesting permanent occlusion. The only consequence of expectant management was the 'annoyance' of a tumescent shaft. Hakim and colleagues conclude that duplex sonography is more accurate than physical examination and arteriography in predicting the existence and persistence of lacunar fistulae. Indeed, all ten patients had a delay in time to presentation from days to years, during which they reported normal or improved sexual activity. These cases are extremely rare; unlike low-flow veno-occlusive priapism there is no need for emergency intervention in high-flow priapism. It is essential to establish the correct classification of priapism by aspiration of bright red blood from the corpora, confirming high oxygen tension. Remote corporal injury may be evident on CDDU by hyperechoic changes within the corpora, a non-specific finding consistent with scar formation. Disruption of the sinusoidal architecture is evidenced by turbulent flow on CDDU, marking the site of an arteriosinusoidal fistula. In the acute phase of injury, unregulated flow may be imaged without vasoactive injection. In follow-up, low-dosage vasoactive injection is needed; the crural bodies must be imaged from the ventrum (transperineally) by frog-legging the patient and lifting the scrotum.

CDDU: staging of Peyronie's disease

Surgical staging of Peyronie's disease must address both penile form and function. The tunica albuginea and dorsal vascular complex are well imaged with CDDU. A standoff wedge increases near-field resolution, bringing dorsal plaques into view. The tunica albuginea is normally hyperechoic compared with the corpora proper. As the corporal bodies distend with blood, the cavernous sinusoids become more hypo-echoic, increasing the contrast between the tunica and corpora. Penile plaques are hyperechoic thickenings of the tunica albuginea. The typical dorsal plaque underlies the dorsal vasculature (Fig. 22.23). Denser plaques cast an acoustic shadow and are well visualized in either the transverse or sagittal planes.

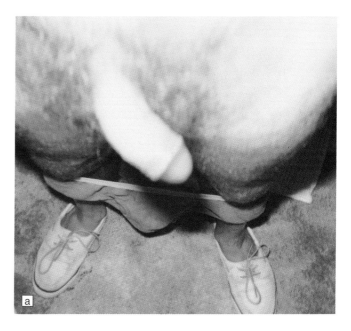

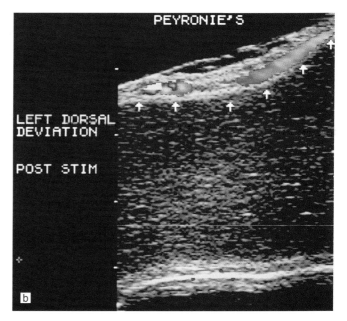

Figure 22.23. (a) The only mandatory imaging in Peyronie's disease is the home photograph of the best erection. (b) Dorsal scan shows Peyronie's deviation in the same patient as in Figure 22.23(a).

Although most plaques localize to the proximal and middle third of the pendulous shaft, distal plaques, even at the level of the corona, may exert minimal curvature. Circumferential narrowing of the corporal bodies by plaque sonographically results in an hour-glass shape to the erection; the patient complains of 'hinging' with erection (Fig. 22.24); the sonographic correlate is a ring of thickened tunica. A similar but focal wedge is seen when penile deviation is lateral. Septal fibrosis is the most technically challenging abnormality to demonstrate. If increased tissue density is discrete, hyperechoic aggregates within the septum are seen. More diffuse septal fibrosis is identified by scanning in a sagittal plane parallel to the septum; from this vantage, the denser septal fibres take on a veil-like appearance with posterior acoustical shadowing. In cases where acoustic shadowing is generated by dense plaques, plain radiographs should follow CDDU.

Potentially, the most useful preoperative staging information is the demonstration of collaterals from the dorsal vascular bundle. Dorsal artery collaterals diving downwards through the tunica to anastomose with the ipsilateral cavernous artery may be in close proximity. Operative mobilization of the neurovascular bundle for plaque excision in these cases would, of necessity, sacrifice the dorsal contribution to cavernous inflow (Fig. 22.25). The author has not been able to visualize

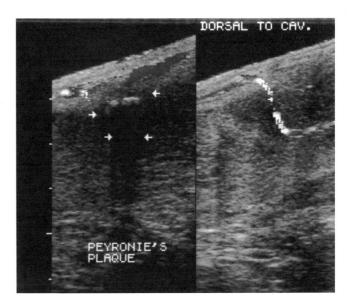

Figure 22.25. Peyronie's plaque of dorsum casts an acoustic shadow; calcification should be suspected. The dorsal artery provides a significant collateral to the cavernous artery; this collateral must be sacrificed on plaque excision.

plaque-associated vein leakage (as some investigators have documented) on dynamic cavernosography, but it is very difficult with current technology to image emissary veins, despite the fact that these are ubiquitous.[91] The author's experience with CDDU suggests that high-resolution sonography not only provides a dynamic non-invasive vascular assessment of erectile function but also can localize penile plaques precisely. Timing must take into account the dynamic phases of erection, the fact that penile pain may pre-empt complete smooth muscle relaxation, and the obstacle that severe penile deviations present to imaging. The plaque should be imaged at 5–10 minutes in the latent/tumescent phase while the penis may still be straightened by the examiner, before rigidity.

■ REFINEMENTS IN PBFS

Age-related changes in erection

As discussed above, age-related decreases in erectile function have long been evident in clinical series and have now been verified in normative community groups, as in the MMAS.[4] Wespes and colleagues[92] have observed an age-related decrease in smooth muscle content, using computerized morphometry of penile biopsies. Comparing young patients with penile

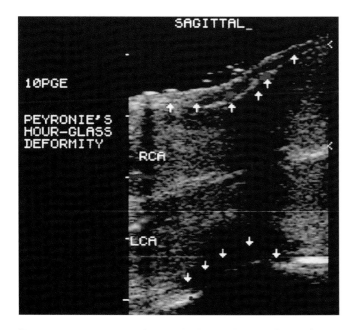

Figure 22.24. Circumferential plaque: hyperechoic plaque (arrows) casts an acoustic shadow.

curvature but haemodynamically adequate erections, with elderly patients with erectile dysfunction, they found that young patients (with penile curvature) have corpora cavernosa composed of 40–52% smooth muscle; patients with corporal veno-occlusive dysfunction have 19–36% smooth muscle and patients with arterial impotence have 10–25% smooth muscle, with collagen content correspondingly increased.

CDDU haemodynamic parameters of a normal erection do seem to vary with age. In a retrospective review of 600 cases, 106 instances where intracavernous challenge with PGE1 produced excellent well-sustained rigidity of at least 20 minutes were documented in patients of various ages. PBFS parameters were recorded 5–10 minutes following PGE1 injection and repeated following privacy and self-stimulation. Mean PGE1 dosages producing excellent erections by age group were as follows: 5μg, (20–49 years); 6μg, (50–59 years); 10μg, (60–79 years). Rigid erection following privacy and self-stimulation was associated with RI/PSV values of: 0.95/54 (cm/s) in 20–29-year-old men; 0.93/45 (cm/s) in 30–49-year-old men; 0.94/33 (cm/s) in 50–69-year-old men; and 0.96/32 (cm/s) in 70–79-year-old men. The data suggest that, in this group of non-vasculogenic patients (neurogenic or psychogenic ED), cavernous arterial flow decreases with age, but normal corporal dynamics permit penile rigidity across a wide range of PSVs. The technique of privacy and self-stimulation should permit safe and effective diagnostic dosing for the typical patient, with 10μg. The RI parameter did not vary with age, suggesting that the dynamics of veno-occlusion are the critical factor in the ageing erectile response.[93]

Power Doppler

CDDU allows precise non-invasive imaging of penile morphology and dynamics, providing direct evaluation of cavernous arterial inflow and indirectly providing evaluation of cavernous venous outflow. The acquisition of data is facilitated by colour assigned to the duplex image based on the Doppler shift. Banya and colleagues[41] identified two circulatory routes within the penis; erection, they maintain, depends on the terminal helicine arteries, which are multiple muscular and corkscrew-shaped arteries opening directly into the cavernous spaces. Montorsi and colleagues[94] have applied a new development in sonography, known as power Doppler, to the study of penile 'morphodynamics'. With this new technology they visualized three orders of distal ramifications originating from the cavernous arteries (Fig. 22.26). In power Doppler imaging, the hue and brightness of the

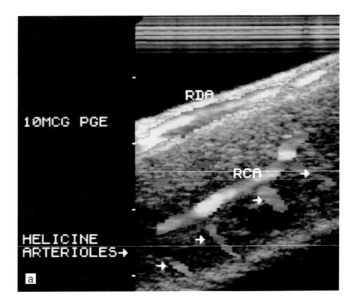

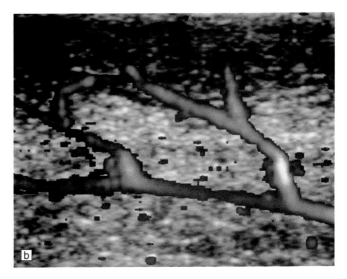

Figure 22.26. (a) Standard colour duplex Doppler scan of the dorsal and cavernous artery (RDA, RCA) with first-order branches of the cavernous artery seen (arrows). (b) Power Doppler scan with three orders of branching seen from the cavernous artery.

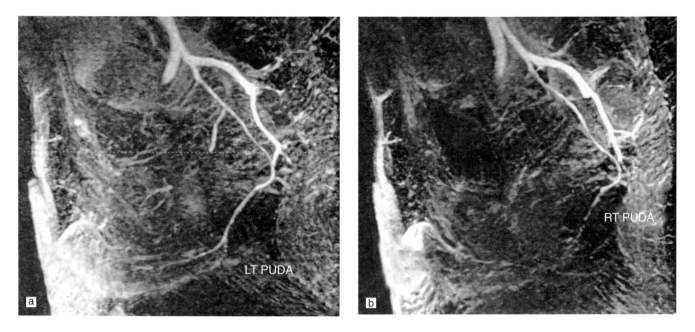

Figure 22.27. (a) Gadolinium-enhanced magnetic resonance angiography in pelvic fracture patient with posterior urethral disruption and impotence. (b) Preoperative imaging 4 months following injury shows pudendal artery flow to perineal and common penile arteries on the left. Right pudendal flow was disrupted by trauma.

signal is a function of the number of flowing red blood cells causing the Doppler shift; the dynamic range of imaging is increased, yielding higher resolution of small vessels with low flows. Further clinical investigations are merited to determine whether this additional 'morphodynamic' information will expand or support the currently utilized classifications of penile vascular disease, which are (a) arterial (PSV < 25 cm/s), (b) veno-occlusive (PSV > 35 cm/s, RI < 0.9) or (c) mixed vascular insufficiency (PSV > 25, < 35 cm/s, RI < 0.9).

Magnetic resonance angiography and pre-penile inflow disease

Numerous studies have documented the accuracy of Doppler imaging in directly diagnosing both penile inflow and penile outflow disease (arterial vs venous impotence). Currently, the author employs angiography only in anticipation of vascular reconstructive surgery, when Doppler imaging suggests that there is a high likelihood of pre-penile inflow disease.

One group of investigators has recently compared penile duplex Doppler with contrast enhanced digital subtraction magnetic resonance angiography (CE-DS-MRA).[95] In 7/11 patients good correlation was seen between the CE-DS-MRA studies and duplex Doppler. MRA localized the disease processes from the iliac down to the IPAs. Of 22 IPAs examined, 27% had occlusions and 23% had stenoses. Resolution of MRA was insufficient to examine penile arteries (cavernous and dorsal), which have diameters of 0.5–1 mm in the erect penis. The clinical utility of non-invasively imaging penile blood supply from the aortic bifurcation down to the IPAs will assume increasing importance when both angiographic correlation and 'angioplastic' therapy are achievable. The author has used this technique in a select number of patients who were undergoing standard magnetic resonance imaging to evaluate the degree of posterior urethral disruption following pelvic fracture, prior to delayed (6 months) posterior urethroplasty. MRA demonstrated an abnormality of pelvic vessels (IPA or common penile artery) in 62% of patients. The lesions were most commonly unilateral in the pelvis, and subsequent CDDU localized the side consistently (PSV < 25 cm/s) (Fig. 22.27).

■ CONCLUSIONS

CDDU is minimally invasive and adds no additional risk to a diagnostic challenge of intracavernous vasoactive agent. CDDU/PBFS should be the first line of testing, if an evidence-based assessment of erectile dysfunction is performed. CDDU/PBFS reveals the penile anatomy as well as corporal haemodynamics. It provides an aetiology-specific diagnosis of vascular erectile dysfunction, differentiating arterial insufficiency from cavernous venous occlusive disease from mixed vascular disease. It is particularly useful in preoperative staging of Peyronie's disease and in selecting candidates for more invasive evaluations (pharmacopenile angiography and DICC). Several important questions about dynamic erectile testing have recently been answered: an intracavernous challenge of 10 µg of PGE1 would appear to be an adequate initial challenge when coupled with genital stimulation or audiovisual stimulation; when pharmacological stimulation alone is used, dosing may need to be higher (20 µg), with redosing after 20 minutes to effect maximal smooth muscle relaxation.

The author's prediction for the future of impotence testing is that men will soon be categorized as having oral-agent-responsive or oral-agent-resistant ED. It is likely that future patients seeking the expertise of urologists will have already tried orally active agents that facilitate erection, such as phosphodiesterase inhibitors, or that promote erection through central nervous system activation, such as apomorphine. These patients will first demand an explanation as to why these agents failed in their cases; ultimately, erectile testing will be relied on to produce 'vascular profiles' for men to predict which single agent or combination of agents will effectively restore their erections.

■ REFERENCES

1. Davis-Joseph B, Tiefer L, Melman A. Accuracy of the initial history and physical examination to establish the etiology of erectile dysfunction. Urology 1995; 45(3): 498–502

2. Lue T F. Intracavernous drug administration: its role in diagnosis and treatment of impotence. Semin Urol 1990; 8(2): 100–106

3. Mellinger B C, Weiss J. Sexual dysfunction in the elderly male. AUA Update Ser 1992; 11(19): 146–152

4. Feldman H A, Goldstein, I, Hatzichristou D G et al. Impotence and its medical and psychosocial correlates: results of the Massachusetts male aging study. Int J Impot Res 1992; 4(suppl2): A17

5. Consensus development conference statement: Impotence. National Institutes of Health. JAMA 1993; 270(1): 83–90

6. Gaskell P. The importance of penile blood pressure in cases of impotence. Cann Med Assoc J 1971; 105: 104

7. Burnett A L, Thayer W S, Allen R P et al. Near infrared diagnosis of vasculogenic impotence. J Urol 1997; 157(4): A693

8. Abelson D. Diagnostic value of the penile pulse and blood pressure: a Doppler study of impotence in diabetics. J Urol 1975; 113: 636

9. Michal V, Kramer R, Pospichal J. External iliac 'steal syndrome'. J Cardiovasc Surg 1978; 19: 355

10. Goldstein I, Siroky M B, North, R I et al. Vasculogenic impotence: role of the pelvic steal test. J Urol 1982; 128–300

11. Schwartz A N, Lowe M A, Ireton R et al. A comparison of penile brachial index and angiography: evaluation of corpora cavernosa arterial inflow. J Urol 1990; 143–510

12. Lue T F, Hricak H, Marich K W, Tanagho E A. Vasculogenic impotence evaluated by high resolution ultrasonography and pulsed Doppler spectrum analysis. Radiology 1985; 155: 777

13. European Perspective on Erectile Dysfunction: Report on a satellite symposium held at the 12th Congress of European Association of Urology, Paris, September, 1996. Pharmacia & Upjohn, UK 8883-0061/3/97

14. Bahren W, Gall H, Scherb W et al. Arterial anatomy and arteriographic diagnosis of arteriogenic impotence. Cardiovasc Intervent Radiol 1988; 11: 195–210

15. Bookstein J J, Lange E V. Penile magnification pharmacoarteriography: details of intrapenile arterial anatomy. Am J Res1987; 148: 883

16. Rajfer J, Canan V, Dorey F J, Mehringer C M. Correlation between penile angiography and duplex scanning of cavernous arteries in impotent men. J Urol 1990; 143: 1128–1130

17. Gall H, Bahren W, Scherb W et al. Diagnostic accuracy of Doppler ultrasound technique of the penile arteries in correlation to selective arteriography. Cardiovasc Intervent Radiol 1988; 11: 225

18. Curet, P, Grellet J, Perrin D et al. Technical and anatomic factors in filling of distal portion of internal pudendal artery during arteriography. Urology 1987; 29: 333

19. Rosen M P, Greenfield A J, Walker T G et al. Arteriogenic impotence: findings in 195 impotent men examined with selective internal pudendal angiography. Radiology 1990; 174: 1043

20. Garibyan H, Lue T F. Anastomotic network between the dorsal and cavernous arteries in the penis. J Urol 1990; 143: 221A

21. Benson C B, Aruny J E, Vickers MA. Correlation of duplex sonography with arteriography in patients with erectile dysfunction. AJR 1993; 160(1): 71–73

22. Bookstein J J. Penile angiography: the last angiographic frontier. AJR 1998; 150(1): 47–54

23. Virag R. Intracavernous injection of papaverine for erectile failure. Lancet 1982; 2: 398

24. Brindley G S. Maintenance treatment of erectile impotence by cavernosal unstriated muscle relaxant injection. Br J Psychiatry 1986; 149: 210

25. Brindley G S. Cavernosal alpha-blockade: a new technique for investigating and treating erectile impotence. Br J Psychiatry 1983; 143: 332–337

26. Zorgniotti A W, Lefleur R S. Auto-injection of the corpus cavernosum with a vasoactive drug combination for vasculogenic impotence. J Urol 1985; 133: 39

27. Ishii N, Watanabe H, Irisawa C et al. Studies on male sexual impotence report 18: therapeutic trial with prostaglandin E1 for organic impotence. Jpn J Urol 1986; 77: 954–962

28. Ishii N, Watanabe H, Irisawa C et al. Intracavernous injection of prostaglandin E1 for the treatment of erectile impotence. J Urol 1991; 146: 1564

29. Bennett A H, Carpenter A J, Barada J H. An improved vasoactive drug combination for pharmacological erection program. J Urol 1991; 146: 1564–5

30. Virag R, Frydman D, Legman M, Virag H. Intracavernous injection of papaverine as a diagnostic and therapeutic method in erectile failure. Angiology 1984; 35–79

31. Lue T F. Impotence: a patient's goal directed approach to treatment. World J Urol 1990; 8: 67

32. Pescatori E S, Hatzichristou D G, Namburi S, Goldstein I. A positive intracavernous injection test implies normal veno-occlusive but not necessarily normal arterial function: a hemodynamic study. J Urol 1994; 151: 1209–1216

33. McMahon C G. An attempt to standardize the pharmacological diagnostic screening of vasculogenic impotence with prostaglandin E1. Int J Impot Res 1995; 7(2): 83–90

34. Broderick G A, Arger P A. Duplex doppler ultrasonography: non invasive assessment of penile anatomy and function. Semin Roentgenol 1993; 28(1): 43–56

35. Landwehr P. Penile vessels: erectile dysfunction. In: Wolf K-J, Fobbe F (eds) Color duplex sonography: principles and clinical application. Stuttgart: Thieme Medical, 1995; 204–215

36. Herbener T E, Seftel A D, Nehra A, Goldstein I. Penile ultrasound. Semin Urol 1994; 12(4): 320–332

37. King B F, Lewis R W, McKusick M A. Radiologic evaluation of impotence. In: Bennett A H (ed) Impotence. Philadelphia: Saunders, 1994; 52–91

38. McAninch J W, Laing F C, Jeffrey R B. Sonourethrography in the evaluation of urethral strictures. J Urol 1988; 139: 294–297

39. Benson C B, Doubilet P M, Richie J P. Sonography of the male genital tract. AJR 1989; 153: 705–713

40. Oates C P, Pickhard P H, Powell P H et al. The use of duplex ultrasound in the assessment of arterial supply to the penis in vasculogenic impotence. J Urol 1995; 153: 354–357.

41. Banya Y, Ushiki T, Takagane H et al. Two circulatory routes within the human corpus cavernosum penis: a scanning electron microscopic study of corrosion casts. J Urol 1989; 142: 879–883

42. Bookstein J J. Cavernosal venocclusive insufficiency in male impotence: evaluation of degree and location. Radiology 1987; 164: 175.

43. Aboseif S R, Lue T F. Hemodynamics of penile erection. Urol Clin North Am 1988; 15: 1–7

44. Andersson K-E, Wagner G. Physiology of penile erection. Physiol Rev 1995; 75(1): 191–236

45. Linet O I, Ogrinc F G. Efficacy and safety of intracavernosal alprostadil in men with erectile dysfunction. N Engl J Med 1996; 334(14): 873–877

46. Schwartz A N, Wang K Y, Mack L A et al. Evaluation of normal erectile function with color flow doppler sonography. AJR 1989; 153: 1155–1160

47. Quam J P, King B F, James E M et al. Duplex and color doppler sonographic evaluation of vasculogenic impotence. AJR 1989; 153: 1141–1147

48. Paushter D M. Role of duplex sonography in the evaluation of sexual impotence. AJR 1989; 153: 1161

49. Collins J P, Lewandowski B J. Experience with intracorporeal injection of papaverine and duplex ultrasound scanning for the assessment of arteriogenic impotence. Br J Urol 1987; 59: 84–88

50. Herbner T E, Seftel A D, Nehra A, Goldstein, I. Penile ultrasound. Semin Urol 1994; 12(4): 320–332

51. Burns P N. Hemodynamics and interpretation of Doppler signals. In: Taylor K J W, Burns P N, Wells P N T. Clinical applications of Doppler ultrasound. New York: Raven Press 1987

52. Burns P N. Physical principles of Doppler ultrasound and spectral analysis. JCU 1987; 15: 567–590

53. Foley W D, Erickson S J. Color Doppler flow imaging. AJR 1991; 156: 3–13

54. Merritt C R. Doppler color flow imaging. JCU 1987; 15: 591–597

55. Broderick G A, Lue T F. The penile blood flow study: evaluation of vasculogenic impotence. In Jonas U, Thon W F, Stief C G (eds) Erectile dysfunction. Berlin: Springer-Verlag, 1991: 126–136

56. Wegner H E H, Andersen R, Knispel H H et al. Evaluation of penile arteries with color coded duplex sonography: prevalence and possible therapeutic implications of connections between dorsal and cavernous arteries in impotent men. J Urol 1995; 153: 1469–1471

57. Paick J S, Won Lee S, Hyup Kim S. Doppler sonography of deep cavernosal artery of the penis: variation of peak systolic velocity according to sampling location. Int J Impot Res 1994; 6(1): A34

58. Chung W S, Park Y Y, Back S Y. The effect of measurement location of the blood flow parameters on their values during Duplex sonography. Int J Impot Res 1994; 6(1): A29

59. Govier F E, Asase D, Hefty T R et al. Timing of penile color flow duplex ultrasonography using a triple drug mixture. J Urol 1995; 153: 1472–1475

60. Meuleman E J H, Bemelmans B L H, Doesburg W H et al. Penile pharmacological duplex ultrasonography: a dose effect study comparing papaverine, papaverine/phentolamine and PGE1. J Urol 1992; 148: 63

61. Fitzgerald S W, Erickson S J, Foley W D et al. Color Doppler sonography in the evaluation of erectile dysfunction: patterns of temporal response to papaverine. AJR 1991; 157: 331–336

62. Patel U, Amin Z, Friedman E et al. Colour flow and spectral Doppler imaging after papaverine induced penile erection in 220 impotent men: study of temporal patterns and the importance of repeated sampling, velocity asymmetry and vascular anomalies. Clin Radiol 1993; 48(1): 18–24

63. Lue T F, Donatucci C F. The combined intracavernous injection and stimulation test: diagnostic accuracy. J Urol 1992; 148: 61–62

64. Montorsi, F, Guazzoni G, Barbieri L et al. The effect of intracorporeal injection plus genital and audiovisual sexual stimulation vs. second injection on penile color doppler sonography parameters. J Urol 1996; 155: 536–540

65. Nehra A, Hakim L S, Abokar R A et al. A new method of performing duplex doppler ultrasonography: effect of re-dosing of vasoactive agents on hemodynamic parameters. J Urol 1995; 153(4): 415A

66. Lue T F, Hricak H, Marich K W, Tanagho E A. Evaluation of arteriogenic impotence with intracorporeal injection of papaverine and the duplex ultrasound scanner. Semin Urol 1987; 3: 43–48

67. Fitzgerald S W, Krysiewicz S, Mellinger C. The role of imaging in the evaluation of impotence. AJR 1989; 153: 1133–1139

68. Golub M, Zia P, Matsuno N, Horton R. Metabolism of prostaglandins A-1 and E-1 in men. J Clin Invest 1979; 59: 1404

69. Hamberg M. Biosynthesis of prostaglandin E1 by human seminal vesicles. Lipids 1976; 11: 249

70. Hedquist P. PGE and prostaglandin synthesis inhibitors of norepinephrine release from vascular tissue. In: Robinson H J, Vane ER (eds) Prostaglandin synthetase inhibitors. New York: Raven Press, 1973: 303

71. Meuleman E F J, Bemelmans B L H, vanAsten W et al. Assessment of penile blood flow by duplex ultrasonography in 44 men with normal erectile potency in different phases of erection. J Urol 1992; 147: 51–56

72. Mellinger B C, Fried J J, Vaughan E D. Papaverine induced penile blood flow acceleration in impotent men measured by duplex scanning. J Urol 1990; 144: 897

73. Lue T F, Tanagho E A. Physiology of erection and pharmacological management of impotence. J Urol 1987; 137: 829

74. Benson C B, Vickers M A. Sexual impotence caused by vascular disease: diagnosis with duplex sonography. AJR 1989; 153: 1149

75. Shabsigh R, Fishman I F, Quesada E T et al. Evaluation of vasculogenic erectile impotence using penile duplex ultrasonography. J Urol 1989; 142: 1469

76. Benson C B, Aruny J E, Vickers M A. Correlation of duplex sonography with arteriography in patients with erectile dysfunction. AJR 1993; 160: 71–73

77. Shabsigh R, Fishman I J, Shottland Y et al. Comparison of penile duplex ultrasonography with nocturnal penile tumescence monitoring for the evaluation of erectile impotence. J Urol 1990; 143: 924

78. Lewis R W, King B F. Dynamic color doppler sonography in the evaluation of penile erectile disorders. Int J Impot Res 1994; 6(1): A30

79. Rhee E, Osborn A, Witt M. The correlation of cavernous systolic occlusion pressure with peak velocity flow using color duplex doppler ultrasound. J Urol 1995; 153: 358–360

80. Schwartz A N, Lowe M A, Berger R E et al. Assessment of normal and abnormal erectile function; color doppler flow sonography vs. conventional techniques. Radiol Sci North Am 1991; 180: 105–109

81. Planiol T, Pourcelot L. Doppler effect study on the carotid circulation. In: de Vlieger M, White D N, McCready V R (eds) Ultrasonics in Medicine. Amsterdam: Excerpta Medica, 1974: 104–111

82. Merckx L A, De Bruyne R M G, Goes E et al. The value of dynamic color duplex scanning in the diagnosis of venogenic impotence. J Urol 1992, 148: 318–320

83. McMahon C G, Daley J. Correlation of duplex ultrasonography, PBI, DICC and angiography in the diagnosis of impotence. Int J Impot Res 1994; 6(1): A32

84. Naroda T, Yamanaka M, Matsushita K et al. Evaluation of resistance index of the cavernous artery with color Doppler ultrasonography for venogenic impotence. Int J Impot Res 1994, 6(1): D62

85. Hinman F, Jr. Priapism, reasons for failure of therapy. J Urol 1960; 83: 420

86. Broderick G A, Lue T F. Priapism and physiology of erection. AUA Update Ser 1988; 7(29): 225–232

87. Broderick G A, Harkaway R. Pharmacologic erection: time-dependent changes in the corporal environment. Int J Impot Res 1994; 6: 9–16

88. Witt M A, Goldstein I, Saenz de Tejada I et al. Traumatic laceration of intracavernosal arteries: the pathophysiology of nonischemic, high flow arterial priapism. J Urol 1990; 143: 129–132

89. Walker T G, Gran P W, Goldstein I et al. High-flow priapism: treatment with superselective transcatheter embolization. Radiology 1990; 174: 1053–1054

90. Hakim L S, Kulaksizoglu H, Mulligan R et al. Evolving concepts in the diagnosis and treatment of arterial high flow priapism. J Urol 1996;155: 541–548

91. Gasior B L, Levine F J, Sowannesian A et al. Plaque associated corporal veno-occlusive dysfunction in idiopathic Peyronie's disease: a pharmacocavernosometric and pharmacocavernosographic study. World J Urol 1990; 8(2): 90

92. Wespes E, deGoes P M, Schulman C. Vascular impotence: focal or diffuse penile disease. J Urol 1992; 148: 1435–1436

93. Broderick G A, Arger P A. Penile blood flow study: age specific reference ranges. J Urol 1994; 151(5): A371

94. Sasteschi L M, Montorsi F, Fabris F M et al. Cavernous arterial and arteriolar circulation in patients with erectile dysfunction: power doppler study. J Urol 1998; 159: 428–432

95. Stehling M K, Liu L, Laub G et al. Gadolinium enhanced magnetic resonance angiography of the pelvis in patients with erectile impotence. Magn Reson Mat Phys Biol Med 1997; 5(3): 247

Chapter 23

Neurophysiological testing in erectile dysfunction

R. Beck and C. J. Fowler

■ INTRODUCTION

Several methods exist that claim to test the integrity of the nerves involved in the erectile pathway but, when examined carefully, none is without limitations. This chapter outlines the methodology and interpretation of the neurophysiological investigations currently available and critically analyses their use in the clinical investigation of erectile dysfunction.

Two major neurological pathways of erection are described, namely psychogenic and reflexogenic. The nerves involved in the initiation and maintenance of an erection via these two pathways are different, although the final vascular events within the penis are the same. Reflexogenic erections are produced by direct stimulation of the genital organs and are a spinal cord reflex, whereas psychogenic erections are the result of cortical activity stimulated by audiovisual or olfactory stimuli, or fantasy.[1] Any condition or injury that impairs transmission of impulses along any of these pathways may be associated with neurogenic erectile dysfunction. The common disorders are listed in Table 23.1.

Although the efferent component of these pathways from spinal cord to cavernosal tissue is autonomic, standard neurophysiological assessment of neurogenic erectile dysfunction relies on tests of the somatic nervous system, such as the bulbocavernosus reflex, the pudendal evoked response and single motor unit evaluation of urethral sphincter electromyography (EMG). Concern about the sensitivity of these investigations in the diagnosis of erectile dysfunction has encouraged some investigators to explore methods of testing the autonomic nervous system. It is this area that has attracted much recent research and has led to

the development of corpus cavernosum EMG (CC-EMG).[2]

The first part of this chapter describes the methodology and assesses the use of the standard neurophysiological

Table 23.1. Disorders commonly associated with neurogenic erectile dysfunction

Intracranial
  Temporal lobe
  Hypothalamus
  Ansa lenticularis

Suprasacral spinal cord disease
  Multiple sclerosis
  Space-occupying lesions
  Trauma

Cauda equina and conus lesions
  Central disc prolapse
  Tethered cord
  Spina bifida
  Vascular malformations

Pelvic nerve damage
  Major pelvic surgery

Small fibre or autonomic neuropathies
  Diabetes
  Amyloid

Multiple system atrophy

tests currently performed in the assessment of erectile dysfunction; the second part explores the theories and controversies surrounding CC-EMG, and other alternative methods of assessing the autonomic nervous system.

PELVIC FLOOR NEUROPHYSIOLOGY

The evaluation of men with erectile dysfunction is not standardized and the indications for the majority of investigations remain controversial. A good history and examination are mandatory and often point towards the cause of the condition. In patients where doubt exists, or no diagnosis is available, further investigation may be performed in some units, although in many cases patients are scheduled to begin on treatment even when the aetiology of their problem remains obscure.

This section covers the neurophysiological tests that may be used to examine the innervation of the genital region. It is divided into parts covering sacral reflex latencies, electromyography and cortical somatosensory evoked potentials.

Sacral reflex testing
Sacral reflexes are reflex contractions of parts of the pelvic floor that occur in response to a stimulus applied either to the perineum, the genitalia or the mucosa of the lower urinary tract. The finding of an absent response, or a response at a prolonged latency, is taken as evidence of neuronal damage in either the afferent or efferent pathways of the reflex arc, or in the cauda equina itself, as the spinal segments that serve these reflexes are S2–S4. The reflexes that can be tested include the bulbocavernosus (BCR), pudendo-anal, vesico-urethral and vesico-anal reflexes. It is only the BCR that has been used extensively in the investigation of erectile dysfunction and it is this test that is described in detail below.

The bulbocavernosus reflex (BCR)
A technique to measure the latency of the BCR was first described by Rushworth in 1967.[3] The dorsal nerve of the penis is repeatedly stimulated with small electrical impulses and the responses recorded using either surface electrodes or a needle electrode in the bulbocavernosus muscle. It is usually easy to elicit the BCR but occasionally the stimulus needed to activate the reflex is too uncomfortable and the test has to be abandoned. Similar responses can be obtained by recording from the striated component of the anal or urethral sphincter.

There are two components to the BCR. The first response, at around 40 ms (Fig. 23.1) is the result of conduction in an oligosynaptic pathway[4] and is the one used clinically; a second, more variable, response is often found at approximately 70 ms. Most investigators have used a concentric needle electrode to record from the bulbocavernosus muscles and report the minimum latency of a number of consecutive raw EMG responses.[5]

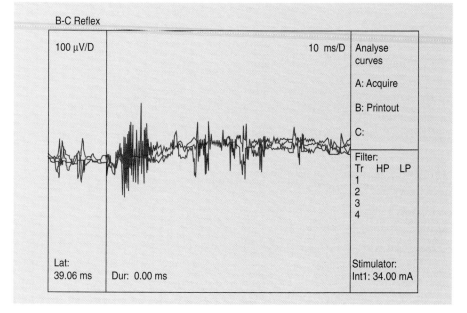

B-C Reflex		
100 µV/D	10 ms/D	Analyse curves
		A: Acquire
		B: Printout
		C:
		Filter: Tr HP LP 1 2 3 4
Lat: 39.06 ms	Dur: 0.00 ms	Stimulator: Int1: 34.00 mA

Figure 23.1. Normal bulbocavernosus reflex (BCR) recorded with a needle electrode inserted into the bulbocavernosus muscle.

Clinical applications

Theoretically, neurophysiological investigation of the BCR might identify both peripheral neuropathic damage to the pudendal nerve and lesions of the cauda equina. However transmission in the autonomic nervous system is not assessed by the BCR and extrapolating from the results of these tests in patients with erectile dysfunction may result in misleading conclusions.

In early studies it was found that many patients with neurogenic impotence due to either cauda equina or lower motor neuron lesions had abnormally prolonged or absent BCR responses (Fig. 23.2).[6,7] However, in some patients with cauda equina lesions the response was normal[8,9] and the sensitivity of the test was not high. In patients with an advanced peripheral neuropathy, latency measurements may be increased or the amplitude of the response decreased. This latter finding is of little clinical significance in the individual patient, however, because the amplitude of a response depends to a large extent on the site of the recording electrode relative to the motor unit, and large variations in amplitude can occur with small changes of needle position.

BCR testing has been used to test diabetic patients with erectile dysfunction,[10–13] and although it is possible to show a delay of the response in some patients (especially those with a severe peripheral neuropathy), in others, also with presumed neurogenic impotence, the test can be normal.[13,14] In a recent study of 300 patients, Ho and colleagues[15] examined the relationship of the BCR response to potency, diabetic status and age. A significant trend towards increasing BCR latency with age was evident but there was no significant correlation with potency, although diabetic men in general were more likely to have a prolonged latency.[15] Furthermore, the response may be prolonged in some men with normal sexual function but with a significant generalized neuropathy, as shown by Vodusek and Zidar when testing patients with hereditary motor and sensory neuropathy.[16]

The value of testing sacral reflexes in patients with suspected neurogenic impotence remains doubtful. The test is useful clinically in confirming the suspicion of a cauda equina lesion in patients with otherwise mild neurological signs. It is a poor test of peripheral neuropathy and does not assess transmission in autonomic fibres at all.

Measurement of cortical evoked responses from the genitourinary tract

An objective assessment of the integrity of the sensory pathways from the periphery to the cortex can be made by recording somatosensory evoked potentials. Measurement of tibial and median nerve evoked potentials have been routine in neurophysiological departments for the last two decades. In 1982, Haldeman and colleagues[17] recorded cortical evoked potentials in response to stimulation of the dorsal nerves of the penis. Other investigators have confirmed the original data and the control values are now well accepted.[18]

Somatosensory evoked potentials are a form of electroencephalographic activity and describe changes in

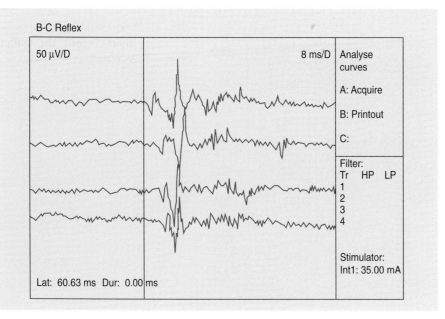

Figure 23.2. Prolonged BCR from a patient with a long-standing cauda equina lesion and impotence.

the electrical potential of neurons in the central nervous system. The cortical electrical response to stimulation of a somatic nerve is of very low amplitude — of the order of 1μV — and cannot on its own be differentiated from the background electroencephalography (EEG). However, by repeating the stimulus to the peripheral nerve at regular intervals many hundreds of times, and averaging the segment of EEG time-locked to the stimulus, the response becomes increasingly obvious and contamination from random background activity diminishes (see Fig. 23.3a). Somatosensory evoked potentials are recorded with EEG electrodes over the sensory cortex.

The waveform of the pudendal evoked potential (PEP) is of similar shape and latency to that of the tibial and consists of a series of consecutive peaks and troughs (Fig. 23.3b). The relative delay in conduction of the pudendal response is thought to occur at both peripheral and spinal cord level, where the sensory information ascends in slower pathways than in the tibial nerves. Difficulty in interpretation can occur, as it can be very easy to miss the small initial response and measure the latency to the second negative deflection. With latencies of 60 ms or greater, clinically apparent spinal cord dysfunction is likely to be present; if not, either the result

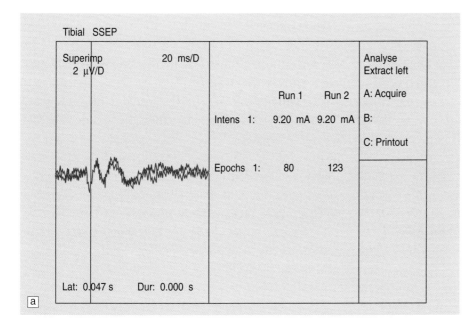

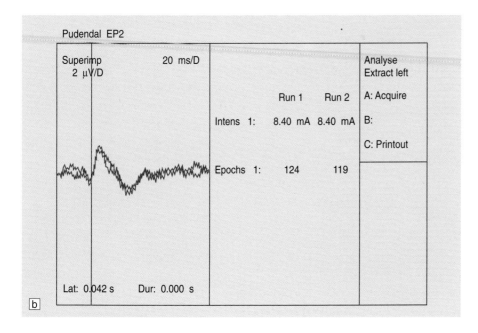

Figure 23.3. Normal tibial (a) and pudendal (b) evoked responses. The shape and latencies of the responses are similar, although the tibial evoked potential is invariably larger and, hence, easier to record.

has been misinterpreted or further detailed tests of spinal cord function are appropriate. Such abnormally prolonged latencies are not found in patients with peripheral neuropathy.[15,19]

Clinical uses

Some urologists have used pudendal evoked response testing as part of their screening tests in the investigation of impotence. Several studies have reported that the latency of the PEP is prolonged in patients with impotence of spinal cord origin: Kirkeby and colleagues[20] found the response abnormal in 26 of 29 impotent men with multiple sclerosis (MS); Betts and colleagues[21] found that 38 of 46 impotent men with MS had prolonged latencies. However, the sensitivity of the test in assessing spinal cord disease is uncertain, as six of the eight patients with normal responses in this series had definite clinical evidence of spinal cord pathology. A further area of controversy is whether the test adds any specific information to what can be obtained by careful clinical examination or measurement of the lower limb evoked potentials that are routinely recorded.

In a recent study, Bemelsman and colleagues[22] found that the PEP was delayed or unrecordable in 21 of 123 patients (17%) with no clinically demonstrable neurological disorder. In only four of these patients was the tibial evoked potential also abnormal. The authors therefore concluded that subclinical peripheral neuropathies were important in the aetiology of impotence but in general it is unusual to find significant abnormalities in evoked potentials in patients with no clinical signs of a sensory neuropathy or myelopathy.

Anal or urethral sphincter EMG

Lesions causing neuronal damage between the anterior horn cells in Onuf's nucleus and the striated portion of the anal and urethral sphincter muscles result in denervation of the sphincter muscle. If the injury is complete, only fibrillation potentials can be recorded electromyographically and the muscle remains electrically silent on attempted recruitment; however, the majority of lesions are incomplete and result in only partial denervation. Subsequent re-innervation of the muscle results in the remaining motor units becoming polyphasic with an increased duration and amplitude. Changes of denervation and re-innervation in the urethral or anal sphincter are indicative of lower motor neuron lesions affecting the S2–S4 myotomes. Damage

may occur in the sacral segment of the spinal cord, the cauda equina or peripherally in the pelvis and may result in erectile dysfunction. Analysis of sphincter EMG has been used to identify somatic nerve injury at all these sites.

Analysis of individual motor units requires recording with a concentric needle electrode or single-fibre needle electrode and an EMG system that has a trigger and delay line facility. Either sphincter can be recorded from: to record from the male urethral sphincter the man lies in the left lateral position and the needle is introduced through the perineum in the midline, approximately 4 cm in front of the anus, being guided towards the apex of the prostate by a finger in the rectum. Accurate positioning of the needle is aided by listening for the tonically firing motor units of the striated muscle activity. Recordings from a normal motor unit are illustrated in Figure 23.4. Both urethral and anal sphincter EMG are abnormal in cauda equina lesions. Clinically, partial cauda equina lesions are easily missed because the resultant sensory loss may be very minor and anal sphincter tone only slightly reduced, yet impotence may still occur. Sphincter EMG is a useful contributory test in these situations and is probably a more sensitive test of denervation than is the BCR. An abnormally prolonged motor unit from a patient with a partial cauda equina lesion secondary to an arteriovenous malformation in the spinal cord is shown in Figure 23.5.

Sphincter EMG has also been used to investigate pudendal nerve injury in patients with erectile and voiding dysfunction following major pelvic surgery.[23] An abnormality either in duration or amplitude was found in 64% of motor units recorded from patients who had undergone pelvic surgery, compared with 8% in the control group. Multiple system atrophy is a degenerative condition of the central nervous system characterized by a combination of impotence, lower urinary tract symptoms, autonomic failure, and extrapyramidal and cerebellar dysfunction.[24] The anterior horn cells of the striated urethral and anal sphincter that lie within Onuf's nucleus are selectively affected by the disease.[25] This results in denervation of both sphincters with subsequent EMG changes of re-innervation on sphincter EMG such that sphincter EMG has become a major tool in the investigation of this disorder, the first symptom of which is often erectile dysfunction.[26]

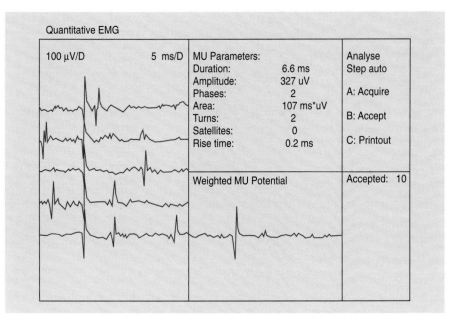

Figure 23.4. Normal motor unit recorded with a needle electrode from the striated part of the external urethral sphincter.

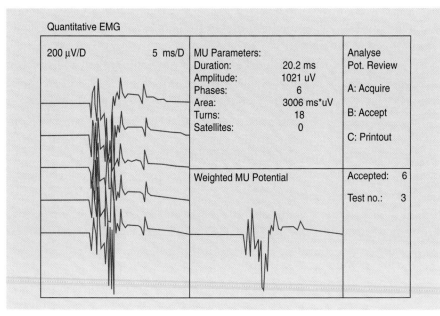

Figure 23.5. Abnormal motor unit from a man with erectile dysfunction secondary to an arteriovenous malformation in the spinal cord. The motor unit is prolonged and polyphasic, compared with the normal unit shown in Figure 23.4.

■ AUTONOMIC FUNCTION TESTING

Clinically, the integrity of the autonomic nervous system is assessed by measuring physiological responses to parasympathetic or sympathetic stimulation, rather than by measuring transmission in the nerves themselves.

In neurological practice, autonomic function testing is used in the diagnosis of generalized autonomic failure and only rarely in the identification of a localized abnormality. Most investigations relate either to the general control of circulation or to sweat production.

Cardiovascular autonomic function tests measure changes in heart rate variability and blood pressure in response to deep breathing, changes in posture from lying to standing, cold stimuli, isometric exercise, sudden inspiratory gasps or Valsalva manoeuvre. These manoeuvres alter autonomic activity so that failure to respond adequately to them is indicative of autonomic impairment. Using a combination of tests, differentiation between generalized cardiovascular sympathetic and parasympathetic failure can be achieved.

The sympathetic nervous system also regulates sweat gland activity, which can be evaluated using techniques that gauge sweat production. One such technique measures the change in voltage on the skin surface secondary to sweat production and is known as the sympathetic skin response (SSR). First described by Tarchanoff at the end of the nineteenth century,[27] the SSR has been used in the investigation of erectile dysfunction. It is described in more detail in conjunction with cavernosal EMG.

AUTONOMIC FUNCTION TESTING IN IMPOTENCE

A correlation exists between the results of certain autonomic function tests and neurogenic erectile dysfunction, although a wide range of variability is reported amongst different studies. Kunesch and colleagues[28] found that, of 30 selected patients with impotence, 53% had abnormal heart rate variability to both deep inspiration and standing, indicating generalized parasympathetic impairment. In a larger study of 542 consecutive impotent men of mixed aetiology, 14% had reduced heart-rate variability.[29] In patients with diabetes this figure rose to over 20% abnormal. Quadri and colleagues[30] reported abnormal cardiovascular responses to deep breathing in 21/38 (55%) men with diabetic impotence, but 26% of potent diabetics also had abnormal results. Robinson and colleagues[31] found that cardiovascular autonomic function testing was not accurate or predictive in identifying neuropathy as a cause of impotence in 50 impotent men.

These tests investigated only generalized cardiovascular autonomic failure and overlooked possible focal or regional abnormalities in peripheral or central autonomic nerve function. It is not surprising, therefore, that abnormal cardiovascular results have been found in some patients with normal erectile function, and vice versa.

Corpus cavernosum EMG and sympathetic skin responses

In 1989, Wagner and colleagues[2] showed that electrical activity could be recorded from the corpus cavernosum using concentric needle electrodes. This bioelectrical activity was termed corpus cavernosum electromyography (CC-EMG). A compressed time-base hindered analysis of individual electrical potentials. An overall decrease in activity was noted in normal subjects in response to visual sexual stimulation, with the conclusion that this represented a reduction in sympathetic activity in the penis allowing for smooth muscle relaxation and penile erection. Stief and colleagues[32] extended the time-base and analysed what originally was thought to be individual cavernosal smooth muscle potentials. This form of recording was given the acronym SPACE — single-potential analysis of cavernosal EMG. In 1992, Stief and colleagues[33] recorded CC-EMG with surface electrodes placed on the penile skin overlying the corpora cavernosa (Fig. 23.6). In seven of eight patients, surface electrical activity was

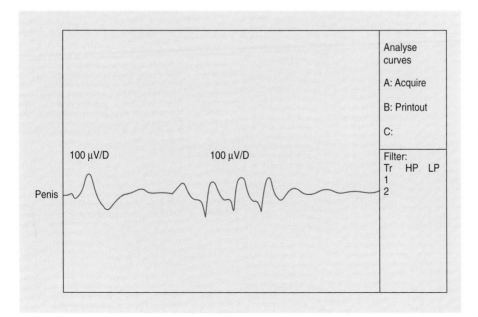

Figure 23.6. CC-EMG recorded with surface electrodes placed on the penile skin using a Dantec Counterpoint. The illustration represents 20 s of the recording at a speed of 1 s per division. The electrical potentials shown were originally termed SPACE — single-potential analysis of cavernosal EMG.

synchronous with needle CC-EMG, and was of similar shape, amplitude and duration. These findings were corroborated by Merckx and colleagues[34] and, together with Stief, they concluded that SPACE recordings were an important part of the armamentarium in the diagnosis of neurogenic impotence. It soon became apparent, however, that the reported bioelectric activity could not represent single cavernosal smooth muscle potentials and therefore the term SPACE was abandoned at the First International Workshop on CC-EMG in 1993.[35] Further controversy followed when Bemelmans and colleagues[36] measured CC-EMG in 40 patients with erectile dysfunction and concluded that, although there did seem to be a physiological basis for the derived potentials, the type and degree of activity did not correlate with any physiological process in the penis itself. Moreover, activity recorded with surface electrodes did not always match that obtained simultaneously from needle electrodes.

Other investigators have shown that potentials similar to CC-EMG can be recorded from surface electrodes placed on the limb of a patient.[37,38] The duration, amplitude and shape of the so-called SPACE waveforms recorded with surface electrodes on the penis were very similar to those obtained when recording perineal, penile and limb sympathetic skin responses (SSRs) (Fig. 23.7). The concept that CC-EMG and SSR are closely related bears further discussion.

The changes in skin resistance that occur following various internally generated or externally applied arousal stimuli result from an increase in sweat gland activity mediated by the sympathetic nervous system, and lead to changes in skin voltage that can be recorded using two surface electrodes. This response is termed SSR.[39] Stimuli used to elicit an SSR have included deep inspiration, startling or painful stimuli or electrical impulses applied to peripheral nerves. When recorded on neurophysiological apparatus, the response appears as a slow depolarization of the skin. This is thought to originate from synchronized activation of sweat glands as a response to a discharge in efferent sympathetic nerve fibres. SSR responses recorded from the limbs can be used in the detection of mixed axonal neuropathies.[40] Ertekin and colleagues[41] were the first to measure the SSR on the genital skin. The recording electrodes were placed on the mons pubis (active) and the dorsum of the penis (reference) and a variety of different stimuli were used to elicit a response, including electrical stimuli to the median nerve at the wrist, the peroneal nerve at the knee and the dorsal nerve of the penis. The SSR could be recorded from the genitalia in normal subjects but the response was absent in some diabetics with erectile dysfunction, both with and without a previously diagnosed polyneuropathy.[42,43]

The similarities between the SSR and CC-EMG suggest that the electrobiological activity claimed as CC-EMG may not originate in cavernosal smooth muscle. The SSR occurs secondary to sudomotor sympathetic nerve activity, with the potential originating from sweat glands and adjacent epidermal and dermal tissues. Some

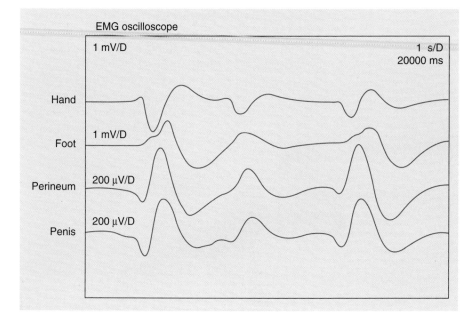

Figure 23.7. Sympathetic skin responses (SSRs) recorded with surface electrodes from the hand, foot, penile skin and perineum using recording parameters identical to those used for recording skin CC-EMG. The recordings from the penile skin are similar in shape and duration to those known to represent SSRs from the limbs.

of the potential is the result of movement of ions across the membrane of sweat gland cells onto the skin surface. The latency, shape and duration of the potential of the SSR (in response to an arousal stimulus) reflects central conduction time, postganglionic peripheral sympathetic conduction, transmission across the neuroendocrine end plate to the sweat gland itself and then the movement of ions from the sweat gland onto the skin surface itself.

Previous studies on CC-EMG both by Stief and colleagues[32] and Merckx and colleagues[34] have recognized that the recorded potentials are sympathetically mediated. Stief showed that mental stimulation increased the frequency of the potentials — a feature known to occur with the sympathetic skin response; Merckx and colleagues commented that the initial 10 min of a CC-EMG recording after cavernosal needle insertion showed excessive activity because of the pain and stress experienced by the subject, and related this to a high degree of sympathetic activity.

Are the recordings of CC-EMG made with surface electrodes actually recordings of sympathetic sudomotor sweat gland activity, or is it possible that two different types of sympathetically induced electrical activity are being recorded on the penile skin simultaneously? While making recordings it may be observed that there are occasions when potentials are present on the genital skin only, with no electrical activity being recorded elsewhere. However, these potentials bear a striking resemblance to the SSR. A possible explanation is that there is a differential autonomic outflow to the various parts of the sudomotor system, so that not all sweat glands are activated simultaneously and it is highly likely that the sweat glands in the perineum have a different role to those elsewhere.

In the authors' minds, these findings raise doubts about the origin of recordings made with surface electrodes and (by inference) also those made by needle electrodes. However, recordings with needle electrodes have been made in vivo following de-gloving of the penis, when it would be expected that no SSR could be recorded. Further research is clearly needed.

Whatever the source of the activity, further scientific evaluation is needed. Meanwhile it must be remembered that there is good evidence that these recordings represent some form of autonomic activity on the genital skin, which is an improvement on many of the other neurophysiological tests used in evaluation of erectile dysfunction.

CONCLUSIONS

Reviewing these various neurophysiological techniques, it becomes clear that there is no single test currently available that will differentiate between neurogenic and psychogenic erectile dysfunction. The standard and well-described pelvic floor tests assess only transmission in the somatic nervous system, whereas the significance of the nature of the responses recorded from the penis by CC-EMG remains controversial.

REFERENCES

1. De Groat W C. Neurophysiology of the pelvic organs. In: Rushton D (ed) Handbook of Neuro-urology. New York: Marcel Dekker, 1993: 55–93
2. Wagner G, Gerstenberg T, Levin R J. Electrical activity of corpus cavernosum during flaccidity and erection of the human penis: a new diagnostic method? J Urol 1989; 142: 723–725
3. Rushworth G. Diagnostic value of the electromyographic study of reflex activity in man. Electroencephalogr Clin Neurophysiol 1967; 25: 65–73
4. Vodusek D B, Janko M. The bulbocavernosus reflex. Brain 1990; 113: 813–820
5. Hassouna M, Lebel M, Abdel-Rahman M, Elhilali M. Evoked potential of the sacral arc reflex: technical aspects. Neurourol Urodyn 1986; 5: 543–553
6. Ertekin C, Reel F. Bulbocavernosus reflex in normal men and in patients with neurogenic bladder and/or impotence. J Neurol Sci 1976; 28: 1–15
7. Dick H C, Bradley W E, Scott F B, Timm G W. Pudendal sexual reflexes: electrophysiological investigations. Urology 1974; 3: 376–379
8. Bilkey W J, Awad E A, Smith A D. Clinical application of sacral reflex latency. J Urol 1983; 129: 1187–1189
9. Blaivas J G, Zayed A A H, Labib K B. The bulbocavernosus reflex in urology: a prospective study of 299 patients. J Urol 1981; 126: 197–199
10. Sarica Y, Karacan I. Bulbocavernosus reflex to somatic and visceral nerve stimulation in normal subjects and in diabetics with erectile impotence. J Urol 1987; 138: 55–58
11. Kaneko S, Bradley W E. Penile electrodiagnosis. Value of bulbocavernosus reflex latency versus nerve conduction velocity of the dorsal nerve of the penis in diagnosis of diabetic impotence. J Urol 1987; 137: 933–935
12. Tackmann W, Porst H, Van Ahlen H. Bulbocavernosus reflex latencies and somatosensory evoked potentials after pudendal nerve stimulation in the diagnosis of impotence. J Neurol 1988; 235: 219–225
13. Desai K, Dembny K, Morgan H et al. Neurophysiological investigation of diabetic impotence. Are sacral response studies of value? Br J Urol 1988; 61: 68–73

14. Siracusano S, Aiello I, Sau G F et al. Bulbocavernosus reflex and somatosensory evoked potential of the pudendal nerve in diabetic impotence. Arch Esp Urol 1992; 45, 549–551

15. Ho K H, Ong B K, Chong P N, Teo W L. The bulbocavernosus reflex in the assessment of neurogenic impotence in diabetic and non-diabetic men. Ann Acad Med Singapore 1996; 25: 558–561

16. Vodusek D B, Zidar J. Pudendal nerve involvement in patients with hereditary motor and sensory neuropathy. Acta Neurol Scand 1987; 76: 457–460

17. Haldeman S, Bradley W E, Bhatia N. Evoked responses from the pudendal nerve. J Urol 1982; 128: 974–980

18. Fowler C J. Pelvic floor neurophysiology. In: Ossleton J (ed) Clinical neurophysiology. Oxford: Butterworth-Heinemann, 1995: 233–252

19. Ziegler D, Muhlen H, Dannehl K, Gries F A. Tibial somatosensory evoked potentials at various stages of peripheral neuropathy in insulin dependent diabetic patients. J Neurol Neurosurg Psychiatry 1993; 56: 58–64

20. Kirkeby H J, Poulsen E U, Petersen T, Dorup J. Erectile dysfunction in multiple sclerosis. Neurology 1988; 38: 1366–1371

21. Betts C D, Jones S, Fowler C G, Fowler C J. Erectile dysfunction in multiple sclerosis. Brain 1994; 117: 1303–1310

22. Bemelmans B L H, Meuleman E J H, Anten B W M et al. Penile sensory disorders in erectile dysfunction. J Urol 1991; 146: 777–780

23. Kirby R, Fowler C J, Gilpin S A et al. Bladder muscle biopsy and urethral sphincter EMG in patients with bladder dysfunction after pelvic surgery. J R Soc Med 1986; 79: 270–273

24. Graham J G, Oppenheimer D R. Orthostatic hypotension and nicotine sensitivity in a case of multiple system atrophy. J Neurol Neurosurg Psychiatry 1969; 32: 28–32

25. Sung J H, Mastri A R, Segal E. Pathology of the Shy–Drager syndrome. J Neuropathol Exp Neurol 1978; 38: 253–268

26. Beck R O, Betts C D, Fowler C J. Genito-urinary dysfunction in multiple system atrophy. A review of 62 cases. J Urol 1994; 151: 1336–1341

27. Tarchanoff J. Uber die galvanischen Erscheinungen an der haut des menschen bei Reizungder Sinnesorgane und bei verschiedenen Formen der psychischen Tatigkeit. Pflugens Arch Ges Physiol 1890; 46: 46–55

28. Kunesch E, Reiners K, Muller-Mathias V et al. Neurological risk profile in organic erectile impotence. J Neurol Neurosurg Psychiatry 1992; 55: 275–281

29. Nisen H O, Larsen A, Lindstrom B L et al. Cardiovascular reflexes in the neurological evaluation of impotence. Br J Urol 1993; 71: 199–203

30. Quadri R, Veglio M, Flecchia D et al. Autonomic neuropathy and sexual impotence in diabetic patients: analysis of cardiovascular reflexes. Andrologia 1989; 21:346–352

31. Robinson L Q, Woodcock J P, Stephenson T P. Results of investigation of impotence in patients with overt or probable neuropathy. Br J Urol 1987; 60: 583–587

32. Stief C G, Djamilian M, Schaebsdau F et al. Single potential analysis of cavernous electric activity — a possible diagnosis of autonomic impotence? World J Urol 1990; 8: 75–79

33. Stief C G, Thon W F, Djamilian M et al. Transcutaneous registration of cavernous smooth muscle electrical activity: noninvasive diagnosis of neurogenic autonomic impotence. J Urol 1992; 147: 47–50

34. Merckx L A, De Bruyne R M, Keuppens F I. Electromyography of cavernous smooth muscle during flaccidity: evaluation of technique and normal values. Br J Urol 1993; 72: 353–358

35. Junemann K P, Buhrle C P, Stief C G. Current trends in impotence research. Conclusions of the first international workshop on smooth muscle EMG recordings. Int J Impot Res 1993; 5: 105–108

36. Bemelmans B L H. Critical appraisal of the electrical activity of cavernous smooth muscles. MD Thesis, 1991

37. Yarnitsky D, Sprecher E, Barilan Y, Vardi Y. Corpus cavernosum electromyogram: spontaneous and evoked electrical activities. J. Urol 1995; 153: 653–654

38. Beck R O. Personal communication, 1995

39. Schondorf R. The role of the sympathetic skin response in the assessment of autonomic function. In: Low P (ed) Clinical autonomic disorders. Evaluation and management. Boston: Little, Brown, 1993: 231–241

40. Shahani B T, Halperin J J, Boulu P, Cohen J. Sympathetic skin response — a method of assessing unmyelinated axon dysfunction in peripheral neuropathies. J Neurol Neurosurg Psychiatry 1984; 47: 536–542

41. Ertekin C, Ertekin N, Mutlu S et al. Skin potentials recorded from the extremities and genital regions in normal and impotent subjects. Acta Neurol Scand 1987; 76: 28–36

42. Opsomer R J, Boccasena P, Traversa R, Rossini P M. Sympathetic skin responses from the limbs and genitalia: normative study and contribution to the evaluation of neuro-urological disorders. Electroencephalogr Clin Neurophysiol 1996; 101: 25–31

43. Ertekin C, Ertekin N, Almis S. Autonomic sympathetic nerve involvement in diabetic impotence. Neurourol Urodyn 1989; 8: 589–598

Chapter 24

Nocturnal penile tumescence and rigidity monitoring for the evaluation of erectile dysfunction

L. A. Levine

INTRODUCTION

Although the evaluation of the impotent male remains a difficult task, which is unlikely to be completed by any single test, nocturnal penile tumescence (NPT) monitoring is considered to be an invaluable tool for the assessment and appropriate management of erectile dysfunction. As an objective, non-invasive measure of erectile activity, NPT is also an integral method in differentiating between psychogenic and organic impotence. Furthermore, NPT testing has become an essential research tool for the objective assessment of various pharmacological therapies and technological advances in the analysis and treatment of the impotent male.

In 1940, NPT was first described in infants by Halverson[1] and, in 1944, a cycle of sleep erections in men aged 20–40 years was characterized by Ohlmeyer.[2] Aserinsky and Kleitman first described rapid eye movement (REM) sleep in 1953 and later recognized that nocturnal erections seemed to correspond with REM periods during normal sleep.[3] It was not until 1965 that Fisher, Karacan and their associates suggested that NPT monitoring can be a valuable resource in the assessment of erectile dysfunction.[4–14] Fisher reported that, in the normal male, three to five erections occur nightly and account for up to 40% of sleep time.[4] In 1966, Karacan reported that 80% of nocturnal erections occurred during REM sleep.[8] In 1975, he described NPT in healthy males between the ages of 3 and 79 years during normal sleep and reported that the amount of NPT was age related.[9–10]

In 1970, Karacan further suggested that NPT testing might provide insight into distinguishing between organic and psychogenic impotence.[11] He assumed that psychological factors inhibiting a sexually induced erection while awake would be inoperative during sleep and, in males with psychogenic causes of impotence, NPT would be present. However, in men with impotence due to neurological and/or vascular factors, the mechanisms responsible for the erectile dysfunction would remain operational and NPT would be absent or diminished. Therefore, NPT could provide an objective measure to differentiate between these two types of impotence. Although some have asserted that NPT monitoring is the best non-invasive means to accomplish this distinction, others have warned that using NPT values alone can be misleading.[15–16] Despite these concerns, NPT testing remains an integral part of the evaluation of the impotent male.[17]

In this chapter, NPT and NPT with rigidity (NPTR) testing in the evaluation of male erectile dysfunction are described. In particular, results of NPTR testing in normal populations and in men with erectile dysfunction, the limitations of NPT testing, such as validity of results and difficulty in establishing normal criteria for a sufficient erection, and current recommendations are discussed.

NPT AND NPTR TESTING

Formal NPT testing, as it was initially introduced and is still often practised, involves continuous penile circumference measurements and repeated measurements of axial rigidity at or near the time of maximum tumescence. Testing is often performed in a sleep laboratory and includes monitoring by electroencephalogram (EEG), electro-oculogram (EOG), and/or electromyogram (EMG). Before penile rigidity testing was routinely practised, change in penile circumference was solely used to determine the adequacy of an erection. It was determined that a change in penile circumference of 20 mm represented a full erection and that a change of 16 mm in circumference or 80% of a full erection would be equivalent to the penile rigidity necessary for intromission.[12] Several studies, however, have shown that direct measurements of penile rigidity are necessary. Studies by Earls and associates demonstrated a significant delay between adequate rigidity based on NPT changes in circumference and the subject's perception of erectile sufficiency for intromission during visual sexual stimulation.[18] Also contributing to the need for direct rigidity measurements are the substantial differences between patients in circumference change associated with a full erection.

Initially, rigidity was measured as a function of buckling pressure when an external device was applied to a full erection. Karacan stated that a buckling pressure of 100 mmHg would be adequate and that a buckling pressure of less than 60 mmHg would be inadequate for vaginal penetration.[13] The limitations of this technique are that buckling force and standard NPT measurements occur during a single isolated event, the measurements are subject to observer error, and the process of detumescence may occur. Further drawbacks with this method include the high cost of the sleep laboratory, the time required, and the anxiety associated with an unnatural setting and procedure.

As a result, other methods to evaluate NPT and NPTR have been developed. In 1980, Barry and colleagues described the use of stamps placed around the base of the penis to measure tumescent activity during sleep.[19] In 1982, the Snap Gauge Band (Urohealth Systems Corporation, Costa Mesa, California, USA, formerly Dacomed Corporation) was developed in which three preset snap-release fasteners with constant release forces of 8, 12 and 16 oz (≈ 224, 336 and 448 g) are placed around the penis. This test was further modified to improve its reliability by replacing the fasteners with a serial arrangement of three plastic elements designed to break at 10, 15 and 20 oz (280, 420 and 560 g).[20] In several studies, the Snap Gauge Band was shown to correlate well with sleep laboratory testing of NPT and

rigidity.[4,21,22] Portable strain-gauge monitors were also found to correlate with tumescence measured in sleep lab settings.[23,24] Although these methods can be used to screen for the presence of NPT, none provides descriptive details of erectile performance such as frequency, duration, or degree of rigidity.

Ultimately, these concerns led to the development of small portable monitors that could measure rigidity continuously as well as record the number and duration of tumescent episodes. The RigiScan, a home monitoring device capable of continuously recording penile circumference and rigidity, was described by Bradley and associates.[25] The RigiScan (Urohealth Systems Corporation) consists of a logging unit strapped to the patient's thigh and two loops placed around the base and tip of the penis proximal to the coronal sulcus (Fig. 24.1). The loops monitor the circumference of the penis and the results are compared with the patient's baseline measurement every 15 s. Penile rigidity is measured every 3 minutes through the application of 2.8 N of radial compression to each loop. When the base loop detects an increase in circumference of more than 10 mm, rigidity measures are increased to every 30 s. When the change in the circumference is less than 10 mm, the device returns to rigidity measurements every 3 minutes. The RigiScan can collect data for three 10 h monitoring sessions, during which the rigidity, tumescence and duration of each event are recorded. The data can then be downloaded and printed in a graphical and numerical display, which provides a composite pattern of base and tip rigidity and tumescence over time.

Previous measurements of penile rigidity, such as buckling pressure, were measures of the response to

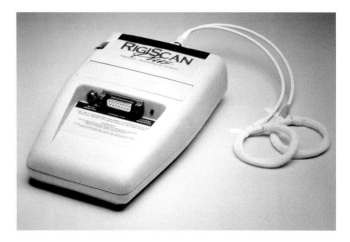

Figure 24.1. RigiScan ambulatory penile tumescence and rigidity monitoring device.

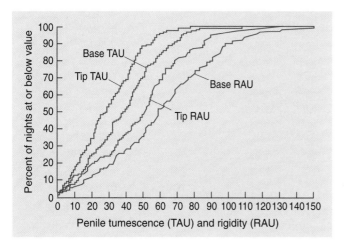

Figure 24.2. Cumulative distribution of penile tumescence activity (TAU) and rigidity activity units (RAU) from 44 potent men. N = 113 nights. Useful for comparison of NPTR results from impotent subjects. (Reproduced from ref. 27 with permission.)

applied axial force, whereas the RigiScan measures rigidity as the response to radial compression. In the RigiScan, rigidity is then expressed as a function of displacement when the loop is tightened around the penis. A rigidity of 100% represents no linear displacement and for each 0.5 mm of loop shortening the rigidity measure is reduced by 2.3%. Frohib and associates compared measurements of axial and radial rigidity at constant corporal body pressures and found that they were functionally related.[26] Furthermore, they demonstrated that these measures correlated with intracavernous pressure, the physiological event considered responsible for penile rigidity.

In 1994, Levine and Carroll described the use of a recent version of RigiScan Summary Analysis software to convert graphic display data of rigidity and tumescence into a more simplified quantitative analysis.[27] An erectile event is defined as a 20% increase in the base loop circumference lasting for a minimum of 3 minutes. Statistical analysis by the software also includes the number of erectile events detected, the cumulative duration of erectile events, average tumescence and rigidity readings during erectile events, and integrated time-dependent measures of tumescence (tumescence activity units, TAU) and rigidity (rigidity activity units, RAU). RAU represents the minutes spent at a given rigidity level multiplied by the rigidity level in decimal form. This value is calculated on a point-by-point basis and summed for the entire erectile event. Similarly, TAU

represents the duration of an erectile event multiplied by the percentage increase of circumference (expressed as a decimal) over the estimated baseline tumescence. RAU and TAU for both tip and base measurements are calculated and evaluated separately. These summary parameters can then be compared with percentile distributions from a normal population (Fig. 24.2).

■ NPTR RESULTS IN NORMAL POPULATIONS

The first normal criteria established for NPTR monitoring with the RigiScan was provided by Dacomed Corporation and based on data from over 500 males with erectile dysfunction studied at the Uro-Center of San Diego.[28] A normal erectile event was described as a minimum increase of 3 cm at the base and 2 cm at the tip of the penis over baseline measurements. Greater than 70% rigidity was considered adequate for vaginal penetration and less than 40% represented a flaccid penis. Measures between 40% and 70% represent varying degrees of penile stiffness. Three to six erections/8 h session or an average of 0.375 erectile events/h lasting an average of 10 minutes was considered normal.

Criteria for sufficient rigidity for vaginal penetration, however, have yet to be universally accepted. In a normal population of potent males, Kirkeby and associates observed that most nocturnal erections fluctuated in rigidity and at least half of the total number of erections recorded were not sufficient for vaginal penetration.[29] This agrees with other estimates that from 23 to 48% of erections, monitored in normal men with adequate nocturnal tumescence, have insufficient rigidity for intromission.[30–32] The issue is further compounded because the concept of adequate rigidity, indicating the ability to accomplish vaginal penetration, should (and yet cannot) account for the subject's particular partner and situation (i.e. vaginal size and lubrication, partner receptivity).[33] Since there is no standard vagina with respect to penetrability, it may be that adequate penile rigidity for an individual should be measured as a relative quantity with respect to his partner's vagina.

Several reports suggest that a measure of at least 70% tip rigidity, as proposed by Dacomed as adequate, may be an overestimate, in which case a man could be incorrectly diagnosed as having organic disease when, in fact, he has normal nocturnal rigidity. In a clinical study of more than

1000 patients with erectile dysfunction, Bain and Guay defined the minimal penile rigidity necessary for vaginal penetration as 60% base rigidity, 50% tip rigidity and a duration of at least 10 minutes.[34] Ogrinc and Linet found that decreasing minimal tip rigidity from 70 to 60%, increased the sensitivity of RigiScan testing from 53.8 to 70.8%.[35] Furthermore, Licht and associates evaluated rigidity with axial loading, RigiScan measurements and assessment of adequate rigidity by a trained observer in the same evening and concluded that a base rigidity of 55% was normal.[36] Clearly, further study is necessary.

RigiScan data are often clinically interpreted through visual analysis of graphic printouts. In an effort to make analysis more objective, Burris and colleagues developed a quantitative approach to RigiScan data analysis in 47 normal potent men.[37] They found that using area-under-the-curve (AUC) as an integrated measure of erectile amplitude and duration was a highly reproducible method to quantify tumescence and rigidity. Significant correlations were also found between tumescence and rigidity ($p<0.001$) and between tip and base measurements ($p<0.001$).

In a study of 44 healthy, potent subjects, Levine and Carroll described the cumulative distribution of the time–intensity measures of tumescence (TAU) and rigidity (RAU).[27] Data from these measures were developed into a nomogram to permit rapid comparison of NPTR findings (Fig. 24.2). The high correlation of tumescence and rigidity was similar to the AUC data described by Burris and colleagues.[37] Although there was a high degree of uniformity for the population as a whole, considerable variability in individual responses during the three nights of monitoring was found (Fig. 24.3). For example, six of the 44 men displayed little or no tip rigidity on at least one of the three nights of monitoring, indicating that at least two nights of monitoring are needed for adequate characterization. However, they concluded that evidence of significant erectile activity during a single night may be sufficient to demonstrate the potential for normal functioning. They also found no simple criteria for a normal RigiScan evaluation such as minimum number of events, duration, or percentage rigidity as has been previously described. Furthermore, they provide an indication of both the reproducibility of these parameters as measures of erectile function and the consistency of the relationship between tumescence and rigidity in normal men. This is further supported by the findings of Bain and Guay, who have shown that NPTR

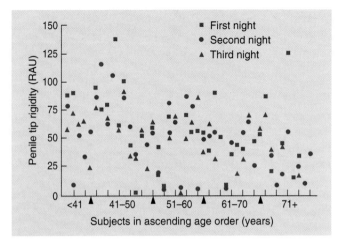

Figure 24.3. Penile tip rigidity measured by rigidity activity units (RAU) arranged by age in 44 potent men. Note intra-individual variation on a nightly basis but only slight downward trend of rigidity with increasing age. (Reproduced from ref. 78 with permission.)

results from RigiScan monitoring are highly reproducible when repeatedly studied in the same patient over time.[38] They found that the initial NPTR pattern was reproducible in 15 of 17 patients and that the two non-reproducible patterns could be explained by febrile illness and alcohol ingestion.

The relationship between erectile activity and ageing has been the subject of numerous studies. Total sleep time has been shown to remain constant between 20 and 50 years of age, as does total rapid eye movement (REM) sleep but total tumescence time decreases with age.[10,13,14] It has also been shown that the average number of erectile episodes decreases with age.[39–41] Buckling forces, however, have been shown to remain stable between 30 and 60 years of age.[41] Another study demonstrated that total tumescence time decreased with advancing age but a significant change in the number of erectile episodes or penile rigidity was not noted.[37] In their study of potent males, Levine and Carroll observed an increase in the number of NPT events with increasing age; however, the duration of each event appeared to decrease with age.[27] This apparent contrast to previous studies may be explained by their definition of an erectile episode as an event lasting for a minimum of 3 minutes, whereas other studies have used a 5 minute criterion to define an erectile episode. They also demonstrated a weak but significant downward trend of tip rigidity with increasing age, although considerable variability was observed in subject responses. Despite multiple patterns of NPT responses in aged populations, there seems to be an overall negative trend with increasing age (Fig. 24.3).

NPTR RESULTS AND ERECTILE DYSFUNCTION

Many investigators agree that NPTR monitoring is the best available objective test to differentiate between erectile dysfunction of organic or psychogenic aetiologies.[42–49] In a study by Davis-Joseph and associates, a high correlation was found between NPTR and final diagnosis based on history, physical examination, biothesiometry, plethysmography, and independent psychological testing.[50] For physicians utilizing the RigiScan, however, interpretation of results can be difficult. Data analysis may consist of a visual review of the graphic printout or an assessment of the single best erectile event over the course of monitoring. Kaneko and Bradley recognized that several NPTR patterns can be visually recognized and associated with impotence.[51] These include (1) dissociation of rigidity between the tip and base of the penis; (2) uncoupling between rigidity and tumescence; (3) shortened episodes of rigidity; (4) low-amplitude rigidity, and (5) no episodes of rigidity and tumescence. This approach allows specific patterns to be recognized but does not take advantage of baseline data obtained from normal potent controls.

The concept of selecting the 'best erection' recorded during NPTR monitoring for quantitative classification of erectile function has been suggested by several authors.[6,7,52,53] By defining the best erection as the erectile event with the highest rigidity and the greatest tumescence, Sohn and colleagues identified a strong correlation between NPTR results and the severity of erectile dysfunction within the various subgroups studied.[53] An additional approach that has proved useful is to determine the percentile rank of highest tip RAU for the night of NPTR monitoring with the highest RigiScan measures.[28,53,54] Three examples of this type of analysis are described below. Graphic printout data, the nomogram, and the highest tip and base RAU and TAU data are shown.

Case 1 (Fig. 24.4) presents the NPTR results for a 42-year-old man with a 1 year history of erectile dysfunction. He has no vascular risk factors. Penile duplex ultrasonography demonstrates a pattern of functional arterial insufficiency (i.e. possibly due to excessive

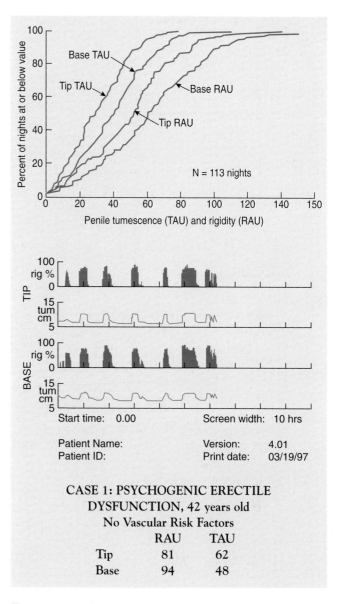

Figure 24.4. Case 1. Comparison of graphic printout and cumulative distribution curve ranking using tip RAU data places this 42-year-old man in the 87th percentile.

adrenergic tone). The mean peak systolic flow velocity was 22.5 cm/s, mean end-diastolic flow velocity was 0 and he experienced a full, lasting erectile response to 60 mg papaverine. Tip RAU data for this patient falls in the 87th percentile, consistent with normal erectile activity in a male with psychogenic erectile dysfunction. Case 2 (Fig. 24.5) presents the study results of a 56-year-old man with a 3 year complaint of progressive erectile insufficiency. He has a history of smoking and hypertension. The NPTR graphic display shows several events of variable duration and rigidity. Evaluation of tip RAU data demonstrates that this individual falls in the

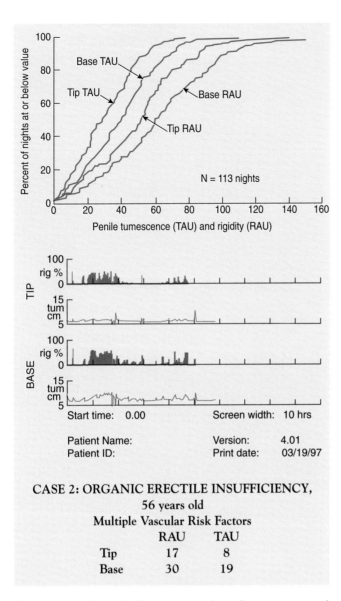

CASE 2: ORGANIC ERECTILE INSUFFICIENCY,
56 years old
Multiple Vascular Risk Factors

	RAU	TAU
Tip	17	8
Base	30	19

Figure 24.5. Case 2. Comparison of graphic printout and cumulative distribution curve ranking using tip RAU data places this 56-year-old male in the 15th percentile.

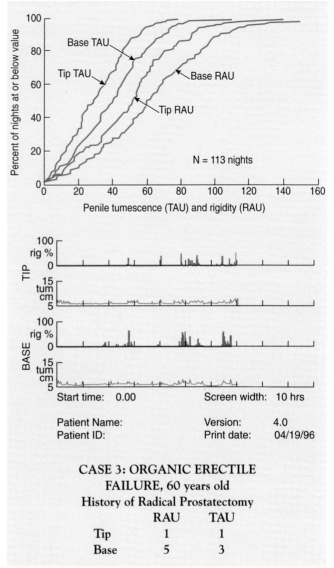

CASE 3: ORGANIC ERECTILE
FAILURE, 60 years old
History of Radical Prostatectomy

	RAU	TAU
Tip	1	1
Base	5	3

Figure 24.6. Case 3. Comparison of graphic printout and cumulative distribution curve ranking using tip RAU data places this 60-year-old male in the 3rd percentile.

15th percentile. Case 3 (Fig. 24.6) demonstrates the NPTR results of a 60-year-old man with erectile failure following radical prostatectomy. His tip RAU reading falls in the 3rd percentile which clearly suggests poor nocturnal erectile activity consistent with an organic aetiology. Therefore, a single-value maximum tip RAU allows a ready comparison of the patient's nocturnal erectile activity with that of a potent population of men.

Frequently, the aetiologies of impotence are complex and combinations of organic and psychogenic causes may be present. NPTR testing has been used in an attempt to unravel these complex issues and to define better the specific subtypes of erectile dysfunction. In 1990, Shabsigh and associates compared the results of penile duplex ultrasound with intracavernous injection of vasoactive drugs with those of NPT monitoring in 50 patients with erectile dysfunction.[17] NPT results were abnormal in vasculogenic impotence but arterial and venous causes could not be differentiated. The nature of vascular insufficiency was more readily detected by duplex ultrasonography with intracavernous injection of vasoactive agents. This was particularly true for patients with pelvic steal syndrome, in whom NPT results are often normal. Conversely, they noted that NPT monitoring was more sensitive in the evaluation of neurogenic impotence.

In contrast, a study by Kirkeby noted that nocturnal erectile rigidity was normal in 11 of 26 patients with a well-established neurological disorder known to affect erectile function (i.e. multiple sclerosis).[55] They recommended that NPTR be used with the following reservations: absence of sufficient rigidity for vaginal intromission during nocturnal erections is found frequently in normal males and, even if performed for several sessions, the presence of NPTR sufficient for vaginal intromission proves the presence of awake erectile capability only in the absence of neurological disorders. In a 1996 study of 16 men with multiple sclerosis and impotence, Staerman and associates utilized stricter criteria for normal NPTR (i.e. rigidity $\geq$ 80% and/or duration > 30 minutes).[56] They concluded that erectile dysfunction in the patient with multiple sclerosis is not always the result of neurological impairment and that a distinction between psychogenic and organic erectile dysfunction is difficult to make in these patients.

In 1991, Montague and colleagues compared the results of infusion pharmacocavernosometry (IPC) with NPTR monitoring in 50 patients with erectile dysfunction.[57] Traditional criteria for IPC resulted in poor correlation between the two, but modified criteria established by logistic regression techniques resulted in a stronger correlation between the two methods. However, Montague and colleagues concluded that the results of either test alone were insufficient to make a specific diagnosis of erectile dysfunction.

Several studies have compared NPT with intracorporal pharmacological (ICP) erection testing. In a study of 37 impotent patients, Allen and Brendler concluded that the response to ICP testing does not accurately distinguish psychogenic from organic impotence.[58] However, the response does correlate well with the degree of erectile impairment. A thorough NPT evaluation provided an accurate prediction of the ICP response but the reverse was not true. They maintain that NPT should be performed before ICP erection testing to avoid unnecessary and inappropriate treatment of psychogenic impotence.

In 1994, Allen and associates compared the results of duplex ultrasound evaluation with NPT evaluation in 40 impotent men.[59] Their results demonstrated that, in men with a history of psychogenic illness, duplex ultrasound is also unreliable. They felt that anxiety and increased sympathetic stimulation resulted in inaccurate responses

to pharmacological stimulation and subsequent duplex ultrasound measurements. They therefore concluded that, in patients suspected of having a psychogenic cause of impotence, NPT testing should be carried out for appropriate treatment recommendations.

■ LIMITATIONS OF NPT

The basic assumption of NPT testing is that the presence of nocturnal erections indicates the capacity to have an awake erection with sufficient rigidity for vaginal penetration. Monitoring of NPT also assumes that the physiological mechanisms for both a nocturnal penile erection and a sexually stimulated erection are similar. Although this assumption has been questioned, it has been suggested that the physiological mechanisms responsible for the development of nocturnal erections are similar to those operative during sexual stimulation.[60] Because of these assumptions, the usefulness of NPT testing has been questioned by various authors. Wasserman and associates agree that NPT monitoring is a useful aid in differentiating organic from psychogenic impotence, but they stress that it has never been validated independent of the NPT measurements themselves.[61] Other groups caution that NPT may not always be a true indication of erectile potential in erotic and sexual circumstances.[16,62]

Another concern regarding NPT is that organic factors may, in fact, alter NPT in the patient with psychogenic impotence. Previously, abnormal results have been demonstrated in 15–20% of patients with no identifiable evidence of organic impotence indicating that subtle, undetectable physiological factors may be operating in these patients.[13] It has also been noted that dreams containing anxiety, aggression and other negative content are associated with abnormal NPT results.[5,8] Another factor that has been shown to affect NPT adversely is depression. Studies by Roose and colleagues[63] and by Thase and colleagues[64,65] have reported on patients with major depression exhibiting a reversible loss of NPT, which was restored when the depression was successfully treated.

A decrease in the number of tumescence episodes, total tumescent time and decreased quality of erections on the first night of sleep laboratory testing, has given rise to the concept of a 'first night effect'.[66] Although wearing the NPT device is unnatural and could presumably interfere with normal sleep, resulting in false NPT readings, a first night effect was not revealed in two recent studies of normal, healthy volunteers using the Rigiscan device.[27,37]

Home monitoring devices, such as the RigiScan, have the additional drawback of the inability to assess the adequacy of sleep. On the other hand, formal NPT monitoring in a sleep laboratory has the drawback of being a costly, inconvenient test for the patient. Conditions such as sleep apnoea, periodic leg movements, and nocturnal myoclonus can negatively affect NPT and thus a diminished NPT result may not be indicative of abnormal erectile function.[67,68] Whereas Bradley has suggested that disturbed sleep impairs the appearance of a spontaneous erectile event, Schiavi has demonstrated that a full erection may not occur in normal potent males despite a normal sleep pattern.[69,70] Several studies have addressed these issues by investigating the usefulness of penile tumescence monitoring during daytime naps. Gordon and Carey monitored NPT during a 3 hour daytime nap in seven healthy male subjects.[71] The subjects were able to fall asleep rapidly, slept well, and experienced REM sleep. More recently, Morales and associates studied 18 impotent men by formal NPT testing during a morning nap session:[72] 16 of the 18 patients (89%) experienced REM sleep and four patients did not experience tumescence during the nap. All four of these patients did not experience nocturnal erections on two separate sessions. Of the 12 patients with documented erections at night, nine also exhibited erectile episodes during napping. Although both of these studies are small, further investigation may indicate that this more convenient and less costly method may provide adequate NPT information for evaluating erectile dysfunction.

A final criticism of NPT monitoring is that radial measures of rigidity, as provided by the RigiScan, may not be accurate when compared with axial measures of rigidity. In a study of 17 men with erectile dysfunction, Munoz and colleagues noted that the RigiScan underestimated rigidity at low levels.[49] This would result in a greater number of patients with potentially normal rigidity, and hence psychogenic erectile dysfunction, being characterized as having organic erectile dysfunction. In contrast, Allen and colleagues found that the RigiScan did not correlate with axial rigidity measurements at high levels of rigidity.[73] This type of error would result in patients with diminished quality of erections due to an organic aetiology being characterized as having psychogenic erectile dysfunction. In a study of 28 men with erectile dysfunction, Licht and colleagues measured radial and axial rigidity and found a strong correlation between base rigidity and buckling pressure.[36] Tip rigidity measurements, however, correlated poorly with axial measurements. This poor correlation may be an indication of disease state, as disassociation between tip and base rigidity has been noted in impotent men.[51] Alternatively, this poor correlation may be the result of using a trained observer as the 'gold standard' to measure rigidity. Furthermore, all of these studies attempt to correlate axial and radial rigidity in populations of men with erectile dysfunction. Further studies are needed in normal, potent populations to determine if these conflicting results are inherent to the design of the RigiScan or are indicative of erectile dysfunction.

■ RECOMMENDATIONS FOR THE USE OF NPTR

Although the use of NPT in all men with erectile dysfunction has been debated and is subject to personal belief, the author's opinion is that men with significant organic factors associated with impotence — such as diabetes mellitus, hypertension, history of smoking, elevated triglycerides or cholesterol, or vascular disease — most probably have an organic aetiology and need not be evaluated by NPT monitoring. On the other hand, it has been shown in several studies that many men with diseases known to affect erectile dysfunction can also have normal NPT as well as adequate sexual function.[27] The patients who will benefit most from NPTR testing are those with no known neurovascular risk factors and who present with a history that arouses suspicion of a psychogenic aetiology. An objective measure of erectile function with NPTR should confirm the diagnosis and aid the physician to guide that patient to the appropriate therapy. Another group of patients who may benefit from NPTR testing are those men with Peyronie's disease, who complain of poor quality erection or softening of the erection distal to the plaque. In these cases an NPTR evaluation may help to determine whether there is underlying organic erectile insufficiency and whether, therefore, the patient would benefit from the placement of a penile prosthesis to ensure adequate rigidity.[74] Some authorities have expressed the opinion that NPT testing should be limited, since office ICP injection provides the quickest, least expensive, and most convincing evidence to demonstrate to a patient the quality of his erection.[75] However, it must be remembered that simply demonstrating to the patient that an erection can be induced by the administration of drug by injection or urethral pellet will not resolve his concern as to why the problem exists. Therefore, more accurate and reliable methods such as NPT monitoring are recommended to distinguish why a patient is dysfunctional and potentially to determine the most appropriate treatment.

The author's approach is to obtain a complete medical history, including medications, and a focused physical examination, including a neurovascular assessment. When a clear psychogenic aetiology is suggested by the history, or neurovascular risk factors are absent, NPTR is recommended. In those patients who present with a complex history, penile duplex ultrasound with pharmacological stimulation is performed first. Patients who present with a recently identified duplex ultrasound pattern, including suboptimal mean peak systolic velocity (less than 30 cm/s), normal mean end-diastolic flow velocity (less than 5.0 cm/s), and a full erectile response to pharmacological stimulation suggest the possibility of excessive adrenergic tone as a potential aetiology. These patients would benefit from further evaluation with NPTR to confirm a psychogenic aetiology associated with excessive adrenergic tone.[76,77] Therefore, NPTR is far less invasive and expensive than phalloarteriography or infusion cavernosometry and will offer more objective data to support a recommendation for psychosexual rehabilitation therapy.

In the author's opinion, the use of 'best erection' criteria addresses nocturnal erectile capacity for full erection rather than the entire nocturnal erectile behaviour as recorded on the one or more nights of study using the RigiScan device. Using the cumulative distribution curve approach with TAU and RAU data allows the comparison of data from one individual to a range of NPTR experience in a potent population rather than a set of unconfirmed criteria.[27] Specifically, it is considered that evaluating the highest tip RAU on the best night of erectile activity as a percentile ranking of normal data provides the most useful impression of erectile function.

Hospital or sleep laboratory NPTR assessment is suggested when a compromise in patient compliance or concerns with the following circumstances occurs: (1) manual dexterity issues preventing the patient from properly applying the RigiScan unit, (2) malingering, (3) dementia, and (4) validity in an outpatient, unobserved setting, particularly in medico-legal testing. Full sleep laboratory evaluation should also be considered when there is a history or suspicion of sleep disturbance.

The author agrees with others that no single test exists that enables the physician to qualify the aetiology and degree of impotence. However, despite its intrinsic weaknesses and limitations, NPTR is a valuable resource in differentiating between psychogenic and organic impotence. The ultimate goal for the practising physician in evaluating erectile dysfunction is to provide useful information and to direct that patient to the most appropriate therapeutic options. For many patients, NPTR provides this information in a rather non-invasive and relatively inexpensive manner.

■ REFERENCES

1. Halverson H M. Genital and sphincter behavior of the male infant. J Gen Psychol 1940; 56: 95–136
2. Ohlmeyer P, Brilmayer H, Hullstrung H. Periodische Vorgange im Schlaf. Pflugers Arch 1944; 248: 559
3. Aserinsky E, Kleitman N. Regularly occurring periods of eye motility and concomitant phenomena during sleep. Science 1953; 118: 273
4. Fisher C, Gross J, Zuch J. Cycle of penile erections synchronous with dreaming (REM) sleep. Arch Gen Psychiatry 1965; 12: 29–45
5. Fisher C. Dreaming and sexuality, In: Loewenstein R M, Newman L M, Schur M et al (eds) Psychoanalysis — a general psychology. New York: International University Press, 1966: 537
6. Fisher C, Schiavi P, Edwards A et al. Evaluation of nocturnal penile tumescence in the differential diagnosis of sexual impotence. Arch Gen Psychiatry 1979; 36: 431
7. Fisher C, Shiavi P, Lear H. The assessment of nocturnal REM erection in a differential diagnosis of sexual impotence. J Sex Marital Ther 1975; 1: 277–290
8. Karacan I, Goodenough D R, Shapiro A et al. Erection cycle during sleep in relation to dream anxiety. Arch Gen Psychiatry 1966; 15: 183–189
9. Karacan I, Williams R L, Thornby J I et al. Sleep related penile tumescence as a function of age. Am J Psychiatry 1975; 132: 932–937
10. Karacan I, Salis P J, Thornby J I et al. The ontogeny of nocturnal penile tumescence. Waking Sleeping 1976; 1: 27–44
11. Karacan I. Clinical value of nocturnal erection in the prognosis and diagnosis of impotence. Med Aspects Hum Sex 1970, 4: 27–34

12. Karacan I, Salis P J, Ware J C et al. Nocturnal penile tumescence and diagnosis in diabetic impotence. Am J Psychiatry 1978; 135: 191

13. Karacan I, Salis P J, Williams R L. The role of the sleep laboratory in the diagnosis and treatment of impotence. In: Williams R L, Karacan I, Frazier S H (eds) Sleep disorders, diagnosis and treatment. New York: J Wiley, 1978

14. Karacan I, Hursch C J, Williams R L. Some characteristics of nocturnal penile tumescence in elderly males. J Gerontol 1972; 27: 39–45

15. Kessler W O. Nocturnal penile tumescence. Urol Clin North Am 1988; 15: 81–86

16. Morales A, Condra M, Reid K. The role of nocturnal penile tumescence monitoring in the diagnosis of impotence: a review. J Urol 1990; 143: 441–446

17. Shabsigh R, Fishman I J, Scott F B. Evaluation of erectile impotence. Urology 1988; 32: 83–90

18. Earls CM, Morales A, Marshall W. Penile insufficiency: An operational definition. J Urol 1988; 139: 536–538

19. Barry J M, Blank B, Boileau M. Nocturnal penile tumescence monitoring with stamps. Urology 1987; 15: 171–172

20. Ek A, Bradley W E, Krane R J. Nocturnal penile rigidity measured by the snap-gauge band. J Urol 1983; 129: 964–966

21. Allen J, Ellis D, Carroll J L, et al. Snap gauge band versus multidisciplinary evaluation in impotence assessment. Urology 1989; 34: 197–199

22. Condra M, Fenemore J, Reid K et al. Screening assessment of penile tumescence and rigidity: clinical test of snap gauge. Urology 1987; 29: 254–257

23. Reid D, Glass C A, Evans C M et al. Screening impotence by home nocturnal tumescence self-monitoring. Br J Clin Psychol 1990; 29: 439–441

24. Kenepp D, Gonick P. Home monitoring of penile tumescence for erectile dysfunction: initial experience. Urology 1979; 19: 261–264

25. Bradley W E, Timm G W, Gallagher J M et al. New method for continuous measurement of nocturnal penile tumescence and rigidity. Urology 1985; 26: 4–9

26. Frohib D A, Goldstein I, Peyton T R et al. Characterization of penile erectile states using external computer-based monitoring. J Biomech Eng 1987; 109: 110–114

27. Levine L A, Carroll R A. Nocturnal penile tumescence and rigidity in men without complaints of erectile dysfunction using a new quantitative analysis software. J Urol 1994; 152: 1103–1107

28. RigiScan: Ambulatory rigidity and tumescence system document no. 750-156-0486. Dacomed Corporation, Minneapolis, MN, USA

29. Kirkeby H J, Andersen A J, Poulsen E U. Nocturnal penile tumescence and rigidity. Translation of data obtained from normal males. Int J Impot Res 1989; 1: 115–125

30. Weinberg J J, Badlani G H. Utility of RigiScan and papaverine in diagnosis of erectile impotence. Urology 1988; 31: 526–529

31. Murray F T, Geisser M, Clark R V et al. Psychological and psychophysiological evaluation in men with diabetes mellitus and organic impotence (abstr). J Androl 1994; 14(suppl): 55

32. Wein A J, Fishkin R, Carpiniello V L et al. Expansion without significant rigidity during penile tumescence testing: A potential source of misinterpretation. J Urol 1981; 126: 343–344

33. Karacan I, Moore C, Sahmay S. Measurement of pressure necessary for vaginal penetration (abstr). Sleep Res 1985; 14: 269

34. Bain C L, Guay A T. Classification of sexual dysfunction for management of intracavernous medication-induced erections. J Urol 1991; 146:1 379

35. Ogrinc F C, Linet O I. Evaluation of real-time RigiScan monitoring in pharmacological erection. J Urol 1995; 154: 1356–1359

36. Licht M R, Lewis R W, Wollan P C et al. Comparison of RigiScan and sleep laboratory nocturnal penile tumescence in the diagnosis of organic impotence. J Urol 1994; 154: 1740–1743

37. Burris A S, Banks S M, Sherins R J. Quantitative assessment of nocturnal penile tumescence and rigidity in normal men using a home monitor. J Androl 1989; 19: 492–497

38. Bain C L, Guay A W. Reproducibility in monitoring nocturnal penile tumescence and rigidity. J Urol 1991; 148: 811–814

39. Kahn E, Fisher C. Amount of REM sleep erection in the healthy aged. Psychophysiology 1968; 5: 226

40. Kahn E, Fisher C. Amount of REM sleep and sexuality in the aged. J Geriatr Psychiatry 1969; 2: 181

41. Reynolds C F, Thase M E, Jennings J R et al. Nocturnal penile tumescence in healthy 20 to 59 year olds: A revisit. Sleep 1989; 12: 368–373

42. Nofzinger E A, Reynolds C F, Jennings J F et al. Results of nocturnal penile tumescence studies are abnormal in sexually functional diabetic men. Arch Intern Med 1992; 152: 114–118

43. Van Nueten J, Verheyden B, Van Camp K. Role of penile nocturnal tumescence and rigidity measurement in the diagnosis of erectile impotence. Eur Urol 1992; 22: 119–122.

44. Nofzinger E A, Fasiczka A L, Thase M E et al. Are buckling force measurements reliable in nocturnal penile tumescence studies? Sleep 1993; 16: 156–162

45. Nofzinger E A, Thase M E, Reynolds C F et al. Sexual function in depressed men. Assessment by self-report, behavioral, and nocturnal penile tumescence measures before and after treatment with cognitive behavior therapy. Arch Gen Psychiatry 1993; 50: 24–30

46. Thase M E, Reynolds C F, Jennings J F et al. Diminished nocturnal penile tumescence in depression: a replication study. Biol Psychiatry 1992; 31: 1136–1142

47. Melman A. The evaluation of erectile dysfunction. Urol Radiol 1988; 10; 119–128

48. Djamilian M, Stief C G, Hartmann U et al. Predictive value of real-time RigiScan monitoring for the etiology of organogenic impotence. J Urol 1993(2); 149: 1269–1271

49. Munoz M M, Bancroft J, Marshall I. The performance of the RigiScan in the measurement of penile tumescence and rigidity. Int J Impot Res 1993; 5: 69–76

50. Davis-Joseph B, Tiefer L, Melman A. Accuracy of the initial history and physical examination to establish the etiology of erectile dysfunction. Urology 1995; 45: 498–502

51. Kaneko S, Bradley W E. Evaluation of erectile dysfunction with continuous monitoring of penile rigidity. J Urol 1986; 136: 1026–1029

52. Wasserman M D, Pollack C P, Spielman A J et al. The differential diagnosis of impotence. The measurement of nocturnal penile tumescence. JAMA 1980; 243: 2038–2042

53. Sohn M H, Seeger U, Sikora R et al. Criteria for examiner-independent nocturnal penile tumescence and rigidity monitoring (NPTR): correlations to invasive diagnostic methods. Int J Impot Res 1993; 5: 59–68

54. Benet A E, Rehman J, Holcomb R G et al. The correlation between the new RigiScan plus software and the final diagnosis in the evaluation of erectile dysfunction. J Urol 1996; 156: 1947–1950

55. Kirkeby H J, Poulsen E U, Petersen T et al. Erectile dysfunction in multiple sclerosis. Neurology 1988; 38: 1366–1371

56. Staerman F, Guiraud P, Coeurdacier P et al. Value of nocturnal penile tumescence and rigidity (NPTR) recording in impotent males with multiple sclerosis. Int J Impot Res 1996; 8: 241–245

57. Montague D K, Lakin M M, Medendorp S et al. Infusion pharmacocavernosometry and nocturnal penile tumescence findings in men with erectile dysfunction. J Urol 1991; 145: 768–771

58. Allen R P, Brendler C B. Nocturnal penile tumescence predicting response to intracorporeal pharmacological erection testing. J Urol 1988; 140: 518–522

59. Allen R P, Engel R M, Smolev J K et al. Comparison of duplex ultrasonography and nocturnal penile tumescence in evaluation of impotence. J Urol 1994; 151: 1525–1529

60. Krane R J. Sexual function and dysfunction. In Walsh P C, Gittes R J, Perlmutter A D, Stamey T A (eds) Campbell's Urology, 5th edn. Philadelphia: Saunders, 1986: 719

61. Wasserman M D, Pollack C P, Spielman A J et al. Theoretical and technical problems in the measurement of nocturnal penile tumescence for the differential diagnosis of impotence. Psychol Med 1980; 42: 575–585

62. Chung W S, Choi H K. Erotic erection versus nocturnal erection. J Urol 1990; 143: 294–297

63. Roose S P, Glassman A H, Walsh B T et al. Reversible loss of nocturnal penile tumescence during depression: a preliminary report. Neuropsychobiology 1982; 8: 284–288

64. Thase M E, Reynolds C F, Glanz L M et al. Nocturnal penile tumescence in depressed men. Am J Psychiatry 1987; 144: 89–92

65. Thase M E, Reynolds C F, Jennings J R et al. Diagnostic performance of nocturnal penile tumescence studies in healthy, dysfunctional (impotent), and depressed men. Psychiatry Res 1988; 26: 79–83

66. Jovanovic U J. Der effect der ersten untersuchungschaft auf die erektionen im schlaf. Psychother Psychosom 1969; 17: 295–308

67. Pressman M R, Fry J M, DiPhillipo M A et al. Avoiding false positive findings in measuring nocturnal penile tumescence. Urology 1989; 34: 297–300

68. Pressman M R, Fry J M, DiPhillipo M A et al. Problems in the interpretation of nocturnal penile tumescence studies: disruption by occult sleep disorders. J Urol 1986; 136: 595–598

69. Bradley W E. New techniques in evaluation of impotence. Urology 1987; 29: 383–388

70. Schiavi R C, Davis D M, Fogel M et al. Luteinizing hormone and testosterone during nocturnal sleep: relation to nocturnal penile tumescent cycle. Arch Sex Behav 1977; 6: 97–104

71. Gordon C M, Carey M P. Penile tumescence monitoring during morning naps: a pilot investigation of a cost-effective alternative to full night sleep studies in the assessment of male erectile disorder. Behav Res Ther 1993; 31: 503–506

72. Morales A, Condra M, Heaton J P et al. Diurnal penile tumescence recording in the etiological diagnosis of erectile dysfunction. J Urol 1994; 152: 1111–1114

73. Allen R P, Smolev J K, Engel R M et al. Comparison of the RigiScan and formal nocturnal penile tumescence testing in the evaluation of erectile activity. J Urol 1993(2); 149: 1265–1268

74. Ganabothi K, Dmochowski R, Zimmern P E, Leach G E. Peyronie's disease: surgical treatment based on penile rigidity. J Urol 1995; 153: 662–666

75. Rajfer J. Editorial: Impotence — the quick work-up. J Urol 1996; 156: 1951

76. Levine L A, Carroll R A, Chapman T N. Identification of a new penile duplex ultrasound vascular flow pattern. J Urol 1995; 153: 331A

77. Tomaszewski C S, Carroll R A, Levine L A. Psychogenic impotence evaluated by penile duplex ultrasonography. Proceedings of the 69th Annual Western Section American Urological Association Meeting, Palm Desert, California, November 1993

78. Levine L A, Lenting E L. Use of nocturnal penile tumescence and rigidity in the evaluation of male erectile dysfunction. Urol Clin North Am 1995; 22(4): 775–778

Chapter 25

Corporal biopsy in the diagnosis of erectile dysfunction

E. Wespes

◼ INTRODUCTION

Erectile impotence may be caused by psychological problems, neurogenic dysfunction, hormonal alterations, or compromised penile blood flow. A better understanding of the erectile mechanism and the development of new investigative techniques have led to dramatic improvement in recognizing the cause of impotence. Results indicate that, in the majority of patients, erectile impotence is due to vascular abnormalities.

At flaccidity, the contracted trabecular smooth muscles allow for venous drainage under conditions of low outflow resistance. During tumescence the smooth muscles are relaxed, producing arterial dilatation and a filling of the lacunar spaces.[1,2] In addition, the intracavernous pressure increases slightly when the penis elongates. The tunica albuginea provides the corpus cavernosum with a fibrous framework and plays a significant role in erectile function. Being rich in elastic fibres, the tunica albuginea is able to resist overstretching of the corpus at raised levels of intracavernous pressure, compressing the subalbugineal venous plexus and promoting the maintenance of erection.

Damage of the smooth muscle cells may induce impotence. Jevitch and co-workers compared the corpora cavernosa of potent and impotent men using electron microscopy.[3] Of the smooth muscle cells, 42.3% from corporal tissues of impotent men showed pronounced thickening of the basal lamina, a paucity of dense bodies and contractile filaments, minimal or no glycogen and fewer vesicles on the surface. By comparison, only 5.4% of the smooth muscle cells from potent men showed similar alterations. The percentage of altered smooth muscle cells in corporal tissues of impotent men was proportional to

the severity of symptoms and clinical findings. Morphometric analysis revealed no significant differences in the relative proportions of the major components of corporal tissue (smooth muscle cells, extracellular matrix, vascular lumina and endothelial cells). Ultrastructural studies on impotent men have produced equivocal results. One study examined ultrastructural changes in penile erectile tissue in 32 patients who underwent penile prosthesis implantation.[4] In patients with severe arterial insufficiency, the cellular structure was markedly altered, the number of intracavernous smooth muscle cells was reduced and the density of the connective tissue separating individual cells was increased. The changes in the smooth muscle cells consisted of contour irregularity with fragmentation and loss of the basal lamina. Similar results have been produced in a study by Karadeniz and co-workers.[5] In contrast, a study by Mersdorf and associates on a similar group of patients showed that a variety of medical conditions produced similar degenerative tissue responses and that no single or specific cause of impotence was manifested by consistent changes in erectile tissue.[6]

An accurate test to assess the intracavernous components is still lacking. The intracavernous structures consist of bundles of smooth muscles, elastic fibres, collagen and loose alveolar tissue with numerous arterioles and nerves. These structures are key to the problem of impotence and demonstration of their alteration could eventually spare patients from reconstructive surgery. Using immunohistochemistry with desmin anti-desmin antibody, the percentage of smooth muscle cells in potent and impotent patients was measured objectively with computerized image analysis.[7] Patients with penile curvature and normal erections were

Table 25.1. Percentage of intracavernous smooth muscle fibres in potent and impotent patients

Patient characteristics	No. of patients	Mean age in years (range)	Percentage of smooth muscle fibres
Penile curvature	5	23 (18–33)	40–52
Venous leakage	20	48 (25–67)	19–36
Arterial insufficiency	10	58 (47–70)	10–25

(From ref. 7 with permission.)

classified as normal controls. The percentage of smooth muscle cells in patients with arterial and venous disease decreased; this was more marked in those with arterial lesions (Table 25.1).

Computerized image analysis has been used to measure the percentage of smooth muscle fibres in penile biopsies from cadavers and men with vascular impotence.[8] No significant difference was observed between the proximal and distal areas, and/or between the peripheral and central areas within each individual corpus cavernosum and between two corpora cavernosa for each patient or cadaver. The percentage of smooth muscle fibres was less in impotent patients than in the cadavers, in whom the erectile status was not known, and this reduction occurred throughout both cavernous bodies. It can be concluded from these data that vascular impotence is a diffuse disease, with the reduction of smooth muscle cells occurring throughout the penis.

In addition, in patients with cavernovenous leak, a significant relation exists between the decrease in smooth muscle cells and the maintenance flow rates. The percentage of smooth muscle cells appears to be the only prognostic factor in evaluating the long-term outcome of venous surgery; patients responding to surgery had more than 29% smooth muscle cells on biopsy.[9] Neither the patient's age nor the maintenance flow rates correspond to the surgical success rate.

■ CAVERNOSAL BIOPSY

Typically, penile biopsies are performed during surgery when the therapeutic decision has already been determined. The recent introduction of the biopty gun (Bard Urological, Covington, Georgia, USA), with its spring trigger mechanism has increased the ability to obtain consistently good samples of cavernosal tissue relatively painlessly. Another benefit is that appropriate therapy can be undertaken after evaluation of the samples. The biopsy is performed by first infiltrating approximately 1 ml lignocaine (lidocaine) into the skin of the penis in the balanopreputial groove on the dorsolateral side. The biopsy needle is introduced longitudinally through the tunica albuginea into the corpus cavernosum. With one hand, the penis is kept stretched and, with the other hand, the needle is fired from an anterior to a posterior trajectory. More than one pass of the needle can be made to obtain adequate tissue.

Needle biopsies have been compared with surgical biopsies taken during penile implants. Cavernous penile arterial Doppler analysis was performed before and after biopsies done with the biopty gun method. In all cases, adequate tissue was obtained for histological analysis and the biopsy tissues were similar to those obtained during surgery. Corpus cavernosum tissue was readily identified, with the intracavernous smooth muscle fibres, arteries, nerves, and collagen. None of the patients experienced pain at biopsy or required any postoperative analgesia. No haematoma or significant bleeding was observed and no lesions were found on the cavernous arteries using Doppler analysis.

A comparative study on patients with erectile dysfunction of various aetiologies again showed that biopty gun specimens were equally as representative as those from open biopsy.[10] Histological analysis of the cavernous bodies in patients with psychogenic impotence revealed normal erectile tissue. In patients with organic impotence, histological lesions were regarded as mild, moderate or severe. The most severe lesions were observed in the erectile tissue and, in particular, in the smooth muscle of the trabeculae and the helicine arteries, which had been reduced and replaced by connective tissue.

Use of the biopty gun to perform penile biopsy under local anaesthesia appears to be a simple and reliable method to obtain sufficient tissue for histological analysis. The site of the needle puncture is important in order to avoid secondary subcutaneous haematoma of the penis. The balanopreputial groove is the preferred site because the glans mucosa of the penile skin adheres closely to the tunica albuginea, making development of haematoma under the skin impossible. The small hole in the tunica albuginea at this point does not damage either the intracavernous artery (as demonstrated by Doppler analysis performed before and after puncture) or the urethra.

This procedure is cost effective and can be done in surgery under local anaesthesia: the procedure usually lasts less than 10 minutes. No complications from the procedure have been observed, but they could include bleeding, infection, or failure to obtain adequate tissue.

■ CONCLUSIONS

Vascular impotence is a diffuse disease. As such, a cavernous body biopsy can be used to study the penile structure in the assessment of vascular impotence. The recently introduced biopty gun method for cavernosal biopsy has several advantages over biopsy performed during therapeutic surgery; principally, patients can be assessed prior to therapy. Further evaluation of the technique is required and histological criteria need to be determined. However, the technique holds promise as a method of selecting patients for penile reconstructive vascular surgery, excluding those with a neurological disorder or smooth muscle atrophy.

■ REFERENCES

1. Lue T F and Tanagho E A. Physiology of erection and pharmacological management of impotence. J Urol 1987; 137: 829–836
2. Krane R J, Goldstein I, Saenz de Tejada I. Impotence. New Engl J Med 1989; 321: 1648–1650
3. Jevitch M J, Khawand N Y, Vidic B. Clinical significance of ultrastructural findings in the corpora cavernosa of normal and impotent men. J Urol 1990; 143: 289–293
4. Persson C, Diederichs W, Lue T F et al. Correlation of altered penile ultrastructure with clinical arterial evaluation. J Urol 1989; 142: 1462–1468
5. Karadeniz T, Topsakal M, Aydogmus A et al. Correlation of ultrastructural alterations in cavernous tissue with the clinical diagnosis of vasculogenic impotence. Urol Int 1996; 57: 58–61
6. Mersdorf A, Goldsmith P C, Diederichs W et al. Ultrastructural changes in impotent penile tissue: a comparison of 65 patients. J Urol 1991; 145: 749–758
7. Wespes E, Goes P M, Schiffman S et al. Computerized analysis of smooth muscle fibers in potent and impotent patients. J Urol 1991: 146: 1015–1017
8. Wespes E, Moreira de Goes P, Schulman C C. Vascular impotence: Focal or diffuse penile disease. J Urol 1992; 148: 1435–1436
9. Wespes E, Moreira de Goes P, Sattar A A, Schulman C C. Objective criteria in the long-term evaluation of penile venous surgery. J Urol 1994; 152: 888–890
10. Malovrouvas D, Petrake C, Constantinidis E et al. The contribution of cavernous body biopsy in the diagnosis and treatment of male impotence. Histol Histopathol 1994; 9: 427–431

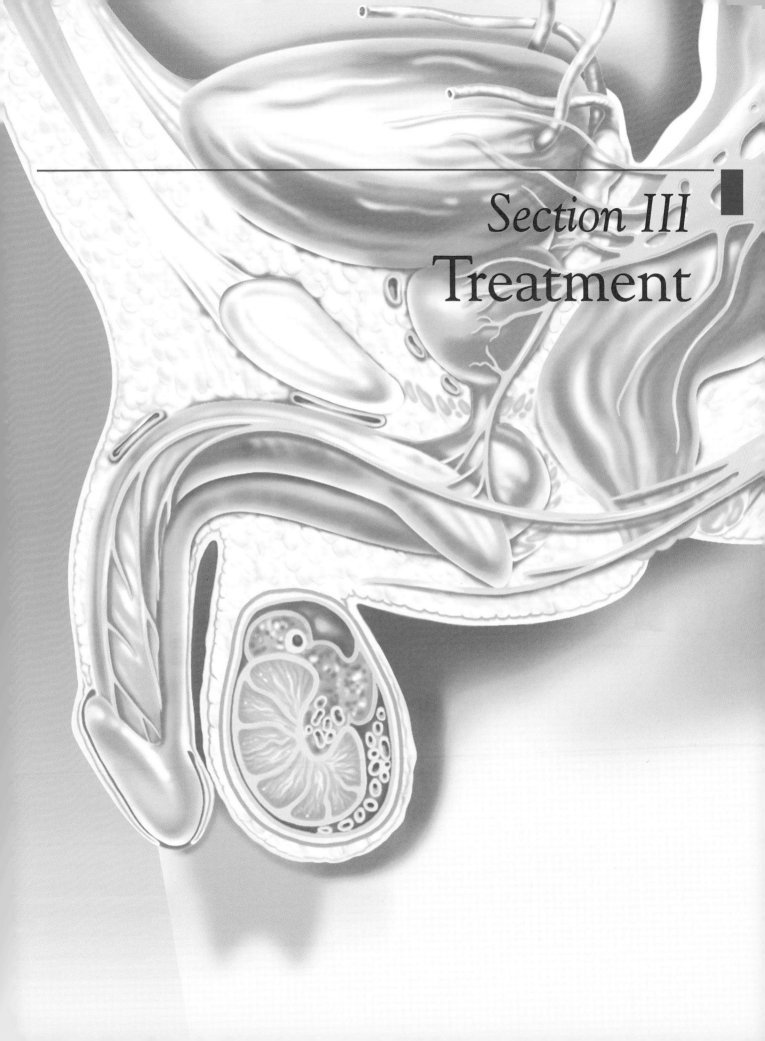

Section III
Treatment

Chapter 26

Sildenafil: a selective phosphodiesterase (PDE)5 inhibitor in the treatment of erectile dysfunction (ED)

I. Osterloh, I. Eardley, C. Carson and H. Padma-Nathan

◼ PDE INHIBITORS AND ED — A HISTORICAL PERSPECTIVE

Although the first orally administered phosphodiesterase (PDE) inhibitor, sildenafil, was only approved as a prescription-only medicine by the Food and Drug Administration and other regulatory authorities in 1998, the potential for this class of agent to revolutionize the treatment of erectile dysfunction (ED) is already apparent. At the 1998 meetings of the American Urological Association (AUA) and the International Society for Impotence Research (ISIR), a considerable volume of clinical data was presented from over 3000 sildenafil-treated patients. This chapter summarizes the currently available data on the biological and clinical effects of sildenafil.

◼ CYCLIC NUCLEOTIDES AND PDE INHIBITION

The cyclic nucleotides cyclic adenosine monophosphate (cAMP) and cyclic guanosine monophosphate (cGMP) are intracellular second messengers that are fundamentally involved in many biochemical and physiological processes. Within the cells of a variety of tissues the levels of both cAMP and cGMP are modulated by PDEs, which control the rate of breakdown (Fig. 26.1). In therapeutic terms, selective targeting of PDE represents an important theoretical locus for drug action. Indeed, for several decades the potential utility of PDE

inhibitors has been hypothesized. However, in general, clinical utility has been limited, owing to the non-selectivity of available agents and/or the occurrence of dose-limiting side effects.

It is now recognized that there is a large and growing family of PDEs, the members of which (also known as isozymes or isoforms) differ with respect to substrate specificity, sensitivity to inhibitors, and organ and subcellular distribution.[1,2] At least nine different gene groups have been identified.[3] The possibility of achieving target organ selectivity, by exploitation of the heterogeneous distribution of PDE isoforms, has led to renewed interest in the clinical potential of a new generation of selective PDE inhibitors. Not surprisingly, therefore, selective inhibitors of the various PDE isoenzymes are under development for a wide variety of cardiovascular, pulmonary and other disorders. Pfizer Inc. (Sandwich, Kent, UK), with sildenafil, have been at the vanguard of research into, and treatment of, one such disorder — ED.

◼ ROLE OF NO/cGMP PATHWAY IN ERECTION AND THE POTENTIAL OF PDE INHIBITORS IN THE TREATMENT OF ED

Figure 26.2 illustrates the molecular basis of the role of NO and cGMP in mediating erections and the mechanism underlying the erectogenic action of PDE inhibitors. There is now unequivocal evidence that NO is

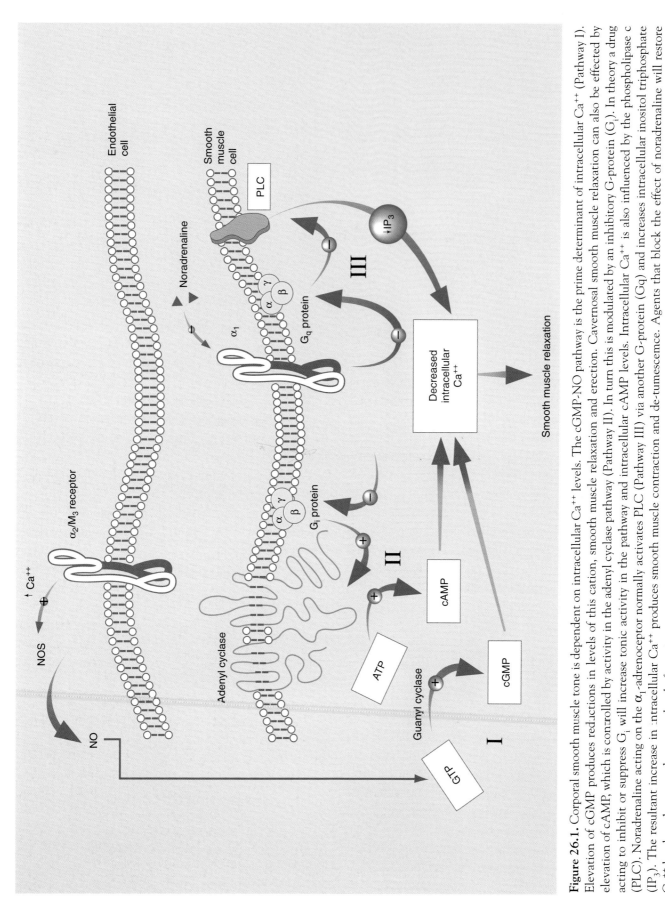

Figure 26.1. Corporal smooth muscle tone is dependent on intracellular Ca^{++} levels. The cGMP-NO pathway is the prime determinant of intracellular Ca^{++} levels (Pathway I). Elevation of cGMP produces reductions in levels of this cation, smooth muscle relaxation and erection. Cavernosal smooth muscle relaxation can also be effected by elevation of cAMP, which is controlled by activity in the adenyl cyclase pathway (Pathway II). In turn this is modulated by an inhibitory G-protein (G_i). In theory a drug acting to inhibit or suppress G_i will increase tonic activity in the pathway and intracellular cAMP levels. Intracellular Ca^{++} is also influenced by the phospholipase c (PLC). Noradrenaline acting on the α_1-adrenoceptor normally activates PLC (Pathway III) via another G-protein (Gq) and increases intracellular inositol triphosphate (IP_3). The resultant increase in intracellular Ca^{++} produces smooth muscle contraction and de-tumescence. Agents that block the effect of noradrenaline will restore Ca^{++} levels and may produce some level of erection.

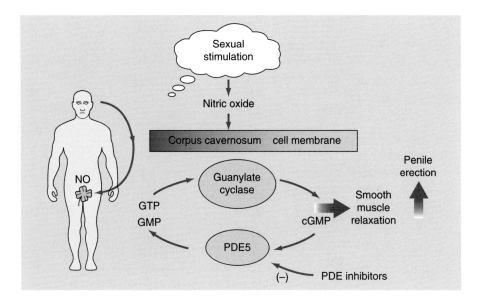

Figure 26.2. Role of NO, cGMP and PDEs in the erectile pathway.

released from the cavernosal nerves during sexual stimulation.[4–11] For more detail see chapter 11 and the review by Naylor.[11] As well as having a primary neurogenic source, NO may also be released from other sites, particularly from the vascular endothelium. Within the cavernosal tissue, NO acts trans-synaptically to activate an enzyme cascade by stimulation of intracellular guanylate cyclase. The resultant elevation in cGMP produces a change in intracellular calcium mobilization and relaxation of corpus cavernosal and vascular smooth muscle.

Selective cGMP-PDE inhibitors will reduce the breakdown of cGMP without affecting cAMP metabolism; levels of the latter, therefore, will be unaffected. This phenomenon is key to the understanding of the effects of sildenafil in man. Thus, in situations associated with low cGMP levels, particularly in ED, an inhibitor will cause an increase in levels of this cyclic nucleotide. As a consequence, corporal smooth muscle relaxation will be induced and an augmented erectile response will be observed. However, in the absence of a sexual stimulus, the intracellular cGMP levels may not be raised to the critical threshold for the production of erections. Equally, in the individual with normal erectile function, PDE inhibitors will have little effect on the steady-state basal cGMP levels in the absence of sexual stimuli.

In marked contrast to the tissue dynamics of cGMP, in several tissues there is substantial basal (background) cAMP production. cAMP activates a similar enzyme cascade of events leading to decreased intracellular calcium and smooth muscle relaxation. On this basis, as there is an appreciable production of cAMP under normal conditions, administration of cAMP-PDE inhibitors may induce erections in the absence of sexual stimulation or, indeed, in normal individuals not suffering ED.

■ PDEs IN THE HUMAN CORPUS CAVERNOSUM AND OTHER ORGANS

In the human corpus cavernosum, PDEs 2, 3 and 5 have been identified,[12] together with PDE4.[13] However, the major cGMP-metabolizing PDE in human corporal tissue has been shown to be the cGMP-specific PDE5.[12] For this reason, agents that inhibit PDE5 should selectively act on the normal physiological pathways in the patient with ED. Several selective and non-selective PDE inhibitors have undergone some level of clinical evaluation.

Papaverine, a non-selective PDE inhibitor, has been successfully used intracavernosally to induce erections, presumably by raising intracellular cAMP levels. However, owing to its non-selectivity and toxicity, papaverine cannot be administered orally. Nevertheless, in several countries the agent is still used intra-cavernosally, with some degree of success, usually in combination with other agents such as phentolamine and/or prostaglandin.

Stief and colleagues have reported that milrinone, a selective inhibitor of PDE3, relaxed human and rabbit corpus cavernosal strips in vitro.[10,14] When milrinone was administered intracavernosally to the rabbit, although slight tumescence and rigidity were observed, dosing was limited, owing to dramatic cardiovascular effects.[14] Nevertheless, at least anecdotally, Stief has also reported that milrinone induced full erections when administered to patients with ED by the intracavernosal route. However, as the actions will not be restricted to cavernosal tissue, it is unlikely that milrinone and other PDE3 inhibitors, which act to raise intracellular cAMP levels, will have potential as oral agents in the treatment of ED. In particular, as PDE3 is also located in cardiac tissue and within the vasculature that would be expected to translate into significant haemodynamic and/or cardiac sequelae.

The clinical utility of any non-selective PDE inhibitor almost certainly will be limited by dose restriction due to side effects produced as a result of enzyme inhibition in a variety of tissues. The use of a selective PDE5 inhibitor, such as sildenafil, may circumvent many of these problems. It is pertinent to note, however, that even in the case of a selective PDE5 inhibitor, theoretically there may be extracorporal manifestations of inhibition of this isoenzyme. In addition to its occurrence in human cavernosal tissue, PDE5 is found elsewhere in the urogenital tract, the gastrointestinal tract, vascular and pulmonary tissue and platelets; only modest amounts are found in brain. An action at any of these loci may be of physiological consequence.

There are published data for only one selective PDE5 inhibitor, sildenafil, which has been administered orally to patients with ED.[12,15–22] Hence, the remainder of this chapter is devoted to summarizing the currently available data on the biological and clinical effects of sildenafil. With respect to treatment of the ED patient, sildenafil has several important features intrinsic in the selectivity of the drug for PDE5. In particular, the localization of PDE5 within the cavernosal tissue, the requirement for sexual stimulation-induced NO production and the intrinsic isoenzyme selectivity of sildenafil would indicate that target organ selectivity is achievable. On this basis, it would be predicted that over the likely therapeutic dose range, sildenafil would have a benign side effect profile.

At the time of preparation of this chapter, sildenafil has been approved in the US and within the EU. It is anticipated that, in most countries, sildenafil will be available at doses ranging from 25 to 100 mg. This chapter cites published articles where relevant but also refers to unpublished data when appropriate.

■ BIOLOGY

Sildenafil is a pyrazolopyrimidine (Fig. 26.3) and its profile of selectivity against the major families of PDE is summarized in Table 26.1. The drug is a potent and selective inhibitor of PDE5.[12,15,16]

Studies in vitro have shown that sildenafil enhances the relaxation of rabbit corpus cavernosum smooth muscle to electrical field stimulation and to exogenous application of nitrates.[17,18] This finding was confirmed with human samples of smooth muscle obtained from patients undergoing implantation of penile prostheses.[19,20] Jeremy and colleagues have shown that sildenafil enhances cGMP levels (but not cAMP levels) in rabbit corpus cavernosum.[15] In a study using cultured human corpus cavernosal smooth muscle cells, Goldstein and colleagues have shown that sildenafil increases cGMP levels with a median inhibitory concentration (IC_{50}) of 2 nM.[16]

In a study in vivo, intravenous sildenafil has been shown to augment the rise in intracavernosal pressure in response to pelvic nerve stimulation in the anaesthetized dog.[21,22] This pro-erectile effect was observed in the absence of any changes in systemic blood pressure and pulse rate and in the absence of any major change in

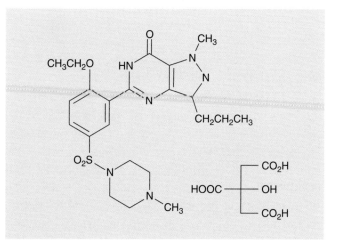

Fig. 26.3. Chemical structure of sildenafil.

Table 26.1. Enzyme-inhibitory profile of sildenafil against human PDE enzymes

PDE isoenzyme family	Substrate specificity	Human source	No. of samples	Geometric mean IC_{50} value (nM)	with 95% confidence interval
PDE 1	cAMP/cGMP	Cardiac ventricle	6	280	(229–337)
PDE 2	cAMP/cGMP	Corpora cavernosa	5	68 000	(31 000–146 000)
PDE 3	cAMP	Corpora cavernosa	4	16 200	(9500–27 800)
		Platelets	3	41 200	(26 100–65 000)
PDE 4	cAMP	Skeletal muscle	3	7200	(4500–11 500)
PDE 5	cGMP	Corpora cavernosa	15	3.5	(2.5–4.8)
		Platelets	3	6.1	(3.0–12.6)
PDE 6	cGMP	Retina — cones	6	34.1	(24.5–47.4)
		Retina — rods	6	37.5	(29.0–48.5)

pudendal blood flow. This finding indicates that the major effect of systemic administration was enhanced relaxation of corpus cavernosal smooth muscle and that any effects on the smooth muscle of the systemic vasculature were clinically insignificant in this model.

Thus, the results of the foregoing studies support the mechanism of action described above and demonstrate that sildenafil exerts its pro-erectile effect via a peripheral mode of action (i.e. acting on the smooth muscle of the corpus cavernosum).

■ PHARMACOKINETICS AND PHARMACODYNAMICS OF SILDENAFIL

Boolell and colleagues have reported on the pharmacokinetics of sildenafil when administered to healthy volunteers at doses ranging from 1.25 to 200 mg.[12] Sildenafil is rapidly absorbed, with maximum plasma concentrations observed within 1 hour after oral dosing in the fasted state. Plasma concentrations decline in a bi-exponential manner with a mean terminal half-life of 3–5 h. Pharmacokinetic simulations predict no significant accumulation of the drug after repeated once-daily dosing. An absolute bioavailability study revealed that sildenafil had a mean plasma clearance of 41 l/h and a mean steady state volume of distribution of 105 litres. The mean absolute bioavailability after oral dosing of a 50 mg capsule was 41%. There were no clinically significant effects on pulse rate, and modest reductions in blood pressure following single administration of oral doses of up to 200 mg. The main adverse effects reported after doses of 90 mg and above were transient headache and flushing. In a separate volunteer study, a high-fat meal has been shown to slow the rate of absorption of oral capsules (mean time to observed peak plasma concentration following administration in the fed state was 2 h) and to reduce the observed peak plasma concentrations by 25%. However, the overall systemic exposure (area under the observed plasma concentration–time curve) was not affected and the clinical significance of these results is unknown. Age >65 years, hepatic impairment and severe renal impairment are associated with increased plasma levels of sildenafil. However, toleration remains similar to that observed in other groups.

Sildenafil is metabolized by cytochrome P450 3A4. Other drugs which inhibit this isozyme (e.g. cimetidine, ketoconazole, erythromyocin) can raise plasma levels of sildenafil. However, in these situations, the dose of sildenafil that patients receive can be adjusted.

In completed interaction studies, no clinically significant interactions have been shown between sildenafil and amlodipine, tolbutamide, warfarin, aspirin, alcohol or antacids in healthy volunteers.

Under experimental conditions (fasted, healthy volunteers positioned at 70 degrees to the horizontal on tilt tables), sildenafil has been shown to enhance the hypotensive effect of glycerol trinitrate. More recently, sildenafil has been shown to enhance the hypotensive effect of glyceryl trinitrate and to enhance the hypotensive effect of isosorbide mononitrate in patients with angina. In view of the magnitude of this effect, sildenafil should not be administered to patients receiving nitrates. This interaction is not surprising, since exogenous nitrates artificially stimulate the NO/cGMP pathway (via release of NO), thus increasing cGMP levels in systemic blood vessels. As sildenafil acts to inhibit the breakdown of cGMP, the response to nitrates will be greatly enhanced and the hypotensive effects may be excessive. Sildenafil has only modest effects on haemodynamic parameters when administered in the absence of nitrates. In clinical trials recruiting patients with ED receiving a variety of concomitant medications, there was no evidence of any interaction between sildenafil and other anti-anginal and antihypertensive agents.

Thus, in healthy-volunteer studies, sildenafil has demonstrated kinetic and dynamic properties that are appropriate for an agent to be administered orally as required prior to sexual activity. These properties include rapid oral absorption and a relatively short plasma half-life of approximately 4 h. Plasma levels are modified by age, certain disease states and concomitant administration of cytochrome P450 3A inhibitors, but the dose of sildenafil can be adjusted, if necessary. Oral doses, within the recommended dose range, have not been shown to have any major effect on cardiovascular haemo-dynamic parameters, including blood pressure and heart rate (except when nitrates are coadministered).

■ CLINICAL EVALUATIONS

The early stage clinical evaluations of sildenafil were designed to determine the magnitude of the response, the dose relationship and toleration. At the outset, a key issue was the definition and determination of efficacy.

Rigiscan® studies

In phase II clinical trials that recruited predominately those men with no known organic cause for ED, sildenafil has been shown to enhance erections in a clinical setting. This effect has been demonstrated objectively by the use of RigiScan® monitoring of penile tumescence and rigidity in response to visual sexual stimulation. In a randomized crossover study, Boolell and colleagues reported that the mean duration of rigidity of more than 80% at the base of the penis during a session viewing erotic videos was 11.2 minutes following a dose of 50 mg sildenafil compared with a mean duration of 1.3 minutes following a placebo.[12] The technique of RigiScan® monitoring during visual sexual stimulation was also used by Eardley and colleagues to investigate the time interval between oral dosing and an erection-enhancing effect.[23] In this randomized, crossover study of 17 semi-fasted patients who started viewing erotic videos 10 minutes after dosing with sildenafil (50 mg dose) or double-blind placebo, the median time to onset of first erection was 19 minutes for the patients responding to sildenafil; the earliest response was seen at 12 minutes. A further RigiScan® study was also performed to assess the time window during which sildenafil can produce an erection in response to sexual stimulation. In this double-blind, placebo-controlled study, sildenafil was still able to produce/enhance an erection in response to sexual stimulation at 2–3 h and at 4–5 h after dose administration.

The RigiScan® device has also been used to explore the potential efficacy of sildenafil in pilot studies of patients with specific organic diseases associated with ED. In a pilot crossover study of 21 patients with diabetes mellitus who underwent visual sexual stimulation and RigiScan® monitoring after 50 and 25 mg doses of sildenafil and double-blind placebo, the mean duration of erection of more than 60% rigidity at the base of the penis was 7.2 minutes, after the 50 mg dose, compared with values of 1.5 and 2.4 minutes after the double-blind placebo and 25 mg doses, respectively.[31]

The potential efficacy of sildenafil has also been investigated in a pilot study of men with documented spinal cord injury.[25] In this study the main recruitment criterion was a requirement to achieve at least a partial erectile response to a vibratory stimulus applied to the penis; in other words, this recruited patients with intact (or at least partially intact) sacral reflexes. The most important exclusion criterion was a spinal injury above the level of T6, since it was considered that patients with high-level lesions would be at risk of autonomic dysreflexia in response to the vibratory stimulus. This study recruited 27 patients who were each monitored during a vibratory stimulus following the oral administration of sildenafil (50 mg) and double-blind placebo in random order. Only two of the 27 patients achieved an erection of more than 60% rigidity at the base of the penis in response to the vibrator following placebo administration; the duration of these erections was 4 and 8 minutes. In contrast, following sildenafil administration, 17 patients achieved an erection of at least 60% rigidity at the base, and the median duration of these erections was 10 minutes.

A further RigiScan® study, which recruited a wide range of patients with a variety of organic diseases associated with ED, also showed that single doses of sildenafil (25, 50 and 100 mg) increased the duration of erection in response to sexual stimulation compared with placebo (unpublished data).

In summary, the technique of RigiScan® monitoring during periods of visual or tactile sexual stimulation has provided objective demonstration of a pro-erectile effect of sildenafil. There is evidence from the dose–response studies that the magnitude of the effect is related to dose. The results suggest that sildenafil has the potential to be effective following the administration of single doses taken as required 30–60 minutes prior to sexual stimulation, and indicate the possibility that sildenafil treatment might be effective in patients with organic causes of ED.

Summary of the early stage clinical evaluations of sildenafil

- The response to sildenafil appears to be dose related over the range 25–100 mg.
- There is no additional benefit to the ED patient at doses above 100 mg and tolerability is reduced.
- Sildenafil is effective in ED patients with organic, psychogenic and mixed organic/psychogenic aetiologies.
- The drug can exert pro-erectile effects 30 minutes to 1 h after administration.
- The effects of sildenafil occur only in response to sexual stimulation.

However, the true effectiveness and utility of sildenafil can only be assessed by trials which allow patients and partners to have sexual activity in the home setting.

Definition and assessment of clinical efficacy: the international index of erectile function (IIEF)

Although objective, quantitative, laboratory-based diagnostic procedures, such as RigiScan® monitoring, are used for evaluating sexual function, they cannot be used in the context of normal sexual activity and are not easily adaptable for large-scale clinical trials. Patient interview techniques have traditionally been difficult to standardize and can be subject to some degree of observer bias. On this basis, sexual function is considered by many to be most relevant when assessed with patient self-report techniques in the home environment using multi-dimensional scales.[26,27,28] Most major clinical trials on sildenafil have employed several self-reported indices of efficacy.

In the majority of studies, particularly the early ones, patients were asked to maintain an event log or diary to record the attempts at intercourse, the degree of success and whether the erections were sufficiently hard for intercourse. Using this scoring system, grade 3 would be 'hard enough for penetration, but not completely hard', whereas grade 4 would be 'completely hard'. In several trials, questions were incorporated to include partner assessment of erections and/or satisfaction with sex life.

In several studies, efficacy was also determined using the International Index of Erectile Function (IIEF)[29] (Appendix 26.1). The IIEF is a brief, reliable, multi-dimensional, self-administered measure for the clinical assessment of ED and treatment outcomes. The questionnaire was specifically developed as an alternative to the complexity of diagnostic tests and the ambiguities associated with patient interviews. In development, all relevant domains of male sexual function were identified across various cultures. The domains were identified as erectile function, orgasmic function, sexual desire, intercourse satisfaction and overall satisfaction. This analysis resulted in the production of the 15-question IIEF that was a major advance in meeting the recommendations of the NIH Consensus Conference, for more robust methodology for determining the symptoms of ED and treatment outcome.[30] Questions 3 and 4 (Table 26.2) are considered to be of particular relevance in the assessment of ability to achieve and maintain an erection sufficient for sexual intercourse — parameters that form an integral part of the definition of ED.[30,31]

Table 26.2. International Index of Erectile Function, questions 3 and 4

Question 3 Over the past 4 weeks, when you attempted sexual intercourse, how often were you able to penetrate (enter) your partner?

Question 4 Over the past 4 weeks, during sexual intercourse, how often were you able to maintain your erection after you had penetrated (entered) your partner?

Subjects respond either by selection 0 ('did not attempt intercourse') or one of the five ordered categorical responses.

1. 'Almost never/never'
2. 'A few times (much less than half the time)'
3. 'Sometimes (about half the time)'
4. 'Most times (much more than half the time)'
5. 'Almost always/always'.

On the basis of a comparison of baseline scores between controls and patients, the IIEF demonstrates a highly significant ability to discriminate between clinical and non-clinical populations[29] (Fig. 26.4). Men with untreated ED had significantly lower scores for all sexual domains of the IIEF except sexual desire, compared with age-matched controls. It is pertinent to note that, of the patients treated with sildenafil, 80% reported improved erections at the end of the study. Further, the domain scores for all sildenafil recipients approached those of age-matched controls without ED.

It is also pertinent to note, however, that during the course of the sildenafil clinical development programme a variety of methods of erectile function evaluation and outcomes analysis have been employed. It is not possible in this chapter to review all the data generated; however, where presented, the data are considered to be representative of the clinical performance of sildenafil in the studies cited. For this reason the bulk of the data presented are based on global efficacy assessment and questions 3 and 4 of the IIEF.

■ MAJOR CLINICAL TRIALS

Background and demographics

Early stage clinical evaluations are designed to determine the potential effective dose range and safety of a potential drug and, as such, may not be entirely reflective of the target population. Two important components of the next phase of clinical evaluation are evaluation in trials that are likely to represent the response in the 'average' ED patient within the community, and the design of trials which are more likely to reflect the clinical setting in which the treatment will eventually be prescribed. Thus, in addition to the eight double-blind, placebo-controlled studies, described earlier, an additional 13 double-blind, placebo-controlled studies have been used to assess efficacy on a self-report basis.

ED is often associated with hypertension, diabetes and depression and the demographic characteristics of the

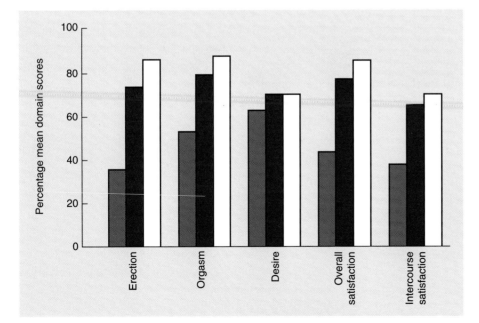

Figure 26.4. Validation of IIEF questionnarie: ■ untreated ED patients at baseline; ■ sildenafil-treated ED patients; □ age-matched controls without ED. Results are from a double-blind, randomized, placebo-controlled study and a non-drug study, both designed to validate the IIEF questionnaire (n = 109–111).

patients receiving sildenafil in clinical trials are shown in Table 26.3.

The use of the questionnaire is exemplified in one phase II study of 233 patients. The design of this study differed from all others. In the initial phase of this study, patients entered a 2-week, single-blind, placebo run-in, followed by a 16-week period of open sildenafil treatment. During this period, patients were started on a dose of 10 mg of sildenafil taken as required prior to sexual activity. The patients visited the investigator at regular intervals, during which the dose could be increased, dependent on toleration and efficacy. At the end of the flexible-dose period, patients were randomized to either placebo or sildenafil. The patients randomized to sildenafil continued on the same dose for another 8 weeks. Efficacy was assessed by global efficacy question, sexual function questionnaire and by diary.

During the open treatment period there were dramatic changes in patient responses to the sexual function questionnaires. Figures 26.6–26.8 illustrate the differences between the baseline and 'end of sildenafil treatment' responses for frequency, hardness and duration of erections. There were similar improvements on other aspects of sexual function. Figure 26.9 represents the difference between baseline and end of treatment for patient assessment of satisfaction with sex life.

The patient population was then subdivided into placebo and sildenafil treatment for an additional 8-week double-blind leg. The response to treatment was maintained in patients taking double-blind sildenafil. However, the frequency, hardness and duration of erection returned to near baseline for patients randomized to double-blind placebo. The data on the differential effects of sildenafil and placebo are summarised in Figures 26.10–26.12. These data confirm that sildenafil is a highly effective treatment for ED arising from a broad spectrum of aetiologies and demonstrate that, for most patients, treatment has to be continued on an 'as required' basis.

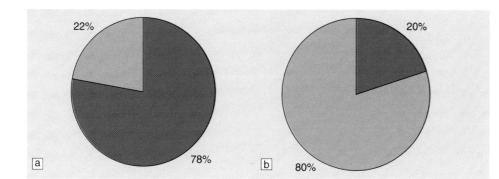

Figure 26.5. Improvement in erections after sildenafil treatment: (a) sildenafil group; (b) placebo group. The results (■ improved; ■ unchanged) are a composite of 3-month and 6-month clinical trial outcomes. These double-blind placebo-controlled, flexible-dose studies were conducted in patients with ED of various aetiologies.

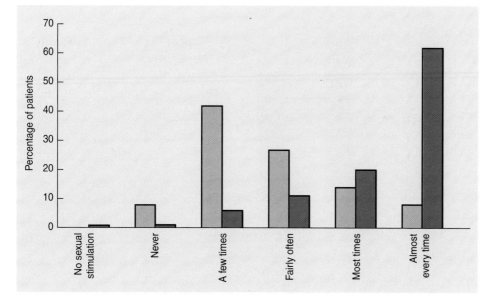

Figure 26.6. Effect of sildenafil on frequency of erections during sexual stimulation: comparison of responses to questionnaire at baseline (■) and at end of 16 weeks' treatment (■). Patients were asked, 'How often did you get an erection during sexual stimulation?'

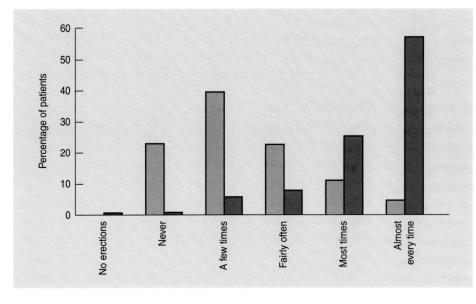

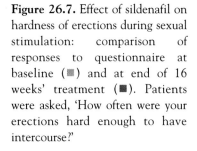

Figure 26.7. Effect of sildenafil on hardness of erections during sexual stimulation: comparison of responses to questionnaire at baseline (■) and at end of 16 weeks' treatment (■). Patients were asked, 'How often were your erections hard enough to have intercourse?'

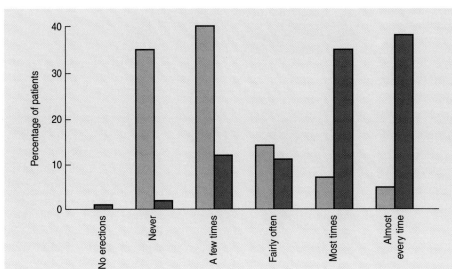

Figure 26.8. Effect of sildenafil on duration of erections during sexual stimulation: comparison of responses to questionnaire at baseline (■) and at end of 16 weeks' treatment (■). Patients were asked, 'How often did your erections last as long as you would have liked?'

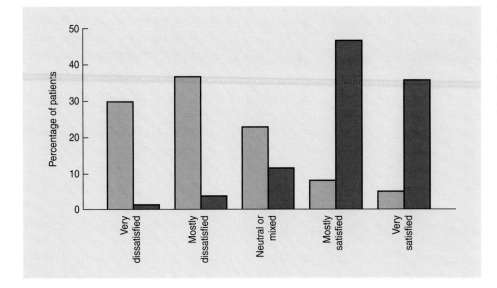

Figure 26.9. Effect of sildenafil on satisfaction with sex life: comparison of responses to questionnaire at baseline (■) and at end of 16 weeks' treatment (■). Patients were asked, 'How satisfied have you been with your sex life?'

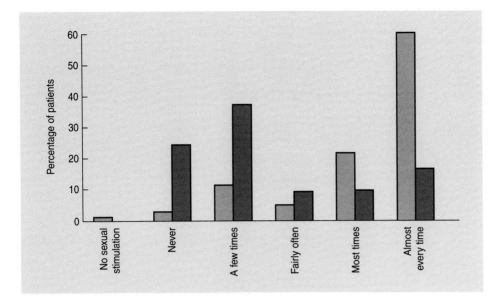

Figure 26.10. Effect of sildenafil (■; n = 95) and placebo (■; n = 103) on frequency of erections during sexual stimulation: responses to questionnaire during 8-week double-blind, placebo-controlled phase. Patients were asked: 'How often did you get an erection during sexual stimulation?'

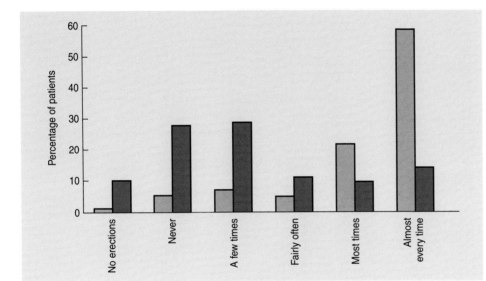

Figure 26.11. Effect of sildenafil (■; n = 95) and placebo (■; n = 103) on hardness of erections during sexual stimulation: responses to questionnaire during 8-week double-blind, placebo-controlled phase. Patients were asked, 'How often were your erections hard enough to have intercourse?'

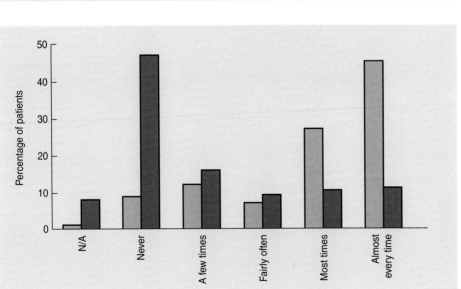

Figure 26.12. Effect of sildenafil (■; n = 94) and placebo (■; n = 101) on duration of erections during sexual stimulation: responses to questionnaire during 8-week double-blind, placebo-controlled phase. Patients were asked, 'How often did your erections last as long as you would have liked?'

Four large, double-blind, randomized, placebo-controlled, multicentre studies of parallel-group design were undertaken to establish the efficacy, tolerability and safety of sildenafil.[32,33,34,35] The main inclusion criteria for these studies were the presence of ED for at least 6 months and the patient being in a stable sexual relationship. Men were excluded if they had penile anatomical defects; a primary diagnosis of another sexual disorder; spinal cord injury; any major psychiatric disorder, not well controlled on treatment; poorly controlled diabetes mellitus; active peptic ulcer disease; a history of alcohol or substance abuse; major renal or hepatic abnormalities; recent (within 6 months) stroke or myocardial infarction; or receipt of regular nitrate therapy. The design and powering of the studies were designed to meet FDA and other regulatory authority requirements. The patient demographics of the approximately 1700 patients, enrolled for 6 months, are shown in Figure 26.13. Over one-half of the patients had ED of organic origin and 29% had mixed organic/ psychogenic aetiology. ED is often associated with hypertension, diabetes and depression. For this reason the efficacy of sildenafil was evaluated in the treatment of ED patients with concomitant disorders, as shown in Table 26.3. Given these patient demographics, it is likely that the patients enrolled in clincial studies of sildenafil will mirror the population in the community at large.

Table 26.3. Demographics of clinical subpopulations in sildenafil studies

Type of study	Number of patients	
Phase I studies	576	
Phase II/III studies	3003	
Long-term extension studies	769	
Other studies	178	
Total	4526	
Hypertension	656	24
Diabetes mellitus	432	16
Cardiovascular disease	378	14
Hyperlipidaemia	389	14
Spinal cord injury	175	6
Depression	132	5
TURP	141	5
Radical prostatectomy	110	4

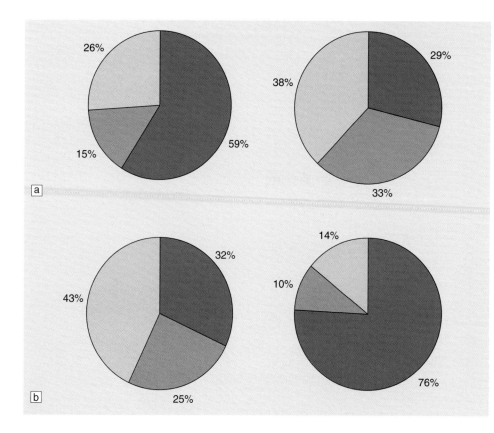

Figure 26.13. Major clinical trials — patient demographics in studies assessed at (left) 3 months and (right) 6 months: (a) fixed-dose studies; (b) flexible-dose studies (■ organic; ■ psychogenic; ■ mixed organic/ psychogenic). For fixed-dose studies, n = 329 and 315, mean age (years) = 59.5 and 54.5, and ED duration (years) = 4.9 and 4.9, respectively. For flexible-dose studies, n = 514 and 532, mean age (years) = 55.7 and 57.6, and ED duration (years) = 4.8 and 3.2, respectively.

In all studies, sildenafil or matching placebo was administered as required, and efficacy was assessed at 3 months and 6 months in the studies of longer duration.

In the flexible-dose studies,[32,34] the dose of sildenafil could be adjusted by the investigator in accordance with the efficacy and tolerability response of the patient. This is considered to be the clinical trial design likely to parallel the use of the drug by the physician: the dose of sildenafil will be adjusted to optimise the balance between benefit and toleration. In one study,[32] shown in Figure 26.14 all patients randomized to receive sildenafil were initiated on 50 mg. The dose could be adjusted to 100 or 25 mg, depending on the patient response and tolerability. At the end, almost three-quarters of patients were on 100 mg and less than 3% on 25 mg.

At the end of 3 months of therapy, the patients were asked if the treatment that they were receiving had improved their erections. Of the patients receiving sildenafil, 78% felt that the treatment had improved erections (Fig. 26.5); the comparable figure in the placebo group was 20%.

The response to the IIEF questions (3 and 4) relating to the ability to achieve and maintain

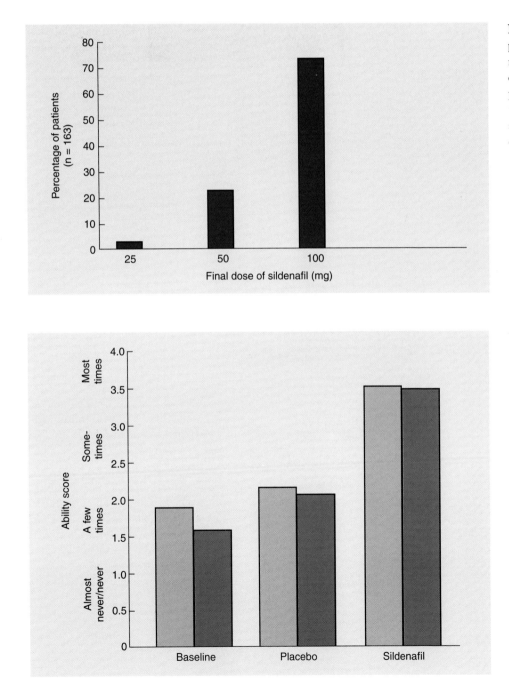

Figure 26.14. Sidenafil: patient preference. Results are from a 3-month, double-blind, placebo-controlled, flexible-dose study. All patients received 50 mg sildenafil initially; the dose could be adjusted to 100 or 25 mg, depending on patient response and tolerability.

Figure 26.15. Patient assessment, using the IIEF questionnaire, of ability to achieve (■) and maintain (■) an erection. Results are from a 6-month, double-blind, placebo-controlled, flexible-dose study. Patients were assessed using questions 3 and 4 of the IIEF (n = 116–254)

erections is shown in Figure 26.15. The mean scores for the sildenafil group, at baseline 1–2, ('almost never/a few times') increased to about 4 ('most times'). Most importantly, there was a good correlation between the IIEF questionnaire data and the number of recorded successful attempts at sexual intercourse (Fig. 26.16).

The effects of sildenafil over the same treatment period (3 and 6 months) were also determined in two fixed-dose studies,[32,35] with patients being randomly assigned to placebo, or to 25, 50 or 100 mg sildenafil, for the duration of the study. The response was dose related (Fig. 26.17). Consistent with the flexible-dose studies, overall 70% (458 of 652) patients reported significant improvements in their erections. Only 26% of patients in the placebo group reported benefit. Once again, the subjective assessment was reinforced by the analysis of data from IIEF questions 3 and 4, from these fixed-dose studies (Fig. 26.18).

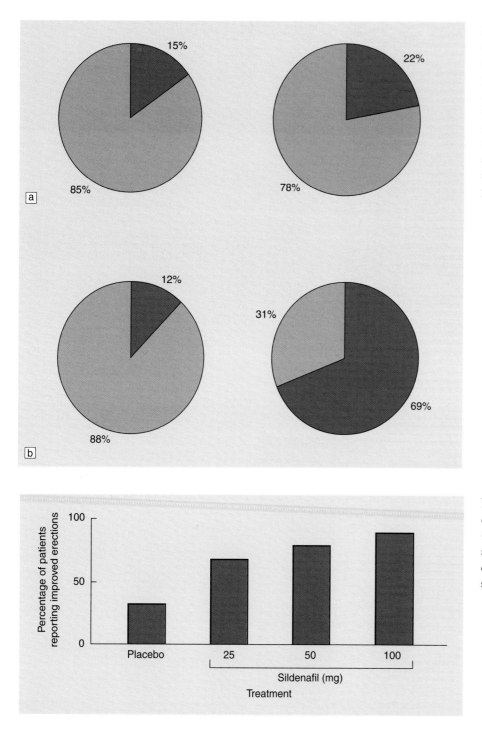

Figure 26.16. Successful (■) or unsuccessful (▨) attempts at intercourse after treatment with (a) placebo (left, baseline; right, final) or (b) sildenafil (left, baseline; right, final). The percentage figures represent the mean percentage of attempts at intercourse that were successful before treatment (baseline) and at the end of a 3-month study period (final): n = 141–157.

Figure 26.17. Improvement in erections after placebo or sildenafil (25–100 mg). Data are from 3-month and 6-month double-blind, placebo-controlled studies (n = 214–223 for sildenafil and 308 for placebo).

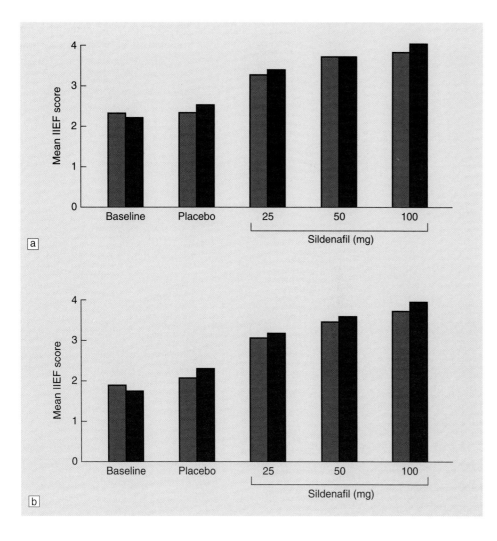

Figure 26.18. Improvement in the ability to (a) achieve and (b) maintain an erection, at the end of a 3-month (■) or 6-month (■) study, as assessed by patients using the IIEF questionnaire (a score of 4 is equivalent to an answer of 'most times' on the questionnaire).

Although a variety of methods of erectile function evaluation and outcomes analysis have been employed during the clinical development programme for sildenafil, certain key features of the drug are apparent. It can be concluded, therefore, from these large studies conducted in the home setting, that sildenafil produces substantial benefit with respect to the ability to achieve and maintain an erection. The response is dose related, much in excess of the placebo response and corroborated by the partner.

Durability of response and need for continued treatment

In the first 12-month study to be completed, of the 292 patients responding to a global efficacy questionnaire, 88% reported that sildenafil improved their erections (Fig. 26.19).[36,37] In addition, 90% of patients indicated that they would continue treatment if sildenafil were widely available.

Two studies conducted separately and described in detail earlier give some insight into the impact of withdrawal of sildenafil treatment.[38,39] At the end of the 16-week open-label study, in which 87% of patients were on 50 or 100 mg sildenafil, patients were randomized to either placebo or active drug at their optimum dose. The results are shown in Figure 26.20. Patients who received open-label sildenafil and were randomized to placebo had mean response scores similar to the overall mean baseline score, recorded at screening prior to treatment. In contrast, the mean scores in patients receiving sildenafil during the double-blind treatment phase were similar to those obtained at the end of a subsequent 12-month open-label study on the drug. The results indicate that most patients will require to continue sildenafil treatment to ensure continued therapeutic benefit.

Studies and analyses of results in population subgroups

From the range of large multicentre studies completed, analyses have been undertaken to evaluate response in

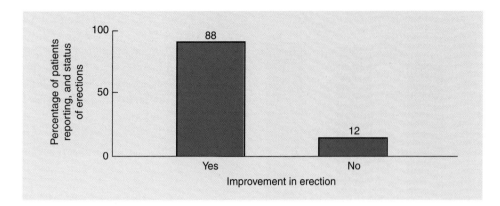

Figure 26.19. Durability of response to sildenafil: results from a 12-month, open-label extension study involving 292 patients, who were asked if their treatment had improved their erections.

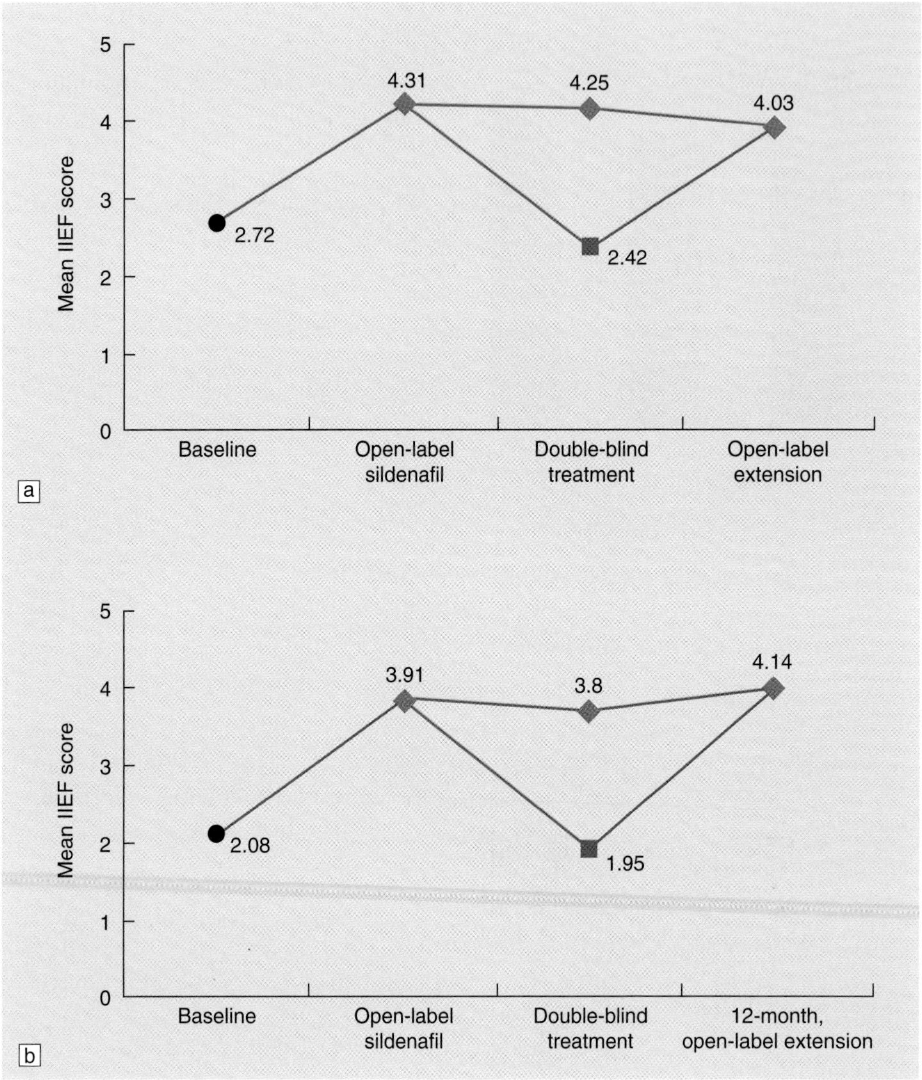

Figure 26.20. Effect of withdrawal of sildenafil treatment, showing (a) frequency of erections and (b) frequency of erections of sufficient duration when patients previously receiving 50 or 100 mg sildenafil were randomly assigned to placebo (■) or active drug (◆). [(●) indicates patients on no drug].

clinically defined subpopulations. In particular, the efficacy and safety of sildenafil has been examined in patients with medical conditions exhibiting co-morbidity with ED; these include diabetes, hypertension and depression.[40]

Diabetes

The efficacy of sildenafil has been examined in patients with type I or type II diabetes with associated organic or mixed organic/psychogenic ED.[32] In one specific study recruiting diabetic patients, the majority of patients

(84%) had type II diabetes. Efficacy assessment was based primarily on IIEF questions 3 and 4. At the end of the 3-month period the majority of patients were on 100 mg.

The response of 57% (Fig. 26.21) was less than in the ED population at large; however, this was partially offset by a lower placebo response (10%) in the diabetic population. A meta-analysis of data obtained from all double-blind placebo-controlled studies indicated that the mean baseline scores were lower in diabetic than in ED patients without diabetes. One interpretation is that the degree of ED is more severe in diabetic patients.

Hypertension

There is a high degree of concomitant ED and hypertension,[40] and some forms of antihypertensive therapy can cause an exacerbation of ED.[41] For this reason, the efficacy of sildenafil was evaluated by meta-analysis of 2195 ED patients subdivided into those who were and were not treated concomitantly with antihypertensives.[42]

Of the patients receiving both treatments, 70% reported that sildenafil improved erections (Fig. 26.21). The magnitude and the nature of the response (determined from IIEF questions three and four) were similar to those ED patients treated with sildenafil but not on antihypertensive medication. The data indicate that sildenafil is effective in treating hypertensive patients on or without medication.

Depression

The efficacy of sildenafil has also been determined in a subpopulation of patients, enrolled in double-blind, placebo-controlled trials, who were diagnosed with concurrent ED and depression.[43] Of the 136 patients, 76% reported an improvement in erections following treatment (Fig. 26.21). This efficacy rate was equivalent to a matched cohort of ED patients not suffering from clinical depression.

Spinal cord injury

A prospective study has been completed in a select patient population in men with ED secondary to spinal cord trauma.[44] For inclusion, the injury had to be sustained at least 6 months prior to entry. The majority of patients had lesions classified as either A or B on the American Spinal Injury Association (ASIA) scale.[45] The study was based on a double-blind, crossover design. Each patient had either placebo or sildenafil for 6 weeks followed by a switch to the other treatment for 6 weeks.

Consistent with the other studies, there was a good correlation with efficacy based on response to the IIEF questions addressing the ability to achieve and maintain erections.

In this trial, 80% of patients reported that sildenafil improved their ability to have intercourse (Fig. 26.22), whereas there was only a 10% response in the placebo group. In addition, of the 118 patients who expressed a

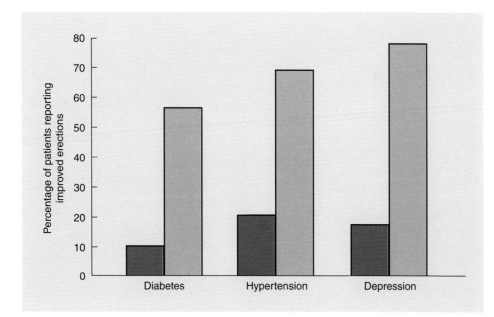

Figure 26.21. Efficacy of sildenafil (▨) or placebo (■) in clinical subgroups (patients with diabetes, hypertension or depression). At the end of the study period (up to 6 months), patients were asked whether their treatment had improved their erections. For the diabetes and depression groups, n = 51–136; the data for the hypertensive group are the result of a subgroup analysis of 1218 patients.

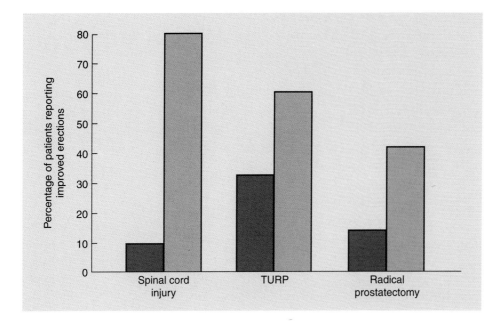

Figure 26.22. Efficacy of sildenafil (■) or placebo (■) in clinical subgroups (patients with spinal cord injury, transurethral resection of the prostate [TURP] or radical prostatectomy). At the end of the study period (6 weeks to 6 months), patients (n = 55–166) were asked whether their treatment had improved their erections.

preference between sildenafil and placebo treatments, 94% preferred sildenafil.

Prostate surgery

The effects of transurethral resection of the prostate (TURP) and radical prostatectomy have been determined by meta-analysis of the clinical trials database.[32] In a subpopulation of patients undergoing TURP, the response to sildenafil was greater than that to placebo (61% and 31%, respectively) and not much less than in an age-matched group (Fig. 26.22).

The efficacy of sildenafil has also been evaluated in a subpopulation of 87% of patients who have undergone a radical prostatectomy (Fig 26.22). Sildenafil was clearly effective in improving erections in some patients. The overall response (43%), although higher than that with placebo (15%), was lower than that in other subpopulations. This relatively low response rate was consistent with a requirement for some degree of residual neuronal activity to ensure a 'full' sildenafil response.

The elderly patient

The relationship of age to response has been measured in clinical trials where one-third of the patients are considered to be elderly (65 years or older):[46] 67% of elderly patients reported that treatment with sildenafil for 3 months improved erections, compared with 75% of patients less than 65 years of age.[46] Response based on IIEF scores was likewise similar to those results, in both groups (Fig 26.23).

Summary of clinical efficacy

Sildenafil has been evaluated in over 3000 patients, aged 19–87 years, in worldwide clinical trials in ED. The mean duration of the ED at trial entry is over 5 years and the disease aetiology has been organic, psychogenic or mixed organic/psychogenic. Prospective studies and retrospective analyses have enabled analysis of response in clinically defined subpopulations: these include ED patients with concurrent diabetes, hypertension, depression or spinal injuries, and those having undergone prostatic surgery and the elderly (>65 years).

- The clinical trials database for sildenafil is likely to be representative of the response in the typical ED patient.
- The results clearly indicate that, although not all individuals will respond, the response rate is substantially better than that to placebo.
- Overall, the response to sildenafil is likely to be about 70%, with an equivalent placebo response of 20–30%.
- Efficacy is maintained for at least a year but treatment must be maintained.
- Sildenafil is effective in patients with organic and psychogenic ED.
- The response in diabetes and post-radical prostatectomy may be less than in other groups.

Adverse events and safety profile

The adverse events reported in clinical trials of sildenafil are usually transient and mild-to-moderate in nature. In

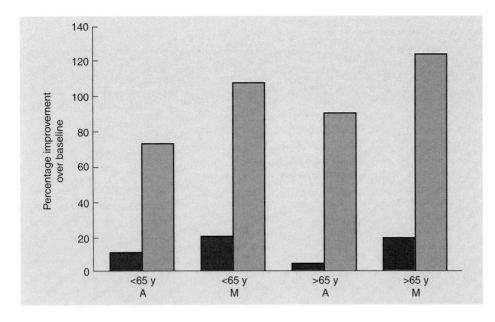

Figure 26.23. Effect of sildenafil (▨) or placebo (■) in the elderly on ability to achieve (A) and maintain (M) an erection. Results are from a subgroup analysis of sildenafil efficacy in non-elderly (< 65 years) and elderly (> 65 years) patients with ED (n = 457–2654).

randomized, double-blind, placebo-controlled trials, over 3000 patients have received sildenafil and 1832 patients placebo, for 6 months or more.[32] In fixed-dose studies, over 190 patients received 200 mg which is twice the maximum-recommended dose, to determine tolerability. In other studies, flexible dosing regimens have been examined. These studies are more likely to reflect actual clinical practice, where the clinician may well attempt dose adjustment to optimize the benefit–tolerability ratio. Overall, the studies have shown that side effects, not unexpectedly, are dose dependent. The flexible-dose studies indicate that the adverse events (of all causalities) in placebo-controlled studies are 60% for sildenafil and 41% for placebo.

The most commonly reported adverse events associated with sildenafil in studies where the dose could be adjusted within the recommended dose range of 25–100 mg are shown in Table 26.4. These are mild and transient headache, flushing, dyspepsia and nasal congestion. Colour vision changes are also reported. Priapism was not reported in clinical trials, although there have been occasional reports of prolonged erections and priapism since launch in the US and other markets.

As can be seen from the placebo response, side effect occurrence in clinical trials is not an unusual feature. More relevant to the physician and patient is the discontinuation due to adverse events,[32] which is shown in Figure 26.24. The overall frequency of discontinuation of sildenafil due to adverse events is very low. In the flexible-dose trials designed to mimic clinical practice, the frequency of discontinuation due to adverse events was comparable in sildenafil and placebo groups (2.3% and 2.1%, respectively). Headache (1.0%), flushing (0.4%) and nausea (0.4%) were the most common treatment-related adverse events resulting in discon-tinuation. Only one patient discontinued treatment at recommended doses due solely to altered vision.

Sildenafil over the effective dose range is an arterio- and venous dilator and will produce modest reductions in blood pressure. There is no evidence, however, that the incidence or severity of side effects is greater in ED patients receiving antihypertensive therapy (Fig. 26.25).

Clinical safety summary

■ Only 1.2% of patients discontinued as a result of treatment-related adverse events.

■ Most common adverse events are headache, flushing, dyspepsia and nasal congestion.

■ Visual effects (colour and brightness perception) have been noted in approximately 3% of patients.

■ Priapism was not reported during clinical trials but has been reported occasionally in post-marketing studies.

■ The incidence of serious adverse events (per 100 man years) was the same for sildenafil and placebo.

■ EFFICACY AND SAFETY POST-MARKETING

The potential for adverse or unexpected events arising from pharmacodynamic or pharmacokinetic interactions is covered earlier in this chapter (see pp. 289–290).

Table 26.4. Adverse events of all causality in placebo-controlled studies

Adverse event	No. of patients reporting an adverse event (%)	
	Viagra (n = 734)	Placebo (n = 725)
Headache	15.8	3.9
Flushing	10.5	0.7
Dyspepsia	6.5	1.7
Nasal congestion	4.2	1.5
Respiratory tract infection	4.2	5.4
Flu syndrome	3.3	2.9
Urinary tract infection	3.1	1.5
Altered vision*	2.7	0.4
Diarrhoea	2.6	1.0
Dizziness	2.2	1.2
Rash	2.2	1.4
Back pain	2.2	1.7
Arthralgia	2.0	1.5

*Mild, transient, predominantly colour tinge to vision, but also increased perception to light or blurred vision. In these studies, only one patient discontinued treatment due to altered vision.

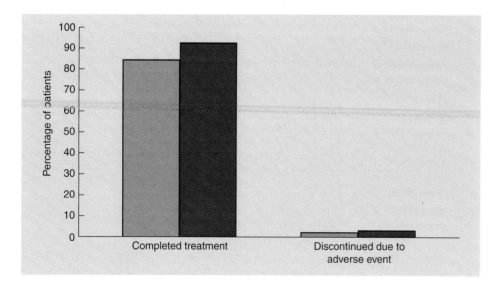

Figure 26.24. Overall rate of discontinuation due to adverse events in placebo (n = 725; ▪) and sildenafil (n = 734; ▪) groups.

At the time of preparation of the manuscript, over three million prescriptions of sildenafil have been written in the US. In general, the reports of efficacy and tolerability match that observed in clinical trials. The most frequently reported

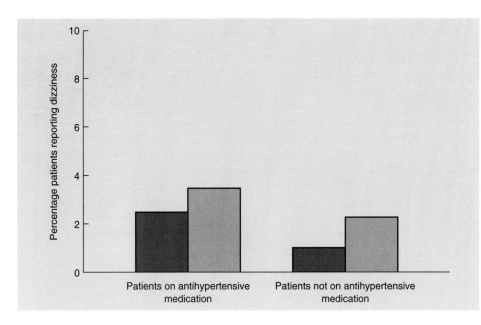

Figure 26.25. Effect of antihypertensive medication on incidence of dizziness while on placebo (■; n = 508 for patients on antihypertensives and n = 1044 for patients not on antihypertensives) or sildenafil (■; n = 885 for patients on antihypertensives and n = 1837 for patients not on antihyper-tensives).

side effects are headache, flushing and dyspepsia. As was the case for both sildenafil and placebo-treated patients in clinical trials, there have been occasional reports of serious adverse events, including myocardial infarction and death. Most of these patients had underlying medical conditions and risk factors for infarction or death, and some were receiving nitrates. Many of the deaths occurred during or shortly after sexual activity. It is impossible to determine unequivocally the cause of these events in these patients. However, the number of serious adverse events is low when considered in relation to that predicted to occur by chance in several million men of comparable age.

Thus, the reports of the efficacy and safety profile of Viagra in the US market are consistent with the findings of the clinical trials. The only exception is that occasional cases of priapism of uncertain cause have been reported.

■ CONCLUSIONS

Sildenafil is a potent and selective inhibitor of PDE5. Inhibition of this enzyme results in augmentation of corpus cavernosal relaxation and thereby restoration of erectile function. The erection-inducing response appears only to occur in ED patients and requires a background of sexual desire and/or stimulation. Based on the results of large, carefully-controlled clinical trials, sildenafil is a simple, effective and well-tolerated treatment of ED in a wide range of patients. The early experience of the introduction of sildenafil to the US market matches the experience in clinical trials.

■ REFERENCES

1. Beavo J A, Reifsnyder D H. Primary sequence of cyclic nucleotide phosphodiaeterase isozymes and the design of selective inhibitors. Trends Pharmacol Sci 1990; 11: 150–155
2. Beavo J A, Conti M, Heaslip R J. Multiple cyclic nucleotide phosphodiesterase. Mol Pharmacol 1994; 46: 399–405
3. Czarniecki M, Ahn H, Sybertz E J. Inhibitors of type I and V phosphodiesterase elevation of cGMP as a therapeutic strategy. Annu Rep Med Chem. 1996; 31: 61–70
4. Burnett A L. Nitric oxide in the penis — physiology and pathophysiology. J Urol 1997; 157: 320–324
5. Raijfer J, Aronson E J, Bush P A et al. Nitric oxide as a mediator of the corpus cavernosum in response to non-cholinergic, non-adrenergic neurotransmission. New Engl J Med 1992; 326: 90–94
6. Burnett A L, Lowenstein C J, Bredt D S et al. Nitric oxide: a physiologic mediator of penile erection. Science 1992; 257: 401–403
7. Burnett A L, Tillman S L, Chang T S K et al. Immunohistochemical localisation of nitric oxide synthase in the autonomic innervation of the human penis. J Urol 1993; 150: 73–76
8. Seftel A D, Ganz M B, Block C et al. Activation of endothelial nitric oxide synthase in endothelium and corporal smooth muscle of human corpus cavernosum mediates relaxation via an NO–K conductance pathway. J Urol 1996; 155: 678A
9. Pickard R S, Powell P H, Zar M A. The effect of inhibitors of nitric oxide biosynthesis and cyclic GMP formation on nerve evoked relaxation of human cavernosal smooth muscle. Br J Pharmacol 1991; 104: 755–759
10. Stief C G, Ückert S, Becker A J et al. Effects of specific phosphodiesterase (PDE) inhibitors on human cavernous tissue in vitro. J Urol 1997; 157: 355 (abstr)

11. Naylor A. Endogenous neurotransmitters mediating penile erection. Br J Urol 1998; 81: 424–431

12. Boolell M, Allen M J, Ballard S A et al. Sildenafil: an orally active type 5 cyclic GMP-specific phosphodiesterase inhibitor for the treatment of penile erectile dysfunction. Int J Impot Res 1996; 8: 47–52

13. Stief C G, Ückert S, Becker AJ et al. Phosphodiesterase isoenzyme of the human cavernous tissue and its functional significance. Aktuel Urol 1995; 26: 22–24

14. Steif C G, Ückert S, Becker A J et al. The effect of specific phosphodiesterase (PDE)-inhibitors on human and rabbit cavernous tissue in vitro and in vivo. Int J Impot Res 1996; 8: 127 (abstr)

15. Jeremy J Y, Ballard S A, Naylor A M et al. Effects of sildenafil, a type 5 cGMP phosphodiesterase inhibitor and papaverine on cyclic GMP and cyclic AMP levels in the rabbit corpus cavernosum in vitro. Br J Urol 1997; 79: 958–963

16. Moreland R B, Goldstein I, Traish A. Sildenafil: a novel inhibitor of phosphodiesterase type 5 in human corpus cavernosum smooth muscle cells. Life Sci 1998; 62: 309–318

17. Tang K, Turner L A, Ballard S A, Naylor A M. Effects of the novel phosphodiesterase type 5 inhibitor, sildenafil, on methacholine induced relaxation of isolated rabbit corpus cavernosum. Br J Pharmacol 1996; 118: 153P (abstr)

18. Ballard S A, Turner L A, Naylor A M. Sildenafil (Viagra™), a potent selective inhibitor of type 5 phosphodiesterase, enhances nitric oxide dependent relaxation of rabbit corpus cavernosum. Br J Pharmacol 1996; 118: 154P (abstr)

19. Ballard S A, Gingell C, Price M E et al. Sildenafil, an inhibitor of phosphodiesterase type 5, enhances nitric oxide mediated relaxation of human corpus cavernosum. Int J Impot Res 1996; 8: 103 (abstr)

20. Ballard S A, Gingell C J, Tang K et al. Effects of sildenafil on the relaxation of human corpus cavernosum tissue in vitro and on the activities of cyclic nucleotide phosphodiesterase enzymes. J Urol 1998; 159: 2164–2171

21. Carter A J, Ballard S A, Naylor A M. Effects of sildenafil on corpus cavernosal responses to pelvic nerve stimulation in the anaesthetised dog. J Urol 1998; 160: 242–246

22. Carter A J, Ballard S A, Naylor A M. Effect of sildenafil (VIAGRA™) on erectile function in the anaesthetised dog. J Urol 1997; 157: 357 (abstr)

23. Eardley I, Brook J, Yates P K et al. Sildenafil (Viagra™), a novel oral treatment with rapid onset of action for penile erectile dysfunction. Br J Urol 1997; 79: 66 (abstr)

24. Price D, Gingell C, Gepi-Attee S et al. Sildenafil (Viagra™): a novel oral therapy for penile erectile dysfunction in patients with diabetes. Diabetic Med 1997; 14: A6 (abstr)

25. Derry F, Gardner B P, Glass C et al. Sildenafil (Viagra™): a double-blind, placebo-controlled, single-dose, two way crossover study in men with erectile dysfunction caused by traumatic spinal cord injury. J Urol 1997; 157: 181 (abstr)

26. Conte H R. Development and use of self-reporting techniques for assessing sexual functioning: a review and critique. Arch Sex Behav 1983; 12: 555–576

27. Stewart A L, Ware J E (eds). Measuring function and well-being: the medical outcomes study approach. Durham: Duke University Press, 1992

28. Andersson B L, Broffitt G. Is there a reliable and valid self-report measure of sexual behaviour? Arch Sex Behav 1998; 17: 509–525

29. Rosen R C, Riley A, Wagner G et al. The International Index of Erectile Function (IIEF); a multidimensional scale for assessment of erectile dysfunction. Urology 1997; 49: 822–830

30. NIH Consensus Development Panel on Impotence. Impotence. JAMA 1993; 270: 83–90

31. Montague D K, Barada J H, Belker A M et al. Clinical guidelines panel on erectile dysfunction: summary report on the treatment of organic erectile dysfunction. J Urol 1996; 156: 2007–2011

32. Data on file, Pfizer Inc., Sandwich, Kent, UK

33. Goldstein I, Lue T F, Padma-Nathan H et al. Oral sildenafil in the treatment of erectile dysfunction. N Engl J Med 1998; 338: 1397–1404

34. Cuzin B, Emrich H M, Meuleman E J H et al. Sildenafil (Viagra™): a 6- month double-blind, placebo-controlled, flexible dose escalation study in patients with erectile dysfunction. Int J Impot Res 1998, in press

35. Montosori F, Morgan R J, Olsson A M et al. Sildenafil (Viagra™): a 3-month double-blind, placebo-controlled, fixed dose study in patients with erectile dysfunction. Eur Urol 1998, in press

36. Guiliano F, Jardin A, Gingell C J et al. Sildenafil (Viagra™), an oral treatment for erectile dysfunction: a 1-year, open-label, extension study. Br J Urol 1997; 80: 93a

37. Buvat J, Gingell C J, Jardin A et al. Sildenafil (Viagra™), an oral treatment for erectile dysfunction: a 1-year, open-label, extension study. J Urol 1997; 157s: 204a

38. Christiansen E, Hodges M, Holingshead M, et al. Sildenafil (Viagra™), a new oral treatment for erectile dysfunction: results of a 16-week, open-label, dose-escalation study. Int J Impot Res 1996; 8: 147a

39. Guirguis W, Dickinson S, Hodges M et al. Sildenafil (Viagra™), a new oral treatment for erectile dysfunction; a 16-week, open-label, dose-escalation, study. Proc R Coll Psychiatrists 1997; 82: 48a

40. Feldman H A, Goldstein I, Hatzichristou D G et al. Impotence and its medical and psychosocial correlates: results of the Massachusetts Male Aging Study. J Urol 1994; 151: 54–61

41. Benet A E, Melman A. The epidemiology of erectile dysfunction. Urol Clin North Am 1995; 22: 699–709

42. Feldman R, and the Sildenafil Study Group. Sildenafil in the treatment of erectile dysfunction: efficacy in patients taking concomitant antihypertensive medication. Am J Hypertens 1998; in press

43. Price D. Sildenafil (Viagra™): efficacy in the treatment of erectile dysfunction (ED) in patients with common concomitant conditions. Int J Impot Res 1998; 10: 53, 254a

44. Holmgren E, Guiliano F G, Hutling C et al. Sildenafil (Viagra™) in the treatment of erectile dysfunction (ED) caused by spinal cord injury (SCI): a double-blind, placebo-

controlled, flexible-dose, two-way crossover study. Neurology 1998; in press

45. Ditunno J F, Young W, Donovan W H, Creasey G. The International Standards Booklet for Neurological and Functional Classification of Spinal Cord Injury. Paraplegia 1994; 32: 70–80

46. Auerbach S, for the Sildenafil Study Groups. Sildenafil (Viagra™) in the treatment of erectile dysfunction in elderly patients. J Am Geriatr Soc 1998; in press

■ APPENDIX 26.1

International Index of Erectile Function (IIEF)[29]

A Multidimensional Scale for Assessment of Erectile Dysfunction

These questions ask about the effects your erection problems have had on your sex life **over the past 4 weeks**. Please answer the following questions as honestly and clearly as possible. In answering these questions, the following definitions apply:

- ■ **sexual activity** includes intercourse, caressing, foreplay, and masturbation
- ■ **sexual intercourse** is defined as vaginal penetration of the partner (you entered your partner)
- ■ **sexual stimulation** includes situations like foreplay with a partner, looking at erotic pictures, etc.
- ■ **ejaculate**: the ejection of semen from the penis (or the feeling of this).

1. **Over the past 4 weeks**, how often were you able to get an erection during sexual activity? *Please check one box only.*
   - ❑ No sexual activity
   - ❑ Almost always/always
   - ❑ Most times (much more than half the time)
   - ❑ Sometimes (about half the time)
   - ❑ A few times (much less than half the time)
   - ❑ Almost never/never

2. **Over the past 4 weeks**, when you had erections with sexual stimulation, how often were your erections hard enough for penetration? *Please check one box only.*
   - ❑ No sexual activity
   - ❑ Almost always/always
   - ❑ Most times (much more than half the time)
   - ❑ Sometimes (about half the time)
   - ❑ A few times (much less than half the time)
   - ❑ Almost never/never

The next three questions will ask about the erections you may have had during sexual intercourse.

3. **Over the past 4 weeks**, when you attempted sexual intercourse, how often were you able to penetrate (enter) your partner? *Please check one box only.*
   - ❑ Did not attempt intercourse
   - ❑ Almost always/always
   - ❑ Most times (much more than half the time)
   - ❑ Sometimes (about half the time)
   - ❑ A few times (much less than half the time)
   - ❑ Almost never/never

4. **Over the past 4 weeks**, during sexual intercourse, how often were you able to maintain your erection after you had penetrated (entered) your partner? *Please check one box only.*
   - ❑ Did not attempt intercourse
   - ❑ Almost always/always
   - ❑ Most times (much more than half the time)
   - ❑ Sometimes (about half the time)
   - ❑ A few times (much less than half the time)
   - ❑ Almost never/never

5. **Over the past 4 weeks**, during sexual intercourse, how difficult was it to maintain your erection to completion of intercourse? *Please check one box only.*
   - ❑ Did not attempt intercourse
   - ❑ Extremely difficult
   - ❑ Very difficult
   - ❑ Difficult
   - ❑ Slightly difficult
   - ❑ Not difficult

6. **Over the past 4 weeks**, how many times have you attempted sexual intercourse? *Please check one box only.*
   - ❑ No attempts
   - ❑ 1–2 attempts
   - ❑ 3–4 attempts
   - ❑ 5–6 attempts
   - ❑ 7–10 attempts
   - ❑ 11+ attempts

7. **Over the past 4 weeks**, when you attempted sexual intercourse, how often was it satisfactory for you? *Please check one box only.*
- ❏ Did not attempt intercourse
- ❏ Almost always/always
- ❏ Most times (much more than half the time)
- ❏ Sometimes (about half the time)
- ❏ A few times (much less than half the time)
- ❏ Almost never/never

8. **Over the past 4 weeks**, how much have you enjoyed sexual intercourse? *Please check one box only.*
- ❏ No intercourse
- ❏ Very highly enjoyable
- ❏ Highly enjoyable
- ❏ Fairly enjoyable
- ❏ Not very enjoyable
- ❏ No enjoyment

9. **Over the past 4 weeks**, when you had sexual stimulation **or** intercourse, how often did you ejaculate? *Please check one box only.*
- ❏ No sexual stimulation/intercourse
- ❏ Almost always/always
- ❏ Most times (much more than half the time)
- ❏ Sometimes (about half the time)
- ❏ A few times (much less than half the time)
- ❏ Almost never/never

10. **Over the past 4 weeks**, when you had sexual stimulation **or** intercourse, how often did you have the feeling of orgasm (with or without ejaculation)? *Please check one box only.*
- ❏ No sexual stimulation/intercourse
- ❏ Almost always/always
- ❏ Most times (much more than half the time)
- ❏ Sometimes (about half the time)
- ❏ A few times (much less than half the time)
- ❏ Almost never/never

The next two questions ask about sexual desire. Let's define sexual desire as a feeling that may include wanting to have a sexual experience (for example masturbation or intercourse), thinking about having sex, or feeling frustrated due to lack of sex.

11. **Over the past 4 weeks**, how often have you felt **sexual desire**? *Please check one box only.*
- ❏ Almost always/always
- ❏ Most times (much more than half the time)
- ❏ Sometimes (about half the time)
- ❏ A few times (much less than half the time)
- ❏ Almost never/never

12. **Over the past four weeks**, how would you rate your level of sexual desire? *Please check one box only.*
- ❏ Very high
- ❏ High
- ❏ Moderate
- ❏ Low
- ❏ Very low or none at all

13. **Over the past 4 weeks**, how satisfied have you been with your overall **sex life**? *Please check one box only.*
- ❏ Very satisfied
- ❏ Moderately satisfied
- ❏ About equally satisfied and dissatisfied
- ❏ Moderately dissatisfied
- ❏ Very dissatisfied

14. **Over the past 4 weeks**, how satisfied have you been with your **sexual relationship** with your partner? *Please check one box only.*
- ❏ Very satisfied
- ❏ Moderately satisfied
- ❏ About equally satisfied and dissatisfied
- ❏ Moderately dissatisfied
- ❏ Very dissatisfied

15. **Over the past 4 weeks**, how do you rate your **confidence** that you can get and keep your erection? *Please check one box only.*
- ❏ Very high
- ❏ High
- ❏ Moderate
- ❏ Low
- ❏ Very low or none at all

Chapter 27
Oral agents in the management of erectile dysfunction

J. P. Mulhall and I. Goldstein

■ INTRODUCTION

The concept of oral agent manipulation of erection is not a novel one, indeed, numerous empiric oral therapies have previously been utilized in an effort to augment the erectile response, most with only minimal benefit over placebo. Much interest is currently focused on the development of newer, more specific, oral agents for the management of the impotent male. In the evaluation of any oral therapy, it is incumbent upon the reviewer to define certain facts concerning the scientific study. First, the exact nature of the study must be critically assessed. Was the study placebo controlled or randomized? What was the sample size evaluated? Second, the exact nature of the population studied must be properly defined. Was the study group predominantly psychogenic or did it represent a random cross-section of the impotence population? Third, what was the endpoint of the study? Was the endpoint any noticeable improvement in erectile function or was it the actual ability to have sexual intercourse? Were parameters of rigidity and duration of erection defined and, if so, how did the criteria compare with those utilized in other studies?

The success of any oral therapy must be based on a thorough knowledge of the cellular mechanisms involved in erection and precise manipulation of these mechanisms. This chapter reviews the basic erectile cellular physiology, in particular, those neurotransmitters known to be involved in erectile tumescence and detumescence.

■ CELLULAR MECHANISM OF ERECTION

At the cellular level, smooth muscle relaxation is mediated through two distinct (though interacting) pathways — namely, the adenylate cyclase/cyclic adenosine monophosphate (cAMP) and guanylate cyclase/cyclic guanosine monophosphate (cGMP) pathways[1] (Fig. 27.1). Adenylate cyclase is activated to

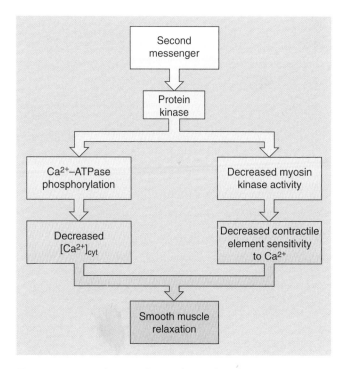

Figure 27.1. Mediation of smooth muscle relaxation.

cleave ATP to 3',5'-cAMP by a variety of stimuli, including calcitonin gene-related peptide, vasoactive intestinal peptide, prostaglandin E1 (CGRP, VIP, PGE1) and forskolin.[2] Guanylate cyclase activation, resulting in 3'5'-cGMP production, results from nitric oxide release from both nerve endings and vascular endothelium. Elevated levels of intracellular second messengers (cAMP/cGMP) result in the movement of intracellular Ca^{2+} into the endoplasmic reticulum, combined with phosphorylation of cellular membrane proteins altering the configuration of the voltage-dependent Ca^{2+} channels.[3–5] These alterations result in the efflux of Ca^{2+} from the cell, which leads to smooth muscle relaxation and penile erection.[6]

■ NEUROTRANSMITTERS

Immunohistochemical studies have demonstrated the existence of neuromediators liberated by nerve fibre endings that are responsible for smooth muscle contraction and relaxation. These neurotransmitters can be subdivided into erection-inducing (erectogenic) and anti-erectile (erectolytic), depending on their effect upon smooth muscle contractility (Table 27.1).

Table 27.1. Neurotransmitters involved in penile erection

Erectogenic	Nitric oxide (NO)
	Serotonin (5HT)
	Dopamine
	Vasoactive intestinal polypeptide (VIP)
	Histamine
	Oxytocin
	Pituitary adenylate cyclase-activating peptide (PACAP)
	Calcitonin gene-related peptide (CGRP)
	Substance P
Erectolytic	Noradrenaline
	Neuropeptide Y
	Gamma-aminobutyric acid (GABA)

Erectogenic neurotransmitters

Acetylcholine

Several authors have demonstrated the presence of muscarinic receptors and acetylcholine synthesis and release in human corpus cavernosum smooth muscle cells.[7–9] Parasympathetic nerve fibre endings appear to elicit their action, not through a direct relaxing effect on erectile tissue itself nor by stimulation of postsynaptic muscarinic receptors, but rather through presynaptic regulation of sympathetic nerve fibre discharge combined with the modulation of nitric oxide release from endothelial cells.[10]

Vasoactive intestinal polypeptide (VIP)

This polypeptide and its receptor have been identified immunohistochemically in human corpus cavernosum smooth muscle and around the helicine arteries.[11] The intracavernosal injection of VIP in impotent patients elicits erection[12] and, when it is combined with acetylcholine, a synergistic effect has been observed.[13] Its primary effect is on G-protein-dependent adenylate cyclase, resulting in the accumulation of cAMP within the smooth muscle cell.

Nitric oxide

Nitric oxide (NO), one of nature's simplest molecules, has been labelled the putative primary neurotransmitter of erection. It is a cleavage product of the amino acid L-arginine[14] and requires the enzyme nitric oxide synthase (NOS) for its production. In vitro, smooth muscle relaxation has been elicited by NO donors and blocked by NO antagonists or NOS inhibitors.[15] Numerous authors have demonstrated the presence of NO in corporal smooth muscle cells. Neural endings with positive immunoreactivity for NOS have been observed in the trabeculae of the corpus cavernosum and around the cavernosal and deep dorsal penile arteries.[15] Following bilateral section of the cavernous nerves in rats, NADPH-diaphorase, a specific marker for NOS, has been demonstrated to diminish in corporal smooth muscle cells.[16]

NO is liberated by both neuronal fibre endings and endothelial cells. Under physiological conditions it has been suggested that neural NO is more important than endothelial NO.[17] Brock and co-workers have postulated that NADPH-diaphorase staining of cavernosal biopsy specimens may add qualitative information about pro-erectile autonomic innervation and may represent a potentially new diagnostic tool for neurogenic impotence.[18]

Calcitonin gene-related peptide (CGRP)

The existence of this peptide has been demonstrated in the neural fibre endings of the human corpus cavernosum.[19] When CGRP is injected intracavernosally combined with subthreshold doses of PGE1, erection is observed.[20] The smooth muscle relaxing effect has also been demonstrated in the bovine model and this effect is believed to be the result of direct corporal smooth muscle relaxation.[21]

Substance P

Substance P has been shown to be present in the human genitourinary tract.[22] In vitro, precontracted strips of corpus cavernosum are relaxed with substance P. This effect may be partially dependent on the presence of endothelial NO release.[23]

Pituitary adenylate cyclase-activating peptide (PACAP)

Hedlund has demonstrated a relaxing effect of this peptide, structurally similar to VIP, upon precontracted strips of corpus cavernosum.[24]

Adenosine triphosphate (ATP)

The intracavernosal or intrarterial injection of ATP relaxes cavernosal smooth muscle and increases intracavernosal pressure in dogs.[13] Precontracted strips of corpus cavernosum are relaxed in vitro by ATP.[25]

Serotonin (5HT)

Steinbusch[26] and Newton and Hamill[27] have demonstrated the close relationship between parasympathetic and 5HT terminations in cavernosal smooth muscle. Several different receptor subtypes exist: 5HT1A, 5HT1B, 5HT1C and 5HT2. The are associated with preganglionic neurons at sacral and thoracolumbar levels and have a role in the regulation and modulation of sympathetic and parasympathetic output. Furthermore, the dorsolateral nucleus of the pudendal nerve exhibits a high density of 5HT1-binding sites. Central receptor stimulation, by intrathecal infusion of 5HT, depresses reflex erection,[28] while peripheral injection of a 5HT agonist (m-chlorophenylpiperazine, mCPP) elicits penile erection.[29]

Dopamine

The hypothalamic medial pre-optic area, rich in dopaminergic receptors, is an important integrating centre contributing to penile erection.[17] Furthermore, dopaminergic stimulation activates serotonergic neurons in the median raphe, improving septo-hippocampal cholinergic transmission, thus promoting erection.[30] However, peripheral intrathecal injection of apomorphine (dopamine agonist) in rats, at the lumbosacral level, was shown to suppress penile reflexes.[31]

Oxytocin

This substance is present in the paraventricular nucleus of the hypothalamus and has been further demonstrated in neurons of the hypothalamic connections to brain-stem and spinal centres involved in autonomic control. There is evidence that oxytocinergic neural terminations may modulate penile erection.[32]

Histamine

A recent study that investigated the relaxant action of histamine on corpus cavernosum in vitro and in vivo (intracavernosal injection in patients with psychogenic impotence), demonstrated that histamine plays a role in human penile erection.[33] The erection-promoting action of histamine appears to be due to H2-receptor activation.

Erectolytic neurotransmitters
Noradrenaline (NA)

Several receptor-binding studies have demonstrated the presence of alpha- and beta-adrenergic receptors in human corpus cavernosum.[19,34,35] It is known that intracavernosal injection of phenoxybenzamine, moxisylate or phentolamine (adrenoreceptor blockers) can elicit erection in man. In contradistinction, intracavernosal injection of beta agonists (e.g. salbutamol) induces penile tumescence.[36] It has been demonstrated that the contractile response to NA, recognized as the main anti-erectile neurotransmitter, was mediated by a heterogeneous population of alpha receptors (alpha-1A, alpha-1B and alpha-1C), which are all expressed in human corpus cavernosum.[34] On the other hand, it seems that presynaptic alpha-2 adrenoreceptors are more involved in the contraction of the cavernous arteries.[19] Furthermore, they exert certain modulating effects on cavernous smooth muscle contraction elicited by alpha-1 adrenoreceptors.[37] Therefore, the pharmacological profile of smooth muscle cells isolated from human penile corpus cavernosum supports the concept of alpha receptors mediating contraction whereas beta receptors mediate relaxation.[38]

Neuropeptide Y (NPY)

This neuropeptide has been documented as occurring in human cavernosal vessels, cavernosal smooth muscle and around the deep dorsal vein of the penis.[39] Arterial injection of NPY diminishes the intracavernosal pressure induced by stimulation of the cavernosal nerve in dogs, inducing penile detumescence.[40]

Gamma-amino butyric acid (GABA)

Magoul demonstrated the presence of GABA-containing spinal nerve fibres, in the vicinity of parasympathetic preganglionic neurons and around the nucleus of the pudendal nerve. Baclofen, a GABA agonist, acts on GABA beta-receptors and inhibits reflex erections in rats, when delivered both peripherally and centrally (intrathecally).[41]

■ CLASSIFICATION OF ORAL AGENTS

This chapter classifies oral agents according to their site/mechanism of action. However, more recently, Heaton and colleagues have introduced a novel taxonomy for therapies in erectile dysfunction based on their mechanism and site of action.[42] Translating that nomenclature to oral therapy, such agents can be subdivided into four main subgroups — central initiators, central conditioners, peripheral initiators and peripheral conditioners. Central initiators have an effect at the central nervous system (CNS) level and thus activate neural events that result in coordinated signalling leading to the initiation of a penile erection. Peripheral initiators, in contradistinction, have their main site of action in the periphery. Central conditioners function to improve the internal milieu in the CNS so that penile erection is enhanced or enabled; similarly, peripheral conditioners enable or enhance penile erection through peripheral action. Conditioners do not initiate erection themselves.

Adrenergic receptor antagonists

Phentolamine

Oral administration of the non-selective antagonist phentolamine has been shown to result in erection.[43] Phentolamine also demonstrates some antiserotonin

actions and a direct non-specific relaxant effect on blood vessels. Zorgniotti demonstrated the efficacy of 50 mg phentolamine in patients with psychogenic and mild arteriogenic erectile dysfunction:[44] there was a 42% rate of functional erection development. These results were confirmed in a non-randomized, non-placebo-controlled multicentre trial where patients used 20–40 mg phentolamine impregnating a strip of filter paper, applied to the buccal mucosa 15 minutes before coitus.[45] In this study, 32% of patients obtained an erection suitable for intercourse versus 13% who had used placebo. More recently, two trials have demonstrated an efficacy of oral phentolamine (Vasomax™) of 60%, when administered 30 min prior to sexual activity. However, a placebo response rate of 40% was cited in the studies.

Yohimbine

This drug is an indole alkaloid with properties as an alpha-2 adrenoreceptor antagonist with central and peripheral effects.[46] Studies have failed to demonstrate any statistically significant benefit of yohimbine over placebo in the treatment of erectile failure.[47,48] Side effects include anxiety, nausea, palpitations, fine tremor and elevations of diastolic blood pressure.[49] The American Urological Association (AUA) erectile dysfunction management guidelines have suggested that yohimbine has never been documented to be effective and offers little benefit. More recently, it has been suggested that the combination of the drug with other agents may prove efficacious.

Delaquamine

This newer alpha-2 adrenoreceptor antagonist is 100 times more selective for the alpha-2 receptor than yohimbine. Delaquamine has good bioavailability, linear pharmacokinetics and a 5–8 h half-life. Data, to date, however, have failed to demonstrate any beneficial effects over placebo.[49]

Dopamine receptor agonist
Apomorphine

Apomorphine has direct central D2 receptor agonist activity. Morales and associates have recently developed a sublingual formulation that appears to be effective in many patients with minimal vasculogenic impotence.[49] Undesirable side effects include persistent yawning, nausea, vomiting and hypotension.[50] In a carefully selected group of patients with psychogenic impotence,

8/12 (67%) experienced durable erections.[49] Phase III trials are ongoing at present, evaluating the efficacy of this agent in the treatment of men with impotence of no certain organic aetiology. The medication is administered sublingually 20–40 minutes prior to sexual relations.

Serotonin receptor agonist
Trazodone

Trazodone is an atypical antidepressant used empirically for the treatment of erectile dysfunction. Besides its serotoninergic activity it has also demonstrated alpha-blocking properties. It has been associated with the development of priapism in approximately 1/10 000–20 000 users.[51] Its mechanism of action in promoting erection is not well known, but it is believed that it exerts its primary effect by stimulation of the 5HT1C receptors through re-uptake inhibition.[52] It may have a secondary effect as an alpha-adrenergic-blocking agent.[53] The medication is used at the dose of 50–200 mg orally at bedtime. One study has cited trazodone's efficacy as being as high as 60%,[54] although this response rate has not been duplicated by others. Synergism has been postulated to exist between yohimbine and trazodone[55] and, although the combination has been used empirically, no scientific study has been conducted evaluating the efficacy of trazodone and yohimbine together.

Phosphodiesterase inhibitor
Sildenafil

This substance (Viagra™), originally used as an anti-anginal agent, is a competitive and selective inhibitor of cGMP type V phosphodiesterase (PDE). This inhibition increases the level of intracellular cGMP and, therefore, results in the efflux of calcium ions from the cell and consequent smooth muscle relaxation. It is administered 1 h prior to sexual activity and at higher doses (50–100 mg) has resulted in improvement in erectile ability in up to 77% of men.[56] It has been associated with minimal side effects, including headache and blurred vision. Recently, this agent has received FDA approval (see Chapter 26).

Nitric oxide donor
L-Arginine

This is the precursor of NO. The only study in the literature is a placebo-controlled trial using large doses of L-arginine (2800 mg daily) for a period of 2 weeks, which reported that 40% of the patients had improvement in their erections.[57] The responders were younger and had better arterial function by haemodynamic investigation than the non-responders.

Hormonal therapy
Testosterone

Testosterone therapy for erectile dysfunction is indicated only in confirmed cases of endocrinopathies and should be reserved for patients with documented hypogonadism. The National Institutes of Health Consensus Conference on Impotence[58] has decreed that oral testosterone preparations are less preferable than intramuscular administration, because of the relatively unpredictable serum levels obtained, the risk of liver toxicity and the elevation of serum lipid levels.[58,59] If given orally, the preparation that is least associated with adverse effects is testosterone undecanoate. Transdermal testosterone has been shown to result in more sustained, even levels of serum testosterone.[60]

Bromocriptine

As a hormonal treatment, this drug has been utilized successfully in hyperprolactinaemia-associated hypogonadism with subsequent improvement in erectile function.[50] It is administered in a starting dose of 1.2 mg once daily and has minimal side effects. It is most useful in the management of microadenomata of the pituitary that have resulted in the development of elevated prolactin levels.

■ THE ROLE OF ORAL AGENTS

There has been an explosion in consumer and industry interest in oral therapy for impotence, following the development of novel oral agents. Consequently, a plethora of data has been released regarding these newer agents. The clinician and scientist must critically evaluate these data before truly defining the role of these agents in the management of the impotent male. Analysis of these data must take into account the nature of the patient population studied, the studies' definition of successful response to therapy and the percentage of men who return to satisfactory sexual relations while on therapy.

The introduction of non-invasive treatments in the form of orally or sublingually administered agents will revolutionize the fashion in which urologists and all physicians approach this problem. Whether or not the soon-to-be-introduced agents demonstrate long-term efficacy in the general population (as opposed to the psychogenic and no-certain-organic aetiology sub-populations), with time, agents will be developed that will certainly be effective in men with vasculogenic impotence. It is likely that oral agents, in the very near future, will come to represent the initial step in the management of all men with erectile dysfunction. It is important, however, that prescribing such medications does not supplant a careful clinical evaluation of the patient, lest some significant and correctable underlying problem be inadvertently missed. The urologist will, in the future, have a responsibility to educate the public as well as primary medical personnel in the true role of oral-agent therapy for impotent men.

■ REFERENCES

1. Lue T F. Physiology of erection and pathophysiology of impotence. In: Walsh P C, Retik A B, Stamey T A, Vaughan E D Jr. (eds) Campbell's Urology, 6th edn. Philadelphia: Saunders 1992: 709

2. Mulhall J P, Gupta S, Traish A et al. Salvaging the failed injection patient with the use of forskolin. J Urol 1997; 158: 1752–8

3. Abe A, Karaki H. Effect of forskolin on cytosolic Ca++ levels and contraction in vascular smooth muscle. J Pharmacol Exper Ther 1989; 249: 895–900

4. Palmer L S, Valcic M, Melman A et al. Characterization of cyclic AMP accumulation in cultured human corpus cavernosum smooth muscle cells. J Urol 1994; 152: 1308–1314

5. Sparwasser C, Drescher P, Will J A, Madsen P O. Smooth muscle tone regulation in rabbit cavernosal and spongiosal tissue by cyclic AMP and cyclic GMP-dependent mechanisms. J Urol 1994; 152: 2159–2163

6. Porst H. The rationale for Prostaglandin E1 in erectile failure: a survey of world wide experience. J Urol 1996; 155: 802–815

7. Blanco R, Saenz de Tejada I, Goldstein I et al. Cholinergic neurotransmission in human corpus cavernosum. II. Acetylcholine synthesis. Am J Physiol 1988; 254: H468–472

8. Godec C J, Bates H. Cholinergic receptors in corpora cavenosa. Urology 1984; 24: 31–33

9. Traish A M, Carson M P, Kim N et al. Characterization of muscarinic acetylcholinergic receptors in human penile corpus cavernosum: studies on whole tissue and cultured endothelium. J Urol 1990; 144: 1036–1040

10. Saenz de Tejada I, Kim N, Lagan I et al. Regulation of adrenergic activity in penile corpus cavernosum. J Urol 1989; 142: 1117–1121

11. Steers W D, McConnell J, Benson G S. Anatomical localization and some pharmacological effects of vasoactive intestinal polypeptide in human and monkey corpus cavernosum. J Urol 1984; 132: 1048–1053

12. Kiely E A, Bloom S R, Williams G. Penile response to intracavernosal vasoactive intestinal polypeptide alone and in combination with other vasoactive agents. Br J Urol 1989; 64: 191–194

13. Takahashi Y, Aboseif S R, Benard F et al. Effect of intracavernous simultaneous injection of acetylcholine and vasoactive intestinal polypeptide on canine penile erection. J Urol 1992; 148: 446–448

14. Rajfer J, Aronson W J, Bush P A et al. Nitric oxide as a mediator of relaxation of the corpus cavernosum on response to nonadrenergic, noncholinergic neurotransmission. N Engl J Med 1992; 326: 90–94

15. Burnett A L, Lowenstein C J, Bredt D S et al. Nitric oxide: a physiologic mediator of penile erection. Science 1992; 257: 401–403

16. Carrier S, Zvara P, Kour N W. The effect of cavernous nerve neurotomy on erectile function and nitric oxide synthase containing nerves in the rat. Int J Impot Res 1994; 6(suppl1): A6

17. Giuliano F A, Rampin O, Benoit G, Jardin A. Neural control of penile erection. Urol Clin North Am 1995; 22: 747–766

18. Brock G, Nunes L, Padma-Nathan H et al. Nitric oxide synthase: a new diagnostic tool for neurogenic impotence. Urology 1993; 42: 412–417

19. Christ G, Maayani S, Valcic M, Melman A. Pharmacological studies of human erectile tissue: characteristics of spontaneous contractions and alterations in alpha adrenoreceptors responsiveness with age and disease in isolated tissues. Br J Pharmacol 1990; 101: 375–381

20. Djamilian M, Stief C G, Kuczyk M, Jonas U. Followup results of a combination of calcitonin gene-related peptide and prostaglandin E1 in the treatment of erectile dysfunction. J Urol 1993; 149: 1296–1298

21. Alaranta S, Uusitalo H, Hautamäk A M. Calcitonin gene-related peptide: immunohistochemical localization in, and effects on, the bovine penile artery. Int J Impot Res 1991; 3: 49–52

22. Alm P, Alumets J, Brodin E et al. Peptidergic (substance P) nerves in the genitourinary tract. Neuroscience 1978; 3: 419–425

23. Kim S C, Oh M M. Norepinephrine involvement in response to intracorporeal injection of papaverine in psychogenic impotence. J Urol 1992; 147: 1530–1532

24. Hedlund P, Alm P, Hedlund H. Localization and effects of pituitary adenylate cyclase-activating polypeptide (PACAP) in human penile erectile tissue. Acta Physiol Scand 1994; 150: 103–104

25. Tong Y C, Broderick G, Hypolite J, Levine R M. Correlations of purinergic cholinergic and adrenergic functions in rabbit corporal cavernosal tissue. Pharmacology 1992; 45: 241–249

26. Steinbusch H W. Distribution of serotonin-immunoreactivity in the central nervous system of the rat-cell bodies and terminals. Neuroscience 1981; 6: 557–618

27. Newton B W, Hamill R W. The morphology and distribution of rat serotoninergic intraspinal neurons: an immunohisto-chemical study. Brain Res Bull 1988; 20: 349–360

28. Mas M, Zahradnik M A, Martino V et al. Stimulation of spinal serotoninergic receptors facilitates seminal emission and suppresses penile erectile reflexes. Brain Res 1985; 342: 128

29. Berendsen H H, Jenck F, Broekkamp C L. Involvement of 5-HT 1C receptors in drug-induced penile erections in rats. Psychopharmacology 1990; 101: 57–61

30. Maeda N, Matsuoka N. Role of dopaminergic, serotoninergic and cholinergic link in the expression of penile erection in rats. Jpn J Pharmacol 1994; 66: 59–66

31. Pehek E A, Thompson J T, Hull U M. The effects of intracranial administration of the dopamine agonist apomorphine on penile reflexes and seminal emission in the rat. Brain Res 1989; 500: 325–332

32. Richard P, Moos F, Freund-Mercier M J. Central effects of oxytocin. Physiol Rev 1991; 71: 331–370

33. Cara A, Lopes-Martins R A, Antunes L et al. The role of histamine in human penile erection. Br J Urol 1995; 75: 220–224

34. Traish A M, Netsuwan N, Daley J et al. A heterogeneous population of alpha 1 adrenergic receptors mediates contraction on human corpus cavernosum smooth muscle to norepinephrine. J Urol 1995; 153: 222–227

35. Levin R M, Wein A J. Adrenergic alpha receptors out-number beta-receptors in human penile corpus cavernosum. Invest Urol 1980; 18: 225–226

36. Domer F R, Wessler G, Brown R L, Charles H C. Involvement of the sympathetic nervous system in the urinary bladder internal sphincter and in penile erection in the anesthesized cat. Invest Urol 1978; 15: 404–407

37. Molderings G J, Gothert M, Van Ahlen H, Porst H. Noradrenaline release in human corpus cavernosum and its modulation via presynaptic alpha-2 adrenoreceptors. Fundam Clin Pharmacol 1989; 3: 497–504

38. Costa P, Soulie-Vassal M C, Sarrazin B et al. Adrenergic receptors on smooth muscle cells isolated from human penile corpus cavernosum. J Urol 1993; 150: 859–863

39. Crowe R, Burnstock G, Dickinson I K, Pryor J P. The human penis: an usual penetration of NPY-immunoreactive nerves within the medial muscle coat of the deep dorsal vein. J Urol 1991; 145: 1292–1296

40. Iwanaga T, Hanyu S, Tamaki M. VIP and other bioactive substances involved in penile erection. Biomed Res 1992; 2: 71–73

41. Leipheimer R E, Sachs B D. GABAergic regulation of penile reflexes and copulation in rats. Physiol Behav 1988; 42: 351–357

42. Heaton J P W, Adams M A, Morales A. Therapeutic taxonomy of treatments for erectile dysfunction: an evolutionary imperative. Int J Impot Res 1997; 9: 115–121

43. Gwinup G. Oral phentolamine in non-specific erectile insufficiency. Ann Intern Med 1988; 109: 162–163

44. Zorgniotti A W. "On demand" oral drug for erection in impotent men. J Urol 1993; 147: 308A

45. Wagner G, Lacy S, Lewis R. Buccal phentolamine: a pilot trial for male erectile dysfunction at three separate clinics. Int J Impot Res 1994; 6(suppl1): D78

46. Grunhaus L, Tiongco D, Zelnik T. Intravenous yohimbine. Selective enhancer of norephinephrine and cortisol secretion and systolic blood pressure in humans. Clin Neuropharmacol 1989; 12: 106–111

47. Reid K, Surridge D H, Morales A. Double-blind trial of yohimbine in the treatment of psychogenic impotence. Lancet 1987; 2: 42–43

48. Susset J G, Tesier C D, Winze J. Effect of yohimbine hydrochloride on erectile impotence: a double-blind study. J Urol 1989; 141: 1360–1363

49. Morales A, Heaton J P, Johnston B, Adams M. Oral and topical treatment of erectile dysfunction: present and future. Urol Clin North Am 1995; 22: 879–886

50. Leonard M, Nickel J C, Morales A. Hyperprolactinemia and impotence: why, when and how to investigate. J Urol 1989; 142: 992–995

51. Pescatori E, Engelman J C, Davis G, Goldstein I. Priapism of the clitoris: a case report following trazodone use. J Urol 1993; 149: 1557–1559

52. Abber J C, Lue T F, Luo J A et al. Priapism induced by chlorpromazine and trazodone: mechanism of action. J Urol 1987; 137: 1039–1042

53. Saenz de Tejada I, Ware J C, Blanco R et al. Pathophysiology of prolonged penile erection associated with trazodone use. J Urol 1991; 165: 60–63

54. Chiang P H, Tsai E M, Chiang C P. The role of trazodone in the treatment of erectile dysfunctin. Kao Hsiung I Hsueh Tsa Chih 1994; 10: 287–294

55. Montorsi F, Strambi L F, Guazzoni G et al. Effect of yohimbine–trazodone in psychogenic impotence: a randomized, double-blind, placebo-controlled study. Urology 1994; 44: 732–736

56. Lue T F, and the Sildenafil Study Group. A study of sildenafil (VIAGRA™), a new oral agent for the treatment of male erectile dysfunction. J Urol 1997; 157: 181 (abstr)

57. Zorgniotti A W, Lizza A F. Effect of large doses of nitric oxide precursor L-arginine, on erectile failure. Int J Impot Res 1994; 6: 33–34

58. NIH Consensus Conference: Impotence. NIH Consensus Development Panel on Impotence. JAMA 1993; 270: 83–87

59. Morales A, Johnston B, Heaton J W. Oral androgens in the treatment of hypogonadal impotent men. J Urol 1994; 128: 1115–1117

60. Meikle A W, Mazer N A, Moellmer J F et al. Enhanced transdermal delivery across non scrotal skin produces physiological concentration of testosterone and its metabolites in hypogondal men. J Clin Endocrinol Metab 1992; 74: 623–628

Chapter 28

Orally active agents: the potential of alpha-adrenoceptor antagonists

M. G. Wyllie and K. -E. Andersson

■ INTRODUCTION

Penile erection is a complicated, integrated, neurally mediated vasomotor response involving both the sympathetic and parasympathetic nervous systems. The pelvic and cavernous nerves carry the parasympathetic outflow. Nitric oxide (NO), released from the neuronal supply, relaxes the corporal smooth muscle, causing a substantial rise in intracavernosal pressure and erection. The sympathetic noradrenergic nervous system is also fundamentally involved in the control of the erectile process, being the prime determinant of cavernosal smooth muscle contraction and detumescence.[1,2] The sympathetic network thereby acts in apposition to the erection-inducing NO-dependent system and, in general, erectile function is dependent on the relative balance of activity in the two major systems. Potentially, therefore, there are several loci whereby drugs active on adrenoceptors could alter erectile function — either directly by altering the action of the neurotransmitter, noradrenaline (norepinephrine), or indirectly by modulation of sympathetic outflow to the cavernosal tissue. In essence, at least anatomically, these can be divided into central (brain and spinal) and peripheral (pre- and post-junctional) sites within the target organ.

This chapter evaluates only the clinical evidence underlying a potential role for alpha-adrenoceptor antagonists (blockers) in the treatment of erectile dysfunction. It does not represent a comprehensive analysis of the molecular biology or pathophysiology of erection, which are covered in more detail elsewhere in this book (Chapter 10). However, to understand the differing clinical profiles, a basic understanding of the dynamics at noradrenergic synapses is required (Fig. 28.1).

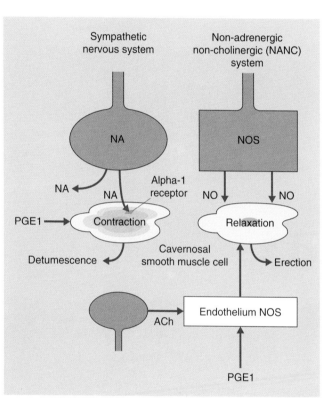

Figure 28.1. Cavernosal smooth muscle tone is the prime determinant of the degree of erection; smooth muscle relaxation produces tumescence and rigidity, whereas detumescence occurs subsequent to smooth muscle relaxation. The predominant neurotransmitter pathways are the sympathetic noradrenergic and non-adrenergic, non-cholinergic (NANC) pathways. Nitric oxide (NO) released from the latter activates an intracellular enzyme cascade culminating in relaxation of the corporal smooth muscle. Acting in apposition to this is the sympathetic nervous system; noradrenaline (NA) released from nerve terminals acts on postjunctional alpha-1-adrenoceptors to produce detumescence. Other transmitter substances or neuromodulators, particularly acetylcholine (ACh) and prostaglandin E1 (PGE1), can directly or indirectly alter smooth muscle tone. NOS = NO synthase.

317

ADRENERGIC NEUROTRANSMISSION

The important features of sympathetic neurotransmission and hence the impact of potential adrenergic agents on erectile function are as follows. Noradrenaline is released from nerve endings and acts on both post-junctional alpha-1 and alpha-2 adrenoceptors. The former are considered to be primarily involved in the control of cavernosal smooth muscle contraction (Chapter 12), although a role for alpha-2 adrenoceptors cannot be dismissed.[3,4] In addition, there are prejunctional alpha-2 adrenoceptors (autoreceptors). Noradrenaline, released into the synapse, activates these to limit further release; this is an example of a negative feedback loop (Fig. 28.2).

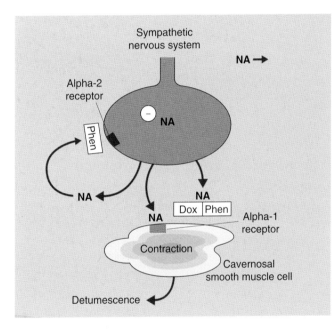

Figure 28.2. Noradrenergic synaptic dynamics within the sympathetic innervation of the corpus cavernosum Noradrenaline (NA) released from the nerve terminals acts on postjunctional alpha-1-adrenoceptors to produce smooth muscle relaxation and detumescence. The selective alpha-1-adrenoceptor antagonist, doxazosin (Dox), and the mixed alpha-1/2-adrenoceptor antagonist, phentolamine (Phen), block this effect. The amount of noradrenaline entering the synaptic cleft and thereby the magnitude of the postjunctional response is controlled by prejunctional alpha-2-autoreceptors for NA. As NA builds up it switches off further release. This process is unaffected by Dox. However, as a consequence of blocking these prejunctional alpha-2-adrenoceptors, Phen enables the build-up of NA to occur in the synapse. The law of mass action would predict that NA would competitively counteract the postjunctional alpha-1-adrenoceptor blocking action of Phen resulting in a diminution of the erectogenic response.

DRUG PROFILES

Drugs active at central adrenoceptors

The *Rauwolfia* alkaloid yohimbine, isolated from the bark of *Pausinystalia yohimbine*, best exemplifies the clinical profile and mechanism of action of this type of drug. Mechanistically, the drug is a relatively selective alpha-2-adrenoceptor antagonist,[5] and is known to increase noradrenaline levels at several neuroeffector junctions.[6] In the synaptic cleft in the presence of yohimbine, noradrenaline can no longer feed back to inhibit its own release; levels build up beyond normal and an augmented post-junctional response occurs. This may be manifest theoretically as a change in affective state (mood or libido) or secondarily as an increased sympathetic drive within the autonomic nervous system.

Although the drug is widely used in the community and under prescription, few data are available from carefully controlled clinical trials. In one study in psychogenic impotence, a response of over 60% was noted which was much higher than in the placebo group.[7] In contrast, however, Morales and co-workers showed in a controlled randomized trial in a population with organic impotence that yohimbine was without effect when administered orally three times a day.[8] More recently, data from double-blind studies show that the clinical response to the drug is equivocal at best.[9–11] It is probably best to conclude that, relative to other agents described elsewhere in this book, improvement is modest and may be restricted to psychogenic impotence. Almost certainly, any benefit accrued is secondary to an effect on libido rather than effect on the erectile process per se, yohimbine having some utility in the treatment of depression.

Apart from the modest response even in clinically defined subpopulations,[7] the utility of yohimbine is limited by its polypharmacology.[5] In addition to blockade of alpha-adrenoceptors, the drug also alters activity at serotonin (5HT), dopamine and histamine receptors, which becomes apparent at high doses and limits toleration. In an attempt to circumvent the problems associated with these non-adrenoceptor actions, more selective alpha-2-adrenoceptor antagonists, e.g. idazoxan and efaroxan, have been developed.[12] Anecdotal information indicates that they offer little advantage over yohimbine with respect to treatment of male erectile dysfunction, and it is unlikely that either agent is now being developed as monotherapy for this indication. However, there is considerable activity within the pharmaceutical industry directed towards the identification of novel alpha-2-adrenoceptor antagonists,[13,14] some of which may eventually be targeted towards impotence. One example of this strategy is the development of delaquamine, an antagonist with 100 times the alpha-1 versus alpha-2 selectivity of yohimbine. Unfortunately, although the compound has good oral bioavailability and pharmacokinetics, the early clinical data in impotence are discouraging; no significant benefit beyond placebo has been observed.[15]

Although other agents, such as apomorphine and trazodone, may act at central adrenoceptors,[5] the contribution of such actions to the overall clinical profile of these agents is unknown.[16,17] It is reasonable to assume, however, that any benefit is more likely to accrue from secondary changes in sympathetic function or mood than as a direct consequence of changes induced in adrenoceptor function. The potential contribution from actions on central adrenoceptors to the overall clinical profile of phentolamine and alpha-1-adrenoceptor antagonists is described below. However, as most drugs cross the blood–brain barrier, albeit to varying extents and at different rates, a central contribution to overall clinical profile can seldom be ruled out, unless the drugs are delivered locally.

Drugs active at peripheral adrenoceptors

The predominant features controlling cavernosal smooth muscle tone are described in detail elsewhere in this volume (Chapter 12).

As mentioned previously, the prime effect of noradrenaline on cavernosal smooth muscle is mediated by the alpha-1-adrenoceptor, although recent evidence, using the selective alpha-2-adrenoceptor agonist UK-14,304 and the selective antagonist idazoxan, indicates that post-junctional alpha-2-adrenoceptors may subserve a component of cavernosal contraction in human tissue in vitro.[3,4] In addition, consistent with the physiological control at other sympathetic neuroeffector junctions, noradrenaline modulates (inhibits) its own release by an action on prejunctional alpha-2-adrenoceptors.[6] On this basis, it can be concluded that the action of alpha-1-adrenoceptor antagonists within the target organ is likely to result from attenuation of the sympathetic nervous system; in contrast, alpha-2-adrenoceptor antagonists could theoretically either attenuate or augment sympathetic responses, depending on the relative contributions from pre- and post-junctional actions (Table 28.1).

Table 28.1. Adrenoceptor affinity and selectivity of selected agents

Antagonist	Binding affinity: pKi Alpha-1	Alpha-2
Doxazosin	8.3	6.1
Terazosin	8.1	6.4
Prazosin	9.1	7.3
Abanoquil	10.7	7.8
Phentolamine	7.3	7.1
Yohimbine	5.6	7.0

Data were obtained from classical radioligand binding studies using 3H-prazosin and 3H-rauwolscine displacements from transfected cell lines to assess alpha-1 and alpha-2 affinities, respectively. It can be seen that doxazosin, terazosin and prazosin are 100-fold selective for the alpha-1 receptor. Abanoquil has similar selectivity but is more potent. Phentolamine has equivalent (balanced) activity at both receptors and yohimbine is approximately 20-fold selective for the alpha-2 receptor

The role of alpha-1-adrenoceptors within the target organ is substantiated with the alpha-1-adrenoceptor antagonist, abanoquil, which is at least 300-fold selective for alpha-1 over alpha-2-adrenoceptors.[18] In clinical trials in organic and psychogenic patient populations, intracavernosal injection of low doses (>100 ng) resulted in tumescence and rigidity equivalent to that with papaverine.[19] Consistent with a local site of action, onset was rapid (<10 minutes). Although this drug entered phase II clinical evaluation as an oral anti-arrhythmic agent,[20] unfortunately, no information is available on drug-induced changes in erectile dysfunction when taken orally. In contrast to the proven effects of local alpha-1-adrenoceptor blockade, a pilot study has shown that direct intracavernosal injection of the selective alpha-2-adrenoceptor antagonist idazoxan was without effect (Fig. 28.3).[21]

There is, however, a relative plethora of data on the intracavernosal activity of the mixed (alpha-1 and alpha-2)-adrenoceptor antagonist, phentolamine. Although the drug has been used as intracavernosal monotherapy,[22] it is more commonly used in combination with either papaverine[23] or vasoactive intestinal

319

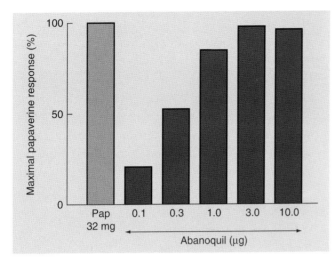

Figure 28.3. The clinical effect of intracavernosal administration of the selective alpha-1-adrenoceptor antagonist, abanoquil, to patients with erectile dysfunction. Efficacy was assessed 15–30 minutes after drug administration using RigiScan technology. Groups of 3–9 patients were pre-evaluated with 32 mg of intracavernosal papaverine (Pap) which was considered to represent the maximal or 100% response shown on the abscissa. Doses of drug administered are total dose and not on a kg basis.

polypeptide (VIP).[24] Like phentolamine monotherapy, VIP alone has only modest activity, whereas combination with phentolamine or papaverine augments activity, when delivered locally.[25] The combination of papaverine and phentolamine is considered to be an effective treatment, producing adequate erections in more than 70% of patients, with greater than 75% satisfaction rate.[26] Although no direct comparative studies are available, the quality of the erection achieved with intracavernosal phentolamine appears to be less than that achieved with abanoquil, particularly with respect to rigidity; when injected alone, although increasing intracorporal blood flow, phentolamine does not result in a significant increase in intracorporal pressure.[27]

On first examination, it is difficult to explain why a mixed (alpha-1 and alpha-2)-adrenoceptor antagonist should produce a lesser clinical response than a selective alpha-1-adrenoceptor antagonist, when delivered locally. It has been hypothesized, however, that phentolamine may negate its own effect and thereby prevent complete sinusoidal relaxation and produce an incomplete erection.[22] This theoretical possibility is based on a consideration of synaptic dynamics. Phentolamine undoubtedly blocks post-junctional adrenoceptors, consequently reducing sympathetic tone. This should result in a diminution of cavernosal smooth muscle contraction and a reduced detumescence, which in turn should manifest as an erection in the patient. In addition, however, owing to the blockade of prejunctional alpha-2-adrenoceptors, in the presence of phentolamine, the concentration of noradrenaline in the synapse rises and reduces the degree of block with phentolamine.[28] Although this has been demonstrated at several autonomic neuroeffector junctions, direct measurement of intracavernosal noradrenergic synaptic dynamics has not been attempted. Alternatively, as has been described for other alpha-adrenoceptor antagonists, contributions of alpha-1 and alpha-2-adrenoceptors within the CNS, ganglia and nerves must be considered.[29] Given the multifactorial aetiology of ED, it is reasonable to assume that benefit may accrue from actions at several loci. Equally drug action at more than one site may be required to produce an optimal clinical profile.

Phentolamine has a major potential advantage over existing therapies, possessing demonstrable oral or buccal activity in the clinic.[30–32] The effect is more consistent and broad spectrum than that observed with yohimbine. Over 700 patients have completed definitive phase III, double-blind, placebo-controlled trials with Vasomax (phentolamine). In these studies, the response to placebo was approximately 20%; the response was elevated by phentolamine to 30–40%. Although parallel trials with sildenafil have not been completed some comparative data are available. Like sildenafil, phentolamine has been found to affect most of the domains of the IIEF except sexual desire (Fig. 28.4). The adverse event profile of phentolamine is likewise consistent with the vasorelaxant properties of the drug (Table 28.2). However, no major systemic cardiovascular haemodynamic changes are observed over the likely therapeutic dose range. There is no evidence of the dyspepsia and visual disturbances associated with sildenafil.

Another adrenoceptor antagonist, moxisylyte (thymoxamine), as anticipated, is effective after intracavernosal administration.[33] Although it is available in Europe as an oral formulation, clinical data are sparse and not directly comparable with the more extensive clinical database of phentolamine.

The relative contributions from alpha-1- and alpha-2-adrenoceptor blockade or peripheral and central blockade to the overall clinical profile of phentolamine, subsequent to oral administration, are not known. However, in this context, there are some limited clinical data on selective

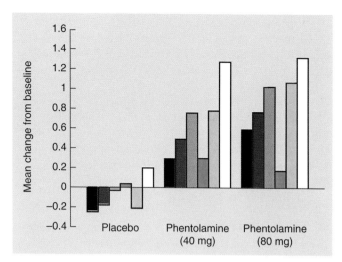

Figure 28.4. Mean change in IIEF domain scores from baseline to end of treatment with phentolamine or placebo for the parallel study group: frequency of penetration (■; p = 0.0012 at 40 mg; p < 0.0001 at 80 mg); frequency of maintaining erection (■; p = 0.0002 at 40 mg; p < 0.0001 at 80 mg); orgasmic function (■; p = 0.0318 at 40 mg; p < 0.0026 at 80 mg); sexual desire (■; p is not significant at 40 or 80 mg); intercourse satisfaction (■; p = 0.0005 at 40 mg; p < 0.0001 at 80 mg); overall satisfaction (□; p = 0.0003 at 40 mg; p < 0.0002 at 80 mg).

Table 28.2. Proportion of patients (%) reporting treatment-related adverse events during the study period

	Phentolamine 40mg	Phentolamine 80mg	Placebo
Rhinitis	7.7	20.9	3.8
Headache	3.1	4.5	1.7
Dizziness	2.0	7.0	0.2
Tachycardia	1.5	7.0	0.6
Nausea	0.7	3.5	0
Hypotension	0.2	2.0	0
Hypertension	0	2.0	0.2

alpha-1-adrenoceptor antagonists. In long-term (4 year) studies in hypertensive patients and in patients with benign prostatic hyperplasia — conditions associated with abnormally high sympathetic drive[19] — the selective alpha-1-adrenoceptor antagonist doxazosin has been shown to reduce the incidence of sexual dysfunction relative to placebo.[34,35] In addition, all males entering the study who were impotent at baseline 'recovered' during the study; the corresponding improvement in the placebo group was only 50%. These effects were not secondary to blood pressure control as other antihypertensive therapies were either ineffective or exacerbated the condition.[36] This may not be a characteristic of the alpha-1-adrenoceptor blocker class, as similar effects have not been observed with terazosin and phenoxybenzamine.[36] The action of doxazosin is thought to be dependent on both peripheral actions in the cavernosal tissue and actions at the spinal cord secondary to changes in the sympathetic outflow to the corpus cavernosum.[29]

Available data on doxazosin may not, however, indicate a potential for new monotherapy; comparative studies using new validated clinical trial methodology including the International Index of Erectile Function[36] would be required to underpin such use. More likely, oral doxazosin could have potential when coadministered to boost the response to agents acting primarily by relaxation of cavernosal smooth muscle tone and, in particular, phosphodiesterase inhibitors and prostaglandin E1 (PGE1). Preliminary studies in 20 patients indicate that doxazosin does, in fact, augment the response of patients who respond poorly to either intracavernosal or intra-urethral PGE1.[37] Similar studies are known to be under way using oral prazosin and locally delivered PGE1. More comprehensive studies will determine whether this represents an additive or synergistic (supra-additive) effect and the potential contribution of such a treatment algorithm to the management of the patient with erectile dysfunction.

■ CONCLUSIONS

Locally-administered adrenoceptor antagonists have proven clinical utility either as monotherapy or in combination. It is likely that the new formulation of phentolamine will achieve widespread use as oral monotherapy. In addition, oral adrenoceptor antagonists may benefit patient subpopulations, or more likely, may be used in combination with other pharmacotherapy.

■ REFERENCES

1. Andersson K-E. Pharmacology of lower urinary tract smooth muscles and penile erectile tissue. Pharmacol Rev 1993; 45: 255–263

2. Andersson K-E, Wagner G. Physiology of penile erection. Physiol Rev 1995; 75: 191–236

3. Traish A M, Moreland R B, Huang Y H, Goldstein I. Expression of functional alpha-2-adrenergic receptor subtypes in human corpus cavernosum and in cultured trabecular smooth muscle cells. Recept Signal Transduc 1997; 7: 55–67

4. Gupta S, Moreland R B, Yang S et al. Corpus cavernosum smooth muscle expresses functional post synaptic alpha-2-adrenoceptors. Br J Urol 1998: in press

5. Hoffman B B, Lefkowitz R J. Catecholamines, sympathomimetic drugs, and adrenergic receptor antagonists. In: Hardman J G, Limbard L L (eds) Goodman and Gillman's The pharmacological basis of therapeutics. New York: McGraw-Hill, 1996: 199–248

6. Langer S Z. Presynaptic regulation of the release of catecholamines. Pharmacol Rev 1981; 32: 337–362

7. Reid K, Surridge D H, Morales A et al. Double-blind trial of yohimbine in treatment of psychogenic impotence. Lancet 1987; 2: 421–423

8. Morales A, Surridge D H, Marshall P G, Fenmore J. Nonhormonal pharmacological treatment of organic impotence. J Urol 1982; 128: 45–47

9. Susset J G, Tessier C D, Wincaze J et al. Effect of yohimbine hydrochloride on erectile impotence: a double-blind study. J Urol 1989; 141: 1360–1363

10. Montague D K, Barada J H, Belker, A M et al. Clinical guidelines panel on erectile dysfunction: summary report on the treatment of organic erectile dysfunction. American Urological Association. J Urol 1996; 156: 2007–2011

11. Vogt H J, Brandall P, Kockott G et al. Double blind, placebo-controlled safety and efficacy trial with yohimbine hydrochloride in the treatment of nonorganic erectile dysfunction. Int J Impot Res 1997; 9: 155–161

12. Benelli A, Arletti R, Basaglia R, Bertolini A. Male sexual behaviour: further studies on the role of alpha2-adrenoceptors. Pharmacol Res 1993; 28: 35–45

13. Hieble J P, Bondinell W E, Ruffolo R R. Alpha- and beta-adrenoceptors: from gene to the clinic. 1. Molecular biology and adrenoceptor subclassification. J Med Chem 1995; 38: 3415–3444

14. Hieble J P, Ruffolo R R. Recent advances in the identification of alpha-1 and alpha-2-adrenoceptor subtypes: therapeutic implications. Expert Opin Invest Drugs 1997; 6: 367–387

15. Morales A, Heaton J P, Johnston B, Adams M. Oral and topical treatment of erectile dysfunction: present and future. Urol Clin North Am 1995; 22; 879–886

16. Heaton J P, Morales A, Adams M A et al. Recovery of erectile function by the oral administration of apomorphine. Urology 1995; 45: 200–206

17. Meinhardt W, Schmidtz P I, Kropman R F et al. Trazodone, a double blind trial for treatment of erectile dysfunction. Int J Impot Res 1997; 9: 163–165

18. Forray C, Bard J A, Wetzel J M et al. The alpha-1-adrenergic receptor that mediates smooth muscle contraction in human prostate has the pharmacological properties of the cloned human alpha-1c subtype. Mol Pharmacol 1994; 45: 703–708

19. Andersson K-E, Wagner G, Wyllie M G. Effects of doxazosin and other alpha-1-adrenoceptor antagonists in sexual function. Fourth International Consultation in BPH. Jersey, Channel Islands: Scientific Communication International Ltd, 1998: in press

20. Voli E, Hull S S, Foreman R D et al. Alpha-1-adrenergic blockade and sudden cardiac death. J Cardiovasc Electrophysiol 1994; 5: 76–89

21. Brindley G S. Pilot experiments on the actions of drugs injected into the human corpus cavernosum penis. Br J Pharmacol 1986; 87: 495–500

22. Juenemann K P, Alken K. Pharmacotherapy of erectile dysfunction: a review. Int J Impot Res 1989; 1: 71–95

23. Zorgniotti A W, Lefleur L S. Auto-injection of the corpus cavernosum with a vasoactive drug combination for vasculogenic impotence. J Urol 1985; 133: 39–41

24. McMahon C G. A pilot study of the role of intracavernous injection of vasoactive intestinal polypeptide (VIP) and phentolamine mesylate in the treatment of erectile dysfunction. Int J Impot Res 1996; 8: 233–236

25. Kiely E A, Bloom S R, Williams G. Penile response to intracavernosal vasoactive intestinal polypeptide alone and in combination with other vasoactive agents. Br J Urol 1989; 64: 191–194

26. Lue T F, Broderick G. Evaluation and non surgical management of erectile dysfunction and priapism. In: Walsh P C, Retik A B, Vaughan E D, Wein A J (eds). Campbell's Urology, 7th edn. Philadelphia: Saunders, 1997; 1181–1214

27. Juenemann K P, Lue T F, Fournier G R, Tanagho E A. Hemodynamics of papaverine- and phentolamine-induced penile erection. J Urol 1986; 36: 158–161

28. Alberts P. Mechanisms of facilitation and muscarinic or alpha-adrenergic inhibition of acetylcholine and noradrenaline secretion from peripheral nerves. Acta Physiol Scand Suppl 1982; 506: 1–39

29. Andersson K-E, Lepor H, Wyllie M G. Prostatic alpha-1-adrenoceptors and uroselectivity. Prostate 1997; 30: 202–215

30. Gwinup G. Oral phentolamine in nonspecific erectile dysfunction. Ann Intern Med 1988; 109: 162–163

31. Zorgniotti A W. Experience with buccal phentolamine mesylate for impotence. Int J Impot Res 1994; 6: 37–41

32. Giuliano F. Treatment per os of disorders of erection. Prog Urol 1997; 7: 108–109

33. Buvat J, Lemaire A, Buvat-Herbaut M K, Marcolin G. Safety of intracavernous injections using an alpha-blocking agent. J Urol 1989; 141: 1364–1367

34. Grimm R H, Granditis G A, Pineas R J et al. Long-term effects on sexual function of five antihypertensive drugs and nutritional hygenic treatment in hypertensive men and women. Hypertension 1997; 29: 8–14

35. Guthrie, R M, Siegel R L. Effect of Cardura (doxazosin) therapy on symptoms of benign prostatic hyperplasia and sexual function in hypertensive patients. Br J Urol 1997; 80: 217

36. Rosen R C, Riley A, Wagner G et al. The international index of erectile dysfunction (IIEF): a multidimensional scale for assessment of erectile dysfunction. Urology 1997; 49(6): 822–830

37. Kaplan S A. Interaction between Cardura and PGE1 on erectile response. J Urol 1998: in press (abstr)

Chapter 29

Intra-urethral and topical agents in the management of erectile dysfunction

H. Padma-Nathan

■ INTRODUCTION

Pharmacological therapies form the cornerstone of management of erectile dysfunction. Intracavernosal pharmacotherapy by self-injection, to this effect, has become a 'gold standard' of such therapy. However, the low long-term utilization of injection therapy is inconsistent with its efficacy and reflects in part the need to inject with a needle.[1] The impetus to develop more minimally invasive pharmacological therapies for the management of erectile dysfunction has led, firstly, to intra-urethral therapy and more recently to topical and oral pharmacological therapies. The oral therapies promise to become first-line therapies that will dramatically influence this field from a medical as well as societal and economic perspective. As the field grows exponentially, intra-urethral and topical therapies may play more of a niche role. This chapter reviews the current data on the efficacy and safety profile of intra-urethral and topical therapies.

■ INTRA-URETHRAL PHARMACOTHERAPY

Pharmacology and mechanism of drug transfer

The principal pharmacological agent utilized in intra-urethral drug delivery has been alprostadil, the synthetic formulation of prostaglandin E1 (PGE1). On administration to the distal urethra, this agent is able to elicit haemodynamic alterations in the corpora cavernosa. The drug transfer appears to occur primarily by venous channels that communicate between the corpus spongiosum and the corpora cavernosa. These vascular channels appear to be variable and increase with age; they may also close early in the erection process. The haemodynamic alterations observed following intra-urethral administration of alprostadil are primarily an increase in arterial dilatation and flow, as shown by a significant increase in peak systolic velocity (PSV) values determined at the time of colour duplex ultrasonography. The PSV values attained following intra-urethral administration of 500 µg MUSE®-alprostadil (VIVUS Inc., Menlo Park, CA, USA) are statistically similar to those seen following a 10 µg injection of alprostadil directly into a corpus cavernosum.[2] However, the degree of veno-occlusion, in comparison, is significantly less following intra-urethral administration, as shown by the elevated end-diastolic velocity values at the same duplex ultrasound examination.[2] This is also clinically correlated with the lesser degree of penile rigidity associated with intra-urethral administration. Similar haemodynamic effects have been observed with a liposomal encapsulation of alprostadil delivered to the navicular fossa — lyophilized liposomal PGE1, LLPGE1® (Harvard Scientific, Irvine, CA, USA).[3]

The absorption of alprostadil administered to the distal urethra is rapid, with only 20% of a 1000 µg dose remaining after 20 minutes.[4] The transfer of drug to the corpora cavernosa, however, appears to be inconsistent and this in turn appears to reflect some systemic dispersion and possibly some urothelial metabolism of alprostadil. The total amount of alprostadil found in an ejaculate following administration of the 1000 µg dose appears to be equal to the total prostaglandin level normally in the ejaculate. This increase in prostaglandin appears to be less than the day-to-day variation of prostaglandin within the ejaculate of an individual.[4] However, nearly 10% of partners report symptoms of vaginitis following intra-urethral alprostadil and thus may be sensitive to this drug when delivered in the ejaculate.

Clinical efficacy and safety

The clinical efficacy and safety of intra-urethral alprostadil in the form of the 'medicated urethral system for erection', or MUSE®, has been established in both clinical reports and regulatory approval (Fig. 29.1).[5,6] The MUSE® formulation of alprostadil is delivered as a semi-solid pellet (3 × 1 mm) to the distal 3 cm of the urethra by an applicator following urination. The urine acts as both a lubricant and a diluent for the pellet. In addition to the MUSE® system, the previously mentioned lyophilized liposomal (trilaminar membrane-covered spherical drug vehicle) PGE1 released in the meatus by a dilute detergent has entered a phase II study. LLPGE1® has a shelf life of 3 years and contains 750 or 1500 μg per delivery dose. The liposomes are delivered to the distal 1.5 cm of the urethra and a detergent (0.1% polyoxyethylene) is employed to release the alprostadil. It is expected that this second intra-urethral approach will result in efficacy and safety almost identical to that observed with MUSE®. The largest clinical trial of intra-urethral alprostadil to date utilized the MUSE® system and involved 1511 men between the ages of 26 and 88 years with complete erectile dysfunction of primarily organic aetiology.[5] The men initially underwent an in-office double-blind dose titration with four different doses (125, 250, 500, 1000 μg) of MUSE®-alprostadil. Nearly 66% (996) of these men had an erection adequate for intercourse. The responders were then randomized to drug at the appropriate dose (as determined in the first phase) or placebo, for a 3 month period of home treatment. The at-home response has been examined from two different perspectives — the percentage of men reporting at least one successful episode of intercourse and the percentage of administrations resulting in successful intercourse. It was observed that, of the 461 men receiving active drug at home, 299 (65%) had successful intercourse at least once; in comparison, only 93 of the 500 men (18.6%) receiving placebo had at least one episode of intercourse (p <0.001). The overall clinical efficacy (in the office and at home) would thus be 43%. However, only 50.4% of administrations resulted in successful intercourse in those men who were in-office responders. If they responded once at home as well, then 69.2% of subsequent administrations were associated with successful intercourse. In contrast, nearly 87% of at-home injections with alprostadil sterile powder (Caverject®, Pharmacia and Upjohn, Kalamazoo, MI, USA) are associated with successful intercourse.[7] In the author's experience, 5–10% of impotent men are able to achieve rigid and consistent erections with intra-urethral alprostadil. It is this population that will continue to preserve a role for intra-urethral therapy with the advent of oral agents. To date, however, it is not possible to pre-identify them clinically. In patients who are responders, there are significant improvements in quality of life, particularly in the domains of self-esteem and sexual and non-sexual aspects of their relationship with their partner.[8]

The long-term safety profile of MUSE®-alprostadil was recently reported in 2595 men, with 684 receiving therapy for over 6 months, 265 for over 12 months, 96 for over 18 months and 57 for over 24 months.[9] This attrition also underscores the high drop-out rate associated with this form of therapy. Pain — including penile, urethral, testicular and perineal pain — was reported by over 50% of men. Hypotension and syncope have been observed in 1.2% to nearly 4% of men,[5,6,8,9] depending on the dose; this effect, although uncommon, can be associated with serious adverse cardiovascular consequences. This therapy should thus be employed with caution in men with such risk profiles and in older men. Minor urethral trauma, prolonged erections and penile

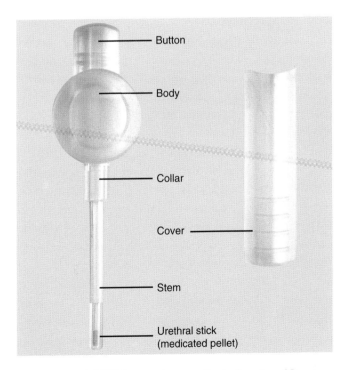

Figure 29.1. MUSE for treating erectile dysfunction. (Courtesy of VIVUS Inc.)

fibrosis appear to be rare but not absent. As previously mentioned, there have been partner-reported adverse events, with about 10% reporting symptoms of vaginal irritation or vaginitis. The overall safety data indicate that MUSE® (alprostadil) is well tolerated.

It has become obvious from the clinical experience since its FDA approval that the intra-urethral administration of alprostadil for the treatment of erectile dysfunction is, although effective, not sufficiently associated with adequate and consistent penile rigidity to maintain its role as a first-line therapy following the advent of more effective oral pharmacological agents. However, within the context of the recent treatment guidelines (Chapter 43) MUSE® could play a major role as second-line therapy in the management of the patient with ED. In addition, an attempt has been made to improve efficacy by polypharmacotherapy with the addition to alprostadil of the alpha-adrenergic antagonist prazosin.[10] This combination therapy has resulted in a minimal increase in efficacy, with 68% of patients reporting successful intercourse following in-office response. However, the incidence of hypotension increased dramatically with combination therapy, being observed in up to 9.2%. The development of a more effective pharmacological approach is, however, clearly the most effective means by which intra-urethral therapy will continue to play a role in this field. Alprostadil is an appealing agent for intra-urethral administration, in comparison to such agents as papaverine, owing to its efficacy at microgram dosages. However, its hyperalgic effects at the doses employed for intra-urethral administration are associated with a high incidence of pain, which frequently limits therapy. The next generation of intra-urethral agents may include other vasoactive agents, including nitric oxide donors, as well as procedures such as nitric oxide synthase gene therapy delivered through this novel approach.[11] A less appealing approach to increase the drug efficacy of intra-urethral alprostadil has been to employ an adjustable penile band (Actis®, VIVUS Inc.) that appears primarily to effect improved erections by mechanical constriction rather than by improved drug transfer (by increasing the spongiosal pressure and by decreasing systemic run-off).[12] If the latter were possible, the addition of a mechanical device for only a short time following drug application would be better accepted by patients than the continuous application of such a device throughout the entire sexual episode — thus mimicking the vacuum device experience.

TOPICAL PHARMACOTHERAPY

Transdermal/transglanular corporal drug delivery

Preliminary trials examining the efficacy of transdermal or transglanular (minoxidil) delivery of nitroglycerine paste,[13] minoxidil with or without a percutaneous absorption enhancer (2-nonyl-1,3-dioxalane) or capsacin,[14] papaverine[15] and PGE1[16] have demonstrated some degree of drug delivery to the corporal smooth muscle sufficient to elicit Doppler-detected increased arterial inflow and penile tumescence. However, rigid erections have been produced only in the rare spinal cord injured neurogenic patient. New drug formulations, absorption enhancers, drug carriers, and iontophoresis may ultimately make this route of drug delivery clinically efficacious. Currently, two proprietary formulations of alprostadil with absorption enhancers are in phase II of clinical development (MacroChem Corp., Lexington, MA and NexMed Inc., Commerce, CA, USA). The most rational site of application is the glans penis and this route may be ultimately more efficacious that the intra-urethral route, since it bypasses the urothelium. Thus, this form of drug delivery may act only to enhance erections in men with mild or moderate erectile dysfunction. However, if effective, it clearly will have a niche because of the appeal to patients of topical agents. Doses up to 4.0 mg prostaglandin appear to be well tolerated by patients and partners and may produce an erection adequate for intromission in 62% of those impotent men previously determined to be excellent responders to intracavernosal injections of low doses of 'tri-mix' (PGE1, papaverine and phentolamine).[17]

CONCLUSIONS

Intra-urethral and topical (transglanular) pharmacotherapy appear to be sufficiently efficacious to play a role following the advent of effective oral pharmacological agents. The oral agents alone or in combination are projected to be effective in 60–70% of men with erectile dysfunction including cases of severe or complete impotence. The second-line pharmacological step will include injectable, intra-urethral and topical agents.

■ REFERENCES

1. Althof S E, Turner L A, Levine S B et al. Why do so many people drop out from auto-injection therapy for impotence? J Sex Marital Ther 1989, 15: 121–129

2. Padma-Nathan H, Keller T, Poppiti R et al. Hemodynamic effects of intraurethral alprostadil: the Medicated Urethral System For Erection (MUSE). J Urol 1994; 151(5): 469 (354A)

3. See J R, Williams J, Sparkuhl A et al. Lyophilized liposomal prostaglandin E1 released by a dilute detergent for intrameatal delivery to treat erectile failure. J Urol 1997, 157:4 (784A)

4. VIVUS Inc. Pharmacokinetic and Toxicological Data. FDA submission

5. Padma-Nathan H, Hellstrom W J G, Kaiser F E et al. Treatment of men with erectile dysfunction with transurethral alprostadil. N Engl J Med 1997; 336(1): 1–7

6. Hellstrom W J G, Bennett A H, Gesundheit N et al. A double-blind, placebo-controlled evaluation of the erectile response to transurethral alprostadil. Urology 1996; 48: 851–856

7. Linet O I, Ogrinc F G. Efficacy and safety of intracavernosal alprostadil in men with erectile dysfunction. N Engl J Med 1996, 334: 873–877

8. Padma-Nathan H and the Vivus MUSE Study Group. Multicenter double-blind, placebo controlled trial of transurethral alprostadil in men with chronic erectile dysfunction. J Urol 1996, 155(5): 496A

9. Spivak A P, Peterson C A, Cowley C et al. Long-term safety profile of transurethral alprostadil for the treatment of erectile dysfunction. J Urol 1997; 157:4 (792A)

10. Lewis R W, Brendler C B, Burnett A L et al. A comparison of transurethral alprostadil and alprostadil/prazosin combinations for the treatment of erectile dysfunction (ED). J Urol 1997; 157: 4(703A)

11. Rehman J, Christ G, Melman A et al. Enhancement of physiologic erectile function with nitric oxide synthase gene therapy. J Urol 1997; 157: 4(782A)

12. Padma-Nathan H, Tam P, Place V et al. Improved erectile response to transurethral alprostadil by use of a novel, adjustable penile band. J Urol 1997; 157: 4(704A)

13. Heaton J P W, Morales A, Owen J et al. Topical glyceryltrinitrate causes measurable penile arterial dilation in impotent men. J Urol 1990; 43: 729–731

14. Cavallini G. Minoxidil and capsacin: an association of transcutaneous active drugs for erection facilitation. Int J Impot Res 1994; 6(1): D71

15. Kim E D, El-Rashidy R, McVary K. Papaverine topical gel for treatment of erectile dysfunction. J Urol 1995; 153: 361–365

16. Kim E D, McVary K. Topical prostaglandin E1 for the treatment of erectile dysfunction. J Urol 1995; 153: 1828–1830

17. Becher E, Momesso A, Borghi M et al. Topical prostaglandin E1 for erectile dysfunction. J Urol 1996; 155: 5(741A)

Chapter 30

Erectile dysfunction: endocrinological therapies, risks and benefits of treatment

N. Burns-Cox and J. C. Gingell

■ INTRODUCTION

Although a wide range of endocrinological conditions can interfere with normal erectile function, it is mainly the roles of androgens and prolactin that are considered in this chapter. Endocrinopathies of thyroxine or cortisol have been associated with erectile dysfunction (ED). There is very little information on their role in ED and therefore they are not mentioned further in this chapter. There is increasing demand from older male patients for androgen replacement/supplement therapies. However, as with all treatments, the potential benefits must be weighed against the risks.

■ ANDROGENS

For thousands of years, people have linked potency with the testis. More recently, in 1889, the eminent French physiologist Brown-Séquard (1817–1894) injected himself with an extract of dog testis, claiming to have been miraculously rejuvenated. In the early 1900s Eugen Steinach noted that vasoligation led to atrophy of the germinal epithelium but hypertrophy of the Leydig cells in the testes. This, it was felt, would lead to an increase in the production of sex hormones; indeed, such was the belief that the Steinach procedure would lead to rejuvenation that, in the 1920s, many Viennese professors, including Sigmund Freud[1] and the Irish poet Yeats[2] underwent the procedure.

Synthesis of androgens

Androgens are C19 steroid hormones and their synthesis begins with hydroxylation of the C21 progesterone (Fig. 30.1).[3] The C20 and C21 side chain is then cleaved to produce the androgen androstenedione; then, by the reduction of the 17-keto group, testosterone is formed. Testosterone is metabolized primarily in the liver and excreted in the urine as androsterone and eliocholanolone. The half-life of free testosterone is 10–20 minutes.

Oestrogens are C18 molecules and are synthesized from androgens by the loss of the C19 methyl group by aromatase activity to give either oestrone or oestradiol (Fig. 30.1).

Secretion

Testosterone is detectable in both the male and female foetus, levels remaining low and constant at about 1.0 nmol/l in the latter. However, in the male, levels increase at 6 weeks, peaking at around 5.5 nmol/l at week 12 (Fig. 30.2). They then decline to levels similar to those in the female foetus.[4] After birth there is another peak of testosterone production between months 2 and 6, returning to baseline levels of less than 1.0 nmol/l until puberty.[5]

At puberty there is an increase in nocturnal pulsatile luteinizing hormone (LH) secretion, leading to maturation of the Leydig cells in the testes and hence to increasing levels of serum testosterone,[6] which reach adult levels around the age of 18 years. The adult male produces 24 μmol

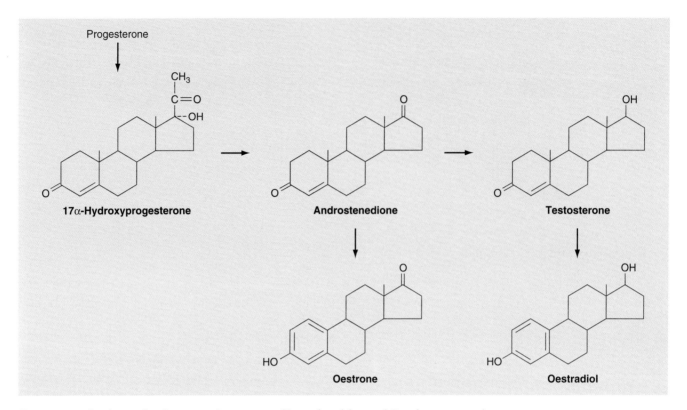

Figure 30.1. Synthesis of androgens and oestrogens. (Reproduced from ref. 3 with permission.)

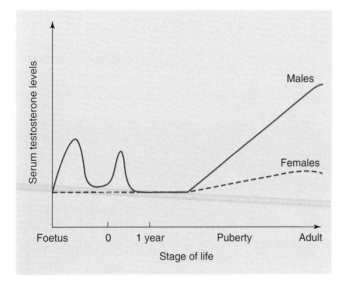

Figure 30.2. Changes in testosterone levels during life. (Reproduced from ref. 6 with permission.)

testosterone daily from the testes and 0.04 μmol/day from the adrenal cortex. The ovaries produce 0.02 μmol/day;[7] however, about one-half of the testosterone in women is produced by conversion of androstenedione in peripheral tissues. Although this does occur in men it is insignificant in comparison to testosterone production by the testes.

Regulation of androgen production is via the homeostatic feedback loop of the hypophyseal–pituitary–adrenal–gonadal axis (Fig. 30.3). In the adult male, secretion follows a circadian rhythm, levels being greatest in the early morning. During the day there are smaller peaks in plasma levels following intermittent rises in LH.

Testosterone suppresses not only LH but also, to a lesser degree, follicle-stimulating hormone (FSH). Oestradiol produced mainly by the action of aromatase on androgens in the peripheral tissue also suppresses LH and FSH. The synthesis of sex-hormone-binding globulin (SHBG) by the liver is decreased by androgens and increased by oestrogens, thereby altering the levels of free testosterone.

Bioavailable testosterone

Testosterone diffuses readily through the cell wall to bind to its cytosol receptors. There is controversy over which portion of circulating testosterone is available to tissues. In men, about 80% of testosterone is bound to SHBG; most of the rest is bound to albumin, and the remainder to cortisol-binding globulin.[6] Only about 2% of testosterone remains unbound and free in men.

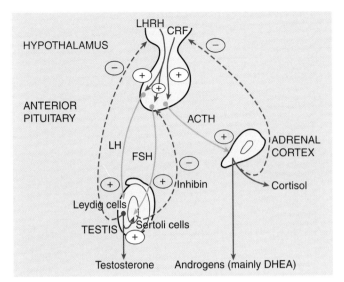

Figure 30.3. Hypothalamic–pituitary–gonadal axis. LHRH = luteinizing hormone; FSH = follicle stimulating hormone; CRF = corticotrophin-releasing hormone; ACTH = adreno-cortico-trophic hormone; DHEA = dihydroepi andro-stenedione.

Testosterone binds strongly to SHBG but weakly to albumin. It is generally accepted that it is the non-SHBG-bound testosterone that is bioavailable. Because of difficulties in measuring unbound testosterone directly, the free or non-SHBG-bound testosterone is usually determined mathematically to give the androgen index from the total serum testosterone and SHBG levels: Androgen Index = (Total testosterone/SHBG) x 100. It seems likely, however, that SHBG itself may be important, as specific receptors to it have been found on tissues and they may communicate directly with intracellular steroid receptors.[8]

Other androgens

Testosterone itself is further converted by the action of 5-alpha-reductase to dihydrotestosterone (DHT). DHT binds more strongly to androgen receptors than testosterone and is thought to be responsible for many of the androgenic actions of testosterone on the prostate, seminal vesicles and external genitalia.

Dihydroepiandrostenedione (DHEA) and its sulphate (DHEAS) are secreted by the zona reticularis of the adrenal cortex and quantitatively are the most important of the steroid hormones (35 mg/day in the young adult male). The physiological role of DHEA is unclear but it is a weak androgen and in the peripheral tissues is converted into testosterone, androstenedione and oestradiol.[9]

Androstenedione is one of the main adrenal androgens and is also formed in the peripheral tissues from DHEA.

Androstenediol and androstenediol glucuronide are produced by 17-beta reduction of DHEA; androstenediol binds to androgen and oestrogen receptors.[10]

■ BIOLOGICAL ACTIONS OF ANDROGENS

Prenatal

On the Y chromosome is a gene that codes for the HY enzyme. This enzyme is responsible for differentiation of the germ cells into Sertoli and Leydig cells around week 6. Testosterone is now secreted, leading to the male phenotype by the development of a phallus, urethral infolding, fusion of the scrotum and migration downwards of the testes.

Sexual function and behaviour

Androgens are necessary for the further development of seminal vesicles, penis, epididymis and prostate at puberty.[8] In the adult, continued secretion of androgens is required for the maintenance and normal function of the above organs. Indeed, in hypogonadal men, testosterone replacement will lead to growth of the prostate to its normal size (Fig. 30.4).[11] Endogenous testosterone is also required for normal spermatogenesis.[12]

Testosterone has an important role in normal sexual function. Suppression of testosterone to castrate levels reduces libido and sexual fantasies in normal young men.[13] Conversely, in hypogonadal individuals testosterone replacement therapy significantly increases sexual interest.[14–16]

It has been shown that castration in the rat induces loss of penile reflexes and a reduction in the erectile response to electric field stimulation (EFS) of the cavernosal nerve. These effects are reversed by testosterone replacement. However, the role of testosterone in erectile function in humans is not clear.[17] In a study of 1709 men there was no difference in the total testosterone levels between those who suffered ED and those who did not.[18] Also, when free and albumin-bound levels of testosterone were studied, once again there was no correlation between the serum levels and the presence or absence of ED.[19]

Hormone replacement, however, in hypogonadal men increases the frequency of nocturnal and spontaneous

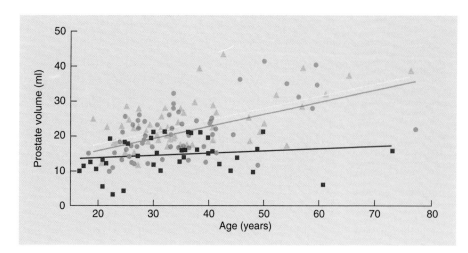

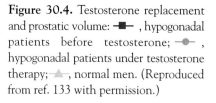

Figure 30.4. Testosterone replacement and prostatic volume: ▬■▬ , hypogonadal patients before testosterone; ▬●▬ , hypogonadal patients under testosterone therapy; ▬▲▬ , normal men. (Reproduced from ref. 133 with permission.)

erections.[14,15,20–22] Nevertheless the role of serum testosterone and erectile activity to external stimuli is less clear and the evidence is contradictory.

Hypogonadal men have been shown to have normal erectile responses to visual erotic stimuli.[20,23] In addition, when a group of sexual offenders underwent medical castration with cyproterone acetate they showed no decrease in erectile response to erotic films;[24] however, suppression of serum testosterone concentrations to castrate levels in normal young men brought about a decrease in spontaneous erections.[13] It has also been reported that men being treated by androgen withdrawal for prostate cancer have an increased rate of developing impotence, increasing from 46% before to 91% after treatment.[25]

In summary, testosterone levels are related to the frequency of nocturnal penile tumescence (NPT) and to spontaneous erections. There is no relationship between the levels of serum testosterone and the presence or absence of ED in the community. The impact on erectile activity to external stimuli of a sudden decrease in testosterone to castrate levels remains unclear from the published data.

Aggressive behaviour is often thought to be an androgenic effect. Indeed, in non-human primates, serum testosterone levels correlate directly with aggressive behaviour.[26] However, in humans no convincing correlation has been shown.[13,21] Administration of methyltestosterone has been reported to increase violent feelings and irritability in young men in the short term,[27] but moderately supraphysiological doses of testosterone ethanoate given for a few months were not associated with increased aggressiveness or irritability.[13,28]

Lean body mass and muscle

Androgens also have an anabolic effect and will cause an increase in nitrogen retention, lean body mass and overall body weight.[29] The increased muscle mass is through increasing muscle cell size rather than number.[8]

Bone

Androgens have an important role in bone metabolism. Androgens stimulate the proliferation of bone cells in vitro.[30] Hypogonadism is known to be a significant risk factor for osteoporosis in men;[31,32] the osteopenia mainly affects trabecular rather than cortical bone. At puberty there is an increase in bone mass, reaching a peak in the mid-20s.[33]

Bone mass declines in men with age, as do testosterone levels; there is also an increase in the rate of fractures associated with osteoporosis.[34] However, it remains unclear as to whether the effects are due directly to androgens or to the oestrogens synthesized from them. Interestingly, there has been one recorded case of a man with oestrogen insensitivity: he presented with severe osteoporosis that did not respond to oestrogen replacement.[35]

Lipids

Men have lower high-density lipoprotein (HDL) and higher low-density lipoprotein (LDL) levels than do premenopausal women.[36] This may, in part, explain the fivefold increase in cardiovascular mortality in men compared with premenopausal women. Androgen administration to boys with delayed puberty and to hypogonadal men causes a decrease in the concentration of HDL.[37]

Haematological effects

Androgens stimulate erythropoietin secretion by the kidney and therefore increase haemoglobin levels.[38] They also enhance fibrinolytic activity[39] by action on the liver, by increasing synthesis of clotting factors, hepatic triglyceride lipase, sialic acid, alpha-1-antitrypsin and haptoglobin. Androgens also cause a decrease in liver synthesis of SHBG, other hormone-binding globulins (e.g. thyroxine-binding globulin), transferrin and fibrinogen.[40]

Hair and skin

The production of sebum is an androgen-dependent process mainly involving the action of DHT on sebaceous glands.[8] Hair growth on the face, chest and upper pubic region requires high levels of testosterone and therefore is a characteristic of the male.

■ TREATMENT WITH ANDROGENS: ANDROGEN PREPARATIONS

Testosterone

A summary of the main types of testosterone preparation and dosage is given in Table 30.1. Testosterone is rapidly metabolized by the liver as part of the first-pass effect.[44] For it to be clinically useful, two modified forms have been developed.

First, testosterone may be esterified at the 17-hydroxy position. These esters are hydrophobic and are therefore injected (except for testosterone undecanoate) in oily vehicles subcutaneously from which the testosterone slowly escapes. It is then hydrolysed at the site of injection to give metabolically active testosterone. Testosterone esters, however, undergo a variable rate of

Table 30.1. Summary of the currently available testosterone compounds for androgen replacement

Type of testosterone	Name (Trade name)	Route of administration	Dose	Frequency
Testosterone esters	Testosterone undecanoate (Restandol®)	Oral capsules	Initially 120–160 mg daily	2–3 divided doses
	Mesterolone	Oral	25 mg	3–4 times a day, reduced for maintenance
	Testosterone propionate (Sustanon®)	Intramuscular injection	40 mg	Every 2 weeks
	Testosterone enanthate	Intramuscular injection	200 mg	Every 10–14 days
17α-alkylated testosterone	Methyl-testosterone	Oral	10–40 mg	Daily
Testosterone	Organon®	Implant	600 mg	6-monthly
Testosterone	Testop® (Testoderm®)	Transdermal on scrotal skin only	3.6 mg	Once daily
Testosterone	Andropatch® (Androderm®, Testoderm TTS)	Transdermal patch placed on any skin that does not cover a bony prominence	5 mg (two patches)	Once daily

hydrolysis, giving a 'saw-toothed' variation in levels, which may be supraphysiological in the first few days and which fall below the required level before the next injection (Fig. 30.5). Testosterone undecanoate has a long aliphatic side chain. This allows its absorption mainly into the lymphatic system from the gut, therefore bypassing the liver and the first-pass effect (Fig. 30.6); it can, therefore, be taken orally.

Secondly, testosterone may be alkylated at the 17-hydroxy position. These alkylated forms are more resistant to hepatic metabolism and can therefore be taken orally. These compounds, however, are generally weaker than the esterified forms and may cause hepatic dysfunction; they should not, therefore, be used.

Transdermal delivery systems

Testosterone patches placed daily on the scrotum have been successful in delivering a physiological level of testosterone in hypogonadal men.[42] However, although this method of delivery has obvious advantages over injections, it does require some men to shave the scrotum

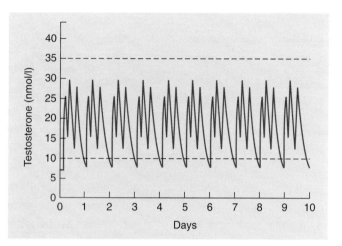

Figure 30.6. Serum testosterone levels after taking oral testosterone undecanoate (3 x 80 mg in hypogonadal men): pharmacokinetic computer simulation assuming basal testosterone levels of 7 nmol/l. Normal range shown by dashed lines. (Reproduced from ref. 133 with permission.)

and in others the scrotum may be too small for adequate application of the patch. Recently, a testosterone patch has become available that can be placed elsewhere on the body, taking care to avoid bony prominences. These daily patches have been shown not only to provide testosterone levels that are physiological but also to follow the circadian rhythm.[43]

Dihydrotestosterone (DHT)

This androgen, synthesized from testosterone by 5-alpha-reductase activity, can also be given as a daily patch.[44]

Dehydroepiandrosterone (DHEA)

With no good evidence to commend it, DHEA is now available over the counter in the USA. Doses used in the two randomized controlled trials to date varied from 50 to 100 mg daily.[45,46]

■ ED: CLINICAL INDICATIONS TO TREAT

Hypogonadism

Documented hypogonadism in men is associated with detrimental effects on lean body mass, bone metabolism, fertility, feelings of well-being, libido, and the development and maintenance of secondary sexual characteristics. For these reasons, men with documented hypogonadism should be started on androgen replacement. It is important, however, to distinguish between primary and secondary

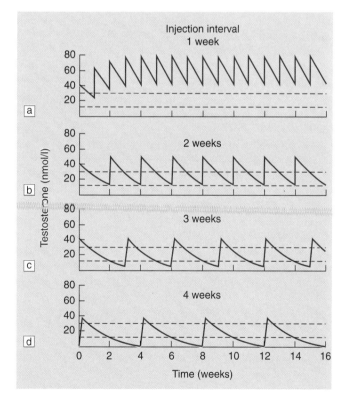

Figure 30.5. Pharmacokinetics of testosterone replacement [250 mg testosterone enanthate i.m. (a) every week, (b) every second week, (c) every 3 weeks or (d) every 4 weeks]: —, pharmacokinetic simulations; ---, range of normal testosterone values. (Reproduced from ref. 133 with permission.)

hypogonadism. In primary hypogonadism, serum levels of testosterone are low but LH and FSH are raised, the abnormality being related to the testicle (e.g. congenital dysgenesis). In secondary hypogonadism the levels of testosterone, LH and FSH are all low, the lesion being related to the hypophyseal–pituitary area. The cause should be determined (Table 30.2), as this will affect the type of treatment required: for example, in secondary hypogonadism a pituitary tumour should be excluded. With regard to prognosis, androgen replacement in men with primary hypogonadism will not restore fertility but replacement with gonadotrophins rather than testosterone may re-establish spermatogenesis in secondary hypogonadism. The favoured form of replacement is testosterone esters such as testosterone enanthate (Table 30.1) which are long acting and have few side effects (see below). However, as described above, supranormal levels are often seen over the first few days and may fall below the normal range prior to the next injection.[47] If these fluctuations are thought to be causing troublesome symptoms in behaviour or function, a smaller dose can be given more frequently (e.g. 100 mg every 7–10 days).[48] Alternatively, serum testosterone levels can be determined immediately prior to the next dose of testosterone; if these are at the upper end of the normal range the dosage interval can be extended and if they are at the lower end of the normal range the interval should be shortened, keeping the dose the same.

■ THE ANDROPAUSE/MALE CLIMACTERIUM/PARTIAL ANDROGEN DEFICIENCY OF THE AGEING MALE (PADAM)

Recently, great interest has developed in the concept of hormone deficiency occurring in the ageing male. This condition has been given many titles — male climacterium, male menopause, PADAM and the andropause. The condition is a poorly defined collection of symptoms including nervousness, depression, inability to concentrate, fatigue, insomnia, reduced libido and hot flushes, first described by Werner in 1939.[49] Erectile dysfunction is also included as part of the condition and there is an increasing demand for hormone supplementation as a proposed treatment. Before a decision can be made as to the validity of hormone supplementation, firstly, the evidence for a deficiency must be determined and secondly, the risks and benefits of treatment must be assessed.

Table 30.2. Causes of hypogonadism

Primary (hypergonadotrophic) hypogonadism
Gonadal defects
    Genetic defects
        Klinefelter's syndrome
        Myotonic dystrophy
        Polyglandular autoimmune disease
        Other genetic syndromes
    Anatomical defect (including castration)
    Defect caused by toxins
        Drugs (cytotoxins and spironolactone)
        Radiation
        Alcohol
    Viral orchitis (mumps most common)
Hormone resistance
    Androgen insensitivity
    LH insensitivity

Secondary (hypogonadotrophic) hypogonadism
Organic causes
    Panhypopituitarism
        Idiopathic
        Pituitary or hypothalamic tumour
        Miscellaneous
            Granulomatous disease
            Vasculitis
            Haemochromatosis
            Infarction
            Trauma
    Hyperprolactinaemia
    Isolated gonadotrophin deficiency
        Kallmann's syndrome and variants
        Idiopathic hypothalamic hypogonadism
        Isolated deficiency of LH or FSH
    Genetic disorder
        Prader–Willi syndrome
        Laurence–Moon–Biedl syndrome
    Systemic disorder
        Chronic disease
        Nutritional deficiency or starvation
        Massive obesity
    Drugs
        Glucocorticoids

Constitutional cause (delayed puberty)

(From ref. 48 with permission.)

Androgens and ageing in the male

Testosterone

There is a progressive decrease in total serum testosterone levels in the male, with age.[50,51] The levels of bioavailable (free) testosterone are determined not only by total testosterone but also by the level of SHBG (Fig. 30.7). There is an increase in serum levels of SHBG with age and therefore a greater fall in the concentration of free testosterone[52–54] reported at a rate of 1% per year (Table 30.3). There is some evidence that this reduction is due to a degree of testicular failure. With advancing age, a decrease in the number of Leydig cells,[55] impaired testicular perfusion,[56] decreased response to beta human chorionic gonadotrophin (beta-HCG)[57,58] and a moderate rise in LH have been shown.[57] There is also evidence, however, that the decrease in testosterone is not all of primary testicular origin, the hypothalamo–pituitary–gonadal axis also being implicated. There is a loss of circadian rhythmicity of serum testosterone[59] and increased

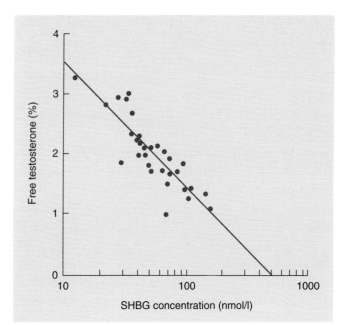

Figure 30.7. Percentage of free testosterone and SHBG levels: $y = 5.56235 - 2.01822 \times \log(x)$; $r^2 = 0.74715$. (Reproduced from ref. 6 with permission.)

Table 30.3. Mean plasma sex hormone levels in 249 healthy men, by age

Age (years)	n	T	FT	SHBG	DHEA	DHEAS	A	E$_2$
25–34	45	21.38 (5.90)†	0.428 (0.098)	35.5 (8.8)	15.91 (6.05)	6.44 (2.29)	3.85 (1.25)	136.8 (50.4)
35–44	22	23.14 (7.36)	0.356 (0.043)	40.1 (7.9)	12.65 (3.69)	6.02 (2.18)	3.81 (1.01)	134.2 (56.3)
45–54	23	21.02 (7.37)	0.314 (0.075)	44.6 (8.2)	11.31 (5.39)	4.75 (2.62)	3.36 (0.90)	142.3 (37.1)
55–64	43	19.49 (6.75)	1.288 (0.073)	45.5 (8.8)	40.20 5.21	3.25 (1.48)	4.66 (1.28)	128.7 (40.4)
65–74	47	18.15 (6.83)	0.239 (0.078)	48.7 (14.2)	7.71 4.15	2.65 (1.68)	4.47 (2.17)	132.3 (38.2)
75–84	48	16.32 (5.85)	0.207 (0.081)	51.0 (22.7)	5.39 (2.76)	1.15 (0.52)	2.18 (1.49)	138.7 (43.4)
85–100	21	13.05 (4.63)	0.186 (0.080)	65.9 (22.8)	3.18 (0.69)	1.23 (0.52)	1.85 (0.91)	136.4 (39.5)

*All values are nmol/1, except for DHEAS (μmol/l) and E: (pmol/); SD in parentheses. T, testosterone; FT, free testosterone; SHBG, sex-hormone-binding globulin; DHEA, dehydroepiandrosterone; DHEAS, dehydroepiandrosterone sulphate; A, androstenedione; E$_2$, oestradiol. (From ref. 10 with permission.)

sensitivity to negative feedback by sex hormones on gonadotrophin secretion.[60]

DHEA

DHEA decreases by 3.1% each year, the most dramatic drop of any of the androgens with age.[52] It is reported that, at the age of 80, the DHEA level will be 20% of that recorded at the age of 20 years.[9,61]

Androstenediol and androstenediol glucuronide

These hormones showed decreases with age of 0.8 and 0.6% per year, respectively.[52]

Androstenedione

The rate of decrease of androstenedione is 1.3% per year — a rate similar to that for free testosterone.[52]

DHT

By contrast to the above androgens, DHT levels do not appear to decrease with age.[52]

'Andropause'

In women, at the menopause there is a complete loss of ovarian function in terms of sex hormones and gamete production. In contrast, in men, although there is a very gradual decrease in testosterone and spermatogenesis,[30] the levels of free and total testosterone do not fall outside the normal range[51] and fertility persists lifelong. It seems, on the evidence available, that an association between the female menopause and the relative decline in androgen levels in the male is not comparable, and the term andropause is not credible in this respect.

■ ANDROGEN SUPPLEMENTATION THERAPY: POSSIBLE BENEFITS

As discussed previously, there are significant decreases in the serum levels of most androgens in the male with age. Age has also been shown to be the strongest predictive variable for the presence of ED.[18] It is this very association that has led to the demand for androgen supplementation therapy for middle-aged and elderly men suffering from ED. There are also an increasing number of reports showing a host of other possible beneficial effects of androgen supplementation. For this reason, current evidence for the effects of androgen supplementation in all areas as well as ED are included.

Testosterone supplementation

Body composition

The link between obesity and a wide range of diseases leading to ill health is accepted[62] and even a modest weight loss of up to 5 kg can produce important health benefits.[63] There is mounting evidence that supplementation can increase lean body mass by reducing fat (mainly visceral in the male) and increasing the amount of muscle.[64-66] In two studies, men with borderline hypogonadism had increases in lean body mass of 5% and decreases in body fat of 6–20% were noted.[67,68] Also, in a group of obese men who underwent 9 months' treatment with testosterone given by gel application, a decrease in visceral fat tissue by 9% on CT scanning was shown.[69] Androgen supplementation may have a significant role to play in reducing obesity; prospective randomized placebo-controlled trials are urgently required.

Bone metabolism

Androgens have an important role in bone metabolism, and hypogonadal individuals have an increased risk of osteoporosis.[31,32] In elderly hypogonadal men, testosterone replacement has led to increases in bone density of 5–13%.[67,70] In the male, as age increases bone mass falls and the chance of a fracture secondary to osteoporosis increases.[34] In a 6 month open prospective trial with 23 eugonadal men with idiopathic primary osteoporosis, a significant increase in bone mineral density was demonstrated in the lumbar spine.[71] Also, in men with testosterone levels at the lower end of the normal range there is evidence of increased bone metabolism and bone density with supplementation.[64,72] However, more information is needed to evaluate this treatment from randomized trials, especially to attempt to demonstrate a decrease in fracture rate with treatment.

Cardiovascular disease and blood lipids

The effects of androgens and their relationship to the increased rate of coronary artery disease in men compared with premenopausal women are complex. Reducing testosterone levels in eugonadal men causes an increase in HDL, giving evidence that it is testosterone — at least in part — that is responsible for the detrimental high LDL/HDL ratio seen in the male after puberty.[73] Conversely, studies in hypogonadal men have shown a potentially advantageous decrease in LDL with testosterone replacement.[64,75,77] This may explain the reported association between coronary artery disease and decreased levels of testosterone.[76,77]

Potentially beneficial increases in fibrinolysis (with the 17-alpha-alkylated androgens only) have also been shown.[78,79] Overall, the role of testosterone supplementation and its benefits to the cardiovascular system remain unclear.

Sexual interest, behaviour and well-being

The importance of testosterone replacement in increasing sexual interest and behaviour in men with hypogonadism is generally accepted, as already cited. A positive correlation between the level of free testosterone (but not of total testosterone) with sexual desire and frequency of masturbation was seen in 77 healthy men aged between 45 and 74 years.[80] In men with an age-related testosterone level at the lower end of the normal range, a number of studies have shown that sexual desire and well-being is increased by supplementation,[64,81-83] however, the improvement is not always deemed adequate by the patient.[83]

Erectile dysfunction

The levels of total and free testosterone are the same in impotent and potent elderly men.[18,19,84] In eugonadal men with an age-related moderately low testosterone level, there have been few controlled trials of testosterone supplementation and ED.[81,83,85] In all these studies no improvement in erectile function was shown. In the eugonadal male, therefore, there is no evidence to date that testosterone supplementation is of proven benefit in the treatment of ED.

DHT supplementation

Circulating (but not necessarily tissue) DHT levels do not seem to decline with age. Because DHT is responsible for many of the actions of testosterone, it could (theoretically) be used in males to supplement low levels of testosterone. DHT cannot be aromatized and therefore supplementation is not associated with an increase in oestradiol levels, which may decrease some of the potential risks of supplementation therapy with testosterone. Supplementation with DHT transdermal patch delivery system has been reported;[44] however, a double-blind placebo-controlled trial is crucial to determine benefit. Remarkably, such a trial has not yet been conducted.

DHEA supplementation

DHEA and its sulphate are quantitatively the most important androgens and the decline in levels with age is certainly the most dramatic.[52] However, DHEA levels show great variation in the male population, and in the only longitudinal study over 15 years, 15 of the 97 men actually showed an increase in DHEA levels.[86]

The physiological role of DHEA is unclear and the implications on health of its decline in level with age are unknown. There have been contrasting claims of an association between DHEA levels and coronary artery disease.[87,88] Animal studies have shown that administration of DHEA inhibits induced tumours of breast, colon, skin and liver in mice and rats.[89] However, results from animal models are notoriously difficult to interpret because these animals do not naturally produce any DHEA themselves. There have been two placebo-controlled studies with older men and women: in the first, which randomized 17 women and 13 men, a dose of 50 mg DHEA was found to increase levels of DHEA to that of healthy young adults; in the men there was an improvement in general well-being but no change in libido.[45] In the other study there was an increase in lean body mass and muscle strength at the knee with supplementation in men.[46] Both papers showed a significant increase in insulin-like growth factor (IGF)-1 of 10–20%. At present there is some information that may indicate some potential benefits of DHEA supplementation. However, further controlled studies are needed and until then the use of DHEA as a supplemental therapy for the middle-aged or elderly should be resisted.

■ POSSIBLE RISKS OF ANDROGEN SUPPLEMENTATION

Testosterone and the prostate

The use of testosterone replacement to provide androgens for patients who are deficient is clinically very important. The benefit, however, of androgen supplementation in the ageing male and in those middle-aged men with erectile failure and low normal levels of testosterone is less clear and is controversial.

Androgens and benign prostatic hyperplasia (BPH)

The incidence of BPH is age related, affecting 13.8% of men aged 40–49 and 43% of men aged 60–69.[90] This increase may, in part, be due to an alteration in the testosterone/oestrogen ratio in favour of the latter. A study to determine whether redressing this balance by administration of an aromatase inhibitor, however, showed no benefit.[91]

It has been known since John Hunter's observations in the 18th century that the prostate undergoes atrophy after castration and that prostate growth and development depend very much upon its hormonal environment. More specifically, it is the testosterone metabolite DHT that has the principal androgenic effects on prostate growth.[92]

In the rare condition of congenital absence of the enzyme 5 alpha-reductase, affected males develop the typical male phenotype at puberty, but the prostate remains vestigial and they never develop BPH.[93] Serum testosterone levels are normal but DHT levels are low. Administration of a 5 alpha-reductase inhibitor has been used therapeutically to treat BPH.[94]

Androgens and prostatic cancer

Adenocarcinoma of the prostate accounts for around 10% of all cancer deaths in the European Community countries[95] and is the second leading cause of cancer death in males in the USA.[96] The incidence of prostate cancer is increasing.[97] Prostate cancer is androgen dependent and advanced disease is treated by removal of androgen support.[98] This is achieved with medical/surgical castration or administration of an anti-androgen, either alone or in combination with an LHRH analogue to achieve 'total androgen blockade'.[99] Furthermore, prostate cancer very rarely occurs in eunuchs or castrated men.[100]

The stimulatory effect that increases in serum testosterone have upon the behaviour of prostatic carcinoma is clearly shown by the phenomenon of 'tumour flare'. Tumour flare occurs 10–12 days after administration of an LHRH analogue for the treatment of prostate carcinoma. As the testosterone levels rise, bony metastases become more painful, spinal cord compression and paraplegia may be precipitated and ureteric obstruction may occur.[101]

Unfortunately, there is very little information available on the safety of androgen supplementation with regard to prostate cancer. Studies to date incorporate a total of less than 300 men and follow-up is usually less than 12 months. This number of men studied is inadequate and a follow-up of at least 10 years would be required to draw any conclusions on the impact of testosterone supplementation on the incidence and behaviour of prostatic carcinoma.

Because of the androgen-dependent nature of prostatic carcinoma it is accepted that its presence is an absolute contra-indication to testosterone therapy. At autopsy, however, the prevalence of histological prostatic carcinoma in 60-year-old men is 32% but the prevalence of clinically defined disease is 4%.[102] It is the potential effect that supplementary androgen will have upon this large number of 'latent' prostatic carcinomas that has led to the use of prostate-specific antigen (PSA) as a screening blood test before starting androgen therapy and in the patient follow-up. To date, in the majority of studies, PSA has not risen significantly in truly hypogonadal[111] and eugonadal[103] men receiving testosterone treatment. In two studies a significant rise in PSA was seen but the level remained below the commonly used 'cut-off' point of 4 ng/l.[64,104] In the authors' opinion, PSA is useful but is not an adequate test for excluding prostate carcinoma before initiating testosterone therapy. First, there is no clear 'cut-off' point and PSA rises with age (Fig. 30.8). Secondly, the ability of PSA with a 'cut-off' of 4 ng/l to identify patients who are truly negative for prostate carcinoma is poor, with a reported specificity of 45.8% in a prospective study of 4962 men over the age of 50.[105] Further evidence for this limitation of PSA testing comes from the Johns Hopkins radical prostatectomy series: of nearly 1000 men with localized prostate cancer, 35% had a PSA value of less than 4 ng/l.[106] Thirdly, in a prospective study of 33 men with hypogonadism and a normal age-adjusted PSA and digital rectal examination (DRE), 26% of men over the age of 60 had prostate cancer on biopsy. This not only

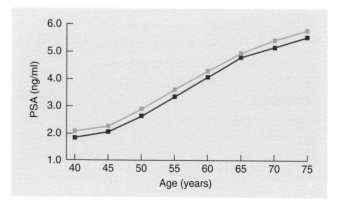

Figure 30.8. Age specific PSA reference ranges: ■, 1992 (n > 49 000); ■, 1993 (n > 53 000). (Reproduced from ref. 134 with permission.)

illustrates the limitation of PSA and DRE but may also indicate that, in hypogonadal patients, the PSA is 'falsely' lowered into the normal range.[107]

If the clinician wishes to determine the presence or absence of prostate carcinoma, then PSA is not adequate and the authors strongly recommend that all men aged 60 and over should undergo transrectal ultrasound (TRUS) and sextant biopsies before commencement of androgen therapy.

Cardiovascular effects

Testosterone seems to have an effect on a number of substances that have a role in the vascular system. Endothelins are a group of peptides produced by a variety of tissues and are potent vasoconstrictors counteracted by nitric oxide, prostacyclin and atrial natriuretic peptide. It has been shown that endothelin levels can be raised by testosterone supplementation and reduced by androgen deprivation in a group of trans-sexual subjects undergoing cross-sex hormone treatment.[108] In addition, testosterone has been shown to decrease the production of prostacyclin (a potent vasodilator and antiplatelet aggregatory compound) in aortic smooth muscle cell cultures[109] and to increase the levels of thromboxane (a potent vasoconstrictor and pro-aggregatory compound) in monkeys.[109,110] These changes may explain the marked atherogenesis reported in female monkeys with androgen supplementation.[111]

The impact of androgens on serum lipids is complex and factors such as route of administration, type of testosterone and hormonal status of the patient are important. For this reason, studies of side effects often seem contradictory and confusing. However, administration of testosterone orally has been shown to reduce HDL levels in hypogonadal men and in women undergoing cross-sex hormone treatment.[73]

There is evidence that, in men who attain supraphysiological levels of testosterone, while taking oral alkylated testosterone, marked decreases in HDL and some increases in LDL are seen,[112,113] with the recognized increase in associated cardiovascular risk.[114] Indeed, sportsmen taking large doses of alkylated testosterone supplements and who suffer myocardial infarction[115] and stroke[116] serve as a warning of their dangers. It must be noted, however, that these are case reports only and that their testosterone levels were supraphysiological. Testosterone esters used within physiological levels do not seem to be associated with marked changes in serum lipid profiles; their overall effect on the cardiovascular system needs further evaluation.

Sodium retention

Androgens lead to an increase in sodium retention and hence an increase in extracellular volume.[117] The effect is small but may be significant in patients with cardiovascular disease, causing an exacerbation of any underlying heart failure.

Sleep apnoea

Androgens have a role in the development of obstructive sleep apnoea and supplementation may exacerbate the condition.[119] These apnoeic events are associated with oxygen desaturation and cardiovascular complications.

Haemopoiesis

Androgen supplementation has been shown to increase the haematocrit in the elderly male by up to 7%.[64] This increase, although small, may be of significance in men with peripheral vascular disease.

Insulin resistance

Insulin resistance and hyperandrogenism have been described mainly in women with polycystic ovary syndrome; improvement in insulin resistance is seen after reversal of the hyperandrogenism.[118] A degree of insulin resistance has been shown in female-to-male trans-sexuals, although the significance of this is unclear.

Liver

Alkylated androgens can cause peliosis hepatitis (haemorrhagic liver cysts). This is a very serious idiosyncratic complication and is unrelated to the dose or duration of androgen treatment.[120] Furthermore, patients with Fanconi's anaemia have an increased risk of hepatic tumours while being treated with alkylated testosterone preparations. However, replacement with testosterone esters is very rarely associated with hepatic dysfunction.[48]

Gynaecomastia

This develops when there is an increase in the ratio of oestrogen to androgen.[121] Supplementation with aromatizable androgens (e.g testosterone) may therefore lead to gynaecomastia. Patients with liver or renal disease may be particularly affected.

Drug interaction of androgens

Androgens interact with anticoagulants, decreasing the dose required by up to 25%.[122] This effect is probably due to an increase in antithrombin III seen with androgen treatment.

■ MONITORING PATIENTS ON HORMONE REPLACEMENT OR SUPPLEMENTATION

The tests and procedures required for monitoring patients receiving hormone replacement or supplementation are summarized in Table 30.4.

■ HYPERPROLACTINAEMIA AND ED

There is good evidence of a strong relationship between hyperprolactinaemia and ED. In a study of 26 men with hyperprolactinaemia, all were suffering from ED[123] and, in another study, 17 of 29 men with raised prolactin complained of ED.[124] The commonest presentation for men with hyperprolactinaemia is low libido and ED.[124–126] In fact, in 22 men with hyperprolactinaemia and ED, 41% also had visual field defects and only 14% had galactorrhoea and/or gynaecomastia.[126] Hyperprolactinaemia is not a common cause of ED and is thought to be significant in only 3–6% of patients presenting with ED.[127,128] Serum

---

Table 30.4. Monitoring patients on androgen replacement or supplementation

Before initiation of treatment

    Clinical examination and DRE

    Serum LH and FSH (to exclude secondary hypogonadism)

    PSA

    Lipid profile

    Haemoglobin

    Liver function tests (LFTs)

    Transrectal ultrasound scan and sextant biopsy (if >60 years old)

Caution: if symptoms of bladder outflow obstruction or suspicion of sleep apnoea
Absolute contraindications: carcinoma of the breast and carcinoma of the prostate

Follow-up

    Initially 6 monthly

    History to assess degree of response and adverse reactions (e.g. increasing urinary symptoms)

    Serum testosterone (on the day and before next IM dose of testosterone is to be given)

    DRE (if >40 years)

    PSA (if >40 years)

    LFTs (only if being treated with 17-alkylated testosterone preparations)

Consider: yearly lipid and haemoglobin serum levels
Care: in patients with: suspicion of sleep apnoea, heart failure, cardiovascular disease, etc.

prolactin determination cannot, therefore, be recommended as part of a routine screen in patients presenting with ED unless there is clinical suspicion.

Prolactin secretion from the anterior pituitary gland is influenced by many factors including stress, sleep, catecholamines, thyrotrophin-releasing hormone and vasoactive intestinal polypeptide, and is inhibited by dopamine secreted by the hypothalamus.[129] The mechanism by which hyperprolactinaemia causes ED is not fully understood, but may well be related to an imbalance of the hypothalamic–pituitary–gonadal axis. Indeed, the majority of patients with hyperprolactinaemia have a low testosterone level.[126,128,130] In 22 men with hypogonadism and hyperprolactinaemia, stimulation of the Leydig cells and pituitary gland by HCG and LHRH analogues, respectively, showed a normal response. From this, the authors hypothesized that the raised prolactin decreased the release of LHRH from the hypothalamus and therefore led to decreased levels of testosterone.[126]

The causes of hyperprolactinaemia are shown in Table 30.5. Drugs that act as dopamine antagonists, such as the phenothiazines (e.g. sulpiride), may lead to hyperprolactinaemia and are associated with low libido and decreased potency. Indeed, in one study the levels of prolactin and sexual dysfunction were proportional to the dose of sulpiride, and restoration of potency and prolactin levels occurred after stopping the drug.[131] Patients with end-stage renal failure who are on haemodialysis commonly have raised prolactin with decreased testosterone levels and complain of ED.[129,132] Hyperprolactinaemia is usually suspected after taking a history and performing a clinical examination. Because prolactin levels are affected by so many factors, including sleep, venepuncture should be performed on three different occasions 2–3 hours after the patient has woken. Management of hyperprolactinaemia depends on the cause (Table 30.5). A pituitary tumour should be excluded by radiological investigations (plain skull X-rays and CT scan) and, if present, surgery may be required. A review of current medication should be undertaken to identify any drugs that antagonize dopamine (Table 30.5) or deplete dopamine levels, which can lead to hyperprolactinaemia.

Treatment

In cases of hyperprolactinaemia secondary to a pituitary adenoma, if surgery is not indicated then bromocriptine is very effective in reducing prolactin levels to within the normal range. Bromocriptine is also effective in increasing libido and improving potency in these patients.[124,125,127,130] Not only does bromocriptine lower the level of prolactin but, in cases with associated hypogonadism, testosterone levels also increase significantly after treatment.[123,124,128] Bromocriptine is also effective in hyperprolactinaemic patients on haemodialysis.[129] The dose of bromocriptine is variable, as are the troublesome side effects such as nausea and hypotension. It is reasonable to start on a small dose of 1.25 mg daily at night. After 2 weeks, prolactin levels can be rechecked, as can clinical progress. Increasing the dose by increments of 1.25 mg should continue until prolactin levels are within the normal range.

Table 30.5. Causes of hyperprolactinaemia in the male

Production by tumours
  Adenoma or more commonly microadenoma of the pituitary gland
Damage to pituitary stalk
  Any non-secreting tumour of pituitary or hypothalamus
  Surgical section
Idiopathic
Severe primary hypothyroidism
Chronic renal failure
Liver failure
Chest injury

Physiological
  Stress
  Rapid-eye-movement sleep
  Coitus

Drug induced
  Phenothiazines
  Metoclopramide
  Cimetidine
  Oestrogens
  Methyldopa
  Haloperidol

■ REFERENCES

1. Gooren L J G. The age-related decline of androgen levels in men: clinically significant? Br J Urol 1996; 78: 763–768

2. Lock S. O that I were young again: Yeats and the Steinach operation. Br Med J 1983; 287: 1964–1968

3. Stryer L. Biochemistry. San Francisco: Freeman, 1975

4. Tappanainen J, Kellokumpu-Liehten P, Pelliniemi L, Huhtaniemi I. Age related changes in endogenous steroids of the human fetal testis during early and mid pregnancy. J Clin Endocrinol Metab 1981; 52: 98–102

5. Forrest M G, de Paretti E, Bertrand J. Hypothalamic–pituitary–gonadal function in man from birth to puberty. Clin Endocrinol 1975; 5: 551–569

6. Wheeler M J. The determination of bio-available testosterone. Ann Clin Biochem 1995; 32: 345–357

7. Jeffcoate S L, Brocks R V, Lim N Y et al. Androgen production in hypogonadal men. J Endocrinol 1967; 37: 401–411

8. Mooradian A D, Morley J E, Korenman S G. Biological actions of androgens. Endocr Rev. 1987; 8: 1–28

9. Weksler M E. Hormone replacement for men. Br Med J 1996; 312: 859–860

10. Vermeulen A. Declining androgens with age. Testosterone replacement therapy advisory panel meeting. (Parthenon Publishing Group Ltd, Carnforth, UK Dec 1995: 3–7

11. Behre H M, Bohmeyer J, Nieschlag E. Prostate volume in testosterone treated and untreated hypogonadal men in comparison to age matched controls. Clin Endocrinol 1994; 40: 341–346

12. Santulli R, Sprando R L, Awonryi C A et al. To what extent can spermatogenesis be maintained in hypophysectomized adult rat testis with exogenously administered testosterone? Endocrinology 1990; 126: 95–101

13. Bagatell C J, Heiman J R, Rivier J E, Bremner W J. Effects of endogenous testosterone and oestradiol on sexual behaviour in normal young men. J Clin Endocrinol Metab 1994; 78: 711–716

14. Davidson J M, Camargo C, Smith E R. Effects of androgens on sexual behaviour in hypogonadal men. J Clin Endocrinol Metab 1979; 48: 955–958

15. Skakkebaek M, Bancroft J, Davidson D, Warner P. Androgen replacement with oral testosterone undecanoate in hypogonadal men: a double blind controlled study. Clin Endocrinol 1981; 14: 49–61

16. Luisi M, Frachi F. Double blind comparative study of testosterone undecanoate and mesterolone in hypogonadal male patients. J Endocrinol Invest 1980; 3: 305–308

17. Lugg J A, Rajfer J, Gonzalez-Cadovid N F. Dihydrotestosterone is the active androgen in the maintenance of nitric oxide-mediated penile erection in the rat. Endocrinology 1995; 136(4): 1495–1501

18. Feldman J A, Goldstein I, Hatzichristou D G et al. Impotence and its medical psychosocial correlates: results of the Massachusetts Male Aging Study. J Urol 1994; 151: 54–61.

19. Schiavi R C, Schreiner-Eugel P, White D, Mandeli J. The relationship between pituitary–gonadal function and sexual behaviour in healthy aging men. Psychosom Med 1991; 55: 363–374

20. Kwan M, Greenleaf W J, Mann J et al. The nature of androgen action on male sexuality: a combined laboratory self report study on hypogonadal men. J Endocrinol Metab 1983; 57: 557–562

21. O'Carrol R, Shapiro C, Bancroft J. Androgens, behaviour and nocturnal erections in hypogonadal men: the effects of varying the replacement dose. Clin Endocrinol 1985; 23: 527–538

22. Bardin W C, Swerdloff R S, Santen R J. Androgens: risks and benefits. J Clin Endocrinol Metab 1991; 73: 4–7

23. Bancroft J, Wu F C. Changes in erectile responsiveness during androgen replacement therapy. Arch Sex Behav 1983; 12: 59–66

24. Bancroft J, Tennent T, Loucas K, Cass J. Control of deviant sexual behaviour by drugs. Behavioural effects of oestrogens and antiandrogens. Br J Psychiatry 1974; 125: 310–315

25. Gilbert H W, Gillatt D A, Desai K M, Gingell J C. Intracorporeal papaverine injection in androgen deprived men. J R Soc Med 1990; 83(March): 161

26. Michael R P, Zupe D. Annual cycles of aggression and plasma testosterone in captive male rhesus monkeys. Psychoneuroendocrinology 1978; 3: 217–220

27. Su T P, Pagliaro M, Schmidt P J et al. Neuropsychiatric effects of anabolic steroids in male normal volunteers. JAMA 1993; 269: 2760–2764

28. Anderson R A, Bancroft J, Wu F C. The effects of exogenous testosterone on sexuality and mood in normal young men. J Clin Endocrinol Metab 1992; 75: 1503–1507

29. Forbes G B. The effect of anabolic steroids on lean body mass: the dose response curve. Metabolism 1985; 34: 571–573

30. Kasperk C H, Wergedal J E, Farley J R et al. Androgens directly stimulate proliferation of bone cells in vitro. Endocrinology 1989; 124: 1576–1578

31. Jackson J A, Kleerekoper M. Osteoporosis in men: diagnosis, pathophysiology and prevention. Medicine 1990; 69: 137–152

32. Finkelstein J S, Klibanski A, Neer R M et al. Osteoporosis in men with idiopathic hypogonadotrophic hypogonadism. Ann Intern Med 1987; 106: 354–361

33. Gilsanz V, Gibbens D T, Roe T F et al. Vertebral bone density in children: effect of puberty. Radiology 1988; 166: 847–850

34. Santavirta S, Konttinen Y T, Heliovaara M et al. Determinants of osteoporotic thoracic vertebral fracture — screening of 57,000 Finnish women and men. Acta Orthop Scand 1992; 63: 198-202

35. Smith E P, Boyd J, Frank G R et al. Estrogen resistance caused by a mutation in the estrogen receptor gene in a man. N Engl J Med 1994; 331: 1056–1061

36. Heiss G, Tamir I, Davis C E et al. Lipoprotein–cholesterol distributions in selected North American populations: the Lipid Research Clinics Program Prevalence Study. Circulation 1980; 61: 302–315

37. Surva R, Kuosi T, Taskinen M R et al. Testosterone substitution increases the activity of lipoprotein lipase and hepatic lipase in hypogonadal males. Atherosclerosis 1988; 69: 191–197

38. Cardner F H, Natham D G, Piomelli S, Cummins J F. The erythrocythaemic effects of androgens. Br J Haematol 1968; 14: 611–615

39. Fearnley G R, Chakrabarti R. Increase of blood fibrinolytic activity by testosterone. Lancet 1962; ii: 128–132

40. Dickinson P, Sinneman H H, Swaim W R et al. Effects of testosterone treatment on plasma proteins and amino acids in men. J Clin Endocrinol Metab 1969; 29: 837–841

41. Wu F C. Testicular steroidogenesis and androgen use and abuse. Baillieres Clin Endocrinol Metab 1992; 6: 373–403

42. Bhasin S. Androgen treatment of hypogonadal men. J Clin Endocrinol Metab 1992; 74: 1221–1225

43. Meikle A W, Mazer N A, Moellmer J F et al. Enhanced transdermal delivery across non scrotal skin produces physiological concentration of testosterone and its metabolites in hypogonadal men. J Clin Endocrinol Metab 1992; 74: 623–628

44. de Lignières B. Transdermal DHT treatment of the 'Andropause'. Ann Med 1993; 25: 235–241

45. Morales A J, Nolan J J, Nelson J C, Yen S C C. Effects of replacement dose of dehydroepiandrosterone in men and women of advancing age. J Clin Endocrinol Metab 1994; 78: 1360–1367

46. Yen S S C, Morales A J, Khurram O. Replacement of DHEA in aging men and women. Ann N Y Acad Sci 1995; 774: 128–142

47. Snyder P J. Clinical use of androgens. Ann Rev Med 1984; 35: 207–217

48. Bagatell C J and Bremner W J. Androgens in men: uses and abuses. N Engl J Med 1996; 334(11): 707–714

49. Werner A A. The male climacteric. JAMA 1939; 112: 1441–1443

50. Hollander M, Hollander Y. The microdetermination of the testosterone in the human spermatic vein. J Clin Endocrinol Metab 1958; 18: 966–970

51. Vermeulen A. The male climacterium. Ann Med 1993; 25: 531–534

52. Gray A, Feldman H A, McKinlay J B, Longcope C. Age, disease and changing sex hormone levels in middle aged men: results of the Massachusetts Male Aging Study J Clin Endocrinol Metab 1991; 73: 1016–25

53. Nahoul K, Rayer M. Age-related decline of plasma available testosterone in adult men. J Steroid Biochem 1990; 35: 293–299

54. Purifoy F E, Koopmans L H, Mayes D M. Age differences in serum androgen levels in normal adult males. Hum Biol 1981; 53: 499–511

55. Neaves W B, Johnson L, Porter J C et al. Leydig cell numbers, daily sperm production and serum gonadotrophin levels in aging men. J Clin Endocrinol Metab 1984; 59: 756–763

56. Sesano M, Ishyo S. Vascular patterns of the human testes with special reference to senile changes. Tohoku J Exp Med 1969; 99: 269–280

57. Rubens R, Dhont M, Vermeulen A. Further studies on Leydig cell function in old age. J Clin Endocrinol Metab 1974; 39: 40–45

58. Mankin H R, Lin T, Muruno E P, Osterman J. The aging leydig cell: III Gonadotrophin stimulation in men. J Androl 1981; 2: 181–189

59. Bremner W J, Vitello M, Prinz P N. Loss of circadian rhythmicity in blood testosterone levels with aging in normal men. J Clin Endocrinol Metab 1983; 56(6): 1278–1281

60. Winters S J, Sherins R J, Truen P. The gonadotrophin suppressible activity of androgens is increased in elderly men. Metabolism 1984; 33: 1052–1059

61. Vermeulen A. DHEA(S) and aging. Ann N Y Acad Sci 1996; 774: 121–127

62. Health Education Authority. Obesity in primary health care. A literature review. London: HEA, 1995

63. Hankey C, Lean M. The benefits of weight reduction and maintenance of weight loss. Royal College of Physicians of Edinburgh Working Group on Obesity, 1995

64. Tenover J S. Effects of testosterone supplementation in the aging male. J Clin Endocrinol Metab 1992; 75: 1092–1098

65. Marin P, Krotkiewski M, Bjorntorp P. Androgen treatment of middle aged obese men: effects on metabolism, muscle and adipose tissue. Eur J Med 1992; 1: 329–336

66. Forbes G B, Porta C R, Herr B E, Griggs R C. Sequence of changes in body composition induced by testosterone and reversal of changes after drug is stopped. JAMA 1992; 267: 397–399

67. Katznelson L, Finkelstein J, Baressi C, Klibanski A. Increase in trabecular bone density and altered body composition in androgen replacement in hypogonadal men. In: Program and Abstracts of the 76th Annual Meeting of the Endocrine Society (USA), abstract 1524, p 581

68. Haddad G, Peachey H, Slipman C, Snyder P J. Testosterone treatment improves body composition and muscle strength in hypogonadal men. In: Program and Abstracts of the 76th Annual Meeting of the Endocrine Society (USA), abstr 1302, p 506

69. Marin P, Holmany S, Gustafsson C et al. Androgen treatment of abdominally obese men. Obesity Res 1993; 1: 245–251

70. Oppenheim D, Klibanski A. Osteopaenia in men with acquired hypogonadism. In: Program and Abstracts of the 76th Annual Meeting of the Endocrine Society (USA), abstract 1070, p 319

71. Anderson F H, Francis R M, Faulkner K. Androgen supplementation in eugonadal men with osteoporosis—effects of 6 months of treatment on bone mineral density and cardiovascular risk factors. Bone 1996; 18(2): 171–177

72. Tomasic P V, Sollock R L, Armstrong D, Shakir K M M. Osteoporosis in men with borderline idiopathic hypogonadotrophic hypogonadism. In: Program and Abstracts of the 76th Annual Meeting of the Endocrine Society (USA), abstract 1043, p 461

73. Asscheman H, Cooren L J G, Megens J A et al. Serum testosterone level is the major determinant of the male–female differences in serum levels of HDL cholesterol and HDL2 cholesterol. Metabolism 1994; 43: 935–939

74. Morley J E, Perry H M III, Kaiser F E et al. Effects of testosterone replacement therapy in old hypogonadal males: a preliminary study. J Am Geriatr Soc 1993; 41: 149–152

75. Ellyin F M. The long term beneficial effect of low dose testosterone in the aging male. In: Endocrine Society 77th Annual Meeting Program and Abstracts, P2-127, p 322 Washington DC: Endocrine Society Press

76. Philips G B, Pinkernell B H, Jing T-Y. The association of hypotestosteronaemia with coronary artery disease in men. Arterioscler Thromb 1994; 14: 701–706

77. Brier C, Muhlberger V, Drexel H et al. Essential role of post heparin lipoprotein lipase activity and of plasma testosterone in coronary artery disease. Lancet 1985; 1242–1244

78. Ansell J E, Tiarks C, Fairchild V K. Coagulation abnormalities associated with the use of anabolic steroids. Am Heart J 1993; 125: 367–371

79. Bonithon-Kopp C, Scarabin P Y, Bara L et al. Relationship between sex hormones and haemostatic factors in healthy adult men. Atherosclerosis 1988; 71: 71–76

80. Shiavi R C, Schreiner-Engel P, Mandeli J et al. Healthy aging and male sexual function. Am J Psychiatry 1990; 147: 766–771

81. Schiavi F C, White D, Mordeli J, Levine A C. Effect of testosterone administration on sexual behaviour and mood in men with erectile dysfuction. Arch Sex Behav 1997; 26: 231–241

82. Matsumato A M. Effects of chronic testosterone administration in normal men: safety and efficacy of high dosage testosterone and parallel dose dependent suppression of luteinizing hormone, follicle stimulating hormone and sperm production. J Clin Endocrinol Metab 1990; 70: 282–287

83. O'Carrol R, Bancroft J. Testosterone therapy for low sexual interest and erectile dysfunction in men: a controlled study. Br J Psychiatry 1984; 145: 146–151

84. Korenman S G, Morley J E, Mooradian A D et al. Secondary hypogonadism in older men: its relation to impotence. J Clin Endocrinol Metab 1990; 71(4): 963–969

85. Cooper A J. A clinical and endocrine study of mesterolone in secondary impotence. J Psychosom Res 1980; 24: 275–279

86. Orentreich N, Brind J L, Rizer R L, Vogelman J H. Age changes and sex differences in serum dehydroepiandrosterone sulphate concentration through adulthood. J Clin Endocrinol Metab 1984; 59: 551–555

87. Barrett-Connor E, Khaw K, Yen S S C. A prospective study of dehydroepiandrosterone sulfate, mortality and cardiovascular disease. N Engl J Med 1988; 315: 1519–1524

88. Hautanen A, Manttarri M, Manninen V et al. Adrenal androgens and testosterone as coronary risk factors in the Helsinki heart study. Atherosclerosis 1994; 105: 191–200

89. Schwarz A G, Pashko L L. Mechanism of cancer preventive action of DHEA: role of glucose-6-phosphate dehydrogenase. Ann N Y Acad Sci 1996; 774: 180–186

90. Garraway W M, Collins G N, Lee R J. High prevalence of benign prostatic hypertrophy in the community. Lancet 1991; 338(8765): 469–471

91. Gingell J C, Knonägel H, Kurth K H et al. Placebo controlled double-blind study to test the efficacy of the aromatase inhibitor Atamestane in patients not requiring operation. J Urol 1995; 154: 399–401

92. Isaacs J T, Coffey D S. Changes in DHT metabolism associated with the development of canine benign prostatic hyperplasia. Endocrinology 1981; 108: 445–453

93. Imperato-McGinley J, Guevro L, Gauteri T et al. Steroid 5α-reductase deficiency in a man: an inherited form of pseudo-hermaphroditism. Science 1974; 186: 1213–1215

94. Stoner E. The clinical effects of a 5α-reductase inhibitor, Finasteride, on benign prostatic hyperplasia. J Urol 1992; 147: 1298–1302

95. Jensen O M, Esteve J, Renard H. Cancer in the European community and its member states. Eur J Cancer 1990; 26: 1167–1256

96. Cancer Facts and Figures—1992. Atlanta: American Cancer Society, 1992

97. Lu-Yao G L, Greenburg E R. Changes in prostate cancer incidence and treatment in USA. Lancet 1994; 343: 251–255

98. Huggins C, Stevens R E Jr, Hodges C V. Studies on prostatic cancer II. The effects of castration on advanced carcinoma of the prostate gland. Arch Surg 1941; 43: 208–223

99. Labrie F, Dupont A, Belanger A et al. A new approach in the treatment of prostate cancer: complete instead of partial withdrawal of androgens. Prostate 1983; 4: 579–594

100. Pienta K J, Esper P S. Risk factors and prostate cancer. Ann Intern Med 1993; 118: 793-803

101. Waxman J, Man A, Hendry W F. Importance of early tumour exacerbation in patients treated with long acting analogues of gonadotrophin releasing hormone for advanced prostate cancer. Br Med J 1985; 291: 1387–1388

102. Shroder F H. Detection of prostate cancer. Br Med J 1995; 310: 140–141

103. Wallace E M, Pye S D, Wild S R and Wu F C W. Prostate specific antigen and prostate gland size in men receiving exogenous testosterone for male contraception. Int J Androl 1993; 16: 35-40

104. Urban F J, Rodenburg Y H, Gilkison C et al. Testosterone administration to elderly men increases skeletal muscle strength and protein synthesis. Am J Physiol 1995; 269: E820–E826

105. Catalona W J, Richie J P, Dekernion J B et al. Comparison of prostate specific antigen concentration versus prostate specific antigen density in the early detection of prostate cancer: receiver operating characteristic curves. J Urol 1994; 152: 2031–2037

106. Partin A W, Pound C R, Clemens J Q et al. Serum PSA after anatomic radical prostatectomy. The Johns Hopkins experience after 10 years. Urol Clin North Am 1993; 20: 71

107. Morgentaler A, Bruning CO III, DeWolf W C. Occult prostate cancer in men with low serum testosterone levels. JAMA 1996; 276: 1904–1906

108. Polderman K H, Stehouwer C D A, Van de Kamp G J et al. Influence of sex hormones on plasma endothelin levels. Ann Intern Med 1993; 118: 429–432

109. Derman R J. Effects of sex steroids on women's health: implications for practitioners. Am J Med 1995; 98(suppl1A): 1375–1343S

110. Ajayi A A. Testosterone increases human platelet thromboxane A2 receptor density and aggregation responses. Circulation 1995; 91: 2742–2747

111. Adams M R, Williams J K, Kaplan J R. Effects of androgens on coronary artery atherosclerosis and atherosclerosis-related impairment of vascular responsiveness. Arteroiscler Thromb Vasc Biol 1995; 15: 562–570

111. Foulks C J and Cushner H C. Sexual dysfunction in the male dialysis patient: Pathogenesis, evaluation and therapy. American Journal of Kidney Diseases, Vol VIII, No 4 (October), 1986: 211–222

112. Zmudia J M, Fahrenbach M C, Yumkin B T et al. The effect of testosterone aromatization on high-density lipoprotein cholesterol level and post heparin lipolytic activity. Metabolism 1993; 42: 446–450

113. Thompson P D, Cullinane E M, Sady S P et al. Contrasting effects of testosterone and stanozolol on serum lipoprotein levels. JAMA 1989; 261: 1165-1168

114. Jacobs D R Jr, Mebane I L, Banydiwala S I et al. High density lipoprotein cholesterol as a predictor of cardiovascular disease mortality in men and women: the follow-up study of the Lipid Research Clinics Prevalence Study. Am J Epidemiol 1990; 131: 32–47

115. McNutt R A, Ferenchick G S, Kirlin P C, Hamlin N J. Acute myocardial infarction in a 22 year old world class weight lifter using anabolic steroids. Am J Cardiol 1988; 62: 164

116. Frankel M A, Eichberg R, Zachariah S B. Anabolic androgenic steroids and a stroke in an athlete: case report. Arch Phys Med Rehabil 1988; 69: 632–633

117. Wilson J D. Androgen abuse by athletes. Endocr Rev 1987; 2: 181–199

118. Shoupe D, Lobo R A. The influence of androgens on insulin resistance. Fertil Steril 1984; 41: 385–388

119. Matsumoto A M, Sandblom R E, Schuene R B et al. Testosterone replacement in hypogonadal men: effects on obstructive sleep apnoea, respiratory drives and sleep. Clin Endocrinol 1985; 22: 713–721

120. Ishaik K G, Zimmerman H J. Hepatotoxic effects of anabolic/androgenic steroids. Semin Liver Dis 1987; 7: 230–236

121. Glass A R. Gynaecomastia. Endocrinol Metab Clin North Am 1994; 23, 825–837

122. Westerholm B C. Sex hormones. In: Dukes M N G (ed) Meyler's Side effects of drugs. Amsterdam: Elsevier, 866–867

123. Spark R F, Wills C A, O'Reilly G et al. Hyperprolactinaemia in males with and without pituitary macroadenoma. Lancet 1982; 2(8290): 129–132

124. Franks S, Jacobs H S, Martin N, Nabarro J D. Hyperprolactinaemia and impotence. Clin Endocrinol 1978; 8(4): 277–287

125. Franks S, Nabarro J D. Prolactin secretion in men with chromophobe adenomas of the pituitary: incidence and presentation of hyperprolactinaemia: results of surgical treatment. Ann Clin Res 1978; 10(3): 157–163

126. Carter N, Tyson J E, Tolis G et al. Prolactin-secreting tumours and hypogonadism in 22 men. N Engl J Med 1978; 299: 847–852

127. El-Beheiry A, Souka A, El-Kamshoushi A et al. Hyperprolactinaemia and impotence. Arch Andrology 1988; 21(3): 211–214

128. Nickel J C, Morales A, Condra M et al. Endocrine dysfunction in impotence: incidence, significance and cost effective screening. J Urol 1984; 132: 40–43

129. Foulks C J, Cushner H C. Sexual dysfunction in the male dialysis patient: pathogenesis, evaluation and therapy. Am J Kidney Dis 1986; 8(4): 211–222

130. Modebe O. Serum prolactin concentration in impotent African males. Andrologia 1989; 21(1): 42–47

131. Weizman A, Moaz B, Treves I et al. Sulpiride induced hyperprolactinaemia and impotence in male psychiatric outpatients. Prog Neuropsychopharmacol Biol Psychiatry 1985; 9: 193–198

132. Mastrogiacomo I, DeBesi L, Zucchetta P et al. Effect of hyperprolactinemia and age on the hypogonadism of uremic men on haemodialysis. Arch Androl 1984; 12: 235–242

133. Nieschlag E, Behre H M. Testosterone therapy. Chapter 15. In: Nieschlag E, Behre H M (eds) Andrology. Berlin: Springer-Verlag, 1997

134. De Antoni E P, Crawford E D. Prostate cancer awareness week. Education service and research in a community setting. Cancer 1995; 75(Suppl.): 1874–1879

Chapter 31

Intracavernosal therapy

M. Spahn, M. Manning and K. P. Juenemann

■ INTRODUCTION

The era of intracavernosal pharmacotherapy and, with it, the breakthrough in impotence research and treatment modalities, began with the first report on an entirely pharmacologically induced penile erection in 1982,[1] and Brindley's spectacular induction of erection by intracavernous self-injection of phenoxybenzamine.[2–4]

Since then, several substances (such as phentolamine, papaverine, prostaglandin E1 [PGE1], vasoactive intestinal peptide [VIP] and nitric oxide [NO] donors) have been introduced, with varying results; not all have become established. To date, pharmacotherapy of erectile dysfunction consists of three highly vasoactive substances — papaverine, phentolamine and PGE1. These three substances have been administered on a long-term basis over the years in diagnostic workup and therapeutic options for impotent patients.

Alternative options in the treatment of erectile dysfunction are either non-invasive (e.g. psychological treatment, oral pharmacotherapy, intra-urethral administration of PGE1, or vacuum pump) or invasive (e.g. penile revascularization surgery, venous ligation or penile prosthesis implantation).

Patient acceptance of oral pharmacotherapy, with less severe side effects, is far better than that of most invasive techniques. Numerous patients must still be evaluated in order to verify the efficacy of this method. Despite minor complications, the main drawback of vacuum devices is poor patient acceptance. There are not, as yet, long-term follow-up data for intra-urethral administration of PGE1, but it is anticipated that many patients will benefit from this treatment option as the complications are comparable to those with injection therapy and the application route is more acceptable to the patients. Surgical intervention results in higher efficacy, but severe complications may arise. In the case of penile revascularization, scrupulous and strict patient selection leads to good results. Penile prosthesis implantation is highly successful, but irreversible damage to cavernous tissue (with consequent complete functional impairment) can occur.

Intracavernosal pharmacotherapy is a well-accepted and successful treatment with an overall (drug-dependent) success rate of about 65%.[5–17] Negative side effects are prolonged erection, painful erection and penile fibrosis of erectile tissue.

■ FUNCTIONAL ANATOMY

The human penis (Fig. 31.1) consists of two corpora cavernosa and the corpus spongiosum. During intracavernous pharmacotherapy, the appropriate substance is injected into one of the two corpora cavernosa. Correct injection technique is very important: the agent must be intrasinusoidally injected, not intratunically, intratrabecularly or intra-urethrally. The best method of injection is from the laterodorsal aspect into the proximal half of the penis (Fig. 31.2), under aseptic conditions. As the two corpora cavernosa are connected — they are apparently separated by an incomplete septum — the injection can be administered to either side, and injection sites can be alternated in order to minimize long-term side effects.

The corpora cavernosa alone evoke penile erection. They consist of a three-dimensional network of connective tissue and smooth muscle cells. Arterial supply of the corpora cavernosa is ensured by the deep penile arteries; venous outflow drains by the circumflex veins and the deep dorsal vein through a subtunical venous network situated at the base of the penis.

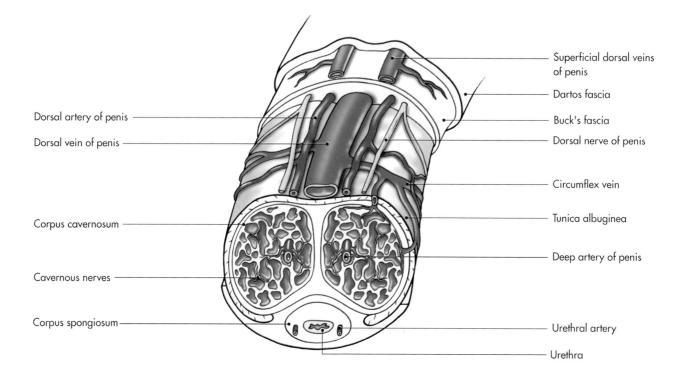

Figure 31.1. Cross-section of the human penis. (From ref. 53 with permission.)

Labels on figure:
Dorsal artery of penis
Dorsal vein of penis
Corpus cavernosum
Cavernous nerves
Corpus spongiosum

Superficial dorsal veins of penis
Dartos fascia
Buck's fascia
Dorsal nerve of penis
Circumflex vein
Tunica albuginea
Deep artery of penis
Urethral artery
Urethra

Erectile tissue innervation is provided by the parasympathetic cavernous nerves (sacral erection centre S2–S4) and sympathetic nerves (hypogastric plexus). Afferent nerves lead from various penile sections via the dorsal penile nerve to the sacral center S2–S4.

ERECTILE MECHANISM

The intracavernous injection of vasoactive substances triggers the erectile mechanism in a manner similar to the physiological process.

In the flaccid penis, the penile arteries are constricted and the smooth muscle cells of the cavernous bodies are contracted. This results in low arterial inflow and high intracavernous resistance, thus enabling free blood efflux via the subtunical veins. Relaxation of the deep penile arteries and the smooth muscle cells leads to increased arterial inflow and decreased intracavernous resistance. Subsequently, filling of the lacunar space with consecutive elongation and enlarged circumference of the

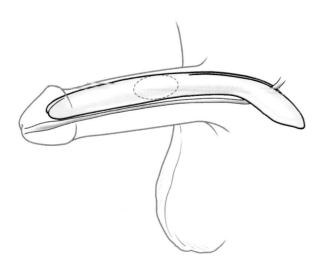

Figure 31.2. Site of intracavernous injection. (From ref. 54 with permission.)

penis results. Further relaxation of the erectile tissue, and blood inflow into the lacunar spaces, lead to venous restriction by compression of the subtunical venules located between the smooth musculature of the corpora cavernosa and inner tunica albuginea layer. During the state of full erection, the intracavernous pressure rises to 80–110 mmHg.

The above-mentioned erectile mechanism, comprising arterial dilatation, cavernous relaxation and venous restriction, is dependent on the smooth muscle relaxation of erectile tissue and can therefore be provoked by any vasoactive agent.

■ INTRACAVERNOUS PHARMACOTHERAPY

Currently, there are over 500 publications on intracavernous pharmacotherapy and reports have been made on approximately 250 000 injections administered to more than 20 000 patients.

Intracavernous administration of erection-inducing agents is most efficacious and has not yet been surpassed by any other form of therapy. Success rates vary between 54% with papaverine, 71% with the papaverine/phentolamine combination, 73% with PGE1 and 75% with the triple-drug combination of these three substances. Various other drugs, such as phenoxybenzamine, moxisylyte, NO donors (linsidomin), VIP or calcitonin gene-related peptide (CGRP) have been introduced but have not yet become established in routine clinical practice.[5,6,18–45]

The first injection should always be performed by the therapist. For practical reasons, the patient should learn to inject himself with a disposable injection system or, even better, with one of the widely used pen multi-injection systems. The injection technique is very important and should be explained and demonstrated in detail to all patients. This should be performed dorsolaterally into the proximal half of the penis under aseptic conditions, changing the injection site each time. Intratunical, intraseptal or intra-urethral injection must be avoided at all costs. Normally, correct injection into the corporal smooth muscle area is possible without a great amount of pressure.

Patient compliance is an important factor in self-injection. Only one injection per day should be made at a predetermined dosage in order to avoid prolonged erection: patients who inject twice or more daily or at higher dosages, are often admitted to hospital with priapism.

Each patient undergoes a series of pharmacotesting for individual dose assessment. If no risk factors, such as cardiovascular decompensation or prolonged erection, are to be expected, this procedure normally starts with one substance, on an outpatient basis. In doubtful cases, patients should be hospitalized for 3–6 hours. Patients who do not comply with treatment conditions, or who are not capable of self-injection, should be excluded from this scheme. All participants must be informed of any eventual side effects or long-term complications such as prolonged erection, bleeding, haematoma, infection, pain, penile fibrosis, penile deviation, definite erectile dysfunction, and systemic side effects (cardiovascular), and advised about therapeutic alternatives. Should any complications arise, then the patient concerned is strongly advised to seek urgent attention at an urological centre.

Each patient must also give signed consent to intracavernous injection; in most European countries and the USA he must be informed that only a few of these substances have recently been granted a licence for this type of treatment.

In the authors' department, testing usually starts at a dosage of 10 μg PGE1. In patients with psychological or neurogenic aetiology of erectile dysfunction, 5 μg PGE1 is sufficient to induce complete erection. If the history and physical examination reveal that the patient suffers from vascular disease with underlying erectile dysfunction (ED), then testing begins at 10 μg or 20 μg and is gradually increased stepwise to a maximum dose of 40 μg. Alternatively, papaverine/phentolamine (15 mg/ml papaverine and 0.5 mg/ml phentolamine) is administered at an initial dose of 0.5 ml and gradually increased to a maximum dosage of 3 ml.

■ DIFFERENT TYPES OF DRUGS

Papaverine

Papaverine was the initial substance used for this purpose and still is the one that is chiefly administered. The poppy *Papaver somniferum* yields an opium alkaloid that has no narcotic action. It exercises a myolytic effect on smooth muscle cells and relaxes all components of the penile erectile tissue, the deep penile arteries and the cavernous sinusoids; it brings about venous constriction by increasing the intracellular cAMP concentration, with a subsequent decrease in calcium concentration.

The first report of papaverine-induced erection was by Virag in 1982.[1] Within 2 years, this substance became the most commonly administered agent by intracavernous injection. Reports have been made on doses ranging from 5 to 160 mg (generally 20–80 mg)[7–12] (Table 31.1), with an average success rate of almost 54%.[7–12] The most frequently observed side effects with papaverine monosubstance were prolonged erections in about 7.4% of patients at the time of testing or 5.1% during the treatment period.[7–12] Other common events, such as intracavernous fibrosis, were found to be long term in 6%.[12] Painful erections are extremely rare and the drop-out rate with intracavernous papaverine injection was 31.3%.

Phenoxybenzamine

Phenoxybenzamine acts as an alpha-adrenoceptor-blocking substance and was the first substance introduced for intracavernous injection.[2–4] Initially, it was thought to be as good as (or even superior to) papaverine, but prolonged erections up to 44 hours, as well as the tendency towards severe fibrosis of the cavernous tissue, made this substance unpopular and not to be recommended.

Papaverine/phentolamine

Phentolamine is a selective alpha-adrenoceptor blocker that avoids contraction of smooth muscle cells. As it acts on the vascular side of the erectile tissue, patients with general vascular disease do not benefit from phentolamine injection. There is a distinct dose-dependent relationship between response rate and the aetiology of ED. Independent of the aetiology of ED, phentolamine, when injected alone, does not generally induce a satisfactory erection.

In 1978, Domer introduced phentolamine[46] and in 1985 Zorgniotti and Lefleurs[47] successfully administered a solution of 30 mg papaverine and 1 mg phentolamine intracavernously. This was considered to be the breakthrough in the treatment of erectile dysfunction and the average success rate was 71% (adequate for intercourse). The common dosages administered vary from 7.5 mg to 30 mg papaverine and 0.25 mg to 1 mg phentolamine (Table 31.2).[13–16] Normally, a solution of 30 mg papaverine and 1 mg phentolamine is administered. During testing, a 0.5 ml solution is administered as an initial dose that is gradually increased up to a maximum dose of 3 ml. Prolonged erections have been reported in about 7.5% of patients during the testing and treatment period, cavernous tissue fibrosis occurred in about 6%[13,15,16] and the drop-out rate was 27%.[15,48]

Prostaglandin E1 (PGE1)

Prostaglandin E1 is a prostanoid that affects various organs in different ways. In the vascular system, PGE1 causes relaxation of the arterioles, thus positively influencing arterial circulation. The pharmacokinetics of this substance are not promising, as 90% is inactivated

Table 31.1. Papaverine: published data

Feature	Reported value
Efficacy	53.9% (average success)
General dosage	20–80 mg
Prolonged erections per patient	7.4% (pharmacotesting) – 5.1% (therapy)
Fibrosis or similar	6.2%
Drop-out rate	31.3%

Table 31.2. Papaverine/phentolamine: published data

Feature	Reported value
Efficacy	70.8% (average success)
General dosage	0.25–7.5 mg to 0.8–30 mg
Prolonged erections per patient	7.5% (pharmacotesting) – 7.7% (therapy)
Fibrosis or similar	6.0%
Drop-out rate	27%

during the first lung passage and is then excreted by the liver and kidneys.

PGE1 causes modulation of adenyl cyclase and an increase in cAMP and subsequent decrease of free calcium concentration via specific receptors of the erectile tissue, finally resulting in relaxation of the smooth muscle cells. Additionally, this substance exercises an anti-adrenergic effect. It was introduced by Ishii and colleagues at the World Meeting on Impotence in 1986[11], and the first clinical results by Stackl and colleagues[17] and by Porst[49] followed, with encouraging success rates.

The most practical dose ranges from 5 μg to 40 μg. PGE1 can be dissolved in 1–2 ml of normal saline and should be administered within a few hours after solution before degradation begins. Testing starts at a dose of 10 μg, gradually increasing stepwise up to 40 μg. If neurological disease is suspected to be the aetiology, then the initial dose should be lowered to 5 μg, taking potential hypersensitivity and the high risk of prolonged erection into consideration.

The success rate with PGE1 injection is high (an average of 73%) with few side effects[5–7,9,10,14,15,17] (Table 31.3).

The most common side effects are a burning sensation during injection, and painful erection; these occur in about 30% of patients during the testing period and in 15% undergoing pharmacotherapy.[17,21,49] Very few cases of prolonged erection have been reported (1%) and fibrosis-like changes arose in only 2.7%.[9,10,15,17,21,42] Today, PGE1 is the most efficient commercially available agent and has become accepted as the 'gold standard' in the pharmacotherapy of erectile dysfunction.

Triple drug

The 'triple drug' is so called because it is a mixture of papaverine, phentolamine and PGE1; it is chiefly administered in the USA. The reported success rate averages 75.5% (up to 100%) and is higher than that for PGE1 alone[14] (Table 31.4).

Painful erections have occurred in 20.6% of patients during testing and in 2.9% during the treatment period. Fibrosis of erectile tissue was observed in only 2.3%.

In the authors' department, the triple drug is administered only as a last resort, when PGE1 and papaverine/phentolamine have failed to take effect.

Other combinations

In several European countries a combination of phentolamine and vasoactive intestinal polypeptide (VIP) has been approved. This combination product (Invicorp, Senetek) appears to produce PGE1-equivalent erections but without pain at the injection site. Data has been accrued from over 2000 patients with efficacy having been evaluated for up to 18 months.

Table 31.3. Prostaglandin E1 (PGE1): published data

Feature	Reported value
Efficacy	73% (average success)
General dosage	5–40 μg
Prolonged erections per patient	1.3% (pharmacotesting) – 1.1% (therapy)
Fibrosis or similar	2.7%
Painful erection	30% (pharmacotesting) – 15% (therapy)
Drop-out rate	42.3%

Table 31.4. Triple drug (papaverine/phentolamine/PGE1): published data

Feature	Reported value
Efficacy	75.5% (average success)
General dosage	8 mg–0.2 mg/10 μg–16 mg/ 0.4 mg–20 μg
Prolonged erections per patient	3.2% (pharmacotesting) – 1.8% (therapy)
Fibrosis or similar	2.3%
Painful erection	20.6% (pharmacotesting) – 2.9% (therapy)
Drop-out rate	24.2%

Neurotransmitters

CGRP is a neurotransmitter/neuromodulator and is not capable of inducing an erection on its own. On the other hand, a solution of 5 µg CGRP and 20 µg prostaglandin E1 is reported to evoke full rigidity suitable for sexual intercourse.[6,32,50] Initial reports have revealed that, in 30% of non-responders to intracavernous therapy, success was achieved with the combination containing CGRP; however, these are only preliminary data.

VIP is another physiological neurotransmitter/neuromodulator that induces tumescence but not full rigidity. In Denmark, a solution of 30 µg VIP and 2 mg phentolamine is the main therapeutic agent. Initial reports are encouraging, with success in almost 100% of patients; however, once again, these data are only preliminary.[23,43]

Linsidomin (SIN-1)

The NO donor linsidomin was introduced in 1992. Experimental and clinical studies have demonstrated that SIN-1 could be a possible physiological mediator of erection in primates and humans. First reports have revealed a success rate of 69% with a dosage of 1 mg and, so far, without any occurrence of prolonged erection or fibrosis-like changes in the erectile tissue. Data at present are preliminary and must be confirmed by further investigations.[5,6,18,19,22,25–38]

Moxisylyte

Moxisylyte is a selective alpha-1-receptor-blocking substance. Initially published data show a success rate of up to 70% with an optimal dosage of 10–30 mg. Only 1% of cases of prolonged erection and 1.5% of fibrosis have been reported.[20,21,24,39] A comparison between moxisylyte and PGE1 showed higher success rates and stronger penile rigidity for PGE1. Moxisylyte caused more systemic side effects, whereas PGE1 resulted in a greater number of painful and prolonged erections.[44,45]

■ SIDE EFFECTS

Short-term side effects

Prolonged erection is the most relevant short-term complication and each patient should be informed of this and the consequences. At present, it is difficult to distinguish precisely between the duration of a normal erection (≤ 3 hours) and that of a prolonged (>3–8 hours) erection.

In clinical practice it is important to distinguish between high-flow and low-flow priapism. High-flow priapism is characterized by an abnormal increase of arterial blood inflow as well as of venous outflow. The P_{O_2}, P_{CO_2} and pH values remain almost normal and damage to erectile tissue is not yet to be expected. High-flow priapism generally resolves during the first 6 hours of prolonged erection after injection of vasoactive substances. So-called low-flow priapism follows high-flow priapism. During low-flow priapism the circulation is arrested and pain caused by ischaemia and time-dependent damage of erectile tissue is to be expected. The onset of fibrosis with subsequent complete functional loss is after 48 hours.

Treatment of prolonged erection

A prolonged erection lasting more than 6 hours after injection is considered to be an emergency and patients are strongly advised to consult a urologist as a matter of urgency.

High-flow priapism can be diagnosed when there is a history of injection within the last 6 hours, no pain, and high arterial flow in deep arteries detected by duplex sonography and blood gas analysis. Vasoconstrictive agents must then be injected intracavernously. The most common substances for this are adrenaline (0.001–0.3 mg), phenylepinephrine (0.02–0.5 mg) and metaraminol (0.5–10 mg).[8,13,16] These drugs are all highly vasoactive and can cause severe side effects such as hypertensive crisis, cardiac arrhythmia, cardiac decompensation and angina pectoris.

Low-flow priapism is characterized by painful erection, low arterial flow in the deep penile arteries shown by duplex scan 6 or more hours after injection, decreased P_{O_2}, increased P_{CO_2} and acid pH values. The corpus cavernosum should be punctured and up to 300 ml blood aspirated until the penis becomes flaccid. If the state of erection returns or remains constant after blood aspiration, then surgical intervention is the last resort: an artificial shunt is created between the corpus cavernosum and the corpus spongiosum (Winther shunt).

Less severe, short-term side effects are haematoma and infection in 2–10% of subjects. These can kept to a minimum by teaching the patient the correct injection technique.

Painful erection caused by prostaglandin is predominantly experienced by patients during the test period and this makes them unsuitable candidates for therapy.

Long-term side effects

Fibrosis or fibrosis-like changes have been observed in 2.1–6.2% of patients.[13,17,21,51] These are drug and injection dependent and are mostly reversible after termination of treatment.

Drop-out rate

Long-term follow-up studies of patients receiving intracavernous injection therapy showed drop-out rates of almost 70% within 5 years. The reasons for discontinuation of therapy were given as the desire for a permanent treatment alternative, fear of injection needles, poor response, lack of a suitable partner and loss of sexual spontaneity.[51,52]

■ COMBINATION OF PHARMACOTHERAPY

Intracavernous pharmacotherapy is currently the most effective treatment for erectile failure. This does not mean that it is limited to severe organic impotence: psychogenically impotent patients may benefit from this type of treatment to initiate later spontaneous erections. In these cases, and in neurogenically impotent patients, the therapist must ensure minimum drug dosage. These latter patient groups should be subjected to pharmacotesting with a dose reduction of at least 50%.

■ FUTURE ASPECTS

The future aim of impotence research is to improve pharmacotherapy. The ideal substance — resulting in high success rates and low complication rates that can be administered in an easy-to-handle manner — has still to be developed. To date, prostaglandin may be considered the most effective substance which may be matched by a combination of phentolamine + VIP. New perspectives opened by such new treatment schemes as intra-urethral application of PGE1 (e.g. the medicated urethral system for erection [MUSE]) and oral therapy with sildenafil or apomorphine will, it is hoped, culminate in both an ideal substance and an ideal method of treatment for erectile dysfunction. Finally, this should be combined with an easy-to-handle method for patients and less severe side effects that ensure detumescence after ejaculation. This will be the main aim of future research into impotence.

■ REFERENCES

This review is based on an evaluation of more than 500 publications dealing with the pharmacotherapy of erectile failure. Because it is impossible to list all the authors who contributed to the database, only the complete list of those publications concerning the drug survey and also the alternative drugs for intracavernous pharmacotherapy is given here, together with particular references cited in the text. For further details, reference can be made to the first review published in 1989,[55] and the review published on PGE1 in 1996.[56]

1. Virag R. Intracavernous injection of papaverine for erectile failure. Lancet 1982; 2: 938
2. Brindley G S. Cavernosal alpha-blockage: a new technique for investigating and treating erectile impotence. Br J Psychiatry 1983; 143: 332–337
3. Brindley G S. Pilot experiments on the actions of drugs injected into the human corpus cavernosum penis. Br J Pharmacol 1986; 87: 495–500
4. Brindley G S. Maintenance treatment of erectile impotence by cavernosal unstriated muscle relaxant injection. Br J Psychiatry 1986; 149: 210–215
5. Porst H. Ten years of experience with various vasoactive drugs — comparative studies in over 4000 patients. Int J Impot Res 1994; 6(suppl.1): D149
6. Stief C G, Wetterauer U, Schaebsdau F H, Jonas U. Calcitonin-gene-related peptide: a possible role in human penile erection and its therapeutic application in impotent patients. J Urol 1991; 146: 1010–1014
7. Kattan S, Collins J P, Mohr D. Double-blind, cross-over study comparing prostaglandin E1 and papaverine in patients with vasculogenic impotence. Urology 1991; 37: 516–518
8. Keogh E J, Watter G R, Earrle C M et al. Treatment of impotence by intrapenile injections: a comparison of papaverine versus papaverine and phentolamine: a double-blind, crossover trial. J Urol 1989; 142: 726–728
9. Liu L C, Wu C C, Liu L H et al. Comparison of the effects of papaverine versus prostaglandin E1, on penile blood flow by color duplex sonography. Eur Urol 1991; 19: 49–53
10. Mahmoud K Z, El Dakhli M R, Fahmi I M, Abdel-Aziz A B A. Comparative value of prostaglandin E1 and papaverine in treatment of erectile failure: double-blind crossover study among Egyptian patients. J Urol 1992; 147: 623–626
11. Ishii N, Watanabe H, Irisawa C et al. Therapeutic trial with prostaglandin E1 for organic impotence. In: Proceedings of the Fifth Conference on Vasculogenic Impotence and Corpus Cavernosum Revascularization. Second World Meeting on Impotence. Prague: International Society for Impotence Research (ISIR), 1986; 11: 2
12. Goonawardena S A, de Silva W A, Ketheeswaran T. Pharmacologically induced penile erections in the assessment

and treatment of erectile impotence: a preliminary study of 100 patients. Ceylon Med J 1997; 42: 72–74

13. Padma-Nathan H, Goldstein I, Payton T, Krane R J. Intracavernosal pharmacotherapy: the Pharmacologic Erection Program. World J Urol 1987; 5: 160–165

14. Padma-Nathan H. The efficacy and synergy of polypharmacotherapy in primary and salvage therapy of vasculogenic erectile dysfunction. Int J Impot Res 1990; 2(suppl2): 257–258

15. Floth A, Schramek P. Intracavernous injection of prostaglandin E1 in combination with papaverine: enhanced effectiveness in comparison with papaverine plus phentolamine and prostaglandin E1 alone. J Urol 1991; 145: 56–59

16. Sidi A, Cameron J S, Duffy L M, Lange P H. Intracavernous drug-induced erections in the management of male erectile dysfunction: experience with 100 patients. J Urol 1986; 135: 704–706

17. Stackl W, Hasun R, Marberger M. Intracavernous injection of prostaglandin E1 in impotent men. J. Urol 1988; 140: 66–68

18. Borges F D. A new approach to the pharmacologic treatment of impotency; Lecture LXXXIX, AUA Congress 1994, San Francisco. J Urol 1994; 151(suppl): 474; 346A

19. Brock G, Breza J, Lue T F. Intracavernous sodium nitroprusside: inappropriate impotence treatment. J Urol 1993; 150: 864–867

20. Buvat J, Lemaire A, Buvat-Herbaut M, Marcolin G. Reduced rate of fibrotic nodules of the cavernous bodies following auto-intracavernous injections of moxisylyte compared to papaverine. Int J Impot Res 1990; 2(suppl2): 299–300

21. Buvat J, Lemaire A, Marcolin G, Buvat-Herbaut M. Comparison of the two second generation drugs for intracavernosal injections moxisylyte and prostaglandin E1. Int J Impot Res 1994; 6(suppl.1): P39

22. Cavallini G. Minoxidil versus nitroglycerin: a prospective double-blind controlled trial in transcutaneous erection facilitation for organic impotence. J Urol 1991; 146: 50–53

23. Gerstenberg T C, Metz P, Ottesen B, Fahrenkrug J. Intracavernous self-injection with vasoactive intestinal polypeptide and phentolamine in the management of erectile failure. J Urol 1992; 147: 1277–1279

24. Hermabessiere J, Costa C F P. Efficacy and safety assessment of intracavernous injection of moxisylyte in patients with erectile dysfunction: a double-blind, placebo controlled study. Int J Impot Res 1994; 6(suppl.1): D147

25. Knispel H H, Wegner H E H, Miller K. The role of linsidomin in diagnosis and treatment of erectile dysfunction. Int J Impot Res 1994; 6(suppl.1): D156

26. Lemaire A, Buvat J, Buvat-Herbaut M, Marcolin G. Erectile response to intracavernous injections of linsidomine in 38 impotent males. Int J Impot Res 1994; 6(suppl.1): D148

27. Martinez-Pineiro L, Lopez-Tello J, Dorrego J M A et al. Preliminary results of a comparative study with intracavernous sodium nitroprusside and prostaglandin E1 in patients with erectile dysfunction. J Urol 1995; 153: 1487–1490

28. Martinez-Pineiro L, Tello J L, Dorrego J A et al. Preliminary results of a comparative study with intracavernous sodium

nitroprusside and prostaglandin E1 in the diagnosis and treatment of penile erectile dysfunction. Lecture LXXXIX, AUA Congress 1994, San Francisco. J Urol 1994; 151(suppl): 910; 455A

29. Meyhoff H H, Rosenkilde P, Bodker A. Non-invasive management of impotence with transcutaneous nitroglycerin. Br J Urol 1992; 69: 88–90

30. Nunez B D, Anderson D C. Nitroglycerin ointment in the treatment of impotence. J Urol 1993; 150: 1241–1243

31. Porst H. Effektivität und Hämodynamik von SIN-1 versus Prostaglandin E1. Lecture XLV DGU Congress 1993, Wiesbaden, Urologe [A] 1993; 32(suppl): S78

32. Schwarzer J U, Pickl U, Kropp W, Hartung R. Schwellkörperautoinjektionstherapie mit Calcitonin Gene Related Peptide. Lecture XLIV, DGU Congress 1992, Munich. Urologe [A] 1992; 31(suppl): A9

33. Stief C G, Djamilian M, Krah H, Jonas U. Die Verwendung des NO-Donors SIN-1 in der SKAT-Therapie der erektilen Dysfunktion; Lecture XLIV, DGU Congress 1992, Munich. Urologe [A] 1992; 31(suppl): A9

34. Stief C G, Holmquist F, Djamilian M et al. Preliminary results with the nitric oxide donor linsidomine chlorhydrate in the treatment of human erectile dysfunction. J Urol 1992; 148: 1437–1440

35. Stief C G, Holmquist F, Krah H et al. Prelimary results with the nitric oxyde (NO) donor SIN-1 in the treatment of human erectile dysfunction. Lecture LXXXVII, AUA Congress 1992, Washington DC. J Urol 1992; 147 (suppl.): 205; 265A

36. Torres L O, Teloken, C, Da Ros C T et al. Nitric oxide donor linsidomine does not produce full erection in men with corporeal veno-occlusive dysfunction. Int J Impot Res 1994; 6(suppl.1): P47

37. Truss M C, Becker A J, Djamilian M H et al. Role of the nitric oxide donor linsidomine chlorhydrate (SIN-1) in the diagnosis and treatment of erectile dysfunction. Urology 1994; 44: 553–556

38. Truss M C, Djamilian M H, Kuczyk M et al. Follow up results of the nitric oxide donor linsidomine chlorhydrate in the diagnosis and treatment of erectile dysfunction. Lecture LXXXIX, AUA Congress 1994, San Francisco. J Urol 1994; 151(suppl): 911; 455A

39. Virag R, Sussman H, Floresco J, Shoukry K. Late results on the treatment of neurogenic impotence by self-intracavernous-injection of vasoactive drugs. World J Urol 1987; 5: 166–170

40. Wegner H E H, Knispel H H, Miller K. Prostaglandin E1 versus SIN-1 versus SIN-1 & urapidil in erectile dysfunction: a double-blind cross over trial. Lecture LXXXIX, AUA Congress 1994, San Francisco. J Urol 1994; 151(suppl): 912; 455A

41. Wegner H E H, Knispel H H. Effect of nitric oxide-donor, linsidomine chlorhydrate in treatment of human erectile dysfunction caused by venous leakage. Urology 1993; 42: 409–411

42. Wegner H E H, Knispel H H, Klein R et al. Prostaglandin E1 versus linsidomine chlorhydrate in erectile dysfunction. Urol Int 1994; 53: 214–216

43. McMahon C G. A pilot study of the role of intracavernous injection of vasoactive intestinal peptide (VIP) and phentolamine mesylate in the treatment of erectile dysfunction. Int J Impot Res 1996; 8: 233–236

44. Buvat J, Costa P, Morlier D et al. Double-blind multicenter study comparing alprostadil alpha-cyclodextrin with moxisylyte chlorhydrate in patients with chronic erectile dysfunction. J Urol 1998; 159: 116–119

45. Buvat J, Lemaire A, Herbaut-Buvat M. Intracavernous pharmacotherapy: comparison of moxisylyte and prostaglandin E1. Int J Impot Res 1996; 8: 41–46

46. Domer F R, Wessler G, Brown R L, Charles H C. Involvement of the sympathetic nervous system in the urinary bladder internal sphincter and in penile erection in the anesthetized cat. Invest Urol 1978; 15: 404–407

47. Zorgniotti A W, Lefleur R S. Auto-injection of the corpus cavernosum with a vasoactive drug combination for vasculogenic impotence. J Urol 1985; 133: 39–41

48. Sidi A A, Cameron J S, Dykstra D D et al. Vasoactive intracavernous pharmacotherapy for the treatment of erectile impotence in men with spinal cord injury. J Urol 1987; 138: 539–542

49. Porst H. Prostaglandin E1 bei erektiler Dysfunktion. Urologe [D] 1989; 28: 94–98

50. Rodriguez Vela L, Gonzalvo Ibarra A, Gil Martinez P et al. Long-term results of the treatment with intracavernous injection of vasoactive drugs. Arch Esp Urol 1996; 49: 257–269

51. Weiss J N, Badlani G H, Ravalli R, Brettschneider N. Reasons for high drop-out rate with self-injection therapy for impotence. Int J Impot Res 1994; 6: 171–174

52. Sundaram C P, Thomas W, Pryor L E et al. Long term follow-up of patients receiving injection therapy for erectile dysfunction. Urology 1997; 49: 932–935

53. Jünemann K-P. Erektionsstörungen. Chapter 12. In: Alken P, Walz P H (eds) Urologie. Weinheim: VCH-Verlag, 1992: 306

54. Truss M C. Schwellkörper-injektionstestung (SKIT). Chapter 3.4. In: Stief C G, Hartmann U, Höfner K, Jonas U (eds) Erektile Dysfunktion. Heidelberg: Springer-Verlag, 1997: 137

55. Jünemann K P, Alken P. Pharmacotherapy of erectile dysfunction: a review. Int J Impot Res 1989; 1: 71–93

56. Porst H. The rationale for prostaglandin E1 in erectile dysfunction: a survey of worldwide experience. J Urol 1996; 155: 802–815

Chapter 32

Future therapeutic alternatives in the treatment of erectile dysfunction

N. F. Gonzalez-Cadavid and J. Rajfer

■ INTRODUCTION

The pharmacological management of erectile dysfunction associated with organic or psychogenic impotence, based on self-injection of vasoactive agents in the penile corpora cavernosa, has become the preferred modality over surgical procedures or mechanical devices, whenever possible, according to the extent of cavernosal compromise.[1-3] This approach has been derived from extensive experimental evidence on the control of cavernosal smooth muscle relaxation, independent of the identification of the main mediator of this process.[4,5] The following discussion is restricted to pharmacological treatment, without ignoring the potential for development of other novel, more effective, procedures.

The first drug shown to be effective for erectile dysfunction, papaverine,[1,3] is the epitome of some of the subsequent clinical agents that relax the cavernosal smooth muscle through their ability to increase or maintain the levels of cyclic nucleotide monophosphates in the cavernosal smooth muscle, and in this way to reduce cytosolic Ca^{2+}. The most commonly used drug, prostaglandin E1 (PGE1),[6-8] coincides in this endpoint by stimulating adenyl cyclase, although the pathway is different because papaverine inhibits cGMP phosphodiesterase (PDE). The other component that is used in the 'trimix' preparations, phentolamine, is an alpha-adrenergic blocker[1-3] that directly inhibits the receptor in the smooth muscle cell.

The new treatments that have just emerged from clinical trials or are under preclinical research are, in general, variations from this basic approach or alternative delivery routes,[9,10] but exciting novel concepts are developing, based on basic research advances, which may

soon translate into a clinical application. This review presents an overview of recently introduced pharmacological treatments of erectile dysfunction, as well as the foundation of frontier therapeutic approaches aimed at the cure or prolonged amelioration of the disorder. Most of these drugs or procedures are still in the experimental phase.

■ CURRENT CONCEPTS OF THE MECHANISM OF ERECTILE DYSFUNCTION

Evidence from the last 8 years[4,11-13] has shown that nitric oxide (NO) is the main mediator of penile erection in man and in experimental animals. NO is synthesized in a variety of tissues and organs in a reaction where the amino acid L-arginine is converted into L-citrulline. The enzyme catalysing this reaction is designated nitric oxide synthase (NOS). NO is released in the penis from the non-adrenergic non-cholinergic (NANC) nerve terminals and possibly (although this is still unproven) from the lacunar endothelium,[14,15] stimulating guanyl cyclase and cGMP synthesis in the corporal smooth muscle. The subsequent effect is similar to that induced by all pharmacological agents in the clinic — namely, the reduction of cytosolic Ca^{2+} that causes relaxation of the corporal smooth muscle.

Two of the three known NOS isoforms have been detected in the rat and human penis: these are the neuronal (nNOS) and the endothelial NOS (eNOS).[16,17] Owing to the difficulties associated with conducting studies in human penile corpora cavernosa from potent subjects, different animal models have been used for this purpose. Whereas testing of pharmacological agents on penile erection in dogs, cats, rabbits, and monkeys is widely conducted, these animals are not useful for studying erectile dysfunction. The best experimental model available so far is the rat, where erectile dysfunction associated with spontaneous diabetes,[16,18] ageing,[19–21] smoking,[17] androgen depletion[22–27] and adrenalectomy[28] is accompanied by a reduction in penile NOS activity and, in chronic or severe conditions,[16,17,28] by a decrease in nNOS content. NOS activity reduction correlates, in most cases, with decreased erectile response to electrical field stimulation (EFS) of the cavernosal nerve,[17–27] and/or penile reflexes.[16]

Although the individual expression of each one of the NOS isoforms has been blocked in NOS gene knockout mice without impairing sexual reproduction,[29–31] this does not imply that physiological erection is not dependent on the NO cascade: it is possible that the remaining NOS isoform(s), non-NO-dependent pathways, or alternative variants of the identified NOS isoforms, may act as compensatory mechanisms for the erectile response in these animals.[29]

Although nNOS has been identified in the nerve terminals of the corpora cavernosa by immunocytochemistry,[32,33] eNOS is difficult to detect in situ.[34] NANC control of this process and of penile erection in vivo indicates that the NO synthesized by nNOS as a neurotransmitter in these nerves is the fundamental mediator, whereas the contribution of the endothelial isoform is less clear. Studies are needed to determine whether eNOS amplifies or potentiates the signal triggered by nNOS activation.

In the ageing rat model, the erectile response to EFS of the cavernosal nerve is considerably decreased, and this is accompanied by a reduction of the response of penile tissue to vasoactive agents and, in very old animals, by decreased penile NOS activity.[19] This suggests that erectile dysfunction results from two factors acting separately or in concert: these are (a) a decrease in penile NOS levels or activity, leading to lower NO synthesis, and (b) a reduction in the compliance of the cavernosal smooth muscle to the relaxation effect of NO. As opposed to the diabetic rat model,[16,18,35] no evidence is available as to whether ageing is accompanied by peripheral neuropathy in the penis that would lead to the destruction of nerve terminals and the reduction of penile nNOS. However, a recent report described the reduction of NOS-containing nerves in the penis of old rats, correlating with the decrease observed (in the same work) in the central and peripheral stimulation of the erectile mechanism.[21]

Studies of the rat penis — particularly in castrated, hypophysectomized and adrenalectomized rats — indicate that NOS activity may be inhibited per se, without a parallel reduction in NOS levels.[23,24,28] The mechanism is unknown, but it may be due to NOS crosslinking by advanced glycosylation end-products (AGEs) similar to the ones observed in diabetes.[36] Collagen-bound AGEs have been found to increase in penile tissue from elderly men.[37] AGEs may also quench NO directly, thus obliterating its effects. Other types of inhibitors of NOS activity may accumulate or bind to NOS more efficiently during erectile dysfunction; these may include putative penile-specific proteins that inhibit NOS (PINs),[38] which have been detected very recently in rat brain and testis tissue.

■ NOVEL DELIVERY ROUTES OF VASOACTIVE AGENTS USED FOR ERECTILE DYSFUNCTION

The major recent developments in the clinical treatment of erectile dysfunction have occurred in the area of new delivery routes for drugs belonging to groups of vasoactive agents with demonstrated value by intracavernosal injection. These approaches have emerged from long-established concepts in the physiology of erection, independent of the current findings on the role of NO in this process. The first innovation is the utilization of a special applicator medicated urethral system for erection (MUSE®) for transurethral delivery of PGE1.[39–41]

A large double-blind placebo-controlled study, of 1577 men from 27 to 88 years of age and suffering from chronic organic impotence, showed that the transurethral route is effective in inducing with PGE1 dose-dependent erections sufficient for intercourse.[40] Two-thirds of men in the physician's office and at home, applying MUSE, responded satisfactorily, apparently with fewer side-effects than found with intracavernosal injection; however, the mean effective transurethral dose of PGE1 is typically ten-fold higher than that administered by injection. This obviously poses a problem, in terms of both cost and pharmacological effectiveness; indeed, recent data from the authors' clinic suggest that transurethral PGE1 is effective in one-third of patients.[42]

Although the transurethral administration procedure has initially been well received by patients, it does not significantly improve the outcome of the therapy, and only time will determine whether it will replace or be preferred to injections. Its main advantage may, perhaps, lie in the slower and more diffuse delivery occurring through columnar cells of the urethral mucosa and submucosal veins that communicate between the corpus spongiosum and the corpora cavernosa. This may be valuable for novel treatments where the goal is not to achieve immediate smooth muscle relaxation but, rather, to allow for prolonged contact with compounds intended to imprint the target corporal tissue, such as gene therapy (see below).

The other alternative route that is currently under intensive clinical evaluation is oral administration. For many years, this has been considered to be a very difficult approach because of the intrinsic systemic effects of vasoactive compounds, mainly hypotension and headaches. Papaverine, the first successful drug for the treatment of erectile dysfunction via intracavernosal injection, inhibits PDE[1,3] but does not discriminate between its several tissue-specific isoenzymes and therefore cannot be used systemically. This lack of specificity has apparently been overcome in the design of a novel agent, sildenafil (Viagra™; UK-92,480), a potent competitive inhibitor of PDE5, which is claimed to be the main cGMP PDE isoenzyme in the human corpora cavernosa.[10,43] This drug does not act on cAMP PDE; it has rapid absorption and a relatively short half-life, and is postulated to require a physiological trigger for the erection, which implies an active cavernosal NO cascade.[44]

Sildenafil would, therefore, have the profile required for a drug to be effective against erectile dysfunction by oral administration. A number of clinical trials have been completed or are in course to test this hypothesis.[45–48] So far, it appears to be effective in impotent patients without an established organic cause, leading to a dose-dependent significantly higher number of erections with adequate rigidity in subjects receiving one single dose, compared with those on placebo. The adverse effects are mild and transient (headaches, dyspepsia, flushing, muscle aches), and the satisfaction with the sexual life appears to improve.

Although the potency in vitro of sildenafil on a molar basis is much greater than that of papaverine,[43] the questions of the tissue specificity of PDE5 and the isoenzyme specificity of sildenafil are still open. The same applies in terms of the quality of the erectile response or the effects of the drug on organic impotence. In a study conducted in monkeys, several PDE inhibitors were shown to prolong the erection rather than to increase intracavernosal pressure, in comparison with sodium nitroprusside.[49] In addition, the most potent PDE inhibitor tested affects also isoenzymes 1 and 4. As in the case of transurethral delivery of PGE1, it is too early to assess whether oral administration of PDE inhibitors will eventually replace intracavernosal injection. A recent multicenter double blind dose–response and open label extension study[108] showed that 69% of attempts at sexual intercourse were successful in impotent men receiving sildenafil as compared with 22% in those receiving placebo, and that the mean number of successful attempts per month was increased considerably by the drug.

Other drugs are being investigated for oral delivery. One, a dopamine agonist, apomorphine,[8,50,51] differs from the peripherally acting vasoactive agents in its mechanism of action. The apomorphine-induced erection has been studied in the rat and shown to be a vascular event primarily mediated via the sacral parasympathetic nerve system and, in cases of injury to the latter, by the thoracolumbar sympathetic pathway. Apomorphine was therefore proposed for the treatment of psychogenic impotence. In a recent clinical trial, an apomorphine preparation reducing emetic effects[52] was reported as increasing the response to erotic stimuli and the number of successful intercourse events. However, the improvement is only moderate, accompanied by nausea in 13% of patients, and, as in the case of sildenafil, it is not entirely clear whether it would be beneficial for the treatment of organic impotence.

In addition to phentolamine, which has been tested for several years in buccal preparations without conclusive results,[8,9,53] antidepressants such as trazodone[54,55] in preclinical and clinical trials have improved the erectile response, but the effects appear to be limited to psychogenic impotence. Their future use, if any, may be in combination therapy with other drugs.[56] The transdermal application of nitroglycerine, PGE1, papaverine, and other drugs, is still being investigated but the clinical effects are not convincing in terms of the quality and frequency of erections.[8,9,56–58]

■ NITRIC OXIDE DONORS AND ANCILLARY NEUROPEPTIDES

Since the discovery of NO as the mediator of penile erection, several synthetic NO donors have been tested in clinical trials or experimental animals,[59–61] on the premise that the release of exogenous NO would be able to stimulate cavernosal guanyl cyclase more physiologically than the other established drugs for the treatment of erectile dysfunction acting by different routes. However, the results so far have been disappointing. This is not surprising, considering that the mechanism of action of NO donors is essentially similar to that of most vasoactive compounds in use for this therapy, i.e. the transient increase of cGMP or cAMP in the cavernosal smooth muscle upon injection, while the kinetics of formation of the active compound (NO in this case) poses more complications. The same applies to the augmentation of cAMP synthesis via forskolin[62] and other agents studied with the expectation of improving the effects induced indirectly by PGE1 or PDE inhibitors. However, novel NO donors continue to be tested,[63] and some combining other types of effects (see below), or a more controllable release, may hold promise.

Prior to the establishment of the role of NO as an NANC neurotransmitter in the corpora cavernosa, other neuropeptides were considered as physiological mediators of penile erection, studied in experimental animals, and even tested clinically. Calcitonin gene-related peptide (CGRP)[64] and vasoactive intestinal peptide (VIP)[65] are two such compounds; they still attract some attention in this respect but, although they may play an ancillary role in erection, it is doubtful whether these drugs or their derivatives have clinical value.

■ SYMPATHETIC INHIBITORS

The erectile mechanism involves the intervention of cavernosal vasoconstrictors that are essential for detumescence and inhibit tumescence, counterbalancing NO.[66] One of the candidates that is being actively studied is endothelin 1, a small peptide belonging to a family of related peptides.[67] Endothelin 1 is released from both endothelium and smooth muscle, and, in contrast to NO, interacts with specific receptors. Both endothelin 1 and its receptors are present in the penis and there is a close connection with NOS, since acute blockade of NOS with Nw-nitro-L-arginine methyl ester (L-NAME) in the rat model leads to enhanced endothelin activity that can be annulled with endothelin-receptor antagonists.[68,69] This has led to the proposal that patients with decreased NOS (older men, diabetic subjects) will be more sensitive to the increased sympathetic activity associated with performance anxiety.

Serum endothelin 1 increases in rats receiving a single dose of radiation to the prostate, and this correlates with a reduced ES erectile response. Both processes can be prevented by endothelin 1 receptor antagonists;[70] some of these drugs, therefore, may warrant clinical pilot studies for psychogenic impotence or as coadjuvants of oral PDE inhibitors. Because of the potency of endothelin 1 as a smooth muscle contractor, it is likely that antagonists for its receptor would be more efficient inhibitors than alpha-1 and -2 adrenoceptor antagonists such as prazosin or rauwolscine.[71] Angiotensin II secretion and receptors have been identified in the human and rabbit corpus cavernosum, and intracavernosal injection of losartan, an antagonist to angiotensin II receptors, increases intracavernosal pressure in dogs in a dose-dependent manner.[72,73]

The interesting approach of combining an alpha-adrenergic blocker with an NO donor has recently been developed in a new series of drugs (NMI-187 and NMI-221), where SNO groups have been introduced into the yohimbine molecule.[74] These compounds were tested with regard to the relaxation of human corpora cavernosa tissue in organ chambers and in vivo on the erectile response of the rabbit to EFS of the cavernosal nerve, and were shown to be superior to the parent molecules.

■ CORRECTION OF CAVERNOSAL TISSUE DEGENERATIVE PROCESSES

The treatments discussed above are merely palliative, aiming to obtain an effect — the controlled relaxation of the corpora cavernosa smooth muscle — without curing the underlying defect. Therefore, a reasonable pharmacological approach is to try to overcome two of the problems frequently associated with erectile dysfunction, namely, cavernosal tissue fibrosis and neuropathy. The first has been shown to be associated with ageing in both the rat[19,75] and human penis,[76] and presumably leads to a reduction of smooth muscle compliance to relaxant agents, both endogenous and pharmacological.

Neuropathy in turn affects 10–15% of diabetic individuals.[77] Two-thirds of men with diabetes and erectile dysfunction have evidence of central and/or peripheral neuropathy including the male reproductive tract. In the other one-third of these patients it is not clear whether the aetiology of the vascular disease is due to diabetes or is secondary to smoking, hyperlipidaemia and/or hypertension. The urogenital sensory neuropathy appears to have a crucial role in the aetiology of diabetic impotence, whereas angiopathy seems to be of secondary importance. The diabetic neuropathy mainly comprises somatic pudendal nerve dysfunction with abnormal bulbocavernosus reflexes that leads to a diminished sensory input from the urogenital tract, is age related, and increases with the duration of diabetes and with the loss of diabetes regulation. In type II diabetes mellitus, patients with primary organic impotence, as defined by diminished nocturnal penile tumescence (NPT) and rigidity, have a decreased conduction velocity of the dorsal penile nerve. This also occurs in BB and BBZ rats with spontaneous diabetes,[35] (the animal models for diabetes mellitus types I and II, respectively), where there is a considerable loss of penile reflexes underlying the erectile dysfunction.

The prevention of both cavernosal fibrosis and decrease in smooth muscle may be an interesting approach to the prophylaxis (and even therapy) of atherosclerotic veno-occlusive erectile dysfunction, and the erectile dysfunction associated with ageing per se.[78,79] Atherosclerotic injury of the iliac arteries leading to corporal ischaemia can be experimentally obtained in a rabbit model with balloon injury of these vessels combined with a high cholesterol diet for 4 months.[80] This process is accompanied by correlative increases in the cavernosal levels of thromboxane A2, a transforming growth factor beta-1 (TGF-β1) stimulator, and of TGF-β1 itself, a growth factor acting as a fibrotic agent that increases in the penis with sexual maturation.[81] This process occurs without affecting PGE2 (a TGF-β1 inhibitor). PGE1 is another inhibitor of the TGF-β1 induction of collagen synthesis, in this case via stimulation of cAMP synthesis.[82] Therefore, prostaglandins and other adenyl cyclase activators, and PDE inhibitors, may find use as antifibrotic agents in the corpora cavernosa, possibly in long-term treatments at doses lower than the ones eliciting cavernosal smooth muscle relaxation.

The reversal or prophylaxis of diabetic neuropathy is being investigated in rats by manipulation of the local nerve environment in vivo through targeted delivery of neurotrophins with mini-osmotic pumps releasing a constant infusion. In streptozotocin-induced diabetes, treatment with insulin-like growth factor I delivered directly to a sciatic nerve ameliorated the impairment of nerve regeneration at a 20-fold lower dose than was needed with systemic administration.[83] The same occurred with acidic fibroblast growth factor in normoglycaemic rats,[84] and it is conceivable that nerve growth factor in slow

release may have similar beneficial effects,[85] as it facilitates restoration of autonomic innervation in the penis of rats submitted to cavernosal nerve ablation. Another possible alternative is the use of Ca^{2+} antagonists, such as nimodipine, which has been shown in long-term i.p. administration to ameliorate diabetic neuropathy in the BB rat[86] (as indicated by sensory and motor nerve conduction velocity), presumably by increasing nerve flow through stimulation of adrenergic responsiveness.

All those approaches are still at an early stage of research and it will take time to show them to be effective in men, either alone or in conjunction with other procedures such as gene therapy.

■ GENE THERAPY OF THE CORPORA CAVERNOSA

The ultimate goals of novel approaches to medical therapy for impotence would be to achieve physiologically elicited erections without resorting to pharmacological treatment immediately prior to the sexual act and eventually to achieve long-term correction of the erectile dysfunction without the need for further intervention. None of the treatments presented so far, with the possible exception of those aimed to prevent or correct cavernosal tissue degeneration, satisfies these requirements, as the patient depends on a pharmacologically induced erection of an intrinsically impaired organ. A truly novel therapy, therefore, should be based on the biological correction of some facets of the defective erectile mechanism.

As discussed above, in the specific case of NO it is assumed that erectile dysfunction results from a reduction in the synthesis of this mediator in the penile nerve terminals and/or endothelium, and/or from impaired mechanical compliance of the target cavernosal smooth muscle to the relaxation induced by NO.[13,19] The studies already mentioned in different rat models of impotence risk factors have led to the proposal that the pharmacological increase of penile NOS content or activity may compensate for the reduction of either the endogenous penile NOS or the compliance of the cavernosal smooth muscle. Therefore, the modulation of endogenous penile NO synthesis may achieve a more stable and biologically controlled effect than that caused by vasoactive drugs injected into the corpora cavernosa.

A promising approach for raising the levels of a critical protein is to introduce its cDNA into the target organ by gene transfer techniques, with the expectation of a sustained expression of the corresponding mRNA and the maintenance of a physiological control of protein activity leading to the correction of the corresponding functional defect ('gene therapy'). This concept is gaining acceptance for a possible treatment of inborn errors of metabolism and cancer,[87] with over 150 clinical trials and numerous preclinical studies in animal models. Vectors are mainly liposomes or adenovirus and adeno-associated virus for non-dividing cells in vivo, and retrovirus for ex vivo modification of tissues or cells to be re-injected into the patient.

Published evidence shows that the transfer of genes to humans is feasible, with expression varying from a few days to several months and years. Cystic fibrosis, adenosine deaminase deficiency and familial hypercholesterolaemia are some of the diseases where a partial correction of some abnormalities has been obtained. Gene therapy studies on urogenital organs such as bladder, prostate, and kidney are being actively pursued with various genes.[88–91] Although the goal of a stable, tissue-specific and efficient production of the recombinant protein is difficult to achieve, prospects are promising.

An obvious candidate for gene therapy of erectile dysfunction is NOS cDNA, on the assumption that the expressed recombinant NOS enzyme is activated only upon physiological stimulation in the penis. This is a likely scenario, based on what is known on the neural control of penile erection and the mechanism of NOS activation. Although the penile-specific activation would occur by a neural signal triggered by sexual stimulus, the degree of control of the transfected gene would be enhanced if a cDNA construct for penile-specific NOS isoform(s) responding to that signal could be used. Recent studies have shown that, indeed, tissue-specific NOS isoforms are expressed, both in the rat and the human penis, and the cDNAs for both the iNOS and nNOS variants have been cloned.[92,93]

Although iNOS does not appear to be expressed in vivo in the rat corpora cavernosa, it may be induced in vitro in cultures of rat penile smooth muscle cells (RPSMC) using cytokine cocktails.[94] The cloned iNOS cDNA, designated RPiNOS, has six base and two amino acid differences from the rat vascular smooth muscle iNOS, which agrees with some functional differences for the RPSMC iNOS. The same applies to its human counterpart, with eight base and six amino acid differences with the human hepatocyte iNOS.[92]

The feasibility of delivering biological modulators in a continuous fashion to the penis and the possibility of correcting ageing-associated erectile dysfunction by manipulation of penile NOS expression was shown in a series of experiments in which penile iNOS was induced in vivo by the infusion of a cytokine mix into the corpora cavernosa using minipumps.[92] This procedure led to the correction of the erectile dysfunction observed in aged rats, and the process was shown to be accompanied by iNOS induction in the corpora cavernosa. Furthermore, a single injection of a construct of the RPiNOS coding region under the control of a strong promoter delivered into the corpora cavernosa as a liposome preparation achieved even better results, with correction lasting for 10–14 days. This suggests that the negligible basal expression of iNOS in the penis of old rats may be increased by local delivery of iNOS inducers or by gene therapy with iNOS constructs (the preferred modality to avoid toxic effects of cytokines). Experiments in vitro confirmed that iNOS protein in the penis appears to remain under physiological control, and it is assumed that a similar situation occurs in vivo, since no priapism is observed, and the activation occurs only when the neural signal is triggered by EFS.

However, the recently discovered penile nNOS variant designated PnNOS,[93] and not iNOS, is the NOS isoform more promising for gene therapy of erectile dysfunction and of other urogenital disorders where NO synthesis may be affected. PnNOS differs from the cerebellar nNOS in the presence of a 34-amino acid stretch that is likely to confer some unique regulatory function related to the role of NO in smooth muscle relaxation. PnNOS is expressed as the predominant or unique nNOS isoform in the prostate and urethra, and is mixed with cerebellar nNOS in the bladder, which strongly suggests that it is the main enzyme in the NO cascade that controls the tone of the whole lower urogenital tract. It is expressed in the human penis, appears to be the product of a second nNOS gene, and may be similar to the form identified in the skeletal and cardiac muscle.[95]

Studies are in progress to determine whether PnNOS gene therapy is more effective than that with iNOS and cerebellar nNOS in eliciting a long-term improvement of erectile dysfunction in aged and diabetic rats. NOS cDNAs have been used experimentally in the rat for gene transfer to the vascular system.[96–98] In the case of the penis, a recent report[99] claims to have stimulated for at least 4 months the erectile response of adult rats by injecting in the corpora cavernosa a plasmid construct of the human cerebellar nNOS, thus indirectly confirming the previous findings with iNOS. However, the cerebellar nNOS results need confirmation, considering the difficulties for human proteins and adenoviral vectors to remain functional in the rat for such prolonged periods. The same group has communicated a promising gene therapy approach with the intracavernosal injection in aged rats of cDNA coding for a subunit of the maxi-K channel, a protein involved in smooth muscle relaxation.[100] Another cDNA, the one encoding the rat androgen receptor, has been directly transfected into the corpora cavernosa and has led to hyperexpression.[101]

A spin-off of the attempts to modulate penile NOS activity by gene therapy is the pharmacological approach based on regulating NO synthesis through more traditional means, such as substrate, cofactor, or inhibitor/stimulator availability in the tissue. A recent contribution[102] has shown that, in the rat, it is possible to correct the age-associated erectile dysfunction measured by EFS of the cavernosal nerve, by long-term administration of high doses of L-arginine. This is accompanied by an increase in the concentration of L-arginine and NOS activity in the serum and penile cytosol of treated rats. Additional experiments may be required before conducting clinical studies[103] based on the oral and topical administration of this substrate, particularly in the case of psychogenic impotence. An earlier (small) clinical trial showed some improvement of the erectile response in impotent men.[104]

The detection in the penis (unpublished) of NOS inhibitors, such as the PIN found in brain and testis[38] that causes the dissociation of the active NOS dimer into an inactive monomer, should provide an alternative strategy based on counteracting the effects of this inhibitor. Another promising avenue is the blockade of AGE formation in the diabetic penis, which is currently being investigated by aminoguanidine administration or metabolic control for other diabetic complications. As mentioned above, AGEs are assumed to inactivate NOS or quench the effects of NO on its targets.

The main doubt regarding the clinical usefulness of gene therapy approaches is related to how efficient, specific and stable the effects may be. Although the liposomal administration may provide only short-term expression of the recombinant protein (be it NOS or another gene), viral constructs will considerably enhance the efficiency and duration of the desired effects. The development of helper-dependent adenoviral vectors, where all sequences coding for viral proteins have been removed except for the packaging signals,[105,106] should help to reduce immunogenicity and increase the duration and intensity of the recombinant protein expression. The adeno-associated virus vectors[107] have in turn the advantage of non-immunogenicity, non-pathogenicity and prolonged expression of the recombinant gene (months/years). In turn, the intracavernosal admini-stration of recombinant genes combined with the use of tissue-specific promoters, or promoters that can be turned on and off by external tissue-specific manipulation, should help to reduce expression in organs other than the penis. Finally, gene transfer with PnNOS may ensure the additional organ specificity provided by the functional significance of its unique amino acid sequence and the signal elicited by sexual stimulus.

■ CONCLUSIONS

In conclusion, from the future therapeutic alternatives discussed above for the treatment of erectile dysfunction, the only one that shows some promise towards ameliorating or curing the underlying disease is gene therapy, and it is likely that, in the near future, clinical trials may be designed with NOS and other genes. The accessibility of the corpora cavernosa for direct delivery of drugs to this organ, and the patient's acceptance of this route of self-administration over long periods, provides a unique advantage for studies of gene therapy of the penis, compared with other organs. If this approach proves successful, it may have three advantages over the intracavernosal treatment with vasoactive agents: (1) it may require single or sporadically repeated administration by the patient, not immediately preceding sexual intercourse; (2) it may facilitate nocturnal penile tumescence and spontaneous erection episodes that may help functional regeneration of the cavernosal tissue; (3) it may evolve into easier local or oral application routes based on new vehicles, vectors and penile targeting promoters.

■ REFERENCES

1. Manning M, Juenemann K P. Pharmacotherapy of erectile dysfunction. In: Hellstrom W J G (ed) Male infertility and sexual dysfunction. New York: Springer, 1997: 440–451

2. Murray F T, Geisser M, Murphy T C. Evaluation and treatment of erectile dysfunction. Am J Med Sci 1995; 309: 99–109

3. Fallon B. Intracavernous injection therapy for male erectile dysfunction. Urol Clin North Am 1995; 22: 833–845

4. Anderson K E, Holmquist F. Regulation of tone in penile cavernous smooth muscle. World J Urol 1994; 12: 249–261

5. Giuliano F A, Rampin O, Benoit G, Jardin A. Neural control of penile erection. Urol Clin North Am 1995; 22: 747–766

6. Gheorghiu S, Godschalk M, Gentili A, Mulligan T. Quality of life in patients using self-administered intracavernous injections of prostaglandin E1 for erectile dysfunction. J Urol 1996; 156: 80–81

7. Godschalk M, Gheorghiu D, Chen J et al. Long-term efficacy of a new formulation of prostaglandin E1 as treatment for erectile failure. J Urol 1996; 155: 915-917.

8. Linet O I, Ogrinc F G. Efficacy and safety of intracavernosal alprostadil in men with erectile dysfunction. The Alprostadil Study Group. N Engl J Med 1996; 334: 873–877

9. Morales A, Heaton J P W, Johnston B, Adams M. Oral and topical treatment of erectile dysfunction. Urol Clin North Am 1995; 22: 879–886

10. Doherty P C. Oral, transdermal, and transurethral therapies. In: Hellstrom W J G (ed) Male infertility and sexual dysfunction. New York: Springer, 1997: 452–467

11. Lugg J, Gonzalez-Cadavid N F, Rajfer J. The role of nitric oxide in erectile function. J Androl 1995; 16: 2–6

12. Burnett A L. Nitric oxide in the penis: physiology and pathology. J Urol 1997; 157: 320–334

13. Gonzalez-Cadavid N F, Rajfer J. Nitric oxide and other neurotransmitters of the corpus cavernosum. In: Hellstrom W J G (ed) Male infertility and sexual dysfunction. New York: Springer Verlag, 1997: 425–439

14. Ignarro L J, Bush P A, Buga G M et al. Nitric oxide and cyclic GMP formation upon electric field stimulation cause relaxation of corpus cavernosum smooth muscle. Biochem Biophys Res Commun 1990; 170: 843–850

15. Rajfer J, Aronson W J, Bush P et al. Nitric oxide as a mediator of relaxation of the corpus cavernosum in response to nonadrenergic, noncholinergic neurotransmission. N Engl J Med 1992; 326: 90–94

16. Vernet D, Cai L, Garban H et al. Reduction of penile nitric oxide synthase in diabetic BB/WOR^{dp} (Type I) and BBZ/WOR^{dp} (Type II) rats with erectile dysfunction. Endocrinology 1995; 136: 5709–5717

17. Xie Y, Garban H, Ng C et al. Long-term passive smoking reduces penile nitric oxide synthase in the rat without impairing the erectile response to electrical stimulation of the cavernosal nerve. J Urol 1997; 157: 1121–1128

18. Garban H, Moody J, Marquez D et al. Normal erectile response to cavernosal nerve stimulation in diabetic BB and BBZ rats with decreased penile nitric oxide synthase. Proc Intl Congr Endocr 1996: 1–189

19. Garban H, Vernet D, Freedman A et al. Effect of aging on nitric oxide-mediated penile erection in the rat. Am J Physiol 1995; 268: H467–H475

20. Garban H, Marquez D, Cai L et al. Restoration of normal penile erectile response in aged rats by long-term treatment with androgens. Biol Reprod 1995; 53: 1365–1372

21. Carrier S, Nagaraju P, Morgan D M et al. Age decreases nitric oxide synthase-containing nerve fibers in the rat penis. J Urol 1997; 157: 1088–1092

22. Lugg J, Rajfer J, Gonzalez-Cadavid N F. DHT is the active androgen in the maintenance of nitric oxide mediated penile erection in the rat. Endocrinology 1995; 136: 1495–1501

23. Penson D F, Ng C, Cai L et al. Androgen and pituitary control of nitric oxide synthase activity and erectile function in the rat penis. Biol Reprod 1996; 55: 567–574

24. Lugg J, Ng C, Rajfer J, Gonzalez-Cadavid N F. Cavernosal nerve stimulation reverses castration-induced decrease in rat penile nitric oxide synthase activity. Am J Physiol 1996; 271: 354–361

25. Mills T M, Reilly C M, Lewis R W. Androgens and penile erection: a review. J Androl 1996; 17: 633–638

26. Mills T M, Stopper V S, Reilly C M. Sites of androgenic regulation of cavernosal blood pressure during penile erection in the rat. Int J Impot Res 1996; 8: 29–34

27. Heaton J P, Varrin S J. Effects of castration and exogenous testosterone supplementation in an animal model of penile erection. J Urol 1994; 151: 797–800

28. Penson D F, Ng C, Rajfer J, Gonzalez-Cadavid N F. Adrenal control of erectile function and nitric oxide synthase in the rat penis. Endocrinology 1997; 138: 3935–3942

29. Nelson R J, Demas G E, Huang P L et al. Behavioral abnormalities in male mice lacking neuronal nitric oxide synthase. Nature 1995; 378: 383–386

30. Huang P L, Huang Z, Mashimo H et al. Hypertension in mice lacking the gene for endothelial nitric oxide synthase. Nature 1995; 377: 239–242

31. Wei X-Q, Charles I G, Smith A et al. Altered immune responses in mice lacking inducible nitric oxide synthase. Nature 1995; 375: 408–411

32. Burnett A L, Tillman S L, Chang T S K et al. Immunohistochemical localization of nitric oxide synthase in the autonomic innervation of the human penis. J Urol 1993; 150: 73–76

33. Beesley J E. Histochemical methods for detecting nitric oxide synthase. Histochem J 1995; 27: 757–769

34. Dail W G, Barba V, Leyba L, Galindo R. Neural and endothelial nitric oxide synthase activity in rat penile erectile tissue. Cell Tissue Res 1995; 282: 109–116

35. McVary K T, Rathnau C H, McKenna K E. Sexual dysfunction in the diabetic BB/WOR rat: a role of central neuropathy. Am J Physiol 1997; 272: R259–267

36. Bucala R, Tracey K J, Cerami A. Advanced glycosylation products quench nitric oxide and mediate defective endothelium-dependent vasodilatation in experimental diabetes. J Clin Invest 1991; 87: 432–438

37. Jiaan D B, Seftel A D, Fogarty J et al. Age-related increase in an advanced glycation end product in penile tissue. World J Urol 1995; 13: 369–375

38. Jaffrey S R, Snyder S H. PIN: an associated protein inhibitor of neuronal nitric oxide synthase. Science 1996; 274: 774–777

39. Hellstrom W J, Bennett A H, Gesundheit N et al. A double-blind, placebo-controlled evaluation of the erectile response to transurethral alprostadil. Urology 1996; 48: 851–856

40. Padma-Nathan H, Hellstrom W J, Kaiser F E et al. Treatment of men with erectile dysfunction with transurethral alprostadil. Medicated Urethral System for Erection (MUSE) Study Group. N Engl J Med 1997; 336: 1–7

41. Hellstrom W J G, Sikka S C, Wang R et al. Effects of transurethral alprostadil on prostaglandin content of human ejaculate and on sperm motility. Int J Impot Res 1996; 8: 103 (abstr 18)

42. Werthman A, Rajfer J. MUSE therapy: preliminary clinical observations. Urology 1997; 50: 809–811

43. Jeremy J Y, Ballard S A, Naylor A M et al. Effects of sildenafil, a type-5 cGMP phosphodiesterase inhibitor, and papaverine on cyclic GMP and cyclic AMP levels in the rabbit corpus cavernosum in vitro. Br J Urol 1997; 79: 958–963

44. Ballard S A, Gingell C J C, Price M E et al. Sildenafil, an inhibitor of phosphodiesterase type 5, enhances nitric oxide-mediated relaxation of human corpus cavernosum. Int J Impot Res 1996; 8:103 (abstr 17)

45. Boolell M, Gepi-Attee S, Gingell J C, Allen M J. Sildenafil, a novel effective oral therapy for male erectile dysfunction. Br J Urol 1996; 78: 257–261

46. Mulhall J. Sildenafil: a novel effective oral therapy for male erectile dysfunction [letter]. Br J Urol 1997; 79: 663–664

47. Virag R, and the Multicentre Study Group. Sildenafil (Viagra™), a new oral treatment for erectile dysfunction (ED): an 8 week double-blind, placebo-controlled parallel group study. Int J Impot Res 1996; 8: 116 (abstr 70)

48. Boolell M, Yates P K, Wulff M B. Sildenafil (Viagra™), a novel oral treatment with rapid onset of action for penile erectile dysfunction (ED). Int J Impot Res 1996; 8: 147 (D101)

49. Piechota H J, Hassan M, Daluns S E et al. Selective phosphodiesterase inhibitors in erection. Int J Impot Res 1996; 8: 127 (D21)

50. Paick J S, Lee S W. The neural mechanism of apomorphine-induced erection: an experimental study by comparison with electrostimulation-induced erection in the rat model. J Urol 1994; 152: 2125–2128

51. Yamaguchi Y, Kobayashi H. Effects of apomorphine, physostigmine and vaso-active intestinal peptide on penile erection and yawning in diabetic rats. Eur J Pharmacol 1994; 254: 91–96

52. Heaton J P W, Adams M A, Morales A et al. Apomorphine SL is effective in the treatment of non-organic erectile dysfunction: results of a multicenter trial. Int J Impot Res 1996; 8: 115 (abstr 64)

53. Zorgniotti A W. Experience with buccal phentolamine mesylate for impotence. Int J Impot Res 1994; 6: 37–41

54. Lance R, Albo M, Costabile R A, Steers W D. Oral trazodone as empirical therapy for erectile dysfunction: a retrospective review. Urology 1995; 46: 117–20

55. Meinhardt W, Kropman R F, de la Fuente R F et al. Oral treatment of impotence, trazodone versus placebo. J Impot Res 1996; 8: 116 (abstr 67)

56. Kim E D, el-Rashidy R, McVary K T. Papaverine topical gel for treatment of erectile dysfunction. J Urol 1995; 153: 361–365

57. Chiang H-S, Lin L-H, Shue M-T. Transdermal study of Prostaglandin E1 and Prostaglandin E1 methylester gel. Int J Impot Res 1996; 8: 130 (D34)

58. Becher E, Momesso A, Borghi M, Montes de Oca L. A double blinded placebo controlled trial of topical Prostaglandin E1 for erectile dysfunction. Int J Impot Res 1996; 8: 148 (D106)

59. Wegner H H, Knispel H H. Effect of nitric oxide-donor, linsidomine chlorhydrate, in treatment of human erectile dysfunction caused by venous leakage. Urology 1993; 42: 409–411

60. Truss M C, Becker A J, Djamilian M H et al. Role of the nitric oxide donor linsidomine clorhydrate (SIN-1) in the diagnosis and treatment of erectile dysfunction. Urology 1994; 44: 553–556

61. Wang R, Hellstrom W J G, Sikka S C, Kadowitz P. Penile erection induced by transurethral administration of sodium nitroprusside. J Urol 1996; 155: 621A (1241)

62. Cahn D, Melman A, Valcic M, Christ G J. Forskolin: a promising new adjunct to intracavernous pharmacotherapy. J Urol 1996; 155: 1789–1794

63. Hellstrom W J G, Wang R, Champion H C, Kadowitz P J. Novel nitric oxide donors can induce penile erections in the cat. Int J Impot Res 1996; 8: 128 (D23)

64. Truss M C, Becker A J, Thon W F et al. Intracavernous calcitonin gene-related peptide plus prostaglandin E1: possible alternative to penile implants in selected patients. Eur J Urol 1994; 26: 40–45

65. Takahashi Y, Aboseif S R, Benard F et al. Effect of intracavernous simultaneous injection of acetylcholine and vasoactive intestinal polypeptide on canine penile erection. J Urol 1996; 148: 446–448

66. Saenz de Tejada I. Commentary on mechanisms for the regulation of the penile smooth muscle contractility. J Urol 1995; 153: 1762

67. Levin A R. Endothelins. N Engl J Med 1995; 333: 356–363

68. Adams M A, Banting J D, Manabe K et al. The major role for nitric oxide in the penis is to regulate the vasoconstrictor actions of endothelins. Int J Impot Res 1996; 8: 124 (D07)

69. Whittingham H A, Banting J D, Manabe K et al. Erectile dysfunction induced by acute NO synthase blockade is reversed by an endothelin receptor antagonist. Int J Impot Res 1996; 8: 100 (abstr 06)

70. Merlin S L, Begin L R, Dion S B et al. Endothelin-1 and radiation-associated impotence. Int J Impot Res 1996; 8: 107 (abstr 31)

71. Gupta S, Daley J, Goldstein I, Traish A M. Lack of selectivity of agents for alpha-adrenergic receptors in human corpus cavernosum. Int J Impot Res 1996; 8: 105 (abstr 25)

72. Kifor I, Williams G H, Vickers M A et al. Tissue angiotensin II as a modulator of erectile function. I. Angiotensin peptide content, secretion and effects in the corpus cavernosum. J Urol 1997; 157: 1920–1925

73. Park J K, Kim S Z, Kim J H et al. Renin angiotensin system in rabbit corpus cavernosum: functional characterization of angiotensin II receptors. J Urol 1997; 158: 653–658

74. Saenz de Tejada I, Cuevas P, Cuevas B et al. S-Nitrosylated alpha blockers as potential drugs for the treatment of impotence. Biological activity of NMI-187 and NMI-221. Int J Impot Res 1996; 8: 103 (abstr 16)

75. Moreland R B, Traish A, McMillin M A et al. PGE1 suppresses the induction of collagen synthesis by transforming growth factor ß-1 in human corpus cavernosum smooth muscle. J Urol 1995; 153: 826–832

76. Conti G, Virag R. Human penile erection and organic impotence: normal histology and histopathology. Urol Int 1989; 44: 303–308

77. Bemelmans B L H, Mueleman E J H, Doesburg W H et al. Erectile dysfunction in diabetic men: the neurological factor revisited. J Urol 1994; 151: 884–889

78. Feldman H A, Goldstein I, Hatzichristou D G et al. Impotence and its medical and psychosocial correlates: results of the Massachusetts Male Aging Study. J Urol 1994; 151: 54–61

79. Benet A, Melman A. The epidemiology of erectile dysfunction. Urol Clin North Am 1995; 22: 699–709

80. Azadzoi K M, Goldstein I, Krane R J, Siroky M B. Ischemia-induced TGF-β1- mediated cavernosal fibrosis is modulated by eicosanoids. Int J Impot Res 1996; 8: 108 (abstr 36)

81. Gelman J, Garban H, Shen R et al. Transforming growth factor β-1 (TGF-β1) and penile growth in the rat during sexual maturation. J Androl 1998; 19: 50–57

82. Moreland R B, Huang Y, Goldstein I et al. Inhibition of TGF-β1-induced collagen synthesis in human corpus cavernosum smooth muscle by cAMP. Int J Impot Res 1996; 8: 102 (abstr 14)

83. Ishii D N, Lupien S B. Insulin-like growth factors protect against diabetic neuropathy: effects on sensory nerve regeneration in rats. J Neurosci Res 1995; 40: 138–144

84. Laird J M A, Mason G S, Thomas K A et al. Acidic fibroblast growth factor stimulates motor and sensory axon regeneration after sciatic nerve crush in the rat. Neuroscience 1995; 65: 209–216

85. Burgers J K, Nelson R J, Quinlan D M, Walsh P C. Nerve growth factor, nerve grafts and amniotic membrane grafts restore erectile function in rats. J Urol 1991; 146: 463–468

86. Kappelle A C, Biessels G, Bravenboer B et al. Beneficial effect of the Ca^{2+} antagonist, nimodipine, on existing diabetic neuropathy in the BB/Wpr rat. Br J Pharmacol 1994; 111: 887–893

87. Crystal R G. Transfer of genes to humans: early lessons and obstacles to success. Science 1996; 270: 404–410

88. Morris B D, Drazan K E, Csete M E et al. Adenoviral-mediated gene transfer to bladder in vivo. J Urol 1994; 152: 506–509

89. Bass C, Cabrera G, Elgavish A et al. Recombinant adenovirus-mediated gene transfer to genitourinary epithelium in vitro and in vivo. Cancer Gene Therapy 1995; 2: 97–104

90. Sanda M G, Ayyagari S R, Jaffee E M et al. Demonstration of a rational strategy for human prostate cancer gene therapy. J Urol 1994; 151: 622–628.

91. Wagner J, Madry H, Reszka R. In vivo gene transfer: focus on the kidney. Nephrol Dialys Transplant 1995; 10: 1801–1807

92. Garban H, Marquez D, Magee T et al. Cloning of rat and human inducible penile nitric oxide synthase. Application for gene therapy of erectile dysfunction. Biol Reprod 1997; 56: 954–963

93. Magee T, Fuentes A M, Garban H et al. Cloning of a novel neuronal nitric oxide synthase expressed in penis and lower urinary tract. Biochem Biophys Res Commun 1996; 226: 145–151

94. Hung A, Vernet D, Rajavashisth T et al. Expression of the inducible nitric oxide synthase in smooth muscle cells from the rat penile corpora cavernosa. J Androl 1995; 16: 469–481

95. Silvagno F, Xia H, Bredt D S. Neuronal nitric oxide synthase-u, an alternatively spliced isoform expressed in differentiated skeletal muscle. J Biol Chem 1996; 271: 11204–11208

96. von der Leyen H E, Gibbons G H, Morishita R et al. Gene therapy inhibiting neointimal vascular lesion: in vivo transfer of endothelial cell nitric oxide synthase gene. Proc Natl Acad Sci USA 1995; 92: 1137–1141

97. Billiar T, Tzeng E, Shears L et al. Gene transfer of the human type II NO synthase: requirements and consequences. Proc 2nd Int Conf Biochem Mol Biol NO, Los Angeles, CA, USA. 1996; 50

98. Chen A F, O'Brien T, Tsutsui M et al. Expression and function of recombinant endothelial nitric oxide synthase gene in canine basilar artery. Circul Res 1997; 80: 327–335

99. Rehman J, Christ G, Melman A et al. Enhancement of physiologic erectile function with nitric oxide synthase therapy. J Urol 1997; 157: 201 (abstr 782)

100. Christ G, Rehman J, Melman A et al. Intracavernous injection of the hSlo maxi-K cDNA: a test of the utility of gene therapy for the treatment of erectile dysfunction. Int J Impot Res 1997; 8: 103 (abstr 15)

101. Gelman J, Shen R, Marquez D et al. Gene transfer of androgen receptor constructs to penile corpora cavernosa. J Urol 1997; 157: 16 (abstr 62)

102. Moody J, Vernet D, Laidlaw S et al. Effect of long-term administration of L-arginine on the rat erectile response. J Urol 1997; 158: 942–947

103. Melman A. L-Arginine and penile erection. J Urol 1997; 158: 686

104. Zorgniotti A W, Lizza E F. Effect of large doses of the nitric oxide precursor, L-arginine, on erectile dysfunction. Int J Impot Res 1994; 6: 33–36

105. Wilson J M. Adenoviruses as gene-delivery vehicles. N Engl J Med 1996; 334: 1185–1187

106. Kochanek S, Clemens P R, Mitani K et al. A new adenoviral vector: replacement of all viral coding sequences with 28 kb of DNA independently expressing both full-length dystrophin and β-galactosidase. Proc Natl Acad Sci USA 1996; 93: 5731–5736

107. Peel A L, Zolotukhin S, Schrimsher G W et al. Efficient transduction of green fluorescent protein in spinal cord neurons using adeno-associated virus vectors containing cell type-specific promoters. Gene Ther 1997; 4: 16–24

108. Goldstein E, Lue T F, Padma-Nathan H et al. Oral sildenafil in the treatment of erectile dysfunction. N Engl J Med 1998; 338: 1397–1409

Chapter 33

Complications of intracavernosal therapy for impotence

C. Evans

■ INTRODUCTION

Intracavernosal injection of vasoactive drugs has, for the last 15 years, made the successful treatment of impotence possible on a large scale, with impotence clinics opening up universally. This method of treatment has revolutionized the management of erectile dysfunction as it has given a good, usable, normal-looking erection, with a remarkable lack of fuss, in a large proportion of patients. There have, however, been problems and complications with the use of these drugs, which have led to a high attrition rate and loss of compliance.

■ DEVELOPMENT OF INTRACAVERNOSAL DRUGS

It was serendipidity that first showed Virag[1] that an intracorporal injection of papaverine caused a good erection, and Brindley,[2] working with phenoxybenzamine, followed closely after. Papaverine in the first instance was the most commonly used intracavernosal agent, although the addition of phentolamine to the armamentation (usually in combination with papaverine) improved the effectiveness of the treatment.[3] There were, however, problems with the use of these agents — pain on injection, prolonged erections and a non-acceptance by the male public that sticking needles into their penises was a sensible thing to do. The initial workers in the field persevered; the number in their ranks (usually urologists) swelled and, in 1987, prostaglandin E1 (PGE1)[4,5] was demonstrated to be not only as effective but more so — and, certainly, initially free of most of the complications, although the occasional report of prolonged erections

filtered through. This new drug was a godsend. The development of PGE1 to the stage where it was licensed and packaged in a user-friendly way took the next 7 years. PGE1 is at present the best vasoactive drug to use as a single agent; other, newer, agents should be studied in controlled trials in comparison before they are marketed as preferable agents. Of the new agents used alone or in combination with PGE1, linsidomine chlorohydrate (SIN-1),[6] calcitonin gene-related peptide (CGRP),[7] moxysylate (Erecnos),[8] vasoactive polypeptide with phentolamine[9] (Invicorp) and nitroprusside[10] have all (except the last) shown promise but are not in widespread use, mainly because they are not as effective as PGE1 or have to be used in combination with other vasoactive agents. Erecnos and Invicorp are now licensed.

Knowledge of the mechanism of action and metabolism of these vasoactive drugs gives some idea of why certain side effects occur.[11] Papaverine,[15] an alpha blocker and smooth muscle relaxant, causes vasodilatation of the cavernosal vessels. It is, however, metabolized in the body and not locally. Because of the pH of the prepared fluid, the injection can be painful. Alprostadil (PGE1) relaxes the cavernosal smooth muscle. When administered intravenously it is rapidly transformed into inactive metabolites: 70–90% is extensively metabolized in a single pass through the lungs, resulting in a metabolic half-life of less than 1 minute.[13] After intracavernosal injection, the concentrations of drug and metabolites are elevated in the cavernosa but not in the peripheral circulation; the drug does not, therefore, have to escape to be metabolized and thus the incidence of prolonged erection is reduced. The cause of pain following use of this agent is unknown.

■ THE ADMINISTRATION OF INTRACAVERNOSAL AGENTS

Much of the worry (and, sometimes, fear) that goes with the thought of intracavernosal drugs should be dispelled by a well and sympathetically run clinic with privacy and time for discussion. Enthusiasm on the part of the staff is essential in order to persuade the patients that the injection is needed.

It should be stressed that, certainly, the initial injection is part of the diagnosis and is best given on the first visit after informed consent, before the patient changes his mind.

It is mooted that the initial dose should be as low as 2.5 μg,[14] but this policy does not allow the patient to have a good erection on the first visit, which is essential if the patient is going to come back with enthusiasm for self-injection on the second visit.

A dosage regime for different aetiologies is suggested (Table 33.1). It is preferable for the first injection to be given with the patient lying supine, as there is a definite (although small) incidence of light-headedness and sweating. Whether this is related to fear of the needle or escape of the vasoactive drug into the general circulation is not well established; certainly it occurs more frequently with papaverine usage and in those patients who were considered to have venous leakage.

After this first injection has been studied by the clinician and the patient, and the result compared with previous erections, the patient should be issued with directions as to what to do if a firm erection is present at 4 hours. If the erection is very good, an oral antidote, terbutaline[15] 5 mg, is provided, to be taken earlier, at 3 hours; the author usually advises the patient to go and use the erection.

■ INITIAL COMPLICATIONS RELATING TO SELF-INJECTION

Initial complications can include the following: dizziness and hypotension; pain; incorrect injection, leading to bruising or bleeding from the meatus; ineffectiveness of the injection and prolonged erection.

Dizziness

Dizziness very rarely occurs as it is probably related as much to apprehension as to the escape of the vasodilator into the general circulation. If the patient is upright performing the technique, then lying down usually resolves this after a few minutes.

Pain

Pain on actual injection may be due to incorrectly injecting into the glans penis, which can be avoided by retracting the prepuce so the glans can be seen and protected by thumb and forefinger (Fig. 33.1). The injection of papaverine using a 26 gauge needle was often

Table 33.1. Suggested initial dose of intracavernosal agents

Diagnosis	Papaverine	Papaverine and phentolamine		PGE1
Neuropathic	5–10 mg			5 μg
Psychological	10–15 mg	30 mg	+ 1 mg	10 μg
Diabetic	30 mg			10 + 10 μg; repeat in 10 min
Atherosclerotic	30 mg + repeat 30 mg in 10 min	30 mg + 30 mg	+ 1 mg	20 μg
Maintenance range	5–60 mg	60 mg	+ 5 mg	5–40 μg

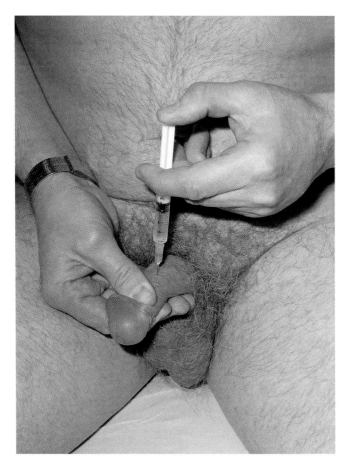

Figure 33.1. Correct technique of intracorporal injection.

uncomfortable but the prepacked syringes with 30 gauge needle used with PGE1 are so very fine that the needle is hardly felt. Injecting into the plaque of Peyronie's disease is also extremely uncomfortable and any nodules should be avoided.

Incorrect injection

Obese men and those with short penises may find self-injection extremely difficult, in which case the use of a mirror may make the technique possible. However, poor hand control, either from intention tremor or in multiple sclerosis, may require the addition of an auto-injector for ease or the use of another pair of hands, for example those of the wife or partner. There are, even despite this, patients who find it difficult to inject. If the needle is too superficial, then bruising will occur; if too posterior, the injection may be given into the corpus spongiosum and the drug will be seen issuing from the meatus. The patient in such a situation should be reassured, reshown the technique and asked to try again. On insertion of the needle against tough cavernous tissue, if subsequent

spillage from the needle syringe gap occurs, this can be rectified by withdrawing the needle very slightly and tightening the needle syringe connection carefully. The use of intracavernous drugs in patients on anticoagulants is no problem if the technique is correct and the clotting times not too prolonged.

Ineffectiveness

Despite careful instruction by nursing staff in the drawing up technique, the procedure is often fiddly and difficult for the patient, especially if it is necessary for the vasoactive agent to be reconstituted from powder. Fluid (and therefore drug) is not drawn up into the syringe. The use of syringes prefilled with some of the agents overcomes this problem. The patient will learn the drawing-up technique with practice, and at home should allow enough time for this, and not rush.

If the effect of the drug is not adequate (and, usually, the erectile response is better at home in a more conducive atmosphere), then the patient may be instructed to increase the dose by small increments,[16] which, if necessary, should be reviewed.

Prolonged erection

A prolonged, painful erection is the most troublesome of the complications of intracavernous drugs. This complication was very soon discovered with papaverine and has been much less common with PGE1. Nevertheless, it can occur (not, it is to be hoped, on the first visit), and it is extremely off-putting for the patient. Care taken to select the initial dose should preclude this; if the patient has good early morning erections he should be given a small dose. It is important to provide terbutaline[17] tablets (5 mg), to be used sublingually at 3 hours and repeated after 15 minutes if necessary, for those patients who get a good, usable erection; in addition, a 4 hour instruction sheet should be provided, with the advice to attend if the erection persists. If the agent is being injected by a non-urologist, arrangements must be in place for the patient to attend a local hospital where aspiration of the penis is possible, or this procedure should be performed by the clinician and team running the impotence clinic.

The technique of aspiration of the penis is simple.[15] As the patient is very uncomfortable and apprehensive, usually about 4–5 hours after injection, a local anaesthesia of the skin near the base of the penis and the tunica albuginea should be used. Under aseptic technique, a large-bore butterfly needle filled with heparinized saline should be inserted into the corpora and used to aspirate, pulling the syringe plunger gently and squeezing the penis full length with the other hand. This often needs two pairs of hands! A volume of about 20–50 ml venous blood will be obtained, relieving the discomfort dramatically. Usually the butterfly needle is left in place to see what happens next. If the penis refills, aspiration should be repeated, the corpora should be flushed with heparinized saline and the use of phenylephrine,[18] up to 500 μg diluted in 2 ml, should be considered; the effect, again, is dramatic. It has been necessary only once in the author's experience to use an alpha-sympathomimetic drug. Metaraminol is not recommended. The patient's blood pressure should be monitored as it may rise. The use of a tourniquet at the base of the penis is not necessary.

Before sending the patient home, enquiry should be made about the dose the patient used and whether it was repeated on the same day; the patient should be advised to use a smaller dose for the next administration, if he has not lost his nerve. If the patient is still using papaverine, changing to an equivalent dose of PGE1 is recommended.

The incidence of prolonged erection varies. In a self-injection programme involving 254 patients, prolonged erections occurred in four (1.6%) with 20 patient episodes (4.7%):[19] four erections resolved spontaneously, but 16 required irrigation and phenylephrine (0.1 ml of 0.1%). The dose of vasoactive agent was reduced and 66% of the patients chose to continue. Those patients with more than three recurrent episodes of erections lasting more than 4 hours were issued with prefilled syringes of phenylephrine to inject at home, if needed.

■ LATE COMPLICATIONS OF INTRACAVERNOUS AGENTS

Late complications can include fibrosis, pain, or loss of effect.

Fibrosis
The incidence of development of corporal fibrosis varies from 1.9[19] to 16%[20]. This takes the form of nodules or plaques, with deviation.[15,21] In the series by Valdevenito and Melman,[19] of 15 patients (5.9%) affected, 12 had palpable nodules and three had plaques; the latter required treatment with a penile implant. These authors noted an increase in scar formation, on using papaverine or mixtures of papaverine, which took up to 18 months to develop; the incidence stabilized after 4 years.

If fibrosis develops, the patient should be advised to stop using that side and use the other; the fibrosis may well resolve. In addition, for patients who develop fibrosis after using papaverine/phentolamine, changing to CGRP and PGE1 has been successful and further fibrosis has not occurred.[7]

In an attempt by Chen and colleagues[20] to elucidate the risk involved in using PGE1, no significant differences were found between those patients who developed scarring and those who did not, regardless of duration of follow-up, injection frequency, PGE1 dose per injection, total number of injections or total dose. Patients with initial penile scarring did not have a higher incidence of further scarring. Chen and colleagues concluded that penile scarring with PGE1 is sporadic and unpredictable.

Pain
Of the later complications, this is the most annoying. With the use of PGE1, significant pain may occur initially in 20–30% of patients.[22] Some patients (7%) complain of pain from the injection itself, 11% of pain during the erection, and 4% on both occasions. The pain is usually burning in quality and, although the erection may be very good, the pain may be sufficient to preclude any thought of sexual intercourse. In other patients the pain is milder and often becomes much less with repeated use, so that the outcome is not affected. The pain usually begins 15 minutes after injection, lasts for 1–2 hours and occurs more frequently in patients with diabetes and neuropathies.[23] The addition of local anaesthetic to the intracavernous solution,[23] or the addition of sodium bicarbonate,[24] has sometimes been successful in reducing the pain. The use of CGRP plus PGE1 can be beneficial in patients who have suffered pain with a larger single dose of PGE1. Also moxisylyte appears to be painless.

Loss of effectiveness
In a few patients, the effect of the intracavernous agents seems to wane with time, especially in older patients. Instructions to revisit the clinician are advisable, rather than increasing the dose haphazardly. Any such patients who are using a maximum dose of agent may benefit from the use of a ring device at the penile base, although this is not universally recommended.[25]

◼ LACK OF COMPLIANCE

There are many causes of lack of compliance. In most cases, the use of intracavernosal drugs depends on the keenness of the patient, but lack of spontaneity is the commonest cause of lack of compliance, followed by lack of interest by the partner, lack of partner and pain.[26] Cost does not appear to be a major consideration when the agents are being provided by the National Health Service, but in private medicine this may limit the frequency of use. In addition, some very elderly patients consider (perhaps with some justification) that the time has come for sexual intercourse to cease.

◼ SPONTANEOUS IMPROVEMENT

Spontaneous improvement in erections is often seen after the first response to the initial injection, as though the mechanism has just 'woken up'. This occurs more often in men who have not been sexually active for a while — for example a widowed middle-aged man who finds that he cannot 'perform' with a new partner. This spontaneous improvement may continue with use, to an extent sufficient to make self-injection unnecessary or needed only occasionally as a 'booster'.

In a study by Marshall and colleagues,[27] spontaneous improvement occurred in 13 of 35 patients (37%). Haemodynamic measurements showed that although the diameter of the intracorporal arteries was unchanged, mean velocity in the right corpus increased from 17.9 to 24 cm/s and in the left from 21.2 to 29 cm/s.

◼ ADJUNCTS TO SUCCESS

The most important adjunct to the success of the drugs is simple seduction; if used in the right context with a willing partner, these drugs are much more successful.

However, the addition of yohimbine (5 mg t.i.d. or five 5 mg tablets given 30 minutes before intercourse) can heighten the response, especially the sensation of ejaculation.[28] This drug can cause excitability and a mild increase in blood pressure.

The use of rings or a combination of a vacuum device and intracavernosal drugs can, in the older patient on a maximum dose, make a simply turgid penis into a distinctly more rigid and usable one. If the effect of the drug is not good and the patient is reluctant to have recourse to surgery or an external device, then multiple drugs are effective.[29] There appears to be pharmacological synergism when using a combination of papaverine, phentolamine, PGE1 and atropine in smaller doses. In the series reported by Montorsi and colleagues,[29] 70% of patients who had vasculogenic impotence were satisfied, 15% dropped out and 4% could not achieve an erection.

◼ LONG-TERM RESULTS

Despite the side effects, complications, lack of compliance and loss of effectiveness, the use of intracavernous vasoactive agents has been successful. In a series of 301 patients injected, 254 (84.4%) responded and were included in a self-injection programme using a variety of agents.[19] Those 47 who had not responded had a vascular aetiology. In those who responded, 56 (22%) had a psychological cause of impotence and in 198 (78%) the cause was organic, of mixed aetiology (vascular 45%, diabetic 22%, neurogenic 36%). In 98 patients (38%), self-injection was discontinued after an average of 10 months (range 1–44 months); of these, 64 were lost to follow-up. Most of the others, usually vascular patients, opted for a penile prosthesis (19), although vacuum devices and other treatments were used.

Althof and colleagues[26] have reported a drop-out rate of 46%. This poor compliance is a waste of clinical time and should be addressed. It might well improve if clinic access was easier and no pre-booked appointment was required. The establishment of more nurse practitioner-led clinics, with more time to spend discussing patient problems, may be the answer; in addition, it is important to stress that other treatment options are available. Those patients who have difficulty in injecting or subsequent pain, or who have developed fibrosis, may well be candidates for one of the newer treatment options, such as transurethral instillation of PGE1 by the medicated urethral system for erection (MUSE®).[30]

Some topical appliances[28] can be effective and the oral preparation sildenafil, a specific GMP phosphodiesterase type V inhibitor, will be available shortly.[31] This drug will reduce the numbers of patients requiring intracorporal drugs and will probably be prescribed by general practitioners. Thereafter, those patients with organic impotence who do not respond to oral therapy will be given intracorporal vasoactive drugs.

■ CONCLUSIONS

In general, the long-term use and the effectiveness of intracavernous agents are good. The treatment is easily available in most developed countries for anyone with genuine erectile problems. These agents have transformed many ailing marriages and relationships and given great happiness.

■ REFERENCES

1. Virag R. Intracavernous injection of papaverine for erectile failure. Lancet 1982; 2: 938

2. Brindley G S. Cavernosal alpha blockade: a new technique for investigating and treating erectile impotence. Br J Psychiatry 1983; 143: 332–337

3. Zorgniotti A W, Lefleur R S. Autoinjection of the corpus cavernosum with a vasoactive combination for vasculogenic impotence. J Urol 1985; 133: 39–41

4 Stackl W, Hanson R, Marberger M. Intracavernous injection of prostaglandin E in impotent men. J Urol 1988; 140: 66–71

5. Stackl N, Hasun R, Marberger M. The use of prostaglandin E1 for diagnosis and treatment of erectile dysfunction. World J Urol 1990; 8: 84–86

6. Stief C G, Holmquist F, Djamilian M et al. Preliminary results with nitric oxide donor linsidomine chlorhydrate in the treatment of human erectile dysfunction. J Urol 1992; 148: 1437–1440

7. Djamilian M, Stief C G, Kuczyk M, Jonas U. Follow up results of a combination of calcitonin gene related peptide and prostaglandin E in the treatment of erectile dysfunction. J Urol 1993; 149: 1296–1298

8. Costa P, Sarrazui B, Bressole F et al. Is the volume injected a parameter likely to influence the erectile response observed after intracavernous administration of an alpha blocking agent? Eur Urol 1993; 24: 43–47

9. Gerstenberg T C, Hetz P, Ollesen B, Fahrenkrug J. Intracavernous self injection with vasoactive intestinal polypeptide and phentolamine in the management of erectile failure. J Urol 1992; 147: 1277–1279

10. Martinez-Pinceiro L, Lopez-Tello J, Alonso Dorrego J M et al. Preliminary results of a comparative study with intracavernous sodium nitroprusside and prostaglandin E1 in patients with erectile dysfunction. J Urol 1995; 153: 1487–1496

11. Van Ahlen H, Peskar B A, Sticht G, Hertfelder H J. Pharmacokinetics of vasoactive substances administered into human corpus cavernosum. J Urol 1994; 151(5): 1227–1230

12. Keogh E J. Pharmacotherapy for impotence. Curr Opin Urol 1994; 4(6): 336–339

13. Pryor J P. Caverject and erectile dysfunction. J Sex Health 1994; (Suppl): S4–5

14. Linet O I, Orinc F G. Efficacy and safety of intracavernosal alprostadil in men with erectile dysfunction. N Engl J Med 1996; 334: 873–877

15. Pryor J P. Management of priapism. Curr Opin Urol 1994; 4(6): 343–345

16. Von Heyden B, Donattucci C F, Kaula N, Lue T F. Intracavernous pharmacotherapy for impotence: selection of appropriate agent and dose. J Urol 1993; 149(5 pt 2): 1288–1290

17. Lowe F C, Jarrow J P. Placebo controlled study of oral terbutaline and pseudo-ephedrine in management of prostaglandin E induced prolonged erections. Urology 1993; 42: 51–54

18. Muruve N, Hosking D H. Intracorporal phenylephrine in the treatment of priapism. J Urol 1966; 155(1): 141–143

19. Valdevenito R, Melman A. Intracavernous self injection pharmacotherapy program: analysis of results and complications. Int J Impot Res 1994; 6: 81–91

20. Chen R N, Lakin M M, Montague D K, Ausmundson S. Penile scarring with intracavernous injection therapy using Prostaglandin E1: a risk factor analysis. J Urol 1996; 155(1): 138–140

21. Chen J, Godschalk M, Katz P G, Mulligan T. Peyronies-like plaque after penile injection of Prostaglandin E. J Urol 1994; 152(3): 961–962

22. Junemann K P, Alken P. Pharmacotherapy of erectile dysfunction: a review. Int J Impot Res 1989; 1: 71–93

23. Keogh E J, Earle C M, Chew K K et al. Experience with self injection in Australia. In: Goldstein I, Lue T F (eds) The role of Alprostadil in the diagnosis and treatment of erectile dysfunction. Princeton: Excerpta Medica, 1993; 155–166

24. Moriel E Z, Rajfer J. Sodium bicarbonate alleviates penile pain induced by intracavernous injections for erectile dysfunction. J Urol 1993; 149: 1299–1300

25. el Saleh J C, Keogh E J, Chew K K et al. Does compression of the base of the penis improve the efficacy of intracavernous injection of prostaglandin E for impotence? A randomised control study. Int J Impot Res 1995; 7(1): 23–31

26. Althof S E, Turner L A, Levin S B et al. Why do so many people drop out from auto injection therapy for impotence? J Sex Marital Ther 1989; 15: 121–129

27. Marshall G A, Breza J, Lue T F. Improved haemodynamic response after long term injection of impotence. Urology 1994; 43(6): 844–848

28. Moralis A, Heaton J P W, Johnstone B. Oral and topical treatment of erectile dysfunction. Urol Clin North Am 1995; 22: 879–886

29. Montorsi F, Guazzoni G, Bergamshi F et al. Effectiveness and safety of multidrug intracavernous therapy for vasculogenic impotence. Urology 1993; 42(5): 554–558

30. Padma-Nathan H, Bennett A, Gesundheit N. Treatment of erectile dysfunction by medicated urethral system for erection (MUSE). J Urol 1995; 153: 472A

31. Gingell C J C, Jardin A, Olsson A M. UK 92,480. A new oral treatment for erectile dysfunction. A double blind placebo controlled once daily dose response study. J Urol 1996; 155: 495A

Chapter 34

Vacuum devices for erectile impotence

N. Oakley, P. Allen and K. T. H. Moore

■ INTRODUCTION

Prolific media attention and the breakdown of sexual taboos has led to an increased awareness in the population of their sexuality, and consequently, to sexual expectation being higher than ever. A decrease in the stigma of impotence, allied to an ageing world population with a prevalence of chronic disorders such as diabetes and vascular disease, means an increasing workload for the andrologist. Consequently, the treatment of sexual dysfunction has attained a higher priority than ever before.[1]

Reflecting the upsurge in interest are the huge strides taken in treatment of impotence, with options ranging from androgen therapy,[2] and medication (e.g. yohimbine),[3] through intracavernosal injection of vasoactive compounds,[4] to surgery such as penile implants[5] or even as far as vascular reconstruction.[6]

The need for a safe, reliable, reversible, non-invasive technique has led to the development of the vacuum/constriction device (VCD)[7] and, more recently, to the constriction band alone as treatment for the impotent patient.

Although such devices were initially seen as no more than 'gadgets that artificially increase the blood supply to the penis'[8] following their introduction in 1982, there subsequently has been a widespread acceptance and awareness of their use by the medical profession; such that it is suggested that by 1991, vacuum devices were prescribed more often than any other successful treatment,[9] becoming an integral part of the urologist's armamentarium.

■ HISTORY

The first report of the principle of negative pressure being applied to the field of erectile insufficiency was by Dr John King,[10] an American physician, who stated in 1874 'when there is impotency with a diminution of size of the male organ the glass exhauster should be applied to the part'. This, however, was simply a vacuum device and it was not until 1917, when a patent was granted to Dr Otto Lederer for his 'surgical device to produce erections with vacuum', that the concept of a 'compression' ring to be used in conjunction with the vacuum device was introduced.[11]

Several patents subsequently have been granted to modifications[12,13] but credit for the popularization of VCD is generally given to a Georgian entrepreneur — Geddins D. Osbon, the grandson of a Pentecostal preacher — who, reluctant to accept his own impotence or enforced abstinence, developed and constructed his 'Youth equivalent device' in the 1960s. After perfecting this on himself for over a decade, it became commercially available in 1974 and was initially marketed as Nu-Potent Inc. However, the sale of equipment and literature was banned by the US postal service, who deemed it to be pornographic. Sales recommenced as Osbon convinced the postal authorities of its value as a marital aid (rather than a sexual toy) and of the medical and educational nature of the accompanying literature. Nevertheless, sales were halted once more in 1976, when the FDA ordered trading to cease because of its concern over the efficacy and safety of the device. Collating data on its usage, Osbon eventually persuaded the FDA of its safety and value and in 1982 was granted FDA permission to market the device, to be known as the Erecaid,[14] as a prescription product — the first of its kind.

Medical acceptance slowly followed, with the work of Drs Roy Witherington and Perry Nadig being instrumental in overcoming early scepticism;[15,16] nevertheless, as late as 1988, it was still seen (even by some of its proponents) as a method to improve partial impotence[17] or as an interim or alternative to first-line therapies.[18] It was thought to have finally gained recognition with Lue's commentary in 1990 that

'I recommend a vacuum constriction device to all of my patients (except those with coagulation disorders and sickle cell disease) as the initial medical option'.[19]

PRINCIPLES OF TREATMENT

The two principles by which these devices work are:

1. A negative pressure (vacuum) device to induce an erection by increasing corporal blood flow.
2. A constriction ring (tension) around the base of the penis to prolong erection by decreasing corporal venous drainage.

The full system incorporates a plastic cylinder, vacuum pump, necessary tubing and constriction bands (Fig. 34.1). The cylinder must be large enough to fit over the erect penis and has an open base with a closed tip, apart from the connection to the vacuum pump.

The pump, penis and constriction rings are lubricated with copious amounts of water-soluble jelly and the rings are fed over a loading cone to the base of the cylinder (Fig. 34.2). The cylinder is then placed over the flaccid penis, pushing firmly against the pubis to obtain an airtight seal (if necessary, scrotal hair may need to be trimmed to effect a seal) and suction is applied with the vacuum pump to effect penile engorgement (Fig. 34.3). This was initially thought to be due to a pure increase in arterial inflow,[20] but recent evidence suggests that there is a variable contribution from back flow of venous blood.[21] Once an

erection-like state has been produced, one or more bands are slipped from the cylinder onto the base of the penis to maintain tumescence, the vacuum is released via a valve and the cylinder is removed (Fig. 34.4). The time taken to obtain an erection varies but has been reported in one study to average 2.5 minutes[22] and within 2 minutes in another study.[23] The bands are left in place for 30 minutes only (Fig. 34.5) and, if intercourse is to be prolonged past this point, the band must be removed, the erection left to subside and the whole procedure repeated. Intermittent pumping may produce a more engorged penis, enabling more satisfactory penetration, and many manufacturers advise patients to pump for 1–2 minutes, release and then pump again for 3–4 minutes[24] (Fig. 34. 6).

VARIATIONS IN EQUIPMENT

There are currently over a half a dozen different makes of VCD on the market, all using essentially the same technique but varying in their method of inducing a vacuum, in their pressure-release valves and in the constriction rings.

The initial Osbon system used mouth suction and elastic rings but, for many years now, the vacuum pumps have either been hand or battery operated, with rings made of soft latex (Fig. 34.7). The cylinder is usually clear plastic, and companies provide either different cylinder sizes or insert rings to modify the internal diameter of the base. The battery pump is generally fitted directly to the end of the cylinder; the hand-held pumps can be similarly fitted or attached to the cylinder via tubing (which tends to be more fiddly and requires two hands). Most manufacturers offer their device with battery or hand pump, although only a few offer both types of hand pump (Fig. 34. 8).

The constriction rings vary widely with regard to their thickness and grips, but some manufacturers have introduced shaped rings with a notch to fit over the urethra in an attempt to reduce ejaculatory difficulties and to concentrate pressure on to the corpora. As the complaint of many patients is an inability to maintain rather than to initiate a normal erection, some manufacturers now offer the constriction ring and applicator separately from the vacuum device[25] (Fig. 34.9).

A novel way of combining the vacuum device and congestion principle appeared briefly in the late 1980s, by using a stiff silicon condom as the vacuum device, with

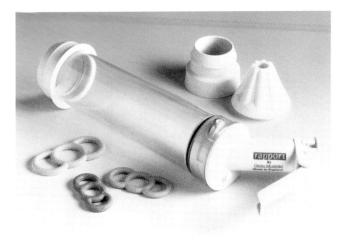

Figure 34.1. A typical VCD with hand pump, constriction rings and loader. (Rapport system; courtesy Owen Mumford Ltd, UK.)

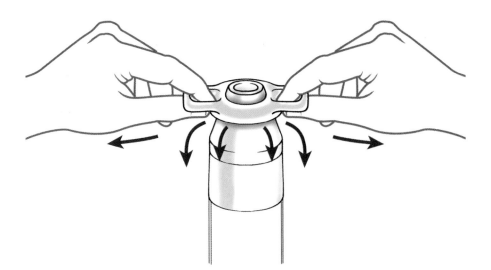

Figure 34.2. Following lubrication, the constriction ring is pulled onto the base of the cylinder with a loading cone.

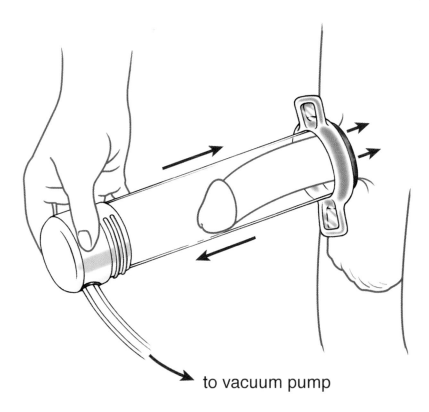

to vacuum pump

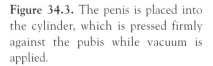

Figure 34.3. The penis is placed into the cylinder, which is pressed firmly against the pubis while vacuum is applied.

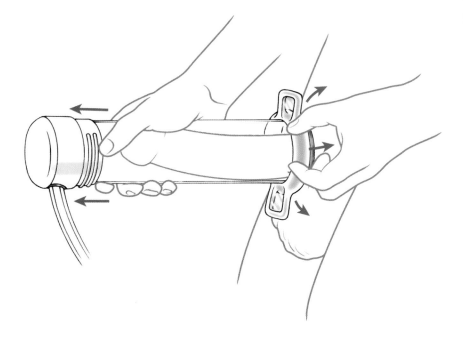

Figure 34.4. Once a satisfactory erection has been achieved, the constriction ring is pulled from the vacuum device onto the base of the penis and the cylinder is removed.

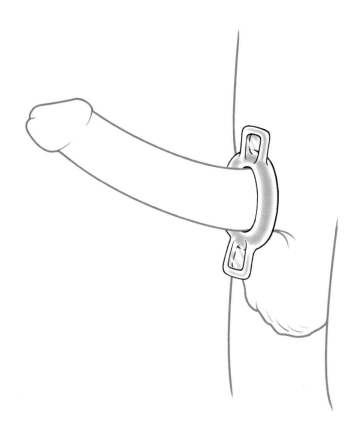

Figure 34.5. The ring maintains the erection but must be removed after 30 minutes.

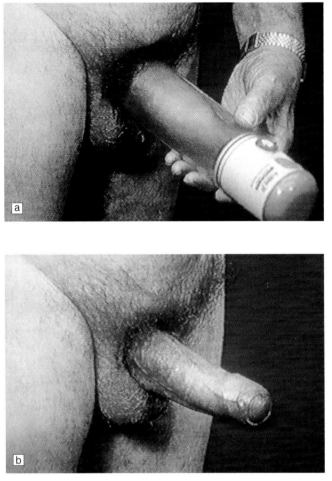

Figure 34.6. (a) Battery-operated VCD in use (Active II, Genesis Medical Ltd, UK); (b) erection showing typical girth increase.

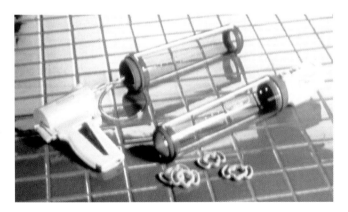

Figure 34.7. Erecaid hand and battery VCD. (Erecaid classic and plus, courtesy of Osbon Medical, UK.)

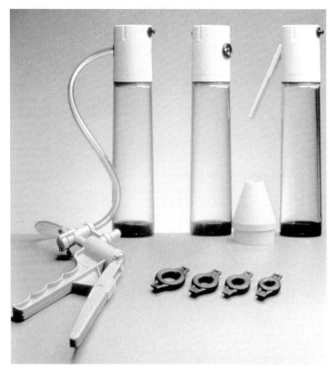

Figure 34.8. One cylinder — three possible pumps. (The 'Response' range, courtesy of Mentor Medical Systems Ltd, UK.)

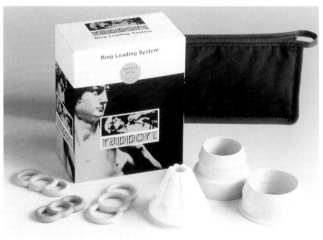

Figure 34.9. The constriction rings and applicator available separately from the vacuum cylinder. (Rapport ring loading system, courtesy Owen Mumford Ltd, UK.)

mouth suction being applied via small tubes to the base of the condom.[26] Being semi-rigid, the condom was kept on once sufficient air had been sucked out to allow penetration to occur, thereby not requiring constriction to prolong erection.[27] Marketed as the 'Correctaid', it was initially developed as treatment for Peyronie's disease after explantation of penile rods. It found little favour when compared with the Osbon technique and was abandoned as a sexual aid in the early 1990s, owing to difficulty in usage, penile irritation, penile enlargement and vaginal discomfort.[28]

■ RESULTS

The initial study on patient satisfaction was presented in 1985 by Witherington,[15] who noted that, of 201 men who were using the Erecaid system, over 90% had erectile quality sufficient for intercourse. The first objective data on the strength of erection obtained were reported in 1986 by Nadig and colleagues,[29] who stated that buckle pressures of 454 g (the minimal criterion for rigidity used by many sleep laboratories) to penile longitudinal rigidity were obtained in 27/35 patients (77%). Bosshardt and colleagues[21] have since shown that a nocturnal penile tumescence rigidity of 80% (70% being sufficient for intercourse)[30] was the norm after 6 months in their group of 26 patients.[21]

The data in the literature tend uniformly to predict successful erections being attainable in 84–95%,[22,31–34] with overall satisfaction with the device slightly less impressive due to side effects but with reported rates ranging from 72 to 94%.[31,32,35,36]

A postal study of 160 couples from the authors' centre in Sheffield confirms that 85% had erectile quality sufficient for intercourse, with 69% being satisfied and continuing to use the VCD at 1 year[37] and 50% at 3 years (personal data).

The largest patient database is held by Osbon (Erecaid), who provide all purchasers of their system with a questionnaire to be returned after 90 days' use. The last update was 1995,[38] with a total of 33 690 users reporting an initial response of 95% with good erections and continued usage of 77% at 3 months. A long-term postal study of Erecaid users by Witherington,[39] with 6902 respondents and follow-up of 2–21 years, quotes 60% satisfied and continuing to use VCD long term. Cookson and Nadig found similar figures in their review of 120 patients, with a 90% chance of attaining good-quality erections and 69% of patients continuing to use VCD 2 years down the line.[33]

Many causes for discontinuation have been cited: 43% of those patients who cease, do so for reasons not related to the device (including decreased libido, return of spontaneous erections and loss of partner); the remainder are troubled by side effects or partner dissatisfaction, or switch to other treatments.[24]

■ SIDE EFFECTS

Differences between a normal and a VCD-induced erection were first outlined by Nadig and colleagues.[29] Plethysmography shows a decreased blood flow to the penis with the band in place, causing a drop in penile skin temperature of almost 1°C. The penile skin becomes cyanosed and girth is larger than a normal erection,[21,31] owing to extracorporal congestion. All turgidity is distal to the constriction band, leaving the potential for pivoting at the base and ejaculate being trapped in the urethra proximal to the band.

Despite these differences, complications are reputed to be minimal with pain the commonest complaint, usually at the beginning of treatment.[40] This either occurs during suction (20–40%) or is related to the ring (45%). These effects are probably linked to unfamiliarity with the pump (e.g. speed and vigour of obtaining the vacuum) or choice of ring, as pain subsides with continued usage and experimentation.[33,34] Pain on ejaculation is reported in 3–16%, with an inability to ejaculate in 12–30%.[22,32,33] Petechiae of the penis is reported in 25–39%, with bruising (especially at the position of the ring) in 6–20%.[33,34] Numbness during erection is reported as a major problem in 5%, as is pivoting in a further 6%.[33]

■ SEX LIFE

Notwithstanding the difference from a normal erection, the majority of patients noted an increase in both quality and frequency of intercourse and orgasm[32] reflected in an improved self-esteem.[32,38,41] This improvement generally occurs rapidly, as 76% of patients can become proficient with the device within 5 days[38] or 4 practice sessions.[22] Despite the constriction ring, 57% said ejaculation was pleasant, with only 23% complaining of a decrease in ejaculatory pleasure.[29,38]

The effect of a compliant partner on the success of the device has long been appreciated.[38,42,43] Overall 6% of partners on the Osbon database expressed unhappiness with the VCD,[38] whereas Cookson quotes higher figures, with 11% unhappy with performance, 7% with the penile temperature and 13% with its appearance.[33]

The majority have noticed not only an improvement in sex life[32] but also an improved marital relationship.[25]

■ DIFFICULT GROUPS

Following success in the general population, the question arises as to the efficacy in potentially difficult groups.

Moul and McLeod looked at 14 patients who had an explanted prosthesis and found that eight had excellent erections with VCD.[31] As size and erectile quality improved with usage, these authors postulated that massage of scar tissue or increased corporal sinus blood flow was a beneficial factor. Interestingly, all patients commented that they wished the VCD had been available as a primary treatment. The VCD has also been shown to be of use to those who have a prosthesis in place but who find erections still unsatisfactory.[44]

Those patients in whom intracavernosal pharmacotherapy has failed and who have subsequently received VCD have been documented in a number of studies. Gould and colleagues[45] reported that 15 of 21 patients (71%) who failed to achieve satisfactory erections by intracavernosal injection subsequently received adequate rigidity and satisfactory erections with VCD. However, although similar efficacy was reported by Gilbert and Gingell[46] in 38 of 45 patients (84%) in their series, only 12 patients were satisfied with the device (27%) and Earle and colleagues[47] report a satisfaction rate as low as 9%.[47] Patient selection often holds the key here, but a further option would be to use a combination of those treatments. Marmar and colleagues[48] used VCD to augment a partial or weak response to intracavernosal injection in 22 patients; of these, 21 (95%) developed satisfactory erections with this combination therapy but few persisted with long-term treatment. Chen and colleagues[49] reported ten patients who failed both injection and VCD subjectively and objectively and in whom satisfactory erections with dramatically increased buckle pressures were obtained by using intracavernosal injections followed by application of the vacuum device without constriction ring.

Those with psychogenic impotence fare no worse than those with organic disease,[33] and others have suggested that, for these patients, it is a useful treatment combined with psychotherapy, with Segenreich and colleagues[50] reporting 12 of 38 (32%) patients eventually achieving normal erections without the pump and 23 (61%) continuing to use a VCD.

Certainly, organic impotence as a whole responds well to this type of therapy,[51] with satisfactory erections expected in at least 70% of diabetic subjects,[36,52,53] 93% of those with arteriopathy, 70% of those with venous leaks[35,54,55] and virtually 100% following radical prostatectomy.[33,44] The elderly can expect results equivalent to those achieved by the general population.[56]

The VCD has also proved popular in those in whom spinal cord injury is the cause of impotence. In such subjects it has had success — in producing erections,[57–59] improving the quality and frequency of intercourse[60] and in long-term usage — similar to that in the general population, often with improvement of the marital relationship.[61] The choice of VCD is a popular one in the spinal cord injured male, with 28/85 opting for this as a first option in a study by Watanabe and colleagues.[62] The main drawback is that, in the presence of penile hypothaesia, there lies the potential risk of leaving the ring on for too long, causing ischaemic injury,[63] or of over-vigorous suction combined with concomitant anticoagulation causing subcutaneous haemorrhage.[64] Most studies bear witness to the efficacy and safety of the procedure[65] if patients are compliant, with the number of reported incidents being low. Lloyd and colleagues[60] note that, although sweating occurred in two of the 13 spinal cord injured men in their study, none of the seven at risk with lesions T5 or above suffered autonomic dysreflexia.

■ DISCUSSION

Vacuum devices have been in use for the last two decades and are well established as a first-line therapy for impotence.[66] Comparisons between the VCD and intracavernosal pharmacotherapy show VCD to be at least as effective in initiating and maintaining an erection,[58,67] with the suggestion that, as venous leakage becomes more severe, so any superior efficacy of VCD becomes more marked.[68] There is also the suggestion that patients find the VCD preferable as a first treatment option: Gould and colleagues[45] showed that 60% of those who have successfully managed intracavernosal injection and subsequently use VCD[45] would continue use of the latter, and the experience of Turner and colleagues[69] is that there appears to be a lower drop-out rate in VCD users.

A major advantage of the VCD lies in its safety, with few serious complications reported. Those complications that are reported are linked to misuse of the device (one instance of skin necrosis, two of Peyronie's disease)[70–72] or to the constriction ring (one case of Fournier's gangrene).[73] Of particular concern is the use of non-prescription devices that are freely available from advertisements in magazines as sex aids and which are rudimentary in design. The vacuum created by VCD pumps can be in the range of 150–300 mmHg,[29] but protection is given in prescription devices by the presence of pressure valves.

The importance of the constriction ring lies in that it must not be inadvertently left in place as, during this time, penile blood flow is noted to decrease significantly[18,29,74,75] and, in one report, stopped completely.[76] Although patients have been advised on a maximum of 30 minutes empirically, evidence has reinforced this with blood gas measurements on cavernosal blood showing the presence of marked ischaemia after this time.[76] The brachial/penile pressure index returns to normal within 60 seconds of removal of the constriction ring.[74]

The authors have found that most patients show good compliance and there remain few contra-indications to a VCD. Patients with bleeding diatheses or who are receiving anticoagulant therapy do not have a significantly raised risk of complications provided that care is taken to use the VCD correctly;[77] it is rare to find those who have such severe arterial disease that they are denied a trial of a VCD. The patient with Peyronie's disease is an exception as he will require corrective surgery before the erect penis will fit into the cylinder. However, the authors generally offer a patient who complains of angulation in combination with a weaker erection a trial of VCD as, in their experience, when the penis is fully turgid minor bends of up to 30 degrees can straighten significantly. It is, of course, a suitable treatment option for those with 'bottle neck' flaccidity at the plication site following Nesbit's procedure.

The use of a vacuum device gives a man total control over his erections, which can be produced and terminated at will. The main disadvantage is the lack of spontaneity in production of an effective erection, and some men complain that the rings act as a reminder of their inadequacy.[69] However with practice and cooperation by both partners, the use of the VCD can be incorporated into foreplay with advantage for the sexual relationship. Unfortunately, the battery-operated pumps can be moderately noisy[41] and, although this is rarely embarrassing, some couples prefer to use background music or change to a hand pump.

The couples that gain most from the use of a VCD are those who are in a comfortable, well-established and mutually loving relationship, and a sense of humour is a great advantage! The authors' experience is that it is usually middle-aged or elderly couples who opt for a VCD rather than one of the more invasive methods of treatment, although they have patients as young as 18 who express satisfaction with the VCD — usually if their impotence is due to an associated disease process, such as multiple sclerosis or diabetes.

One of the disadvantages of vacuum devices is their not-inconsiderable cost (£150–300) which, in general, must be borne fully by the patient: currently, these devices are not generally available on free prescription in the UK. Although the purchase price of a VCD is comparable to the cost of 30 injections of PGE1 and thus is ostensibly financially appealing to the long-term user, drop-out rates may be lower if couples have to make the financial commitment.[41]

Understandably, many patients are unwilling to buy a VCD before they have decided that this is the treatment that they prefer. The authors find it important that couples who present to the Male Sexual Dysfunction (MSD) clinic in Sheffield are therefore given full information as to all the various options available, including full counselling by a clinical nurse specialist with considerable expertise in the field, opportunity to view videos and printed material on VCD and intracavernosal pharmacotherapy, and the opportunity to talk to psychosexual counsellors if appropriate.

Once a patient decides to try VCD, he may borrow a device for up to a month free of charge from the authors' stock of over 100 available for loan from a selection of manufacturers. The choice of VCD is a very personal thing, with couples placing emphasis on many different factors such as ease of use, telephone support and 'feel' of the device.[78] In the authors' opinion, this approach leads to better long-term usage as the majority otherwise tend to discontinue within 3 months.[33] Any difficulties can be discussed with one of the visiting representatives and, as the choice of VCD is very personal, many devices may be tried before the couple decide to buy — or, indeed, to try some other method. As a result of this scheme, the authors have a much higher usage of VCD in their clinic than is found in most MSD clinics.

Once the VCD has been selected, the authors now advise the patient to use the VCD on a daily basis as a penile exerciser, whether intercourse is attempted or not. This has the benefit of maintaining dexterity and making its use a part of a more 'natural' routine — and possibly increases natural potency.[79]

■ FUTURE PROSPECTS

In order to reduce side effects further and improve efficacy, interest has focused on modifying the technique, especially with regard to the use of the constriction band. Whereas manufacturers have worked on self-releasing devices, the efforts of clinicians have included the use of Doppler imaging to select rings that do not prevent arterial inflow,[65] while others have suggested that the vacuum device can be used as an initiator, with intracavernosal injection,[80] topical minoxidil[81] or intra-urethral PGE1[82] for prolongation. Initial experience is promising, with topical minoxidil removing the need for a ring in 12/18 (67%) and intra-urethral PGE1 in 19/19 (100%) of patients.

Further use of the vacuum device has turned full circle to King's original description without a constrictor.[10] Following reports that spontaneous erections have returned in 8–25% of patients following prolonged use of the VCD,[33,34,38,40,41] and that natural erections have significantly improved in many more,[32,34,50] speculation has been raised by Colombo and colleagues[79] in using the vacuum as a form of 'erectile trainer' to restore natural potency. They have reported a series of 52 patients in whom daily use of the vacuum without constriction ring, unrelated to intercourse, led to an improvement in spontaneous erections in 31 (60%).[79] It undoubtedly produces larger erections than normal,[21,31] and has certainly been effective in numerous patients seen in the Sheffield clinic. Indeed, the authors have a number of patients with microphallus all of whom use the vacuum alone, with improved size of both the flaccid and the erect penis.

The mechanism behind these changes is unclear but is a combination of breaking the vicious cycle of performance anxiety[50] allied to a physical effect. Arterial calibre has been shown to be improved,[76,83] but there have been conflicting reports as to whether there is an improvement in brachial/penile pressure indices.[29,56] Whether the effect needs to be maintained, and whether treatment of incipient impotence in a high-risk group such as those with diabetes can delay onset of intractable impotence raises interesting possibilities.

CONCLUSIONS

Use of a vacuum/constriction device is a safe, effective form of therapy and is one of the three treatments recently recommended by the clinical guidelines panel of the American Urological Association as those that should be offered as first-line therapy for impotence.[84] Certainly, patients themselves prefer non-invasive to surgical treatment.[85] Careful and adequate counselling, and the possibility of a home trial before making a financial commitment, are important factors in gaining patient acceptance.

REFERENCES

1. Kirby R S. Impotence: diagnosis and management of male erectile dysfunction. Br Med J 1994; 308: 957–961
2. Bancroft J, Wu F C. Changes in erectile responsiveness during androgen replacement therapy. Arch Sex Behav 1983; 12: 59–62
3. Reid K, Sturridge D H C, Morales A et al. Double blind trial in treatment of psychogenic impotence. Lancet 1987; ii: 421–423
4. Padma-Nathan H, Goldstein I, Payton T, Krane R J. Intracavernosal pharmacotherapy: the Pharmacologic Erection Program. World J Urol 1987; 5: 160–165
5. Wilson S K, Wahman G E, Lange J L. Eleven years' experience with the inflatable penile prosthesis. J Urol 1988; 139: 951–952
6. Goldstein I. Arterial revascularisation procedures. Semin Urol 1986; 4: 252–258
7. Nelson R P. Non-operative management of impotence. J Urol 1988; 139(1): 2–5
8. Baum N. Treatment of impotence — non-surgical methods. Postgrad Med J 1987; 81(7): 133–136
9. Hoffman J A S. External vacuum therapy for erectile dysfunction. An historical and clinical review. Product monograph series. Osbon Medical Systems. 1996
10. King J. The American Physician — domestic guide to health. Indianapolis: Streight & Douglass, 1874: 384
11. Lederer O. Specification of letter patent. United States Patent Office #1,225,341. Application filed Nov 29, 1913; serial No 803,853. Granted May 8 1917
12. Sell F W. Erector. US patent No 2,874,698. Feb 24 1959
13. Wilson F M. Apparatus for obtaining artificial erection. US patent No 3,744,486. July 10 1973
14. Osbon G D. Erection aid device. US patent 4,378,008. Mar 29 1983
15. Witherington R. The Osbon ErecAid system in the management of erectile impotence. J Urol 1985; 133: 190A
16. Nadig P W. Evaluation of a non-invasive device to produce and maintain an erection-like state. AUA South Central Section Meeting, 6–9 Nov 1983, St Louis MO, USA (abstr)
17. Witherington R. Suction device therapy in the management of erectile impotence. Urol Clin North Am 1988; 15(1): 123–128
18. Aloui R, Iwaz J, Kokkidis M J, Lavoisier P. A new vacuum device as alternative treatment for impotence. Br J Urol 1992; 70: 652–655
19. Lue T F. Editorial comment on Clinical experience of vacuum tumescence enhancement therapy for impotence from Int J Impot Res 1990; 1(suppl2): 191–196. In: J Urol 1991; 145: 1112
20. Diedrichs W, Kaula N F, Lue T F, Tanagho E A. The effect of subatmospheric pressure on the simian penis. J Urol 1989; 142: 1087–1989
21. Bosshardt R J, Farwerk R, Sikora R et al. Objective measurement of the effectiveness, therapeutic success and dynamic mechanisms of the vacuum device. Br J Urol 1995; 75: 786–791

22. Witherington R. Vacuum constriction device for management of erectile dysfunction. J Urol 1989; 141: 320–322

23. Sidi A A, Becher E F, Zhang G, Lewis J H. Patient acceptance of and satisfaction with an external negative pressure device for impotence. J Urol 1990; 144: 1154–1156

24. Lewis R W, Witherington R. External vacuum therapy for erectile dysfunction: use and results. World J Urol 1997; 15: 78–82

25. Althof S E, Turner L A, Levine S B et al. Through the eyes of women: the sexual and psychological responses of women to their partner's treatment with self-injection or external vacuum therapy. J Urol 1992; 147(4): 1024–1027

26. Osopa R, Williams G. Use of the 'Correctaid' device in the management of impotence. Br J Urol 1989; 63: 546–547

27. Zasler N D, Katz P G. Synergist erection system in the management of impotence secondary to spinal cord injury. Arch Phys Med Rehabil 1989; 70(9): 712–716

28. Ryder R E, Close C F, Moriarty K T et al. Impotence in diabetes: aetiology, implications for treatment and preferred vacuum device. Diabetic Med 1992; 9(10): 893–898

29. Nadig P W, Ware J C, Blumoff R. Non invasive device to produce and maintain an erection-like state. Urology 1986; 27(2): 126–131

30. Kessler W O. Nocturnal penile tumescence. J Clin Psychol 1990; 29: 439–441

31. Moul J W, McLeod D G. Negative pressure devices in the explanted prosthesis population. J Urol 1989; 142: 729–731

32. Turner L A, Althof S E, Levine S B et al. External vacuum devices in the treatment of erectile dysfunction: a one-year study of sexual and psychosocial impact. J Sex Marital Ther 1991; 17(2): 81–93

33. Cookson M S, Nadig P W. Long term results with vacuum constriction device. J Urol 1993; 149: 290–294

34. Baltaci S, Aydos K, Kosar A, Anafarta K. Treating erectile dysfunction with a vacuum tumescence device: a retrospective analysis of acceptance and satisfaction. Br J Urol 1995; 76(6): 757–760

35. Vrijhof H J, Delaere K P. Vacuum constriction devices in erectile dysfunction: acceptance and effectiveness in patients with impotence of organic or mixed aetiology. Br J Urol 1994; 74(1): 102–105

36. Price D E, Cooksey G, Jehu D et al. The management of impotence in diabetic men by vacuum tumescence therapy. Diabetic Med 1991; 8(10): 964–967

37. Rosario D J, Allen P A, Moore K T M. A twelve month study of external vacuum devices for the treatment of erectile dysfunction. Presented to BAUS Annual Meeting, 28–30 June 1994, Birmingham, UK

38. User survey report 1995. Data on file. Osbon Medical Systems, Augusta, GA, USA

39. Witherington R. Long term follow up (2–21 years) of users of external vacuum devices for treatment of impotence. Proceedings AUA New York Section Meeting. 9–13 Oct 1995, Istanbul, Turkey

40. Turner L A, Althof S E, Levine S B et al. Treating erectile dysfunction with external vacuum devices: impact upon sexual, psychological and marital functioning. J Urol 1990; 144(1): 79–82

41. Bodansky H J. Treatment of male erectile dysfunction using the active vacuum assist device. Diabetic Med 1994; 11: 410–412

42. Villeneuve R, Corcos J, Carmel M. Assisted erection follow-up with couples. J Sex Marital Ther 1991; 17(2): 94–100

43. Segenreich E, Israilov S R, Shmueli J et al. Psychotherapy combined with use of the vacuum constrictive device for erectile impotence. [in Hebrew] Harefuah 1994; 126(11): 633–636, 692

44. Korenman S G, Viosca S P. Use of a vacuum tumescence device in the management of impotence in men with a history of penile implant or severe pelvic disease. J Am Geriatr Soc 1992; 40(1): 61–64

45. Gould J E, Switters D M, Broderick G A, deVere White R W. External vacuum devices: a clinical comparison with pharmacologic erections. World J Urol 1992; 10: 68–70

46. Gilbert H W, Gingell J C. Vacuum constriction devices: second-line conservative treatment for impotence. Br J Urol 1992; 70(1): 81–83

47. Earle C M, Seah M, Coulden S E et al. The use of the vacuum erection device in the management of erectile impotence. Int J Impot Res 1996; 8(4): 237–240

48. Marmar J L, DeBenedictis T J, Praiss D E. The use of a vacuum constrictor device to augment a partial erection following an intracavernous injection. J Urol 1988; 140(5): 975–979

49. Chen J, Godschalk M F, Katz P G, Mulligan T. Combining intracavernous injection and external vacuum as treatment for erectile dysfunction. J Urol 1995; 153(5): 1476–1477

50. Segenreich E, Israilov S R, Shmueli J, Servadio C. Vacuum therapy combined with psychotherapy for management of severe erectile dysfunction. Eur Urol 1995; 28(1): 47–50

51. Almara Schiavo R, Pomerol Monseny J M. Penile erection using vacuum devices: our experience with 100 impotent patients with organic pathology. [in Spanish] Arch Esp Urol 1993; 46(10): 901–904

52. Kaplan F J, Levitt N S, Stevens P J, Phillips C. Non-invasive management of organic impotence. S Afr Med J 1995; 85(4): 276–278

53. Wiles P G. Successful non-invasive management of erectile impotence in diabetic men. Br Med J [Clin Res] 1988; 296: 161–162

54. Blackard C E, Borkon W D, Lima J S, Nelson J. Use of vacuum tumescence device for impotence secondary to venous leakage. Urology 1993; 41(3): 225–230

55. Kolettis P N, Lakin M M, Montague D K et al. Efficacy of the vacuum constriction device in patients with corporeal venous occlusive dysfunction. Urology 1995; 46(6): 856–858

56. Korenman S G, Viosca S P, Kaiser F E et al. Use of a vacuum tumescence device in the management of impotence. J Am Geriatr Soc 1990; 38(3): 217–220

57. Heller L, Keren O, Aloni R, Davidoff G. An open trial of vacuum penile tumescence: constriction therapy for neurological impotence. Paraplegia 1992; 30(8): 550–553

58. Chancellor M B, Rivas D A, Panzer D E et al. Prospective comparison of topical minoxidil to vacuum constriction device and intracorporeal papaverine injection in treatment of erectile dysfunction due to spinal cord injury. Urology 1994; 43(3): 365–369

59. Seckin B, Atmaca I, Ozgok Y et al. External vacuum device therapy for spinal cord injured males with erectile dysfunction. Int Urol Nephrol 1996; 28(2): 235–240

60. Lloyd E E, Inder M D, Toth L L. Vacuum tumescence: an option for spinal cord injured males with erectile dysfunction. SCI Nurse 1989; 6(2): 25–28

61. Denil J, Ohl D A, Smythe C. Vacuum erection device in spinal cord injured men: patient and partner satisfaction. Arch Phys Med Rehab 1996; 77(8): 750–753

62. Watanabe T, Chancellor M B, Rivas D A et al. Epidemiology of current treatment for sexual dysfunction in spinal cord injured men in the USA model spinal cord injury centers. J Spinal Cord Med 1996; 19(3): 186–189

63. LeRoy S C, Pryor J L. Severe penile erosion after use of a vacuum suction device for management of erectile dysfunction in a spinal cord injured patient. Case report. Paraplegia 1994; 32(2): 120–123

64. Rivas D A, Chancellor M B. Complications associated with the use of vacuum constriction devices for erectile dysfunction in the spinal cord injured population. J Am Paraplegia Soc 1994; 17(3): 136–139

65. Aloni R, Heller L, Keren O et al. Noninvasive treatment for erectile dysfunction in the neurogenically disabled population. J Sex Marital Ther 1992; 18(3): 243–249

66. National Institutes of Health. NIH Consensus statement. Impotence 1992; 10(4): 21–22

67. Wada H, Sato Y, Suzuki N et al. A study on the erectile response with the vacuum constriction device compared with intracavernous injection of a vasoactive drug. [in Japanese] Jpn J Urol 1995; 86(2): 321–324

68. McMahon C G. Nonsurgical treatment of cavernosal venous leakage. Urology 1997; 49(1): 97–100

69. Turner L A, Althof S E, Levine S B et al. Twelve-month comparison of two treatments for erectile dysfunction: self-injection versus external vacuum devices. Urology 1992; 39(2): 139–144

70. Meinhardt W, Kropman R F, Lycklama a Nijeholt A A B, Zwartendijk J. Skin necrosis caused by use of negative pressure device for erectile impotence. J Urol 1990; 144: 983

71. Hakim L S, Munarriz R M, Kulaksizoglu H et al. Vacuum erection associated impotence and Peyronie's disease. J Urol 1996; 155(2): 534–535

72. Kim J H, Carson C C III. Development of Peyronie's disease with the use of a vacuum constriction device. J Urol 1993; 149: 1314

73. Theiss M, Hofmockel G, Frohmuller H G. Fournier's gangrene in a patient with erectile dysfunction following use of a mechanical erection aid device. J Urol 1995; 153(6): 1921–1922

74. Marmar J L, DeBenedictis T J, Praiss D E. Penile plethysmography on impotent men using vacuum constrictor devices. Urology 1988; 32(3): 198–203

75. Katz P G, Haden H T, Mulligan T, Zasler N D. The effect of vacuum devices on penile hemodynamics. J Urol 1990; 143(1): 55–56

76. Broderick G A, McGahan J P, Stone A R, White R D. The hemodynamics of vacuum constriction erections: assessment by color Doppler ultrasound. J Urol 1992; 147(1): 57–61

77. Limoge J P, Olins E, Henderson D, Donatucci C F. Minimally invasive therapies in the treatment of erectile dysfunction in anticoagulated cases: a study of satisfaction and safety. J Urol 1996; 155(4): 1276–1279

78. Salvatore F T, Sharman G M, Hellstrom W J. Vacuum constriction devices and the clinical urologist: an informed selection. Urology 1991; 38(4): 323–327

79. Colombo F, Cogni M, Deiana G et al. Vacuum terapia. [Vacuum therapy]. [in Italian] Arch Ital Urol Nefrol Androl 1992; 64(3): 267–269

80. Bellorofonte C, Dell'Acqua S, Mastromarino G et al. Dispositivi esterni: a quali pazienti proporli? [External devices: for which patients?] [in Italian] Arch Ital Urol Nefrol Androl 1995; 67(5): 293–298

81. Cecchi M, Sepich C A, Felipetto R et al. Vacuum constriction device and topical minoxidil for management of impotence. Arch Esp Urol 1995; 48(10): 1058–1059

82. John H, Lehmann K, Hauri D. Intraurethral prostaglandin improves quality of vacuum erection therapy. Eur Urol 1996; 29(2): 224–226

83. Donatucci C F, Lue T F. The effect of chronic external vacuum device usage on cavernous artery function. Int J Impot Res. 1992; 4: 149–155

84. Montague D K, Barada J H, Belker A M et al. Clinical guidelines panel on erectile dysfunction: summary report on the treatment of organic erectile dysfunction. American Urological Association. J Urol 1996; 156(6): 2007–2011

85. Dewire D M, Todd E, Meyers P. Patient satisfaction with current impotence therapy. Wis Med J 1995; 94(10): 542–544

Chapter 35

Treatment of venous leakage: techniques and outcomes

J. A. Vale

■ INTRODUCTION

There can be few areas of andrology that provoke such heated debate and such polarized views as the treatment of veno-occlusive dysfunction. Some argue that it fails to address the primary pathology — which is probably a failure of cavernosal smooth muscle relaxation or elasticity — and therefore do not advocate surgery on this basis. Others have recommended increasingly sophisticated surgical approaches directed at the site of venous drainage diagnosed on cavernosography. A third group believe that there is a role for ligation of the deep dorsal vein to increase venous resistance, on the grounds that, although this may not address the primary pathology, it is an intermediate day-case operation with a success rate of 40–50% at 1 year in a group of patients in whom the only other options are a vacuum device or penile implant surgery.

Before discussing surgical options, it is important to review the basic venous anatomy of the penis, the physiology of venous mechanisms in erection, and the pathophysiology of veno-occlusive dysfunction.

■ PENILE VENOUS ANATOMY

Venous drainage of the penis is via three main venous systems — the superficial system, which drains the skin and subcutaneous tissues, the intermediate system, which drains the pendulous portion of the penis, and the deep system, which drains the proximal corpora cavernosa and the crura.[1]

Superficial system

This is the least important route of venous drainage in functional terms. Multiple superficial veins run on the dorsolateral surface of the penis between Buck's and Colles' fasciae and unite at the base of the penis to drain into one (usually the left) or both saphenous veins (Fig. 35.1).

Intermediate system

This is based on the deep dorsal vein (DDV). The DDV arises from multiple small veins (five to eight) emerging from the glans penis — the retrocoronal plexus. As it runs proximally, the DDV has multiple tributaries — the circumflex veins — that usually number three to 12 (Fig. 35.2). These arise from the emissary veins, which pass through the tunica albuginea, carrying blood from the endothelial-lined lacunar spaces of the corpora cavernosa.

The circumflex veins can be seen running dorsolaterally on the surface of the tunica albuginea and may communicate with each other, with their contralateral counterparts and the lateral veins of the penis.

The DDV is usually a single large channel running in the groove between the corpora cavernosa, and it enters the pelvis by passing through the suspensory ligament. It drains into the periprostatic plexus and thence into the perivesical plexus and internal iliac veins. The DDV usually has three to eight bicuspid valves along its entire length.[1,2]

In cadaveric studies,[1] the most common anatomical variant of the intermediate system is branching of the DDV in the proximal half of the penis into two or more veins draining separately into the periprostatic plexus. Communication between the intermediate and superficial venous systems is also found, and not infrequently there is a communication with the cavernous veins deep to the suspensory ligament.

Deep venous system

Emissary veins in the proximal one-third of the penis join to form two to five large cavernous veins, which themselves unite to form one or two larger veins on the dorsomedial surface of each corpus cavernosum. These run deep and medial to the cavernosal arteries, pass between the urethral bulb and crura, and then course laterally for 2–3 cm to drain into the internal pudendal veins (Fig. 35.3). As with the DDV, variations are common: there are often connections between the cavernous veins and the periprostatic plexus and with the contralateral cavernous veins.

In most men, three or four small crural veins arise from the dorsolateral surface of the crus on each side and coalesce to form a single large channel draining into the internal pudendal vein.

■ PHYSIOLOGY OF THE PENILE VENOUS SYSTEM

In the flaccid penis, the trabecular smooth muscle of the corpora cavernosa is contracted and venous drainage occurs relatively freely in a situation of low outflow resistance.[3] During tumescence the cavernosal smooth muscle relaxes, permitting filling of the lacunar spaces with blood. The resulting rise in intracavernous pressure causes compression of the subtunical venous plexus against the tunica albuginea (Fig. 35.4), increasing outflow resistance.[4] As the intrapenile blood pressure increases towards systolic blood pressure, the penis

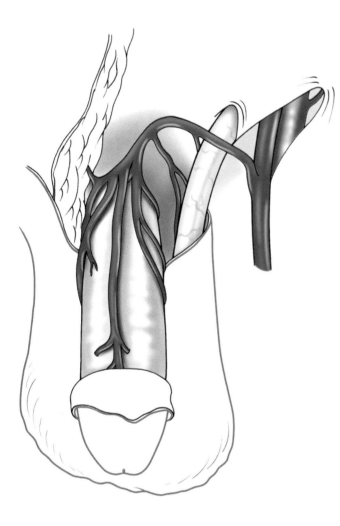

Figure 35.1. Superficial venous system. This comprises multiple prominent veins on the dorsolateral surface of the penis, running between Colles' and Buck's fasciae.

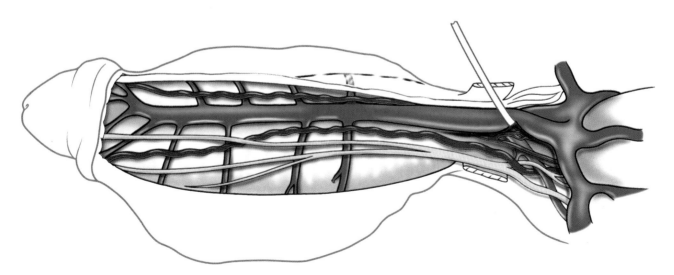

Figure 35.2. Intermediate venous system. This lies deep to Buck's fascia, and includes the deep dorsal vein (DDV) and circumflex veins. The latter arise in the distal two-thirds of the penis and drain into the deep dorsal vein.

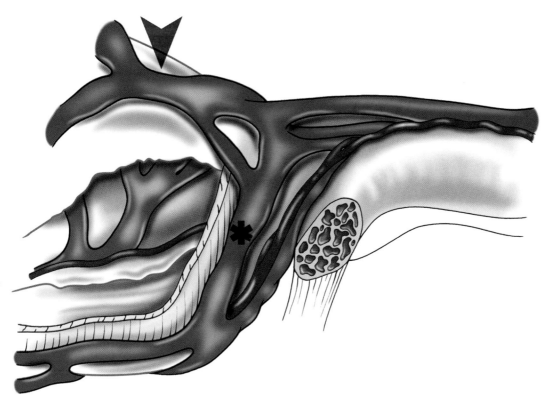

Figure 35.3. Lateral view of the base of the penis showing the DDV draining into the periprostatic plexus (arrowhead) and the cavernous veins draining into the internal pudendal vein (*).

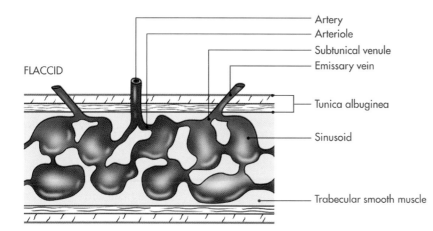

Figure 35.4. Diagrammatic representation of the corpus cavernosum in the flaccid and erect state. During erection the trabecular smooth muscle is relaxed, the sinusoids are filled with blood and the resulting rise in intracavernosal pressure compresses the subtunical venules against the tunica.

becomes rigid and this passive venous compression is maximal. At full erection, the emissary veins are probably also occluded by stretching of the tunica albuginea. Although compression of the subtunical and emissary veins is a passive phenomenon, the primary process leading to venous occlusion is relaxation of the trabecular smooth muscle of the corpora cavernosa. This smooth muscle relaxation is under the control of nerves derived from the pelvic neural plexus.[5]

Penile erection therefore represents an equilibrium between arterial inflow and venous outflow. Detumescence occurs when vasoconstrictive (probably adrenergic)[6] impulses cause contraction of the arterial smooth muscle and the trabecular smooth muscle. This leads to a reduction in intracavernous pressure, and permits the subtunical and emissary veins to open.

VENOUS LEAKAGE AND IMPOTENCE

It was recognized in the early 1900s that there are three critical steps in the development of an erection: these are relaxation of trabecular smooth muscle, arterial dilatation and venous compression.[7] It was further demonstrated that ligation of the dorsal vein of the penis could improve erectile ability. However, this seminal work was largely ignored until the 1980s, when it was shown that venous return from the penis was reduced when men watched erotic films.[8] Subsequent physiological studies (dynamic cavernosometry) have put this beyond doubt,[9–12] with some patients requiring high infusion rates to produce and sustain an erection owing to a low outflow resistance — a failure to store.

Closure of venous channels during an erection is a passive phenomenon, and venous leakage is probably not due to any primary venous abnormality. Excised veins usually show no discernible histological change; if any change is noted, it is usually one of fibrosis, which may develop secondary to increased flow and pressure resulting from a failure of veno-occlusion.[13] The latter occurs as a result of a failure of trabecular smooth muscle relaxation; smooth muscle from patients with venous leakage shows fragmentation/loss of the basal lamina, nuclear changes and a reduction in contractile elements within the cytoplasm.[14,15] An overall reduction in smooth muscle content measured objectively using computerized image analysis has also been reported.[16,17] Organ bath studies of cavernosal smooth muscle from patients with venous

impotence have demonstrated a marked impairment of the normal relaxation response to electrical field stimulation.[18]

Of course, it is possible that the aetiology of venogenic impotence may be multifactorial, with some patients having a primary trabecular smooth muscle dysfunction and some patients having a true failure of venous occlusion. Using single potential analysis of cavernous electrical activity (SPACE), it was shown that patients who had normal penile electrical activity and proven venous leakage had a good postoperative outcome from venous leak surgery, whereas patients with abnormal electrical activity did poorly.[19] Although SPACE and its significance remain highly controversial, SPACE abnormalities are believed to correlate with pathology of the cavernosal smooth muscle or its neural supply. This study would suggest that patients with normal smooth muscle activity and venous leakage are a good prognostic group for venous leak surgery; their pathology may be one of primary venous disease. Further studies will be necessary to elucidate this.

INDICATION FOR TREATMENT OF VENO-OCCLUSIVE DYSFUNCTION

Penile venous ligation or embolization reduces the number of channels for venous outflow from the penis and therefore increases venous resistance. This has been confirmed by clinical studies in which cavernosometry has been repeated following successful therapy.[20,21] Intervention can be considered in any patient with physiological evidence of venous leakage — poor (or no) response to intracavernosal vasoactive agents and a requirement for a high infusion rate to develop and sustain an erection on pharmacocavernosometry. Prior to surgery or embolization, a functional assessment of arterial inflow should be obtained; mixed vasculogenic erectile failure will respond poorly to a procedure that simply increases vascular resistance. This is particularly important in the older patient, where erectile failure is often multifactorial.[22]

TREATMENT OPTIONS FOR VENOUS LEAKAGE

Surgery
Some enthusiasts believe that the surgical objective should be to ligate all venous channels opacified on

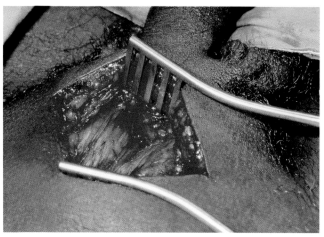

Figure 35.6. Infrapubic skin incision for penile venous ligation.

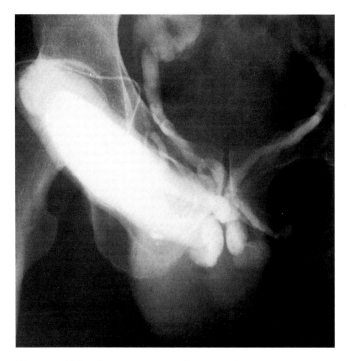

Figure 35.5. Cavernosogram demonstrating gross venous leakage, predominantly via the deep dorsal venous system.

cavernosography (Fig. 35.5), whereas others adopt a more pragmatic view and centre their surgery on ligating and dividing the DDV. The former may seem more anatomical, but it is a more major procedure and the purpose of surgery is physiological — an increase in venous resistance. The author favours an approach in which the DDV is ligated and excised together with any other large dilated veins accessible through an infrapubic incision; this will sometimes include the cavernous veins. The procedure is performed under general anaesthesia with the patient supine.

Detailed description

A transverse infrapubic incision (approximately 5 cm) is made at the base of the penis (Fig. 35.6), and the vertically running superficial veins encountered at this point are ligated with vicryl and divided. Scarpa's fascia is incised until the penis can be inverted through the wound by blunt dissection outside Buck's fascia. This is facilitated by placing a sling or Jacques' catheter around the ventral surface of the penis. This dissection is extended proximally to the suspensory ligament of the penis, which is then divided in order that the DDV can be followed as far proximally as possible; there are frequently further venous connections at this level.

Buck's fascia is then opened longitudinally in the midline to avoid damage to the deep dorsal arteries and nerves. The DDV is sometimes difficult to identify as it may be compressed by connective tissue within the angle between the two corpora cavernosa. It becomes more prominent as this tissue is gently stroked with a scalpel; the vein starts to bulge through the fascia (Fig. 35.7). Once the vein has been clearly identified, it is carefully dissected from its origin a short distance below the glans (Fig. 35.8). Assisted magnification can be helpful to find small tributaries that require careful ligation and division. As far as possible, it is best to avoid diathermy on the tunica albuginea of the corpus cavernosum; first, it is often ineffectual because the veins retract into the spongy tissue; secondly, the arteries and nerves (contained within Buck's fascia) are close to each side of the trench from which the deep vein is being removed. The DDV is

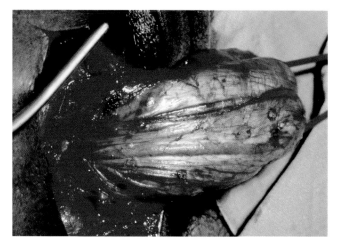

Figure 35.7. DDV exposed in the midline after incising Buck's fascia. The dorsal arteries and nerves are clearly visible laterally.

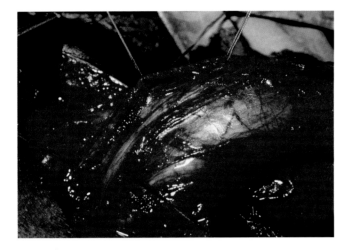

Figure 35.8. Dissection of the DDV from its origin at the retrocoronal plexus to its entry into the pelvis beneath the suspensory ligament. The circumflex veins are carefully ligated and divided as they enter the DDV.

ligated and divided as deeply as possible in the infrapubic space. Sometimes it appears to divide or receive tributaries at this level; these must be ligated also.

Before the wound is closed, any large accessory or communicating veins visible are ligated and divided. The suspensory ligament is re-approximated and a Minivac drain is inserted. The wound is extensively infiltrated with plain bupivacaine and closed in layers.

The entire procedure takes approximately 40–45 minutes, and can be performed on a day-case basis. The Minivac drain is removed at 12–24 hours. Some patients develop a minor degree of penile oedema, which settles over 2–4 weeks, and about one-half of patients experience some penile numbness, which normally resolves by 3 months.

Results of this surgical approach

In a carefully selected group of patients with normal arterial function confirmed by colour Doppler imaging and veno-occlusive dysfunction confirmed by pharmaco-cavernosometry/cavernosography,[23] 64% of patients were able to have sexual intercourse 1 year after surgery, although one-third of these required papaverine or prostaglandin self-injection. None of these patients had been able to have intercourse (with or without papaverine) prior to surgery and, when asked whether they would undergo the procedure again, 65% of patients responded positively. Interestingly, patients responding positively were not necessarily those who had a favourable outcome from surgery, illustrating the point that these patients are frequently desperate and the only

other available options — use of a vacuum device or insertion of a penile prosthesis — are less than ideal.

The infrapubic approach described above can be used for a more extensive operation in which the cavernous veins are ligated, and some of the upper crural veins may also be accessible.[24] This requires dissection of the crura from the inferior pubic rami, and can be difficult in overweight patients without perineal extension of the incision as an 'inverted J'. Alternatively, the crural veins can be approached via a separate midline perineal incision, behind the scrotum similar to that used for bulbar urethroplasty.[25] Through this incision, each crus can be felt against the inferior pubic ramus and ligated by passing a non-absorbable suture on a round-bodied needle around the crus, in apposition to the periosteum of the inferior pubic ramus superolaterally. However, this is a blind technique and there is a risk — theoretically, at any rate — of damaging the penile arteries.[1]

Debate remains as to the most appropriate surgical procedure: some say that it is mandatory to take the cavernous veins;[1] others believe that all veins identified on cavernosography should be ligated; a third group perform a procedure similar to that of the author, on the basis that it achieves the desired physiological effect. After all, in the absence of a full erection at high infusion rates, can any credence be placed on the apparent site of leakage on cavernosography, given the passive nature of venous closure mechanisms? In the author's experience, the minimalist approach achieves results comparable to those of any other group (Table 35.1).

Perhaps the most rational approach is to perform an operation limited to the DDV and then to repeat on-table cavernosometry. If the infusion rate necessary to induce and maintain an erection is still abnormal, the dissection can be extended to ligate the cavernous veins and cavernosometry repeated. If there is still significant venous incompetence, then the crural veins can be accessed by extending the incision or making a separate perineal incision.

Embolization

This would seem to be an ideal non-operative treatment option for veno-occlusive dysfunction, allowing treatment to be directed anatomically to the main venous systems. It can be performed under local anaesthesia and via one of two routes: antegradely via the DDV (transpenile) and retrogradely via the femoral vein. In the transpenile procedure, a 1–3 cm incision is made over the

Table 35.1. Outcome studies of venous leak surgery

Approach	Reference	Outcome			
		Good (%)*	Improved (%)**	Initially good (%)	Follow-up (months)
DDV	32	80		n/a	1
DDV, cavernous, crural	33	69		n/a	4
Directed by cavernosogram	34	24	24	64	15 (mean)
DDV	35	33	30	–	12 (mean)
Directed	36	24	17	74	>12
DDV, cavernous, crural	37	61		94	>12
DDV, cavernous	38	40	23	93	>12
DDV	39	45	18	70	>12

* Good outcome: spontaneous erections sufficient for intercourse.
** Improved: erections sufficient for intercourse with the aid of intracavernosal injection.
DDV, deep dorsal vein.

midline of the penis and the DDV is cannulated under direct vision. The retrograde technique is performed by standard puncture of the femoral vein and appropriate guidewires to direct a catheter into the deep pelvic venous system. Contrast is injected to delineate the anatomy, and platinum coils and sclerosant are introduced as necessary. The technique is directed to the sites of leakage shown on the pre-operative cavernosogram.

Embolization is technically possible in up to 90% of patients,[21,26] and post-procedure cavernosometry has confirmed a reduction in the infusion rate necessary to maintain an erection in patients with a successful outcome.[21] In terms of potency, results have been broadly comparable with those of surgery, with return of spontaneous erections in 25–40% of patients.[21,26] However, currently there is a paucity of long-term follow-up data.

Some have tried to combine surgery with embolization, inserting a cannula into the DDV at the time of ligation and then placing coils into any remaining points of leakage in the deep perineum/pelvis. This produced only minimal improvement, compared with the results of surgery alone.[27]

■ INVESTIGATION AND MANAGEMENT OF TREATMENT FAILURES

With a success rate of only 50% at 1 year, it is important to have a strategy for the management of treatment failures (Fig. 35.9). Failure may arise from inadequate patient selection, although it is hoped that, with the use of some form of pre-operative arterial assessment, patients with mixed vasculogenic disease will have been counselled against this surgery. Other causes of failure include failure to raise venous resistance sufficiently by tying off insufficient venous channels, the opening up of venous collaterals, or progression of the primary disease which, as stated earlier, is likely to be a change in cavernosal elasticity/contractility.

In the first instance it is important to ascertain response to pharmacotherapy, as patients who have been converted from non-responders to responders can be managed using this modality; they are really 'partial successes'. If the patient fails to respond to intracavernosal injection of a vasodilator, then logically a further cavernosometric/graphic study should be

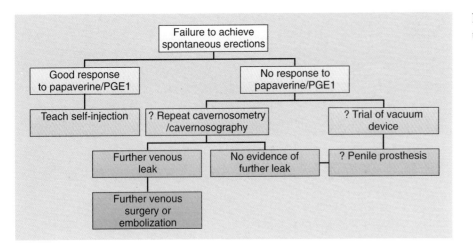

Figure 35.9. Treatment algorithm for the management of treatment failures.

conducted to identify the site of leakage. However, further investigation is justified only if an additional procedure is under consideration — and there is really a law of diminishing returns, with the likelihood of success decreasing with each additional failed procedure. This should be discussed with the patient, and some patients and many surgeons prefer to consider some alternative treatment modality such as penile implant surgery, or trial of a vacuum device/penile constriction ring. In theory, the latter should enable the patient to have intercourse, and it is a useful temporizing manoeuvre while the patient considers the more drastic alternatives.

If postoperative cavernosography is performed, the most common site of ongoing leakage appears to be cavernous–spongiosal,[28,29] and this can be corrected by spongiolysis.[30] This is carried out through a circumcision incision, and the glanular corpus spongiosum is carefully dissected from the distal limits of the corpora cavernosa, ligating any veins encountered. Any other sites of leakage can be approached in the ways discussed previously.

THE FUTURE

It is possible that surgery will become an outdated treatment for this condition if the primary problem is a failure of cavernosal relaxation. Sildenafil potentiates cavernosal smooth muscle relaxation by inhibiting type V phosphodiesterase and causing an accumulation of cGMP.[31] It may well be effective in patients with veno-occlusive dysfunction, although none of the sildenafil papers published to date have addressed this particular group.

CONCLUSIONS

Ligation and division of the DDV of the penis attempts to increase venous resistance in patients with veno-occlusive dysfunction, enabling 70% of patients to return to intercourse in the short term. Although longer-term results are less satisfactory, this minor surgical procedure still has a role, because alternative treatment options — such as penile implant surgery — are far from perfect. More extensive venous operations have not been widely adopted as they have not resulted in a dramatic improvement in outcome. After all, the purpose of surgery is to increase vascular resistance, not to prevent all venous outflow from the penis.

Unlike penile implant surgery, venous ligation does not prevent patients from benefiting from any future developments: if sildenafil is effective in veno-occlusive failure, postoperative patients will have as high a chance — if not a higher one — of responding.

REFERENCES

1. Breza J, Aboseif S R, Orvis B R et al. Detailed anatomy of penile neurovascular structures: surgical significance. J Urol 1989; 141: 437–443

2. Fitzpatrick T J, Cooper J F. A cavernosogram study on the valvular competence of the human deep dorsal vein. J Urol 1975; 113: 497–499

3. Wespes E, Schulman C. Venous impotence: pathophysiology, diagnosis and treatment. J Urol 1993; 149: 1238–1245

4. Fournier G R Jr, Juenemann K P, Lue T F, Tanagho E A. Mechanism of venous occlusion during canine penile erection: an anatomic demonstration. J Urol 1987; 137: 163–167

5. Juenemann K P, Luo J A, Lue T F, Tanagho E A. Further evidence of venous outflow restriction during erection. Br J Urol 1986; 58: 320–324

6. Brindley G S. Neurophysiology. In: Kirby R S, Carson C, Webster G D (eds). Impotence: diagnosis and management of male erectile dysfunction. Oxford: Butterworth–Heinemann, 1991: 27–31

7. Wooten J S. Ligation of the dorsal vein of the penis as a cure for atonic impotence. Texas Med J 1903; 18: 325–328

8. Wagner G, Uhrenholdt A. Blood flow measurement by clearance methods in the human corpus cavernosum in the flaccid and erect states. In: Zorgniotti A, Rossi G (eds). Vasculogenic impotence (Proceedings of the First International Conference on Corpus Cavernosum Revascularization). Springfield: Charles C. Thomas, 1980: 42–48

9. Lue T F, Takamura T, Schmidt R A et al. Haemodynamics of erection in the monkey. Urology 1983; 130: 1237–1241

10. Lue T F, Hricak H, Schmidt R A, Tanagho E A. Functional evaluation of penile veins by cavernosography in papaverine-induced erection. J Urol 1986; 135: 479–482

11. Aboseif S R, Breza J, Lue T F, Tanagho E A. Penile venous drainage in erectile dysfunction. Anatomical, radiological and functional considerations. Br J Urol 1989; 64: 183–189

12. Eardley I, Vale J A, Holmes S et al. Pharmacocavernometry in the assessment of erectile impotence. J R Soc Med 1990; 83: 22–25

13. Hirsch M, Lubetsky R, Goldman H et al. Dorsal vein sclerosis as a predictor of outcome in penile venous ligation surgery. J Urol 1993; 150: 1810–1813

14. Persson C, Diederichs W, Lue T F et al. Correlation of altered penile ultrastructure with clinical arterial evaluation. J Urol 1989; 142: 1462–1468

15. Jevitch M J, Khawand N Y, Vidic B. Clinical significance of ultrastructural findings in the corpora cavernosa of normal and impotent men. J Urol 1990; 143: 289–293

16. Wespes E, Moreira de Goes P, Schiffmann S et al. Computerized analysis of smooth muscle fibers in potent and impotent patients. J Urol 1991; 146: 1015–1017

17. Wespes E, Moreira de Goes P, Sattar A A, Schulman C. Objective criteria in the long-term evaluation of penile venous surgery. J Urol 1994; 152: 888–890

18. Pickard R S, King P, Zar M A, Powell P H. Corpus cavernosal relaxation in impotent men. Br J Urol 1994; 74: 485–491

19. Stief C G, Djamilian M, Truss M C et al. Prognostic factors for the postoperative outcome of penile venous surgery for venogenic erectile dysfunction. J Urol 1994; 151: 880–883

20. Yu G W, Schwab F J, Melograna F S et al. Preoperative and postoperative dynamic cavernosography and cavernosometry: objective assessment of venous ligation for impotence. J Urol 1992; 147: 618–622

21. Schild H H, Muller S C, Mildenberger P et al. Percutaneous penile venoablation for treatment of impotence. Cardiovasc Intervent Radiol 1993; 16: 280–286

22. Mulligan T, Katz P G. Why aged men become impotent. Arch Intern Med 1989; 149: 1365–1366

23. Vale J A, Feneley M R, Lees W R, Kirby R S. Venous leak surgery: long term follow up of patients undergoing excision/ligation of the deep dorsal vein of the penis. Br J Urol 1995; 76: 192–195

24. Williams G. Venous leak and its correction. In: Kirby R S, Carson C, Webster G D (eds). Impotence: diagnosis and management of male erectile dysfunction. Oxford: Butterworth–Heinemann, 1991: 177–183

25. Bar-Moshe O, Vandendris M. Treatment of impotence due to perineal venous leakage by ligation of crura penis. J Urol 1988; 139: 1217–1219

26. Schwartz A N, Lowe M, Harley J D, Berger R E. Preliminary report: penile vein occlusion therapy: selection criteria and methods used for the transcatheter treatment of impotence caused by venous–sinusoidal incompetence. J Urol 1992; 148: 815–820

27. Fowlis G A, Sidhu P S, Jager H R et al. Preliminary report — combined surgical and radiological penile vein occlusion for the management of impotence caused by venous–sinusoidal incompetence. Br J Urol 1994; 74: 492–496

28. Kerfoot W W, Carson C C, Donaldson J T, Kliewer M A. Investigation of vascular changes following penile vein ligation. J Urol 1994; 152: 884–887

29. Rajfer J, Mehringer M. Cavernosography following clinical failure of penile vein ligation for erectile dysfunction. J Urol 1990; 143: 514–517

30. Gilbert P, Stief C. Spongiolysis: a new surgical treatment of impotence caused by distal venous leakage. J Urol 1987; 138: 784–786

31. Jeremy J Y, Ballard S A, Naylor A M et al. Effects of sildenafil, a type-5 cGMP phosphodiesterase inhibitor, and papaverine on cyclic GMP and cyclic AMP levels in the rabbit corpus cavernosum in vitro. Br J Urol 1997; 79: 958–963

32. Wespes E, Schulman C C. Venous leakage: surgical treatment of a curable cause of impotence. J Urol 1985; 133: 796–798

33. Williams G, Mulcahy M J, Hartnell G, Kiely E. Diagnosis and treatment of venous leakage: a curable cause of impotence. Br J Urol 1988; 61: 151–155

34. Lewis R W. Venous surgery for impotence. Urol Clin North Am 1988; 15: 115–121

35. Treiber U, Gilbert P. Venous surgery in erectile dysfunction: a critical report on 116 patients. Urology 1989; 34: 22–27

36. Freedman A L, Neto F C, Mehringer C M, Rajfer J. Long-term results of penile vein ligation for impotence from venous leakage. J Urol 1993; 149: 1301–1303

37. Montague D K, Angermeier K W, Lakin M M, Ignaut C A. Penile venous ligation in 18 patients with 1 to 3 years of follow up. J Urol 1993; 149: 306–307

38. Hwang T I, Yang C. Penile vein ligation for venogenic impotence. Eur Urol 1994; 26: 46–51

Chapter 36

Microvascular arterial bypass surgery for arteriogenic erectile dysfunction

J. Mulhall, M. D. LaSalle and I. Goldstein

■ INTRODUCTION

Erectile dysfunction (ED) is defined as the consistent inability to achieve or maintain a penile erection satisfactory for sexual performance.[1] Community epidemiological studies have revealed that 52% of non-institutionalized, free-living, community-based men between the ages of 40 and 70 years have self-reported minimal (17%), moderate (25%), and complete (10%) forms of erectile dysfunction.[2] Non-surgical treatment alternatives for ED include psychological, endocrinological, neurological, pharmacological and external device interventions.[3–17] While newer forms of pharmacological treatments continue to evolve, including oral,[18,19] topical[19] and intra-urethral delivery agents,[20] surgical interventions for ED still have an important role in management.

Surgical interventions have consisted primarily of penile prosthesis insertion and microvascular arterial bypass surgery.[21] Venous leak surgery for corporal veno-occlusive dysfunction, popular among urologic surgeons in the mid 1980s to early 1990s, has been associated with poor long-term success rates and this surgical procedure is no longer widely utilized. The American Urological Association Clinical Guidelines Panel on Erectile Dysfunction has recommended only one surgical treatment alternative as standard care for the patient with acquired organic ED — that is, the use of implantation of penile prostheses.[22] These guidelines still consider arterial surgery to be experimental. Currently, penile re-vascularization is the only treatment modality with the capability of permanently restoring fully natural penile erections without the necessity for external mechanical devices, chronic use of vasoactive medication or surgical placement of internal penile prosthetic devices.

Historically, the first cases of penile arterial bypass surgery for ED were reported by Michal in the early 1970s using the inferior epigastric artery as the donor vessel.[23,24] Subsequent modifications by Virag and others resulted in a multitude of procedures that included the use of the deep dorsal vein as the recipient vessel.[25–28] It is documented that there are over 100 different variations of surgeries entitled 'penile revascularization surgery'. Lack of standardized techniques and selection criteria may have contributed to the current low popularity of arterial revascularization such that no one procedure has been universally accepted. Follow-up of patients undergoing microvascular arterial bypass surgery for impotence has been limited. It is the purpose of this chapter to re-assess the role of microvascular arterial bypass surgery for arteriogenic ED.

The ultimate goal of microvascular arterial bypass surgery for ED is to provide an alternative arterial pathway beyond obstructive arterial lesions in the iliohypogastric–cavernous arterial bed. Utilizing this technique, cavernosal arterial perfusion pressure and arterial inflow can be increased, thereby offering a potential cure to patients with ED secondary to pure arterial insufficiency. A successful outcome will improve erectile haemodynamics during sexual stimulation, by conferring a more rigid (increased arterial perfusion pressure) and more spontaneous (increased arterial inflow) penile erection.[29–31] New objective follow-up data to examine the safety and efficacy of a specific type of microvascular arterial bypass surgery for the cure of arteriogenic ED are presented in this chapter. In this light, it may be shown that, under certain conditions, arterial surgery is a safe and effective treatment opportunity.

HISTORY OF PENILE REVASCULARIZATION SURGERY

Donor artery–recipient tunica albuginea procedures

The origin of small-vessel surgery to restore erectile potency is derived from the work of the Czechoslovakian vascular surgeon Vaclav Michal.[23,24] In 1973 (interestingly, also the year of the report of the first inflatable penile implant by Scott), Michal reported that he had performed a series of end-to-side anastomoses between the inferior epigastric artery and a defect made in the side of the tunica albuginea of the corpus cavernosum (Michal I procedure) as treatment for erectile dysfunction.[23,32] The most problematic aspects of the Michal I procedure were initial priapism and/or poor long-term patency of the arterial–tunical anastomosis. Occlusion of the anastomosis between the inferior epigastric artery and the tunica was most commonly encountered. Nevertheless, the initial work by Michal was significant because it opened the door for the first time to the possibility of using small-vessel microvascular bypass surgery as a treatment to cure ED without artificial mechanical devices.

Donor artery–recipient artery procedures
Donor artery–recipient dorsal penile artery

In the continuing clinical research by Michal, a Michal II procedure was developed. In 1980, he reported a new series of vascular reconstructive procedures in which the inferior epigastric artery was anastomosed end-to-side to the dorsal artery of the penis.[33] As was not the case in the original procedure, Michal experienced patients with long-term patency of the vascular anastomoses. Others who performed the Michal II also observed good results.

Several authors reported their series of Michal II variations. Such surgeries involved anastomosis of the inferior epigastric artery to the dorsal penile artery, either end-to-end in the proximal direction, end-to-end in the distal direction or end-to-side. These procedures were performed when there was an obstruction proximal to the bifurcation of the internal pudendal artery into its cavernous and penile branches.[34] Sharlip in 1984 introduced his modification to Michal II by anastomosing the inferior epigastric artery to the proximal dorsal penile artery, end-to-end fashion.[35] Carmignani and colleagues in 1987 reported a series of patients in whom an end-to-end anastomosis of the

inferior epigastric artery to the proximal stump of the transected dorsal penile artery was performed.[36] Optimal distal perfusion was also achieved by a cross end-to-side anastomosis of the distal stump of the dorsal artery to the contralateral dorsal penile artery. Few complications were reported in any series by those who used the Michal II approach. Austoni in 1992 anastomosed the inferior epigastric artery to both the distal and the proximal divided ends of the dorsal penile arteries.[37] Lund in 1995 retrieved the inferior epigastric artery laparoscopically prior to microsurgical anastomosis to the recipient vessel.[38]

Donor artery–recipient cavernosal penile artery

Crespo, an Argentinian vascular surgeon, and his colleagues in 1982 described a procedure in which he utilized the femoral artery as the neoarterial inflow source, and the recipient penile vessel was one or both of the cavernosal arteries.[27] Crespo tunnelled a reversed saphenous vein subcutaneously in the groin to accomplish the bypass. Sharlip, in 1981, had unsuccessful results with the Crespo technique, as did several others who attempted this surgery.[35] MacGregor and Konnak (1982) reported on another variant.[39] They anastomosed the inferior epigastric artery, instead of the reversed saphenous vein, directly to the cavernous artery, as did Shaw and Zorgniotti in 1984.[40] These procedures required the inferior epigastric artery to be passed through the tunica albuginea and the surrounding erectile tissue to be dissected to obtain proximal and distal control of the cavernosal artery.

Donor artery–recipient vein procedures

Ronald Virag, a French vascular surgeon, performed a series of operations (Virag I–VI) designed to revascularize the corpus cavernosum by retrograde flow of blood through the dorsal vein of the penis.[25,41] These procedures were designed to achieve revascularization in the same fashion as an arterialized vein graft for revascularization of the lower extremities or the myocardium. In the Virag I procedure, the anastomosis was between the inferior epigastric artery and the deep dorsal vein (DDV) end-to-side, with the proximal vein not ligated. In Virag II, the proximal DDV was ligated. In the Virag III procedure, the anastomosis between the inferior epigastric artery and the DDV was fashioned in an end-to-end manner. In Virag procedures IV, V and VI, a direct shunt between the DDV and the tunica albuginea of the corpus body was added to the Virag I, II and III procedures. This latter surgical manoeuvre was performed especially when vein values were encountered in the emissary veins preventing retrograde flow into the corporal bodies.

A similar operation was devised by Hauri in 1986 in which the inferior epigastric artery was anastomosed both to the dorsal penile artery and to the DDV.[26] The rationale for the surgery was that the dorsal artery and dorsal vein anastomoses together were better than individual anastomoses because the combined procedure would offer neo-arterial inflow in both the antegrade and retrograde fashion. Few others have performed this procedure. Hauri has published several articles claiming that the use of his procedure, even in diabetic patients, resulted in a high rate of success, with restoration of erectile rigidity. Juenemann in 1992 modified the Hauri procedure by creating three arteriovenous fistulae instead of one, to improve clinical results.[42] Benhathismou, in 1985, developed an alternative venous arterialization procedure.[43] This indirect revascularization of the corpora cavernosa involved the inferior epigasteric artery anastomosed end-to-side to the DDV followed by a series of side-to-side anastomoses between that vein and the corpora cavernosa. He reported satisfactory results in a limited number of patients followed up for a mean period of 12 months. In 1994, Shah and colleagues developed a new procedure (Shah–Parulkar ADVA procedure) in which the distal half of the dorsal vein was completely mobilized, divided near the glans and then flipped to lie upon the symphysis pubis where it was anastomosed end-to-end to the inferior epigasteric artery.[44]

Other procedures

Shafik in 1995 performed pudendal canal decompression through a perineal approach and reported an improvement in cases with obstruction of the internal pudendal artery on both sides with poorly visualized or non-visualized penile arteries.[45] Among others, DePalma and colleagues in 1988 attempted to restore penile erections in those with vasculogenic impotence using aorto-iliac reconstruction.[46] Such surgery did not involve anastomoses of an inflow source to a recipient penile vessel: the aorto-iliac reconstruction utilized such manoeuvres as endarterectomy of atherosclerotic plaque from the aorta, common or internal iliac artery. In 1979, Michal and colleagues reported on saphenous or prosthetic Gore-Tex (polytetrafluoroethylene) grafts from the aorta directly to the internal iliac or internal pudendal arteries to bypass large vessel arterial occlusions.[47]

■ REPORTED OUTCOMES OF PENILE REVASCULARIZATION SURGERY

The historic results of penile revascularization are difficult to compare as there are many differences in: (a) the selection of patients, (b) the choices of the procedures performed and (c) the means of assessing efficacy outcome.

Artery–tunica procedures

Metz and colleagues used the Michal I technique and reported in 1983 that the long-term results of this procedure were unsatisfactory in a study of nine patients.[48] This report did not select patients by presence or absence of accompanying corporal veno-occlusive dysfunction, nor was there any mention of the method used to assess clinical outcome.

Artery–artery procedures

Michal reported in 1980 that the success with his procedure was 78% in 138 patients followed for more than 6 months.[33] McDougal and Jeffrey, using this Michal technique, reported in 1983 that six of eight patients had long-term successful results.[49] Carmignani and colleagues in 1987 reported 80% success in five patients with pudendal or common penile artery obstruction; these authors performed end-to-end anastomosis of the inferior epigastric artery to the proximal stump of the transected dorsal penile artery.[36] Zorgniotti and Lizza subsequently rated the success of revascularization surgery as good if the patient was able to achieve satisfactory erections resulting in intercourse in 50% of attempts without using intracavernous injection.[30] In a series of 38 patients, they reported a 68% success rate at 3 months which fell to 29% at 2 years. In none of the above-mentioned reports were patients selected by presence or absence of accompanying corporal veno-occlusive dysfunction, and in none was there any mention of the means utilized to assess clinical outcome.

In 1984, Sharlip reported a 30% success rate in a series of ten patients, all of whom had arterial occlusive pathology based on a traumatic aetiology.[50] No success from revascularization surgery was found among those with cavernosal arterial insufficiency (failure to fill) from systemic atherosclerosis. In 1990, the same author reviewed the results of 45 patients with arteriogenic impotence and showed that the best results were obtained in the group that had retrograde revascularization of the dorsal penile artery (70% success and improved).[51] He found that patients with isolated arterial disease were better candidates for penile revascularization than those with diffuse arterial disease. By 1994, Lotfy and colleagues, in a study of five patients with pure arterial insufficiency, were able to report 80% success with the inferior epigastric artery anastomosed to the proximal segment of one or both dorsal arteries.[52] They recommended this procedure for patients with pure arterial insufficiency and no evidence of corporal veno-occlusive dysfunction.

Goldstein and Padma-Nathan in 1990 reviewed the results of 130 procedures of different types of revascularization with follow-up of 2 months to 5 years; they found an overall success rate of 54%.[53] Those impotent patients whose underlying arterial pathology was based on a crush injury from blunt perineal or pelvic trauma had an 81% rate of success. Goldstein and his team subsequently studied 226 patients who underwent penile revascularization and postoperative follow-up dynamic infusion cavernosometry.[54] They concluded that patients with pure arteriogenic impotence had an increased equilibrium intracavernosal pressure (intracavernosal pressure after administration of vasoactive agents) postoperatively and this improvement was correlated with a subjective improvement in erectile function postoperatively. Patients with corporal veno-occlusive dysfunction had no change in postoperative equilibrium pressure and thus were not considered candidates for microvascular arterial bypass surgery.

Jarow and Defranzo in 1996 evaluated the long-term results of arterial bypass surgery in impotent men carefully selected for non-atherosclerotic arterial vascular surgery.[55] They reported initial and final success rates of 82% and 62%, respectively, with an average follow-up of 50 months. They performed inferior epigastric to dorsal artery bypass in nine patients. In 1994, Fitch and colleagues had reported that their study of 170 patients with penile microvascular revascularization procedures suggested that patients who were smokers, had diabetes, were abusers of alcohol and who demonstrated corporal venous leakage have less chance of a successful surgical

outcome,[56] whereas patients with a history of pelvic trauma appeared to have a greater chance of excellent results.

Artery–vein procedures

Virag in 1982 reported 42% success in 12 patients with DDV arterialization and 33% showed overall improvement.[41] Grasso and colleagues, 12 years later, reported 55% success in 12 patients for whom inferior epigastric artery–DDV anastomosis was performed.[57] Neither of these reports selected patients by presence or absence of accompanying corporal veno-occlusive dysfunction, nor was there any mention of the means utilized to assess clinical outcome. Sohn and colleagues in 1990, using a combination of Hauri and Virag techniques in 20 patients, reported a 95% success rate at 3 months which fell to 80% at 12 months.[58] They defined success as the ability to have regular satisfactory intercourse. Wespes and colleagues had earlier reported 58% graft patency up to 21 months after surgery in 12 patients who underwent DDV arterialization; however, only four patients developed almost normal erections.[59] Shaw et al. in 1984 reported five successful outcomes of 12 patients in their series.[40] Furlow and colleagues reported 27 successful outcomes from 29 patients, using a modified Virag V procedure.[60] The modification was in the form of both proximal and distal ligation of the DDV.

Hauri in 1986, in 44 consecutive patients, identified an 89% success rate, including seven of seven patients with impotence associated with diabetes mellitus.[26] Melman and Riccardi in 1991 reported seven cured and four improved in a group of 18 patients with anastomosis of the inferior epigastric artery to DDV, and six cured and four improved in an 18-patient group with inferior epigastric artery anastomosed to both DDV and dorsal artery.[61] In 1991, Floth and colleagues created three different types of bypasses in an animal model:[62] the inferior epigasteric artery was anastomosed either to the dorsal penile artery, or to the dorsal artery and the dorsal vein (Hauri procedure), or to the dorsal vein alone (Virag). In the first group they found patent anastomosis without anticoagulants in three of four animals. With erection, the flow in the inferior epigastric artery and the dorsal artery increased significantly. In the combined group, the run-off was demonstrated only to the venous system. The resistance in the dorsal artery was higher and preferential neoarterial flow did not pass into this arterial system. Arterial bypass to the dorsal vein increased outflow resistance in the animal model and improved intracorporal pressure during erection in four animals. The procedure also increased the resting intracavernosal pressure which might be deleterious to corporal smooth muscle in the long term. Kaufman and Fitch in 1995 reported 46.1% excellent and 38.5% improved results in 16 patients with DDV arterialization using the dorsal artery as a neoarterial source.[63]

Other procedures

Shafik in 1995 performed pudendal canal decompression through a perineal approach.[45] He reported an improvement in 80% of cases with obstruction of the internal pudendal artery on both sides with poorly or non-visualized penile arteries. DePalma and colleagues in 1988 reported that 6–7% of impotent patients became candidates for vascular intervention by aorto-iliac reconstruction.[46] About 70% of these men were functional after operation including those functioning with intracavernous injection. They reported also that these men undergoing aorto-iliac reconstruction had a significantly higher rate of spontaneous function than those undergoing microvascular procedures. Such large vessel procedures were initially reported as successful but in the long term results were poor. The most likely explanation was that these procedures did not address the presence of distal small vessel pathology in the common penile or cavernosal arteries. In addition, most of these patients were older and had diffuse atherosclerotic vascular disease. On direct testing of the veno-occlusive mechanism, the majority of these impotent men were found to have not only the arterial abnormalities but also the presence of a 'venous leak'. It would not be expected that aorto-iliac surgery would correct this latter haemodynamic abnormality.

■ SUMMARY OF HISTORIC REVIEW OF PENILE REVASCULARIZATION PROCEDURES

The review of the literature suggests that 131 microvascular penile revascularization procedures have been reported and are theoretically possible (Table 36.1). This extensive list of procedures nevertheless excludes large vessel (aorta, common and internal iliac artery) reconstruction.

Where the tunica albuginea is the recipient structure, the two potential neoarterial inflow sources are the inferior epigastric artery or the arterialized saphenous vein. There is one anastomosis to the tunica — end-to-side.

Where the dorsal penile artery is the recipient vessel, the two potential neoarterial inflow sources are the inferior epigastric artery or the arterialized saphenous vein. There are multiple types of single anastomoses to the dorsal artery including end-to-side, end-to-end in the proximal direction, and end-to-end in the distal direction.

Where the cavernosal artery is the recipient vessel, there are three potential neoarterial inflow sources — the inferior epigastric artery, the arterialized saphenous vein and the dorsal penile artery. There are multiple types of single anastomoses to the cavernosal artery including end-to-side, end-to-end in the proximal direction, and end-to-end in the distal direction.

Where the dorsal vein is the recipient vessel, the three potential neoarterial inflow sources are the inferior epigastric artery, the arterialized saphenous vein and the dorsal penile artery. There are multiple types of single anastomoses to the dorsal vein including end-to-side and end-to-end in the proximal direction. Combinations of these may be performed. Additional variations include proximal ligation of the dorsal vein (to prevent early escape of arterialized blood to the systemic circulation), distal ligation of the dorsal vein (to prevent glans hyperaemia) or anastomosis of the arterialized deep dorsal vein directly to the tunica albuginea (to increase retrograde flow of arterialized blood to the corpora cavernosa). Additional procedures to increase venous outflow resistance may include cavernosal vein ligation with or without crural ligation, plication or banding.

Where the combination of the dorsal vein and the dorsal artery (Hauri procedure) are the recipient vessels, the two potential neoarterial inflow sources are the inferior epigastric artery or the arterialized saphenous vein. There are multiple types of single anastomoses to the dorsal vein, including end-to-side, end-to-end in the proximal direction, and end-to-end in the distal direction.

In all the above procedures, where there are multiple possible types of single anastomoses, combinations of these may be performed. Additional procedures to increase venous outflow resistance may be performed concomitantly, including deep dorsal and/or cavernosal vein ligation with or without crural ligation, plication or banding.

Table 36.1. Reported and theoretical variations of penile revascularization procedures (total 131)

Donor vessel	Recipient vessel	Anastomoses/others*	n
Inferior epigastric artery	Tunica albuginea	E–S	1
Arterialized saphenous vein	Tunica albuginea	E–S	1
Dorsal artery	Tunica albuginea	E–S	1
		DDV/CV ligation	6
		Crural plic./lig./banding	3
Inferior epigastric artery	Dorsal artery	E–S, E–E (prox), E–E (dist)	3
Arterialized saphenous vein	Dorsal artery	E–S, E–E (prox), E–E (dist)	3
		DDV/CV ligation	18
		Crural plic./lig./banding	6
Inferior epigastric artery	Cavernosal artery	E–S, E–E (prox), E–E (dist)	3
Arterialized saphenous vein	Cavernosal artery	E–S, E–E (prox), E–E (dist)	3
Dorsal artery	Cavernosal artery	E–S, E–E (prox), E–E (dist)	3
		DDV/CV ligation	27
		Crural plic./lig./banding	9
Inferior epigastric artery	Deep dorsal vein	E–S, E–E (prox)	2
Arterialized saphenous vein	Deep dorsal vein	E–S, E–E (prox)	2
Dorsal artery	Deep dorsal vein	E–S, E–E (prox)	2
		Dist/prox DDV ligation	12
		CV ligation	6
		Tunica – DDV anast.	6
		Crural plic./lig./banding	6
Inferior epigastric artery	Dorsal artery/dorsal vein	E–S	1
Arterialized saphenous vein	Dorsal artery/dorsal vein	E–S	1
		DDV/CV ligation	4
		Crural plic./lig./banding	2

*E–S, end-to-side; E–E, end-to-end; prox, proximal; dist, distal; DDV, deep dorsal vein; CV, cavernosal vein; plic., plication; lig., ligation; anast., anastomosis

RATIONALE FOR ANASTOMOSIS OF THE INFERIOR EPIGASTRIC ARTERY TO THE DORSAL PENILE ARTERY

Vickers and Vickers, in 1996, in the *International Journal of Impotence Research*, addressed similar concerns about the objectivity of outcome assessment of penile revascularization procedures.[64] They also reported that the efficacy of arterial bypass surgery was questionable. They noted that initial surgical success rates were not duplicated by subsequent studies with a larger number of patients, longer and more frequent follow-up periods, and multimodal and multimethod physiological measurements. These authors concluded that the efficacy of penile microvascular arterial bypass surgery had not yet been evaluated by outcome studies that had utilized the criteria of any ideal experiment. They further reported that, in several studies, the subject's outcome assessment was not accurately predicted by the postoperative physiological studies. For example, whereas arteriography might have demonstrated a patent penile vascular anastomosis, the patient stated that he had remained impotent. Conversely, arteriography might detect the blockage of the anastomosis, despite the patient's assertion that the operation had successfully cured his impotence. Other studies have found complete agreement between the predictive values of the physiological test and the subjective outcome claimed. The Vickers paper supports the need for objective assessment of penile revascularization surgery as a treatment for male ED.

Of note, the Vickers article was accompanied by an editorial comment by DePalma.[65] He reported that the problems with the early efforts at penile artery bypass surgery were that the patients were poorly chosen, workups were inadequate and follow-ups were sporadic. Certain revascularization procedures were neither well based physiologically nor well done. DePalma noted that the finding that sometimes potency was restored after graft closure was similar to experiences in vascular surgery: here, ischaemia and threatened limb loss were improved by bypass surgery providing temporary limb nutrition. Such bypasses, even though late patency was not achieved, could result in limb salvage.

What is the type of revascularization surgery associated with the least complications and most efficacy?

Donor artery–recipient tunica procedures

Attempts to create anastomoses between the neoarterial inflow source and the tunica albuginea have been abandoned because of associated complications and the low long-term success rates. It should not be surprising that the Michal I procedure led to the development of a form of high-flow arterial priapism. The usual form of high-flow priapism was from a lacerated cavernosal artery secondary to, for example, blunt perineal trauma after a fall onto a bicycle bar. By definition, high-flow priapism occurs with the presence of unregulated arterial inflow to the erectile tissue, bypassing the physiological regulation of the helicine arterioles.[66] Thus, the basic definition was fulfilled with the Michal I operation, that is, unregulated arterial inflow bypassing physiological helicine arterioles and passing directly to lacunar spaces. Successful patients from the Michal I procedures were similar to patients with high-flow priapism, in that they did not report

painful erections. These erections were approximately two-thirds of a full rigid erection and were able to be increased in rigidity with sexual stimulation.

The most likely explanation for long-term failure of the anastomosis of the donor artery to the tunica was that it violated an important vascular surgical principle: this principle dictates that the requirement of long-term patency of a vascular anastomosis is that an endothelial surface from one vascular structure is anastomosed to another endothelial surface of another vascular structure. Since the tunica albuginea is composed of connective tissue collagen and elastin and is not a defined vascular structure with an endothelial cell layer surface, there was no possibility of long-term patency.

The 'health' of the endothelial cells in the region of the anastomosis will dictate vascular patency. Endothelial cells that are injured or are exposed to thrombogenic surfaces will release vasoconstrictive factors dedicated to occlude the vascular anastomosis.

Hatzichristou and colleagues, in 1994, evaluated 194 blood vessel segments in 111 patients in an effort to enhance understanding of the pathophysiological mechanisms of vascular graft failure.[67] They concluded that the inferior epigastric artery is an ideal inflow source, especially in patients without vascular disease. Intimal changes of varying degrees, as well as frequencies of occurrence have been documented in vessels used as grafts during microvascular artery bypass surgery and exposure to systemic vascular risk factors of patients with a history of trauma was associated with more frequent pre-existing penile vessel vasculopathy.

Donor artery–recipient artery procedures

Donor artery–recipient dorsal penile artery
Attempts to create anastomoses between the neoarterial inflow source and the dorsal artery have been associated with the most success and the fewest complications.

Donor artery–recipient cavernosal penile artery
Attempts to create anastomoses between the neoarterial inflow source and the cavernosal arteries have been abandoned because of associated complications and low success rate. The most important complication was that this form of penile revascularization surgery possibly exacerbated the overall condition of impotence. In this procedure, dissection around the cavernosal artery was necessary, which caused permanent scarring of the erectile tissue around the cavernosal artery. Such scarring

led to site-specific corporal veno-occlusive dysfunction and potential worsening of the ED. The most likely explanations for the long-term failure of these reconstructive procedures are as follows. First, the tunical defect, through which the arterialized saphenous vein graft or inferior epigastric passed, required closure. Without an intact closed tunical system surrounding the erectile tissue, there would be inability to obtain penile rigidity and increased intracavernosal pressure. Thus, closure of the tunica defect often led to obstruction of the inflow artery precisely at the location of the artery passing through the tunica defect. In addition, in the case of the arterialized saphenous vein graft, the arterial outflow through the graft was too low, owing, in part, to the resistance of the helicine arterioles downstream. The slow arterial inflow led to occlusion of the entire saphenous vein graft. Finally, the diameter of the cavernosal artery is smaller than that of the dorsal artery, making it highly likely that endothelial cells in and around the area of the anastomosis would be injured during the procedure.

Donor artery–recipient vein procedures

Attempts to create anastomoses between the neoarterial inflow source and the deep dorsal veins have lost popularity because of the low success rate and potential complications. The most important complication of this form of penile revascularization surgery is glans hyperaemia. This painfull swelling of the glans is caused by an excess of blood, and has been reported to lead to urethral obstruction and tissue death of the glans. Glans hyperaemia has resulted when arterialized veins to the glans penis caused raised tissue pressures within the glans tissue. Ultimately, the elevation in glans tissue pressure prevented venous return, which then led to absent arterial inflow. In fact, the irony of glans hyperaemia is that there is ischaemia of the glans despite the presence of high arterial flow in the veins draining the glans. To help prevent glans hyperaemia, the distal end of the DDV is ligated.

The overall problem with venous arterialization surgery has been the lack of control of where the arterialized blood flows once the anastomosis has been completed. The goal was to allow the arterial blood to revascularize the corpora; the arterialized vein, however, transfers the blood to the pathway of least haemodynamic resistance — that is, more commonly to the systemic venous circulation. Postoperative arteriograms have commonly shown closure of the anastomosis, especially if venous valves have prevented egress of blood from the dorsal vein. Alternatively, such arteriograms have shown patency of the arteriovenous anastomosis but the contrast has rarely revealed arterialized blood entering the erectile tissue. Arterialized blood usually has been seen to enter the systemic venous circulation. On the basis of the literature evaluated, the form of revascularization surgery associated with the best and most consistent clinical outcome with the least complications has been anastomosis of the donor artery to the dorsal penile artery.

In summary, the type of revascularization surgery associated with the least complications and most efficacy is donor artery–recipient dorsal penile artery.

What patient characteristics are associated with most efficacy in re-establishing erectile potency?

The patient characteristics associated with most efficacy in re-establishing erectile potency were in young impotent men whose vasculogenic impotence was based solely on cavernosal arterial insufficiency from blunt pelvic or perineal trauma and not from systemic atherosclerosis. Such perineal trauma may result from a myriad of events such as a fall onto a bicycle bar, a kick during a sporting event or a pelvic fracture. The distal internal pudendal, common penile and cavernosal arteries lie in apposition to the bony pelvis. Blunt trauma may injure the vascular endothelium at a site-specific location and thus induce immediate or delayed arterial-occlusive pathology.

Younger impotent patients with a history of blunt perineal or pelvic trauma appear to be ideal candidates for microvascular arterial bypass surgery using donor artery–recipient dorsal penile artery for several important reasons. First, young patients are at the beginning of their sexual lives and have the desire to achieve restored natural spontaneous erectile function without the need for external or internal mechanical devices or pharmacological administration. Second, young patients are also less likely to have systemic conditions adversely affecting penile tissue, penile nerves or penile corporal veno-occlusive function. Third, young impotent patients have discrete arterial occlusive lesions in the distal internal pudendal, common penile or cavernosal arteries on selective internal pudendal arteriography. Finally, young patients do not tolerate well the possibility of experiencing any complications from the surgery (such as glans hyperaemia associated with donor artery to dorsal vein surgery) or the possibility of reduction of erectile function from their preoperative capabilities (such as erectile tissue scarring associated with donor artery to cavernosal artery surgery).

In summary, the patient characteristics associated with the most efficacy in re-establishing erectile potency include being young and having suffered blunt perineal or pelvic trauma without evidence of systemic vasculopathy.

What haemodynamic diagnosis is associated with the most efficacy in re-establishing erectile potency?

On the basis of the literature evaluated, it appears that the donor artery to recipient dorsal artery form of penile revascularization surgery is associated with the best clinical outcome when patients with ED have pure arterial insufficiency and absence of corporal veno-occlusive dysfunction — that is, the clinical syndrome of 'failure to fill' or pure arteriogenic impotence. Such patients have a history characterized by (a) a consistent reduction in erectile rigidity during sexual activity and (b) poorly spontaneous erections, often taking much effort and excessive time to achieve the poorly rigid erectile response. Patients with pure arteriogenic impotence often lose the partial erection during preparatory sexual stimulation prior to penetration or soon after penetration, secondary to the anxiety of the delayed partially rigid erection with the associated increased sympathomimetic response. They characteristically possess an ability to achieve a more rigid, longer-lasting erection upon awakening in the morning. The frustration with the slow-developing sexual erection is not appreciated with the nocturnal erection, since the latter occurs during sleep. The increased ability to sustain the morning erection reflects the fact that such patients have underlying normal corporal veno-occlusive function if their trabecular smooth muscle is completely relaxed.

The aim of penile microvascular arterial bypass surgery for impotence is to provide, in those patients with pure cavernosal arterial insufficiency, an alternative arterial pathway beyond obstructive arterial lesions. Impotent patients with failure-to-fill ED have the pathology that is able to meet the primary objective of the bypass surgery — that is, to increase the cavernosal arterial perfusion pressure and blood inflow. A successful surgical result in a patient with cavernosal artery insufficiency will yield improved erectile haemodynamics during sexual stimulation, giving a more rigid (increased arterial perfusion pressure), more spontaneous (increased arterial inflow) penile erection. It is imperative that the diagnostic evaluation in these patients should include provocative testing in the dynamic state of erection. Such testing must reveal pure arteriogenic impotence without any evidence of corporal veno-occlusive dysfunction, or of neurological or endocrinological factors. Arterial bypass surgery cannot improve any of these latter clinical problems.

In particular, there is no objective evidence to date that arterial surgery has any long-term success in the presence of corporal veno-occlusive dysfunction.[54] Erectile haemodynamics differ from those of other vascular organs in that function is dependent not only on arterial inflow and perfusion but also on the development of adequate venous outflow resistance. There is no physiological basis for improvement of corporal veno-occlusion through arterial bypass surgery. Patients with systemic atherosclerotic disease or arterial occlusive disease secondary to atherosclerotic vascular risk factors, (such as ageing, hypertension, cigarette smoking, diabetes mellitus and hypercholesterolaemia) are not ideal candidates for microvascular arterial bypass surgery. These latter patients have generalized vascular disease and commonly have an associated corporal veno-occlusive dysfunction with abnormal compliance of the erectile tissue.[67–70] This may be secondary to an excess ratio of collagen to trabecular smooth muscle, dysfunctional endothelium or abnormalities of the tunica albuginea preventing adequate elongation and compression of the subtunical venules despite complete trabecular smooth muscle relaxation. It is, therefore, unusual for patients with atherosclerotic vascular risk factors to meet the strict selection criteria — that is, to have pure arterial insufficiency with normal corporal veno-occlusive function, without neurological or endocrinological factors. If the selection criteria are met, independent of the history of vascular risk factors, such patients may be considered for vascular reconstruction although they may have diffuse (especially distal cavernosal) arterial disease that will ultimately hinder successful restoration of erectile function.

Those impotent patients who are candidates for microvascular arterial bypass surgery using the donor artery to dorsal artery, and who have pure cavernosal artery insufficiency and normal corporal veno-occlusive function, may exhibit a long-lasting erection of varying rigidity quality (depending on the magnitude of the cavernosal artery occlusion pressure) following office intracavernosal injection testing. The clinician may erroneously conclude that such patients are not appropriate candidates for surgery, since 'they achieved a rigid erection to vasoactive agent administration — they must have psychogenic impotence'. It must be understood that a positive (rigid) office intracavernosal injection test may exist in the presence of clinically significant arterial insufficiency. In a study published in the *Journal of Urology*, 19% of patients with positive in-office intracavernosal injection tests and rigid erectile response were found to have abnormal gradients between the cavernosal and the brachial artery systolic occlusion pressure, some even exceeding 80 mmHg.[71]

What is the basis for abnormal cavernosal arterial haemodynamics and arterial occlusive disease in the presence of a positive injection test? The answer lies in the relationships between (1) the systemic systolic arterial blood pressure (peak pressure in an individual), (2) the cavernosal systolic arterial blood pressure (actual cavernosal pressure) and (3) the threshold cavernosal systolic arterial blood pressure (prerequisite cavernosal pressure to achieve a positive injection test in a low-outflow state). Ideally, there should be no gradient between the systemic and cavernosal systolic arterial blood pressure values. The systemic systolic arterial blood pressure should be transferred without energy loss to the cavernosal artery via an intact hypogastric–cavernous arterial bed. This peak pressure should then be transferred to the closed-outlet erectile chamber through relaxed helicine arterioles. If a systemic–cavernosal systolic arterial blood pressure gradient is identified, this reflects the presence of pressure energy loss, that is, arterial inflow occlusive disease within the hypogastric–cavernous arterial bed. The key is that, as long as a threshold cavernosal pressure is achieved in a low-outflow state, a positive injection test will result, independent of any difference between systemic (peak) and cavernosal (actual) systolic arterial blood pressure. In other words, the positive injection test is, at worst, a threshold erectile response. The positive injection test may or may not indicate the maximum erection response as determined by the systemic pressure in an individual case.

In summary, the haemodynamic diagnosis associated with the most efficacy in re-establishing erectile potency is pure cavernosal artery insufficiency with normal corporal veno-occlusive function. The underlying pathology of the cavernosal artery insufficiency is traumatic and not atherosclerotic.

BASIC MICROSURGICAL PRINCIPLES

Four basic clinical principles for microvascular arterial bypass procedure involving a donor artery to dorsal penile artery have been identified.[28,34,58,72–75]

The first surgical principle is to perform anatomically oriented arterial bypass procedures. The primary objective of the arterial bypass surgery is to increase the cavernosal arterial perfusion pressure and blood inflow to the erectile tissue. This goal is best achieved by designing the vascular reconstruction to the individual's specific arteriographic findings. The four most important radiological discoveries on selective internal pudendal arteriography are (1) confirmation of the existence of arterial-occlusive disease within the hypogastric–cavernous arterial bed previously only suspected by history and erectile function testing, (2) identification of the presence of a good-quality, long-length donor artery, (3) identification of the presence of a recipient dorsal penile artery, and (4) identification of the location of communicating arterial pathways from the dorsal penile to the cavernosal artery to justify an anastomosis of the inferior epigastric artery to the dorsal penile artery. According to the arterial anatomy, increased arterial blood flow to the lacunar spaces may be accomplished by increasing the flow in the cavernosal arteries through arterial communications that emanate from the distal or proximal aspect of the dorsal artery. Failure to identify communicating cavernosal branches off the proximal or dorsal aspect of the dorsal artery will not meet anatomical considerations for the success of the bypass. Selective internal pudendal pharmacoarteriography is, at present, the most effective method available to provide the necessary anatomical information for surgical strategy-making.

The second surgical principle is to utilize an endothelium-preserving microvascular technique. The surgical technique should embody modern endothelium-sparing vascular and microvascular surgical principles similar to those applied for occlusive disease within other peripheral vascular beds. Long-term bypass patency is based on four microvascular principles: (1) prevention of ischaemic, mechanical or thermal injury to the vascular endothelium of the donor or recipient vascular structures; (2) transmission of systolic neoarterial inflow pressures and flow; (3) technically accurate arterial anastomoses, and (4) low recipient vascular outflow resistances. The prevention of endothelial injury is critical during surgical preparation of the vessels for anastomoses, using technically sound 'no touch' techniques in order to improve long-term vascular patency. The presence of healthy vascular endothelium is essential. The endothelium releases numerous endothelium-derived relaxing factors, which act not only as potent vasodilators but also as strong inhibitors of platelet adhesion and aggregation.[76–79]

The third surgical principle is to avoid injury to the neurovascular bundle, with careful dissection under microscopic magnification. Permanent neuropathic penile pain and diminished penile sensation from injury to the nearby dorsal nerve must be avoided with careful technique. In addition, injury to the suspensory and fundiform ligaments must be avoided; loss of compliance of these ligaments postoperatively may lead to diminished penile length.

The fourth surgical principle is to allow for anastomotic healing postoperatively. Mechanical disruption of the microvascular anastomosis and subsequent uncontrolled arterial haemorrhage may occur from blunt trauma in the first few postoperative weeks, following coitus or masturbation or from accidents. For a substantial period (6 weeks) postoperatively, patients should abstain from sexual activities involving the erect penis.

In summary, there are four surgical/microsurgical principles associated with the least complications and most efficacy. The first is to use an anatomically oriented arterial bypass procedure in which the selective internal pudendal arteriogram reveals four specific findings — the existence of common penile/cavernosal arterial occlusive disease, the presence of a donor artery, the presence of a recipient dorsal penile artery and the location of communicating arterial pathways from the dorsal penile to the cavernosal artery. The second principle is to use endothelium-preserving microvascular techniques; the third is to avoid injury to the neurovascular bundle, including the fundiform ligament, and the fourth is to allow for healing in the postoperative period.

■ INFERIOR EPIGASTRIC ARTERY ANASTOMOSIS TO DORSAL PENILE ARTERY: OPERATIVE TECHNIQUE

Routinely, the patient's arteriograms are brought to the operating room for intra-operative review, if necessary. General endotracheal or regional anaesthesia may be used for the procedure. Before the start of the operation, one dose of intravenous broad-spectrum antibiotic (such as cephalosporin) is administered. The patient is positioned supine on the operating table with the legs in a 'frog-leg' orientation. As the procedure may take more than 5 or 6 hours, great care must be taken in the positioning and padding of the limbs, in particular of the neurovascular points on the upper and lower limbs. The authors have had one patient who developed a transient postoperative ulnar palsy due to protracted pressure on his medial epicondylar area. It now is their policy to instruct the anaesthesiologist to move the arms around and to alternate the position of the blood-pressure cuff periodically throughout the procedure, to avoid this complication.

The patient's abdomen and perineum are carefully shaved, and a 5 minute Betadyne scrub is performed. Once the patient has been prepared and draped, a sterile 16 Fr Foley catheter is inserted into the bladder and left to closed drainage throughout the operation. The operative procedure is in three stages: (1) scrotal exploration and dorsal artery dissection; (2) inferior epigastric artery harvesting, and (3) microsurgical anastomosis.

Scrotal exploration and dorsal artery dissection
Inguinoscrotal incision (Fig. 36.1)
Using a scalpel with a 15 blade, a curvilinear incision is made, generally opposite the side of the planned abdominal incision, for inferior epigastric artery harvesting. The incision is made two finger-breadths from the penoscrotal junction, extending from the area opposite the ventral root of the stretched penis to the midline scrotal raphe. The dartos layer is opened using electrocautery; the numerous advantages of this approach include (1) excellent exposure of the penile neurovascular bundle, (2) the ability to identify and preserve the suspensory and fundiform ligaments and (3) the avoidance of unsightly postoperative scars on the penile shaft or at the base of the penis. During dissection, a Scott ring retractor with its elastic hooks maximizes operative exposure of the penis with a minimum of assistance.

Penile inversion (Fig. 36.2)
Using blunt dissection, the tunica albuginea of the corpora cavernosa is subsequently identified at the mid-penile shaft level. The urethra is identified in the midline and avoided. With the penis stretched, blunt finger

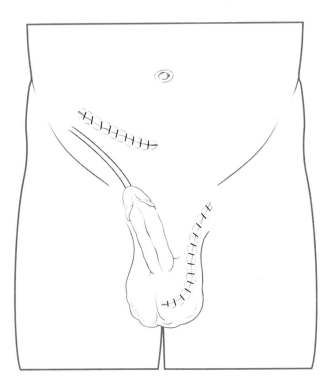

Figure 36.1. Inguinoscrotal and transverse abdominal incisions utilized for microvascular arterial bypass surgery.

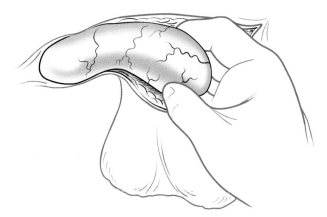

Figure 36.2. Penile inversion to prevent injury to the fundiform ligament.

dissection along the tunica albuginea and below Buck's fascia is performed on the lateral aspect of the penile shaft to the level of the coronal sulcus. Using this approach, dissection is completed in a distal direction deep to the spermatic cord structures and the fundiform ligament. By carefully pushing directly on the glans, the penis can be inverted through the scrotal skin incision. Penile tumescence must be avoided during this manoeuvre. If a partial erection is present, direct intracavernosal alpha-adrenergic agonist (100 μg phenylephrine) should be administered. Once the penis is in the inverted position, careful blunt finger dissection can establish a plane between Buck's fascia and Colles' fascia at the level of the distal penile shaft. A Penrose drain is placed to secure this plane.

Preparation of the recipient dorsal arteries

Exposure of the neurovascular bundle and, in particular, the right and left dorsal penile arteries, is now performed. First, the dorsal vein is identified in the midline of the mid-penile shaft with the dorsal arteries seated on either side. Complete isolation and preparation of the dorsal penile arteries required for arterial bypass surgery is unnecessary at this stage of the procedure. Ischaemic, mechanical and thermal trauma to the dorsal penile arteries is minimized with limited dissection. Topical papaverine hydrochloride irrigation is applied frequently to the dorsal arteries in order to avoid injurious vasospasm. In this way, preservation of endothelial and smooth muscle cell morphology during dorsal artery preparation is ensured. This process is very critical as the room temperature of the operating room, the use of irrigating solution at room temperature, and even the skin incision, can induce vasoconstriction, spasm and possible endothelial cell damage. For intraluminal irrigation, a dilute papaverine, heparin and electrolytic solution is used, as it is thought that this inhibits the early development of myointimal proliferative lesions during surgical preparation.

The course of the right and left dorsal penile arteries is followed proximally underneath the fundiform ligament, with care being taken to leave the fundiform ligament intact. A fenestration is fashioned in the fundiform ligament proximally, usually near the junction of the fundiform and suspensory ligaments at a location where the pendulous penile shaft becomes fixed proximally (Fig. 36.3). Blunt dissection is performed under the proximal aspect of the fundiform ligament above the pubic bone toward the external ring. This dissection enables the inferior epigastric artery to pass from its abdominal location to the appropriate location in the penis while simultaneously preserving the fundiform ligament.

Harvesting of the inferior epigastric artery
Abdominal incision (Fig. 36.4)

The inguinoscrotal incision is temporarily closed with staples after the penis is inverted back to its normal

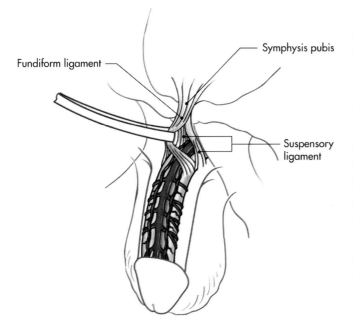

Figure 36.3. The fundiform ligament is the extension of Scarpa's fascia onto Buck's fascia. Preservation of the fundiform ligament diminishes postoperative shortening and penile numbness.

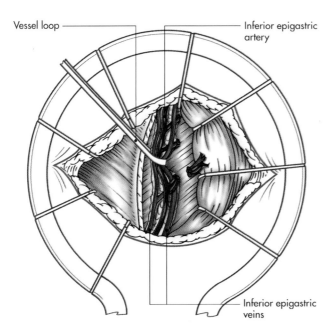

Figure 36.4. Transverse abdominal incision with vertical incision in rectus fascia enables exposure of inferior epigastric bundle.

anatomical position. A unilateral (transverse or paramedian) abdominal incision is made with a scalpel (15 blade). The transverse incision provides excellent operative exposure of the inferior epigastric artery and heals with a more cosmetic scar than those observed with paramedian skin incisions. The transverse incision starting point is approximately one-quarter of the total distance between the umbilicus and the pubic bone in the midline. The incision extends laterally along the natural skin lines for approximately four finger-breadths. The subcutaneous tissue and Scarpa's fascia are opened in a similar direction with electrocautery; however, the rectus fascia is vertically incised in a paramedian location. The rectus muscle is reflected medially after maximal pharmacological skeletal muscle relaxation is obtained. The junction between the rectus muscle and underlying pre-peritoneal fat is identified and the pre-peritoneal space is entered.

Inferior epigastric artery dissection

The inferior epigastric artery and its two accompanying veins are located beneath the rectus muscle in the pre-peritoneal plane. The Scott ring retractor is again utilized to maximize operative exposure. Harvesting sufficient length during the inferior epigastric artery dissection is critical in order to prevent tension on the microvascular anastomosis. Again, topical papaverine is routinely applied to the inferior epigastric artery throughout the dissection in a effort to minimize vasospasm. Thermal injury is avoided using low current microbipolar cautery set at the minimum level necessary for adequate coagulation. The vasa vasorum are preserved by dissecting the artery en bloc with its surrounding veins and fat. The inferior epigastric artery is dissected inferiorly to its origin at the level of the femoral artery to a point cephalad at the level of the umbilicus. The artery usually bifurcates at this level, and the authors usually attempt to preserve the bifurcation to allow anastomoses to both dorsal arteries, if needed.

Inferior epigastric artery transfer (Fig. 36.5)

The abdominal transfer route of the neoarterial inflow source to the scrotum is prepared prior to transecting the vessel distally. The temporary scrotal staples are removed and the penis is re-inverted. The internal ring on the side of the harvested artery is identified lateral to the origin of the inferior epigastric artery. Using blunt finger dissection through the inguinal canal, a long, fine, vascular clamp is passed through the fenestration in the fundiform ligament, the external and the internal inguinal rings. A Penrose drain is brought through to protect this transfer route.

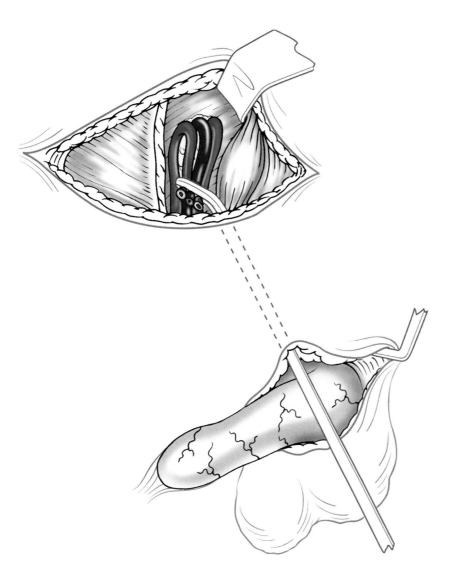

Figure 36.5. Transfer of inferior epigastric bundle to base of the penis through inguinal canal.

Transection of the donor vascular bundle is completed at the level of the umbilicus between two Ligaclips. The ligated site is carefully inspected for any proximal bleeding points. The harvested vessel is irrigated with papaverine solution and a small Ligaclip is then placed on the distal aspect of the vessel prior to vessel transfer. The long, fine, vascular clamp is brought through the internal inguinal ring again, this time to grasp the end of the transected inferior epigastric artery. The inferior epigastric vascular bundle is transferred to the base of the penis. The artery should be briskly pulsating and of adequate length. The origin of the inferior epigastric artery should be inspected for kinking or twisting prior to abdominal closure. Once complete haemostasis has been noted, the abdominal wound is closed in three layers. The rectus fascia is closed utilizing two running 0 polyglycolic acid sutures (i.e. one suture started at either end of the

incision). The subcutaneous tissue and Scarpa's fascia are then closed with a running 2/0 polyglycolic suture, and finally, the skin edges are reapposed using skin staples.

Microvascular anastomosis
Vessel preparation (Fig. 36.6)
The Scott ring retractor and the associated elastic hooks are utilized once again, on the inguinoscrotal incision and the fenestration of the fundiform ligament, to gain exposure of the proximal dorsal neurovascular bundle. The pulsating inferior epigastric artery is placed against the recipient dorsal penile artery/arteries and a convenient location is selected for the vascular anastomosis. Creation of the anastomosis (or anastomoses) is based on the arteriographic findings. An end-to-side anastomosis is best under conditions where dorsal penile artery communications exist to the cavernosal artery. Furthermore, an end-to-side

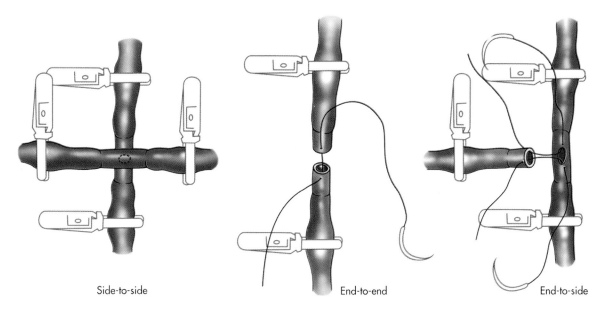

Side-to-side   End-to-end   End-to-side

Figure 36.6. Inferior epigastric artery anastomosis to dorsal penile artery.

anastomosis protects arterial blood flow in the distal direction to the glans penis. In the authors' experience, however, ligation of both dorsal penile arteries to perform bilateral proximal end-to-end anastomoses has never caused ischaemic injury to the glans penis.

The appropriate dorsal penile artery segment is freed from its attachments to the tunica albuginea, care being taken to avoid injury to any communicating branches to the cavernosal artery. Vascular haemostasis of this segment of the dorsal penile artery may be achieved with either gold-plated (low-pressure) aneurysm vascular clamps or vessel loops under minimal tension and duration. In order to avoid causing subsequent thrombosis, the adventitia must be carefully removed at the site of the vascular anastomosis, i.e. the distal end of the inferior epigastric artery and the selected region of the dorsal penile artery. Patency of the anastomosis is jeopardized when segments of adventitia enter the anastomosis, because adventitia activates clotting factors from the extrinsic clotting system. The remaining adventitia in the vessels should be preserved, as the vasa vasorum provide nutrition for the vessel wall. The preservation of the adventitia is additionally important in terms of vessel innervation.

Anastomotic technique

Under microscopic control at ×5–10 magnification, a 10/0 suture (single-armed, 100 μm/149-degree curved needle) is placed along the longitudinal axis of the dorsal penile artery

in a 1 mm segment in the region of the intended anastomosis. After tension has been placed on the suture, an oval section of the artery wall is excised with curved micro-scissors, resulting in a 1.2–1.5 mm horizontal arteriotomy (Fig. 36.7). The authors use a coloured plastic background material to aid vessel visualization under the microscope. A temporary 2 Fr Silastic stent is placed within the arteriotomy for clearer definition of the vessel lumen.

An end-to-side anastomosis is performed between the inferior epigastric artery and the dorsal artery, using interrupted 10/0 nylon sutures under the ×5–10 magnification. The sutures are placed initially at each apex of the anastomosis and then subsequently three to five interrupted sutures are placed into each side wall

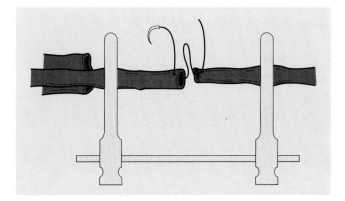

Figure 36.7. Multiple 10/0 microvascular sutures are placed in an interrupted fashion to anastomose the inferior epigastric artery to the dorsal penile artery.

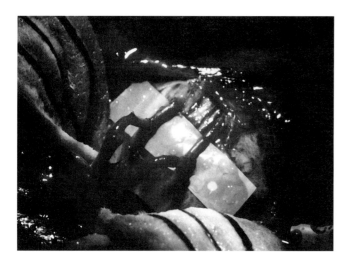

Figure 36.8. Actual intra-operative photograph of an end-to-side anastomosis between the right and left dorsal penile arteries.

(Fig. 36.8). All sutures used to complete the anastomosis are inserted equidistant from each other to avoid an uneven anastomosis. One side of the anastomosis is completed before the other side is started. If a temporary vascular stent is used, it is removed following placement of all sutures. The use of such a stent enables careful inspection of the vessel back wall. Following release of the temporary occluding vascular clamps (or vessel loops) on the dorsal penile artery, the anastomosed segment should reveal arterial pulsations along its length and retrograde in the inferior epigastric artery; such an observation implies a patent anastomosis. At this time, the inferior epigastric artery gold-plated aneurysm clamp may be removed. The intensity of the arterial pulsations in the anastomosis usually increases. Occasionally, the application of a small amount of haemostatic material may be needed to help to promote haemostasis from suture needle holes in the vessel walls. After complete haemostasis has been achieved and correct instrument and sponge counts are ensured, closure of the inguinoscrotal incision may begin. The dartos layer is reapproximated using a 3/0 polyglycolic acid suture in a running fashion. The skin edges are closed with skin staples. The Foley catheter is left to closed-system gravity drainage overnight.

The procedure described above may be modified. The most common alternative arterial anastomosis is an end-to-end anastomosis between the inferior epigastric artery and the ligated proximal end of the dorsal penile artery. Depending on the site of the arterial communication from the dorsal penile artery to the cavernosal artery, the end-to-end anastomosis may also be anastomosed to the distal ligated end of the dorsal penile artery. It is also most common to anastomose the opposite dorsal penile artery to the inferior epigastric artery. This can be done with an appropriately sized distal branch of the inferior epigastric artery end-to-side, as previously described.

OUTCOMES

Complications

During the first few postoperative weeks, any trauma in the region of the anastomosis can cause mechanical disruption of the microvascular anastomosis, resulting in uncontrolled arterial bleeding. Arterial injury can occur following coitus, masturbation or accidents, and, as previously mentioned, the authors therefore recommend abstention from any sexual activities or vigorous activity involving the erect penis until postoperative week 6.

Penile pain and diminished penile sensation from injury to the nearby dorsal nerve have also resulted from penile microvascular arterial bypass.[30] Other complications, such as loss of compliance of the suspensory and fundiform ligaments postoperatively, may lead to diminished penile length. Careful identification and preservation of these two ligaments during surgery has markedly minimized those complications in the authors' series. Glans hyperaemia, once a complication seen when inferior epigastric artery to DDV anastomoses (dorsal vein arterialization) were performed, is no longer seen since this is a complication exclusively seen in arterializations of the deep dorsal vein. Poor arterial run-off with failure of the microvascular arterial bypass may be due to inadequate arterial inflow or technical errors during the microvascular procedure. Poor arterial run-off can be minimized by proper patient selection, good microvascular surgical technique and preoperative arteriographic presence of communicating branches between the dorsal penile arteries and the cavernosal tissue.

A recent complication, of indirect inguinal hernias, occurred in two patients at the authors' institution when the internal inguinal ring and adjacent medial transversalis fascia were opened and excessively dilated to accommodate passage of the inferior epigastric vessels to the scrotum during microvascular arterial bypass. In both cases, open inguinal surgical repair was necessary, with placement of mesh to correct the hernia defect. Surgical scarring in this region with incorporation of the inferior epigastric artery obviates the need for the urologist familiar with the course of the inferior epigastric vessels to be present during hernia repair. Intraoperative Doppler ultrasound was utilized during hernia repair to avoid vascular injury. This method of excessive inguinal canal dilatation and transfer of the harvested inferior epigastric vessels to the scrotum has been abandoned.

OPERATIVE RESULTS

We have previously reported on the objective postoperative haemodynamic status, including steady-state equilibrium intracavernosal pressures and veno-occlusive and arterial function tests, in patients in whom successful as well as unsuccessful clinical results were achieved following microvascular arterial bypass surgery for impotence.[54] Of the 226 patients who underwent penile microvascular arterial bypass surgery from 1985 to 1992, 68 (30%) (mean age 34 ± 10 years) underwent both preoperative and postoperative pharmacocavernosometry/graphy. The mean duration between the bypass procedure and follow-up postoperative testing was 8 ± 6 months. Surgical bypasses in these 68 patients included 65 inferior epigastric artery to dorsal penile artery including 30 with dual dorsal arterial anastomoses. There were, in addition, nine artery to DDV anastomoses, including six performed in conjunction with an arterial anastomosis. Of these 68 patients, 49 (72%) had concomitant venous surgery for veno-occlusive dysfunction (46 deep dorsal vein excisions, 35 crural plication, 19 cavernosal vein ligations and three spongiolyses).

Twelve patients (18%) with pure arteriogenic impotence had a postoperative mean increase in steady-state equilibrium intracavernosal pressure of 25.1 ± 12.3 mmHg (range 13 ± 45 mmHg). Of the remaining 56 patients, 49 had concomitant venous surgery. There was no significant change in mean steady-state equilibrium intracavernosal pressure (38 ± 20 mmHg preoperative vs 43 ± 17 mmHg postoperative), mean pressure decay in 30 seconds (67 ± 9 mmHg preoperative vs 64 ± 26 mmHg postoperative) or mean flow-to-maintain values (38 ± 36 ml/min preoperative vs 28 ± 28 ml/min postoperative). The remaining seven patients, who did not undergo venous surgery, had normal veno-occlusive function pre- and postoperatively; however, the postoperative intracavernosal pressure did not increase (54 ± 22 mmHg preoperative vs 58 ± 27 mmHg postoperative).

Variable long-term success rates ranging from 30 to 84% have been reported following penile revascularization.[55] Unfortunately, accurate interpretation of these data is limited since definitions of success following the procedures have no standardization. Historically, successful outcomes have been variably defined by questionnaire, patient interview and haemodynamic evaluation. Furthermore, the patient populations have been heterogeneous with varying numbers of patients with venogenic impotence. The authors no longer perform this type of surgical intervention in any patient with veno-occlusive dysfunction. Another pitfall relating to data interpretation is the inclusion in many reported series of dorsal vein arterialization procedures. Success rates for this specific technique are inferior to those for procedures utilizing pure arterial anastomoses. Finally, short postoperative follow-up periods ranging from 16 to 36 months are reported. The most recent study had a short-term success rate of 80% and long-term (up to 5 years) success rate of 64%, utilizing strict patient selection criteria.

The authors recently studied the results of postoperative arteriography in order to determine the neoarterial anastomosis integrity and outcomes of microvascular arterial bypass surgery.[80] Twenty-two patients (mean age 35 ± 12, range 24–51 years) underwent postoperative flush iliac arteriography on the same side as the harvested inferior epigastric artery, using local anaesthesia and without vasodilators for pharmacological erections. Three groups of patients were identified prior to microvascular arterial bypass procedure. The inferior epigastric artery was anastomosed end-to-side to the DDV (group 1; n = 6), to the dorsal penile artery without any distal communicating branches to the cavernosal tissue (group 2; n = 7), and to the dorsal penile artery with distal communicating branches to the cavernosal tissue (group 3; n = 9). All patients had comparison of pre- and postoperative arteriograms at 6 months postoperatively. Two patients in group 1 required earlier studies secondary to complaints of glans hyperaemia.

Group 1 patients had a mean follow-up of 4 ± 4 months. Brisk visualization of the anastomosis of the inferior epigastric artery into the dorsal vein was noted on the arteriogram in 66% of cases, but no patient demonstrated arterial run-off into the corporal tissue. Group 2 patients (mean follow-up of 9 ± 2 months) had poor or no visualization of the arterial anastomosis in all seven cases, with no communicating branch to the cavernosal tissue. Group 3 patients (mean follow-up 10 ± 3 months) showed arteriographic evidence of brisk visualization of the neoarterial anastomosis with run-off into cavernosal tissue in all cases studied. The findings of the study emphasized the importance of preoperative arteriographic evidence of communicating branches off the recipient dorsal penile artery to the cavernosal tissue distal to the site of anatomical obstruction. These anatomical radiographic findings are present in approximately 75% of patients undergoing arteriogram prior to microvascular arterial bypass and have become a prerequisite for proper patient selection. Utilizing strict inclusion/exclusion criteria, long-term microvascular patency as well as clinical outcomes can be maximized. On the basis of these results, it is now the authors' routine practice not to perform any microvascular arterial bypass procedure on recipient DDVs or dorsal penile arteries without communicating branches.

With the advent of minimally invasive surgical techniques to minimize patient morbidity, newer advances in penile microvascular arterial bypass procedures, including laparoscopy-assisted penile revascularization, are now being reported.[81-83] Although more advanced surgical and diagnostic modalities may contribute to improved outcomes, only limited numbers of patients with long-term follow-up have been reported. To evaluate this operation further as a valid management strategy, prospective analyses of patient outcomes are essential. Standardization of the definitions for successful outcomes, and longer postoperative follow-up, are necessary when comparing postoperative outcomes.

■ CONCLUSIONS

Microvascular arterial bypass surgery can achieve the goal of increasing cavernosal arterial inflow and perfusion pressure. Young male patients exhibiting arteriogenic ED with a normal corporal veno-occlusive mechanism are appropriate candidates for surgical cure of ED. If strict haemodynamic and arteriographic criteria are used, each patient offered such treatment can have a safe and effective means to restore normal erectile function naturally. The goal of the operation is to restore natural, spontaneously occurring erections (without the aid of any internal or external means) to young men with ED. Much research needs to be performed to define the reasons why a significant number of men continue to fail to respond to penile revascularization.

■ REFERENCES

1. NIH Consensus Development Panel on Impotence. Impotence. JAMA 1993; 270: 83–90
2. Feldman H A, Goldstein I, Hatzichristou D G et al. Impotence and its medical and psychosocial correlates: results of the Massachusetts Male Aging Study. J Urol 1994; 151: 54–61
3. Krane R J, Goldstein I, Saenz de Tejada I. Impotence. N Engl Med J 1989; 321: 1648–1659
4. Lerner S E, Melman A, Christ, G J. A review of erectile dysfunction. J Urol 1993; 149: 1246
5. Jeffery N W, Rose R C U, Gopal H B. Intracavernous pharmacotherapy in psychogenic impotence. Urology 1991; 5: 437–441
6. Korenman S G, Morley J F, Mooradian A D. Secondary hypogonadism in older men: its relation to impotence. J Clin Endocrinol Metab 1990; 71: 963–969
7. Brindley G S. Cavernosal alpha-blockade. Br J Psych 1983; 143: 332
8. Virag R. Intracavernous injection of papaverine for erection failure. Lancet 1982; 2: 938
9. Virag R, Frydman D, Legman M, Virag H. Intracavernous injection of papaverine as a diagnostic and therapeutic method in erectile failure. Angiology 1984; 35: 79
10. Junemann K P, Alken P. Pharmacotherapy of erectile dysfunction. Int J Impot Res 1989; 1: 712
11. Lue T F, Tanagho E A. Physiology of erection and pharmacological management of impotence. J Urol 1987; 137: 829
12. Mahmoud K Z, El Dakhli, M R, Fahmi I M, Abel-Aziz A B. Comparative value of prostaglandin E1 and papaverine in treatment of erectile failure: double-blind crosssover study among Egyptian patients. J Urol 1992; 147: 623–626
13. McMahon C G. A comparison of the response to the intracavernosal injection of a combination of papaverine and phentolamine, prostaglandin PGE1 and a combination of all three agents in the management of impotence. Int J Impot Res 1991; 3: 113–121
14. Nadig M. Vacuum erection devices. A review. World J Urol 1990; 8: 114–117
15. Sidi A, Becher E F, Zhang G, Lewis J H. Patient acceptance of and satisfaction with an external negative pressure device for impotence. J Urol 1990; 144: 1154–1159
16. Witherington W. Suction device therapy in the management of impotence. Urol Clin North Am 1988; 15: 123
17. Witherington W. External penile appliances for the management of impotence. Semin Urol 1990; 8: 124
18. Mulhall J. Sildenfil: a novel effective oral therapy for male erectile dysfunction. Br J Urol 1997; 79: 663–664
19. Morales A, Condra M, Owen J A. Oral and transcutaneous pharmacologic agents for the treatment of impotence. In: Tanagho E A, Lue T F, McClure R D (eds) Contemporary management of impotence and infertility. Baltimore: Williams and Wilkins 1988: 178

20. Padma-Nathan H, Helstrom W J, Kaiser F E et al. Treatment of men with erectile dysfunction with transurethral alprostadil. Medicated Urethral System for Erection (MUSE) Study Group. N Engl J Med 1997; 336: 1–7

21. Goldstein I. Arterial revascularization procedures. Semin Urol 1986; 4: 252

22. Montague D K, Barada J H, Belker A M et al. Clinical guidelines panel on erectile dysfunction: summary report on treatment of organic erectile dysfunction. J Urol 1996; 156: 2007–2011

23. Michal V, Kramar R, Popischal J, Hejhal L. Direct arterial anastomosis on corporal cavernosa penis in therapy of erectile dysfunction. Rozhl Chir 1973; 52: 587–590

24. Michal V, Kramer R, Popischal J. Femoropudendal bypass, internal iliac thrombendarterectomy and direct arterial anastomosis to the cavernous body in the treatment of erectile impotence. Bull Soc Int Chir 1974; 33: 341–345

25. Virag R, Zwang G, Dermange H, Legman M. Vasculogenic impotence: a review of 92 cases with 54 surgical operations. Vasc Surg 1981; 15: 9–17

26. Hauri D. A new operative technique in vasculogenic erectile impotence. World J Urol 1986; 4: 237–249

27. Crespo E, Soltanik E, Bove D. Treatment of vasculogenic sexual impotence by revascularizing the cavernous and/or dorsal arteries using microvascular techniques. Urology 1982; 20: 271–275

28. Hatzichristou D G, Goldstein I. Arterial bypass surgery for impotence. Curr Opin Urol 1992; 1: 114

29. Frohrib D A, Goldstein I, Payton T R et al. Characterization of penile erectile states using external computer-based monitoring. J Biomech Eng 1987; 109: 110–113

30. Zorgniotti A W, Lizza E. Complications of penile revascularization. In: Zorgniotti A W, Lizza E F (eds) Diagnosis and management of impotence. Philadelphia: Decker, 1991:

31. Junemann K P, Persson-Juneman C, Alken P. Pathophysiology of erectile dysfunction. Semin Urol 1990; 8: 80–93

32. Scott F B, Bradley W E, Timm G W. Management of erectile impotence. Urology 1973; 2: 80

33. Michal V, Kramar R, Pospichal J. Vascular surgery in the treatment of impotence: its present possibilities and prospects. Czech Med 1980; 3: 213–217

34. Goldstein I. Penile revascularization. Urol Clin North Am 1987; 143: 805

35. Sharlip I. Penile arteriography in impotence after pelvic trauma. J Urol 1981; 126: 1981

36. Carmignani G, Pirozzi F, Spano G et al. Cavernous artery revascularization in vasculogenic impotence: a new simplified technique. Urology 1987; 30: 23–26

37. Austoni H. Penile revascularization. In: Mulcahy J J (ed) Diagnosis and management of male sexual dysfunction. New York, 1992; 1281

38. Lund J. Penile revascularization. In: Mulcahy J J (ed) Diagnosis and management of male sexual dysfunction. New York, 1995: 1281

39. MacGregor R J, Konnack J W. Treatment of vasculogenic erectile dysfunction by direct anastomosis of the inferior epigastric artery to the central artery of the corpus cavernosum. J Urol 1982; 127: 136–9

40. Shaw W S, Zorgniotti A W. Surgical techniques in penile revascularization. World J Urol 1984; 5: 104–110

41. Virag R. Revascularization of the penis. In: Bennet A H (ed) Management of male impotence. Baltimore: Williams and Wilkins, 1982: 219–237

42. Juenemann K P. Penile revascularization. In: Mulcahy J J (ed) Diagnosis and management of male sexual dysfunction. New York, 1992: 1282

43. Benhathismou A C. Technique for the indirect revascularization of corpus cavernosum in sexual impotence from distal arterial origin by double epigastro-veno-cavernous fistula. Presse Med 1985; 14: 691–693

44. Shah R S, Parulkar B, Kulkarni V. Antegrade dorsal arterialization (Shah-Parulkar procedure) for penile revascularization. Int J Impot Res 1994; 6:

45. Shafik A. Pudendal artery syndrome with erectile dysfunction: treatment by pudendal canal decompression. Arch Androl 1995; 34: 83–94

46. DePalma R G, Edwards C M, Schwab F J, Steinberg D L. Modern management of impotence associated with aortic surgery. In: Bargan J J, Yao S T (eds) Arterial surgery: new diagnostic and operative techniques. Orlando: Grune and Stratton, 1988: 337–348

47. Michal V, Kramar R, Hejhal L, Firt P. Aortoiliac occlusive disease. In: Zorgniotti A W, Rossi G (eds) Vasculogenic impotence. Proceedings of the first international meeting on the corpus cavernosum revascularization. Illinois: Thomas Springfield, 1979: 203–214

48. Metz P, Frimodt-Moller C. Epigastrico-cavernous anastomosis in the treatment of arteriogenic impotence. Scand J Urol Nephrol 1983; 17: 271–275

49. McDougal W S, Jeffrey R F. Microscopic penile revascularization. J Urol 1983; 129: 517–521

50. Sharlip I. Retrograde revascularization of the dorsal penile artery for arteriogenic erectile dysfunction. J Urol 1984; 131: 232A

51. Sharlip I D. The role of vascular surgery in arteriogenic and venogenic impotence. Sem Urol 1990; 8: 129–137

52. Lotfy K, Elgabrawy M, Bayoumi S, Madi M. Pathological study and surgical management of vasculogenic impotence. MD thesis, Urology Department, Faculty of Medicine, Tanta University, Egypt, 1994

53. Goldstein I, Padma-Nathan H. Venous evaluation of impotence. In: Rajfer J (ed) Infertility and impotence. Chicago: YBMP, 1990: 269–275

54. Goldstein I, Nehra A, Dimitrios G. Objective assessment of hemodynamic outcome from microvascular arterial bypass surgery. Int J Impot Res 1994; 6:

55. Jarow J P, DeFranzo A J. Longterm results of arterial bypass surgery for impotence secondary to segmental vascular disease. J Urol 1996; 156: 982

56. Fitch I, Kaufman J, Borges F. Effect of risk factors upon microsurgical penile revascularization post-operative results. Int J Impot Res, Suppl. 1994

57. Grasso M, Lania C, Castelli M, Rigatti P. Inferior epigastric artery–deep dorsal vein anastomosis in the treatment of vasculogenic impotence. Int J Impot Res 1994; 6

58. Sohn M, Sikora R, Bohndorf K, Deutz F J. Selective microsurgery in arteriogenic erectile failure. World J Urol 1990; 8: 104–107

59. Wespes E, Corbusier A, Delcour C et al. Deep dorsal vein arterialization in vascular impotence. Br J Urol 1989; 64: 535–540

60. Furlow W L, Fisher J, Knoll L D. Penile revascularization: experience with deep dorsal vein arterialization: the Furlow-Fisher modification with 27 patients. In: Proc 6th Biennial Int Symp for Corpus Cavernosum Revascularization and Third Biennial World Meeting on Impotence. Boston: International Society of Impotence Research (ISIR), 1988

61. Melman A, Riccardi R. The success of microsurgical penile revascularization in treating arteriogenic impotence. Int J Impot Res 1993; 5: 47–52

62. Floth A, Paick J S, Suh J K, Lue T F. Hemodynamics of revascularization of the corpora cavernosa in animal model: a preliminary report. Urol Res 1991; 19: 281–284

63. Kaufman J, Fitch W. Deep dorsal vein arterialization in arteriogenic impotence: use of the dorsal artery as a neoarterial source. Int J Impot Res 1995; 7: 73–84

64. Vickers K E, Vickers MA. Has the efficacy of penile arterial by-pass surgery in the treatment of arteriogenic erectile dysfunction been determined? Int J Impot Res 1996; 8: 247–251

65. DePalma R G. Editorial comment on paper by Vickers K E, Vickers M A: Has the efficiency of penile arterial by-pass surgery in the treatment of arteriogenic erectile dysfunction been determined? Int J Impot Res 1996; 8: 251–252

66. Witt M A, Goldstein I, Saenz de Tejada I et al. Traumatic laceration of intracavernosal arteries: their pathophysiology of nonischemic, high flow, arterial priapism. J Urol 1990; 143: 129

67. Hatzichristou D G, Goldstein I, Quist W C. Pre-existing vascular pathology in donor and recipient vessels during penile microvascular arterial bypass surgery. J Urol 1994; 151: 1217–1224

68. Azadzoi K M, Goldstein I. Atherosclerosis-induced corporal leakage impotence. Surg Forum 1987; 38: 647

69. Goldstein I. Vascular diseases of the penis. In: Pollack H M (ed) Clinical urography. Philadelphia: Saunders, 1992: 2231–2252

70. Rosen M P, Greenfield A J, Walker T G et al. Cigarette smoking as an independent risk factor for atherosclerosis in the hypogastric–cavernous bed of men with arteriogenic impotence. J Urol 1991; 145: 759–763

71. Pescatori E S, Dimitrio G, Hatzichristou G et al. A positive intracavernous injection test implies normal veno-occlusive but not necessarily normal arterial function: a hemodynamic study. J Urol 1993; 151: 1209

72. Guity A, Young P H, Fisher V W. In search of the 'perfect' anastomosis. Microsurgery 1990; 11: 5–11

73. Hatzichristou D C, Goldstein I G. Microvascular arterial bypass surgery for arteriogenic impotence. In: Whitehead D, Nagler H (eds) Management of impotence and infertility. Philadelphia: J B Lippincott, 1994: 55–72

74. Microvascular surgery. In: Shaw W W (ed) Vascular surgery: principles and techniques. Norwalk: Appleton–Century–Crofts, 1988: 289–308

75. Siemionow M. Evaluation of different microsurgical techniques for arterial anastomosis of vessels of diameter less than one millimeter. J Reconstr Microsurg 1987; 3: 333–340

76. Ignarro L J, Bush P A, Buga G M. Nitric oxide and cyclic GMP formation upon electrical stimulation cause relaxation of corpus cavernosum smooth muscle. Biochem Biophys Res Commun 1990; 170: 843

77. Burnett A L, Lowenstein C J, Bredt D S. Nitric oxide: a physiologic mediator of penile erection. Science 1992; 257: 401–403

78. Kim N, Azadzoi K M, Goldstein I, Saenz de Tejada I. A nitric oxide-like factor mediates nonadrenergic-noncholinergic neurogenic relaxation of penile corpus cavernosum smooth muscle. J Clin Invest 1991; 88: 112

79. Sattar A A, Schulman C C, Wespes E. Objective quantification of cavernous endothelium in potent and impotent men. J Urol 1995; 153: 1136–1138

80. Sadeghi-Nejad H, Abdel-Moneim A, Reid S K et al. Post-operative arteriography in microvascular bypass surgery for impotent. J Urol 1997; 158: abstract

81. Moon Y T, Kim S C. Laparoscopic mobilization of the inferior epigastric artery for penile revascularization in vasculogenic impotence. J Korean Med Sci 1997; 12: 240–243

82. Hatzinger M, Seemann O, Grenacher L, Rassweiler J. Laparoscopy-assisted penile revascularization: a new method. J Endourol 1997; 11: 269–272

83. Trombetta C, Liguori G, Siracusano S et al. Laparoscopically assisted penile revascularization for vasculogenic impotence: 2 additional cases. J Urol 1997; 158: 1783–1786

Chapter 37

Unitary inflatable, mechanical and malleable penile implants

J. J. Mulcahy

■ INTRODUCTION

A quarter of a century has passed since the introduction of effective penile implants. Almost simultaneously the three-piece inflatable[1] and Small–Carrion[2] models were introduced in the early 1970s. Shortly thereafter the Finney Flexirod[3] came on the scene and in 1980 the Jonas malleable rod[4] was brought to this country. In the early days of prosthetics for impotence, the rod-like devices, which were contained completely within the erectile bodies, outsold their three-piece inflatable counterparts by a 3 to 1 margin. Experienced implanters were few and far between and most surgeons felt more comfortable inserting the simpler devices. Hydraulic problems such as fluid leaks, tubing kinks and cylinder aneurysms were problems not seen with the rod-like devices. As urologists gained experience in dealing with hydraulic problems of inflatable devices, and as the manufacturers changed construction of their implants to decrease the incidence of fluid leaks and other malfunctions, a shift in the market was seen towards a preference for the three-piece inflatable devices because they gave a better quality of erection and a more natural flaccid state.

In an attempt to combine the features of the current rods and inflatables, American Medical Systems (AMS) introduced the Hydroflex prosthesis in 1985.[5] This device consisted of paired inflatable cylinders placed entirely within each of the erectile bodies. Inflation and deflation were accomplished by pressing on different portions of the cylinders located distally in the subglandular area of the penis. The cylinders were supplied in two fixed widths, 13 mm and 11 mm diameter, and the fluid was transferred back and forth between the proximally located reservoir and the central chamber to give alternating flaccidity and rigidity. Many patients experienced difficulty in inflating and deflating this prosthesis, especially with the deflation, and the device was redesigned to obviate some of the problems of the original model.

■ THE DYNAFLEX PROSTHESIS

In 1990 this revised version of the Hydroflex was introduced as the Dynaflex. It consists of two paired cylinders with all operating components contained within each device. The device is composed of three main parts — distal pump, central inflatable chamber and proximal reservoir (Fig. 37.1). Squeezing the pump pushes fluid into the central chamber and, as the pump is released, negative pressure draws fluid from the proximal reservoir, through a series of small channels located outside the central chamber, into the pump. Bending the cylinder 55 degrees or more from the horizontal and holding it for 10 seconds or longer operates a pressure switch and opens a passageway for fluid to flow from the central chamber to the proximal reservoir. This degree of angulation and time-frame are designed to prevent spontaneous deflation during sexual activity. During flaccidity the central chamber remains almost completely full. Only 1–2 ml fluid pumped into the central chamber are needed to change from the flaccid to the erect state. Two width diameters are available, 11 mm and 13 mm, with lengths in 2 cm increments between 14 and 18 cm for the 11 mm width and between 16 and 22 cm for the 13 mm width device. The differences in length between the cylinder and measured total corporal length may be adjusted by adding rear tip extenders which are supplied in 0.5 cm

413

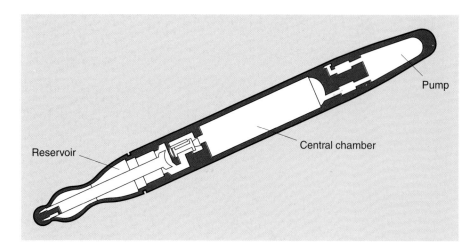

Figure 37.1. Cross-section of the Dynaflex prosthesis (courtesy of American Medical Systems, Minnetonka, MN, USA).

sizes and attached to each other and to the proximal end of the cylinder as 'pop beads'. Each cylinder comes filled with isotonic saline, prepackaged, and sterile in a saline medium. If contaminated, it should be returned to the manufacturer for partial credit and should not be resterilized.

The best rigidity with hydraulic penile implants is achieved when the cylinder completely fills the corporal body, as an inner tube fills a bicycle tyre. If a loose fit occurs, shifting of the cylinder will result and a tendency to buckle during intercourse. Patients with a broad penis that is incompletely filled by even the wider Dynaflex cylinders would obtain better rigidity from a device which gives a more accurate width fit. Patients who have had both a three-piece inflatable prosthesis and a Dynaflex will almost always prefer the rigidity and flaccidity of the three-piece device. Those with decreased finger-to-finger coordination or who have difficulty in learning even simple tasks will be frustrated with the inflation mechanism of the Dynaflex: of all the implants on the market it remains the most difficult to inflate. A reliable technique to help with complete cylinder inflation is to instruct the patient to place the thumb and index finger between the two cylinder distal tips and pump from the middle of the penis outward. Alternating back and forth, pumping one cylinder and then the other two or three times, will ensure complete inflation, which is necessary for optimal rigidity. The distal pump length is 4 cm and is not bendable. An additional 2 cm is needed for proximal hinge effect of the central chamber and so patients with an exposed penis shorter than 2 inches will have a less optimal flaccid appearance in the deflated state. Since the pumping mechanism is located distally, patients with a previous distal urethral erosion of an implant would be

exerting pressure during inflation of a Dynaflex over an area of weakened tissue, and might be better served by an alternative model prosthesis.

After the healing process has been completed, patients should be encouraged to cycle the prosthesis on a regular basis. Leaving the prosthesis inflated continuously will result in encapsulation of the reservoir portion, making deflation difficult, and a tendency towards autoinflation.

■ MECHANICAL PENILE IMPLANTS

Omniphase and Duraphase

In 1984, Dacomed Corporation (Minneapolis, MN, USA) introduced the Omniphase prosthesis.[6] This consisted of two rod-like cylinders composed of a series of polysulphone segments that articulated in a ball and socket arrangement held together by a central cable attached to a spring. Bending the cylinders would alternately shorten and lengthen the cable, thus allowing the rods to become taut as the segments abutted against each other or flaccid as the segments separated. Cable breakage, difficulty in cylinder selection, and problems with activation and deactivation gave a short market life to this device. The intent was to provide a prosthesis that gave the rigidity of a malleable device but with superior bendability for positioning during intercourse and good downward positioning without springback.

A derivative of the Omniphase was the Duraphase, which contained the same polysulphone segments without the activation–deactivation switching mechanism.[7] The device was easy to insert, very easy to manipulate, provided reasonably good rigidity, and was easy to conceal without the springback seen with the other semi-rigid implants. It became a very popular prosthesis, but segment wear and cable breakage necessitated replacement of many of these devices sooner than had been expected.

Dura II prosthesis

To increase the life span of the Duraphase, segment material was changed to high-molecular-weight polyethylene, which was five times more durable than polysulphone. In addition, the cable was redesigned with smaller and more numerous strands which, in bench testing, showed no fatigue after 8 million bends. This improved cylinder was renamed the Dura II prosthesis. The body segments are held together by a cable attached to a fixed post at each end by a spring. A polytetrafluoroethylene sleeve covers the segments and a thin silicone membrane covers the entire device to prevent adherence to body tissues. This implant is supplied in two width diameters — 10 mm and 12 mm. Each cylinder in both widths is 13 cm long. The segments are positioned at the point of bending, the penoscrotal junction, and proximal and distal tips of varying lengths are attached at each end and screwed in place with a stainless steel set screw. A grid combining glans pubis distance and total corporal length determines which size of proximal and distal tips to use. When measuring the glans pubis distance, the distal point should be at the proximal one-third of the glans. The proximal end of the measuring tool should rest without pressure against the skin over the pubis. In the heavy-set patient this may be some distance from the bone, but it is more accurate in determining the best bending location of the segments. If a discrepancy in intracorporal length between the two sides is observed, the difference in cylinder length should be adjusted by inserting proximal tips of different sizes: this will ensure the preservation of symmetric bending of the device. The Dura II cylinders can actually be bent more than the limits of the corporal anatomy will allow (Fig. 37.2). This is the prosthesis of choice for patients with little or no manual or mental ability to manipulate the device (Fig. 37.3). As with the Dynaflex implant, patients with a very broad penis will achieve suboptimal axial rigidity during penetration for intercourse with the Dura II. The shortest cylinder implantable is 15 cm long and hence patients with a very short penis, or with scarring from removal of a previous implant, may not be candidates for this prosthesis.

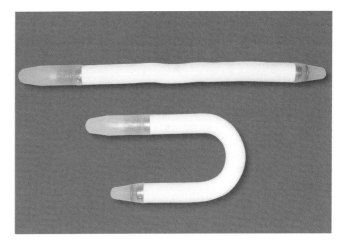

Figure 37.2. Dura II prosthesis (courtesy of Imagyn Co., Los Angeles, Ca, USA).

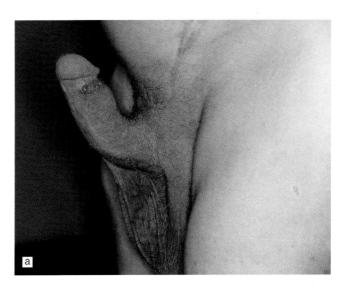

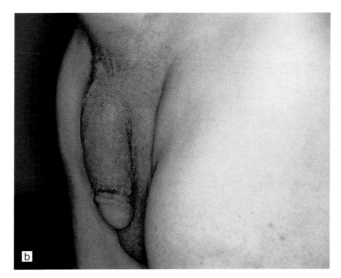

Figure 37.3. Bendability of the Dura II in the (a) upward and (b) downward positions.

■ MALLEABLE IMPLANTS

Jonas and AMS 600 prostheses

The first malleable implant, the Jonas prosthesis, offered good rigidity; however, breakage of the braided silver wire eventually resulted in many of these devices giving inadequate support for intercourse. In 1983, AMS introduced a similar malleable, the AMS 600, with twisted stainless steel wire as the central support surrounded by solid silicone.[8] A trimmable outer jacket of pliable silicone enabled this device to be placed as 13 mm or 11 mm diameter cylinders. This device was very durable with very few mechanical problems noted. The stainless steel wire was difficult to bend and exhibited significant springback, especially with the outer silicone jacket left intact.

AMS 650

The manufacturer redesigned the core wire, making the strands finer and more numerous with a spiral configuration without increasing the total girth, and enclosing it in a three-layered polyester covering. This covering was then encased in a solid silicone body. This resulted in a rod that bent more easily and with less springback and was introduced in 1996 as the AMS 650 (Fig. 37.4). Like its precursor the AMS 600, it was supplied in the 13 mm width with a trimmable outer jacket that could be removed to provide a cylinder of 11 mm girth, and in three lengths of 12, 16 and 20 cm with appropriate rear tip extenders for accurate length sizing

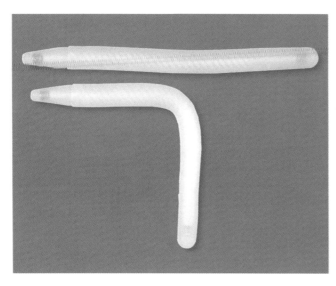

Figure 37.4. AMS 650 prosthesis (courtesy of American Medical Systems, Minnetonka, MN, USA).

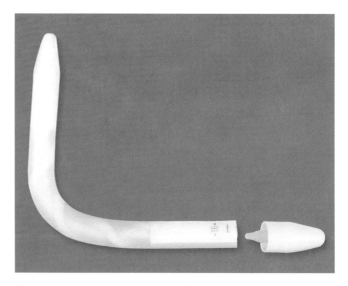

Figure 37.5. AccuForm prosthesis (courtesy of Mentor Corporation, Goleta, CA, USA).

within 0.5 cm. A narrower version, the AMS 600M, maintains the original wire configuration and is more malleable than the AMS 600. No enhancement of bendability or concealment was thought to be needed and this model is still available in 12, 14, 16 and 18 cm lengths with an 11.5 mm diameter reducible to 9.5 mm by removal of the pliable outer silicone sheath.

Mentor Malleable and AccuForm prostheses

Mentor Corporation (Goleta, CA, USA) markets two semi-rigid prostheses, the Malleable and the AccuForm.[9] The difference between the two is the configuration of the silver wire, which is arranged as a single spiral in the former and an outer helical wire surrounding a central wire core in the latter device to give more bendability with less springback after ventral positioning. Both versions are covered by a silicone elastomer and provided in three widths (9.5, 11 and 13 mm diameter). Cylinder lengths between 14 cm and 27 cm can be created by trimming a portion of the cylinder and adding a cap to provide a smooth tapered end (Fig. 37.5).

■ PRE-OPERATIVE PREPARATION

Patients are encouraged to bathe with a strong soap and thoroughly cleanse the genital area on the 3 days prior to surgery. The urine should be sterile, although this is sometimes difficult to achieve in patients with indwelling catheters or those with a neurogenic bladder. In such patients bladder and urethral washings with povidone-iodine and antibacterial solutions are used during the surgical preparation. Aggressive preparation with concentrated povidone-iodine, however, may irritate the mucosal lining of the lower urinary tract.

Antibiotic cover is started after the intravenous line has been placed before the induction of anaesthesia. The rationale for using systemic antibacterials is to provide adequate tissue levels while the wound is open during surgery and until the wound has sealed, usually up to 48 hours postoperatively. A number of antibiotic combinations have been used and recommended. Coverage against staphylococcal skin contaminants, and Gram-negative rods is desired and a combination of vancomycin and an aminoglycoside achieves this goal.[10] Antibiotics are commonly used in conjunction with prosthetic surgery, although no valid study has been performed that demonstrates their superiority in preventing intra-operatively acquired infections. Frequent irrigation of the wound with antibiotics is another feature that helps to reduce wound infection.

The patient's genital area is shaved after the induction of anaesthesia and a thorough skin preparation (usually with povidone-iodine scrub, paint, and spray) is completed prior to draping. The incidence of infection associated with prosthesis insertion has been low. In the face of infection the prosthesis may be removed, the wound thoroughly irrigated with antiseptic solutions and a new implant placed at the same setting, with success in the range of 85%.[11]

■ SURGICAL APPROACH

The Dynaflex can be inserted through any standard corporotomy — subcoronal, penoscrotal, dorsal penile or infrapubic — as it is easily bendable in the flaccid state. The Dura II and the malleables are not as bendable and, if a mid-shaft approach is used, a longer corporotomy is needed to place these devices. A very convenient incision to place all unitary cylinders is the ventral penile approach and local anaesthesia can also be used (Fig. 37.6).[12] A penile block using 1% lignocaine (lidocaine) without adrenaline is placed circumferentially at the base of the penis, as in performing a circumcision. A tourniquet is placed snugly around the base of the penis and 25 ml 1% lignocaine without adrenaline is injected intracorporally as an artificial erection. Bupivacaine

should not be used intravascularly as it may be cardiotoxic in large doses. In 2 minutes the tourniquet is released, allowing the anaesthetic to flow proximally to anaesthetize the entire length of the corpora cavernosa.

A midline skin incision is made on the proximal half of the penile shaft ventrally and carried down to the corpus spongiosum (Fig. 37.7). A vein retractor is used to pull the distal skin incision towards the glans penis and Buck's fascia is dissected from the tunica albuginea of the corpus cavernosum about two-thirds of the way down the shaft towards the glans. Two stay sutures for retraction of the edge of the corporotomy and for reference points during corporal measurement are placed in each corpus

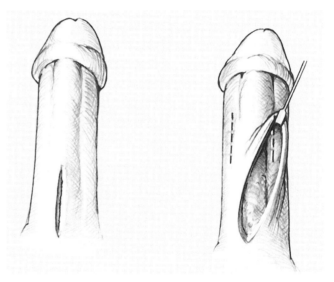

Figure 37.6. Diagram of the ventral penile incision for placing unitary prostheses.

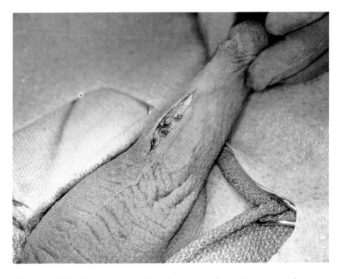

Figure 37.7. Skin incision for the ventral penile approach.

417

cavernosum lateral to the corpus spongiosum. A 3 cm incision is made between the stay sutures (Fig. 37.8) and the plane of dissection is made under the tunica albuginea, first proximally to the ischial tuberosities (Fig. 37.9) and then distally to the subglandular area with Metzenbaum scissors. Dilators starting with size 8 or 9 mm diameter are passed in each direction (Fig. 37.10). All unitary cylinders come in two fixed widths and during insertion the question arises which width to use. This should be done prior to opening the sterile package containing the device, rather than contaminating two sets of cylinders. To determine which of the two would be the better fit, two dilators of the smaller width are placed simultaneously side by side into each corporal body, first proximally and then distally. After each placement, the thumb should be apposed to the index finger between the dilators (Fig. 37.11). Slight separation between the dilators would indicate an ideal width fit. If no separation is noted, a snug fit with that size cylinder will result. If the thumb can easily touch the index finger between the dilators, a relatively loose fit will be achieved with that size of paired rods. The corporal cavities should then be dilated one size wider than the cylinder width to be inserted, to allow easy passage of the device in both directions. The corporal length is then measured in each direction with a stay suture used as the reference point (Fig. 37.12) and the two dimensions added to give the total corporal length. For the Dynaflex, the length inserted should be the length measured. For the Dura II and the malleables, inserting a rod about 0.5 cm shorter than the measured corporal length will give better bendability and less discomfort.

When too long a pair of Dynaflex cylinders has been inserted, the corporal bodies will take on an 'S' configuration. If excessively long, rigid rod pairs have been placed, a similar 'S' configuration will be noted, as well as excessive springback during ventral bending.

Once the appropriate size length and width have been determined, the cylinder is removed from its sterile package and appropriate tips or extenders applied. The prosthesis is inserted proximally to the ischial tuberosities (Fig. 37.13). A vein retractor is then used to pull the distal end of the corporotomy over the distal end of the rod (Fig. 37.14). The Dynaflex may first be deflated; the Dura II and malleables need not be bent during insertion using this technique. If desired with the Dynaflex, the suture through the end of the cylinder can first be brought through the glans penis using a Keith needle and

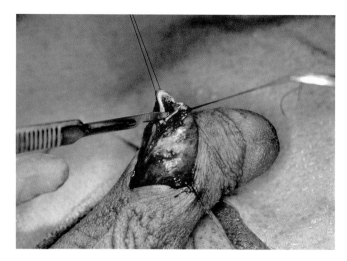

Figure 37.8. Corporotomy incision between two stay sutures.

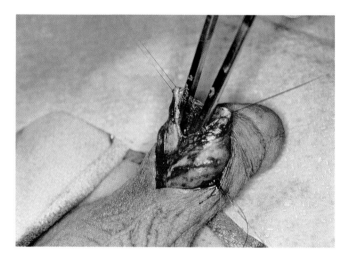

Figure 37.9. Proximal dissection to ischial tuberosity with Metzenbaum scissors.

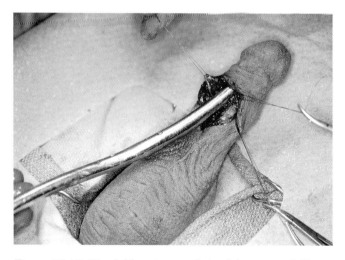

Figure 37.10. Distal dilatation to subglandular area with Hegar dilator.

418

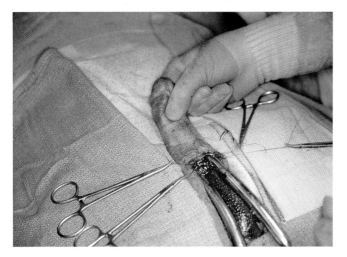

Figure 37.11. Width sizing — thumb apposed to index finger between two Hegar dilators.

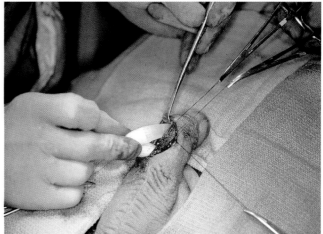

Figure 37.14. Distal placement of cylinder.

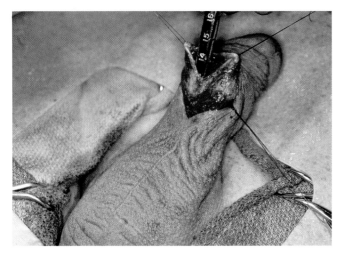

Figure 37.12. Corporal length measured proximally.

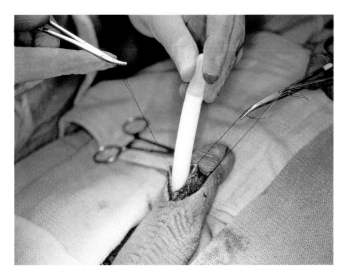

Figure 37.13. Proximal placement of cylinder.

insertion tool, although in the author's experience this has not been necessary using this approach. The wound is then closed in three layers —corporotomy, subcutaneous tissue and skin. The advantages of this incision include preservation of foreskin in the uncircumcized patient and the avoidance of overlapping suture lines.

POSTOPERATIVE CARE

The patient is discharged from the recovery room on the day of surgery or from the hospital the following morning. Antibiotics are continued for 48 hours after surgery, until the wound has sealed. No urethral catheter is usually placed during the surgery or afterwards, although some urologists favour its use until the morning after the procedure. The Dynaflex is kept slightly inflated and pointing cephalad. The Dura II and malleables are left in any comfortable position, usually upward to prevent rubbing of the head of the penis against the undergarments. Cycling and use of the device for intercourse is begun at about 5–6 weeks postoperatively.

TROUBLE SHOOTING

The Dynaflex prosthesis has been more durable than its precursor the Hydroflex although, with repeated bending, wear in the crease created at the bend angle of the penis has been seen. In 1996 the manufacturer, AMS, reinforced the entire outer layer of this device, making leakage at this site less likely to occur. Slow spontaneous deflation has occurred rarely with this device, due to malfunction of the valves internally.

The durability of the Dura II has also been superior to that of its precursor, the Duraphase. Segment wear may occur with time, so that there remains little or no tension on the springs attaching the cable to each post. The rods then lose rigidity and the penis appears floppy.

Wire breakage of the malleable rods has been very unusual. Whenever these mechanical problems occur, the cylinders can easily be replaced by a surgical approach similar to that used for insertion. The ventral penile approach using local anaesthesia on an outpatient basis is commonly used.

All three manufacturers of penile implants have a lifetime replacement policy for these devices in the USA.

■ SATISFACTION AND RELIABILITY

Despite the availability of less-invasive alternative treatments of erectile dysfunction, penile implants have maintained their share of the market. In 1996, about 21 000 implants were sold in the United States and 5000 internationally. Over the preceding 2 years a modest yearly growth in the range of 4% in sales was seen. The US domestic market is heavily weighted with inflatable devices, with greater than an 80% share.

Kabalin and Kuo compulsively surveyed 62 patients in whom a Dynaflex prosthesis was placed:[13] mean follow-up was 50 months and a mechanical failure rate of 10% was noted; mean time to cylinder failure was 40 months. Difficulty with the inflate–deflate mechanism was seen in 8%, despite apparent careful preoperative patient selection and postoperative instruction. Unsuccessful outcomes due to patient dissatisfaction occurred in an additional 16%. Of the 42 living patients with a functioning Dynaflex, 88% were satisfied when interviewed. Wilson and his colleagues did not have as positive an experience with the Dynaflex, reporting a mechanical failure rate of 26% and patient dissatisfaction rate also of 26%.[14] Kearse and colleagues, in a multicentre evaluation of the Dura II prosthesis up to 2 years after implantation, noted no mechanical failures and patient satisfaction rates in the range of 80%.[15]

Fallon and Ghanem[16] found overall satisfaction of about 90% in a series of 142 patients with an inflatable or a malleable implant: 18% of the rod group and 6% of those with an inflatable device believed that they had chosen the wrong prosthesis; 26% thought that their prosthesis did not meet expectations, in that it was too short or not stiff enough; 80% of partners were happy with the results. Krauss and associates[17] completed a prospective study of 19 malleable implant recipients and their partners, and found that both groups were generally satisfied with the prosthesis: 85% of patients and 70% of spouses were pleased with the function of the device. The frequency of sexual intercourse increased during the follow-up period but there were no changes in sexual desire. A total of 92% of patients and 90% of partners indicated that they would choose the implant surgery if faced with the same option again. The size of the penis postoperatively was a major disappointment to many patients, although with time and acclimatization to the new device this became less of a concern. Dorflinger and Bruskewitz[8] evaluated 57 patients implanted with an AMS 600 malleable implant: 91% of patients were satisfied with their decision and 66% reported no difficulty with concealment.

■ SILICONE ISSUE

The recent furore and legal publicity that breast implants have experienced has now turned to penile implants. No increased incidence of autoimmune disease has been found in patients with breast implants when compared with age-matched controls.[18] Barrett and associates[19] looked at silicone particle shedding and migration of silicone in genito-urinary prosthetic devices: 18 of 25 patients (72%) had silicone particles in the periprosthetic capsule and a few patients had silicone particles in inguinal and peri-aortic lymph nodes. Adjuvant disease was not seen in any of these patients. The Food and Drug Administration has made it mandatory for the manufacturers of inflatable implants to conduct prospective clinical trials to document the safety, efficacy and patient satisfaction with these devices. Attempts to combine instances of penile implant malfunction as class action lawsuits have so far been unsuccessful.

■ CONCLUSIONS

Unitary hydraulic and semi-rigid rod penile implants continue to play a significant role in the treatment of erectile dysfunction. Ease of insertion, low malfunction rate, lower cost and simplicity of operation have made them popular choices in many circumstances. Satisfaction rates in the range of 80% are consistently higher than those of other, less invasive, treatments. The predictable and reliable result which these devices afford adds to the patient's confidence in his ability to perform sexually. His overall outlook on life, productivity and body image are consequently enhanced.

■ REFERENCES

1. Scott F B, Bradley W E, Timm G W. Management of erectile impotence: use of implantable inflatable prosthesis. Urology 1973; 2: 80–82

2. Small M D. Small–Carrion penile prosthesis: a report on 160 cases and review of the literature. J Urol 1978; 119: 365–368

3. Finney R P. New hinged silicone penile implant. J Urol 1977; 118: 585–587

4. Jonas U, Jacobi G H. Silicone–silver penile prosthesis: description of approach and results. J Urol 1980; 123: 865–867

5. Mulcahy J J. The Hydroflex penile prosthesis. Urol Clin North Am 1989; 16(1): 33–38

6. Krane R J. Omniphase penile prosthesis. Semin Urol 1986; 4: 247–251

7. Mulcahy J J, Krane R J, Lloyd L K et al. Duraphase penile prosthesis: results of clinical trials in 63 patients. J Urol 1990; 143: 518–519

8. Dorflinger T, Bruskewitz R. AMS Malleable penile prosthesis. Urology 1986; 28: 480–485

9. Mulcahy J J. Overview of penile implants. In: Mulcahy J J (ed) Diagnosis and management of male sexual dysfunction. New York: Igaku-Shoin, 1997: 218–230

10. Carson C C. Infections in genitourinary prostheses. Urol Clin North Am 1989; 16: 139–147

11. Brant M D, Ludlow J K, Mulcahy J J. The prosthesis salvage operation: immediate replacement of the infected penile prosthesis. J Urol 1996; 155: 155–157

12. Wahle G R, Mulcahy J J. Ventral penile approach in unitary component penile prosthesis placement. J Urol 1993; 149: 537–538

13. Kabalin J N, Kuo J C. Long term follow-up and patient satisfaction with the self-contained inflatable penile prosthesis. J Urol 1997; 158: 456–459

14. Wilson S K, Cleves M, Delk J J II. Long term results with Hydroflex and Dynaflex penile prosthesis: device survival, comparison to multicomponent inflatables. J Urol 1996; 155: 1621–1623

15. Kearse W S, Sago A L, Perets S J et al. Report of a multicenter clinical evaluation of the Dura II penile prosthesis. J Urol 1996; 155:1613–1616

16. Fallon B, Ghanem H. Sexual performance and satisfaction with penile prostheses in impotence of variouse etiologies. Int J Impot Res 1990; 2: 35–42

17. Krauss D J, Lantinga L J, Carey M P et al. Use of the Malleable penile prosthesis in the treatment of erectile dysfunction: a prospective study of postoperative adjustment. J Urol 1989; 142: 988–991

18. Sherine G E, O'Fallon W M, Kurland L T et al. Risk of connective tissue diseases and other disorders after breast implantation. N Engl J Med 1994; 330: 1697–1702

19. Barrett D M, O'Sullivan D C, Malizia A A et al. Particle shedding and migration from silicone genitourinary prosthetic devices. J Urol 1991; 146: 319–322

Chapter 38
Inflatable penile prostheses

C. C. Carson

INTRODUCTION

Although the problem of erectile dysfunction (ED) has been recognized since ancient times, adequate treatment has been available only for the last half of the 20th century. In the early 20th century, attempts to design surgical procedures to provide rigidity of the penis for sexual activity and to recreate the os penis of lower animals was unsuccessfully attempted by a variety of surgeons and investigators. In 1902, Wooten[1] reported the restoration of erectile activity by ligation of the dorsal penile vein, while Steinach in 1906 suggested that bilateral vasectomy might be a surgical procedure used for the cure of ED.[2] The Steinach procedure remained popular until an objective study by Macht and Teagarden in 1923[2] demonstrated that bilateral vasectomy and placebo treatment were fully as effective in treating patients with ED.[2] The first attempts at penile prosthesis implantation were in the 1930s, when Bogaras described the use of a tailored section of rib cartilage to produce penile rigidity in a fashion similar to that provided by the os penis of walruses, squirrels and other animals.[3] These tailored grafts, however, were unsatisfactory, and cartilage reabsorption, infection, extrusion and progressive angulation resulted in abandonment of this procedure. Bergman and co-workers in 1948 reported the use of a rib graft with similar complications.[4]

Development of newer synthetic materials in the 1950s and 1960s propelled the advancement of prosthetic devices in the treatment of a variety of medical conditions, including ED. Early reports by Goodwin and colleagues[5] in 1952 suggested that synthetic materials could produce satisfactory results when implanted into the penis for ED. The era of modern penile prosthetic devices began with the development of silicone-based prosthetic materials in the late 1960s as a result of the

space programme.[6] Lash and colleagues[7] in 1968 reported 28 patients using single silicone prosthetic devices with good results and Pearman[8] designed a single silicone silastic prosthetic rod placed beneath Buck's fascia in 126 patients in 1972 (Fig. 38.1). Although these devices increased the success of penile prosthesis implantation, their placement beneath Buck's fascia provided little stability, significant discomfort, and a non-physiological penile shape. Extrusion rates were also high with these initial attempts at penile prosthesis design.

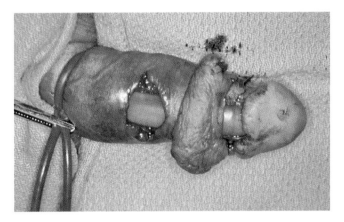

Figure 38.1. Pearman penile prosthesis placed beneath Buck's fascia through dorsal penile incision.

TYPES OF PENILE PROSTHESES

Modern penile prosthetic devices were first developed in the early 1970s when Scott and colleagues,[9] together with Small and colleagues,[10] reported the implantation of penile prosthetic devices into the corpora cavernosa to fill the corpora cavernosa and to provide a physiological functional erection with good cosmetic results. The development of semi-rigid rod prostheses for which the

Small–Carrion device is a prototype, was previously described (Chapter 37). Scott and colleagues in 1973 described the second group of penile implants, which are inflatable. These devices have undergone multiple revisions and new designs between the early prosthetic devices and the currently implanted inflatable penile prostheses. The initial device consisted of four components including an inflation pump, deflation pump, reservoir, and two implantable cylinders. The current device has combined the inflation and deflation pump into a single pump. There are currently three varieties of hydraulically inflatable penile prostheses, including self-contained, two-piece, and three-piece penile prostheses. Early three-piece inflatable penile prostheses were widely used, with excellent erections and a physiologically flaccid-appearing penis between uses. Mechanical malfunction rates in these early devices, however, were reported in excess of 60% of cases.[11–13] Current inflatable prosthetic devices, however, have a greatly improved mechanical reliability.[14,15] These current devices (Table 38.1) can be divided into multiple-component inflatable penile prostheses, of which two- and three-piece models are available. There are also single-rod inflatable penile prostheses, which have been termed the 'hydraulic hinge' penile prostheses. Because these latter prostheses do not provide a significant increase in penile girth and frequently are limited in flaccidity, their classification as true inflatable penile prostheses remains controversial.

The three-piece inflatable penile prostheses are currently available from American Medical Systems (AMS; Minnetonka, MN, USA) as the AMS 700 CX, Ultrex, and Ultrex Plus, as well as the Mentor Alpha-1 prostheses (Fig. 38.2). The newer design cylinders from AMS consist of a three-layer construction, with an inner layer of silicone, middle layer of limited-expansion Dacron mesh in the CX cylinders and middle layer of Lycra in the Ultrex cylinders, with an outer layer of silicone to prevent tissue adherence from the middle-layer mesh.[16] Whereas the CX cylinders have controlled expansion capabilities, the Ultrex cylinders permit girth expansion to 18 mm and elongation by as

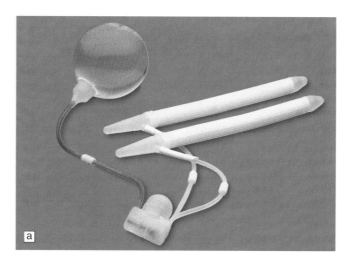

Table 38.1. Current penile prostheses

Semi-rigid rods
    AMS 600 (AMS)
    Jonas Bard
    Malleable (Mentor)

Inflatable
    700 CX (AMS)
    700 Ultrex (AMS)
    Alpha 1 (Mentor)
    GFS (Mentor)
    Ambicor (AMS)

Self contained
    Dynaflex (AMS)

Mechanical
    Duraphase (Osbon)

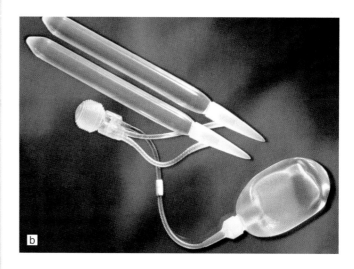

Figure 38.2. Multiple component inflatable penile prostheses. (a) AMS 700 Ultrex Plus penile prosthesis. (Courtesy of American Medical Systems, Inc., Minnetonka, MN, USA. Illustration by Michael Schenk.) (b) Alpha-1 penile prosthesis. (Courtesy of Mentor Corporation, Santa Barbara, CA, USA.)

much as 20% in length to allow increased filling of the corporal bodies and possible axial expansion.[17,18] The prosthetic cylinders of the Mentor Alpha-1 prosthesis are constructed of Bioflex material (Mentor Corporation, Goleta, CA, USA) which expands to 20 mm in girth without axial elongation.[15] As a result of its single-layer design, more rigid wall and resilient construction, the Bioflex material appears to be more durable than single-layer silicone although the currently available triple-layer silicone prostheses appear to have durability equivalent to that of Bioflex cylinders.[19] Aneurysmal dilatation is rare with both of these cylinder designs but has been reported.[18-21] Similarly, other design changes, including replacement of stainless steel connectors with plastic connectors, addition of non-kinked tubing, single-design construction, Teflon cylinder input sleeves and multiple-layer cylinders have improved the longevity of these devices. Because the cylinder portion of the inflatable system functions at significantly higher pressure than the reservoir portion, most complications occur where pressure maintenance is important. Therefore, strengthening or eliminating connectors, strengthening cylinder materials and input tubes have decreased mechanical malfunction rates from more than 30% to less than 5%.

The three-piece inflatable penile prostheses continue to be the most satisfactory prostheses once they are implanted and while they remain functional.[22-29] These prosthetic devices produce the most natural-appearing erection in girth and length, and impart satisfactory rigidity and excellent flaccidity for optimal concealment. They also have advantages for many patients with complex penile implantations, since the flaccid position removes pressure from the corpora cavernosa and decreases the possibility of erosion in these highly difficult implantations. Pressure within the corpus cavernosum is reflected upon the layers of the tunica albuginea. The thinnest portion of the tunica albuginea appears to be the ventral aspect, which lacks longitudinally directed outer bundles of collagen and corresponds to the area of most common penile prosthesis extrusion.[30] In situations such as where patients have had previous extrusion, infection, severe diabetes or peripheral neuropathy, or in patients with severe corpus cavernosum fibrosis or reconstruction, the inflatable penile prosthesis may be the optimum choice.[22,25,29]

To improve ease of surgical implantation and to remove a portion of the prosthesis placed within the abdominal region, two-piece prostheses were designed[31] (Fig. 38.3). These currently include the Mentor GFS

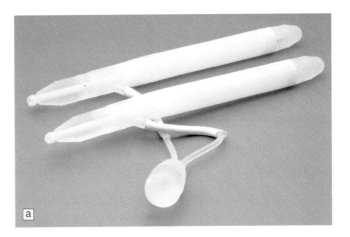

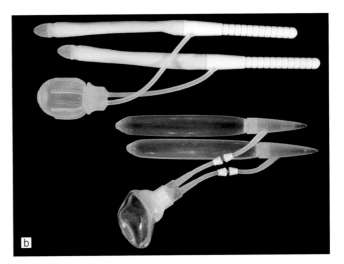

Figure 38.3. Two-piece inflatable penile prostheses. (a) Ambicor inflatable penile prosthesis. (Courtesy of American Medical Systems, Inc., Minnetonka, MN, USA. Illustration by Michael Schenk.) (b) Top: Surgitek Uniflate 1000 inflatable penile prosthesis (Courtesy of Dacomed). Bottom: GFS Mark II inflatable penile prosthesis. (Courtesy of Mentor Corporation, Santa Barbara, CA, USA.)

Mark II and the AMS Ambicor prostheses. The previously available Uniflate 1000 (Surgitech) is still frequently encountered in patients implanted with these devices in the early 1990s.[32] Because these two-piece inflatable prostheses remove the separate reservoir, additional fluid is available either by a larger scrotal pump (GFS Mark II) or by a combination of proximal cylinder and pump reservoir (Ambicor). The GFS Mark II combines the Alpha-1 Bioflex cylinders with a large 'resipump'.[31] The Ambicor (AMS) combines cylinders similar to those of the Dynaflex prosthesis with a separate scrotal pump/reservoir. Although these devices provide adequate erection in many patients, the limited reservoir capacity

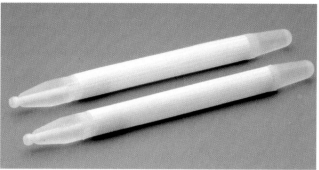

Figure 38.4. Dynaflex single piece inflatable prosthesis. (Courtesy of American Medical Systems, Inc., Minnetonka, MN, USA. Illustration by Michael Schenk.)

decreases flaccidity and may, in some patients, diminish rigidity. These prostheses are especially difficult to deflate in patients with small penises and frequently provide inadequate rigidity for patients with longer penises. In these devices, instead of recycling the full device, 15–20 ml fluid are transferred and at least 5–10 ml fluid remain within the cylinders between uses. This difference in cycled volume may decrease flaccidity and be objectionable to some patients. Although they are less optimal than three-piece devices, these two-piece implants may be ideal for patients in whom reservoir placement is difficult or contra-indicated. Such patients as renal transplant recipients and those who have undergone significant radical pelvic exenteration procedures may benefit from two-piece devices.

Single-piece inflatable cylinder prostheses, also known as the 'hydraulic hinge', are available as the Dynaflex (AMS) (Fig. 38.4). These devices are even simpler than the two-piece devices for implantation and are implanted in a fashion similar to that for semi-rigid rod prostheses. They require inflation by pressure on the distal portion of the penis with penile shaft deflection for deflation. Although full inflation results in a firm shaft, there is no increase in girth or length. Deflation, likewise, may be less than optimal because of the pump portion of the device located in the distal penis. Because of limitations of rigidity and flaccidity, use of these devices should be reserved for patients with average-size penises and for specific indications.[33]

■ PATIENT SELECTION

Although there are a variety of penile prosthesis designs currently available for implantation, not all patients with

ED are candidates for penile prosthesis implantation. Careful counselling of patients before penile implant procedures avoids many of the problems with postoperative dissatisfaction. Despite careful counselling, however, many patients enter penile prosthesis procedures with expectations that cannot be met by penile prosthesis surgery. Complaints about decreased penile length compared with pre-implant state, decreased penile sensation, and 'coolness' of the penis and glans penis, as well as chronic pain and partner dissatisfaction, are among the complaints that patients may voice despite adequate surgical implantation and satisfactory mechanical functioning. Fortunately, these complaints are unusual and more than 90% of patients report satisfaction with their prostheses.[24,34] Many patients who are dissatisfied with their penile prostheses will benefit from sexual counselling or continued counselling assistance from the implanting surgeon to be sure that they are able to operate the device satisfactorily and understand its use.[27] Most patients' dissatisfaction results from difficulty with functioning and unrealistic expectations. Discussions with patients should include the concept that penile prostheses do not create normal erections but only support the penis for sexual activity. Penile prosthesis surgery brings about the ability to resume sexual functioning and vaginal penetration, but decreased penile sensation, length and engorgement may result.[35] Furthermore, patients should be made aware of the possibility of mechanical malfunction, infection and other common complications that may compromise the results of their penile implant. Patients should also be advised that a penile prosthesis will not improve libido or ejaculation. Patients frequently report delayed or difficult ejaculation initially following penile prosthesis surgery. This delay is primarily a result of inadequate preparation, stimulation and psychological adjustment to the prosthesis. Most patients require 3–6 months of prosthesis use, with careful attention to presexual stimulation, before ejaculation routinely returns to pre-operative levels.[32] Because the prosthesis neither improves nor detracts from pre-operative ejaculatory ability, patients must be counselled regarding their pre-operative ejaculatory ability before prosthesis placement.

Once the discussion and demonstration of penile implant varieties has been carried out, patients can be counselled about the most appropriate penile prosthesis for their individual use. Patients may choose a specific prosthetic type based on their needs and preferences. Younger patients with normal manual dexterity often choose a three-piece inflatable penile prosthesis because appearance in the flaccid position is important, particularly for patients who wear stylish, form-fitting, athletic clothing or who shower in public at a health club or other athletic facility. For these patients, implantation of a semi-rigid rod penile prosthesis requires a significant lifestyle change and they are better served with an inflatable-type prosthesis. Similarly, patients with Peyronie's disease, secondary implantation, or significant peripheral neuropathy such as occurs in severe diabetes, are best served with an inflatable penile prosthesis because interior tissue pressures are diminished between uses and the possibility of extrusion is diminished.[36–38] For patients in whom the convenience of inflation and deflation are not important, the risks of mechanical malfunctions may outweigh the disadvantage of a malleable penile prosthesis. Such patients as paraplegics who require an external urinary collection device, those with inadequate manual dexterity, or those with significant obesity may be better served with a malleable penile prosthesis.

SURGICAL IMPLANTATION OF PENILE PROSTHESES

Surgical implantation of penile prostheses can be carried out using a variety of surgical approaches and incisions. Single-rod inflatable prostheses of the hydraulic hinge variety are implanted in a fashion similar to that for semi-rigid rod prostheses, as described by Mulcahy in Chapter 37. Multiple-piece prostheses, however, can be implanted by the infrapubic or penoscrotal approach. Although individual surgeons have a variety of rationales for each of these approaches, there does not appear to be any clear advantage in patient satisfaction or outcome of either of the two approaches.[39] Patient anatomy may dictate the appropriate choice: patients with previous abdominal surgical procedures, where reservoir placement is difficult, may be better served with an infrapubic approach, whereas patients with massive obesity may be better approached through a penoscrotal incision. Two-piece devices (because no separate reservoir is present) are best implanted through a penoscrotal incision.

The infrapubic approach is usually carried out with a horizontal incision approximately one finger-breadth above the symphysis pubis allowing implantation with an easily concealed incision once the pubic hair regrows (Fig. 38.5). In patients with significant obesity or a previous midline incision, however, midline incision carried out

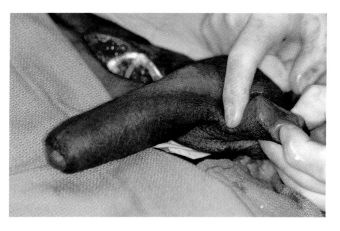

Figure 38.5. Infrapubic incision for penile prosthesis insertion.

just to the base of the penis facilitates exposure of the corpus cavernosum and improves the ability for corpus cavernosum dilatation. Because the penoscrotal approach requires differentiation from the corpus spongiosum during resection, initial placement of a Foley catheter is necessary. The infrapubic approach allows more direct section of the corpora cavernosa; however, because of the dorsal neurovascular bundle, injury is possible, resulting in decreased distal penile sensation in some patients.

Infrapubic approach

Surgical implantation of a multipiece inflatable penile prosthesis is by the infrapubic approach, which begins with a (usually) horizontal incision one finger-breadth above the pubic symphysis. In obese patients, however, a midline incision may facilitate dilatation by improving exposure of the corpora cavernosa. Similarly, if a patient has a previously healed midline incision, this incision can again be used for the infrapubic approach to penile prosthesis implantation. After incision of the subcutaneous tissue, the section is continued to the rectus fascia. The rectus fascia is sized horizontally and dissected cephalad for approximately 2–3 cm. A midline separation of the rectus muscles is carried out and, using sharp and blunt dissection, a pouch is created beneath the rectus muscles to insert the inflatable reservoir comfortably without compression. This step is eliminated by the use of a two-piece penile prosthesis.

The section is then carried out over the corpora cavernosa. Sharp and blunt dissection is begun on either side of the fundiform ligament, identifying the dorsal neurovascular bundle. It should be noted that the dorsal nerves of the penis lie approximately 2–3 mm lateral to the deep dorsal vein. Once Buck's fascia has been dissected free from the tunica albuginea, the shiny white tunica albuginea is fixed with traction sutures.

A corporotomy incision is then carried out between the traction sutures and the corpora cavernosa entered. The corporotomy incision can be carried out with scalpel or electrocautery. Metzenbaum scissors are then used carefully to initiate the tunnelling of the corpora cavernosa, gently spreading the cavernosal tissue both proximately and distally until the ischial tuberosities and crura are encountered, and distally palpating the glans penis to identify the most distal aspect of dilatation. Hagar dilators can be used (size 9–12) or Brooks, Pratt, or Dilamezinsert dilators can be used (Fig. 38.6). If fibrosis is encountered, Rosillo cavernotomes can be used to dilate to size 12. Once dilatation has been adequately carried out bilaterally, the Furlow is introduced or Dilamezinsert is used to measure the length of the corpora cavernosa, using a traction suture as a central point of reference. The proximal and distal measurements are added to identify total corporal length and obtain appropriate-sized inflatable cylinders. A length slightly less than this measurement is usually selected to permit comfortable positioning of the cylinders. Rear tip extenders of size 1, 2, or 3 cm, or combinations thereof, are placed on the proximal cylinder end to adjust length.

Once the measurement has been obtained, interrupted sutures can be placed for later corporotomy closure. The advantage of this technique is the elimination of suture needles close to the area of the inflatable cylinder, diminishing the possibility of cylinder damage during corporotomy closure. Other methods of corporotomy closure include running sutures with or without a locking technique. Once the interrupted sutures are placed in the cavernosotomy incision, cylinders are positioned within the dilated corpora cavernosa using the inserting tool with distal needle to pull the cylinders into position. Once the cylinders are positioned, it is essential to visualize each one within the corpus cavernosum to ensure that no kinking is seen and complete proximal and distal seating has taken place. The cavernostomy incision should be placed proximal enough to allow easy exit of the input tube and to minimize cylinder/input tube contact. Closure of the corpus cavernosum incision is carried out with traction on the cylinder placement suture to maintain it in a flat non-kinking position and to ensure adequate seating. Following placement of cylinder and closure of the corporotomy incision, cylinder inflation can be tested by placing fluid in each of the cylinders through the input tubes, gently inflating the prosthesis to identify any abnormalities in position, any curvature, or other problems.

A finger is then placed in the most dependent portion of the scrotum lateral to the testicle on the right or left side. The finger is then pushed to the area of the external inguinal ring and adipose tissue in this area is dissected free using sharp and blunt dissection to expose the dartos fascia, which is thoroughly cleaned to allow pump placement. Following development of a subcutaneous pouch for the pump, the pump is positioned in the most dependent portion of the scrotum and temporarily fixed into position using a Babcock clamp. The inflatable reservoir is then placed in the previously constructed sub-rectus pocket and filled with an appropriate volume of normal saline or water/radiographic contrast medium. Tubing connection is then carried out using quick connectors, or suture tie plastic connectors. The snap-on connectors are used for the Mentor prosthesis. In a 'redo' prosthesis, in which a residual tubing segment is connected to a new device piece, suture tie plastic connectors must be used. Connection is carried out by tailoring tubing to eliminate excessive length but allow for adequate pump positioning. Rubber-shodded clamps are used to compress the tubing, and the ends of the tubing, once tailored, are flushed with inflation fluid to eliminate small particles and blood clots. After connection, the adequacy of the connection is tested. All rubber-shodded clamps are removed and the device is inflated and deflated on multiple occasions to ensure adequate location, placement, and erection.

Following testing, thorough irrigation with antibiotic solution is carried out and the rectus fascia is closed with

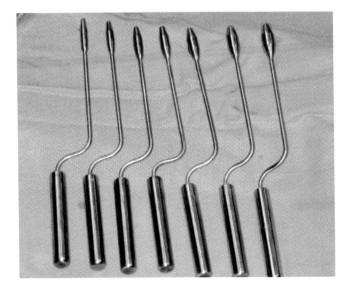

Figure 38.6. Brooks corporal dilators.

interrupted sutures. The wound is then closed in the standard fashion with two layers of subcutaneous tissue and a subcuticular skin suture. A dry sterile dressing is applied, a Foley catheter is placed if necessary, and an ice pack applied. Suction drains may be used at the surgeon's discretion.

Postoperatively, patients are instructed to maintain their penis in a Sutherland position for 4–6 weeks. Tight underwear and athletic supports are not used, in an effort to maintain the pump in its most dependent position.

Penoscrotal approach

Three-piece inflatable penile prostheses can be implanted by a transverse or vertical penile scrotal incision (Fig. 38.7). This approach has distinct advantages in obese patients and is widely used for routine penile prosthesis implantation. An incision is begun in the upper portion of the scrotum following placement of a Foley catheter. The Scott retractor facilitates exposure with this incision. Once the skin incision has been carried out, the section is continued lateral to the corpus spongiosum and urethra to expose the corpora cavernosa. Incision and closure of the corpora cavernosa are similar to those described previously for the infrapubic incision. Pump placement is likewise in the most dependent portion of the scrotum just above the Dartos fascia, with positioning using a Babcock clamp. The section for reservoir placements, however, can be carried out with a second separate infrapubic incision but is more commonly performed through the penoscrotal incision. The scrotal skin incision is retracted to the areas of the external inguinal ring and dissection is carried out medial to the spermatic cord. The transversalis fascia is identified and incised sharply using Metzenbaum scissors placed against the pubic tubercle. Dissection is carried out using a combination of sharp and blunt dissection. A reservoir insertion tool can be passed through the inward canal to allow balloon placement. More often, however, dilatation is carried out with the index finger after incision of the transversalis fascia and with gentle blunt dissection using a large Kelly clamp. The reservoir balloon is then positioned over the index finger and placed in the perivesical space. Inflation of the reservoir is carried out with care that no back-pressure on the fluid is observed. If refilling of the syringe occurs, the reservoir should be removed and further reservoir pocket dissection must be carried out. Once the reservoir is placed and inflated, and the tubing connected as previously described, the device is tested in inflation and deflation (Fig. 38.8). Closure is carried out with a subcuticular suture in the standard fashion.

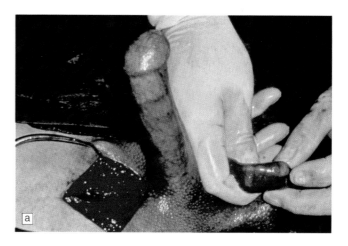

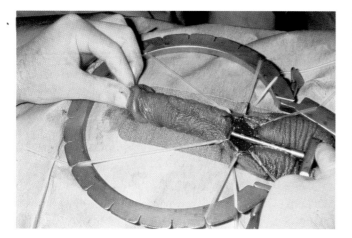

Figure 38.7. Penoscrotal incision with Scott retractor for penile prosthesis insertion.

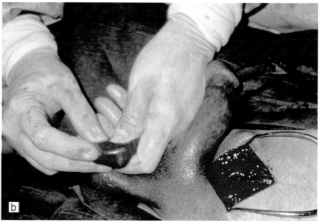

Figure 38.8. (a) A surgeon inflating an AMS inflatable penile prosthesis placed through an infrapubic approach. (b) Prosthesis deflation.

ANAESTHESIA

The choice of anaesthesia for penile prosthesis implantation varies with surgeon and patient preference. Although the majority of penile prostheses are placed with general, spinal, or epidural anaesthesia, some implanting surgeons have had success with local anaesthesia.[40,41] Candidates for local anaesthesia must be carefully selected, as corporal dilatation, even after infusion of local anaesthetic agents, may be somewhat uncomfortable. The author prefers general and regional anaesthesia, since patients are less likely to move during surgery and describe the implantation procedure as more satisfactory in postoperative interviews.

PERI-OPERATIVE CARE

Peri-operative antibiotic treatment is critical in reducing the incidence of peri-operative infection and prosthetic removal.[22] An initial peri-operative dosage of an agent effective against the most common infectious pathogens should be administered 1–2 hours prior to surgery and continued for 48 hours postoperatively.[23] Choice of an aminoglycoside with a first-generation cephalosporin, a cephalosporin alone, vancomycin or a fluoroquinolone is appropriate for prophylaxis of the most common infections from Staphylococcus epidermidis.[24] Patients are discharged for 7 days of continued antibiotic therapy. The penile prosthesis remains deflated for 4 weeks while healing occurs. Prior to activation, the patient is advised to retract the pump into his scrotum on a daily basis and tight underwear and athletic supports are avoided to maintain pump position. A return office visit for activation of the device is carried out once discomfort has resolved. Patients are advised to inflate and deflate the device on a daily basis for 4 weeks to allow tissue expansion around the prosthesis. Most patients can then begin use of their device immediately.

POSTOPERATIVE COMPLICATIONS

The most worrisome postoperative complication is postoperative infection. Fortunately, this complication occurs in fewer than 10% of all patients. Perioperative prosthetic infections can, however, occur at any time in the postoperative period in patients with penile or other prosthetic devices. Patients continue to be at risk for haematogenously seeded infections from gastrointestinal, dental or urological manipulations as well as remote infections. Patients must be counselled to request antibiotic cover if remote infections occur.[42] Most periprosthetic infections are caused by Gram-positive organisms such as Staphylococcus epidermidis but Gram-negative organisms such as E. coli and Pseudomonas are also common culprits.[43,44] Severe gangrenous infections with a combination of Gram-negative and anaerobic organisms have also been identified and frequently result in significant disability and tissue loss.[45–47] Patients at increased risk for perioperative infections include those with diabetes, patients undergoing penile straightening procedures or circumcision with prosthetic implantation, patients with urinary tract bacterial colonization and immunocompromised patients such as post-transplant patients.[48,49] Although these patients are at increased risk, the risk of infection continues to be less than 10% and is, in most cases, quite acceptable.[49] Spinal cord injury patients have also been reported to have a specially increased risk of infections with rates reported as high as 15%.[43] Because of a decrease in sensation, an increased risk of extrusion of semi-rigid prostheses has been reported in this group of patients. Diabetic patients with poor control may be evaluated with glycohaemoglobin studies prior to surgery to enhance diabetic control prior to prosthesis implantation and, perhaps, decrease the possibility of infection.[50]

Appropriate treatment of periprosthetic infections requires early and immediate identification with institution of parenteral antibiotic therapy and early prosthesis removal.[51] Conservative treatment would dictate a healing period of 3–6 months followed by repeat prosthesis implantation. Satisfactory results with prosthesis removal and a 5–7-day course of antibiotic irrigation, followed by additional replacement, has been reported for selected patients.[52–55] Reports have also suggested that immediate replacement of the prosthesis following intraoperative irrigation may be successful.[56,57] Several reviews of the problem of penile prosthesis infection and its treatment have been published.[44,51,57]

The most common complication of penile prosthesis function is mechanical malfunction.[11,58] Mechanical malfunction has declined from rates as high as 61% to levels below 5% since the 1970s[59,60] (Fig. 38.9). Aneurysmal dilatation of inflatable cylinders, both AMS

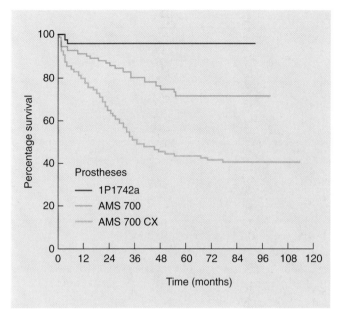

Figure 38.9. Penile prosthesis survival of different American Medical System penile prosthesis models (Kaplan–Meier curve): ——, 1P1742a; ——, AMS 700; ——, AMS 700 CX.

CONCLUSIONS

The implantation of inflatable penile prostheses is commonly performed throughout the world. This successful procedure restores erectile function in most men in whom implantation is carried out. The knowledge of the types of prostheses available, together with their advantages, disadvantages and implantation techniques, is necessary for the skilled prosthetic management of ED. Careful discussion of these factors and the potential risks optimizes patient satisfaction. Patients should be allowed to choose a prosthesis from each of the classifications of prostheses available. With careful patient selection, prosthesis choice, and with currently available reliable prosthetic devices, the urologist can expect excellent patient and partner satisfaction with low morbidity.

and Mentor, tubing kinking, reservoir leakage and pump malfunction have been limited by device modifications.[61–63] Fluid leak, however, continues to be a problem in many inflatable penile prostheses. These mechanical malfunctions require replacement of the leaking portion of the inflatable portion of the prosthesis.[63] If a non-functioning prosthesis has been in place more than 4 years, however, the author usually replaces the entire device in order to reduce further mechanical malfunction.

Semi-rigid rod penile prostheses are associated with few mechanical problems and the most common complication associated with these prostheses is cylinder erosion through skin or urethra.[32] Prosthesis fracture or breakage has been reported and patients may return, 6–8 years after implantation with complaints of decreased rigidity of their semi-rigid rod, indicating fracture of central prosthetic cylinder wires.[64] These wire fractures cannot usually be appreciated radiographically unless the prosthesis is put on stretch once it has been explanted. Replacement of these devices is indicated when patients note decreased rigidity. Prosthesis extrusion or erosion is most common in patients with diabetes and spinal cord injury, especially those requiring urinary management with catheter placement or condom collection.

REFERENCES

1. Wooten J S. Ligation of the dorsal vein of the penis as a cure for atonic impotence. Texas Med J 1902; 18: 325–327

2. Macht D, Teagarden E. Rejuvenation experiments with vas ligation in rats. J Urol 1923; 10: 407–411

3. Kim J H, Carson C C. History of urologic prostheses for impotence. Prob Urol 1993; 7: 283–288

4. Bergman R T, Howard H, Barnes R W. Plastic reconstruction of the penis. J Urol 1948; 59: 1177–1179

5. Goodwin W E, Scardino P L, Scott W W. Penile prosthesis for impotence: case report. J Urol 1981; 126: 409

6. Habal M B. The biologic basis for the clinical application of silicones. Arch Surg 1984; 119: 843–854

7. Lash H. Silicone implant for impotence. J Urol 1968; 100: 709–712

8. Pearman R O. Treatment of organic impotence by implantation of a penile prosthesis. J Urol 1967; 97: 716–719

9. Scott F B, Bradley W E, Timm G W. Management of erectile impotence: use of implantable inflatable prosthesis. Urology 1973; 2: 80–84

10. Small M P, Carrion H M, Gordon J A. Small–Carrion penile prosthesis: a new implant for management of impotence. Urology 1975; 5: 479–485

11. Carson C C. Inflatable penile prosthesis: experience with 100 patients. South Med J 1983; 76: 1139–1145

12. Malloy T R, Wein A J, Carpiniello V L. Improved mechanical survival with revised model inflatable penile prosthesis using rear tip extenders. J Urol 1982; 128: 489–499

13. Nickas M E, Kessler R, Kabalin J N. Long term experience with controlled expansion cylinders in the AMS 700 CX

inflatable penile prosthesis in comparison with earlier versions of the Scott inflatable penile prosthesis. Urology 1994; 34: 400–403

14. Woodworth B W, Carson C C, Webster G D. Long term survival of inflatable penile prosthesis. Urology 1991; 38: 533–540

15. Seinkohl W B, Leach G E. Mechanical complications associated with Mentor inflatable penile prosthesis. Urology 1991; 38: 32–36

16. Montague D K, Lakin M M. Early experience with a controlled girth and length expanding cylinder of the American Medical Systems Ultrex penile prosthesis. J Urol 1992; 148: 1444–1446

17. Montague D K, Angermeier K W, Lakin M M, Ingerright B J. AMS 3-piece inflatable penile prosthesis implantation in men with Peyronie's disease: Comparison of CX and Ultrex cylinders. J Urol 1996; 156: 1633–1635

18. Wilson S K, Cleves M A, Delk J R. Ultrex cylinders: problems with uncontrolled lengthening (S shape deformity). J Urol 1996; 155: 135–137

19. Lewis R W. Long term results of penile prosthetic implants. Urol Clin North Am 1995; 22: 847–856

20. Nickas M E, Kessler R, Kabalin J N. Long term experience with controlled expansion cylinders in the AMS 700CX inflatable penile prosthesis in comparison with earlier versions of the Scott inflatable penile prosthesis. Urology 1994; 44: 400–403

21. Garber B B. Mentor Alpha-1 inflatable penile prosthesis cylinder aneurysm: an unusual complication. Int J Impot Res 1995; 7: 13–16

22. Kowalszyk J J, Mulcahy J J. Penile curvatures and aneurysmal defects with the Ultrex penile prosthesis corrected with insertion of the AMS 700 CX. J Urol 1996; 156: 398–401

23. Garber B B. Mentor Alpha-1 inflatable penile prosthesis: patient satisfaction advisory liability. Urology 1994; 43: 421–427

24. Goldstein I, Bertero E B, Kaufman J M et al. Early experience with first pre-connected 3-piece inflatable penile prosthesis: the Mentor Alpha-1. J Urol 1993; 150: 1814–1818

25. Quesada E T, Light J K. The AMS 700 inflatable penile prosthesis: long term experience with controlled expansion cylinders. J Urol 1993; 149: 46–48

26. Gerstenberger D I, Osborne D, Furlow W L. Inflatable penile prosthesis: follow-up study of patient–partner satisfaction. Urology 1986; 14: 239–244

27. Steege J F, Stout A L, Carson C C. Patient satisfaction in Scott and Small–Carrion implant recipients: a study of 52 patients. Arch Sex Behav 1986; 15: 393–396

28. Walen R K, Murrill B C. Patient satisfaction with Mentor inflatable penile prosthesis. Urology 1991; 37: 531–536

29. Bandru P E, Wilson S, Mobley D et al. Clinical experience with Mentor Alpha-1 inflatable penile prosthesis. Report on 333 cases. Urology 1993; 42: 305–308

30. Shu G L, Brock G, Martinez L et al. Anatomy and strength of the tunica albuginea: its relevance to penile prosthesis extrusion. J Urol 1994; 151: 1205–1208

31. Engel R M, Fein F L. Mentor GFS inflatable prosthesis. Urology 1990; 35: 405–406

32. Carson C C. Current status of penile prosthesis surgery. Probl Urol 1993; 7: 289–297

33. Wilson S K, Cleves M, Delk J R. Long term results with Hydroflex and Dynaflex penile prostheses: device survival comparison to multi-component inflatables. J Urol 1996; 155: 1621–1623

34. McLaren R H, Barrett B M. Patient and partner satisfaction with AMS 700 penile prosthesis. J Urol 1992; 147: 62–65

35. Garber B B. Mentor Alpha-1 inflatable penile prosthesis: patient satisfaction and device reliability. Urology 1994; 43: 214–217

36. Eigner E B, Kabalin J N, Kessler R. Penile implants and treatment of Peyronie's disease. J Urol 1991; 145: 69–75

37. Carson C C, Hodge G B, Anderson E E. Penile prosthesis and Peyronie's disease. Br J Urol 1983; 55: 417–422

38. Montague D K, Angermeier K W, Lakin M M, Inggeright B J. AMS 3-piece inflatable penile prosthesis implantation in men with Peyronie's disease: comparison of CX and Ultrex cylinders. J Urol 1996; 156: 1633–1635

39. Candela J V, Helstrom W J. 3-Piece inflatable penile prosthesis implantation: a comparison of penoscrotal and infrapubic surgical approaches. J La State Med Soc 1996; 148: 296–301

40. Martin-Morales A, Del Rosal Samaniego J M, Marchal-Escalona C, et al. Penile prosthesis: implantation under local anesthesia. Arch S Esp Urol 1994; 47: 791–795

41. Dos Reis J M, Goina S, Da Silva M F, Furlan V. Penile prosthesis surgery with a patient under local, regional anesthesia. J Urol 1993; 150: 1179–1181

42. Carson C C, Robertson C N. Late hematogenous infection of penile prosthesis. J Urol 1988; 139: 112–116

43. Kessler R. Complications of inflatable penile prostheses. Urology 1981; 18: 470–481

44. Licht M R, Montague D K, Angermeir K W, Lakin M M. Cultures from genitourinary prostheses at re-operation: questioning the role of Staphylococcus epidermidis in periprosthetic infection. J Urol 1995; 154: 387–390

45. Bejny D E, Perito P E, Lustgarten M, Rhamy R K. Gangrene of the penis after implantation of penile prosthesis: case reports, treatment recommendations and review of the literature. J Urol 1993; 150: 190–191

46. McClellan D S, Masih B K. Gangrene of the penis as a complication of penile prosthesis. J Urol 1985; 133: 862–865

47. Walther P J, Andriani R T, Mhaggi M I, Carson C C. Fournier's fascia gangrene: a complication of penile prosthetic penile implantation in a renal transplant patient. J Urol 1987; 137: 299–304

48. Radmoski S B, Hershorn S. Risks factors associated with penile prosthesis infection. J Urol 1992; 147: 383–385

49. Carson C C. Management of penile prosthesis infection. Probl Urol 1993; 7: 368–380

50. Bishop J R, Moul J W, Saihelnik S A et al. Use of glycosylated hemoglobin to identify diabetics at high risk for penile preprosthetic infections. J Urol 1992; 147: 386–388

51. Montague D K. Periprosthetic infections. J Urol 1987; 138: 68–74

52. Fishman I J. Corporeal reconstruction for penile prosthesis implantation. Probl Urol 1993; 7: 350–367

53. Fishman I J, Scott F B, Selim A M. Rescue procedure: an alternative to complete removal for treatment of infected penile prosthesis. J Urol 1987; 137: 202–208

54. Mulcahy J J, Steidle C P. Erosion of penile prosthesis: a complication of urethral catheterization. J Urol 1989; 142: 736–739

55. Teloken C, Souto J C, DaRos C et al. Prosthetic penile infection: rescue procedure with Rifamycin. J Urol 1992; 148: 1905–1906

56. Brant M D, Ludlow J K, Mulcahy J J. The prosthesis salvage operation: immediate replacement of the infected penile prosthesis. J Urol 1996; 155: 155–157

57. Carson C C. Infections in genitourinary prostheses. Urol Clin North Am 1989; 116: 139–152

58. Merrill D C. Mentor inflatable penile prosthesis. Urol Clin North Am 1989; 16: 51–64

59. Bertero E B, Goldstein I. Inflatable penile prosthesis: experience with the Mentor Alpha-1. Probl Urol 1993; 7: 334–341

60. Lewis R W. Long term results of penile prosthetic implants. Urol Clin North Am 1995; 22: 847–856

61. Garber B D. Mentor Alpha-1 inflatable penile prosthesis cylinder aneurysm: an unusual complication. Int J Impot Res 1995; 7: 13–16

62. Seinkohl W B, Leach G E. Mechanical complications associated with Mentor inflatable penile prosthesis. Urology 1991; 38: 32–36

63. Lewis R W, McLauren R. Re-operation for penile prosthesis implantation. Probl Urol 1993; 7: 381–401

64. Agastin E H, Farrer J H, Raz S. Fracture of semirigid rod prosthesis: a rare complication. J Urol 1986; 135: 376–377

Chapter 39

Complications of penile prostheses and complex implantations

C. C. Carson

■ INTRODUCTION

Penile prosthesis implantations, previously procedures performed only at large medical centres, are now performed by most urologists throughout the world.[1] Although these procedures result in a high rate of patient satisfaction and usually function without difficulty, unique complications occur with these procedures that are not encountered with other urologic operations.[2,3] Similarly, unique conditions of the penis and secondary implantations challenge the urologic surgeon to use creativity and problem-solving in ways not required with other surgical endeavours. It is of critical importance, prior to penile prosthesis implantation for any indication, to discuss the procedure — its risks, expectations, and caveats — thoroughly with each patient. The alternative devices available for penile prosthesis implantation should be discussed. Patients should be aware that pain and discomfort are usually present for 3–4 weeks and may be present for as long as 12 weeks postoperatively in severe diabetics.

■ INTRA-OPERATIVE COMPLICATIONS

Most of the difficulties with penile prosthesis implantation arise from placement of the cylinders within the corpora cavernosa, most often characterized by challenges in corpus cavernosum dilatation. Inadequate dilatation can occur but more often problems arise from perforation of the corpus cavernosum proximally, distally, or crossing over from one corpus cavernosum to the other. These perforations are frequently caused by misdirection of a dilator, over-aggressive dilatation or erosion through a weakened tunic albuginea from previous surgery or associated conditions. It is most important to identify these perforations or ruptures intra-operatively and to take appropriate measures to correct them at the time of initial surgical intervention. It is not always possible to identify these changes and occasionally the results of perforation are identified only in the postoperative period.

Initial corpus cavernosum dilatation should be carried out carefully to prevent perforation. Initial dissection should be done gently with Metzenbaum scissors or Hegar or Brooks dilators size 8 or larger. As a result of their very sharp ends, smaller dilators are more likely to cause perforation. Similarly, dilatation beyond size 13 may cause rupture or weakening of the corpus cavernosum. The subsequent discussion on dilatation in patients with corpus cavernosum fibrosis (pp. 438–40) elucidates some of the techniques for difficult corpus cavernosum dilatation.

Corporal crossover

Perforation of the septum between the corpora cavernosa is easily done, as the corpus cavernosum septum in the distal portion of the penis is little more than a gossamer membrane. Beginning dilatation by maintaining a lateral and not medial course in the corpus will limit crossovers. These crossovers do occur, however, surprisingly frequently. Distal crossover, the most common problem, can be suspected when both dilators reside on one side of the penis and positioning of the cylinders is difficult with retraction of one cylinder after placement of the contralateral cylinder. Distal crossover can be easily corrected by redilatation of the corpus cavernosum, maintaining a lateral course. This can be facilitated by maintaining a small Hegar dilator in the contralateral corpus cavernosum while dissection is carried out. This will identify the contralateral corpus cavernosum and guide ipsilateral dissection. It is not necessary surgically to repair or suture the septal perforation as this will compromise the corporal lumen and is not necessary for satisfactory prosthesis function.

Proximal crossover, although rare, is suspected when proximal dilatation or proximal cylinder placement is difficult. As with distal crossover, the diagnosis can easily be confirmed by placing two dilators, one in each dilated cylinder. If these dilators meet, proximal crossover can be suspected. Redilatation with a dilator in the contralateral corpus cavernosum facilitates this dissection. Both proximal and distal crossover should be suspected in patients requiring different-length cylinders on each side. Although this discrepancy can occur in a natural, normal condition, it is most common in septal crossover or inadequate dilatation. If a measured difference greater than 1 cm is found, or if there is significant curvature on inflation, cylinder crossover must be suspected. It is important to recognize this crossover intra-operatively as the postoperative result will be penile curvature, pain on inflation, or significant penile deviation.

Corporal perforation

Corporal perforation may occur proximally, distally, or per urethram. Proximal or crural perforation usually occurs following vigorous proximal corporal dilatation, most often in patients with significant corpus cavernosum fibrosis. If proximal dilatation is difficult and requires excessive force, initial sharp dissection using Metzenbaum scissors should be considered. Extending the corporotomy incision proximally will allow further dilatation to be carried out under fingertip control, decreasing the chances of proximal perforation. Should proximal perforation occur, it can be diagnosed by inadequate dilator seating or a difference in measurement of more than 1 cm. If perforation has occurred with scissor dissection or an 8 or 9 dilator, continued dilatation can be carried out with a large 12 Hegar or Brooks dilator with subsequent reinforcement of the proximal crus.

Correction of a proximal perforation can be carried out with a variety of techniques.[2,4] If a multicomponent penile prosthesis with rear tip extenders is implanted, the cylinder input tubing will frequently secure the prosthesis in place if the input tube is carefully anchored to the tunica albuginea on closure of the cavernosotomy incision. With the AMS 700 cylinders, the polytetrafluoroethylene (PTFE) tubing sleeve can be selectively and carefully sutured to the tunica albuginea to secure the cylinder in place. Because a scar tissue envelope is formed around the entire prosthesis, the defect will be closed during healing. An additional reasonable choice is to suture the rear tip extender of the prosthesis to the tunica albuginea or pelvic bone, using monofilament permanent suture material. For all penile prosthetic types, reconstruction of the proximal corpus cavernosum can be carried out with creation of a wind-sock using Gor-Tex or Dacron material (Fig. 39.1). Fascia lata or rectus fascia can also be used if synthetic materials are not available. Once placed, this wind-sock is secured to the tunica albuginea of the corpus cavernosum of the ipsilateral corpus cavernosum, using non-absorbable sutures. The choice of autologous fascia may be best in some patients, as it has been suggested that the introduction of additional synthetic materials increases the risk of penile prosthesis infection.[4]

Primary reconstruction of the proximal crura is difficult because of extensive difficult perineal exposure and inadequate recurrence. A primary suture line of the proximal crus is likely to fail with time and result in cylinder migration. Reinforcement using a rear tip extender or wind-sock requires less surgical exposure and is more likely to be successful in these patients.

Intra-operative recognition of proximal corpus cavernosum perforation is important, because this perforation may result in proximal cylinder migration with possible penile prosthesis infection or poor glans penis support (termed SST deformity).

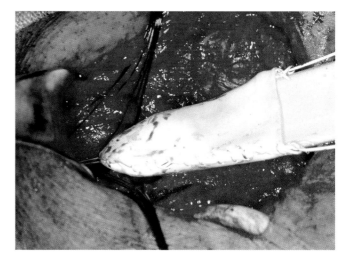

Figure 39.1. Gore-Tex wind-sock inserted to reinforce distal corporal extrusion.

Urethral perforation

Urethral perforation occurs rarely, most often with corpus cavernosum fibrosis or other difficult dilatations (Fig. 39.2). The urethral laceration that occurs during corporotomy incision as a result of an excessively medial corporotomy incision can be treated by ending the procedure, placement of a single contralateral cylinder, or repair of the urethral incision primarily. These surgical incisions into the urethra, although rare, do occur; if they are identified at an early stage and are repaired with interrupted multiple-layer absorbable sutures over a small Foley catheter stent, will usually heal without difficulty. The Foley catheter is left indwelling for 3–5 days and suprapubic drainage is not usually necessary.

More often, however, laceration of the urethra occurs with dilatation when a dilator is seen to exit through the meatus, or can be suspected when urethral bleeding is noticed during or following dilatation procedures. If urethral perforation is suspected, it can be confirmed by irrigation of both corpora cavernosa following dilatation. If irrigation fluid is seen exiting the urethra, the side that has been perforated is identified and allowed to heal for 4–6 weeks with repeat cylinder placement at that time. Repair of the urethral laceration in this circumstance is not recommended because of difficulty of exposure, inadequate repair and risk of infection.

Delayed urethral lacerations occur and usually present with cylinder erosion at the urethral meatus or into the proximal urethra. Cylinder injury and erosion can also occur following endoscopic procedures such as direct-vision internal urethrotomy.[5]

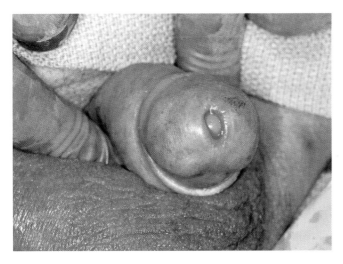

Figure 39.2. Urethral extrusion of inflatable penile prosthesis cylinder 4 weeks after insertion.

Urethral cylinder extrusion, either delayed or immediate, is best treated by removal of the ipsilateral cylinder and retention of the contralateral cylinder. Frequently, patients can be functional with a single cylinder and require no further surgical intervention. If the single cylinder is inadequate, however, delayed re-implantation of a new pair of cylinders is best carried out at least 4–6 weeks following extrusion and prosthesis removal. If extrusion is associated with purulent drainage from an infection, however, prosthesis removal and delayed re-implantation of the entire prosthesis is a better choice.

Prevention of corporal perforation is of critical importance. Careful dilatation beginning with gentle spreading and insertion of Metzenbaum scissors rather than initial passage of a dilator allows controlled tunnelling of the corpora cavernosa. Dilatation can then be carried out using Hegar dilators on the Dilamezensert. Brooks dilators, however, are more easily controlled and somewhat simpler to use, with blunter tips decreasing the chance of proximal or distal crural injury. If dilatation is difficult distally, a second circumcoronal incision and corporotomy incision at the level of the distal corpus cavernosum allows for controlled dilatation and decreases the chance of distal corpus cavernosum injury. If a question of crural crossover occurs, placement of a single dilator in one corpus cavernosum with dilatation of the contralateral corpus cavernosum will allow controlled dilatation of the appropriate corpus cavernosum.

■ PENILE PROSTHESIS EROSION

Erosion of the cylinders through the corpus cavernosum proximally or distally, or extrusion, is usually characteristic of prosthesis infection. Erosion can occur, however, from the corpus cavernosum beneath the skin of the penis distally, producing pain and discomfort in the distal portion of the corpus cavernosum and the distal penis. These erosions are most commonly identified in patients with semi-rigid rod prostheses and in patients with compromised tissues such as those with diabetes or post-infection implantations. Although they are less common with inflatable penile prostheses, they do occur with these multipiece prostheses (Fig. 39.3). Erosions are also frequently seen in patients with voiding dysfunction requiring condom catheterization or self-intermittent catheterization, especially if genital sensation is

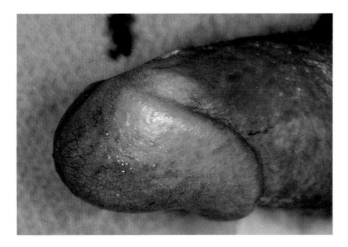

Figure 39.3. Penile prosthesis erosion through the distal corpus cavernosum beneath the skin, causing penile curvature and pain on inflation and coitus.

diminished.[6] The signs and symptoms of intra-urethral erosion include difficulty with catheterization, induration, erythema, and tenderness of the penile prosthesis cylinders, passage of blood or purulent material from the urethral meatus, and exposure of a penile cylinder. If extrusion and erosion result in exposure of the prosthetic cylinder, this cylinder should be removed as previously described. If erosion remains beneath the skin, repositioning of the prosthetic cylinder can be performed safely.[7,8]

With distal erosion beneath the skin (Fig. 39.3), a circumcoronal incision and distal corporotomy can be performed. The base of the surgical capsule around the corpus cavernosum is incised longitudinally and redilatation of the corpus cavernosum can be carried out to return the cylinder to its normal position. This is performed approximately 2 cm proximal to the distal corpus cavernosum to prevent further erosion and migration of the prosthetic cylinder. Once redilatation has been carried out, the prosthetic cylinder is replaced distally and the corpus cavernosum is closed with polyglycolic acid (PDS) suture.

GLANS BOWING (SST DEFORMITY)

Glans bowing or SST deformity can occur as a result of inadequate prosthesis sizing or distal dilatation, but often occurs as a result of anatomical changes providing poor support to a small glans penis (Fig. 39.4). SST deformity is named for the supersonic transport (SST) which is

characterized by a deflected tip. Irrespective of the aetiology, repair of glans bowing or SST deformity is easily carried out. Initially, dilatation should be checked to be sure that it is adequate and the cylinders have not been undersized. If size or dilatation are a problem, these can be corrected at the time of initial surgery. One must also be aware that proximal cylinder migration or proximal corpus cavernosum disruption has produced this inadequate cylinder length and glans penis support. While occasionally this problem may require glans fixation, after initial penile prosthesis implantation, it is most appropriate to allow postoperative healing and scar formation to provide glans penis fixation. If SST deformity persists, precluding comfortable vaginal penetration, however, postoperative glans fixation may be easily carried out.[9,10]

Glans fixation begins with a circumcoronal incision halfway around the penis. A dorsal incision is chosen for downward bending while a ventral incision is chosen for upward bowing. Care is taken to avoid the neurovascular bundle. Buck's fascia is dissected free from the tunica albuginea and proximal dissection beneath the foreskin is then continued beneath the glans penis to allow sutures to be placed on the underside of the glans. Although many authors suggest permanent suture material, the present author's experience has been excellent using 3/0 PDS suture. Sutures are placed with the prosthesis deflated to avoid cylinder injury. Suturing is performed with two interrupted sutures on either side of the midline away from the neurovascular bundle dorsally and the urethra ventrally. While sutures are placed, the deflated cylinders can be reflected away from the area of suture

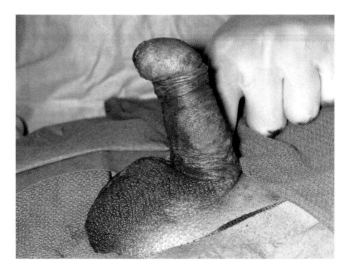

Figure 39.4. SST deformity on inflation of inflatable penile prosthesis.

placement by the surgeon's finger. Once placed, the sutures are tied and the prosthesis inflated to be sure that cylinder injury has not occurred and that adequate fixation has been obtained. Skin closure is in the standard fashion for circumcision.

■ POST-PROSTHESIS PENILE CURVATURE

Penile prosthesis curvature following placement of an inflatable or non-inflatable penile prosthesis can occur following implantation for Peyronie's disease, after implantation for corporal fibrosis, or in patients with other fibrotic aetiologies. Correction of this curvature can be accomplished by several techniques. The simplest, least morbid, and most straightforward is the modelling procedure described by Wilson and Delk.[11] This procedure can be performed without additional incisions or surgical manipulations. After placement of the prosthesis and closure of corporotomies, the penile prothesis is maximally inflated, rubber-shod clamps are applied to the input tubes of the cylinders to protect the pump from damage, and modelling is begun. This is carried out by bending the penis in a direction opposite to the curvature, holding pressure in this direction for approximately 90 s (Fig. 39.5). Repeat modelling can be carried out for persistent curvature. Between modelling procedures, additional fluid is added to the cylinders in an effort to straighten the penis further. During this straightening procedure, lysis of scar tissue can be felt between the surgeon's hands. If curvature is less than 30 degrees, modelling can be successfully achieved in almost 90% of patients.[11] If adequate straightening has not been obtained with three trials of modelling, incisional procedures should be considered.[12]

To perform modelling safely, high-pressure penile prosthesis cylinders are necessary. As a result, it is recommended that AMS 700 CX or Mentor Alpha 1 cylinders be used. Because of the multidirectional expansibility of Ultrex cylinders, aneurysmal dilatation may result from modelling of these cylinders and may exaggerate penile curvature.[13] Although this procedure is usually safe and frequently effective, complications include urethral erosion in 4% of patients and tunica albuginea injury in 2% of patients. If penile modelling is insufficient for penile straightening, a contralateral corpus plication similar to a Nesbit procedure can be carried out. In this situation, it is best to remove elliptical wedges of

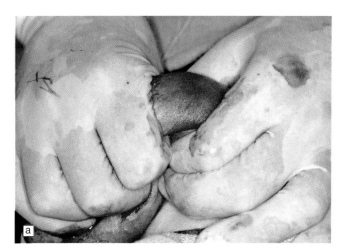

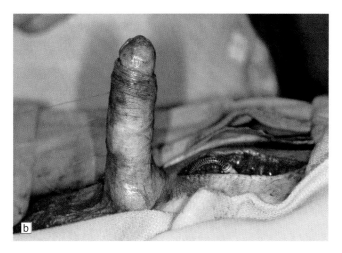

Figure 39.5. (a) Modelling a penile curvature after placement of an inflatable penile prosthesis. It is important to clamp input tubes before modelling, to protect the pump. (b) Post-modelling result is straight and functional.

tunical albuginea on the side opposite the curvature and to place absorbable 3/0 PDS sutures to provide straightening. When performing this straightening procedure, it is important to avoid injury to the prosthetic cylinders during placement of sutures and to maintain the prosthesis in a deflated position for at least 6 weeks to allow thorough and complete healing before inflation places pressure on the Nesbit ellipse or plications.

More significant curvature is best approached by incision or excision of the curvature or Peyronie's plaque, to allow complete straightening and restoration of some penile length.[12] Exposure of the area of curvature is critical during this manoeuvre. For distal or mid-shaft curvatures, a circumcoronal incision with retraction of the penile skin will provide excellent exposure. If curvature is ventral, a ventral or penoscrotal incision can

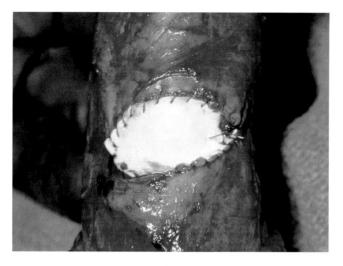

Figure 39.6. Gore-Tex patch placed to reinforce defect in corpus cavernosum after incision of curvature.

be used to expose the area of curvature. Once the area of curvature is exposed, dorsal exposure of the curved area should begin by dissecting away from the dorsal neurovascular bundle to decrease the possibility of distal glans sensation problems. It is best to ligate the deep dorsal vein, dissect through its bed and carefully elevate the dorsal nerves from the area to be incised. Even careful dissection of the dorsal neurovascular bundles, however, may lead to decreased penile sensation in some cases because of severe fibrosis around the dorsal nerves. Similarly, ventral curvatures should begin by placement of a Foley catheter, and dissection, identification and protection of the urethra. Once the area of curvature has been dissected free, electrocautery is best for incision since it can be performed with less chance of injury to the prosthetic cylinders. While the American Medical Systems (AMS) silicone rubber cylinders are best suited for this purpose, successful incision over the Mentor Bioflex cylinders has also been reported.[14] In order to correct curvature adequately, the prosthesis is fully inflated, the area of curvature is incised, and incision continued until complete straightening is observed. This frequently requires incision of an area of the septum between the corpora which produces the maximum tethering in many curvatures. Once straightening has been confirmed, the defect in the corpus cavernosum must be assessed to consider the possibility of patch placement to cover the prosthesis. In these curvature repairs, Ultrex cylinders should not be used because of the possibility of aneurysmal dilatation and herniation through the area of incision. If a large defect has been

created from correction of curvature, a patch graft reinforcement will provide the best cosmetic result and reinforce the corpus cavernosum for strength and cylinder protection. This patch grafting can be created using a Gore-Tex, Dacron, dermis, or fascial patch graft. Gore-Tex (polytetrafluoroethylene), because of its ease of availability, ease of suturing, and excellent postoperative results, provides excellent reinforcement in these situations. A tailored segment of 0.06 mm Gore-Tex can be sutured and placed with 3/0 Gore-Tex suture with excellent results (Fig. 39.6).

■ PENILE PROSTHESIS INFECTION

The most disastrous complication of penile prosthesis implantation is infection (Table 39.1). Infections can range from superficial wound infections, easily treated with local care and antibiotics, to penile gangrene, a disastrous complication associated with penile tissue loss. The majority of penile prosthesis infections, if identified early, can be treated effectively with removal and subsequent re-implantation of a penile prosthesis and expected return of prosthetic function.

Most penile prosthesis infections begin with bacterial organisms entering the wound during surgery. Because normal skin is colonized by organisms such as *Staphylococcus epidermidis* and other Gram-positive organisms, as well as Enterobacteriaceae from the perineum and genitalia, prosthetic infections can be caused by Gram-positive or Gram-negative organisms. The introduction of anaerobic bacteria to these infections may result in the gangrenous infections reported.

All foreign bodies will potentiate infection if bacteria are present. This concept has been well established since the identification of staphylococcal infection stimulation by the presence of silk sutures.[15] These studies documented a 100-fold decrease in the number of bacteria necessary to produce infection in the presence of braided silk suture acting as a foreign body. It was subsequently demonstrated that the more reactive an implanted material, the more enhancement of infection could be expected.[16]

It has also been suggested that implanted foreign materials may weaken host defence mechanisms. The implanted foreign bodies may activate the complement system, enhance phagocytosis, and possibly even trigger microvascular thrombosis and release of cytotoxic

Table 39.1. Penile prosthesis infection

Author (Year)	Patients	Infections	Percentage
Rod prostheses			
Small (1978)	140	1	0.7
Kramer (1979)	76	1	1.3
Finney (1980)	100	1	1.0
Kaufman (1982)	1207	19	1.6
Small (1984)	900	15	1.6
Benson (1985)	100	3	3.0
Montague (1987)	169	1	0.6
Kabalin (1988)	125	3	2.4
Fallon (1989)	156	3	1.9
Kearce (DuraII) (1996)	196	5	2.6
Total	3169	52	1.6
Inflatable (multiple component)			
Furlow (1979)	175	6	3.4
Malloy (1975)	93	2	2.2
Kessler (1981)	128	1	0.8
Carson (1982)	100	1	1
Fishman (1984)	1100	24	3.1
Engel (1987)	202	2	1.
Thomella (1987)	150	12	8.9
Montague (1987)	246	9	3.7
Kabalin (1988)	292	6	2.1
Brooks (1988)	137	3	2.2
Furlow (1988)	120	1	0.8
Wilson (1988)	245	11	4.5
Merrill (1988)	301	12	4.0
Fallon (1989)	270	8	2.9
Knoll (1990)	94	3	3.2
Goldstein (1993)	112	3	2.6
Randrup (1993)	333	4	1.2
Quesada (1993)	214	7	3.0
Garber (1994)	50	1	2.0
Fein (1994)	138	2	1.4
George (1995)	50	2	4.0
Randrup (1995)	180	9	5.0
Wilson (1996)	1251	67	5.0
Total	5981	196	3.3

Table 39.1. (cont'd)

Author (Year)	Patients	Infections	Percentage
Inflatable (self contained)			
Thomella (1987)	37	3	8.1
Montague (1987)	29	1	3.4
Stanicik (1988)	23	1	4.3
Mulcahy (1988)	100	3	3.0
Stanicik (1989)	22	1	4.5
Total	211	9	4.3
Grand total	9361	257	2.7

enzymes.[17] Because of the nature of currently available implantable materials, this host defence reaction fails to cause damage to the implanted device but, rather, is turned on itself and to some extent injures the normal defence mechanisms of the host. It has been suggested, therefore, that these foreign bodies act in a fashion similar to bacteria in the process of inducing an abscess. Thus, a prosthetic device can be associated with the infection and a very small inoculum of bacteria as a result of the presence of the prosthetic material itself will limit host defences.[17]

Furthermore, bacteria present around prosthetic devices tend to adhere to the device securely and this adherence is critical in the formation of prosthesis-associated infections.[18,19] Bacteria have been demonstrated to adhere to the surfaces of prosthetic materials including both silicone elastomer, used in AMS penile prostheses, and Bioflex, used in Mentor penile prostheses.[20] This binding is promoted and enhanced by the production of a mucopolysaccharide matrix by the bacteria. This biomass formation is most likely to occur with infections caused by *Staphylococcus aureus* and *Pseudomonas aeruginosa* and may also occur with *Staphylococcus epidermidis*.[18,20] While the exact process of bacterial adherence and biomass production is unclear, the surface charge of bacteria and prosthetic material may differ, allowing attraction of these bacterial cells to prosthetic surfaces. This biofilm production and formation has been documented in all prosthetic systems including penile prostheses. Neither prosthetic material appears to be more or less likely to

attract bacteria and support biofilm formation. This glycocalyx matrix protects the bacteria from antibiotic activity and from the host natural defence mechanisms of antibodies and phagocytosis.

Bacteria most commonly colonize prostheses at the time of initial implantation.[21] Bacteria may also contact the periprostatic space through haematogenous or lymphatic spread.[22,23] Carson and Robertson have demonstrated that the haematogenous route of infection occurs frequently and may be responsible for late infections.[31] Fishman and colleagues, however, believe that haematogenous infection is less common and that bacterial biofilm may allow infection to be quiescent for many years prior to clinical demonstration.[24] Licht and colleagues[25] have questioned the role of *S. epidermidis* in prosthesis infections, demonstrating these organisms on prostheses removed for mechanical problems without known infection. There is little question, however, that the majority of infections occur as a result of colonization at the time of original implantation. The experience of Fishman and colleagues has demonstrated that 56% of prosthesis infection occurred within 7 months of implantation, 36% between 7 and 12 months, and 2.6% occurred after 5 years.[24]

Pathogenic organisms

Staphylococcus epidermidis is the most common organism implicated in penile prosthesis infection. It has been isolated from between 35 and 56% of infected penile prosthesis patients. It has also been identified as the most common pathogen in infections of orthopaedic prostheses, prosthetic heart valves, and intracranial shunts and reservoirs. *S. epidermidis* and other staphylococcal species have an enhanced ability to produce glycocalyx biofilm that potentiates their infectious capacity.[20,21,26]

Gram-negative enteric bacteria are also frequently identified as pathogens in prosthetic infections. Thomalla and colleagues studied 23 patients who had penile prostheses removed following infection. In addition to the most common staphylococcal pathogens, Gram-negative organisms included *Proteus mirabilis* in six patients, *Pseudomonas aeruginosa* in four patients, *Escherichia coli* in two and *Serratia marcescens* in two patients.[27] Montague found that Gram-negative bacteria accounted for 20% of penile prosthesis infections in his series.[28] Infections caused by these Gram-negative organisms were more likely to occur at an earlier time, with the average time to infection with Gram-negative organisms less than 1 month after implantation compared with 5.75 months in those patients infected with staphylococcal organisms. Occasionally, Gram-negative infection with or without associated anaerobic organisms such as Bacteroides may progress to gangrene of the penis.[29,30]

Nelson and Gregory have presented two cases of penile prosthesis infection caused by *Neisseria gonorrhoea*.[31] The origin of these neisserial infections is probably previous urethral infection with subsequent prosthesis inoculation.

Prosthesis risk factors

Significant risk factors can be identified in those patients with infected penile prostheses. Prolonged hospitalization with change in skin flora is a risk factor that can be reduced by hospital admission on the day of surgery. Other host factors will also place patients at higher risk for these prosthetic infections. Fallon and Ghanem have reported that diabetes mellitus increases infection risk by more than threefold when compared with other aetiologies of erectile dysfunction.[32] Likewise, circumcision at the time of penile prosthesis implantation significantly increased the risk of infection in their series. They and others were, however, unable to identify any significant change in infection risk when comparing prosthesis type, first or repeat operations, or other aetiologies.[32] The author has noted significant increases in infection when any other surgical procedure is combined with penile prosthesis implantation. This

includes simultaneous inguinal hernia repair, circumcision, penile straightening, and other simultaneous manipulations.[12,32] Other investigators have demonstrated little increase in risk in patients with diabetes when carefully treated with perioperative antibiotics.[33,34]

Patients with paraplegia or spinal cord injury also appeared to be at increased risk for prosthesis infections. An increased incidence of infection from 8 to 33% has been recorded for patients with spinal cord injury. Diokno and Sonda, however, have demonstrated no increase in infection in patients with spinal cord injury and neuropathic bladder undergoing penile prosthesis implantation, who continued to practise safe and well-informed clean intermittent self-catheterization.[35] It seems, therefore, that maintenance of urinary hygiene with self-catheterization can be safely practised following penile prosthesis implantation.

Patients with other causes of immunocompromise, such as transplantation, appear to be at some (but minimal) increased risk for prosthetic infection (Fig. 39.7). Whereas Walther and associates[30] have reported a case of Fournier's gangrene of the penis and scrotum following penile implantation in a renal transplant patient. Whereas Fallon and Ghanem[32] identified no increased risk in those patients with repeat surgical procedures and, in fact, had a somewhat diminished incidence of infection in those revision patients, Thomalla and associates[27] as well as Kabalin and Kessler[36] identified a higher incidence of infection in patients undergoing repeat implantations.[27,32,36]

There is little question that there is some appreciable increase in risk in patients who are immunocompromised,

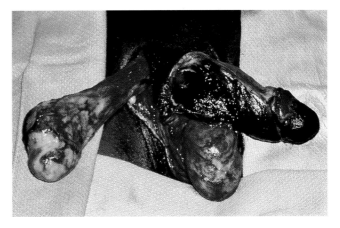

Figure 39.7. Penile gangrene in an immunocompromised transplant patient after semi-rigid rod penile prosthesis removal.

in those with severe poorly controlled diabetes, and in those patients undergoing multiple surgical procedures. This risk, however, continues to be statistically small and does not contraindicate penile prosthesis implantation. These increased risk factors do, however, strongly support increased attention to the principles of infection prevention.[21,37]

Prevention of infection is better than infection treatment. Special precautions during any prosthetic implantation include skin shaving in the operating room, broad-spectrum perioperative antibiotics aimed at the organisms most likely to produce infection, and careful preoperative skin preparation. A 10 minute skin scrub using iodiophore is important and the avoidance of penile prosthesis implantation in patients with remote infections is critical. If a patient has a remote skin infection, dental abscess, or urinary tract infection, this infection should be treated and eradicated prior to penile prosthesis implantation. Ostomies should be carefully draped and sealed from the operative field prior to skin preparation. Perioperative antibiotics should be administered approximately 1–2 h prior to surgery, using a fluoro-quinolone, aminoglycoside with or without a beta-lactam agent or vancomycin for Gram-positive coverage. Recent studies have documented the excellent corpus cavernosum penetration of fluoroquinolone antibiotic agents, suggesting that intravenous or oral treatment with these agents may be excellent perioperative preparation.[38,39] Prophylaxis begun in the perioperative period should be continued for at least 48 h following surgery. No benefit has been demonstrated from prophylactic antibiotic administration after 48 h.[26] Intra-operative irrigation with antibiotic solution containing bacitracin 50 000 units and kanamycin 1 g or gentamycin 80 mg/l normal saline is effective in intra-operative antibiotic irrigation.[21,40] Despite careful preoperative preparation and intra-operative procedures, penile prosthesis infections occur in all reported series. The incidence of prosthesis infections varies from 1 to 8%, with the majority of series reporting a 3% infection rate.[26,40–42] Infections increase with additional surgical procedures and immunocompromise and, in many series, are increased in patients with diabetes. Although the issue of diabetic control continues to be controversial, recent studies have demonstrated that monitoring of haemoglobin A1C is not an esssential predictor of infection in diabetic patients, as previously had been suggested.[43,44]

Penile prosthesis infections can be suspected postoperatively if patients have an increased or persistent postoperative pain beyond the usual resolution time. Additionally, periprosthetic erythema and induration, fever, fluctuance, wound drainage or erosion suggest penile prosthesis infection. Similarly, fixation of the scrotal pump to the scrotal skin postoperatively may be an early sign of prosthesis infection. While symptoms are frequently subtle and the diagnosis difficult, white blood cell count and sedimentation rate may, in some cases, suggest the presence of an infection when signs and symptoms are unclear. In some equivocal situations, a gallium-67 scan may confirm the clinical suspicion of prosthesis infection.[45] Although surgical exploration is usually necessary for these patients, a trial of long-term broad-spectrum antibiotics may be effective in some early patients. Since fluoroquinolones have been identified as penetrating the corpus cavernosum effectively, oral fluoroquinolones are frequently used for 4–6 weeks in these situations.[38] Although resistance to these antibiotics is more frequently identified once the infection is established, early antibiotic intervention may eliminate later surgical intervention.

When an infection is suspected, surgical exploration may be necessary through the previously healed incision. If no purulent exudate is encountered, a Gram stain of the area around the prosthesis can be obtained. If purulence is identified, complete removal or replacement may be considered. If extensive erosion of the prosthesis has occurred or a patient is immunocompromised, removal of all components with placement of drains and subsequent wound closure with re-implantation 4–6 months later is a conservative approach. In these situations, with severe infection, the author removes all portions of the penile implant and places Jackson–Pratt drains in the area where all penile prosthesis parts reside. Antibiotic irrigation is then carried out with a solution containing vancomycin and gentamycin, every 8 h for 3–5 days; drains are then removed and the patient is discharged. Re-implantation is delayed for 4–6 months. A second option in less severe infections has been proposed in several reports.[24,46,47] This early salvage and rescue procedure may be successful in many patients and should be carried out for minimal to moderate infections. After removal of the infected penile prosthesis and all its parts, multiple wound irrigations are carried out with solutions. Brant and colleagues suggest the use of the 'water pik' pressure irrigator to irrigate, beginning with 5 l vancomycin–gentamycin solution and placing a rubber catheter in each area for thorough irrigation.[47] It is critical that no portion of the old prosthesis be left behind, as the bacteria-containing biofilm that envelops the entire infected penile prosthesis will be continuous throughout the portions of penile implant and will colonize a future penile prosthesis. Brant and colleagues report success of irrigation and re-implantation of a new penile prosthesis in as many as 80% of patients. Prosthesis salvage procedures are worthwhile because they maintain penile length and sensation, decrease subsequent corpus cavernosum fibrosis and eliminate subsequent difficult re-implantation procedures. These procedures should be avoided, however, in patients with significant purulent corpus cavernosum drainage, insulin-dependent diabetes, or immunocompromise.

Postoperative infections should be avoided by careful antibiotic coverage of all patients undergoing surgical procedures after their prosthesis implantation. Although the issue of postoperative prosthesis colonization continues to be controversial, studies in orthopaedics and urology have documented colonization of penile prostheses by remote infections postoperatively.[23]

The most disastrous penile prosthesis complication is that of penile gangrene and necrosis caused by severe penile prosthesis infection. Although the incidence of gangrene is rare, several cases have been reported.[29,30,48,49] These severe infections occur chiefly in patients with immunocompromise and are often a result of symbiotic infections with Gram-negative and anaerobic organisms. Progression from initial symptoms to ultimate necrosis occurs rapidly within hours of presentation and must be aggressively treated as a lifesaving measure. Frequently in these cases the infection behaves like Fournier's gangrene. Patients who present with new-onset severe penile pain, excessive penile or scrotal oedema, or colour change in the glans penis or penile shaft, should be suspected of having early penile gangrene. These changes can be encountered when postoperative compression dressings around inflated prostheses are used with indwelling catheters, and should be avoided in all patients.

Once there is a suspicion of penile gangrene, early surgical intervention to remove the prosthesis is critical. Broad-spectrum antibiotics to include coverage of anaerobic organisms should be initiated immediately, the prosthesis removed and devitalized tissue débrided. The use of hyperbaric oxygen has been suggested, but the author's experience has not demonstrated significant benefit from hyperbaric oxygen in these patients. Urinary diversion with a suprapubic cystostotomy may be helpful. Subsequent phallic reconstruction is delayed for at least 6 months to allow complete penile healing.

■ MECHANICAL MALFUNCTION

Although all penile prostheses including semi-rigid rods can suffer from mechanical malfunction, multipiece inflatable prostheses are at significantly higher risk. The majority of reoperations for penile prostheses are for mechanical malfunction.[50] Modifications of these inflatable penile prostheses have substantially increased the survival of penile prostheses.[51,52] The modification of the AMS prosthesis to include a three-piece cylinder design and the introduction of the polyurethane material Bioflex by the Mentor Corporation (Goleta, CA, USA) have decreased mechanical malfunction to less than 5% in many series. Most hydraulic prosthesis malfunctions result in fluid leakage or inadequate inflation. Fluid leakage is most likely to occur in the high-pressure portion of the device from pump to cylinders rather than from pump to reservoir, a lower-pressure system.[53] Cylinder aneurysm formation, while most common in AMS Ultrex cylinders, also occurs in the Mentor Alpha 1 cylinders (Fig. 39.8).[2,13,53,54] Whereas, previously, connector problems and tubing kinking occurred frequently, with newer designs these mechanical malfunctions are rare. Since most penile prosthesis mechanical malfunctions currently occur more than 4 years beyond original implantation, the author's policy is

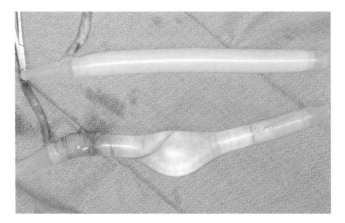

Figure 39.8. AMS Ultrex penile prosthesis cylinder aneurysm.

to replace all parts of the penile prosthesis if it is more than 3 years old. If a prosthesis is less than 3 years old and a confined mechanical problem such as a connector malfunction occurs, focused repairs using new connectors, new cylinders, or replacement parts can be considered. Inadequate inflation of a cylinder, especially Ultrex cylinders, may result from S-shaped deformities of these cylinders.[55] These can be diagnosed readily by magnetic resonance imaging investigation of the penis and prosthesis.[55] Successful treatment of these Ultrex S-deformities or aneurysmal dilatation can be performed by removal and implantation of AMS 700 CX cylinders.[56]

Penile prosthesis revision is begun by re-entry of the original healed incision. The prosthesis parts are explored by following input tubing to the various portions of the prosthesis using electrocautery dissection, since electrocautery will not injure the prosthesis. If the location of the leak is unclear, the entire prosthesis should be replaced. Previously, the author has used ohmmeter resistance testing to identify leaking areas. This has been abandoned because of occasional inaccuracies and the improved outcome of re-implantation of an entire new prosthesis when necessary. Once all portions of penile implant have been removed, the prosthesis is replaced where the parts were removed if they were satisfactory. A pump can be replaced, if not easily palpable by the patient, or a capsule can be lysed around the reservoir if the patient has sustained autoinflation. Prosthesis revision, however, must be conducted with the caveat that increased infections, especially in patients with diabetes, have been reported in many series. With these revision procedures and dissections, it must be borne in mind that fibrosis and scarring are frequently encountered, and special care must be taken to avoid the neurovascular bundles if approaching the prosthesis infrapubically or the urethra if approaching penoscrotally. Because identification of all portions of the prosthesis is difficult when using an incision that differs from the original implantation, revisions should be carried out through the original approach.

Other assorted postoperative problems can occur, including scrotal haematoma in the early postoperative period and autoinflation in the postoperative period. Scrotal haematoma can be avoided by meticulous attention to haemostasis and careful closure of the corporotomy incision. The majority of scrotal haematomas occur from leakage of blood from the corporotomy incisions. If a scrotal haematoma appears to be occurring in the early postoperative period, the prosthesis can be inflated temporarily to tamponade this leakage. The author's practice is to use a Jackson–Pratt drain placed in the scrotum for 24 h to further decrease the chances of scrotal haematoma or oedema. The use of drains after prosthesis implantation, favoured by some authors and not by others, does not seem to increase the incidence of prosthesis infection.

Autoinflation occurs when pressure around the reservoir of three-piece devices is sufficient to push fluid through the pump mechanism and into the cylinders. Usually, this complication occurs 3–6 months postoperatively or in patients in whom the prosthesis has remained inflated in the early postoperative period. Treatment of autoinflation is first attempted conservatively, with patients asked to deflate their device actively two or three times daily to enlarge the capacity of the capsule surrounding the reservoir. Active deflation is carried out by having the patient hold the deflation portion of the pump and squeeze actively on the penis to expel all fluid into the reservoir. If this fails to produce the desired results, surgical lysis of the periprosthetic capsule may be required. In this situation, the prosthesis is explored, the capsule identified and multiple stellate incisions carried out to lyse the capsule. The prosthetic reservoir is then replaced and the prosthesis remains deflated for at least 3 weeks postoperatively to allow capsule formation to accommodate the reservoir.[57]

■ CORPUS CAVERNOSUM FIBROSIS

The most difficult penile prosthesis implantations occur in patients with corpus cavernosum fibrosis, which is usually caused by previous penile prosthesis infection. Other conditions such as priapism, Peyronie's disease, pharmacological erections, penile trauma or penile fracture may produce significant fibrosis. Replacement of the prosthesis is difficult in corporal dilatation and placement of the penile prosthesis cylinders. When attempting penile prosthesis replacement in these clinical situations, it is important to have downsized inflatable penile prosthesis cylinders available when choosing inflatable prosthetic devices. These devices, available from Mentor and AMS as the AMS 700CXM, permit placement of a prosthesis in a seriously fibrotic corpus cavernosum.[58] A vacuum erection device may be used preoperatively to increase penile length and soften corporal fibrosis. Patients are asked to apply vacuum two or three times weekly without a constriction ring for 8–12 weeks.[59] Use of a vacuum device with a prosthesis in place has been reported but may result in damage to an implanted device.[60]

If re-implanting a prosthesis in a patient with previous infection, changing incisions and exposure may provide non-fibrotic corpus to dilate. Thus, if an infected penile prosthesis has been removed from a patient by an initial initial penoscrotal approach, an infrapubic incision should be chosen as a second alternative and vice versa. In the event of significant corpus cavernosum fibrosis, the operator must be prepared to undertake multiple cavernosotomies, to dilate with a variety of techniques, and to reconstruct the corpus cavernosum with synthetic material if necessary. After initial corporotomy is performed, dissection is begun with blunt-tipped Metzenbaum scissors, carefully dissecting and spreading in each direction. Dissection should be carried out well away from the urethra and the Foley catheter should always be placed prior to initiation of dissection. Further dilatation with Hegar, Brooks or Dilamezinsert dilating tools is then begun gently. In severe fibrosis, dilatation may continue to be difficult and additional incisions may be necessary. Because the distal portion of the corpus cavernosum is frequently fixed, a distal corporotomy incision will allow safe dilatation under direct vision without excessive pressure and risk of distal extrusion and erosion. If dilatation continues to be difficult, other techniques must be employed. A large Kelly or Bridge clamp may be placed and opened actively to dilate the channel created by Metzenbaum scissors. Once this is performed, the fibrotic tissue may be relaxed using an Otis urethrotome (Fig. 39.9). The urethrotome is placed in the initial channel in the corpus cavernosum with incisions of the fibrotic corpus cavernosum well away from the urethra. Once the urethrotome is placed, it is opened maximally and the blade used to incise the fibrosis in multiple directions sharply. Further dilatation is then carried out using a Bridge clamp followed by Brooks or Hegar dilators. Care must be taken with the Otis urethrotome to avoid incision of the tunica albuginea. An additional device that has been useful in this difficult situation is the Rosillo cavernotome, a dilator designed like a rasp to remove fibrotic tissue as it dilates (Fig. 39.10). These cavernotomes are sized from 9 to 12 mm, with rasp teeth on three sides. By advancing and retracting the cavernotomes actively, fibrous tissue can be incised or removed to allow for placement of prosthetic cylinders.

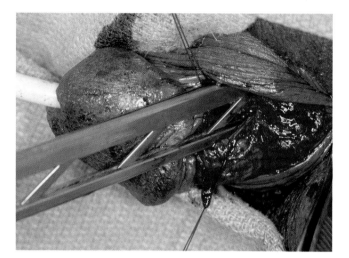

Figure 39.9. Otis urethrotome placed in the corpus cavernosum to incise corporal fibrosis during dilatation.

If these techniques are unsuccessful, longitudinal incision of the corpus cavernosum can be carried out with dissection of the fibrotic tissue from the corpus cavernosum. This is a difficult procedure and requires significant care to avoid the urethra, neurovascular bundle and other structures of the penis. Once it has been performed, however, a prosthetic cylinder can be placed in the open dissected area and covered with tunica albuginea or a Gore-Tex graft (Fig. 39.11). Entire reconstruction of the corpus cavernosum may not be necessary and only the most fibrotic portion of the corpus cavernosum may require this extensive dissection. Under very difficult circumstances, a single cylinder may be

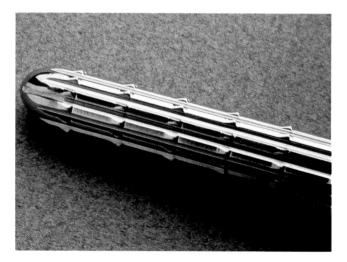

Figure 39.10. Rosillo cavernotome. Dilators designed for dilatation of fibrotic corpora may also be helpful in cylinder placement for Peyronie's disease.

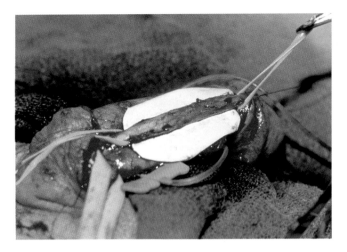

Figure 39.11. Gore-Tex patch used to reconstruct a long segment of fibrotic corpus and to cover a penile prosthesis cylinder. These patches and reconstructions are useful in placement of full-sized cylinders in severe fibrosis.

placed or small cylinders placed to act as tissue expanders, with a subsequent surgical procedure to upsize the prosthetic device 3–6 months later.[4,12,61,62]

The use of synthetic material may be necessary if the tunica albuginea cannot be closed over the corpus cavernosum or if significant curvature is encountered, as previously described. In this situation, Gore-Tex or Dacron may be used to reconstruct the corpus cavernosum.[4,12,61,62] These patches can be used as described in the wind-sock procedure or to reconstruct portions of the corpus cavernosum.[63] In many patients with severe corpus cavernosum fibrosis, penile shortening may be problematic. Penile enhancement by incision of the suspensory ligament with resection of suprapubic adipose tissue may improve the postoperative result in selected patients.[64,65]

■ PATIENT DISSATISFACTION

Perhaps one of the most frustrating complications of penile implants is difficulty with patient dissatisfaction despite an apparently successful surgical procedure. Avoidance of this distressing problem is best approached preoperatively with discussion of the patient's expectations, sexual function and results of penile implants. The surgeon must allow the patient to choose the most appropriate prosthesis, and a trial of conservative medical therapy prior to implantation may help the patient's decision regarding prosthesis implantation. Generally, however, penile prosthetic implantation is the best-

tolerated and most satisfactory method for restoration of erectile function, in studies reported.[51,66–68]

Nevertheless, patients should be warned that the erection achieved with a penile prosthesis will differ somewhat from the natural erection. The erection will be of shorter length, sometimes of decreased warmth, and may be associated with decreased penile sensation, ejaculatory dysfunction and compromised flaccidity. Patients must be cautioned that the implantation of a penile prosthesis will not affect a diminished libido, a compromised orgasm, or a dysfunctional marital relationship. Because many patients have difficulty with orgasm and ejaculation postoperatively, they should be counselled to increase foreplay, precoital lovemaking and stimulation prior to use of the prosthesis. In many patients, 3–9 months are required to regain orgasm on a regular basis.

■ CONCLUSION

Penile prosthesis complications, although rare, require vigilance and attention. Intra-operative complications can usually be addressed if identified and postoperative complications can be treated with a successful outcome. The urologic surgeon must first counsel his patient regarding the possibility of these complications and be prepared to identify them at the time of surgery or to care for them in the postoperative period, to obtain a satisfactory result with a functional penile prosthesis.

■ REFERENCES

1. Carson C C. Current status of penile prosthesis surgery. Probl Urol 1993; 7: 289–297
2. Wilson S K, Delk J R. Prevention and treatment of complications of inflatable penile prosthesis surgery: a review article. Arch Esp Urol 1996; 49: 306–311
3. Lewis R W. Long term results of penile prosthetic implants. Urol Clin North Amer 1995; 22: 847–856
4. Carson C C. Management of corpus cavernosum extrusion after penile prosthesis placement. Contemp Urol 1998; 10: 13–17
5. Carson C C. Inflatable penile prosthesis cylinder rupture after internal urethrotomy. Urology 1988; 31: 510
6. Steidle C S, Mulcahy J J. Erosion of penile prosthesis: a complication of urethral catheterization. J Urol 1989; 142: 736–739

7. Mulcahy J J. Distal corporoplasty treatment of penile prosthesis extrusion. Int J Impot Res 1996; 8: 121

8. Carson C C. Increased infection risk with corpus cavernosum reconstruction and penile prosthesis implantation with corporal fibrosis. Int J Impot Res 1996; 8: 155

9. Ball T P. Surgical repair of penile SST deformity. Urology 1980; 15: 603

10. Stefani S D, Simonato A M, Caponi M et al. The benefit of glans fixation in prosthetic penile surgery. J Urol 1994; 152: 1533–1534

11. Wilson S K, Delk J R. A new treatment for Peyronie's disease: modeling the penis over an inflatable penile prosthesis. J Urol 1994; 152: 1121–1123

12. Bertram R A, Carson C C, Altaffer L F. Severe penile curvature following implantation of inflatable penile prosthesis. J Urol 1988; 139: 743

13. Wilson S K, Cleves N A, Delk J R. Ultrex cylinders: problems with uncontrolled lengthening (the S-shaped deformity). J Urol 1996; 155: 135–137

14. Hakim L S, Kulaksizoglu H, Hammill B K et al. A guide to safer corporotomy incisions in the presence of underlying inflatable penile cylinders: results of in vitro and in vivo studies. J Urol 1996; 155: 918–923

15. Elek S D, Conin P E. The virulence of Staphylococcus pyogenes for man: the study of the problems of wound infection. Br J Exp Pathol 1957; 38: 573

16. James R C, McLeod C J. Induction of staphylococcal infection in mice with small inocula introduced on sutures. Br Exp Pathol 1961; 42: 266

17. Dougherty S H, Simmons R L. Infections and bionic man: the pathophysiology of infections and prosthetic devices. Curr Probl Surg 1982; 19: 217

18. Gristina A G, Costerton J W. Bacteria laden biofilms: a hazard to orthopedic prostheses. Infect Surg 1984; 3: 655

19. Nickel J C, Heaton J, Morales A, Costerton J W. Bacterial biofilm in persistent penile prosthesis associated infections. J Urol 1986; 135: 586

20. Roberts J A, Fussell E N, Lewis R W. Bacterial adherence to penile prostheses. Int J Impot Res 1989; 1: 167

21. Carson C C. Management of penile prosthesis infection. Probl Urol 1993; 7: 368–380

22. Ainscow D A, Denhem R A. The risk of hematogenous infection in total joint replacements. J Bone Joint Surg [Br] 1984; 66: 580

23. Carson C C, Robertson C N. Late hematogenous infection of penile prosthesis. J Urol 1988; 139: 50

24. Fishman J J, Scott F B, Selim A M. Rescue procedure: an alternative to complete removal for treatment of infected penile prosthesis. J Urol 1987; 137: 202a

25. Licht M R, Montague D K, Angermeier K W, Lakin M M. Cultures from genitourinary prostheses at re-operation: questioning the role of Staphylococcus epidermidis in periprosthetic infection. J Urol 1995; 154: 387–390

26. Carson C C. Infections and genitourinary prostheses. Urol Clin North Am 1989; 16: 139–152

27. Thomalla J V, Thompson R G, Mulcahy J J. Infectious complications of penile prosthesis implants. J Urol 1987; 138: 65

28. Montague D K. Periprosthetic infections. J Urol 1987; 138: 68

29. McLellan D S, Masih B K. Gangrene of the penis as a complication of penile prosthesis. J Urol 1985; 143: 862–863

30. Walther P J, Andriani R T, Carson C C et al. Fournier's gangrene: a complication of penile prosthesis implantation in a renal transplant patient. J Urol 1987; 137: 299–300

31. Nelson R P, Gregory J C. Gonococcal infections of penile prostheses. Urology 1988; 31: 391

32. Fallon B, Ghanem H. Infected penile prostheses: incidence and outcomes. Int J Impot Res 1989; 1: 175

33. Benson R C, Patterson D E, Barrett D M. Long term results with Jonas malleable penile prosthesis. J Urol 1985; 134: 899

34. Persky Y L, Luria S, Porter A. Staphylococcus epidermidis in diabetic urologic patients. J Urol 1986; 136: 466

35. Diokno A C, Sonda L P. Compatibility of genitourinary prostheses and intermittent self catheterization. J Urol 1981; 125: 659

36. Kabalin J N, Kessler R. Infectious complications of penile prosthesis surgery. J Urol 1988; 139: 953

37. Chodak G W, Plant N E. Systemic antibiotics for prophylaxis in urologic surgery: a critical review. J Urol 1979; 121: 695

38. Schwartz B F, Swanzy S, Thrasher J B. A randomized prospective comparison of antibiotic tissue levels in the corpora cavernosa of patients undergoing penile prosthesis implantation using gentamycin plus cefazolin versus oral fluroquinolone for prophylaxis. J Urol 1996; 156: 991–994

39. Walters F P, Neal D E, Rege A B et al. Cavernous tissue antibiotic levels in penile prosthesis surgery. J Urol 1992; 147: 1282–1284

40. Wilson S K, Delk J R. Inflatable penile implant infection: predisposing factors and treatment suggestions. J Urol 1995; 153: 659–661

41. Jarow J P. Risk factors for penile prosthetic infection. J Urol 1996; 156: 402–404

42. Parsons C L, Stein P C, Dobke M K et al. Diagnosis and therapy of subclinical infected prostheses. Surg Gynecol Obstet 1993; 177: 504–506

43. Wilson S K, Carson C C, Cleves M A, Delk J R. Quantifying risk of penile prosthesis infection with glycosylated hemoglobin. J Urol: in press

44. Bishop J R, Moul J W, Asiahelink S A et al. Use of glycosylated hemoglobin to identify diabetics at high risk for penile periprosthetic infections. J Urol 1992; 147: 386–388

45. Better N, Ahn C S, Drum D E, Tow D E. Identification of penile prosthetic infection on gallium-67 scan. J Urol 1994; 152: 475–476

46. Furlow W L, Goldwasser B. Salvage of the eroded inflatable penile prosthesis: a new concept. J Urol 1987; 138: 312–315

47. Brant M D, Ludlow J K, Mulcahy J J. The prosthesis salvage operation: immediate replacement of the infected penile prosthesis. J Urol 1996; 155: 155–157

48. Kardar A, Pettersson B A. Penile gangrene: a complication of penile prosthesis. Can J Urol 1995; 29: 355–356

49. Bejany D E, Perito P E, Lustgarten M, Rhamey R K. Gangrene of the penis after implantation of penile prosthesis: case reports, treatment recommendations, and review of the literature. J Urol 1993; 150: 190–191

50. Lewis R W, McLaren R H. Re-operation for penile prosthesis implantation. Probl Urol 1993; 7: 381–401

51. Garber B B. Mentor Alpha 1 inflatable penile prosthesis: patient satisfaction and device reliability. Urology 1994; 43: 214–217

52. Woodworth B W, Carson C C, Webster G B. Inflatable penile prosthesis: effect of device modification on functional longevity. Urology 1991; 38: 533

53. Pescatori E S, Goldstein I. Intraluminal device pressures in 3-piece inflatable penile prostheses: the pathophysiology of mechanical malfunction. J Urol 1993; 149: 295–300

54. Garber B B. Mentor Alpha 1 inflatable penile prosthesis cylinder aneurysm: an unusual complication. Int J Impot Res 1995; 7: 13–16

55. Mancada I, Jara J, Llado E et al. Prolonged penile pain after prosthesis implant is due to buckling of cylinders. Int J Impot Res 1996; 8: 121

56. Kowalczyk J J, Mulcahy J J. Penile curvatures and aneurysmal defects with the Ultrex penile prosthesis corrected with insertion of the AMS 700CX. J Urol 1996; 156: 398–401

57. Wilson S K, Delk J R. Excessive periprosthetic capsule formation of the penile prosthesis reservoir: incidence in various prostheses and simple surgical solution. J Urol 1995; 153: 359a

58. Knoll L D, Furlow W L, Benson R C, Bilhartz D L. Management of non-dilatable corpus fibrosis with the use of a downsized inflatable penile prosthesis. J Urol 1995; 153: 366–367

59. Moul J W, McLeod D G. Negative pressure device in the explanted penile prosthesis population. J Urol 1989; 142: 729–731

60. Koremman S G, Vioca S P. Use of vacuum tumescence device in the management of impotence of men with a history of penile implant or severe pelvic disease. J Am Geriatr Soc 1992; 40: 61–64

61. George V K, Shah G S, Mills R, Dhabuwala C B. The management of extensive penile fibrosis: a new technique of minimal scar tissue excision. Br J Urol 1996; 77: 282–284

62. Hershschorn S, Ordorica R C. Penile prosthesis insertion with corporal reconstruction with synthetic vascular graft material. J Urol 1995; 154: 80–84

63. Fishman J J. Corporal reconstruction for penile prosthesis implantation. Probl Urol 1993; 7: 350–367

64. Knoll L D, Fisher J, Benson R C et al. Treatment of penile fibrosis with prosthetic implantation and flap advancement with tissue debulking. J Urol 1996; 156: 394–397

65. Knoll L D. Use of penile prosthetic implants in patients with penile fibrosis. Urol Clin North Am 1995; 22: 857–863

66. McLaren R H, Barrett D M. Patient and partner satisfaction with the AMS 700 penile prosthesis. J Urol 1992; 147: 62–65

67. Steege J F, Stout A L, Carson C C. Patient satisfaction in Scott and Small–Carrion penile implant recipients. Arch Sex Behav 1986; 15: 393–397

68. Jarow J P, Nana Sinkam P, Sabbagh M. Outcome analysis of goal directed therapy for impotence. J Urol 1996; 155: 1609–1612

Chapter 40

Psychotherapy in the treatment of erectile dysfunction

B. Daines and Tricia Barnes

■ INTRODUCTION

All medical conditions involve both biophysical and psychosocial processes and, in any illness, it can be useful to consider both. With a syndrome such as erectile dysfunction (ED), which has such clear psychological and relationship aspects, it is essential to consider psychosocial processes.[1] It can be important, for example, to ask why a patient reports ED in the way that he does and presents when he does. Daines et al.[2] point out the way in which symptoms are framed by the patient 'will be informed by his view of the world and his place within it, by the views of others in his life, and by his previous experiences of seeking medical or psychological help (p.38)'. Therefore, ED may be perceived by a patient as physical illness, a reaction to stress or resulting from an unhappy marriage, *irrespective of the true cause or causes*, and these perceptions may need careful attention as a part of treatment or in order to facilitate it.

ED, and other sexual problems, have traditionally been characterized as emerging predominantly within three distinct systems — physical, psychological and relationship. However, clinical experience shows that ED can be better understood by seeing sexual difficulties as emerging at the boundaries of these systems and within identified subsystems. The particularly relevant subsystems are the male sexual organs and relevant physiological mechanisms related to sexual functioning (within the physical system), sexual identity (within the psychological system) and the sexual relationship (within the relationship system).

The erectile response can therefore be seen as a complicated expression of a functioning physical system (cardiovascular, hormonal, neuronal, side effects of drugs), the psychological system (the individual's sexual identity and sense of well-being) and the relationship system (the context for a sexual relationship). To give examples by way of clarification, looking at the effect of ED with an identifiable physical aetiology on a relationship would be an exploration of the interface between two main systems — the physical and the relationship. On the other hand, viewing the erectile dysfunction in the context of concerns about sexual identity would be an example of working at the interface between a subsystem (sexual identity) and the main psychological system. An example of working with subsystems from different main systems would be looking at the effect of the ED (subsystem of physical system) on the couple's sexual relationship (subsystem of relationship system).

It therefore follows that, in many instances, ED cannot be most effectively treated exclusively by physical means, or just by working psychotherapeutically with the individual or the couple's relationship. Rather, it is best approached with a combination of two or more of these — that is, by working at the interface between systems. It is no surprise, therefore, that aspects of individual and couple psychotherapies are often used by practitioners of sex therapy in treating ED. In this chapter the focus is on presentations of ED where a psychotherapeutic approach may constitute the main treatment of choice. This will be the case where either the prime cause of the dysfunction, or behaviours and dynamics that contribute to maintaining the sexual problem, are firmly located in the areas addressed by these kinds of therapy.

Competent assessment is needed to determine when this is the case and where other treatments may be needed as an adjunct. The focus of a practitioner's professional work will always influence views on appropriate

451

treatment, but it is important that all who work with ED have a basic understanding of the main psychotherapeutic approaches and are able to make appropriate referrals to agencies or individuals offering such help.

HISTORICAL RELATIONSHIP BETWEEN PSYCHOTHERAPY AND SEX THERAPY

The treatment of couples with sexual difficulties was revolutionized by the work of Masters and Johnson.[3,4] However, the background to their work is to be understood within the context of sexology rather than psychotherapy with individuals or couples. Belliveau and Richter's authorized account of their work[5] lists only one psychologically minded antecedent, Freud,[6] among the five that they identify. The others are Ellis,[7–10] (a physician), Van der Velde[11] and Dickinson[12,13] (gynaecologists), and Kinsey[14,15] (a zoologist). The discipline of sexology has continued, particularly in the United States, as an interdisciplinary science involving a wide range of professionals including sociologists, anthropologists, biologists, lawyers and educators, as well as medical doctors and psychologists.

Therefore, although cognitive and behavioural techniques can be clearly seen in Masters and Johnson's work,[3,4] they are not identified as such. Bancroft[16] considers that their original descriptions conveyed, by default, a predominantly behavioural model, but that their subsequent writing revealed that there was much more to their treatment approach. In Britain, the work of Dicks[17] was very influential in the '60s in establishing a strong psychodynamic emphasis in couples work and since then many practitioners have integrated Masters and Johnson's sensate focus techniques into such an approach. More recently, influences on sex therapy from family therapy have been evident, in particular the importance of systems approaches.[18–20]

UNDERSTANDING AND TREATING ED WITHIN A PSYCHOTHERAPEUTIC FRAMEWORK

From a psychosocial point of view, a man's relationship to his ED can be construed in a number of ways. Three approaches are presented below, each of which offer an understanding of the possible causes and treatment options. The understandings arrived at within each are not necessarily mutually exclusive:

1. Unconscious processes (analytic and psychodynamic psychotherapies);
2. Beliefs and behaviour (cognitive and behavioural psychotherapies);
3. Relationship processes (systems psychotherapies).

Analytic and psychodynamic psychotherapies
Formulation of erectile dysfunction
Analytic and psychodynamic psychotherapies view many of the patterns of longings, fears and fantasies in marriage (or equivalent committed relationships) as stemming from each partner's infantile and childhood experiences. The motivations that underlie the choice of partners, sustain relationships and give them their particular qualities are related as much to unconscious factors as to conscious ones.

Traditionally within psychoanalysis, sexual problems have been seen as a result of an unresolved Oedipus conflict. This is 'a group of largely unconscious ideas and feelings centred around the wish to possess the parent of the opposite sex and eliminate that of the same sex.'[21] Sexual feelings towards parents have fear and guilt associated with them and the idea is that, if these remain unresolved, sexual excitement stirs up these incestuous wishes and the associated anxiety and guilt are re-evoked.

Within this framework, ED can be seen as a defence against these desires and feelings, a way of avoiding experiencing them. Part of the Oedipus complex, according to Freud, is a fear of castration by the father and therefore ED is to be understood in terms of unresolved castration anxiety — the man fearing that he will be punished if he is sexually potent. It may be that the mechanism by which ED happens is, in fact, the failure to control these feelings, especially of anxiety.

The classical psychoanalytic understanding of ED needs to be understood within the context of such an understanding of the various other common psychosexual problems, as described by Kaplan.[22]

1. Premature ejaculation as expressing unconscious sadistic feelings towards women in soiling and defiling the woman and depriving her of pleasure;
2. Non-ejaculation as an expression of castration anxiety, the man believing that he will be injured or harmed in some way if he ejaculates into the vagina;

3. Vaginismus as an hysterical or conversion symptom — a symbolic expression of psychic conflict where envy and hostility to men exists because of unresolved penis envy;

4. Orgasmic difficulties where penis envy impedes a transition from the clitoris to the vagina and can lead to no orgasm at all.

Each of these formulations is controversial and special notoriety has surrounded the explanation of orgasmic problems, in particular the idea of the inferiority of the clitoral orgasm and the existence of a distinctive and 'mature' vaginal orgasm.

More recent psychodynamic formulations have been in more general terms,[23] looking at sexual difficulties in terms of a number of possible mechanisms, all of which may be relevant to understanding ED:

1. *Unconscious motivations in partner choice.* A common example of this is selecting a partner who resembles a significant other, often the opposite gender parent. This frequently turns out to be the case even when the apparent choice is of someone who superficially appears to be significantly different.

2. *Connections between partner choice and unconscious needs.* An example of this would be a man who chooses a woman to meet his mothering needs, but then cannot obtain an erection when making love to her because of incestuous anxieties.

3. *The expression of defences or potential defences contained within the couple (or potential couple) relationship.* A common defence is idealization, and sometimes men will idealize their partner to the point where sex with her would be seen as a defiling. The breakdown of idealization can result in anger that the partner has not lived up to expectations and is a common process behind domestic violence.

4. *An expression of individual problems and defences.* It is clear that such features as anxiety states, depression and paranoid tendencies can be very disruptive both of couples' general and sexual relationships.

Hiller[24] suggests a psychoanalytic understanding of erectile dysfunction based on the work of Ogden,[25] which is founded on failures in the secure development of male sexual identity:

I suggest that the collapse of the physiological reflex of the erectile response represents an internal collapse into a dyadic relationship with the mother of the pre-genital early holding environment: the inability to sustain an erection to intra-vaginal containment represents the lack of containment in the transitional oedipal relationship for the boy's secure attribution of phallic meaning to his penis: the fear of sexual failure represents the failure of the parental environment to facilitate adequate male sexual identification, either with the mother's unconscious oedipal father or with the actual father at a later stage of development (p.17).

Such processes can be seen as a possible explanation for a psychological predisposition to erectile failure, but does not necessarily explain onset or maintenance of the problem.

Analytic and psychodynamic techniques in therapy

- The work is often with both partners.
- The therapist gives insights into the man's internal psychological dynamics and the dynamics of the couple relationship.
- Therapy is based on attempts to understand processes of interaction rather than applying a set of techniques.
- The therapist tries not to avoid the clients' pain and anger by giving premature reassurance or responding to pressure to take charge, provide easy answers or give advice.
- The overall aim of treatment is to provide a safe enough environment whereby the individual or couple can increasingly give expression to their feelings and perceptions.
- Reflections by the partners and the therapists on the feelings between them (transference and counter-transference) and on what is being communicated and experienced in the sessions enables unconscious conflicts to be brought into awareness, perceptions to be altered and problems to be resolved.
- The therapist does not structure the sessions but rather responds to what clients bring, because what is talked about has an important unconscious purpose.

Case example using analytic and psychodynamic techniques

Referral and assessment

Mr and Mrs C were referred by their family doctor who had excluded physical causes for Mr C's erectile dysfunction and Mrs C's loss of interest in sex. Both these problems had been gradually developing since the birth of their second child a year before. Both Mr and Mrs C were in their early 30s and had another child, aged 4 years.

Taking a full history revealed that Mrs C had pursued a career as a pharmacist before having children. She had carried on working after the first child was born, but felt she had to give up her job when the second, unplanned, child was born. To have carried on working would have made her feel guilty that she was not being a proper mother to them in not giving them enough of her time and attention. However, she was angry and resentful to find herself in a traditional 'housewife and mother role', one which her mother had seemingly happily embraced all her life, but which she had been determined to avoid.

Mr C had been referred to a urologist, but investigations had revealed no physical cause for the problem. His family background included a mother who was dominant in the family and, through his teenage years in particular, he had worked hard to avoid her disapproval, but his attempts to please her always failed. He now felt in a similar situation with his wife, feeling guilty about 'making her pregnant' even though it was a result of a coil failure. He now had a resentful wife whom he tried to appease and please, but without success.

Formulation

The psychodynamic formulation of the problem was that both partners were unconsciously re-enacting unresolved conflicts from relationships in their families of origin. Mrs C had invested a great deal in being different from her mother, but identification with her made her sabotage her career, possibly from fears of disloyalty and a sense that perhaps her mother was not as happy as she seemed and would have liked a career herself. Mr C wanted someone who would treat him as a partner very differently from the way his mother did, but found himself in a repetition of unresolved issues of whether he could be 'good enough' for a woman.

Therapy

The therapist's understanding of the problem was shared with the couple, who experienced some relief at being given an explanation of what was happening in their marriage and sexual relationship. Over the course of the treatment, various themes emerged during the sessions, including Mrs C's feelings of being trapped, and Mr C's guilt and feelings of failure. It was probably important that their therapist was a woman, as it made it possible to work through in the transference some of the issues. For example, the therapist could be for Mr C a woman with whom he did not have to work hard to gain acceptance

and approval. Similarly, with Mrs C some of the issues surrounding women having a career and being a mother were worked through in an environment where judgements were not perceived to be made.

As therapy progressed, issues of sexuality were processed more explicitly. Mrs C came from a family where sexual matters were discussed only obliquely and where women were not expected to be sexual. Mr C had grown up in a climate where women were romantically idealized and seen as frail by men and this made it hard for him to think of them wanting a robust sexual relationship. Working through these and similar issues, together with the work on their general relationship, led to them beginning to resume their sexual relationship, which had been non-existent for some months. Mrs C's interest began to return and Mr C became less anxious about his erection failing. By the end of therapy their sexual relationship was much better, but still not as good as they thought it should and could be. However, they both felt that it was time to end therapy and identified the changes in their relationship generally as the most important outcome. They expressed confidence that, as their relationship continued to improve, this would be paralleled by further improvements in their sexual relationship.

Discussion

The assumption tends to be made that a psychodynamic approach to sexual difficulties is less cost effective than the alternatives, in particular behavioural approaches. The discrediting of traditional psychoanalytic understandings has tended to prejudice exploration of the use of more modern analytic understandings and there is a need for research in this area to establish whether the assumptions made about psychodynamic therapy in relation to sexual problems are true. For a number of reasons, most therapists working psychotherapeutically with ED became interested in exploring cognitive–behavioural psychotherapies, which are considered below. The reasons for this include the following:

1. The comparative ease with which the effectiveness of a cognitive–behavioural approach, as opposed to analytic and psychodynamic psychotherapies, can be investigated and researched. This is partly because the aims, methods and outcome measures are more easily defined and quantified;
2. The charisma surrounding Masters and Johnson's work and the treatment methods associated with it;

3. Analytic and psychodynamic psychotherapies have been perceived as longer term and therefore less cost effective;
4. Analytic and psychodynamic psychotherapies have been seen as more difficult to integrate with allied helping activities, such as education and medical interventions;
5. The political and cultural climate of the last 20 years, with its emphasis on immediate gratification, has often not been conducive to more reflective approaches, which were more in line with the culture of the '60s and '70s.

Although it does not deal directly with the treatment of erectile problems, Scharff's book, *The Sexual Relationship*,[26] provides a useful survey of sexual development and sexuality in general from a psychodynamic viewpoint. Hiller's[24] article on psychoanalytic concepts and psychosexual therapy is also to be recommended.

Cognitive and behavioural therapies
Formulation of erectile dysfunction
These therapies are based on detailed models of the cognitive and behavioural factors involved both in successful functioning and in creating and maintaining problems and symptoms. Within this context, successful couple relationships are seen to be those in which both partners are flexible enough to be able to adjust expectations and behaviour so that change does not lead to significant decrease in satisfaction with each other.[27] ED is to be viewed against a background of early learning and sexual experiences and the beliefs and ideas that provide the context for sexual activity.

Within the cognitive–behavioural perspective, the onset and maintenance of ED is understood in terms of recognition and a learned anticipation of performance anxiety and sexual failure. Within the Masters and Johnson programme, the sensate focus exercises were specifically formulated to address these issues, and relieve the couple from such pressures. However, this approach does not seem to address the individual's perceptions and interpretations of his physiological and psychological functioning. Understanding such cognitive processes and the inevitable distortions affecting information, beliefs, and feelings is the initial task of the cognitive therapist, who then helps the client (and partner) to find alternative ways of viewing the sexual difficulty and adapting sexual responses.

Men with ED typically experience some or all of the following responses:

- An increasing urge to penetrate as soon as possible before any partial or semi-rigid erection subsides;
- The experience of anxiety surrounding all aspects of the problem and an increasing preoccupation with this;
- The focus of attention changes from that of a participant to that of an observer and 'monitor', and from erotic cues to anticipated failure;
- Feelings of humiliation in front of a partner;
- An irrational fear, particularly in the context of a new or uncommitted relationship, that this 'secret' will be revealed leading to more public humiliation; and
- A fear that a relationship will, de facto, end because of the lack of satisfactory sex.

For some men the anxiety is so high that they visualize the whole structure of their lives collapsing, including the probability that no-one would ever want to be in a long-term relationship with them, that they will not be able to have children, and so on.

Other relevant issues for consideration include:

- A loss of sexual interest as a response to experiencing conflict, a manifestation of which can be secondary ED or premature ejaculation;
- ED as a direct consequence of painful first experiences of intercourse. Thereafter there is a learned avoidance response of which the man is fully aware but is unable to overcome. The fear of associated psychological pain leads to a flaccid penis, which ensures avoidance of the anticipated pain. This pattern of response inevitably reinforces the maintenance of the problem;
- A possible consequence is absent, or infrequent, sexual opportunities in which to learn how to function successfully with a partner;
- A misperception that the erection is lost too quickly, when this is actually a consequence of loss of control over ejaculatory inevitability (premature ejaculation);
- A fear of making a partner pregnant.

Following on from the work of Masters and Johnson some therapists, clearly identifying themselves as practising within the cognitive–behavioural field, developed therapeutic techniques to deal with sexual fears and phobias, increase behavioural repertoires and change irrational beliefs.[28–31] The application of cognitive behavioural principles has continued to develop[32,33] and in general has been particularly effective in clinical settings in managing anxiety[34] and depression.[35]

There has also been considerable interest in using behavioural and cognitive approaches in a group setting for the treatment of ED.[36–40] Some have focused specifically on the group treatment of gay and bisexual men.[41,42] Elaborations of the use of behavioural principles with individuals have introduced humanistic[43] and feminist[44] elements.

Cognitive and behavioural techniques in therapy

There are a number of techniques for both the individual and the couple that can be used to assist them in adapting their patterns of response. Such approaches usually involve an element of listening and monitoring behaviours more accurately, and directly testing out clients' assumptions and interpretations.

In work with an individual the therapist's task is to do the following:

- Challenge and correct existing information and belief systems by education and dialogue. Books and other educational materials are particularly useful with those people who require evidence to support alternative ways of thinking.
- Teach techniques for reducing anxiety and excessive monitoring of sexual activity.
- Address unhelpful cognitive patterns, such as tendencies to exaggerate and/or minimize certain responses, blaming, and not being able to differentiate between the responsibility of one's own sexual pleasure and that of one's partner.

In work with a couple, the therapist facilitates the couple's understanding of the self in relation to the other person and much of the focus is on communication:

- To reverse self-defeating patterns of withholding rewards, by increasing awareness of existing rewards and increasing the frequency of positive behaviours;
- To identify unhelpful or poor communication patterns and offer interpersonal skills training;
- To teach problem-solving skills, differentiating between assertion and aggression and enabling couples to perceive such resolution as a positive solution rather than mediocre compromise;

- To facilitate compromises by using contingency contracting, a specific contractual agreement between the couple that specifies the particular rewards to be given when one partner's behaviour is in direct response to a request by the other;
- To help couples to tolerate or accept the notion of difference — sex may differ significantly from how it used to be but perhaps it can improve to the point of satisfaction;
- To help couples accept that change does not necessarily have the same meaning and impact on both partners: for example, the man may state that his erection is always soft and penetration cannot be achieved, whereas the partner may say that sometimes it is hard enough for penetration.

Case example using cognitive and behavioural techniques

Referral and assessment

Mr S, a 52-year-old man, was referred by his family doctor after complaining of difficulty in achieving erections and premature ejaculation, which he had experienced for the past 20 years. He had experienced a few short-term relationships, but had never had any lasting a significant time. He came for help because he had just got married to a woman 12 years his junior, with whom he had experienced a whirlwind romance. Neither partner had been married before, they were both orthodox Jews, and both wanted to have children as soon as possible.

The doctor described Mr S as highly anxious. He had investigated him fully and all the tests were normal. He prescribed yohimbine to augment his sexual responsiveness and possibly assist his erectile response, and lorazepam for his anxiety; he also advised him to see a therapist. There was no other relevant medical history.

Formulation

Associations and dynamics of the home territory Upon marriage, Mrs S moved into his house, which was the home in which he grew up and shared with his mother until her death a few years previously. She completely redecorated the house and made it into their home, both partners saying how happy they were living in it. Her mother also came to live with them, which they both agreed was not intrusive. However, this clearly continued the strong association for both of them of having a maternal figure living under the same roof, which is where, historically, most of their sexual experiences had occurred. Mr S had no awareness that this may contribute to sexual inhibition.

Sexual naïvety Both partners were inexperienced sexually, Mrs S. being a virgin upon marriage, and so, for their ages, they lacked sexual confidence and had few reference points from which to gauge current experiences. Their level of sexual knowledge was very basic and Mr S in particular was uncertain as to what he was 'meant to be feeling and experiencing'. He was convinced, however, that the erectile difficulties would resolve with time. Mrs S was very willing to learn how to arouse her partner, but felt that he was 'withholding something'.

Anxiety Mr S had extremely high levels of generalized anxiety, accompanied by physical symptoms easily recognizable of an anxious state. He acknowledged anxiety only at the thought of penetrative sex, but levels of sexual desire were high, which drove him to attempt sex daily. It seemed as though they were both trying to make up for lost time. They were experiencing feelings of both anger and sadness at the obstacle to their new-found sexual enjoyment but were unable to express this for fear of inflicting hurt or blame on the other.

Communication Mr S was a traditional and proud man who believed in shouldering responsibilities as a husband, and had not had the experience or opportunity of sharing or talking about these before. Prior to marriage he had a coronary infarct, of which he had not informed his wife as he felt that he was fully recovered and therefore it was irrelevant. It was only during therapy that he was able to recognize the power and potential anxiety of holding such a secret, and was encouraged to share with his wife such a personal and significant life event. Mrs S, on the other hand, was very open, in touch with her thoughts and feelings, and could be very challenging when she felt her husband was holding something back from her.

Therapy The couple were seen separately for assessment but together for the therapy sessions. They responded well to a structured approach, which was initially focused on enabling them to learn about their own sexual arousal and responses and communicate these in a non-threatening manner. Mr S was helped to understand and accept that the thought of sex provoked enormous anxiety in him, and recognized that this was principally in the form of having to impregnate his wife as soon as

possible. He also felt pressure to communicate to his wife in a manner which was unfamiliar to him, which she was utilizing as a sign of his commitment to her. They both were apprehensive of their ability to sustain a relationship, but unable to acknowledge this.

Permission was given to enjoy giving and receiving sexual pleasure, and to learn to ask for what they wanted sexually. Mr S's early experiences had done little to validate his sense of self and, although he was comfortable with the idea of emotional nurturing, he was confused when there were expectations on him that he did not know how to meet. After six sessions they reported that sex was enjoyable, that Mrs S was orgasmic, but that Mr S was not able to ejaculate intravaginally, although he did so externally. This is a clear example of how the dynamics can shift in therapy, and the problem became one of response and control, rather than fear and arousal.

The couple decided to commence infertility treatment to assist conception, but they continued therapy sessions to explore issues that were impacting on both the sexual and general relationship. They learned to identify feelings, to express some of them much more effectively, and to have more respect and trust for one another as a result. This was particularly evident as a dynamic when Mr S told his wife about his coronary infarct, as she was not scared by the information as he had anticipated, but received it as a gift of intimacy, knowing how difficult this was for him to share it. Although they were very much in love and excited by the relationship, they achieved a greater sense of trust and intimacy through this.

Mr S became able to enjoy sex free from concerns about his erections, but retained control over the ejaculatory phase. It is interesting to note that he complained initially to his male GP of ED and premature ejaculation, symptoms which he had experienced for 20 years. Neither of these were perceived to be problem areas by Mr S, or his wife, after only six sessions of therapy. The persistence of a problem over a long period does not necessarily represent resistance to treatment, but other underlying issues may manifest themselves at the point of 'success'.

Discussion

When there are coexisting sexual disorders presented by the patient or his partner, one of the most taxing decisions that the clinician has to make is whether it is necessary or desirable to focus the treatment strategy on a single disorder, or to tackle the sexual difficulties more comprehensively. In the case above, the single approach was selected because the premature ejaculation was seen to be secondary to the erectile disorder, and had a good chance of improving when sexual confidence and experience was achieved, and the patient saw sexual pleasure as a valid goal for himself. If the secondary disorder does not resolve, one can always move on to focus on that after a period of consolidation. The key elements in this decision are that the couple have a strong commitment to staying together, have reasonable communication with one another, and that they perceive the risk of changing existing behaviour as worth taking to attain the desired behaviour.

It has been suggested that behavioural approaches will be most successful where its methods of understanding problems and working with them, match couples' perceptions and concepts about their problems.[45] Those wishing to learn more of this approach to erectile problems should consult *Sex Therapy: a practical guide*[46] and *Psychosexual therapy: a cognitive–behavioural approach*.[32]

Kaplan[22,47] introduced a psychodynamic under-standing alongside the behavioural and can also be seen as pioneering a sequential approach to the use of theory, whereby one therapy is tried first and another moved on to if this is unsuccessful. Whereas Kaplan used a behavioural–psychodynamic axis, more recently Crowe and Ridley[48] have developed a behavioural–systems therapy. It has been recognized that some individuals and couples will sabotage the tasks set within cognitive–behavioural therapy and that systems therapies can offer powerful ways of dealing with such situations.

Systems psychotherapies
Formulation of erectile dysfunction
Systems therapists base their ideas about the generation and treatment of problems on general systems theory, which was originally developed to explain biological systems and is pervasive within physiology and medicine. Techniques devised for work with families have been adapted for use with individuals and couples. Within this framework, ED can be understood in terms of a process going on between the couple, in the family or within wider systems. Important concepts in understanding ED from this perspective include the following:

1. *Communication processes*, whereby an erection problem might be seen as a blocking of general interaction patterns in the relationship. For example, an erectile problem may enable a couple to avoid communication about sex, because for them it is too sensitive an issue to talk about.

2. *Homeostasis*, which refers to the tendency for a system (e.g. the couple system) to have self-regulatory elements within it that resist attempts at change by re-introducing the original state of affairs. This mechanism can help us to understand why attempts to resolve erectile difficulties, by whatever means, may be sabotaged by the individual or his partner. For example, where an erectile problem is enabling a couple to lessen their intimacy, solving this problem may result in his partner losing interest in sex, thus restoring the status quo sexually.

3. *Symptom function*, whereby symptoms serve a purpose that is not immediately obvious. In the above example, the man's ED deals with both partners' anxieties about too much intimacy in their relationship, and loss of control. By keeping the disorder in place, at least both partners can predict their thoughts, reactions and feelings, and therefore do not have to face the unknown, however appealing it may seem.

4. *Symptom substitution*, where another symptom replaces the treated symptom. For example, in ED, if the erection becomes reliable due to a specific treatment, then loss of desire or an ejaculatory disorder may appear. Its purpose is to regulate the couple functioning back to where it was when the ED was 'serving its purpose' in the overall structure.

5. *Collusive maintenance of roles* from, and loyalties to, family of origin. Often, couples will have difficulties in their sexual relationship at the same stage of their relationship that their parents had similar difficulties or discontinued sex.

Probably, the most common conceptualization of sexual difficulties such as ED is as a regulator of intimacy for the couple. There can also be ways in which the couple or family express certain difficulties, as when they become expressions of couples' overall system of relating, e.g. the 'impotent' man and the 'castrating' woman.

Systems techniques in therapy
Systems techniques are wide and varied but some of the main ones are outlined below and some are illustrated in the case example.

Working with alliances, boundaries and hierarchies

Within the couple, appropriate alliances, boundaries and hierarchies are said to be essential for a healthy functioning family system. The therapist observes existing alliances and their functions and from this develops a working hypothesis. There is an assumption that a firm boundary needs to be maintained around the parental couple. In order for this to happen there needs to be a sound parental alliance and a workable distance between parents and children. Many couples need to establish boundaries, and in doing so, not only improve their own relationship, but also offer a more functional role model. An example of this is in the case history that follows.

Working with closeness and distance

Within the couple relationship and the family, there needs to be a balance between connectedness and separateness in order to avoid the extremes of enmeshment and disengagement. A common presentation is one where one partner desires and/or needs more intimacy than another and this frequently leads to a 'chase'. ED can become part of such a 'chase', as the woman presses for more intimacy and the man avoids it through erectile failure.

Structural interventions

The aim of structural interventions is to enable the couple to experience a different way of relating to each other in the session. One type of intervention is to encourage arguments over trivial matters in the session which helps to increase the mutual exchange of emotional messages, and proves that the situation does not necessarily lead to the feared outcome. One situation in which structural intervention is useful is where modesty or inhibition hold the relationship static. An example of this is where the woman states that the loss of erection 'does not matter', thus 'helping' her partner feel less shamed. However, the avoidance of conflict blocks off the expression of sexual desire in the relationship and perpetuates the problem.

Using messages, formulations, tasks and timetables

These are designed to change the current interaction of the couple. A message to a couple may consist of a positive statement about the couple or the individual, reflections on the work done in the session, or some aspect of the therapist's understanding or formulation of their relationship. Tasks may be added, sometimes within the framework of a timetable, the function of which is to change the interactions of the couple in a way that overcomes a presenting problem.

Case example using systems techniques

Referral and assessment

Mr T and his wife were referred by his family doctor because Mr T had experienced difficulties in obtaining an erection for the previous three years. They were both in their late 50s at the time of referral, with two sons in their mid-20s (living at home), and a 10-year-old daughter. The situation had come to a head after a recent holiday, when Mrs T became concerned that her husband might begin an affair with a family friend because she had seen them flirting with each other in a pub.

His doctor had investigated the erectile problem and found no physical cause. Mr T had experienced increasing stress in his work as a self-employed decorator in recent years and the doctor speculated in his referring letter that this might have been the original triggering factor.

After taking a full history, a behavioural approach to the sexual problem was initially considered to be the most appropriate, and the therapist explained a treatment process that would involve them carrying out a sensate focus programme at home aimed at reducing anxiety and moving the focus away from achieving particular goals in lovemaking. It soon became clear, however, that such an approach could not work because of the lack of privacy in their house, including their bedroom, and in their lives generally.

Mr and Mrs T were clearly the centre of an 'extended' family, and family members and friends would expect to be able to call in on them at any time unannounced. Additionally, their bedroom was not a private space, and there was an expectation that the bedroom door would be kept open at all times, and that their sons or daughter could shout to them from downstairs, or come to see them, more or less at any time. There was, understandably, a particularly close bond between Mrs T and her daughter, who was included in nearly all activities, which resulted in the marital couple never having time together — except in bed.

Formulation

This couple's problems were re-formulated systemically as follows (Fig. 40.1):

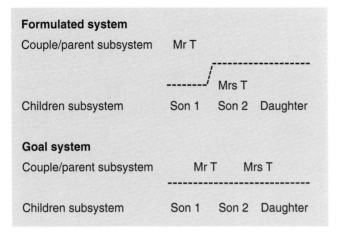

Figure 40.1. Formulated system and goal system (----- denotes a boundary between subsystems).

- There was a lack of boundary between the couple subsystem and the family, and between the family and extended family-and-friends systems;
- A particularly strong bond existed between Mrs T and the family, and this tended to leave Mr T isolated and lacking the attention he wanted and required;
- Mr T responded to this situation with the erectile problem and the 'flirtation' which produced an instability in the system that provoked the referral.

Therapy
The therapy initially tackled helping the couple to mark and establish clearer boundaries, both physically and emotionally. They were encouraged to consider closing their bedroom door once they went to bed and to ask the children to knock before entering their room. These ideas were initially resisted, but were overcome by the message that the children needed the same privacy in return. This reframing meant that, instead of the couple seeing the suggestion as selfish and rejecting of their children, it was seen as one that also met their children's needs. There was also the need for some examination and rewriting of family myths and scripts about what families should be like and how much closeness and distance is allowed.

The establishment of this physical boundary was important in creating some physical space in which their relationship could operate without fear of interruption. This then made it easier to help them to sometimes say 'no' to family members and friends, and made further opportunities for their relationship to be re-established.

The possibility of Mr T flirting with the 'other woman' still caused Mrs T anxiety, as she feared that it would continue. Obtaining further information about the way that Mr T had always related to women and learning that this particular woman tended to flirt with men anyway, made the therapist think that it was unlikely to be a realistic goal to end the flirtatious exchanges completely. The therapist was successful in helping them to treat such flirtations in a less serious way, creating a kind of secret conspiracy between them by acknowledging together when this woman was being, or had been, 'a flirt'.

This re-framing changed a threat of intimacy with someone else into an intimate exchange between them about the issue. This seemed to work well and they both felt confident that such a situation in the future would not produce unresolvable tensions between them. Within this context, the erectile problem was quite easily resolved by practical advice about managing sexual contact in a non-pressurizing way that enabled confidence about his erections to be established. Alongside these changes, the therapist had also asked them to use their private time and space for sexual contact, initially with a ban on attempts at intercourse, but ending this once Mr T's erections became more reliable.

During the course of the therapy the possibility was considered that the erectile problem, the family arrangements, and the issue of the 'other woman' were all operating as distance regulators for the couple and that therefore direct attempts to change these might be resisted. In the event, however, the interventions designed to change these patterns and produce more intimacy were not resisted.

Discussion
The development of systems approaches to sexual problems is in its early stages, but the work done so far indicates considerable potential. One of the main features and strengths of a systems perspective is the avoidance of splitting off the problem or part of the relationship. This approach seeks to gain an understanding of a symptom in terms of wider processes. For those who wish to follow up this approach further, Crowe and Ridley[48] explain in detail the application of systems techniques to sexual problems. Alongside an interest in applying systems theory to general couples work, there is a growing body of writing on the application of systems theory specifically to sexual difficulties, using concepts such as distance regulation to understand problems and techniques to treat them that have been adapted from family therapy.[20,49–53]

■ CONCLUSIONS

It is commonly believed that, at best, the worth of psychotherapy in sexual dysfunction has not been proved and, at worst, it has been discredited. Research into the effectiveness of psychotherapy is complex, but progress has been made in recent years in tackling some of the difficulties such as defining a 'good' outcome and the need to take into account the variations in practice between psychotherapists, even within a particular orientation. Many emphasize the importance of a 'horses for courses' approach in relation to allocating patients to different forms of psychotherapy.[54]

Oatley[54] usefully surveys the development of research into the outcome of psychotherapy since the Second World War. Two noteworthy conclusions are, first, that people 'are not things to whom technical solutions are to be applied' and, secondly, that the psychotherapist 'hopes to make a difference, but he is not the cause of change' (pp. 73–87). Lambert and Bergin[55] conclude:

Many psychotherapies have been subjected to empirical study and have been shown to have demonstrable effects on a variety of clients. These effects are not only statistically significant but also clinically meaningful (p. 180).

Roth and Fonagy[56] comprehensively survey research findings on psychotherapy. In relation to ED, their main conclusion is that behavioural and cognitive–behavioural approaches aimed at reducing sexual anxiety and improving communication have been shown to be clearly effective. However, they do note that the outcome literature relevant to the treatment of sexual disorders is small, and that there is therefore 'a need for well-designed, large, controlled trials with specific dysfunctions and specified therapies' (p. 244).

There are three clinical presentations where the physician may consider an assessment and possible treatment for ED from a psychotherapeutic perspective. In the first of these, significant psychological issues can be identified that underlie the onset and/or maintenance of the dysfunction and predominantly affect the male partner. Examples of such presentations include men in whom generalized or specific forms of anxiety can be identified, those who suffer from features of depression, or cases where obsessional, ritualistic or phobic behaviours associated with sexual identity, orientation and behaviour are evident. Life events or other externalized pressures can also impact on an individual's sexual functioning. These include high stress factors (frequently related to work or financial considerations) and the experience of trauma (sexual abuse, physical abuse, post-traumatic stress disorder, postoperative complications), all of which can contribute to low self-esteem and a poor self-image.

The second presentation is where additional psychological help is required after other treatments have been tried. An example of such a case is a man who, despite a positive response to Caverject in a clinical situation, cannot (or chooses not to) use the treatment successfully in practice. This effectively leaves him impotent although, in theory, he has the choice of what is usually considered artificial erectile functioning.

The third presentation is where psychotherapy is required to help the patient (or couple) come to terms with absent or limited sexual functioning, which cannot be helped further by any medical intervention. A typical example would be a young man whose sexual responses are severely compromised by a venous leak or trauma and in whom further surgery is not recommended, and other treatment options are resisted.

There are additional issues that affect the couple and family system, as opposed to the individual, and that need to be taken into account. If there is evidence of chronic, or acute but severe, difficulties in a couple's relationship, such as communication problems, hostile behaviour, power imbalances and struggles, it is unlikely that any 'cure' will be effective until these matters are partially resolved. It is very common for conflict in a relationship to be played out in a sexual arena, and therefore an understanding of the role of the symptom is relevant when selecting an appropriate solution; if not, the symptom will simply be substituted. Additional commonly held fears and behaviours that can affect the wider system include fear of pregnancy and unsatisfactory contraception arrangements, the effect of secrets, affairs, and coping with illness and/or the ageing process.

In summary, a variety of treatment options can be considered when treating ED, that can be used separately or in combination. Where there are identifiable issues that affect the functioning of the individual, the couple, and possibly the wider family, short-term focused psychotherapy can be very effective. It is certainly a valuable consideration for men who do not have a partner, or who do not wish to disclose or involve their partner in couple sex therapy. Longer-term psychotherapy would not usually be considered for the treatment of ED, unless the history suggested that more general work was indicated.

■ REFERENCES

1. Usherwood T. Responses to illness — implications for the clinician. 1990; 83: 205–207
2. Daines B, Gask L, Usherwood T. Medical and psychiatric issues for counsellors. London: Sage, 1997
3. Masters W H, Johnson V E. Human sexual response. Boston: Little Brown and Co, 1966
4. Masters W H, Johnson V E. Human sexual inadequacy. Boston: Little, Brown & Co, 1970
5. Belliveau F, Richter L R. Understanding human sexual inadequacy. London: Hodder and Stoughton, 1971
6. Freud S. Three essays on the theory of sexuality. In: The standard edition of the complete works, Volume 7. London: Hogarth Press, 1953: 135–243
7. Ellis H. Man and woman. Boston: Houghton Miflin, 1929
8. Ellis H. Studies in the psychology of sex. New York: Random House, 1936
9. Ellis H. Sex and marriage. New York: Random House, 1952
10. Ellis H. Psychology of sex, 2nd edn. New York: Emerson Books, 1954
11. Van der Velde T H. Ideal marriage. New York: Covici-Friede, 1930
12. Dickinson R L, Pierson H H. The average sex life of the American woman. JAMA 1925; 85: 1113–1117
13. Dickinson R L. Human sex anatomy. Baltimore: Williams and Wilkins, 1933
14. Kinsey A C, Pomeroy W, Martin C. Sexual behaviour in the human male. Philadelphia: Saunders, 1948
15. Kinsey A C, Pomeroy W, Martin C, Gebhard P. Sexual behaviour in the human female. Philadelphia: Saunders, 1953
16. Bancroft J. Sexual problems. In: Clark D M, Fairburn C G (eds) Science and practice of cognitive behaviour therapy. Oxford: Oxford University Press, 1997: 243–257
17. Dicks H V. Marital tensions. London: Routledge and Kegan Paul, 1967
18. Bubenzer D L, West J D. Counselling couples. London: Sage, 1993
19. Crowe M J. Marital therapy: a behavioural-systems approach. Indications for different types of interventions. In: Dryden W (ed) Marital therapy in Britain. London: Harper and Row, 1985; Vol 1: 312–338
20. Crowe M J, Ridley J. The negotiated timetable: a new approach to marital conflicts involving male demands and female reluctance for sex. Sex Marital Ther 1986; 1: 157–173
21. Rycroft C. A critical dictionary of psychoanalysis. Harmondsworth: Penguin, 1972
22. Kaplan H. The new sex therapy. New York: Brunner/Mazel, 1974
23. Daniell D. Marital therapy: the psychodynamic approach. In: Dryden W. Marital therapy in Britain, London: Harper and Row, 1985: 169–194
24. Hiller J. Psychoanalytic concepts and psychosexual therapy. Sex Marital Ther 1993; 8: 9–26
25. Ogden T. The primitive edge of experience. London: Jason Aronson, 1991
26. Scharff D E. The sexual relationship. London: Routledge, 1982
27. Mackay D. Marital therapy: the behavioural approach. In: Dryden W (ed) Marital therapy in Britain. London: Harper and Row, 1985: 222–248
28. Heiman J R, Lopicollo L, Lopicollo L. Becoming orgasmic: a sexual growth program for women. Englewood Cliffs, NJ: Prentice Hall, 1976
29. Zilbergeld B. Men and sex. Boston: Little, Brown, 1978
30. Quadland M C. Private self-consciousness, attribution of responsibility, and perfectionistic thinking in secondary erectile dysfunction. J Sex Marital Ther 1980; 6: 47–55
31. Munjack D J, Schlacks A. Sanchez V C et al. Rational–emotive therapy in the treatment of erectile failure: an initial study. J Sex Marital Ther 1984; 10: 170–175
32. Spence S H. Psychosexual therapy: a cognitive–behavioural approach. London: Chapman and Hall, 1991
33. Baker C D. A cognitive–behavioural model for the formulation and treatment of sexual dysfunction. In: Ussher J M, Baker C D (eds) Psychological perspectives on sexual problems. London: Routledge, 1993: 110–128
34. Wells A, Butler G. Generalised anxiety disorder. In: Clark D M, Fairburn C G (eds) Science and practice of cognitive behaviour therapy. Oxford: Oxford University Press, 1996: 155–178
35. Williams J G. Depression. In Clark D M, Fairburn C G (eds) Science and practice of cognitive behaviour therapy. Oxford: Oxford University Press, 1996: 259–283
36. Lobitz W C, Baker E L Jr. Group treatment of single males with erectile dysfunction. Arch Sex Behav 1979; 8: 127–138
37. Reynolds B S. Psychological treatment models and outcome results for erectile dysfunction: a critical review. Psychol Bull 1977; 84: 1218–1238
38. Mills K H, Kilmann P R. Group treatment of sexual dysfunctions: a methodological review of the outcome literature. J Sex Marital Ther 1982; 8: 259–296
39. Reynolds B S, Cohen B D, Schochet B V et al. Dating skills training in the group treatment of erectile dysfunction for men without partners. J Sex Marital Ther 1981; 7: 184–194
40. Kilmann P R, Milan R J Jr, Boland J P et al. Group treatment of secondary erectile dysfunction. J Sex Marital Ther 1987; 13: 168–182

41. Reece R. Group treatment of sexual dysfunction in gay men. J Homosex 1981/2; 7: 113–129

42. Everaerd W, Dekker J, Dronkers J et al. Treatment of homosexual and heterosexual sexual dysfunction in male-only groups of mixed sexual orientation. Arch Sex Behav 1982; 11: 1–10

43. Gillan P. Sex therapy manual. Oxford: Blackwell, 1987

44. Dickson A. The mirror within. London: Quartet Books, 1985

45. Duncan B L, Parkes M B. Integrating individual and systems approaches: strategic–behavioural therapy. J Marital Fam Ther 1988; 1(2): 151–161

46. Hawton K. Sex therapy: a practical guide. Oxford: Oxford University Press, 1985

47. Kaplan H. Disorders of sexual desire. New York: Brunner/Mazel, 1979

48. Crowe M J, Ridley J. Therapy with couples. Oxford: Blackwell, 1990

49. Byng-Hall J. Symptom bearer as marital distance regulator: clinical implications. Family process, 1980: 19: 355–365

50. Divita Woody J. Treating sexual distress. London: Sage, 1992

51. Foreman S, Dallos R. Inequalities of power and sexual problems. J Fam Ther 1992; 14: 349–369

52. Rampage C. Power, gender and marital intimacy. J Fam Ther 1994; 16: 125–137

53. Speed B. The use of the Milan approach in sex therapy. In: Campbell D, Draper R (eds) Applications of systemic family therapy. New York: Grune and Stratton, 1985: 127–134

54. Oatley K. Selves in relation: an introduction to psychotherapy and groups. London: Methuen, 1984

55. Lambert M J, Bergin A E. The effects of psychotherapy. In: Handbook of psychotherapy and behaviour change. New York: Wiley, 1994: 143–189

56. Roth A, Fonagy P. What works for whom: a critical review of psychotherapy research. New York: Guilford Press, 1996

Chapter 41

Integrated sex therapy: the interplay of behavioural, cognitive and medical approaches

Tricia Barnes

■ INTRODUCTION

This chapter outlines current perspectives in sexual and relationship therapy in the treatment of erectile dysfunction (ED). The treatment approach is predominantly a cognitive–behavioural one, with a strong biomedical aspect. This is in contrast to the psychotherapeutic approach outlined in the previous chapter, which focuses more on psychodynamic and interpretative principles, although certain elements are common to both. Three different but related contexts for understanding the man with erectile problems are presented, providing a foundation from which to make treatment decisions.

First, particular cognitive processes that highlight the known differences between sexually functional and non-functional men are reviewed. A knowledge of these processes may assist understanding of why certain men appear to respond to some treatments, and others do not.

Secondly, there is discussion of sexual functioning in the intrapersonal sexual context, which includes gender identity, object choice, and sexual intention and the four phases of sexual desire, arousal, orgasm and satisfaction. This model is then positioned alongside the model of sexual functioning of the partner to obtain a sense of the interpersonal and sexual dynamics of the couple.

Thirdly, a sexual arousal circuit is described, providing a model for observing where the different treatments for ED target the system. All current therapeutic, mechanical and medical interventions are presented within this system.

The final section goes on to look at sex therapy outcomes in the treatment of ED, providing some guidelines for prognosis and improved outcome adopting an integrated approach to sex therapy.

Definition of erectile dysfunction

Producing an operational definition of a sexual dysfunction can be difficult and sometimes controversial, especially where there is reference to normal levels of activity, interest or sexual orientation. The identification of ED as a separate class of disorder within the DSM-IV can give a misleading impression of homogeneity, as well as leaving the clinician and researcher with the role of ascertaining co-morbidity. One of the most clinically satisfying definitions of ED is by Rowland and colleagues:[1] 'self-reported failure to obtain an erection sufficient for vaginal intromission at least 50% of the time without ejaculation, or loss of erection following intromission without ejaculation at least 50% of the time'. This definition not only takes into account the subjective nature of the problem and the ultimate concern with rigidity, but also differentiates it clearly from any ejaculatory control difficulties.

A diagnosis is helpful only if it embraces both the physiological and subjective aspects of the arousal disorder and is subclassified in terms of onset, the context and specific situations in which it manifests itself. Interviewing the partner can frequently reveal a significantly different perspective on the dysfunction. The findings of a study by Tiefer and Melman[2] suggest that clinicians alter their diagnosis and treatment options as much as 58% of the time if taking the partner's views into account. Certainly, if a patient's current partner is willing to be interviewed, then her (his) contribution is desirable. In urology settings it is usual for the male to attend on his own, both for assessment and treatment. In psychotherapeutic environments it is frequently the female who initially presents on her partner's behalf. Male presenters have usually been referred by their GP or a urologist, but generally indicate a preference to talk about their problems with a female therapist.

Prevalence

There is a paucity of systematic or reliable data regarding the prevalence of sexual dysfunctions, and the majority of studies reflect a heterosexual sample, as do the classified definitions of ED. Spector and Carey[3] reviewed 23 studies of incidence and prevalence in community samples, suggesting a current prevalence for ED of 4–9%. Hawton[4] states similar figures for surveys conducted among patients attending medical clinics. Variables that significantly affect the incidence of ED in specific populations include age, diabetes and chronic illness. Slag and colleagues[5] reported a 5% incidence at 40 years, 15–25% at 65 years and 50% at 76 years and older. Ellenberg[6] reports that approximately 50% of diabetic men have ED. It is not known whether the incidence of ED differs significantly in exclusively heterosexual, homosexual or bisexual populations.

Co-morbidity

Sexual problems do not usually arise in isolation from other psychological difficulties, nor are their effects limited to the sexual arena. There is evidence of associated relationship difficulties, reduced self-esteem, anxiety and depression. In such cases it is not always easy to distinguish cause from effect, particularly in desire phase disorders. A relatively high proportion of patients exhibit psychiatric symptoms and suffer psychiatric disorders requiring active drug therapy.[4] Judging the primary nature of presenting problems is crucial to the assessment process and will influence treatment strategies by defining prognosis rather than diagnosis.

Clinical presentation

Single men

For treatment purposes, single men with erectile difficulties fall into three broad categories:

- Those men who have never had a partner;
- Those men without a current partner; and
- Those men without a regular sexual partner but who have transient sexual encounters with one or more partners.

There are significant differences in how these groups of men define their sexual problems, their expectations of desired sexual performance and of the help they require to restore their functioning. Their problems can also include social skills deficits, fear of intimacy and commitment, excessive fear of sexual failure (equating it with failure as a human being), and a profound lack of self-belief. Clearly, all these concerns can also affect homosexual males, although less has been published about the incidence, prevalence and treatment of ED in gay men. Paff[7] reported an incidence of 50% of arousal phase disorders in a sample of 500 gay men, and an in-depth study of 22 gay men noted that 45% reported erectile difficulties that were likely to be secondary or situational in nature. The HIV and AIDS epidemic has affected the perceptions and behaviours of gay men, which can alter over time. It has also probably influenced erectile responsiveness both in terms of withdrawal or abstinence as well as indulging in high-risk behaviours. However, this review is limited to studies in heterosexual men.

Men with a regular partner

This is a complex and heterogeneous group, consisting of men who have a regular partner but who may or may not be married, monogamous, or in a stable or satisfactory relationship. Depending on whether the female partner is unaware or uninvolved in the help-seeking process, the treatment options may be very different.

The functioning of the couple unit can contribute significantly to the onset, maintenance and successful treatment of ED. Couples with strong committed relationships and reasonable communication skills have a higher chance of successful treatment outcome, as they are able to process issues of intimacy, trust, anger, control and lack of desire.

Couples who create and experience a lot of conflict in their relationship, whether that be loud or silent, will need to process those issues in couple therapy before attempting sexual reconciliation. The power struggles between such couples can ensure that treatment is sabotaged — whether the focus is predominantly psychosexual or a physical treatment.

■ EARLY SEX THERAPY INTERVENTIONS

Individual and couple therapy approaches for the treatment of erectile dysfunction have developed considerably since the early days of the behaviourists,[8] and Masters and Johnson[9] focused on desensitizing the individual or couple to increasingly sexual and erotic experiences while alleviating feelings of anxiety. Many sex therapists attempted to replicate the Masters and Johnson programme on different clinical populations, but the results were disappointing relative to expectations. Those practising in the field at the time attempted to tease out which variables were essential to the effectiveness of the treatment programme, and tinkered with the model, testing out possible essential elements, the timing of sessions, the mode of presentation, and the number and gender of therapists. Very few of these treatment variables seemed to relate to outcome, although trends were observed. The studies had small samples and methodological flaws, but nevertheless the information gathered suggested that, although there was a relatively high attrition and drop-out rate, if couples persisted with treatment there was a very reasonable chance of success.

With specific reference to the treatment of ED, it became clear that the misbehaving penis was only part of the problem. Attempts at reducing performance pressures by encouraging a man to relax and enjoy being massaged, to define what sexual pleasure consisted of to him and a partner, and to share the responsibility of giving and receiving sexual experiences, certainly helped many couples to regain their confidence and ability to enjoy sex. When the process worked it seemed like magic; however, it did not address the issues of those men who required a certain level of anxiety to become aroused, those who found their levels of anxiety heightened at the thought of the exercises, couples who just felt too awkward or those who found that the process exposed vulnerabilities in their relationships and made them feel less safe.

The therapeutic options available to the single male with sexual difficulties were limited, although a few groups were set up that enabled men to feel less alone, learn coping strategies, and obtain social skills training.[10] The only alternative was the use of a surrogate, which had its own set of complicated issues for both the patient and the clinician.[11]

■ COGNITIVE PROCESSES IN SEXUALITY

Although behavioural aspects of sensate focus and guided techniques to overcome performance fears remain in use,

in the last decade significant advances have been made in cognitive,[12] systemic[13] and medical areas, which are relevant to the understanding and treatment of sexual drive and erectile disorders. The cognitive approach to the treatment of anxiety and depression has received much attention and is now a well-established part of the management of these disorders. Psychological problems are conceptualized in terms of three interrelated, but largely independent systems — behavioural, cognitive and physiological. The focus of treatment is understanding the role of cognitions in interpreting, exaggerating, minimizing or misinterpreting the physiological changes that often accompany the emotional state in anxiety, and cognitions and affect in relation to depression.[14] The focus of treatment for depression is understanding the interplay of cognitions and affect on the depressive illness.

More recently, cognitive behavioural principles have been applied to sex therapy techniques, as part of this experimental process, but only after more analytic interpretations and counselling techniques had been explored.[15] In the light of the variability in outcome, both Bancroft[16] and Hawton[17] have described psychotherapeutic procedures and concepts to enable the individual or couple to overcome the blocks of the traditional behavioural sex therapy approach. The three-tier system approach, which has served other areas so well, is only beginning to be applied in a co-ordinated way to the area of sexual health and dysfunction. Data are now accumulating on the relationship between cognitive elements and sexual responsiveness in both functional men and men with erectile dysfunction.

The interplay between attentional and emotional variables

Current conceptualizations of sexual response emphasize the importance of attentional and emotional processing in a sexual situation. Within this framework, an individual's level of arousal is measured concurrently with the extent of *absorption* (the degree to which they attend to, and become immersed in, a sexual situation) and *subjective emotion* (whether the experience is associated with pleasant emotions). This information processing approach has been adopted by several researchers since the 1980s.

Functional vs dysfunctional subjects

In their clinical research, Beck and Barlow[18,19] measured erectile response to erotic stimuli when manipulating cognitive (awareness) or affective (feelings) states. They found that functional subjects responded differently from dysfunctional subjects on certain key variables, giving a different profile to the two groups. The results are summarized below, and suggest that an individual's response to sexual stimulation is mediated by attentional and emotional processing of the stimulation. Sexual dysfunction is therefore a consequence of a neutral or negative emotional reaction to erotic stimulation, which in turn becomes the focus of attention. Two distinct themes emerged from Barlow's work — distraction and the amplifying effect of arousal.

In functional subjects, sexual response was *enhanced* by either inducing states of anxiety, imposing 'performance' demands or increasing arousal in non-specific ways and then measuring penile response. Subjects correctly perceived their degree of sexual response or exaggerated it, and this response was clearly impaired by a deliberate non-erotic distraction. Barlow interpreted the negative effect of distraction as evidence of the importance of attention to sexual cues to elicit an erectile response in functional men. Any form of arousal will amplify the information being processed, and therefore if information cues are interpreted as sexual, then the sexual response will be enhanced. Equally so, if the attentional focus is on non-erotic or anti-erotic cues, such as a preoccupation with failure, then this effect will be exaggerated.

In the dysfunctional sample, sexual responses were *impaired* by the introduction of an anxiety state, imposing sexual 'performance' demands, or increasing arousal in non-specific ways. These subjects tended to underestimate the degree of their sexual responses, showing some negative cognitive distortion in the way they judged and perceived themselves. Non-erotic distraction did not affect their sexual responses negatively, and occasionally even assisted it. Barlow suggested that distractions are adopted by this group as a means of avoiding focusing on erotic cues, which are perceived to be threatening and heighten anxiety rather than producing sexual arousal, as in the case of functional subjects. It is possible that the experimental non-erotic distractions were less distracting than those adopted automatically in sexual situations, and so their sexual responses may have been slightly improved. Barlow's explanations have been valuable in leading sex therapists to focus on the cognitive processes involved in observing, interpreting and reacting to both sexual and non-sexual cues, which are also affected by current cultural and sub-cultural influences.

Dekker and Everaerd[20,21] also found that subjects' sexual arousal in response to erotic text, slides and sexual fantasy was greater if they attended to both the sexual situations presented (stimulus focus) *and* the sexual feelings associated with the events (the emotional focus), compared with attending only to the sexual stimulation. This finding was significant for both males and females.

The cognitive processes in sexual arousal are summarized in Figure 41.1.

Misattribution: effect on physical and emotional responses

Cranston-Cuebas and Barlow[12] examined the possibility of influencing sexual arousal by interfering with information processing. They gave a placebo tablet to both functional and dysfunctional groups of men, informing one group that it would increase their sexual response while looking at erotic stimuli, and another group that it would decrease their sexual response. Any sexual response was therefore, misattributed to the effect of the pill. The functional men responded in line with their understanding of the drug's action, the effect being noticeable in actual erectile responses, but not the subjective report of arousal. This finding in functional men was replicated by Janssen and Everaerd.[22] The dysfunctional group also showed decreases in physical responses when told the pill would have that effect, whereas their subjective reports of sexual arousal were unaffected; however, when told that the pill would have an enhancing effect, their responses were no different to

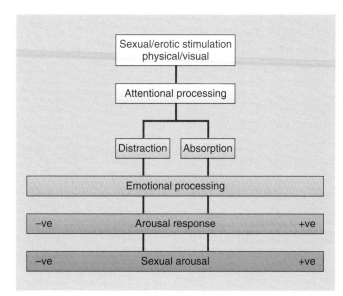

Figure 41.1. Cognitive processes in sexual arousal.

placebo, which was in marked contrast to the functional pill-enhancing group. This study demonstrated the clear effect of the misattribution procedure on the physiological erectile response, and the concurrent lack of effect on the subjective response or self-rating of sexual arousal.

In 1997, Koukounas and McGabe[23] conducted similar attentional studies, using an erotic film depicting vaginal sexual intercourse or oral sex combinations. They found that the degree to which subjects became absorbed in the erotic scenarios depicted was associated with their assessment that the material was entertaining and emotionally appealing and that subjects had previously engaged in sexual fantasy during masturbation or heterosexual intercourse. An interesting finding was that the men and women differed in their attentional and emotional processing of the erotica: females reported more disgust, but also higher levels of curiosity. Socialization and cultural factors do play a role in information processing of erotica, shown here by the fact that respondents were simultaneously angered and disgusted by the film, yet sexually aroused and curious to watch the material. The authors concluded that the magnitude of subjective sexual arousal was predicted largely by the separate groupings of state measures, both appetitive (absorption, pleasure, entertainment, curiosity) and aversive (anxiety, anger, disgust) rather than trait measures. This is contrary to the findings from Rosen and Beck's study,[24] where there was no identified gender difference in absorption and appetitive nature of the material presented.

Information processing: effect on a central inhibitory mechanism

Bancroft[25] presented an interesting explanation for the difference between the responses of the functional and non-functional men. He suggested that the altered expectation produced by the misattribution effect was associated in functional men with a reduction in the usual level of inhibitory tone. As this is an effect that one is unaware of, it therefore would not lead to any change in subjective states. In contrast, he suggests that dysfunctional men process the information differently, so that inhibitory tone is not reduced and may well be increased. Thus he is proposing that cognitive mechanisms can mediate a central inhibitory mechanism. A proportion of men with ED, of assumed psychological origin, fail to respond to an intracavernosal injection intended to relax the smooth muscle of the sinusoidal spaces of the corpus cavernosum. It is possible that some inhibitory mechanism, triggered cognitively, overrides or counteracts the effects of the injection.

Buvat and colleagues[26] suggested that the inhibition is a result of increased circulating levels of noradrenaline resulting from anxiety associated with the injection. It is the noradrenergic tone in the smooth muscle that is responsible for penile flaccidity, which is inhibited or switched off during REM sleep, allowing the erectile response to occur. In line with this notion, Kim and Oh[27] found significantly higher levels of noradrenaline in the penile blood of men who fail to respond to intracavernosal injection (ICI) than in that of responders. This suggests that some specific noradrenergic mechanism within the erectile tissue is involved; it does not, however, imply that these men are aware of feeling anxious.

These findings may shed some light on why some men are unable to respond during the sensate focus exercises in a standard sex therapy programme. This may be despite apparently ideal, private, sexual situations which they describe as exciting and stimulating, with their partner optimally enhancing their arousal. In theory, all pressure to perform is removed by the ban on specifically sexual activities, and subjects are in control of what stimulation they receive in a relaxed environment. However, for some men it is not at all a relaxing experience, and others become concerned that they cannot become aroused despite feeling relaxed. It is not unreasonable to assume that the emotional processing of physical, mental or visual stimulation as neutral, unappealing or negative, and the removal of obvious anxiety associated with sexual expectations, are not sufficient to release the inhibitory mechanisms.

Interplay between attentional and physical variables

Janssen and Everaerd[22] and Jansen[28] compared the erectile response in both functional and non-functional men, with two types of stimulation — vibration applied directly to the penis with and without accompanying erotic stimulation. With vibration alone, the dysfunctional men showed significantly less erectile response than the functional men, suggesting that the 'need to respond' produced an inhibitory response in the former group which overrode the effect of the physical stimulation, however pleasurable. However, this difference disappeared when the cognitive element was introduced, suggesting that viewing an erotic film allowed the dysfunctional men to alter the focus of their cognitions.

Several authors have acknowledged a need for concomitant physiological indices of sexual arousal to be measured in conjunction with measures of information processing of erotic stimulation. Over and Koukounas[29] identified an eye-blink startle reflex as a way of measuring the nature of emotional processing during erotic stimulation. This primary task was measured by the magnitude of the eye-blink startle response to an unexpected intense auditory stimulus (the secondary task probe) presented during stimulation. When the attention and the auditory probe matched in affective content, the eye-blink response increased; when they differed in emotional content, the eye-blink response decreased. With repeated erotic stimulation the subjects found the material boring and/or aversive, and more difficult to attend to, as indexed by a faster response to the secondary task presented during stimulation.

■ COGNITIVE–INTERPERSONAL TREATMENT MODEL FOR ERECTILE DYSFUNCTION

Males with long-standing erectile problems typically present with distorted cognitions about the nature of sexual arousal, sexual skills and their partner's feelings regarding the sexual experiences. These beliefs and expectations can lead to increased anxiety about sexual performance and to low self-regard; if prolonged, they can generalize to a negative self-worth and clinical depression and relationship breakdown. The psychological and interpersonal consequences of the problem can, therefore, be very serious.

The cognitive processes involved during sexual arousal are depicted in Figure 41.2, indicating typical pathways for men with and without sexual dysfunctions.

Partner-specific erectile dysfunction

If a man has situational ED in a long-term relationship, where the sexual scenario and the partner are very familiar, he may label this as predictable, safe and uninteresting, and so be easily distracted from the sexual process. If presented with new, unpredictable sexual cues, he may well interpret these as exciting and challenging. Thus, the two significant variables of attention and emotional interpretation are positive and reinforce each other, and he can become sexually aroused. This group of situationally dysfunctional men present with ED with their long-term partner, but are usually functional with masturbation and/or another partner.

However, if he is able to focus on sexual cues but interprets sexual advances as threatening, aversive, or unappetizing, he may feel anxious or angry, or not allow himself to feel anything at all, and so the arousal response is inhibited. It is important to discover how the attentional and accompanying emotional responses vary between different partners, as this gives the clinician significant information for future treatment suggestions.

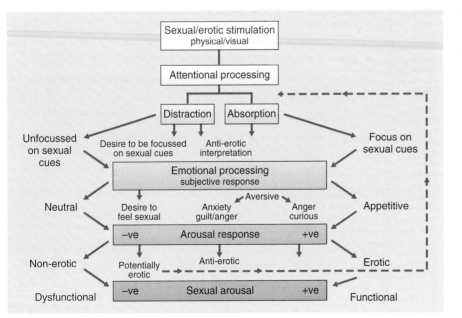

Figure 41.2. Cognitive processes of the dysfunctional and functional man during sexual arousal.

Situational erectile dysfunction

Many domestic, social and relationship situations can provoke ED, probably involving changes in the attentional and emotional labelling processes. Examples would include fear of commitment, anger, fertility issues, the short-term effect of alcohol and certain pharmacological agents, as well as illicit drugs. Such cases of ED are usually reversible when the cognitive processes and affect are re-aligned again after processing the other issues.

Treatment model for erectile dysfunction

Rosen and colleagues[30] developed a treatment model for ED, intended principally for use with heterosexual couples but adaptable to homosexual and bisexual men. The programme consisted of five basic components and was designed to be implemented in 12–16 weeks.

Psycho-educational and cognitive interventions

Distorted cognitive patterns are identified and the patient is taught to monitor and reconstruct dysfunctional cognitive errors. These typically include catastrophizing, overgeneralization, disqualifying the positive, mind-reading a partner's reactions, and predicting the future with regard to sexual behaviours.

Sexual and performance anxiety reduction

Sexual anxieties can be very broad, such as fear of intimacy, commitment or physical contact, or more focused onto specific fears of loss of erection or premature ejaculation.

Sexual script modification

This concerns the overt performing sexual script between the partners, and the ideal fantasized script of each individual partner. A sexual script has four dimensions — complexity, rigidity, conventionality and satisfaction. Couples experiencing ED typically present with restricted, repetitive, and inflexible sexual patterns or scripts, usually offering unreliable or minimal satisfaction. These difficulties can precede the onset of a specific dysfunction, or can develop as a consequence of it.

Conflict resolution and relationship enhancement

Dynamics of the relationship, including intimacy conflicts, power and control struggles and trust issues, need to be addressed in any psychological intervention for ED. The partner's emotional reaction over time to living with ED usually changes from being very supportive and encouraging, to feeling sexually undesired herself, losing her confidence, feeling frustrated and impotent that she cannot 'fix it', to becoming critical and demanding, or rejecting of sexual advances.

Relapse prevention

Previous research has shown a high rate of relapse or return of the sexual difficulties originally complained of. McCarthy[31] recommended strategies for prevention of relapse with addictive and compulsive behaviours and adapted specific strategies for the treatment of sexual disorders, as follows:

- The scheduling of regular non-demand pleasuring sessions, along the lines of Masters and Johnson[9] sensate focus exercises, in order to maintain intimacy and flexibility in the relationship.
- Regular communication and information gathering so that actual sexual experiences can be tailored to realistic expectations regarding sexual performance and satisfaction.
- Couple communication to address issues of trust, intimacy, control, dominance, and management of conflict or difference.
- Encouraging a wider range of intimate, sensual and erotic experiences between a couple, which encourages spontaneity, flexibility, and an element of unpredictability (a wider sexual script).
- Partner cognitive feedback exercises to encourage sexual self-esteem, confidence as a lover, resisting cognitive distortions.
- The development of techniques to manage absent, negative, mediocre or disappointing sexual experiences.
- Arranging short- and long-term follow-up appointments with the therapist, so that patients do not feel abandoned at termination of treatment, and defined times are provided when it is legitimate to solve any ongoing difficulties, without making the patient feel a failure.
- Problems should be labelled as 'lapses' to be learned from, and not as 'relapses' to be feared.

THE LARGER PICTURE: THE INTER- AND INTRAPERSONAL CONTEXT OF SEXUAL FUNCTIONING

Understanding sexual functioning in terms of the cognitive and arousal circuits presented is a critical part of the assessment. However, the larger picture must also be viewed — that is, the intrapersonal and interpersonal sexual contexts in which sexual functioning or dysfunctioning occur. Althof[32] provides an extremely useful model of sexuality, enabling us to view sexual desire, arousal, orgasm and satisfaction in the broader context of gender identity, object choice and sexual intention. This provides a complete context of functioning of the individual, which can then be interpreted alongside a similar framework for his partner (Fig. 41.3).

Gender identity

Gender identity is the person's subjective sense of himself or herself as male or female. It is possible that primary erectile failure, or paraphilic behaviours, indicate a mismatch between what someone feels and how they are labelled by others in terms of their gender identity. These may be relatively rare clinical presentations, but the clinician has to consider the effect on the patient and his partner of facilitating a 'cure'. An intracavernosal injection may well provide the erection, but may contribute significantly to the inner conflicts that can only be explored in psychotherapy. Sometimes the answer may well be not to intervene, or certainly not too enthusiastically.

Object choice

Object choice describes the source of the person or object to which one is attracted, and with whom or which one engages in sexual behaviour. The concept includes attractions to inanimate objects as well as animate ones, exclusively heterosexual through to exclusively homosexual. Many people are aware of their sexual urges, desires and needs, but if they feel that the source of this is inappropriate or unacceptable, they deliberately choose

an object of desire that they believe others will find acceptable. For example, a male who has homosexual desires but aligns himself with a suitable female sexual partner is likely to feel trapped. He has placed himself in a position of having to perform sexually, where the conditions for desire and arousal are constrained. For some males the perhaps more honest route cannot be tolerated. They marry, have children and attempt to rationalize the conflict by being seen to be heterosexual or 'ordinary'. This does not necessarily offer resolution in sexual terms. This is not the case for a bisexual male who feels sexually comfortable in either sexual environment.

It is essential to ask every male patient the varied sources of his intellectual, physical, emotional and fantasy attractions, and to what extent these are met by the partner or object of choice. If an incompatibility is clear, then the clinician is ill-advised to offer quick solutions to erectile difficulties without once again understanding the implications and likely repercussions of such interventions, both in the short and long term.

Sexual intention

Sexual intention is simply an awareness of what one wants to do at a behavioural level, to satisfy one's sexual desires or impulses. Gender differences can be very apparent here. Women frequently state they want affection, warmth and intimacy, and this provides the context to allow themselves to become sexually active and responsive. Many men perceive this as a phase of lovemaking they have to go through to achieve their sexual intentions. Male sexual behaviour often involves some form of assertion, domination or aggression to oneself or to one's partner. Men who predominantly rely on these forces for arousal may experience sexual difficulties if these needs are not met; many women are unwilling to partake in fear-provoking behaviours.

The therapist needs to ask whether the partners understand each other's sexual intentions. Is it penetrative sex? What is the function of the erection in the context of known intentions, both in the short and long term? Experience in clinical practice suggests that males and females do not necessarily have the same sexual intentions. Any differences need to be aired before embarking on a sex therapy programme, or any other form of treatment.

In the consulting room, these three aspects of sexuality may not seem of critical importance relative to the presenting flaccid or semi-flaccid penis, but understanding their contribution to the problem may

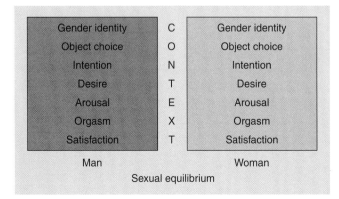

	Man			Woman	
	Gender identity	C		Gender identity	
	Object choice	O		Object choice	
	Intention	N		Intention	
	Desire	T		Desire	
	Arousal	E		Arousal	
	Orgasm	X		Orgasm	
	Satisfaction	T		Satisfaction	

Sexual equilibrium

Figure 41.3. Sexual equilibrium: a model for understanding the context of sexual functioning. (From ref. 32 with permission.)

make the difference between restored satisfactory sexual functioning and dissatisfaction with treatment. Hawton[4] has developed a very useful system, which examines three sets of factors that contribute to the onset and continuation of the problem — factors that predispose, precipitate and maintain the sexual problem in the individual. The causes of origin, if known, are not always the ones maintaining the problem in its current form, and this may become obvious as treatment progresses and resistances begin to develop. A typical example is when the male begins to regain confidence about his erectile responses, and the partner becomes less tolerant of the difficulties and expresses her anger. He immediately retreats and is afraid to attempt less than successful sexual encounters, and so the couple have retrieved homoeostasis in their relationship. At some level the improvement has proved to be intolerable. Change in one partner has repercussions for the couple and alters the context in which the partner functions, sexually and otherwise. Although enhanced erectile functioning may appear positive to the clinician, and be the identified target area for change, tolerating change is not easy for some couples and can threaten the relationship.

THE SEXUAL CIRCUIT

A very useful six-phase model, informally known as the Sexual Circuit,[33] assists thinking about the relationship between sexual drive (sexual appetite), sexual desire (the notion of having sex with someone specific) and sexual arousal (physiological and cognitive responses to sexual excitement), sexual response (orgasm), resolution (the body reverting back to baseline measures) and sexual satisfaction. Looking at the circuit (Fig. 41.4), the area of specific initial interest when assessing ED is the triangle connecting sexual drive to sexual desire, manifested by a specific sexual or sensual behaviour or communication, which in turn feeds the sexual arousal part of the circuit, both from a physiological (vasocongestion) and cognitive (awareness of sexual excitement) perspective. Evidence of arousal in turn feeds the awareness of being sexual driven, and so the circuit reinforces itself if the appropriate responses are secured. The sexually functional male has thoughts about penetration fairly early on in the arousal process, can rely on obtaining and maintaining his erection and usually, once intercourse has been achieved, ejaculates, has a sense of sexual satisfaction and the arousal–response circuit has been completed.

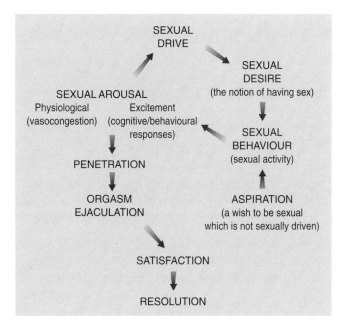

Figure 41.4. The sexual arousal circuit. (From ref. 33 with permission.)

For the man with ED, understanding the current characteristics of each process and the clear differences between them is essential. For some people there is an aspiration at a cognitive level that they want or need to be engaged in a sexual activity, but it is definitely not sexually driven. This is a fairly common experience for men who have an identifiable hormonal deficiency or medical problem which results in impaired sexual functioning (e.g. prostatectomy), but also can exist in non-organic cases. An example would be men who are involved directly or indirectly in infertility treatment and are required to perform sexually according to the calendar, and lose all sexual desire. It is also reported by men who are enjoying regular sex outside the marriage and feel duty bound to have sexual intercourse within the marriage, but feel no particular desire to do so. The sexual drive of the majority of men with ED with no identifiable organic aetiology remains intact. They do experience the desire to be sexual, but the circuit breaks, often at the commencement of sexual activity, or specifically at the thought of penetration. It is important to crystallize the exact point of anticipated failure, and to assess whether this is predominantly associated with erectile or ejaculatory difficulties. The perspective of the partner is critical in the understanding of the problem as *she* experiences it, her comprehension of what it feels like for her partner, and what both their expectations of sex are.

■ TREATMENT OPTIONS AND THE AROUSAL CIRCUIT

The circuit also allows us to see where psychosexual and medical interventions have their impact on the system (Fig. 41.5).

Non-medical treatment options

What are the current non-medical treatment options available to the therapist? Clearly, this depends on a patient's profile, and to some extent that of their partner. Some patients require minimal help in the form of information and sex education, but respond to a large dose of permission and encouragement. Most therapists operate on the basis of offering psychotherapeutic assistance, in conjunction with — if not followed by — more invasive physical procedures.

The job of the therapist is to outline all the options and, if there is a medical or psychological recommendation, to state the reasoning behind it. Some patients will request a specific treatment and the therapist has to be clear about her/his own boundaries when challenged. All approaches can be contra-indicated in certain circumstances, even psychological ones. The traditional Masters and Johnson approach has its limitations and only the experienced therapist will know the likelihood of certain recommendations being helpful or effective. The typical regime accepted by most couples is to start with the varied psychological approaches, focusing on sexual and relationship issues, and, if necessary, to add more physically invasive treatments.

Vacuum constriction devices

Vacuum constriction devices provide a mechanical, reversible and simple means of inducing an erection. The data suggest that, for those who persist with this form of treatment, there is a high degree of patient and partner satisfaction.[34] These devices are generally well tolerated and can be used with a variety of neurogenic, vasculogenic and psychogenic problems. Female partners

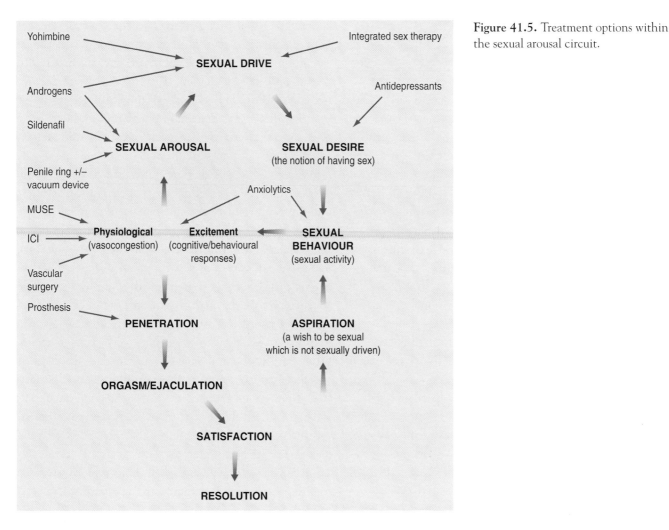

Figure 41.5. Treatment options within the sexual arousal circuit.

tend to favour the least-invasive forms of treatment and generally prefer a vacuum device to drug treatments. The initial expense is justified if the device is used regularly. However, early drop-out rates are relatively high, owing to problems such as desensitization of the glans, decrease in orgasmic quality, pain with the constriction ring, lack of spontaneity, a colder penis and ejaculatory discomfort, but problems are less likely to occur if used with devices that have a vacuum-limiter.

The device may be an unrealistic option for single men without a familiar and supportive partner, who cannot conceive of using such an intrusive and unwieldy method of producing an erection. However, for men who can obtain but not maintain an erection, the rings on their own have been used successfully. Their presence can be explained in terms of keeping a condom in place.

Medication

Oral medication is readily accepted by the majority of men, can be kept secret, and is effectively marketed as a treatment for sexual difficulties. It is often used in conjunction with therapy, or as a second-line treatment approach.

Testosterone

Male patients frequently request oral medication, usually testosterone, with the belief that it is completely safe. Female partners are far less enthusiastic about drug treatments for their partners. There are conclusive studies showing a correlation between testosterone withdrawal and a decline in sexual interest, which is dose related and reversible.[35] The relationship between androgens and ED is clear in hypogonadal men who display improved nocturnal and waking erections. Decreased serum levels of testosterone do not necessarily predict good outcome of testosterone treatment for ED. The purpose of the study by Rakic and colleagues[36] was to determine which men with ED and decreased serum levels might benefit from treatment. They found that good treatment outcome was associated with several variables but only high levels of luteinizing hormone (LH) and low values of the T/LH (testosterone/LH) ratio consistently emerged as significant correlates for predictors of effective treatment. Bancroft and Wu[37] found that erections in response to erotic fantasy were not androgen dependent. Schiavi and colleagues[38] conducted a double-blind, placebo-controlled, crossover study to assess the effect of testosterone administration on sexual behaviour, mood and psychological symptoms in healthy men with ED. They found that the androgen regimen had no effect on any of the mood or psychological symptoms measured, nor was there any improvement of erectile rigidity; the increase in sexual activity reflected a higher sexual drive and more frequent sexual play rather than enhanced erectile function.

Yohimbine

For over 70 years, yohimbine has been assumed to have aphrodisiac properties,[39] and animal studies have revealed positive effects on sexual arousal and motivation. In man, however, the results are very mixed. It is usually administered on a daily basis for 4–10 weeks, 5.4 mg t.d.s., and is generally well tolerated. Although some authors state there is a delay in therapeutic effect of a few weeks after drug commencement,[40] clinical experience suggests that some men respond beneficially if the drug is taken an hour before anticipated intercourse. Rowland and colleagues[1] conducted a double-blind, placebo-controlled crossover study, using 30 mg yohimbine daily, on a group of men with ED and a sexually functional group. The results indicated no effect on most aspects of sexual response measured in the functional men. More mixed effects were reported in the dysfunctional group, but the increases in sexual arousal and masturbation did not translate to sexual intercourse, and the authors concluded that a positive effect with yohimbine was more probable in the absence of the sexual partner. Mann and colleagues[41] conducted a similar study and global assessment revealed, beyond placebo effect in both organic and non-organic patients, therapeutic effect (at 15 mg daily) in the subgroup of non-organic patients. There was a significantly greater improvement in the yohimbine group compared with the placebo group, but no such effect was found in the organic group. All the findings were on a subjective level and had no correlate in nocturnal penile tumescence and rigidity (NPTR) recordings, suggesting that yohimbine primarily stimulates those neural pathways subserving erotically induced erections. This agent was not effective in the management of patients with mixed vasculogenic ED.[42] In a UK trial involving men with mixed aetiology, 37% reported good stimulated erections after 8 weeks on yohimbine, compared with only 13% on placebo.[43] When placebo was replaced by the active drug, this percentage increased to 42%, but there was no effect on morning erections, ejaculation, sexual interest or sexual thoughts.

The findings of these studies suggest that the therapeutic effect of yohimbine is unreliable. Nevertheless, the drug is probably worth considering as a proportion of patients report a definite subjective improvement, and this may well facilitate enhanced erectile functioning without further assessment or medical treatments.

Sildenafil

Sildenafil, and similar oral compounds which will inevitably become available, will have popular appeal and good compliance will enhance its therapeutic effectiveness.[44] Other modes of delivery, such as the injections, are less acceptable but will be persisted with if the result compensates for the procedure, or alternatives prove to be less effective for the individual. There is no doubt that the management of ED will be significantly altered by the introduction of these new oral medications, but the issue of partner desire remains to be addressed. A women who knows her partner has to take a pill to be able to have penetrative sex with her is likely to feel fundamentally undesired sexually, and that may have consequences for her self-esteem, her sexual responsiveness and the relationship. Such issues need to be identified and processed in assessment, treatment and follow-up phases. This requires a willingness and ability to focus on cognitive and relationship functioning, and understand the potential impact of successful treatment of ED on the partner and the couple.

Intracavernosal injection therapy (ICI)

Major developments have occurred in the last few years, not only in terms of the range and type of drugs but also in the loading and the delivery systems. Injection programmes have been devised with educational videos and brochures to enable patients to become more comfortable with self-injection. Its utility with men with irreversible ED is proven, but problems frequently remain as a result of inadequate training, lack of confidence in self-administration and misconception about the drug. It is important that patients and partners understand that intracavernosal administration of vasoactive drugs produces an erection, but does not induce sexual drive, desire or arousal, unless these were inhibited solely because of the erectile dysfunction. The case for ICI with predominantly psychogenic ED is more confused. Men want a 'quick fix' answer, but the treatment is not without risk, and research shows that injection therapy is accepted by only 40–50% of men referred for this treatment.[45] In

Wylie's study,[46] ICI therapy had a higher initial take-up rate than a vacuum device, but also a higher 6- and 12-month drop-out rate. These preference rates may well reflect the presentation of specific treatments available to patients at specific clinics, or the type of patient seen within a clinic, for example diabetic patients. The cost of ICI is considerable but if the procedure is well tolerated, a major advantage is that it is less visibly intrusive than the vacuum device and rings. This is particularly attractive to single men. There is no doubt that in selected cases it combines well with sex therapy interventions in the short term, enabling the man to bypass certain blocks, and he remains functional upon slow withdrawal of the injection therapy.[47]

Transurethral alprostadil (MUSE: Medicated Urethral System for Erection)

Early clinical trials suggest that transurethral alprostadil is effective, producing erections lasting 30–60 minutes,[48] with a low risk of priapism or fibrosis. Some patients may be reluctant to accept the treatment because the insertion of an applicator in the urethra is associated with pain and treatment of infectious sexual diseases, and the most common side effects so far reported include burning sensation in the urethra; aching in the penis, testicles, legs and perineum; and minor urethral bleeding or spotting due to improper administration. However, for some men it will be more appealing than a penile injection but its use will be compromised in the context of oral preparations.

Surgery

In some cases there is no alternative to surgical treatments for ED. These treatments fall into two broad categories. The first is surgical correction of certain potentially reversible conditions (Peyronie's disease, arterial insufficiency) and the procedures are generally associated with a high success rate. Surgery for 'venous leakage' is more controversial, particularly in the longer term. The second category is prosthetic implantation for irreversible ED. On the basis of their own follow-up study of 406 patients, Melman and colleagues[49] and Tiefer and colleagues[50] concluded that there were no significant differences in satisfaction levels between the different types of implant, and that the device can be as relevant to a patient's self-esteem as to his sexual functioning. There is clearly a role for counselling couples prior to surgery, in particular assessing the risks of mechanical failure, the possibility of postsurgical infection, changes in the size of the penis, and addressing the questions and concerns the partner may have as she has rarely been included in any of the investigations and discussions. Most men who have surgery are relieved to have been diagnosed with an identifiable organic problem, and believe that a medical procedure will offer a cure. Even though they have been told about risk factors, they may only be able to see a positive outcome, see no other acceptable alternative, and are bitterly disappointed and angry when their sex life does not match up to their expectations. This may be particularly true if there has been a history of sexual avoidance, sexual problems in the partner, poor communication, or relationship difficulties. Men do tend to blame many of their difficulties on their sexual failure, and when this has been corrected and sexual intimacy does not return, both parties feel resentful. The careful selection and preparation of patients and an awareness and willingness to confront the complex psychological and interpersonal impact of these procedures will assist most couples in resuming a satisfactory sexual life, which they would otherwise be denied.

Deciding what is the optimal treatment for a man presenting with ED is a balancing act between the actual and perceived invasiveness of the treatment, whether it will be well tolerated physically, psychologically and emotionally, is reasonably cost-effective, relatively discreet, allows an element of sexual spontaneity, does not shame the participants and facilities satisfactory, if not pleasurable, sexual intercourse.

■ FACTORS ASSOCIATED WITH OUTCOME

Jarow and colleagues[51] reviewed the outcome of treatment in 377 impotent men, both at the start and end of treatment; in 90% of cases, patients initially chose the less-invasive forms of therapy. As an example, almost 80% of the men chose an oral medication initially but the ultimate satisfaction rating was only 28%. In contrast, less than 2% of men initially selected surgery, but this treated group had a satisfaction rate of 94%, the highest of all therapies.

Sexual satisfaction is a complex notion, comprising both physiological and emotional constructs. The biological act is complete once resolution has been achieved and the body has regained its equilibrium. However, for many men their sense of satisfaction is entwined with how they perceive their partner's enjoyment, and particularly her orgasmic responsiveness. Haavio-Mannila and Kontula[52] conducted a survey looking at correlates of increased sexual satisfaction. They found that many social factors are connected to sexual satisfaction, and there are gender differences in these predictors. The importance of sexuality in life, love and the use of sexual materials are directly connected to sexual satisfaction in men, but only indirectly in women. Young women who are sexually assertive, use many sexual techniques, frequently engage in sexual intercourse and often achieve orgasm in intercourse are sexually as satisfied as men with similar characteristics. They concluded that sexual dissatisfaction in women is, at least to some extent, due to their late start of sexual life, conservative sexual attitudes, low importance of sexuality in life, lack of sexual assertiveness and not using versatile sexual techniques.

In the field of sex therapy, several key issues have become associated with positive outcome, although the number of adequately controlled outcome studies in the field is small. Assessment of outcome is problematic, as definitions of the diagnostic and outcome criteria, assessment measures, treatment techniques and follow-up evaluations have been so varied and unsystematic. Attempts to identify prognostic variables have been limited to retrospective case-note studies or a by-product of treatment outcome studies examining different variables in treatment approaches.[53] Follow-up studies suggest that approximately two-thirds of couples derive and maintain significant benefits in the initial months following sex therapy,[54,55] but there has been limited review of outcome over a longer period. Hawton and Catalan[56] attempted systematically to identify prognostic factors, as the success rates achieved by the behavioural sex therapists adopting the Masters and Johnson approach were not replicable or sustainable.

Reviewing the outcome of therapy specifically for ED, Masters and Johnson[9] reported only 26% of cases of secondary ED as treatment failures after therapy, with a relapse rate of 11% five years later. De Amicis[57] noted that over a 3 year follow-up period, increased overall satisfaction was maintained and significant improvements in maintaining erections during intercourse were reported, but not in obtaining them prior to intercourse. LoPiccolo and colleagues[58] also reported greater gains in the area of enhanced satisfaction rather than symptom remission. Hawton and colleagues[59] reported a positive treatment outcome in 70% of couples attending for sex therapy for ED. Positive outcome was associated with good pre-treatment communication and general sexual adjustment, early completion of homework assignments and, in the female partner, an interest in and enjoyment of sex and an absent positive psychiatric history. Another study in the UK to look at prognostic factors prospectively in men presenting with psychogenic ED has recently been completed by Wylie.[46] The men were offered brief modified modern sex therapy with additional behavioural–systems couple therapy if required. The only factor found to predict outcome was a history of psychiatric illness in the male, which was predictive of a poor outcome. Factors found to predict drop-out were poor marital inventory scores for both males and females.

A basic dilemma frequently facing therapists is whether couple conflicts need to be addressed in couple therapy as a prior or adjunctive treatment to tackling specific sexual tensions and dysfunctions. Sex therapy is unlikely to be successful if the following issues are not dealt with in the therapeutic process:

- The couple are unable to offer an unequivocal commitment to each other;
- The degree of marital conflict is high and persistent;
- There is a current and active extramarital relationship;
- There is a serious and unstable medical and/or psychiatric illness;
- There are external pressures or life events influencing the sexual relationship (e.g. infertility treatments).

Several key factors appear consistently to be affected by therapeutic interventions and are worthy of independent comment across the studies. These include relationship factors, mode of patient presentation at the clinic, psychiatric illness, and gender and ethnicity issues.

Relationship conflict

The role that sexual dysfunction plays in the maintenance of homeostasis in the general relationship has been described by LoPiccolo[60] and the systemic marital therapists, described more fully in the previous chapter. Leiblum and Rosen[61] identified four problem areas of a couple's relationship that are frequently implicated in the development and/or maintenance of erectile dysfunction. They observed that any of the four can be involved in a given case, regardless of the presence of other organic or psychological factors. The four topics are (1) status and dominance issues, (2) intimacy and trust, (3) sexual attraction and desire, and (4) sexual scripts, which refers to both the organization of sexual activity and the circumstances under which it occurs.

Speckens and colleagues[62] investigated the female partners of men with both organic and no identified organic cause for ED. They found relationship problems and pre-existing psychosexual dysfunctions of vaginismus and dyspareunia, and reported that higher levels of sexual interest were more common in the partners of men with non-organic ED. These three factors may well contribute to the onset, exacerbation and maintenance of ED in this group and could imply that they are predisposing factors in the development of ED, as well as appearing to be important prognostic factors regarding sex therapy.

In the study by Hawton et al,[60] mentioned above, one variable associated with good treatment response was a female partner who showed an interest in and enjoyment of sex and a commitment to carry out the homework assignments. In Wylie's study,[46] relationship factors were found to predict drop-out from therapy if the male reported poor adjustment on the Golombok Rust Inventory of Marital State (GRIMS scale 1988).[63] This suggests that males have little investment in persisting with therapy while their relationship is perceived to be unstable. Drop-out was also associated when the female reported good adjustment, which suggests that her perceived need for attending therapy is lessened if she places less emphasis on the importance of sexual activity and more on the general relationship.

RELATE, the national organisation for relationship counselling, is also the most consistent provider of traditional sex therapy in the UK, adopting psycho-therapeutic and behavioural interventions. McCarthy and Thoburn[64] reported on 3693 cases entered on a national database between the years 1992 and 1994. This information is compared with an analysis conducted by Crowhurst in 1981,[65] revealing a change in the pattern of male sexual problems. In this earlier report, premature ejaculation was the most commonly diagnosed complaint, presenting in 30% of males. The most common difficulty presenting 15 years later is erectile failure — secondary ED (25%), primary ED (2%), premature ejaculation (19%) and male inhibited sexual desire (7%). Unpublished figures for 1998 see the pattern changing yet again: from 1818 cases they are secondary ED (38%), primary ED (3%), premature ejaculation (29%) and male inhibited sexual desire (19%).

The assessment procedure at RELATE is a staged one with an initial assessment, followed by history-taking interviews and a final round-table interview where, if psychosexual therapy is indicated, the contract is formulated; 53% of the couples did not progress to this final assessment stage, showing what a highly selected group of clients RELATE counsels. Of those who started sex therapy, 62% completed the programme, with a mean of 11 sessions. The principal reason stated by therapists for drop-out from therapy was relationship problems or lack of commitment to the relationship. In terms of outcome, 53% of men and 73% of women reported increased sexual satisfaction. With reference to the 365 men with ED, 33% reported no change, 2% had deteriorated, and positive changes were recorded by 65%. These were graded in four bands of improvement, 54% in the lower two bands, and 11% in the upper bands. What is apparent from RELATE's current data is that, despite the wide-ranging nature and complexities of the cases presenting to therapists and the defined, non-medical approach of counsellors, 62% of accepted clients for sex therapy complete therapy. An important variable affecting selection for and potential outcome of treatment is whether the complaint is viewed by the patient(s), referrer and/or therapist as residing in the individual or the couple. Partners who view themselves as asymptomatic may not wish to be involved in the therapeutic process and frequently present in treatment only after the relationship has broken down.

Relationship problems may pass unrecognized by professionals concerned about biological or other individual factors. Rust and colleagues[66] found that 30% of a random sample of patients attending their general practitioner (GP) or physician for non-sexual problems had significant marital difficulties that had not been detected.

Psychiatric illness

Concurrent psychiatric illness or personality disorder in the presenting patient or partner tends to affect sex clinic treatment outcome,[67] although the evidence is conflicting. Hawton and colleagues[59] reported a positive outcome in couples attending sex therapy for ED with the absence of a positive psychiatric history in the female partner. In his study, a history of psychiatric illness in the female was related to non-completion of therapy. Wylie,[46] found that the only factor to predict poor outcome of brief couple therapy in psychogenic ED was a history of psychiatric illness in the male, and suggests that individual therapy is more suited to such patients.

Understanding the organic, psychological and emotional effects of psychiatric illness, perhaps particularly depression in the context of sexual dysfunctions, is extremely complex. Both the patient and the partner are affected by living with the illness itself and, in terms of sexuality, the illness affects both sexual drive and sexual arousal, which impacts on both parties. The side-effects of psychotropic medication on sexual functioning are well documented,[68] and restoring erectile functioning in this context needs great care to maintain balance in the system.

Mode of clinic attendance: individual or couple

Sexual relationships are inherently interpersonal and it is not unreasonable to assume that couples attending treatment together have a better chance of addressing the erectile problem in the context of the relationship, as well as other contributing factors affecting either partner, than if the individual is treated alone. However, it is also a clinical reality that many men with sexual difficulties prefer to seek help in a medical setting and present on their own for what they see as their individual problem. Hirst and Watson[69] conducted a retrospective case-note study on 830 cases of attenders at a sex and relationship clinic in Central London. Completed data sets on 189 subjects were examined to explore the extent to which outcome was related to the mode of clinic attendance — as an individual without a partner, or as an individual with a partner who did (or did not) also attend the clinic. ED was the commonest problem (49% of the 189 cases), although there was twice the incidence among patients attending alone — whether they currently had a partner (49%) or not (41%) — compared with those patients who attended with their partners (23%).

Of the 55 single patients who attended the clinic alone, just over 17% described themselves as of homosexual orientation; they were more likely to be younger, never married and childless. They were the largest group (26%) to be offered intracavernosal injection, compared with the 18% of men with non-attending partners, and 5% with attending partners.

The 82 patients with partners who attended alone, tended to be older and more likely to be having multiple relationships or in their second or third marriages. Half of this group were born outside the UK and, for nearly 25%, English was not their first language. Thus, cultural and religious expectations and pressures originating outside the UK were potentially relevant in this group. The most common problem was again ED, but was assessed as being of predominantly psychological origin in 68% of cases. This group has the worst outcome of all, with a high rate of premature termination of therapy. Other authors have suggested that treatment drop-out may be predicted by relationship instability and heightened conflict. However, the problems of both these groups of single presenters were more likely to be rated by the assessment team as of largely or completely organic aetiology than the problems of those attending as a couple.

Of the 38 couples who attended together, the dysfunction most commonly presenting was female low sexual desire (28%), followed by ED (23%). The attrition rate was much lower in this group, 77% not missing a single appointment in a daytime clinic, compared with 47% of solo attenders.

Hirst and Watson[69] concluded that 'the most significant predictor of good outcome was the mode of attendance, being found in 90% of patients without a relationship, 84% of patients with attending partners, but only 51% of patients whose partners did not attend' (p. 329). Within this latter group, outcome was improved if the problem aetiology was putatively organic (85%) compared with a mixed aetiology (47%) and if there was no significant relationship conflict identified, and the partner at home was supportive.

These findings point to the appropriateness of seeing and treating individuals without partners for sexual and relationship problems, acknowledging that they are more likely to be offered, and accept, pharmacological treatments. The expectation is that the success rate will improve as the mode of delivery systems of the drugs becomes more acceptable. However, improved sexual performance or symptom reversal does not constitute treatment success in the longer term if the intention is to enhance sexual and relationship functioning. The relationship context is all-important, and clinicians should attempt to gauge the viability of any existing relationships. Valuable resources are wasted if patients do not continue attending the clinic, of if interventions are used that have been identified as improving sexual responses in the clinical environment but that are not useful in their daily lives.

Ethnicity and gender issues

Cultural and religious factors affect patterns of seeking help, clinical methods and treatment outcome. Ethnic differences between therapists and patients are suggestive of higher drop-out rates,[70] although no consistent preferences are expressed for therapist colour. Bhui and colleagues[71] found 60% of British patients had a single attendance only at a psychosexual clinic, compared with 75% for a matched Asian group. Many factors may have contributed to this, but clearly language is a significant variable in assessment and treatment. In a retrospective case-note study of 189 completed cases of attenders at a psychosexual clinic, 41% were diagnosed with ED.[69] 'While 84% had a good outcome, a significant predictor of bad outcome was the minority ethnic status of the partner of the presenting patient; 33% and 94% of ethnic minority and white couples respectively had a good outcome' (p. 334). Hirst and Watson[69] state that these findings were unexpected and may be an artefact of the data of a relatively small sample group.

Men

Men prefer to understand their problems in terms of physical disorder and initially are more likely to seek medical help, anticipating a physical solution. The physician they encounter is likely to be male, particularly in the urology setting. Clinical evidence suggests that men find it more comfortable to talk to female clinicians about the emotional and psychological impact of living with erectile difficulties on themselves, current and potential partners. Harley[72] suggests that white and black male and female patients would all prefer to see female, rather than male, therapists.

When male patients are asked about their expectations, they commonly declare that they require a sizeable, hard penis that will function automatically and reliably. Zilbergeld's fantasy model of sex describes a model of Western societal sexuality which became the blueprint for men and women, believing that, 'the penis is two feet long, is as hard as steel and can go on all night' (p. 30).[73] The media, in all its forms, feed this message, particularly when portraying sexuality. There are not many small or micro-penises in X-rated films, pornographic materials or fashionable current publications. Female editors are equally responsible for feeding the mythology to the female populations they target in their magazines. In the same way, female breasts are usually large, round and full (but not with milk), if they are to be seen as erotic. The male quest is therefore for penile rigidity and men will consider any treatment which will facilitate this response.

Although most men are unaware of it, the sexual model that they have been indoctrinated into and accepted forces them to play against a stacked deck. Everything — pleasing their partners, success and failure, self esteem and respect, their very identity as men — hinges on the performance of an organ that they cannot directly control and that is adversely affected by a large number of physical and emotional factors. (Zilbergeld,[73] p. 34)

Women

Women, on the other hand, are less concerned about rigidity but demand intimacy. A non-erect or semi-erect penis is interpreted initially as a sign that the woman's partner does not find her attractive or exciting enough, that he does not love her, or that she does not have the skill to 'turn him on' and therefore the woman assumes that she is partially, if not fully, responsible for the lack of response. Men find this difficult to accept, as they too feel responsible for the absent or partial erection. If no acceptable explanation can be found, the woman will tease out other theories, questioning whether there is anything else wrong in the physical or general relationship, if her partner is having sex elsewhere, is in another relationship, or if he is bisexual or gay.

Whatever the specific interpretation, she is not going to feel good about herself. And this in turn will cause her to exert pressure on him at some stage — overt or covert, subtle or blatant — to get hard. Women do not need an erection to experience orgasm and sexual satisfaction, so the problem is not the physical need for an erection, but the emotional meaning of its presence or absence.

Women are used to seeking help for matters related to sex, fertility and procreation, and are far less reluctant to talk about sexual difficulties in themselves or their partners. They are therefore more likely to seek advice from a therapist or gynaecologist, who may well be female. When eliciting their expectations, they report that they want to be able to have sex for the intimacy and closeness it brings, as well as the sexual pleasure. For many women there is not a direct connection between arousal and orgasm, and frequently their only orgasmic release is through masturbation or oral stimulation, when an erection is superfluous. The erection is related to a feeling of sexual empowerment, that she has some influence over her partner's arousal and response. For some women, in certain sexual positions, the sensation of the erect penis intravaginally can trigger heightened sensations, possibly leading to orgasm, if the stimulation is sustained. The balancing of all these variables is a delicate one, timing often being the deciding factor.

A favourable outcome is more likely if there is a previous history of unproblematic sexual functioning and pleasure derived from sexual experiences. Hawton and colleagues[59] found that a positive outcome was particularly associated with the female partner's interest in and enjoyment of sex, and a willingness of the couple to engage in sex therapy homework assignments. The shorter the problem has been tolerated, the less fixed are perceptions of poor self-esteem and motivations can be mobilized more readily. The mutual attraction of partners is helpful in this process. If there is an ongoing relationship, effective communication facilitates and speeds up the therapeutic process of understanding both partners' sexual agendas and enabling them to ask for, and therefore increase the likelihood of getting, what they want from the relationship. The prognostic significance of a good general relationship has been identified in several studies.[59,74] If couples engage in three or more therapy sessions, the outcome is likely to be favourable with regard to symptom reversal and increased sexual satisfaction.[75] Factors that suggest that a couple are unsuitable for standard sex therapy are a poor relationship, poor motivation, current severe psychiatric illness, a current affair engaged in by either partner, and pregnancy. Not to be underestimated is the nature of the therapeutic relationship, which can facilitate a more positive outcome, particularly as difficulties in the treatment are experienced.

■ SUMMARY

Increasing numbers of men are seeking help for ED, with expectations that a 'cure' is available, owing to the high media profile given to this particular sexual problem. Current trends in the medical arena indicate 'more clinical trials and approvals for new medications, development of less invasive treatments, increasing interest in the management of ED by the urological community and perhaps by non-urologists, and the availability of diverse treatment options with good efficacy and safety profiles'.[76] Recent years have seen the arrival of new products, as well as new and improved delivery systems. Within the next few years, new oral medications, heralded by sildenafil, will become available, revolutionizing not only our treatment options, but also the perception of treatment for ED by the general public. One can only hope that the media will present an informed and accurate picture, not sensationalizing the drugs and their effects, and thereby reducing the risks of uncontrolled use and misuse of the drugs. As knowledge of sexual physiology becomes more sophisticated, there will be further technological developments in the medical evaluation of erectile disorders. New generations of medical and surgical treatments will inevitably emerge. The experiments mentioned have begun the search for understanding how information-processing and neurophysiological responses affect one another. Future research needs to establish the precise cognitive mechanisms that trigger inhibitory effects of a central mechanism as well as its peripheral manifestations, resulting in blocking the sexual response.

Our continued understanding of the relevant intrapsychic, cognitive, interpersonal and systemic mechanisms, have enabled sex therapy to become a more integrated, sophisticated and effective process. Part of the cognitive revolution in psychotherapy has been the inclusion of an evaluation of a patient's cognitions regarding sexual issues. Assisting the patient to process unrealistic expectations, negative self-images, distorted views of the opposite sex's needs and requirements, and tendencies towards catastrophic thinking became an integral part of therapy. LoPiccolo[60] has been influential in promoting a 'post-modern' view to ED, arguing that erectile failure represents a complex, over-determined psychophysiological problem. He identified three critical elements: the functional analysis of the positive value that ED may have for a couple and the individual partners, the diagnosis of both physiological and psychological contributions to erectile impairment and, finally, the actual sexual behaviour patterns engaged in by the couple. He states that 'Although unitary approaches may make for elegantly simple theory, they are also likely to result in ineffective clinical practice with many of our patients who struggle with erectile failure. We owe each patient and his partner a thorough assessment of the factors involved in their unique case, and a treatment plan individualised for maximum possibility of therapeutic success' (p. 196).

A fairly recent and significant development in the professionalization of sex and relationship therapy has been the accreditation of therapists (by the British Association for Sexual and Marital Therapy in the UK).

This is a licence to practice and is a statement about the identified training and clinical competency of the individual therapist. It is renewable every 5 years, requiring evidence for the updating of skills, training and education in related fields including medical interventions, and adequate levels of supervision. The medical profession and the public need to be aware of the difference between accredited and non-accredited therapists, as it is the only current means we have of setting minimum standards. Shared care (joint medical and psychological assessment and treatment) is the recommended way of managing the patient presenting with ED. Mutual understanding and respect for the different disciplines is the only way we can identify, monitor and address the needs of the man with ED and his partner, who also lives with the problem.

■ REFERENCES

1. Rowland D L, Kallan K, Slob A K. Yohimbine, erectile capacity and sexual response in men. Arch Sex Behav 1997; 6: 49–62

2. Tiefer L, Melman A. Interview of wives: a necessary adjunct in the evaluation of impotence. Sex Disabil 1983; 6: 167–175

3. Spector I P, Carey M P. Incidence and prevalence of the sexual dysfunctions: a critical review of the empirical literature. Arch Sex Behav 1990; 19: 389–408

4. Hawton K. Sex therapy: a practical guide. Oxford: Oxford University Press, 1985

5. Slag M R, Morley J E, Elson M K, Trence D L. Impotence in medical clinic outpatients. JAMA 1983; 249: 1736–1740

6. Ellenberg M. Sexual function in diabetic patients. Annals of Internal Medicine, 1980; 92(2): 331–333

7. Paff B A. Sexual dysfunction in gay men requesting treatment. J Sex Marital Ther 1985; 11: 3–18

8. Wolpe J. Psychotherapy by reciprocal inhibition. Stanford, CA: Stanford University Press, 1958

9. Masters W H, Johnson V E. Human sexual inadequacy. Boston: Little Brown, 1970

10. Zilbergeld B. Male sexuality. New York: Bantam, 1978

11. Cole M. Surrogate sex therapy. In: Dryden W (ed) Marital therapy in Britain, Vol 2. London: Harper and Row, 1985: 93–122

12. Cranston-Cuebas M A, Barlow D H. Cognitive and affective contributions to sexual functioning. Annu Rev Sex Res 1990; 1: 119–161

13. Crowe M J, Ridley J. Therapy with couples: the behavioural-systems approach to marital and sexual problems. Oxford: Blackwell Scientific, 1990

14. Clark D M, Fairburn C G. Science and practice of cognitive behaviour therapy. Oxford: Oxford University Press, 1997

15. Kaplan H S. The new sex therapy. London: Baillière Tindall, 1974

16. Bancroft J. Human sexuality and its problems. Edinburgh: Churchill Livingstone, 1989

17. Hawton K. Sexual dysfunctions. In: Hawton K, Salkovkis P M, Kirk J, Clark D M (eds) Cognitive behaviour therapy for psychiatric problems. Oxford: Oxford University Press, 1989

18. Beck J G, Barlow D H. The effects of anxiety and attentional focus on sexual responding: physiological patterns in erectile dysfunction. Behav Res Ther 1986; 24: 9–17

19. Beck J G, Barlow D H. The effects of anxiety and attentional focus on sexual responding: cognitive and affective patterns in erectile dysfunction. Behav Res Ther 1986; 24: 19–26

20. Dekker J, Everaerd W. Attentional effects on sexual arousal. Psychophysiology 1988; 25: 45–54

21. Dekker J, Everaerd W. A study suggesting two kinds of information processing on the sexual response. Arch Sex Behav 1989; 18: 435–447

22. Janssen E, Everaerd W. Determinants of male sexual arousal. Annu Rev Sex Res 1993; 4: 211–245

23. Koukounas E, McGabe M. Sexual and emotional variables influencing sexual response to erotica. Behav Res Ther 1997; 35(3): 221–231

24. Rosen R C, Beck J G. Patterns of sexual arousal: psychophysiological processes and clinical applications. New York: Guilford Press, 1988

25. Bancroft J. Sexual problems. In: Clark D M, Fairburn C G (eds) Science and practice of cognitive behaviour therapy. Oxford: Oxford University Press, 1997

26. Buvat J, Buvat-Herbaut M, Lemaire A et al. Recent developments in the clinical assessment and diagnosis of erectile dysfunction. Annu Rev Sex Res 1990; 1: 265–308

27. Kim S C, Oh M M. Norepinephrine involvement in response to intracorporeal injection of papaverine in psychogenic impotence. J Urol 1992; 147: 1530–1532

28. Janssen E. Provoking penile responses: activation and inhibition of male sexual response. D.Phil thesis, University of Amsterdam, 1995

29. Over R, Koukounas E. Habituation of sexual arousal: product and process. Ann Rev Sex Res 1995; VI: 187–223

30. Rosen R C, Leiblum S R, Spector I P. Psychologically based treatment for male erectile disorder: a cognitive-interpersonal model. J Sex Marital Ther 1994; 20(2): 67–85

31. McCarthy B W. Relapse prevention strategies and techniques in sex therapy. J Sex Marital Ther 1993; 19: 142–147

32. Althof S E. Psychogenic impotence: treatment of men and couples. In: Leiblum S R, Rosen R C (eds) Principles and practice of sex therapy: update for 1990s, 2nd edn. New York: Guildford Press, 1989: 237–265

33. Riley A J, Athanasiadis L. Impotence and its non-surgical management. Br J Clin Pract 1997; 51(2): 99–103, 105

34. Turner L A, Althof S E, Levine S B et al. Treating erectile dysfunction wtih external vacuum device: impact upon sexual, psychological and marital functioning. J Urol 1990a; 144(1): 79–82

35. Skakkebaek N E, Bancroft J, Davidson D W, Warnes P. Androgen replacement with oral testosterone undecanoate in hypogonadal men: a double blind controlled study. Clin Endocrinol 1981; 14: 49–61

36. Rakic Z, Starcevic V, Starcevic V P, Marinkovic J. Study to determine which men with erectile dysfunction and decreased serum testosterone levels might benefit from testosterone treatment. Arch Sex Behav 1997; 26(5): 495–504

37. Bancroft J, Wu F C. Changes in erectile responsiveness during replacement therapy. Arch Sex Behav 1983; 12: 59–66

38. Schiavi R C, White D, Mandeli J et al. Effect of testosterone administration on sexual behaviour and mood in men with erectile dysfunction. Arch Sex Behav 1997; 26(3): 231–241

39. Hunner M. A practical treatise on disorders of the sexual function of the male and female. Philadelphia: Davis, 1926

40. Morales A, Condra M, Owen J A et al. Is yohimbine effective in the treatment of organic impotence? Results of a controlled trial. J Urol 1987; 137: 1168–1172

41. Mann K, Klinger T, Noe S et al. Effects of yohimbine on sexual experiences and nocturnal penile tumescence and rigidity in erectile dysfunction. Arch Sex Behav 1996; 25(1): 1–16

42. Knoll L D, Benson R C, Bilhartz D L et al. A randomised crossover study using yohimbine and isoxsuprine versus pentoxifylline in the management of vasculogenic impotence. J Urol 1996; 155(1): 144–146

43. Riley A J, Goodman R E, Kellett J M, Orr R. Double blind trial of yohimbine hydrochloride in the treatment of erection inadequacy. Sex Marital Ther 1989; 4: 17–26

44. Boolell M, Gepi-Attee S, Gingell J C. Sildenafil: a novel-effective oral therapy for male erectile dysfunction. Br J Urol 1996; 78: 257–261

45. Althof S E, Turner L A, Levine S B et al. Long-term use of self injection therapy or papaverine and phentolamine. J Sex Marital Ther 1991; 17(2): 101–112

46. Wylie K. Treatment outcome of brief couple therapy in psychogenic male erectile disorder. Arch Sex Behav 1997; 26(5): 527–545

47. Kaplan H S. The combined use of sex therapy and intrapenile injections in the treatment of impotence. J Sex Marital Ther 1990; 16: 4

48. Padma-Nathan H, Hellstrom W J, Kaiser F E et al. Treatment of men with erectile dysfunction with transurethral alprostadil. Medicated Urethral System for Erection (MUSE) Study Group. N Engl J Med 1997; 336(1): 1–7

49. Melman A, Tiefer L, Pedersen R. Evaluation of the first 406 patients in urology department based center for male sexual dysfunction. Urology 1988; 32: 6–10

50. Tiefer L, Pederson B, Melman A. Psychological follow-up of penile prosthesis implant patients and partners. J Sex Marital Ther 1988; 14: 184–201

51. Jarow J P, Nana-Sinkam P, Sabbagh M, Eskew A. Outcome analysis of goal-directed therapy for impotence. J Urol 1996; 155(5): 1609–1612

52. Haavio-Mannila E, Kontula O. Correlates of increased sexual satisfaction. Arch Sex Behav 1997; 26(4): 399–419

53. Whitehead A, Matthews A. Attitude change during behavioural treatment of sexual inadequacy. Br J Soc Clin Psychol 1977; 16: 275–281

54. Bancroft J, Coles L. Three years' experience in a sexual problems clinic. Br Med J 1976; 1: 1575–1577

55. Crowe M J, Gillan P, Golombok S. Form and content in the conjoint treatment of sexual dysfunction: a controlled study. Behav Res Ther 1981; 19: 47–54

56. Hawton K, Catalan J. Prognostic factors in sex therapy. Behav Res Ther 1986; 24: 377–385

57. De Amicis L A, Goldberg D C, LoPiccolo J et al. Clinical follow-up of couples after treatment for sexual dysfunction. Arch Sex Behav 1985; 14: 467–489

58. LoPiccolo J, Heiman J R, Hogan D R et al. Effectiveness of single therapist versus cotherapy teams in sex therapy. J Consult Clin Psychol 1985; 53: 287–294

59. Hawton K, Catalan J, Fagg J. Sex therapy for erectile dysfunction: characteristics of couples, treatment outcome and prognostic factors. Arch Sex Behav 1992; 21(2): 161–175

60. LoPiccolo J. Postmodern sex therapy for erectile failure. In: Rosen R, Leiblum S (eds) Erectile disorders, assessment and treatment. New York: Guilford Press, 1992

61. Leiblum S R, Rosen R C. Couples therapy for erectile disorders: observations, obstacles, and outcomes. In: Leiblum S R, Rosen R C (eds) Erectile disorders, assessment and treatment. New York: Guilford Press, 1992

62. Speckens A E, Hengeveld M W, Lycklama à Nijeholt G et al. Psychosexual functioning of partners of men with presumed non-organic erectile dysfunction: cause or consequence of the disorder? Arch Sex Behav 1995; 24(2): 157–172

63. Rust J, Bennum I, Crowe M, Golombok S. The Golombok–Rust Inventory of Marital State (GRIMS). Windsor: NFER-NELSON, 1988

64. McCarthy P, Thoburn M. Psychosexual therapy at RELATE: a report on cases processed between 1992 and 1994. Relate Centre for Family Studies, University of Newcastle upon Tyne, 1996

65. Crowhurst H M. The NMGC client in sexual dysfunction clinics. Marriage and Family Trust, National Marriage Guidance Council, now RELATE, 1981

66. Rust J, Golombok S, Pickard S. Marital problems in general practice. Sex Marital Ther 1987; 2: 127–130

67. Catalan J, Hawton K, Day A. Couples referred to a sexual dysfunction clinic: psychological and physical morbidity. Br J Psychiatry 1990; 156: 61–67

68. Barnes T R E, Harvey C A. Psychiatric drugs and sexuality. In: Riley A, Peet M, Wilson C (eds) Sexual pharmacology. Oxford: Clarendon Press, 1993

69. Hirst J F, Watson J P. Therapy for sexual and relationship problems: the effects on outcome of attending as an individual or as a couple. Sex Marital Ther 1997; 12(4): 321–337

70. Boddington J A. Factors associated with drop-out from a couples therapy clinic. Sex Marital Ther 1995; 10: 321–328

71. Bhui K, Herroit P, Watson J P. Asians presenting to a sex and marital therapy clinic. Int J Soc Psychiatry 1994; 40(3): 194–204

72. Harley E. Therapist ethnicity and gender preferences of patients attending a sexual and relationship problems clinic. Unpublished MSc dissertation. London: United Medical and Dental Schools, 1997

73. Zilbergeld B. The man behind the broken penis: social and psychological determinants of erectile failure. In: Rosen R, Leiblum S R (eds) Erectile disorders: assessment and treatment. New York: Guilford Press, 1992

74. Snyder D C, Berg P. Predicting couples' response to brief directive sex therapy. J Sex Marital Ther 1983; 9: 114–120

75. Becker P S. Comparative treatments for sexual problems: couple therapy, group therapy, postal therapy. Unpublished PhD thesis. London: Guy's Hospital, 1980

76. Shabsigh R. Impotence on the rise as a urological subspeciality. J Urol 1996; 155: 924–925

Chapter 42

Shared care management: the primary care perspective

M. G. Kirby

■ INTRODUCTION

Impotence or erectile dysfunction (ED) is the inability to maintain an erection sufficiently long to fulfil sexual activity. It has been estimated that up to 10% of the adult male population suffer from this disorder.[1] Further, only a small subfraction asks for help. The condition is age-related with an incidence at age 65 of 25%.[2] The incidence can be affected by other risk factors or associated conditions. In particular 35–50% of diabetics may experience ED.[3] Traditionally men with ED have been referred to specialists e.g. urologists, psychiatrists and diabetologists/endocrinologists, often with long waiting lists. The referral period can be highly dependent on the country and there can even be considerable regional variations. Increasingly, however, several factors will lead to an increasing number of men presenting to their primary care physician:

- The advent of Viagra and other simple safe and effective treatments.
- Increasing media coverage of ED.
- A change in the traditional reluctance to seek advice.
- The 'greying' of the population.
- Limited specialist access in most healthcare environments.

On this basis the primary care physician must gear up to be able to provide appropriate diagnosis, disease management and long-term follow-up and counselling. Although ED does not affect mortality it can have a major negative effect on patient and partner well being and quality of life. The primary care physician and supporting local infrastructure is ideally placed to provide appropriate advice and/or medical and non-medical treatment and support.

ED will appear in most men at least once in their life. It is considered significant only if it occurs on more than an occasional basis, such that it interferes with normal sexual functioning. The problem may also affect a man's interactions with his family and associates, and the problem tends to be compounded by unrealistic expectations of continuing sexual prowess, particularly as a result of most men's reluctance to admit to the problem, or even to discuss it with their peers. The situation is often not discussed with the partner and some men may hide their difficulties, which may make the relationship worse, because apparent lack of sexual interest may be misinterpreted as a sign of unfaithfulness.

An open approach is most important and some couples are prepared to accept impotence as an inevitable consequence of the passage of years. However, increasing press and television coverage of this subject is removing some of the traditional reluctance to consult. With increasing life expectancy of men, those in their 70s no longer feel old and often wish to continue with an active sex life. Some of these men may have younger partners and are now requesting medical help to resolve the problem.

With the advent of Viagra and other simple, effective and safe therapies, there is an increasing awareness within the community of the improved prospects of the patient with ED. However, the bulk of the increasing number of males is looking for a quick fix and does not necessarily wish to engage in psychosexual counselling. On this basis, the advent of orally active agents such as Viagra and injectables (various prostaglandin preparations) would be particularly attractive and encourage patient presentation.

It is perfectly natural that elderly couples should wish to continue to share an active sex life. This may be less related to sexual drive and more related to the giving of comfort and security that comes as a result of intimacy. It is not uncommon for older people to report that their sex life is more satisfying than it was in their younger days and this naturally has beneficial effects on both physical and psychological health. There are several factors that predict the continuance of sexual activity past 70 years:

- Greater importance of sex in their younger days.[5]
- Better psychological health.[6]
- Earlier age at first intercourse.[7]
- Better subjective health in women.[8]
- A stronger sexual drive in men in their 20s.[5]

The wider availability and use of hormone replacement therapy (HRT) for women will almost certainly have an impact on the enthusiasm for sexual activity in the older woman. The genital consequences of oestrogen deficiency, especially dyspareunia and urinary symptoms, are significant factors in women withdrawing from sexual activity. It has been shown that, in women continuing sexual activity in the second half of their lives, there is a reduced risk of genital atrophy.[9]

These factors have led many primary care physicians to consider the advisability of setting up an in-house service for ED. This may be partly due to a desire to develop new multidisciplinary skills that would benefit such patients and to be able to offer the patient assessment and appropriate treatment in a non-hospital setting. There are advantages in using existing communication skills based around an established doctor/patient relationship which is integral with the knowledge of the patient's physical, social and psychological history.

There may be financial advantages to the practice in terms of a reduction in unnecessary referrals to outpatient urology departments. When expertise is developed there may be opportunities to assess and treat patients of other primary care physicians in the area as a local provider unit. The use of trained nurses will keep waiting times comparatively short and it is important to have a line of communication with local psychosexual therapists.

NORMAL MECHANISMS

The knowledge of the physiological mechanisms of ED has resulted in the development of various realistic treatment options. Erection of the penis depends on the adequate filling of the corpora cavernosa with blood at systolic pressure. Arterial blood enters from the paired cavernosal arteries, which are the terminal branches of the internal iliac arteries. The mechanism of the erection is controlled by the autonomic nervous system. Parasympathetic nerves from S2–S4 are the principal mediators of erection while sympathetic nerves from T11–L2 control ejaculation and detumescence. Basic research into the smooth muscle physiology of the erectile tissue and the identification of neurotransmitters such as nitric oxide and acetylcholine has opened the pathway to new treatments (Fig. 42.1).

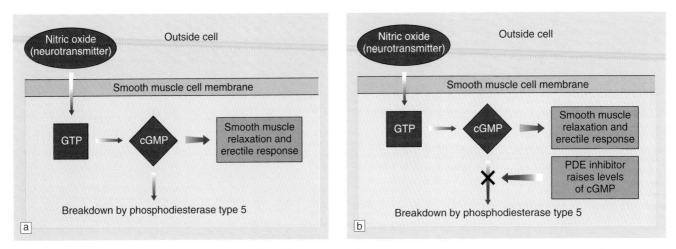

Figure 42.1. (a) The erectile mechanism is mediated by nitric oxide via a second-messenger system involving cyclic guanosine monophosphate (cGMP). Detumescence results from breakdown of cGMP by phosphodiesterase type 5. It has been hypothesized that ED results from reduced tissue cGMP levels. (GTP, guanosine triphosphate.) (b) Phosphodiesterase (PDE) type 5 inhibition e.g. by sildenafil prevents cGMP breakdown and thereby enhances the normal erectile response in a patient with ED. (From ref. 31 with permission.)

■ CAUSES

The human sexual response is extremely complex; problems with potency are often multifactorial and there is a need for an integrated approach that may have to be multidisciplinary, involving the primary care physician, urologist, psychologist or psychiatrist and specialist nurse. The causes of ED can be divided into six groups — psychogenic, neurogenic, endocrine, arteriogenic, drugs and miscellaneous. A summary is given in Table 42.1.

Psychogenic impotence

Psychogenic stimuli can inhibit erection, mainly through stimulation of the sympathetic nervous system: the increased sympathetic tone interferes with the mechanism of smooth muscle relaxation that underlies erection. Once failure has occurred, the problem is self-perpetuating, with each failure increasing anxiety. Psychogenic impotence is the commonest cause of intermittent erectile failure in young men. However, it is usually secondary to some organic dysfunction in middle-aged and elderly men.[10] Diagnostic clues include the following:

- Life event at time of onset.
- No physical illness.
- Baseline tests normal.
- Early morning and nocturnal erections intact.
- Normal erection during masturbation.
- Intermittent, depending on partner.
- Sudden onset.

Neurogenic impotence

ED may be caused by changes in the central nervous system, at the level of either the brain, the spinal cord or the peripheral nervous system, and there are usually other clinical signs of neurological involvement. For example, a prolapsed intervertebral disc may cause pressure on the cauda equina and peripheral neuropathies (usually caused by diabetes or alcoholism) may affect the S2–S4 segment. Upper motor neuron lesions dissociate the sacral reflex arc from the midbrain, hypothalamic and cortical controlling mechanisms. Diagnostic clues include the following:

- Inability to masturbate.
- Absent or infrequent morning or nocturnal erections.
- Postural hypotension.

Table 42.1. Causes of erectile dysfunction[*]

Psychogenic

> Anxiety
> Depression

Neurogenic

> Trauma
> Myelodysplasia (spina bifida)
> Intervertebral disc lesion
> Multiple sclerosis
> Diabetes mellitus
> Alcohol
> Pelvic surgery

Endocrine

> Hormone deficiency — low testosterone and raised SHBG; high prolactin
> Thyrotoxicosis

Arteriogenic

> Hypertension
> Smoking
> Diabetes
> Hyperlipidaemia

Venous

> Functional impairment of the veno-occlusive mechanism

Drugs

> Central and/or direct effect (most commonly implicated, antihypertensives, antidepressants and LHRH analogues)

Miscellaneous

> Peyronie's disease
> Penile trauma
> Opiate use
> Lack of exercise
> Obesity
> Drug abuse

[*]These conditions are not mutually exclusive — many cases of ED are multifactorial.

- Urinary symptoms.
- Diminished sweating in lower limb.
- Intermittent attacks of diarrhoea.
- Loss of orgasmic sensation.
- Absent cremasteric, anal or pubocavernosal reflexes.
- Diminished testicular sensation.

Endocrinological impotence

Endocrinological impotence may result from abnormalities in serum testosterone, prolactin or thyroxine. Free serum testosterone concentrations fall progressively with age because the testes produce less hormone and more androgens are bound to sex-hormone-binding globulin (SHBG), the concentration of which increases with age. Falling free testosterone concentrations are associated with a loss of libido and reduced frequency of erections. Diagnostic clues include the following:

- Beyond middle age.
- Progressive loss of erections under all circumstances.
- Recent loss of libido.
- No spontaneous sexual fantasies.
- Feminization.
- Gynaecomastia or testicular atrophy.
- Low testosterone.
- Raised levels of SHBG.
- Raised gonadotrophins.
- Raised prolactin.
- Diminished beard growth.

Raised prolactin concentration is also associated with reduced circulating free testosterone, and decreased potency may be an early feature of raised serum prolactin levels.[11] This may be idiopathic or due to drug use, renal failure or a pituitary tumour.

Vascular impotence

Erection may be impaired by either arterial insufficiency or a disorder of the veno-occlusive mechanism, but often both are present. In older patients, arteriosclerosis is the most common cause.[12,13] Changes in the fibroelastic components of the lacunar trabeculae may cause venous leakage and Peyronie's disease may be associated with a venous leak. Diagnostic clues include the following:

- Insidious onset.
- Inability to masturbate.

- No morning or nocturnal erections.
- Evidence of poor blood supply to fingers, feet or penis.
- Angina.
- Worsened by the use of small amounts of alcohol.
- Smoking.

Medication

Drug therapy is not an uncommon contributory factor in ED.[14,15] Slag and colleagues[16] showed that, in a group of over a thousand men attending medical outpatients, 34% were suffering from ED and, of those investigated, medication was thought to be the cause in 25%.

As the patients grow older they are much more likely to be receiving a variety of drugs and it is important to review their medication, as this simple intervention can result in the return of normal sexual function.[17,18] Antihypertensives are the group of drugs most commonly associated with this problem. These drugs are often used in combination, which may compound the effect. The incidence of ED is higher in untreated hypertensive men than in normotensive individuals, probably owing to arteriosclerosis. The association between beta blockers and ED is well known,[14,15] and a change to one of the more cardioselective beta blockers may be helpful. Centrally acting antihypertensives such as methyldopa and clonidine may also cause problems, but alpha blockers such as doxazosin are much less troublesome and may even improve the situation. Thiazide diuretics may also be a problem.

The MRC trial[18] showed a rate of 36% ED in patients on bendrofluazide, and withdrawal of diuretic often led to an improvement in sexual function. Spironolactone is an aldosterone antagonist and acts as a potassium-sparing diuretic. There are many reports of its association with gynaecomastia, reduced libido and an incidence of between 4 and 30% of ED. This drug may act as an anti-androgen by inhibiting the binding of dihydrotestosterone. Antipsychotics, antidepressants and anxiolytics may all cause problems due to their central effect, anticholinergic effect and effect on the hypothalamus. The increasing use of anti-androgen drugs, particularly for the treatment of hormone-sensitive prostate cancer, leads to a major incidence of ED.

It is impossible to be comprehensive in this text as there is an ever-increasing list of drugs associated with this problem. The mechanisms are complex but there is often a relation to reduced libido. The common offenders are cimetidine, digoxin, nicotine, alcohol and opiates.

Miscellaneous conditions

Obesity, lack of exercise and general lack of fitness, drug and alcohol abuse may often be contibutory factors in patients presenting with ED. Peyronie's disease, other penile deformities and penile trauma can also cause discomfort, leading to loss of function.

■ MANAGEMENT OF ED IN THE PRIMARY CARE SETTING

The advent of more widespread disease awareness and the availability of orally active agents have prompted the development of guidelines to be used specifically as the potential basis for patient management in the primary care setting (Chapter 43). The guidelines include diagnosis and treatment, both medical and non-medical involving lifestyle modification.

Diagnosis

A careful history and physical examination are required to help elucidate the cause of ED and to decide whether the problem is psychogenic or organic in origin. There may be clinical signs of recognized risk factors. Men with ED usually have normal libido and unimpaired ejaculatory function.

Psychogenic ED may begin suddenly, following some life event. Early morning, self-stimulated and spontaneous nocturnal erections are often preserved. By contrast, organic impotence is characterized by a progressive loss of erectile function; it is consistently present and associated with loss of early morning and nocturnal erections. A detailed psychosocial and psychosexual history is required to explore sources of relationship difficulties, sources of anxiety or stress and to establish whether the partner is sympathetic towards the problem. Specific questions, such as the following, may be helpful:

■ When did you last have successful sexual intercourse?
■ How frequently do you have problems with your erections?
■ What sort of problems have you had with your erections?
■ Have you discussed this matter with your partner?
■ Do you have any relationship problems?
■ Have you heard of any treatments which may help your problem?
■ How interested are you in sex and how often do you have sexual desires?

■ Do you have any current physical problems?
■ What were your childhood experiences and parents' attitude to sexuality?
■ Did you have any abnormal sexual experiences during adolescence?
■ Are you content with your sexual relationship?
■ How do you rate yourself as a sexual partner?

Focused examination

1. Examine the size and shape of the penis, in the flaccid state and, where appropriate, in the erect state, to observe any bowing or distortions.
2. Look for any inflammation under the foreskin and determine whether the foreskin retracts normally.
3. Examine the testes with regard to size, shape and consistency and palpate the epididymis and vas deferens to detect any abnormal swelling or varicocoeles.
4. The prostate should be of the same rubbery consistency as the tip of the nose. The presence of induration or a palpable nodule should raise the suspicion of prostate cancer.

General examination should include the endocrine, vascular and neurological systems. Look for loss of secondary sexual characteristics, and for signs of liver disease such as gynaecomastia, palmar erythema, spider naevae and leuconychia. Vascular assessment should include measurement of blood pressure, cardiac status and lower extremity pulses. Look for arterial bruits, poor capillary return and signs of diabetes. Examination of the fundi may reveal changes of hypertension or diabetes, such as haemorrhages, cotton-wool spots or arteriovenous nipping. A brief neurological examination should be made to exclude abnormal reflexes, muscular tone or motor loss. The S2–S4 dermatomes should be evaluated by testing the perineal sensation and anal sphincter tone (Fig. 42.2).

Summary

Decide: What is the likely cause of the complaint? What are the expectations and motivations of the man and his partner for further diagnostic tests and treatment?

Refer if: Evidence of significant peripheral vascular disease.
An organic cause in a young man.
Hypogonadism in a young man.
Severe psychosexual problems.

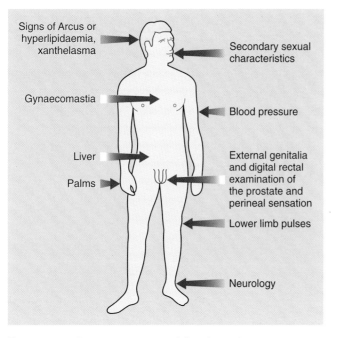

Figure 42.2. Important aspects of the physical examination in men with ED. (Adapted from ref. 31 with permission.)

Investigations

It is important to exclude undiagnosed diabetes mellitus with the urine dipstick test, which may also indicate proteinuria or suggest the presence of infection. Blood investigation, where necessary, may include one or any of the following tests depending on history and clinical findings:

■ Full blood count.
■ Liver function tests.
■ Renal function tests.

■ Thyroid function tests.
■ Blood sugar.
■ Testosterone.
■ Sex hormone binding globulin (SHBG).
■ Prolactin.
■ Luteinizing hormone.
■ Fasting lipid profile.

Self-administered tests of nocturnal erections may be made with the snap gauge band[19] and the Rigiscan device (Dacomed, Minneapolis, MN, USA). Unless the problem is obviously psychogenic, a trial injection of an intracavernosal vasoactive agent will be helpful and will distinguish responders from non-responders and help select candidates for self-injection treatment.

More specialized investigations need be performed only when a detailed knowledge of the cause of ED is required. These include colour Doppler imaging and pharmacocavernosography.

Psychosexual counselling

There are many psychological causes that diminish the capacity for erectile response (Table 42.2). These include anxiety, depression, relationship problems, negative experiences and sexual technique problems. Psychosexual therapy began at the beginning of this century with the use of Freudian psychoanalysis. In 1970, Masters and Johnson described a treatment programme involving a combination of behavioural and psychotherapeutic elements and they reported a 70% success rate after 5 years of follow-up. Current day therapy concentrates on the behavioural aspects and aims to reduce performance

Table 42.2. Differential diagnosis of psychogenic and organic ED

Psychogenic	Organic
Sudden onset	Gradual onset — age 50+
Specific situation	Normal libido
Normal nocturnal and early morning erections	All circumstances and every occasion
Relationship problems	Absent nocturnal and early morning erections
Problems during sexual development	Normal libido and ejaculation
Premature ejaculation	
Life event at the time of onset	Normal sexual development

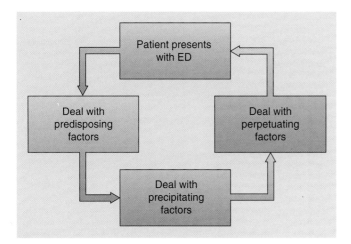

Figure 42.3. Breaking the cycle of erectile failure.

anxiety by means of a programmed relearning of a couple's sexual behaviour. This aims to break the vicious circle of erectile failure that is reinforced by the anticipation of failure the next time (Fig. 42.3). Sex therapy consists of a graduated programme of homework assignments combined with education and follow-up to overcome barriers to progress:[20]

1. Dealing with predisposing factors;
   - Underlying problems
   - Education
   - Communication skills
   - Giving permission.

2. Dealing with precipitating factors;
   - Emotional support
   - Physical treatments.

3. Dealing with perpetuating factors;
   - Patient confidence building
   - Redefining success
   - Allowing expression of feelings
   - Partner — open discussion — must be supportive
   - Interpersonal communication
   - Breakdown problems with intimacy
   - Easing pressure — stress management
   - Joint responsibility for the partner with the difficulty.

Medical management

Ever since the advent of penile prostheses, there has been a continuous improvement in the availability of user-friendly, reliable and dependable interventions with potential in the management of ED. Traditionally in any ED healthcare management system patient education and training is rate limiting and expensive. In the primary care system; at least, this can be overcome with the help of trained nurse practitioners. Under these circumstances although training in vacuum devices and injection therapy is time consuming, in motivated patients the success rate can be high. The advent of sildenafil, however, is likely to change radically the patient–healthcare provider interface.

The enthusiasm for taking a pill for the treatment of ED has been traditionally shown by the OTC use of various homeopathic remedies including yohimbine.[26]

Sildenafil (Viagra) has recently been approved in the US and worldwide approval is anticipated within the next year. This agent is a selective inhibitor of phosphodiesterase type 5. Inhibition of this isoenzyme elevates cavernosal cGMP that produces an erection in ED patients with little effect on normal sexual activity. This drug has been shown to be effective in organic and psychogenic impotence and in diabetics and spinal injury patients. Some degree of success is also observed in post radical prostatectomy patients with surgery-induced ED. Given the reliability of the response to Viagra and the side effect profile, the drug may in fact become a diagnostic for ED in the primary care setting. One can imagine the scenario that only when an inadequate or poor response to Viagra is observed, would specialist referral be required. However, as with any new class of agent, care should be taken on prescribing Viagra. In addition to an absolute contra-indication for nitrates the full side effect profile of Viagra may only become known after several years of further investigation. It remains, however, that the advent of Viagra represents for many patients a quantum leap in the management of ED.

The biggest problem with the management of this condition in primary care is lack of time and this may be overcome with the help of trained nurses. Teaching vacuum or injection therapy is time consuming but the careful selection of highly motivated patients is rewarding. Both these techniques are well tried and tested and have good success rates, but only if the technique is properly taught.

Intracavernosal injection (ICI)

This method of treatment (Chapter 31) was introduced in the early 1980s and was a significant advance in the treatment of ED.[21]

Papaverine, alone or in combination with phentolamine, and prostaglandin E1 (PGE1) (alprostadil) are the agents

Table 42.3. Suggested doses for penile injections

Drug	Initial dose (neurological disorder)	Initial dose (standard dose)	Maximum dose
Alprostadil (Caverject)	2.5 µg	5 µg	20 µg increasing to 40 µg
Papaverine	10 mg	10 mg	80 mg increasing to 120 mg

most widely used (Table 42.3). Alprostadil has also been studied as an intra-urethral preparation, given by means of a unique applicator.[22] There appears to be a good response to intra-urethral alprostadil; systemic effects are uncommon and complications such as priapism and penile fibrosis are less common than when the drug is given by penile injection. Papaverine and PGE1 are both muscle relaxants and probably have a similar mode of action in ED. PGE1 is a naturally occurring substance, metabolized locally following ICI in cavernosal tissue with little systemic penetration. The risk of priapism (defined as an erection lasting more than 4 hours) is very low. Occasionally it does cause a dull throbbing ache in the penis and occasional giddiness and nausea has been reported.

Moxisylyte (Erecnos®) is an alternative intracavernosal injection that has recently been introduced. It facilitates an erection in men with ED (Table 42.4). Erecnos® is a selective alpha-1 blocker that facilitates tumescence within 10 minutes. In a study including more than 300 men with ED, 90% of those receiving Erecnos® reported an erectile response, sufficient for penetration in 50% of cases.[23]

If a programme of penile injection therapy is commenced, it is necessary to obtain informed consent from the patient, warning him about the risk of priapism; clear instructions should be given regarding what to do should this occur,[24] and if so, it is essential to instruct him to return to the GP concerned or to go to the local hospital for treatment. In the event of a prolonged erection, detumescence may be achieved by inserting a butterfly needle into one of the corpora, aspirating 20–40 ml of blood. This may take approximately 20 minutes and may be complemented by the concomitant administration of an alpha-adrenergic antagonist.

Patients should also be warned of the long-term risk of scarring at the site of injection, and instructed to use the injections no more than twice a week. This treatment should be used with particular caution in men under the age of 50 and in those with neurological disease or where psychological features predominate. Larger doses may be necessary in patients with hypertension, peripheral vascular disease or hyper-cholesterolaemia (Fig. 42.4).

Vacuum devices
Vacuum devices are a non-invasive, inexpensive and simple treatment for a man who does not respond to intracavernosal injection.[25] The penis is placed inside a cylinder where a pump is used to create a vacuum that pulls blood into the penis. A rigid erection is produced

Table 42.4. Erecnos® for the treatment of ED

Active ingredient	Moxisylyte hydrochloride
Presentation	Powder plus diluent in dual-chamber, prefilled syringes. Available in 10 mg/ml and 20 mg/ml strengths
Dosage	10 mg by intracavernous injection, increasing to 20 mg for subsequent injections if the response is inadequate. Up to 3 doses can be given per week, with a minimum interval of 48 hours
Contra-indications	Patients with systolic blood pressure less than 100 mmHg, penile implants, or conditions predisposing them to priapism, such as sickle-cell anaemia, multiple myeloma or leukaemia

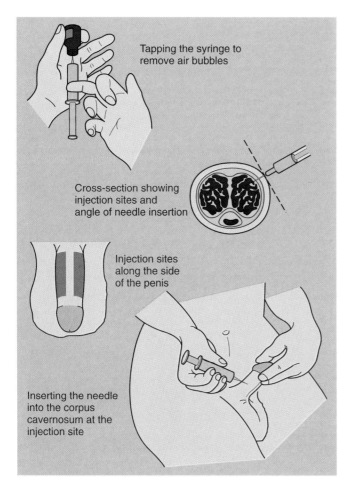

Figure 42.4. Self-injection technique. (From ref. 31 with permission.)

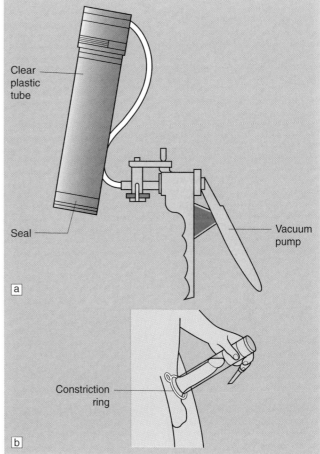

Figure 42.5. A typical vacuum erection device (a), which is placed over the penis and used to induce an erection that is maintained with a constriction ring (b). (From ref. 31 with permission.)

within minutes. A tension ring is then pulled off the cylinder onto the base of the penis, where it remains during sexual activity. Some patients complain that the erection produced is cold and lifeless and the tension ring may cause discomfort, especially during ejaculation. The technique requires good manual dexterity on the part of the patient and the partner. The ring should be removed after 30 minutes of use. Various devices are available (Chapter 34), ranging in price from £150 to £250. They are usually available with a money-back guarantee and are particularly useful in older and less fit men (Fig. 42.5).

Follow-up studies have demonstrated disappointing long-term benefit from vacuum devices or ICI, despite a good initial response. This may be due to any of the following:[28]

■ Ineffectiveness.
■ Side effects.
■ Lack of spontaneity.
■ Partner dislike.
■ Failure to engage partner at an early stage.
■ Interpersonal problems.

If the patient is shown to be hypogonadal, androgens can restore both libido and potency.[29] There is no useful therapeutic effect in patients whose free testosterone concentrations are within the normal range. Oral testosterone supplements are less effective than parenteral preparations and are known to have hepatotoxic side effects. Testosterone patches may be a useful alternative. Clinical and biochemical evaluation of the prostate with prostate-specific antigen (PSA) and monitoring of blood lipids is necessary when treating men with testosterone.

Topically acting vasodilating drugs

The use of these drugs is not new (Chapter 29). Glyceryl trinitrate has been used with some limited success.[30]

Where there is loss of tumescence following penetration, caused by the pelvic steal syndrome or in the presence of a venous leak, improvement may be achieved using a constrictor ring in addition to intra-urethral alprostadil.

Surgical treatment

Men who do not respond to the self-injection technique, or the vacuum device, may benefit from surgery. Many of these patients will have significant arterial or venous disease or penile corpus cavernosum fibrosis. There are three surgical options available: vascular bypass surgery for arterial or venous abnormalities (Chapter 36), ligation for venous incompetence (Chapter 35) or implantation of a penile prosthesis (Chapters 37–39).

■ CONCLUSIONS

The management of ED has been revolutionized by the development of new therapies and it can now be undertaken by any physician with an interest in this subject. In the UK this is usually a urologist but may also be a diabetologist, specialist nurse or primary care physician. With the advent of intra-urethral therapy and oral therapy, it is likely that there will be a huge increase in demand for treatment and the emphasis may swing towards the primary care physician. There will be cost concerns for purchasers in the current climate of limited resources and there will be challenges to primary care in terms of how they deliver new physical treatments and investigate these patients. This may be overcome by setting up in-house clinics run by specialist nurses.

What patients want is a sympathetic interview with a clear explanation of the problem and expert advice about self-administered treatments. This condition has serious adverse effects on the quality of life and to address the problem doctors need to be able to discuss sexual matters with their patients.

It should not be forgotten that this problem affects not only the men but also their partners, and ED can lead to considerable marital disharmony. Primary care physicians can be supportive by providing accurate, unbiased and realistic information for men and their partners. This can help to counter the effect of this disability and help to dispel the inaccurate and misleading information that patients have so often received through the media and friends and family.

■ REFERENCES

1. Stakl W. The use of prostaglandin E1 for the diagnosis and treatment of erectile dysfunction. World J Urol 1990; 8: 84–86

2. Krane R J, Goldstein I, Saenz de Tejada I. Impotence. N Engl J Med 1989; 321(24): 1648–1654

3. Drugs and Therapeutics Bulletin. Help for erectile impotence. 1989; 27(16): 61–64

4. Fieldman H A, Goldstein I, Hatzichristou D et al. Impotence and its medical and psychological correlates. Results of the Massachusetts Male Aging Study. J Urol 1994; 150: 54–61

5. Bretshneider J G, McCoy N L. Sexual interest and behaviour in healthy 80 to 120 year-olds. Arch Sex Behav 1988; 17: 109–129

6. Nilsson L. Sexuality in the elderly. Acta Obstet Gynecol Scand 1987; 140(suppl): 52–58

7. Vallery-Masson J, Valleron A J, Poitrenaud J. Factors related to intercourse frequency in a group of French pre-retirement managers. Age Ageing 1981; 10: 53–59

8. Persson G. Sexuality in a 70 year old urban population. J Psychosom Res 1990; 24: 335–342

9. Leiblum S, Bachmann G, Kemmann E et al. Vaginal atrophy in the post-menopausal woman. JAMA 1983; 249: 2195–2198

10. Krane R J, Goldstein I, Saenz De Tejada I. Medical progress: impotence. N Eng J Med 1989; 321: 1648–1659

11. Franks S, Jacobs H S, Martin N, Nabarro J D. Hyperprolactinaemia and impotence. Clin Endocrinol 1978; 8: 277–287

12. Troy K, Cuttner J, Reilly M et al. Tartrate-resistant acid phosphatase staining of monocytes in Gaucher disease. Am J Hematol 1985; 19: 237–244

13. Michael V. Arterial disease as a cause of impotence. J Clin Endocrinol Metab 1982; 11: 725–748

14. Brock G B, Lue T F. Drug induced male sexual dysfunction. Drug Safety 1993; 8(6): 414–426

15. Horowitz J D, Gobel A J. Drugs and impaired male sexual function. Drugs 1979; 18: 206

16. Slag M F, Morley J E, Elson M K et al. Impotence in medical outpatients clinic. JAMA 1983; 249: 1736–1740

17. Bansal S. Sexual dysfunction in hypertensive men: a critical review. Hypertension 1988; 12: 1–10

18. Medical Research Council Working Party on Mild to Moderate Hypertension. Adverse reactions to bendrofluazide and propranolol for the treatment of mild hypertension. Lancet 1981; 2: 539–543

19. Ek A, Bradley W E, Krane R J. Nocturnal penile rigidity measured by the snap-gauge band. J Urol 1983; 129: 964–966

20. Hawton K. Treatment of sexual dysfunction by sex therapy and other approaches. Br J Psychiatry 1995; 167(3): 307–314

21. Junemann K P. Pharmacotherapy for impotence: where are we going? In: Lue T F (ed) World Book of Impotence. London: Eldred Smith Gordon, 1992: 181–188

22. Padma-Nathan H, Hellstrom W J, Kaiser F E et al. Treatment of men with erectile dysfunction with transurethral alprostadil. N Engl J Med 1997; 336: 1–7

23. Costa P, Mottet N. Efficiency and side effects of intra-cavernosal injections of moxisylyte in impotent patients: a double blind, placebo controlled study. Proc Am Urol Assoc 1995; 153(suppl): 472A

24. Andersson K E, Holmquist F, Wagner G. Pharmacology of drugs used for treatment of erectile dysfunction and priapism. Int J Impotence Res 1991; 3: 155–172

25. Witherington R. Vacuum constriction device for management of erectile impotence. J Urol 1989; 141: 320–322

26. Susset J G, Tessier C D, Wincze J et al. Effect of yohimbine hydrochloride on erectile impotence. A double-blind study. J Urol 1989; 141: 1360–1363

27. Boolell M, Allen M, Ballard S et al. Sildenafil: an orally active type 6 cyclic GMP specific phosphodiesterase inhibitor for the treatment of penile erectile dysfunction. Int J Impot Res 1996; 8: 47–52

28. Althof S E, Turner L A, Levine S B et al. Why do so many people drop out from autoinjection therapy for impotence? J Sex Marital Ther 1989; 15: 121–129

29. Bancroft J, Wu F C. Changes in erectile responsiveness during androgen replacement therapy. Arch Sex Behav 1983; 12: 59–62

30. Class H, Baert I. Transcutaneous nitroglycerine therapy in the treatment of impotence. Urol Int 1989; 44: 309–312

31. Holmes S, Kirby R, Carson C. Male Erectile Dysfunction. Fast Facts Series. Oxford: Health Press Ltd., 1997

Process of care model for the management of erectile dysfunction in the primary care setting

R. Rosen, H. Padma-Nathan and I. Goldstein

INTRODUCTION

The field of male sexual health, and in particular, erectile function and dysfunction, is dynamic and is continuously evolving.[1-6] As recently as 25 years ago, this field was considered to be the exclusive domain of psychologists and/or endocrinologists. The advent of penile prosthesis insertion in 1973 and other, non-surgical, therapies such as vacuum constriction devices and local self-injection of therapeutants in the 1980s brought the urologist to the forefront of clinical practice. This speciality, in conjunction with many other clinical experts and basic scientists, has contributed greatly to current understanding of the physiology of the erectile process, the pathophysiology of erectile dysfunction (ED) and diagnostic and therapeutic options in patient management. Not surprisingly, from the therapeutic perspective alone, there has been, and continues to be, considerable improvement in the availability of user-friendly, reliable and dependable interventions in the arena of male sexual health.[1-6]

Despite the prevalence of ED,[6] fewer than one in ten men seek treatment for this disorder, and even within this sub-population, a high drop-out rate is routinely observed.[1-5] Reasons advanced include the fact that treatment is relatively invasive/intrusive in nature or artificial, has associated risks, may be irreversible and is expensive. On this basis, the general availability of effective and safe oral therapeutants for the management of ED will have a considerable and far-reaching impact on the management of male sexual health issues. In particular, primary care physicians will become the front line in the management of patients complaining of sexual disorders.

The advent of more widespread disease awareness and the availability of orally active agents have prompted the development of the process of care model to be used specifically as the potential basis for patient management in the primary care setting. It was also designed to facilitate dialogue between physicians, patients and, increasingly, the initial health care provider in issues relating to male sexual health.

METHODOLOGY AND PROCESS

The objectives in the development of the model were as follows:

1. To utilize contemporary research and epidemiological data to develop a consensus-based, step-care algorithm to be used in treatment design and patient education;
2. To help to define the relative roles and synergy between the primary care physician and the specialist;
3. To enhance the knowledge and training of the primary care physician in the field of male sexual health.

To this end, a multidisciplinary panel of 11 experts in primary care, internal medicine, endocrinology, psychology and urology in the field of male sexual medicine (Table 43.1) was convened. Prior to the initial meeting, panellists were provided with a selection of key peer review articles.[1-5] Each study was used to develop the

Table 43.1. Process of care panellists

Panellist	Affiliation
Raymond Rosen, PhD	Professor of Psychiatry, University of Medicine and Dentistry of New Jersey (Panel Chairperson)
Irwin Goldstein, MD	Professor of Urology, Boston University School of Medicine
Julia Heiman, PhD	Professor of Psychiatry, University of Washington School of Medicine
Stanley Korenman, MD	Professor of Medicine, University of California, Los Angeles
Milton Lakin, MD	Professor of Medicine, Cleveland Clinic Foundation
Tom Lue, MD	Professor of Urology, University of California, San Francisco
Drogo Karl Montague, MD	Professor of Surgery, Cleveland Clinic Foundation
Harin Padma-Nathan, MD	Associate Professor of Urology, University of Southern California
Richard Sadovsky, MD	Professor of Family Medicine, State University of New York, Brooklyn
R. Taylor Segraves, MD, PhD	Professor of Psychiatry, Case Western Reserve
Ridwan Shabsigh, MD	Associate Professor of Urology, Columbia University School of Medicine

model with regard to patient history, physical examination, laboratory tests and specialized tests. The most pertinent literature provided the framework for devising a contemporary algorithm. However, the preliminary model was refined on the basis of additional input from additional multidisciplinary expert panel discussions and decision-making. The groups focused on methodology concerning definitions and classifications, diagnostic studies and therapeutic options. The ultimate model also included input from several panel member subcommittees charged with bringing further definition to ED history and physical examination, patient education, psychosocial issues, medication, ageing and step-care issues. In essence, therefore, the process consisted of three meetings and separate focus group discussions with physicians in primary care and internal medicine, culminating in the generation of the consensus-based algorithm (Fig. 43.1).

Recommendations and guidelines

The process of care model consists of clinical guidelines for the assessment and management of ED in the primary care setting. The essential principles of the model are as follows:

1. Identification and recognition of ED and the associated concomitant medical and psychological conditions are implicit and the need emphasized strongly.
2. The model is goal orientated, directly addressing patient and partner requirements and preferences.
3. Patient and partner education and dialogue are essential requirements during all phases of patient management, i.e. during assessment, treatment and follow-up.
4. The underlying tenet of the model is a stepwise approach to patient management. This covers both

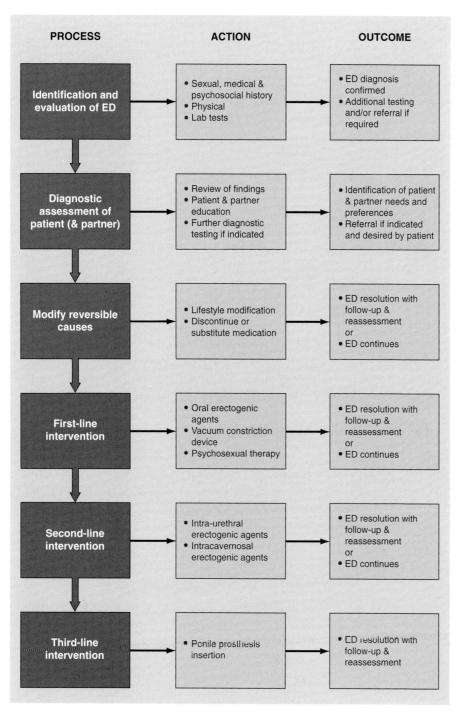

Figure 43.1. A process of care model for the management of erectile dysfunction (ED).

the degree of invasiveness of diagnostic and treatment procedures and the degree of involvement of non-primary-care specialities.

5. The model (Fig. 43.1) provides explicit guidelines for follow-up and referral.

The following represents the nucleus of the new guidelines for the management of ED in a primary care setting, formulated from the process care model.

Definition of erectile dysfunction

The consensus panel definition of ED (formerly termed impotence) was as follows: erectile dysfunction is the persistent or repeated inability for 3 months' duration or more to attain and/or maintain an erection sufficient for satisfactory sexual performance.

The performance definition is based upon the patient's self-report in conjunction with medical, psychological and sexual history assessments. Duration may be modified in special circumstances, for example after prostatectomy.

Classification of erectile dysfunction

Classification may be based on severity, aetiology or onset.

When classified on a severity basis, ED can be stratified as mild, moderate or severe, depending on the ability to attain and/or maintain an erection with either intermittent (mild), infrequent (moderate) or absent (severe) satisfactory sexual performance.

Although the conditions frequently coexist, on the basis of aetiology, ED is defined as either psychological or organic. The former definition is used when there is clear-cut evidence of a psychological precipitant and/or determinant. Organic ED is considered to be that which occurs as the result of an acute or chronic physiological precipitant and/or determinant, including underlying endocrinological, neurological or vascular aetiologies.

Using onset as the criterion, ED is classified as either primary or secondary. The former, which is uncommon, is that which occurs in men who have never had the ability to attain and/or maintain an erection. The potential causes include deep-seated psychological conflicts or perineal/pelvic trauma. Secondary ED is that which is acquired following a period of satisfactory sexual performance.

Diagnosis and assessment of erectile dysfunction

As with any medical condition, the ideal foundation for the management of ED is a careful clinical evaluation. As a minimum, thorough medical and psychological histories, physical examination and focused laboratory testing are recommended. More specialized diagnostic tests (e.g. nocturnal penile tumescence and rigidity or penile vascular studies) are available and can be justified in individual patients. However, it should be stressed that the cornerstone of clinical assessment remains a detailed sexual, medical and psychological history. This accomplishes several goals, including characterization of the problem and identification of patient and partner needs and priorities, as well as fostering a good relationship between physician and patient. Although this is not always possible on the first visit, every effort should be made to involve the patient's partner early in the process.

The underlying principle throughout the whole process of evaluation is the determination of whether the patient meets the consensus definition of ED i.e. has a repeated inability (over a 3-month period) to attain and/or maintain an erection sufficient for sexual intercourse. Subsequent issues relate to whether intervention is warranted and whether ED is the primary complaint or is associated with other sexual dysfunction such as premature ejaculation or hypoactive desire.

The next phase of the evaluation, following problem identification, is the obtaining of a comprehensive sexual, medical and psychological history (Table 43.2). In addition to the usual concerns in medical history taking, clinicians should pay special attention to the sensitivity of the topic, as well as the opportunity to initiate patient and partner education and communication (Table 43.3).

Well within the remit and capability of the primary care physician is arrangement for supportive laboratory evaluations. Of particular importance is an evaluation of the hypothalamic–pituitary–gonadal axis via assessment of serum testosterone (and dihydrotestosterone) and prolactin levels. Abnormalities of either may correlate with diminished libido and reduced sex glandular mass. Also of merit are evaluations of serum lipids, which can be predictive of vasculogenic (atherosclerosis-based) ED and other evaluations including prostate-specific antigen.

Specialized diagnostic testing may be indicated in several circumstances, as follows: (a) if the initial laboratory assessment reveals abnormalities potentially warranting further evaluation to enable a more precise diagnosis; (b) if the selected treatment option requires more specialized diagnostic assessment (e.g. penile ultrasound and angiography prior to penile revascularization) prior to decision-making; (c) if the patient would prefer a more comprehensive evaluation and understanding prior to selection of a treatment option; (d) for medico-legal reasons.

Specialized diagnostic tests for ED include a wide range of vascular, neurological and endocrinological studies. Although specialists, often in gaining insight into the underlying pathophysiology, may routinely use these tests, their use should be reserved for selected cases in the primary setting. Although useful knowledge can be gained, their utility may be limited by expense and associated risks. However, nocturnal penile tumescence and rigidity (NPTR) testing is widely and increasingly used and may assist in the discrimination of organic and psychogenic dysfunction. NPTR studies can be conducted in a sleep-laboratory or, more commonly, in an ambulatory setting. Also of interest, and certainly feasible in the office

Table 43.2. Patient evaluation

Sexual history	Medical history	Physical examination
Erectile dysfunction (onset, duration, progression; sexual activity, a.m., p.m., masturbatory)	Chronic conditions (diabetes, anaemia and renal failure)	General appearance and secondary sexual characteristics
Penile sensation (pain, numbing)	Concurrent drugs (antihypertensives, antidepressants, alcohol, nicotine)	Cardiovascular system (peripheral pulses, occlusive and aneurysmal disease)
Penile curvature and shortening	Vascular risk factors (diabetes, hypertension, hypercholesterolaemia or familial background)	Neurological (penile sensation and bulbocavernosus reflex)
Altered libido, ejaculation or orgasm	Pelvic/perineal/penile trauma (penile fracture or bicycling injury)	Urogenital system (penile, testicular and rectal examination)
Partner's sexual function	Previous surgery (radical prostatectomy, laminectomy, coronary artery bypass graft	
	Neurological illness (spinal cord injury, multiple sclerosis)	
	Endocrine disease (hypogonadism, hyperprolactinaemia or thyroid disorders)	
	Psychiatric illness (depression or anxiety)	
	Sexually transmitted disease	

evaluation, is the use of intracavernosal injection of pharmacological agents (such as prostaglandin E1 (PGE1) or 'trimix') to determine functional assessment of penile arterial inflow and veno-occlusive integrity.

It is likely, particularly with the advent of effective and safe orally active agents, that an increasing amount of diagnostic evaluation will take place in the primary care environment. However, more complex evaluation, particularly of poor or non-responders to therapeutic agents, will be necessary. It is almost certain that this will involve dialogue with, and referral to, a specialist to ensure the ultimate in patient care management.

Indications for referral
Most patients with ED can be managed within the primary care environment. However, in specific circumstances,

Table 43.3. Patient and partner education

- Anatomy and physiology of sexual response and erection

- Pathophysiology of erectile dysfunction, risk factors and lifestyle determinants

- Review of initial assessment and diagnostic testing results

- Assessment and modification of patient/partner expectations

- Review of lifestyle changes and treatment options

- Continued education and communication during follow-up

referral to a specialist may be required for additional diagnostic testing, patient management or indeed surgery. The need for referral or consultation may arise at any time from initial evaluation, i.e. prior to or during the course of treatment or follow-up. When referring patients, care should be taken to ensure that patients are fully informed about the reasons for referral, the evaluations to be undertaken and the potential outcomes. Equally, after referral, results should be carefully reviewed with the patient.

Specific indications for specialist referral include the following:

1. When additional laboratory evaluations are ambiguous or to identify the need for more comprehensive evaluation;
2. In instances of primary ED, e.g. in young patients with a history of pelvic/perineal trauma;
3. In patients with significant penile curvature (e.g. Peyronie's disease and congenital deformity);
4. When there is a request from a patient or a medico-legal requirement for further evaluation.

Specialist referrals will be to urologists, psychiatrists, endocrinologists, sex therapists, or vascular-reconstructive or neurosurgeons, as appropriate.

Patient management

Options for patient management can be subdivided into lifestyle modification and treatment interventions. The latter, in turn, can be considered as first-line (primary), second-line (secondary) or third-line (tertiary) options. The process of care model (Fig. 43.1) is based on a step-wise approach to disease management and therefore treatment would normally follow the above order.

Epidemiological analysis shows that a number of risk factors and lifestyle issues can contribute to the occurrence of ED. In keeping with a stepwise approach, risk-factor modification may often represent the least minimally invasive and therefore the first approach. In the present era of cost containment, although quantification of risk-factor modification on ED is lacking, good clinical practice mandates that this is an initial focus perhaps in conjunction with more direct (i.e. therapeutic) intervention. By analogy to the general systemic circulation, as the penis is a modified vascular bed, modification of cardiovascular risk factors would represent an obvious starting point; these include hyperlipidaemia and hypertension. Environmental factors such as cigarette smoking and alcohol abuse may also contribute to cardiovascular disease and/or ED. Equally, modification of several other self-destructive behaviours relating to interpartner relationships and sexual behaviours and conflicts may be of benefit. Finally, many patients presenting with ED have a history of prescription and non-prescription drug use and abuse. On this basis, in many instances ED may have an iatrogenic origin. This association is described in more detail elsewhere (Chapter 15). One viable treatment option could involve withdrawal or replacement of existing agents. Obviously, however, caution should be exercised to ensure that primary therapeutic activity is not compromised.

The next level of patient management would involve therapeutic, device or surgical intervention. Three levels of treatment intervention are apparent when stratified on the clinical criteria of: ease of administration, reversibility, invasiveness and cost. Efficacy is an underlying assumption for all interventions designated as first-line (primary), second-line (secondary) and third-line (tertiary).

First-line interventions include oral erectogenic agents (e.g. sildenafil, phentolamine, yohimbine and apomorphine), vacuum erection devices and psychosexual therapy. In addition to meeting the above criteria, the primary interventions all have relatively low risk profiles, which make them particularly important considering the heterogeneity of patients in the primary care setting. Within the primary category, the selection of individual agents or strategies will be dependent on patient profile and need, medical indications and contraindications, as well as cost and reimbursement. In specific instances (e.g. documented endocrine abnormality), hormone replacement therapy may be also considered as first-line therapy.

Second-line treatment interventions are selected on the basis of (a) failure or insufficient response or adverse effects associated with one or more of the above primary therapies, and (b) patient preference. These interventions are based on local (intra-urethral or intracavernosal) delivery of pharmacological agents. In general, vasoactive agents and other agents such as PGEs are employed as monotherapy, in combination or as drug cocktails. Although widely used, drug administration by these routes is subject to more variable efficacy than observed via more conventional routes, high patient discontinuation rates, side effects (local and systemic), concerns regarding long-term safety and trauma, and a moderately high cost.

Although historically the first option, surgical implantation of semi-rigid or inflatable penile prostheses is now considered tertiary intervention. The surgery is highly invasive and is associated with potential complications; it is essentially irreversible and as such is now reserved for select cases of severe, treatment-refractory ED. However, despite these concerns and the high cost, penile prostheses have been associated with a high rate of patient satisfaction in several studies.

In summary, there are several advantages and disadvantages associated with all current treatments of ED. Available treatment options vary widely in the degree of invasiveness, level of efficacy and side effects, patient acceptability and compliance, and cost. Paramount in the selection of treatment modality is patient and partner preference. Ultimately, the long-term success of any therapy is intimately associated with appropriate patient use and compliance and requires sustained monitoring and follow-up by the physician.

■ CONCLUSIONS AND PROSPECTS

It is recognized that the advent of proven effective orally active agents will have a major impact on the treatment of erectile dysfunction. It is likely that many more patients will seek advice (currently 10%). Of these, the majority will present to the primary care physician. In an attempt to legislate for increased demand for diagnosis and management of erectile dysfunction in the primary care setting, the process of care model has been developed as a potential treatment algorithm (Fig. 43.1) as we enter the 21st century. The field of male sexual health is, however, still dynamic and continuously undergoing change. Through time, with the advent of other agents and greater experience of existing agents and a better scientific understanding of erectile dysfunction, other options will become available. However, although the algorithm is derived on the basis of contemporary knowledge, it should provide a framework for eventual incorporation of new treatment modalities.

■ REFERENCES

1. NIH Consensus Conference on Impotence. JAMA 1993; 270: 83–90

2. Krane R J, Goldstein I, Saenz de Tejada I. Impotence. N Engl J Med 1989; 321: 1648–1659

3. Lue T. Impotence: a patient's goal-directed approach to treatment. World J Urol 1990; 8: 67–74

4. Hatzichristou D G, Bertero E B, Goldstein I. Decision making in the evaluation of impotence: the patient profile-oriented algorithm. Sex Disabil 1994; 12: 29–37

5. Korenman S G. Advances in the understanding and management of erectile dysfunction. J Clin Endocrinol Metab 1995; 80: 1985–1988

6. Feldman H A, Goldstein I, Hatzichristou D G et al. Impotence and its medical and psychological correlates: results of the Massachusetts Male Aging Study. J Urol 1994; 151: 54–61

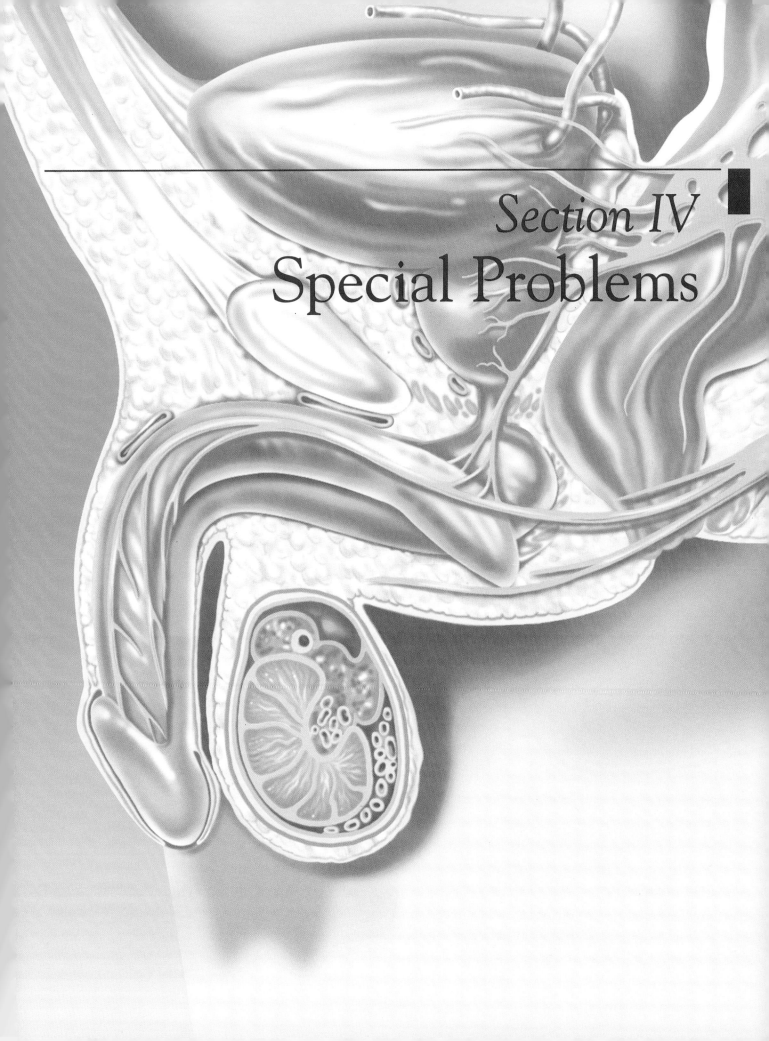

Section IV
Special Problems

Chapter 44

Risks, complications and outcomes of penile lengthening and augmentation procedures

H. Wessells and J. W. McAninch

■ INTRODUCTION

Elongation of the penis has been contemplated since antiquity,[1] but only since 1971 has it been carried out as a reconstructive surgical technique for congenital and acquired shortening of the penis.[2–6] Cosmetic penile enlargement began with girth enhancements in Miami in the late 1980s, but it was the Chinese surgeon Long who in 1990 described division of the suspensory ligament and penile skin advancement as a cosmetic procedure to increase penile length.[7,8] Since then, over 10 000 men have undergone penile lengthening and girth enhancement, although no peer-reviewed paper has reported a reliable description of the techniques or results. The risks, both cosmetic and medical, have never been described by the proponents of the operations, and the complication rate is unknown.[9] Interest in the procedures remains intense,[8] despite action by the California Medical Board against one of the major proponents.[10] A full understanding of penile enlargement is therefore necessary for urologists and plastic surgeons, who may be called upon to treat the complications of these procedures. This chapter reviews the indications, techniques, risks, complications, and results of penile lengthening and girth enhancement, and discusses considerations in the reconstruction of failures.

■ INDICATIONS

Penile lengthening procedures have traditionally been reserved for patients who suffer severe shortening of the penis as a result of epispadias, trauma, Peyronie's disease, or failed penile implant. The definition of micropenis in the neonate is established as greater than 2.5 standard deviations below normal, or 2.5 cm stretched length.[11] In adults, controversy exists as to the definition of a penis small enough for lengthening.[12,13] It is unclear whether the flaccid or erect length is an appropriate guideline, or whether normal men should be considered for the procedure, since even men with the smallest most deformed penises can have appropriate sexual relationships.[14] However, despite such arguments, penile enlargement surgery continues unabated for aesthetic reasons and to improve self-esteem. Anecdotally, most men desire increase in flaccid length and girth, in response to a 'locker room' mentality, but erect length is mentioned as motivation by others.[15,16] It is unlikely that these procedures will go away; rather, with improvements in technique, they may become routine cosmetic surgical procedures.

■ TECHNIQUE

The detail in this section on technique is meant to give the reader enough familiarity with the methods of penile enlargement to allow patient counselling and to guide reconstruction of failed operations. The authors' experience with penile lengthening comes not in physically normal men, but only in those men with traumatic loss of penile length.

Penile lengthening

Early reports of penile lengthening describe division of the suspensory ligament and mobilization of the proximal crura off inferior pubic rami. Because of the risk of injury to the neurovascular structures of the penis, cosmetic surgery for penile lengthening relies on division of the suspensory ligament and skin flap advancement to increase the pendulous penile length. The corpora cavernosa, fused along the distal three-quarters, are attached to the pubic symphysis by the suspensory ligament; this structure, a condensation of Buck's fascia, maintains penile position during coitus.[17]

Division of the ligament can be accomplished through a variety of infrapubic incisions, but the technique is straightforward. By dissecting just below the pubic bone, hugging the periosteum, the relatively broad, dense fibrous tissue can be released while avoiding injury to the cavernous arteries and nerves. The more superficial fundiform ligament is encountered prior to identification of the suspensory ligament, but does not contribute to the position of the penis.

Choice of incision is more important from the perspective of skin flap advancement and wound healing than exposure of the suspensory ligament. Long described an M-shaped skin incision, while Roos developed an inverted V–Y flap for skin advancement, which was 'modified for the Western male' to deal with problems of angulation (Fig. 44.1).[18,19] Rosenstein has the distinction of popularizing the inverted V flap in the United States and with starting the risky but profitable industry of penile enlargements.[8,20] This incision has several drawbacks: these include poor healing at the intersection of the limbs of the inverted Y due to excess tension; advancement of hair-bearing skin onto the shaft, resulting in 'scrotalization' of the penis; and dog-ears on the scrotal margins. Experience in treating complications of the V–Y plasty led Alter to adopt a double-Z plasty to expose the suspensory ligament and advance skin onto the penile shaft without tension (Fig. 44.2).[21] He also advocates the insertion of autologous or synthetic material to fill the dead space created by release of the ligament, preventing re-attachment of the penis in its original location.

Girth enhancement

Enlarging the girth of the penis may be aesthetically desirable if penile length is also increased, thus maintaining the normal aspect ratio of the penis.[22] Two methods have been

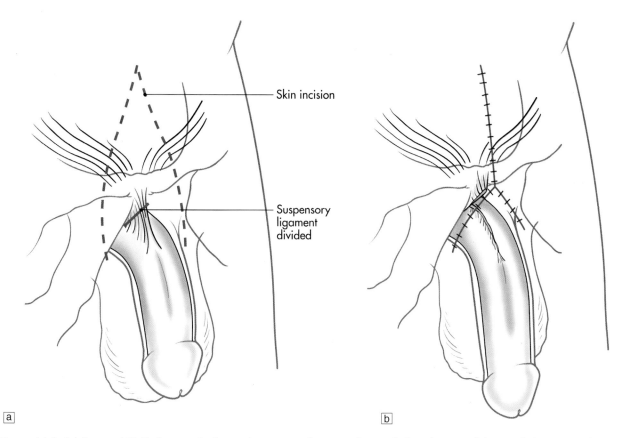

Skin incision

Suspensory ligament divided

[a]

[b]

Figure 44.1. (a) Inverted V–Y plasty and release of suspensory ligament for penile lengthening; (b) intended outcome. (From ref. 9 with permission.)

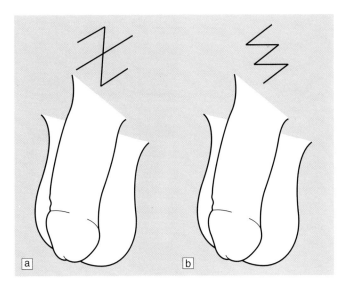

Figure 44.2. Double-Z plasty skin advancement: (a) initial incision; (b) after skin closure.

proposed to enhance penile girth — injection of harvested autologous liposuction specimen and surgical placement of a dermal-fat composite free graft around the penis.

Injection of liposuctioned fat from the abdominal wall or inner thighs was popularized by Rosenstein, but has several potential pitfalls.[20] The harvested fat is injected into the dartos fascia through several small incisions at the base or corona. Distribution of fat may be irregular, or the fat may migrate in the early postoperative period, leading to nodular deposits of fat with resultant penile deformity (see Complications). Human fat grafts lose weight and volume over time, with as little as 10% remaining after 1 year.[23,24] Thus reabsorption of fat is also likely, causing loss of girth and, if not uniform, penile distortion.

In an attempt to provide more uniform and persistent girth augmentation, combined grafts of dermis with attached fat have been placed between the twin graft beds of the dartos fascia and Buck's fascia. The dermal surface of the graft is placed facing up towards the dartos for a smooth contour, and theoretically each side of the graft undergoes neovascularization from its respective fascial covering. Harvest sites for these dermal grafts may be from the groin or bilateral gluteal creases. Grafts of 1.0 cm thickness are considered ideal.[15] The harvesting is more time consuming and requires closure of the donor site, but graft-take and cosmetic appearance are considered to be superior. The graft is sutured at the corona and base of the penis and anchored on either side of the urethra, to avoid a fully circumferential graft that may contract and cause constriction. Placement of the graft may be achieved by inverting the penis through the infrapubic incision used for penile lengthening; if only girth enhancement is desired, a circumferential incision below the corona is sufficient.

THEORETICAL RISKS

No operation is without risk, especially when the technique is not standardized or described in the literature. Within the last year, excellent descriptions of penile enlargement procedures have been published by Alter, which should allow better understanding of the surgery and, it is hoped, reduce the incidence of complications.[15,21] Significant bleeding from the procedure is rare, although in 1992 a Miami lounge singer died after penile enlargement while on anticoagulation.[8] Other potential risks of penile augmentation include infectious complications, downward deflection of the penis due to release of the suspensory ligament,[25] resorption of fat grafts, and injury to the neurovascular bundle with resultant erectile dysfunction or penile numbness. Failure to increase penile length or girth is a notable possibility as well.

ACTUAL COMPLICATIONS

Rosenstein in 1995 reported postoperative problems of pain, discharge, oedema, dehiscence, flap loss, phimosis, paraphimosis and infection. Long-term fat loss and encapsulation were also reported and, in 10% of patients, additional surgery was necessary.[20] Another source of information on complications is reports of patients seen after penile augmentation surgery by other physicians.[9,26] Dissatisfaction with the cosmetic result is the most common complaint and may be due to lengthening or girth augmentation. These cases represent only a small percentage of men who have undergone penile augmentation; the denominator is unknown and thus a verifiable complication rate may never be available.[9]

The most common complaint related to lengthening procedures is scrotalization of the penile shaft, in which the advancement of hair-bearing skin onto the penis after V–Y plasty leads to an undesirable result (Fig. 44.3). The skin advancement can also lead to a picture of phimosis; circumcision should be undertaken with caution, since later reversal of the V–Y plasty may not be possible, owing to lack of shaft skin.[26] A thick, hypertrophic scar, most prominent at the apex of the Y plasty, is another frequent complaint (Fig. 44.4). It is the authors' opinion that this

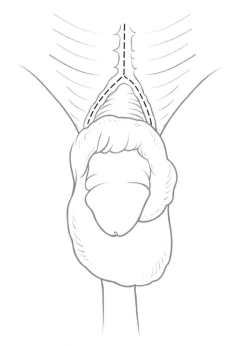

Figure 44.3. Scrotalization of penile shaft skin after penile lengthening via inverted V–Y flap advancement. (From ref. 9 with permission.)

relates to excess tension due to inadequate mobilization of the lateral skin flaps rather than keloid formation. Wound infections requiring hospitalization, abscess formation and wound separation also have been described.

Girth enhancement using autologous fat injection can lead to irregular residual fat nodules that cause patients to seek treatment (Fig. 44.5). Some have undergone repeat 'touch-up' injections in an attempt to smooth the contour. Difficulty with intromission may occur, owing to excessive fat deposits on the shaft, as well as a decrease in shaft sensation over especially large nodules. Complete loss of the graft over time may occur.

Sexual function may be impaired by the development of erectile dysfunction (ED), loss of penile sensation due to neurological injury, painful erections, ventral penile deflection, or failure to address pre-existing ED.[9]

RESULTS

Interpretation of results is difficult, since most practitioners of penile enlargement do not use standardized techniques to measure length before and after surgery. Ideally, flaccid length from penopubic skin to meatus, stretched length, and erect length would be measured by a single observer. Rosenstein reported a mean

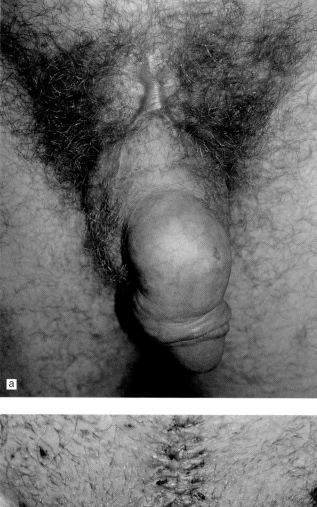

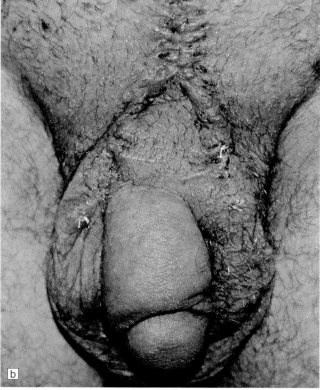

Figure 44.4. Patients with poor cosmetic outcome of skin incision: (a) hypertrophic scar; (b) scrotal dog-ears and scrotalization incompletely reversed by the original surgeon. (From ref. 9 with permission.)

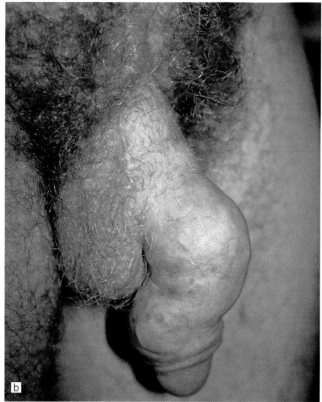

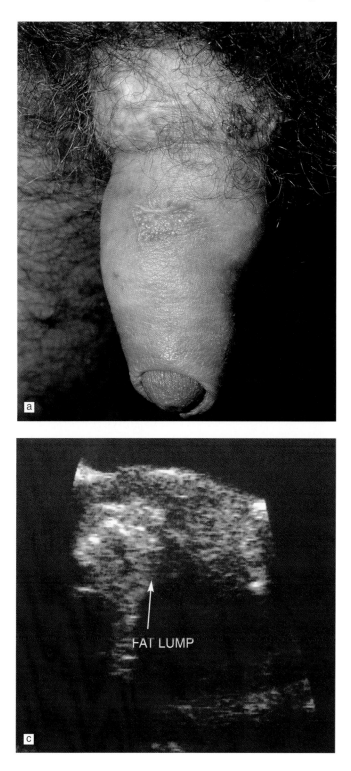

Figure 44.5. Patients with irregular deposition of autologous fat harvested with liposuction and injected into the penis: (a) excessively broad base; (b) nodule of fat due to shifting in early postoperative period; (c) sonographic appearance of fat deposit. (From ref. 9 with permission.)

increase in length of 2.1 inches, but he did not specify whether flaccid or erect and, most importantly, based measurements on photographs of the patients.[20] Long reported a mean increase in length of 3.8 cm, but the measurements were taken in the operating room immediately after surgery, which makes their interpretation suspect. The only reliable English-language report on

penile length after release of the suspensory ligament was a study performed on cadavers: Bondil and Delmas[27] found that division of the suspensory ligament alone increased penile length by 0.5 cm, while addition of a skin advancement increased the gain in length to 1.6 cm.[27]

Division of the suspensory ligament can certainly give the appearance of greater penile length, with more dangle, but the literature does not support these observations with numerical data.[28] Likewise, girth enhancement clearly increases penile circumference, but the exact amount of increase and durability are unproven at the present time. Until a prospective study measuring penile dimensions before and after surgery is completed, it must be concluded that no evidence exists to support claims that penile augmentation is effective. To support the use of these procedures to increase self-esteem, a validated questionnaire should be developed to measure this construct and to show that penile augmentation increases self-esteem in a statistically significant manner.

■ CORRECTION OF COMPLICATIONS

The two main complaints that lead patients to seek reversal of their penile augmentation are scrotalization of the penile shaft and irregular fat deposits. Since 1994, the authors have operated on 20 men to correct these complications, and Alter has reconstructed another 17 men.[26,29] The successful correction of these penile deformities is very challenging, both from a technical point of view and because of the demanding nature of the patient population. These men have suffered disfiguring genital complications from surgery that they themselves requested. As a result, many have to resolve shame, guilt, and self-recrimination before they can seek help. Once it has been determined that the patient desires correction of the deformities, choosing the timing of the procedure becomes one of the key decisions for the surgeon. To avoid tissue ischaemia and flap loss, the authors advise waiting at least 6 months until all the oedema and induration has resolved.

Reversal of the V–Y plasty usually will correct scrotalization of the penis and any dog-ears. Patients should expect to lose any gain in length from the original operation, and if they are not willing to accept this risk the procedure should not be undertaken. Paucity of shaft skin may prevent a complete reversal, but in most men, opening up the full extent of the Y incision allows mobilization and reattachment of the apex of the flap, re-creating the inverted V (Fig. 44.6). If penile deflection or instability has occurred, formal re-attachment of the tunica albuginea to the pubis should be performed with an absorbable suture. When advancing the inferior skin flap back up to the superior aspect of the Y, dermal sutures should be placed from beneath the flap to the pubis or Scarpa's fascia in order to anchor the proximal aspect of the shaft skin, thus re-creating the penopubic skin junction. A multilayer closure and closed suction drainage are recommended.

Resection of irregular fat deposits should not be considered easy, since the fat is extremely adherent to the penile shaft skin. If care is not taken, the penile skin can be devascularized and may slough. Patients should be counselled that it may not be possible to remove all the fat in a single procedure, and that a staged approach may be indicated. If reversal of the V–Y incision is planned, the fat can be removed through that incision

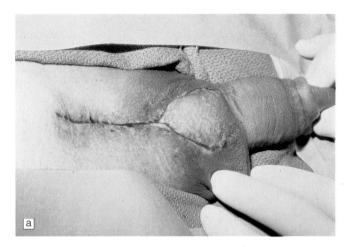

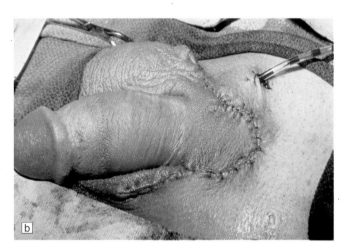

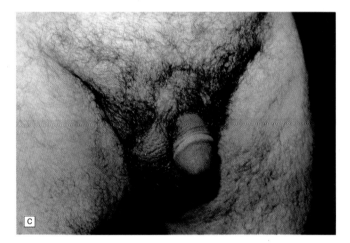

Figure 44.6. Reversal of deformity shown in Figure 44.3. (a) Incision through original scar; (b) re-approximation of apex of flap into a V; (c) final result after 3 months. (From ref. 9 with permission.)

by inverting the penis. When fat excision alone is desired, a distal incision can be performed below the corona: a partial circumference incision may be preferable to retain as much collateral blood supply as possible.

Complications occurred rarely with reversals. Of the authors' 20 patients, one developed a haematoma and another developed significant induration and oedema of the penile skin which took 6 months to resolve, which was attributed to embarrassment of the skin circulation after resection of fat. Alter reported one haematoma and one inadequate reversal in 25 reconstructive operations.[26]

CONCLUSIONS

Penile augmentation techniques have been described in reputable publications, but supporting data to prove the effectiveness of these procedures are lacking. No clear-cut indications have been developed, although guidelines for what is considered a normal adult penile length have been proposed.[13,22] Division of the suspensory ligament is a straightforward technique that has been used along with other methods to increase penile length. Nevertheless, complications from skin advancement manoeuvres are devastating to patients, who expect results without risk. Likewise, girth enhancement can increase circumference, but the simpler technique of autologous fat injection should be considered discredited at the present time. A significantly higher level of skill is needed to perform dermal-fat grafting successfully, and long-term data on this technique are not yet available. Treatment of complications should be undertaken with caution, after allowing the existing wounds to mature, by reversal of the V–Y plasty and resection of aberrant fat deposits.

Penile augmentation is an unregulated cosmetic procedure that is not reimbursed by insurance companies; nevertheless, it must be efficacious if it is to be performed. Comparisons between penile enlargement and breast augmentation are not appropriate, since breast augmentation, for all its potential risks, does increase the size of the breast in a statistically significant fashion. The results of penile lengthening and girth enhancement are unproven, whereas the complications are well described, implying that a risk–benefit analysis cannot be carried out. For these reasons, the authors consider penile augmentation to be still experimental.[30]

REFERENCES

1. Van Gulik R H. Sexual life in Ancient China. Vol. 1. Leiden: Brill, 1974
2. Kelly J H, Eraklis A J. A procedure for lengthening the phallus in boys with exstrophy of the bladder. J Pediatr Surg 1971; 6: 645–649
3. Johnston J H. Lengthening of the congenital and acquired short penis. Br J Urol 1974; 46: 685
4. Horton C E, Dean J A. Reconstruction of traumatically acquired defects of the phallus. World J Surg 1990; 14: 757–762
5. Kabalin J N, Rosen J, Perkash I. Penile advancement and lengthening in spinal cord injury patients with retracted phallus who have failed penile prosthesis placement alone. J Urol 1990; 144: 316–318
6. Rigaud G, Berger R E. Corrective procedures for penile shortening due to Peyronie's disease. J Urol 1995; 153: 368–370
7. Long D C. Elongation of the penis. Chung Hua Cheng Hsing Shao Shang Wai Ko Tsa Chih [Chinese Journal of Plastic Surgery and Burns] 1990; 6: 17–19
8. Bannon L. Growth industry: how a risky surgery became a profit center for some L.A. doctors. Wall St J; 1996: 1
9. Wessells H, Lue T F, McAninch J W. Complications of penile augmentation seen at one referral center. J Urol 1996; 156: 1617–1620
10. Judge halts 'penile enlargements: Culver City plastic surgeon accused of gross negligence. San Francisco Chron 1996: A5
11. Aronson I. Micropenis: medical and surgical implications. J Urol 1995; 155: 4–14
12. Bondil P, Salti A, Sabbagh R et al. Is the erect penile length < 7 cm a reliable guideline for penile lengthening? Int J Impot Res 1995; 7: S58
13. Wessells H, Lue T F, McAninch J W. Penile length in the flaccid and erect length: guidelines for penile lengthening. J Urol 1996; 156: 995–997
14. Woodhouse C R J. The sexual and reproductive consequences of congenital genitourinary anomalies. J Urol 1994; 152: 645–651
15. Alter G J. Penis enhancement. AUA Update Ser XV, 1996.
16. Lue T F. Personal communication, 1995
17. Hinman F Jr. Atlas of urosurgical anatomy. Vol. 1. Philadelphia: Saunders, 1993
18. Roos H, Lissoos I. Penile lengthening. Int J Aesthetic Restorative Surgery 1994; 2: 89
19. Roos H, Constantinides C, Lissoos I. Penis lengthening. Int J Impot Res 1995; 7: S33
20. Rosenstein M. Penile enlargement surgery. Presented at Western Section AUA 71st Ann Meet, Scottsdale, Ariz., USA. November 1995
21. Alter G. Penile enhancement. Adv Urol 1996; 9: 225–254
22. Wessells H, McAninch J W. Penile size: what is normal? Contemp Urol 1997; 9: 85
23. Peer L A. Loss of weight and volume in human fat grafts. Plast Reconstr Surg 1950; 5: 217–230

24. Ersek R A. Transplantation of purified autologous fat: a 3-year follow-up is disappointing. Plast Reconstr Surg 1991; 87: 219

25. Kropman R F, Venema P L, Pelger R C. Traumatic rupture of the suspensory ligament of the penis. Case report. Scand J Urol Nephrol 1993; 27: 123

26. Alter G J. Reconstruction of deformities resulting from penile enlargement surgery. J Urol 1997; 157:(suppl 4): 362

27. Bondil P, Delmas V. Is the section of the suspensory ligament of penis really efficient for penile lengthening? Preliminary results of an anatomical study. Int J Impot Res 1995; 7: S32

28. Jordan G H. Personal communication, 1997

29. McAninch J W. Unpublished data, 1997

30. Sharlip I D. Personal communication, 1995

Chapter 45
Peyronie's disease

D. J. Ralph and J. P. Pryor

■ INTRODUCTION

Peyronie's disease is a benign condition of the penis of unknown aetiology that predominantly afflicts middle-aged men. The disease is characterized by its insidious, and often painful, onset with the formation of fibrous tissue plaques that envelop the cavernous tissues of the penis. There is usually a penile deformity and a subsequent degree of erectile dysfunction. Although first observed in 1561 by Fallopius and Vesalius, it was not until 1743 that the disease was fully described by Francois Gigot de la Peyronie in his paper entitled 'Some Obstacles Preventing the Normal Ejaculation of Semen'.[1]

■ CLINICAL FEATURES

Incidence and age

The apparent increase in the number of men presenting with Peyronie's disease has been confirmed in Rochester although this might reflect a greater readiness of men to seek medical advice.[2] The incidence was found to increase from 4.3 per 100 000 men aged 20–29 years to a peak incidence of 66 per 100 000 men aged 50–59 years. Approximately two-thirds of patients will be between 40 and 60 years with the youngest reported patient being 18 years and the oldest being 80 years.[3,4]

Presenting symptoms

The presenting symptoms of Peyronie's disease are shown below:

1. Presence of a plaque or induration.
2. Penile curvature during erection.
3. Penile pain.
4. Erectile dysfunction.

All patients have either a well-defined plaque or an area of induration that is palpable on physical examination, even though 38–62% of patients are unaware of this.[5–8] The plaque is usually located on the dorsal surface of the penis with a corresponding dorsal penile deformity. Lateral- and ventral-sited plaques are not as common but result in more coital difficulties as there is a greater deviation from the natural coital angle. Multiple plaques located on opposite sides of the penis, or plaques appearing in the pectinate septum, may not cause a penile deformity. Penile pain may be persistent in the inflammatory stage of the disease but is usually present only during erection. The pain is not usually severe but may interfere with sexual function, although spontaneous improvement usually occurs as the inflammation settles.

■ HISTOPATHOLOGICAL REVIEW

In the early stages of Peyronie's disease, an inflammatory infiltrate is present in the vascular loose areolar connective tissue sleeve between the corpus cavernosum and the tunica albuginea[9] (Fig. 45.1). Focal areas of fibrous tissue are laid down in this subtunical layer which is eventually completely replaced by fibrous tissue. The fibrous tissue may, in advanced cases, differentiate and become calcified or ossified.[9,10] The cellular infiltrate consists of T lymphocytes, macrophages and plasma cells surrounding the small vessels in the subtunical layer[6,11] (Fig. 45.2). The cellular infiltration can also be seen extending out into the erectile tissue and the tunica albuginea, with the cells showing evidence of immune activation[11] (Fig. 45.3). The inflammatory infiltrate, with its activated cytokine network, is eventually replaced by hyalinized fibrosis extending from the tunica albuginea into the erectile tissue[12] (Fig. 45.4). The cause of this inflammation is unknown but the finding of fibrin deposition within the

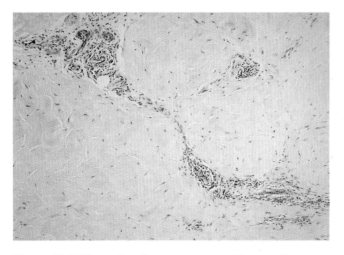

Figure 45.1. The early inflammatory stage of Peyronie's disease. A perivascular inflammatory infiltrate can be seen. (H&E × 100.)

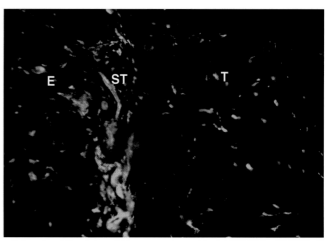

Figure 45.3. Marked cellular immune activation in early Peyronie's disease. The inflammation extends from the tunica (T) into the erectile tissue (E) but is maximal in the subtunical space (ST). (Immunofluorescence for HLA class-2 expression, magnification × 100.)

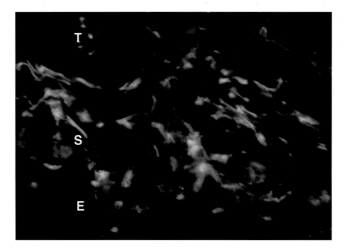

Figure 45.2. The inflammatory infiltrate shown to be maximal in the subtunical space surrounding the small vessel vasculature: T, tunica albuginea; S, subtunical space; E, erectile tissue. (Double immunofluorescence, macrophages green, endothelium red.)

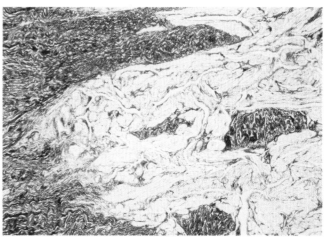

Figure 45.4. Long-standing Peyronie's disease. Section shows extension of fibrous plaque into erectile tissue.

plaque in 95% of cases may suggest a microvascular injury as a cause of the initial inflammation.[13]

Calcification of the Peyronie's plaque occurs adjacent to vascular areas and can occur in 30% of patients (Fig. 45.5). These patients tend to be young and have severe disease.[14] Osteoblasts have also been found near the endothelial cells involved.[15] Cell culture studies of the Peyronie's plaque have shown that the normal cellular process of contact inhibition is lost, allowing the cells to grow in a random criss-cross fashion.[16] These cells also tend to have an abnormal chromosomal content in 60% of cases, although this may be

a result of the disease and not a cause of it.[17] Although an increased amount of actin has been found in the plaque tissue, myofibroblasts responsible for contraction have not been identified.[16,18] Within the plaque itself there are disordered collagen and elastic fibres,[19] and these have also been shown to occur in the tunica not directly affected by the Peyronie's plaque.[20] Collagen abnormalities have also been found during the progression of the disease, with excessive immature collagen deposition, predominately type III, in the tunica albuginea with elastogenesis between the collagen bundles.[21,22] Electron microscopy has demonstrated endothelial disruption with the presence of electron-dense material being engulfed by mast cells and macrophages, with a few Gram-negative bacilli found in the tunica.[18]

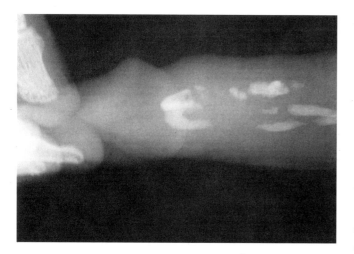

Figure 45.5. Plain radiograph showing that there is a calcification associated with Peyronie's disease.

■ AETIOLOGY

Peyronie was the first to report a suggested aetiology for the disease in 1743.[1] He considered that the disease was caused by a combination of frequent chronic irritation induced by sexual abuse, the venereal diseases gonorrhoea and syphilis, and tuberculosis also being a contributing factor. Many other theories have subsequently been suggested and are discussed in turn below.

Trauma
The initial theory, of repeated minor sexual trauma, is today still considered the most likely cause of the disease. Furey expressed the opinion that rupture of small vessels caused small haematomas which were then replaced by fibrous tissue, this being more common in ageing connective tissue.[23] This is supported by the finding of fibrin within 18 of 19 plaques that were biopsied but not in control tunica,[24] indicating microvascular injury. In addition, the dorsal and ventral stresses that are more common during sexual activity would account for the usual dorsal position of the plaque following hyperextension injuries that result in minor tears of the tunica albuginea.[25,26] It is also known that in ageing tunica albuginea there is a reduced elastic fibre content and this has also been found in patients with Peyronie's disease.[27,28]

Smith puts the case for a relation between the repeated minor sexual trauma of coitus and the development of penile fibrotic plaques, on more scientific grounds. He performed a histological study on 100 penises obtained at autopsy: in 23 of the penises there was a mild inflammatory change in the loose areolar connective tissue sleeve and in several there was fibrosis forming nodular areas, both features compatible with the recognized histology of Peyronie's disease. There was no common denominator in these 23 men in terms of admitting illness, cause of death or autopsy findings, and to find Peyronie's disease in such a large percentage of men was suggestive of a simple common aetiological factor.[29]

However, despite this evidence, the majority of patients do not give a history of sexual trauma. Trauma occurred in only nine of 250 patients examined by Chesney and in 4–11% in other series.[5,6,9,10] In the largest series of 408 patients, 21.5% gave a history of trauma although only 6.4% sustained this during sexual intercourse.[4]

Although acute penile injuries may result in plaques indistinguishable from those of Peyronie's disease, experimental trauma of dogs' penises did not cause a condition similar to Peyronie's disease.[30,31] If trauma is an aetiological factor, it is unlikely to be the sole factor involved, as the expected incidence of Peyronie's disease would be much higher than is currently recorded. It has therefore been suggested that the patients must also have an inherited predisposition for the disease.[25]

Genetic predisposition
Evidence to suggest that there is a genetic predisposition for Peyronie's disease has been gathered. A family history of Peyronie's disease may be expected in 2% of patients[4] and there is a significant association with Dupuytren's palmar fibromatosis (a disease with a known inherited autosomal dominant trait) in 16–20% of patients.[4,6,32] Other studies have shown associations with certain tissue types — HLA-B27,[33] HLA-A1 and HLA-DQw2,[34] and HLA-DQ5.[35] The combination of these findings with the discovery of anti-elastin antibodies in the sera of patients with Peyronie's disease,[36] and features of cell-mediated immunity within the Peyronie's tissue,[37] may indicate an underlying autoimmune basis for the disease.

Infection
Peyronie first suggested that venereal disease was a contributory factor to the disease, but there has been no support for this theory in any modern series. Electron-microscopic studies of the plaque have revealed the presence of a few Gram-negative bacilli within the

tunica,[18] and Smith found bacteria in the peri-urethral glands in seven of 23 cases examined histologically.[29] Urine and urethral cultures are usually negative and, despite an extensive search for an infective agent, including cultures and bacterial antibodies, no infective cause has been found.[6,33] The connection between urethral manipulation and Peyronie's disease is unclear. In two series, 9% of patients gave a history of urethral instrumentation including urethral catheterization, dilatation, cystoscopy and transurethral resection of the prostate.[4,6] As the plaques were not in an expected ventral position and 10% of patients undergoing urethroscopy did not have any urethral abnormality, it is difficult to see how the urethra can play a role in the pathological process.[6]

Arterial disease

The incidence of arterial disease in Peyronie's disease is 30%, and of diabetes with associated small vessel disease is 2.7–12% in patients with Peyronie's disease.[4] Premature atherosclerosis has been proposed as a factor that initiates the vasculitis that occurs in the initial stages of the disease,[29] and others have suggested that the premature ageing of the vascular connective tissue is more susceptible to repeated minor trauma.[38] Patients with retroperitoneal fibrosis secondary to periaortitis have been shown to have circulating antibodies to ceroid, an oxidized lipid found in atherosclerotic plaques.[39] These antibodies are present only when there is a breach of the media, thereby exposing the atheromatous material to the adventitia. This may explain the associated atherosclerosis, trauma and the inflammation that occurs in the initial stages of Peyronie's disease.

■ INVESTIGATIONS

The majority of patients with Peyronie's disease may be managed without investigation. Patients usually give an accurate description of their deformity to within 10–20 degrees and it is, therefore, often unnecessary to obtain clinical confirmation of this, either with a photograph or an intracavernosal injection of a vasoactive agent.[40–42]

When the site and size of the Peyronie's plaque needs to be assessed, ultrasound usually will suffice[43] (Fig. 45.6). For visualization of the detailed anatomy prior to surgical intervention in extensive Peyronie's disease, contrast-

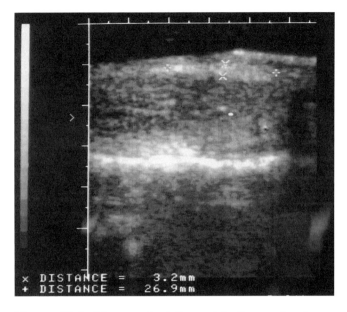

Figure 45.6. Ultrasound of Peyronie's disease showing a dorsally sited plaque.

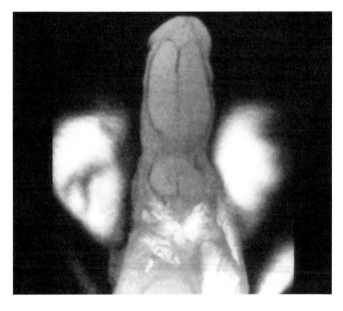

Figure 45.7. Magnetic resonance image of Peyronie's plaque in body of penis.

enhanced magnetic resonance imaging is the investigation of choice[44] (Fig. 45.7).

In patients who also complain of an impaired erection, further evaluation is essential and this should be with a combination of colour Doppler ultrasound and dynamic infusion cavernosometry[40,45] (Fig. 45.8).

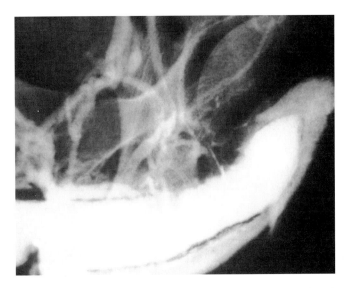

Figure 45.8. Cavernosogram showing extensive dorsal Peyronie's plaque with site-specific venous leak.

■ ERECTILE DYSFUNCTION IN PEYRONIE'S DISEASE

The reported incidence of erectile dysfunction in Peyronie's disease is variable. Bystrom and Rubio reported that 52% of 106 patients had coital difficulties and 17% had poor penile rigidity distal to the plaque.[6] However, only 8% of patients described coital difficulties at the initial presentation, suggesting that this was probably a late feature of the disease. Stecker and Devine found abnormal nocturnal penile tumescence in 29% of patients with Peyronie's disease with suspected organic impotence, although in only 5% of patients could the Peyronie's disease plaque have been the sole cause of the dysfunction.[46] Other series have reported an incidence of erectile dysfunction (ED) of 19%.[8] Amin discovered that, of 208 patients investigated routinely by colour Doppler ultrasound for ED, 20% had undiagnosed Peyronie's disease.[47] It is clear, therefore, that ED in Peyronie's disease is common and is usually due to one of four factors, as follows:[48]

1. *Psychological (performance anxiety)*. The physical abnormality of the penis can cause anxiety that may be severe enough to interfere with the ability to obtain or maintain an erection.
2. *Deformity preventing coitus*. The penile deformity may be so severe that penetration is made difficult or even impossible. This is more likely to occur if the deformity is in a ventral or lateral direction, where

deviation from the normal angle of vaginal entry is maximal. The pain that is sometimes experienced in Peyronie's disease may also interfere with the erectile capacity.

3. *Flail penis*. There is a small group of patients with extensive Peyronie's disease who also have cavernosal fibrosis. Tumescence is absent from this segment and, if extensive, may result in an unstable penis.
4. *Impaired erection*. It is often difficult to decipher the cause of the impaired erectile capacity. It may be due to concomitant vascular disease, which occurs in 30% of patients with Peyronie's disease,[4] or to veno-occlusive dysfunction (VOD).[49,50] Most studies have used both colour Doppler ultrasound and cavernosometry to investigate the impaired erection in Peyronie's disease. Lopez showed that, of 76 patients, 36% had arterial disease and 59% had VOD.[51] Others have also suggested there is a mixture of arteriogenic and venogenic factors.[52,53] It is thought that the venous leakage may occur through the emissary veins that pass through the Peyronie's plaque into the dorsal vein of the penis.[51] The reduced compliance of the tunica albuginea of the plaque prevents the normal compression of these veins during rigidity and therefore does not inhibit the venous flow. This site-specific VOD has also been found in 15 of 19 patients with an impaired erection secondary to trauma, one of the suggested aetiological factors in Peyronie's disease.[54]

The finding that there is reduced elastic fibre content of the tunica and an increased type III collagen content also supports the finding that Peyronie's disease is associated with VOD, as these pathological abnormalities can also be seen in patients with VOD disease without Peyronie's disease.[22,27]

Patients may present with only a flaccid distal portion of the penis or a soft glans penis, the proximal segment being normal. There is controversy as to the mechanism of this, be it arterial, venous or fibrotic in nature. One study has shown that this feature is likely to be of mixed pathology, in that patients are likely to have extensive cavernosal fibrosis that impedes the distal arterial flow as measured on colour Doppler ultrasound.[4] This would be supported by the fact that the inflammation in the early stage of Peyronie's disease and the fibrosis in the latter stages can extend into the erectile tissue.[11] Patients with a soft glans only are likely to have extensive dorsal plaques, with interference of the dorsal neurovascular bundle.[4]

■ MANAGEMENT

The treatment of Peyronie's disease can be based only on the knowledge of its natural history. A recent questionnaire sent to 98 patients with Peyronie's disease revealed that 42% had progression of their disease, predominately an increased penile curvature. Only 13% of patients thought that their condition had improved and 45% thought that the condition had remained stable from the time of initial presentation.[60] Many patients have little in the way of symptoms, and reassurance — particularly that the palpable lump is not cancer — is all that is necessary. Treatment is indicated only when penile pain — an indication of early disease — or deformity is troublesome.

Conservative treatment

As the aetiology of the inflammatory infiltrate in Peyronie's disease remains obscure, it is not surprising that many treatment options have been tried for this condition[3,14,56–76] (Table 45.1). Current options include tamoxifen, which has been shown to affect the secretion of transforming growth factor beta from human fibroblasts in vitro and should inhibit the inflammatory response.[77] Some improvement has been shown in 20 of 36 patients (55%) treated with tamoxifen, 20 mg b.d. for 3 months. Patients with early disease were more likely to respond and, in those with biopsy-confirmed inflammation, three-quarters had an excellent response.

Colchicine may decrease collagen synthesis and induce collagenase and was found to be useful in fibromatosis.[78] In a series of 24 men with Peyronie's disease, it was found to produce an improvement in plaque size in 12 and an improvement in pain in seven of the nine patients where this symptom was present.[81] Gelbert and colleagues[79] injected collagenase directly into the Peyronie's plaque and, in a prospective double-blind randomized controlled trial in 49 men, found a significant benefit over placebo, although there was little improvement in the erectile deformity. Levine and colleagues[75] injected the calcium-channel-blocking agent verapamil into the plaque on the basis that calcium-channel blockers alter the metabolism of fibroblasts to inhibit collagen formation. In a study of 14 men, 12 completed the 6 month course of treatment: the pain improved in ten of the 11 men in whom it was present and the deformity improved in five (42%). The improvement in pain always has to be observed against the natural history of the disease.

Duncan and colleagues[80] showed that interferons alpha, beta and gamma are all capable, during culture in vitro, of inhibiting fibroblast proliferation and collagen production as well as increasing the production of collagenase by Peyronie's tissue. Benson[73] reported favourable clinical results but in another study there was improvement in only one of 25 patients.[81]

The new methods of treatment all attempt to interfere with fibroblast activity and might be expected to be useful during the early stages of disease. Their efficacy has to be seen against the natural history of the disease and the knowledge that discomfort on erection rarely persists beyond 6 months.[55,82] Vitamin E is the traditional treatment of choice for Peyronie's disease: it is easy to take, cheap, free of side effects and better than placebo for treating the pain.[83] Para-aminobenzoate (Potaba) is more expensive, is unpleasant to take, has more side effects and needs to be taken for 12 months.[84,85] This allows time for the disease to stabilize and patients with persisting symptoms may then be candidates for surgery. Beneficial results of low-dosage radiotherapy are still being reported,[86,87] but it is probably best avoided in men under the age of 60 years as it has also been reported as the cause of extensive penile fibrosis.[88]

Surgical management

The surgical management of Peyronie's disease consists of either correction of the penile deformity, once the disease is fully stable, or the insertion of a penile prosthesis in those patients who have a concomitant impaired erection. The various operations are discussed below but, in general terms, the choice rests between a Nesbit-type procedure, the implantation of a penile prosthesis or, possibly, in the much-shortened penis, a Lue procedure. It is meddlesome to operate just because there is a lump or a minor erectile deformity.

Plaque excision and dermal graft

The surgical management of Peyronie's disease was unsuccessful until Devine and Horton[89] in the United States and Bystrom and colleagues[90] in Scandinavia described the operation of plaque excision and dermal graft replacement of the defect in the tunica albuginea. Bystrom and colleagues[91] reported that, despite good initial results, the late results were disappointing, with only six of 17 men having a good result after 10 years. Personal experience,[92] and a subsequent review of the literature,[93] confirmed that many patients had poor

Table 45.1. The non-surgical treatment of Peyronie's disease

Therapy	Author	Date
Mercury + mineral water	de la Peyronie[1]	1743
Potassium iodide	Ricord*	1844
Electricity	Van Buren*	1864
Bromides + hyperthermia	Hodgen*	1876
Sulphur	Dubuc*	1890
Copper sulphate	O'Zoux*	1896
Salicylates + thiosinamin	Sachs*	1901
Arsenic	Passover*	1902
Fibrolysin	Mendel*	1907
Ionization	Lavenant*	1910
Milk	Van der Pool*	1911
X-radiation	Lavenant*	1911
Ultraviolet light	LeFur*	1912
Trypsin injection	Sonntag*	1922
Radium	Kumer	1922
Diathermy	Wesson[56]	1943
Vitamin E	Scardino and Scott[57]	1949
Cortisone injection	Teasley[58]	1954
Hyaluronidase + steroid injection	Bodner et al.[59]	1954
Potassium *para*-aminobenzoate	Zarafonetis and Horrax[60]	1959
Histamine iontophoresis	Whalen[61]	1960
Prednisolone	Chesney[62]	1963
Ultrasound	Heslop et al.[63]	1967
Dimethyl sulphoxide	Persky and Stewart[64]	1967
Steroid iontophoresis	Rothfeld and Murray[65]	1967
Procarbazine	Aboulker and Benassayag[66]	1970
Parathyroid hormone injection	Morales and Bruce[67]	1975
Orgotein	Bartsch et al.[68]	1981
β-Aminopropionitrile	Gelbard et al.[69]	1983
Collagenase injection	Gelbard et al.[14]	1985
Laser ablation	Puente de la Vega et al.[70]	1985
Prostacyclin	Strachan and Pryor[71]	1988
Lithotripsy	Bellorofonte et al.[72]	1989
Interferon α2b	Benson et al.[73]	1991
Tamoxifen	Ralph et al.[74]	1992
Verapamil	Levine et al.[75]	1994
Colchicine	Akkus et al.[76]	1994

*Cited in ref. 3.

results with this operation. This has been confirmed in a recent large series of 418 men treated by plaque excision and a dermal graft operation.[94] It was found that 17% of patients required further surgery for curvature and that 20% of patients had significant impairment of erection. ED following plaque excision is due to a combination of factors, including damage to the underlying erectile tissue adherent to the plaque, loss of compliance of the dermal graft, new venous channels forming to give VOD[95] and a deterioration of the underlying aetiological factors. It is now recognized that the histological changes of Peyronie's disease are not confined to the plaque but may also be seen in the normal tunica albuginea excised during the Nesbit procedure.[20,28] It is for these reasons that the authors consider plaque excision and grafting to be an obsolete operation.

The Nesbit procedure

Reed Nesbit[96] described the correction of erectile deformities due to congenital abnormalities by shortening the opposite side of the penis using plication or the excision of an ellipse of tunica albuginea. The technique was applied to Peyronie's disease with good initial success[92] and, in 359 men operated upon between 1977 and 1992, 295 (82%) had good results and were able to have intercourse.[97] Operative treatment is performed only when the disease has stabilized — usually at least a year after its onset — and when the deformity makes intercourse difficult or impossible.

The operation is performed through a circumglandular incision — circumcising the man if necessary in order to prevent a secondary phimosis. An artificial erection is induced by injecting saline from a rapid transfusion apparatus and no tourniquet is used, as it sometimes makes for inaccurate assessment of the bend (Fig. 45.9). It is also essential to observe the bend at the time of full erection, otherwise the deformity may be underestimated. The site of maximum bend is marked with a stay suture. Buck's fascia is incised longitudinally and dissected medially to bare the tunica albuginea. This technique permits elevation of the corpus spongiosum ventrally, or the dorsal vascular bundle and the nerves, without appreciable damage (Fig. 45.10). The Nesbit ellipse is marked out opposite the site of maximum deformity and, for every 10 degrees of bend, the ellipse is 1 mm wide (Fig. 45.11). In a retrospective study it was found that the mean width of the ellipse was 7 mm and the angle of deformity was 68 degrees.[97] When in doubt, it is possible to apply two Alliss

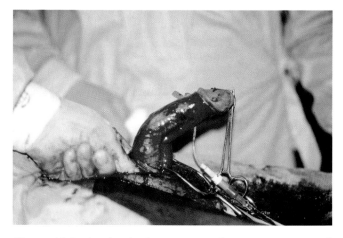

Figure 45.9. Artificial saline erection demonstrating ventral deformity due to Peyronie's disease.

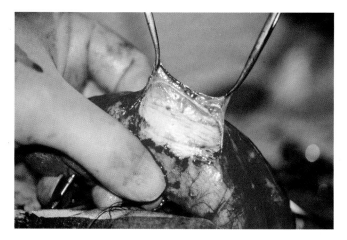

Figure 45.10. Buck's fascia completely elevated to enable mobilization of either the urethra or dorsal neurovascular bundle.

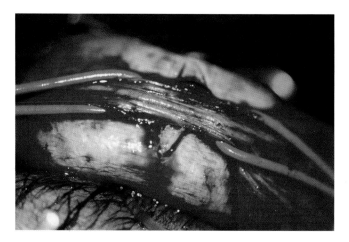

Figure 45.11. The dorsal neurovascular bundle has been mobilized and a Nesbit ellipse marked.

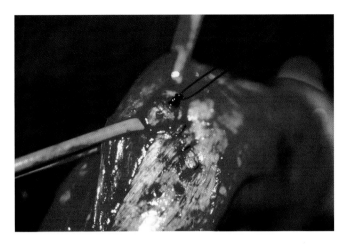

Figure 45.12. The ellipse is closed with interrupted 0 PDS suture, knots buried.

Table 45.2. Results of Nesbit procedure for Peyronie's disease

Result	Year 1977–1984	Year 1985–1992	Total
Excellent	101 (58)*	136 (73)	237 (66)
Satisfactory	27 (16)	31 (17)	58 (16)
Poor	46 (26)	18 (10)	64 (18)
No. of men	174	185	359

*Percentages in parentheses.

forceps to the tunica albuginea (when the penis is flaccid) and then inflate the penis to check the correction. The ellipse is excised with minimum disturbance to the underlying muscle of the corpus cavernosum and the defect closed with 0 PDS sutures with the knots on the inside (Fig. 45.12). Finally, an artificial erection is induced to check that the penis has been straightened.

The results of the Nesbit technique are very satisfactory (Table 45.2). Some of the poor initial results in the period 1977–1983 have been eliminated by preoperative assessment with intracavernous drugs, either alone or combined with colour Doppler ultrasound examination.[98] A literature review has confirmed the favourable results,[93] as have more recent studies.[99,100]

A variety of corporoplasties that may be regarded as variants of the Nesbit procedure have been introduced and these usually give good results.[101–105] Some authors favour a simple plication technique,[106,107] but the problem with this procedure is that the correction is dependent upon the strength of the suture material, and this probably accounts for the unfavourable results of some authors[100] and the late failure in others (as high as 24% in one series).[107]

The alleged drawback of the Nesbit procedure is penile shortening. In Peyronie's disease the penis is shortened by scar tissue and the operation straightens the penis by shortening the unaffected side. In reality, the shortening is rarely troublesome and was only more than 2 cm in 17 of 359 men and intercourse was possible in 15 of these.[20] The past 5 years have seen attempts to lengthen the penis by incising the fibrous plaque[108–116] (Fig. 45.13; Table 45.3) and covering the defect with a

Table 45.3. Plaque incision and graft replacement of the tunica albuginea in the surgical treatment of Peyronie's disease

First author	Year	No. of men	Graft technique
Sampaio[108]	1992	7	Dura
Brock[109]	1993	18	Vein
Faerber[110]	1993	9	Dacron
Moriel[111]	1994	10	Vein
Ganabathi[112]	1995	16	Gore-Tex
Gelbard[113]	1995	30	Temporalis fascia
Kim[114]	1995	7	Laser and vein
Krishnamurti[115]	1995	17	Pedicled dermal flap
Rigaud[116]	1995	5	Dermal graft

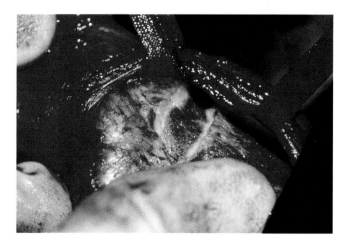

Figure 45.13. Following mobilization of the neurovascular bundle the Peyronie's plaque is incised to gain extra length.

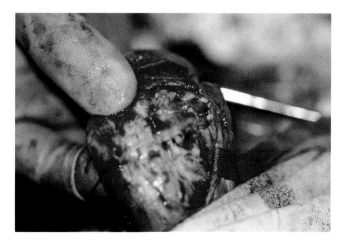

Figure 45.14. Following plaque incision, the defect is covered with a long saphenous vein graft.

graft that does not contract. Dorsal penile, or saphenous vein graft (Fig. 45.14) would seem to be the simplest but, in the uncircumcised man, the pedicle dermal graft of Krishnamurti[115] is a good alternative. These procedures would seem to have a role to play in those men with an already shortened penis, but longer-term follow-up is still required. Early recurrence of deformity after the Nesbit procedure is due to the sutures cutting out, whereas poor results stemming from the use of absorbable sutures occur after 3 months. Recurrent deformity due to progression of the disease is not usually apparent for 9–15 months.

Implantation of a penile prosthesis
In those men where there is an appreciable element of vasculogenic impotence, it is sensible to implant a penile

prosthesis. These have always given excellent results,[93] provided that the men have a realistic expectation from the operation. The plaque may cause some narrowing of the corpus cavernosal space but this seldom makes for difficulties. A malleable prosthesis usually corrects the deformity but with an inflatable prosthesis it may be necessary to incise the plaque. Operative moulding of the penis[117] over a prosthesis may look and sound horrible but gives a good result in correcting any deformity. The mechanical reliability of modern multipart inflatable prostheses has improved so much that failure is now more likely to be due to surgical error.[118]

■ CONCLUSIONS

The aetiology of Peyronie's disease is unknown, corresponding to the poor results of its medical management in the early stage. In the majority of patients reassurance is all that is necessary, and surgery should be reserved for those patients in whom the deformity interferes with sexual function. It is imperative to investigate patients who also have an impaired erection, as these patients should undergo insertion of a penile prosthesis. In the future, with the increased knowledge obtained from basic scientific research in understanding the possible aetiology and disease mechanism, the medical management should be improved, with fewer patients needing surgery.

■ REFERENCES

1. de la Peyronie F. Sur quelques obstacles qui s'opposent a l'éjaculation naturelle de la semence. Mem Acad R Chir 1743; 1: 425

2. Lindsay M B, Schain D M, Grambsch P et al. The incidence of Peyronie's disease in Rochester, Minnesota, 1950 through 1984. J Urol 1991; 146: 1007–1009

3. Poley H J. Induratio penis plastica. Urol Cut Rev 1928; 32: 287–308

4. Chilton C P, Castle W M, Westwood C A, Pryor J P. Factors associated in the aetiology of Peyronie's disease. Br J Urol 1982; 54: 748–750

5. Burford C E, Glen J E, Burford E H. Fibrous cavernositis: further observation with report of 31 additional cases. J Urol 1943; 49: 350–356

6. Bystrom J, Rubio C. Induratio Penis Plastica: clinical features and aetiology. Scand J Urol Nephrol 1976; 10: 12–20

7. Williams G, Green N A. The non-surgical treatment of Peyronie's disease. Br J Urol 1980; 52: 392–395

8. Furlow W L, Swenson H E, Lee R E. Peyronie's disease: a study of its natural history and treatment with orthovoltage radiotherapy. J Urol 1975; 114: 69–71

9. Smith B H. Peyronie's disease. Am J Clin Pathol 1966; 45: 670–678

10. Chesney J. Peyronie's disease. Br J Urol 1975; 47: 209–218

11. Ralph D J, Mirakian R, Pryor J P, Bottazzo G F. The immunological features of Peyronie's disease. J Urol 1996; 155: 159–162

12. Davis C J Jr. The microscopic pathology of Peyronie's disease. J Urol 1997; 157: 282–284

13. Somers K D, Dawson D M. Fibrin deposition in Peyronie's disease plaque. J Urol 1997; 157: 311–315

14. Gelbard M K, Lindner A, Kaufman J. The use of collagenase in the treatment of Peyronie's disease. J Urol 1985; 134: 280–283

15. Vandeberg J S, Devine C J, Horton C E et al. Mechanisms of calcification in Peyronie's disease. J Urol 1982; 127: 52–54

16. Somers K D, Dawson D M, Wright G L et al. Cell culture of Peyronie's disease plaque and normal penile tissue. J Urol 1982; 127: 585–588

17. Somers K D, Winters B A, Dawson D M et al. Chromosomal abnormalities in Peyronie's disease. J Urol 1987; 137: 672–675

18. Vandeberg J S, Devine C J, Horton C E et al. Peyronie's disease: an electron microscopic study. J Urol 1981; 126: 333–336

19. Brock G, Hsu G L, Nunes L et al. The anatomy of the tunica albuginea in the normal penis and Peyronie's disease. J Urol 1997; 157: 276–281

20. Anafarta K, Beduk Y, Uluoglu O et al. The significance of histopathological changes of the normal tunica albuginea in Peyronie's disease. Int Urol Nephrol 1994; 26: 71–77

21. Somers K D, Sismour E N, Wright G L et al. Isolation and characterization of collagen in Peyronie's disease. J Urol 1989; 141: 629–631

22. Chiang P H, Chiang C P, Shen M R et al. Study of the changes in collagen of the tunica albuginea in venogenic impotence and Peyronie's disease. Eur Urol 1992; 21: 48–51

23. Furey C A. Peyronie's disease: treatment by the local injection of meticortelone and hydrocortisone. J Urol 1957; 77: 251–266

24. Somers K D, Dawson D M. Fibrin deposition in Peyronie's disease plaque. J Urol 1997; 157: 311–315

25. Hinman F. Etiologic factors in Peyronie's disease. Urol Int 1980; 35: 407–413

26. Devine C J Jr, Somers K D, Jordan S G, Schlossberg S M. Proposal: trauma as the cause of the Peyronie's lesion. J Urol 1997; 157: 285–290

27. Akkus E, Carrier S, Baba K et al. Structural abnormalities in the tunica albuginea of the penis: impact of Peyronie's disease, ageing and impotence. Br J Urol 1997; 79: 47–53

28. Iacono F, Barra S, De Rosa G et al. Microstructural disorders of tunica albuginea in patients affected by Peyronie's disease with or without erectile dysfunction. J Urol 1993; 150: 1806–1809

29. Smith B H. Subclinical Peyronie's disease. Am J Clin Pathol 1969; 52: 385–390

30. Pryor J P, Hill J T, Packham D A, Yates-Bell A J. Penile injuries with particular reference to injury to the erectile tissue. Br J Urol 1981; 53: 42–46

31. Horton C E, Devine C J. Peyronie's disease. Plast Reconstr Surg 1973; 52: 503–510

32. Ling R S M. The genetic factor in Dupuytren's disease. J Bone Joint Surg (UK) 1963; 45: 709–718

33. Ralph D J. Schwartz G, Moore W et al. The genetic and bacteriological aspects of Peyronie's disease. J Urol 1997; 157: 291–294

34. Rompel R, Weidner W, Mueller-Eckhardt G. HLA association of idiopathic Peyronie's disease: an indication of autoimmune phenomena in etiopathogenesis? Tissue Antigens 1991; 38: 104–106

35. Nachtsheim D A, Rearden A. Peyronie's disease is associated with an HLA class II antigen HLA-DQ5, implying an autoimmune etiology. J Urol 1996; 156: 1330–1334

36. Stewart S, Malto M, Sandberg L, Colburn K K. Increased serum levels of anti-elastin antibodies in patients with Peyronie's disease. J Urol 1994; 152: 105–106

37. Ralph D J, Mirakian R, Pryor J P, Bottazzo G F. The immunological features of Peyronie's disease. J Urol 1996; 155: 159–162

38. Desanctis P N, Furey C A. Steroid injection therapy for Peyronie's disease: a 10 year summary and review of 38 cases. J Urol 1967; 97: 114–116

39. Parums D V, Brown D L, Mitchinson M J. Serum antibodies to oxidized low-density lipoprotein and ceroid in chronic periaortitis. Arch Pathol Lab Med 1990; 114: 383–387

40. Ralph D J, Hughes T, Lees W R, Pryor J P. Pre-operative assessment of Peyronie's disease using colour Doppler sonography. Br J Urol 1992; 69: 629–632

41. Kelami A. Classification of congenital and acquired penile deviation. Urol Int 1983; 38: 229–233

42. Desai K M, Gingell J C. Out-patient assessment of penile curvature. Br J Urol 1987; 60: 470–471

43. Hamm B, Friedrich M, Kelami A. Ultrasound imaging in Peyronie's disease. Urology 1986; 6: 540–545

44. Helweg G, Judmaier W, Buckberger W et al. Peyronie's disease: MR findings in 28 patients. AJR 1992; 158: 1261–1264

45. Jordan G H, Angermeier K W. Preoperative evaluation of erectile function with dynamic infusion cavernosometry/cavernosography in patients undergoing surgery for Peyronie's disease: correlation with postoperative results. J Urol 1993; 150: 1138–1142

46. Stecker J F, Devine C J. Evaluation of erectile dysfunction in patients with Peyronie's disease. J Urol 1984; 132: 680–681

47. Amin Z, Patel U, Friedman E P et al. Colour Doppler and duplex ultrasound assessment of Peyronie's disease in impotent men. Br J Radiol 1993; 66: 398–402

48. Pryor J P. Peyronie's disease and impotence. Acta Urol Belg 1988; 56: 317–321

49. Metz P, Ebbehoj J, Uhrenholdt A, Wagner G. Peyronie's disease and erectile failure. J Urol 1983; 130: 1103–1104

50. Gasior B L, Levine F J, Howannesian A et al. Plaque-associated corporal veno-occlusive dysfunction in idiopathic Peyronie's disease: a pharmacocavernosometric and pharmacocavernosographic study. World J Urol 1990; 8: 90–96

51. Lopez J A, Jarow J P. Penile vascular evaluation of men with Peyronie's disease. J Urol 1993; 149: 53–55

52. Montorsi F, Guazzoni G, Bergamaschi F et al. Vascular abnormalities in Peyronie's disease: the role of colour Doppler sonography. J Urol 1994; 151: 373–375

53. Levine L A, Coogan C L. Penile vascular assessment using color duplex sonography in men with Peyronie's disease. J Urol 1996; 155: 1270–1273

54. Penson D F, Seftel A D, Krane R J et al. The hemodynamic pathophysiology of impotence following blunt trauma to the erect penis. J Urol 1992; 148: 1171–1180

55. Gelbard M K, Dorey F, James K. The natural history of Peyronie's disease. J Urol 1990; 144: 1376–1379

56. Wesson M B. Peyronie's disease, causes and treatment. J Urol 1943; 49: 350–356

57. Scardino P L, Scott W W. The use of tocopherols in the treatment of Peyronie's disease. Ann N Y Acad Sci 1949; 52: 390–396

58. Teasley G H. Peyronie's disease: a new approach. J Urol 1954; 71: 611–614

59. Bodner H, Howard A H, Kaplan J H. Peyronie's disease: cortisone–hyaluronidase–hydrocortisone therapy. J Urol 1954; 72: 400–403

60. Zarafonetis C J D, Horrax T M. Treatment of Peyronie's disease with potassium para-aminobenzoate (POTABA). J Urol 1959; 81: 770–772

61. Whalen W H. A new concept in the treatment of Peyronie's disease. J Urol 1960; 83: 851–852

62. Chesney J. Plastic induration of the penis: Peyronie's disease. Br J Urol 1963; 35: 61–66

63. Heslop R W, Oakland D J, Maddox B T. Ultrasonic therapy in Peyronie's disease. Br J Urol 1967; 39: 415–418

64. Persky L, Stewart B H. The use of dimethyl sulfoxide in the treatment of genitourinary disorders. Ann N Y Acad Sci 1967; 141: 551–554

65. Rothfeld S H, Murray W. The treatment of Peyronie's disease by iontophoresis of C21 esterified glucocorticoids. J Urol 1967; 97: 874–875

66. Aboulker P, Benassayag E. Traitement de l'induration plastique des corps caverneux par la procarbazine (Natulan). J Urol (Paris) 1970; 76: 499–503

67. Morales A, Bruce A W. The treatment of Peyronie's disease with parathyroid hormone. J Urol 1975; 114: 901–902

68. Bartsch G, Menander-Huber K B, Huber W, Marberger H. Orgotein: a new drug for the treatment of Peyronie's disease. Eur J Rheumatol Inflamm 1981; 4: 250–259

69. Gelbard M K, Lindner A, Chvapil M, Kaufman J. Topical beta-aminopropionitrile in the treatment of Peyronie's disease. J Urol 1983; 129: 746–748

70. Puente de la Vega A, Calvo-Mateo M A, Domenech M S. Laser therapy in Peyronie's disease. Actas Urol Esp 1985; 9: 107–108

71. Strachan J R, Pryor J P. Prostacyclin in the treatment of painful Peyronie's disease. Br J Urol 1988; 61: 516–517

72. Bellorofonte C, Ruoppolo M, Tura M et al. Possibility of using piezoelectric lithotriptor in the treatment of severe cavernous fibrosis. Arch Ital Urol Nefrol Androl 1989; 61: 417–422

73. Benson R C Jr, Knoll L D, Furlow W L. Interferon-α2b in the treatment of Peyronie's disease. J Urol 1991; 145(suppl): 1342 (abstr)

74. Ralph D J, Brooks M S, Bottazzo G F, Pryor J P. The treatment of Peyronie's disease with tamoxifen. Br J Urol 1992; 70: 648–651

75. Levine L A, Merrick P F, Lee R C. Intralesional verapamil injection for the treatment of Peyronie's disease. J Urol 1994; 151: 1522–1524

76. Akkus E, Carrier S, Rehman J et al. Is colchicine effective in Peyronie's disease? A pilot study. Urology 1994; 44: 291–295

77. Colletta A A, Wakefield L M, Howell F V et al. Venogenic impotence following dermal graft repair for Peyronie's disease. J Urol 1990; 146: 849–851

78. Dominguez-Malagon H R, Alfeiran-Ruiz A, Chavanna-Xicotencatl P. Clinical and cellular effects of colchicine in fibromatosis. Cancer 1992; 69: 2478–2483

79. Gelbard M K, Jones K, Raich P, Dovey F. Collagenase versus placebo in the treatment of Peyronie's disease: a double blind study. J Urol 1993; 149: 56–58

80. Duncan M R, Berman B, Nseyo U O. Resolution of the proliferation and biosynthetic activities of cultured human Peyronie's disease fibroblasts by interferon-alpha, -beta and -gamma. Scand J Urol Nephrol 1991; 25: 89–94

81. Wegner H E H, Andresen R, Knipsel H H, Miller L. Local interferon alpha 2b is not an effective treatment in early stage Peyronie's disease. Eur Urol 1997; 32: 190–193

82. Williams J L, Thomas C G. The natural history of Peyronie's disease. Br J Urol 1970; 103: 75–76

83. Pryor J P, Farell C F. Controlled clinical trial of vitamin E in Peyronie's disease. Prog Reprod Biol 1983; 9: 41–45

84. Shah P J R, Green N A, Adib R S et al. A multicentre double-blind controlled clinical trial of potassium para-aminobenzoate (Potaba) in Peyronie's disease. Prog Reprod Biol 1983; 9: 47–60

85. Ludwig G. Evaluation of conservative therapeutic approaches to Peyronie's disease (fibrotic induration of the penis). Urol Int 1991; 47: 236–239

86. Rodrigues C I, Njo K H, Karim A M. Results of radiotherapy and vitamin E in treatment of Peyronie's disease. Int J Radiat Oncol Biol Phys 1995; 31: 571–576

87. Viljoen I M, Goedhals L, Dom M J. Peyronie's disease: a perspective on the disease and the long term results of radiotherapy. S Afr Med J 1993; 83: 19–20

88. Hall S J, Basile G, Bertero E B et al. Extensive corporeal fibrosis after penile irradiation. J Urol 1995; 153: 372–377

89. Devine C J, Horton C E. Surgical treatment of Peyronie's disease with a dermal graft. J Urol 1974; 111: 44

90. Bystrom J, Johansson B, Edsmyr F, Körlof B, Nylén B. Induratio penis plastica (Peyronie's disease): the results of the various forms of treatment. Scand J Urol Nephrol 1972; 6: 1–5

91. Bystrom J, Alfthan O, Gustafson H, Johansson B. Early and late results after excision and dermo-fat grafting for Peyronie's disease. Prog Reprod Biol 1972; 9: 78–84

92. Pryor J P, Fitzpatrick J M. A new approach to the correction of the penile deformity in Peyronie's disease. J Urol 1979; 122: 622–623

93. Pryor J P. Peyronie's disease. In: Hendry W F (ed) Recent advances in urology, Vol 4. London: Churchill Livingstone, 1987: 245–261

94. Austoni E, Colombo F, Mantovani F et al. Chirurgia radicale e conservazione dell'erezione nella malattia di La Peyronie. Arch Ital Urol Nefrol Androl 1995; 67: 359–364

95. Dalkin B L, Carter M F. Venogenic impotence following dermal graft repair for Peyronie's disease. J Urol 1991; 146: 849–851

96. Nesbit R H. Congenital curvature of the phallus: report of three cases with description of corrective operation. J Urol 1965; 93: 230

97. Ralph D J, Al-Akraa M, Pryor J P. The Nesbit operation for Peyronie's disease: 16-year experience. J Urol 1995; 154: 1362–1363

98. Ralph D J, Hughes T, Lees W R, Pryor J P. Pre-operative assessment of Peyronie's disease using colour Doppler sonography. Br J Urol 1992; 69: 629–632

99. Sulaiman M N, Gingell J C. Nesbit's procedure for penile curvature. J Androl 1994; suppl: 545–565

100. Poulsen J, Kirkeby H J. Treatment of penile curvature — a retrospective study of 175 patients operated upon with plication of the tunica albuginea or with the Nesbit procedure. Br J Urol 1995; 75: 370–374

101. Yachia D. Modified corporoplasty for the treatment of penile curvature. J Urol 1990; 143: 80–82

102. Saissine A M, Wespes E, Schulman C C. Modified corporoplasty for penile curvature: 10 years experience. Urology 1994; 44: 419–421

103. Geertsen U A, Brok K E, Andersen B, Nielsen H V. Peyronie curvature treated by plication of the penile fasciae. Br J Urol 1996; 77: 733–735

104. Licht M R, Lewis R W. Modified Nesbit procedure for the treatment of Peyronie's disease: a comparative outcome analysis. J Urol 1997; 158: 460–463

105. Rehman J, Benet A, Minsky L S, Melman A. Results of surgical treatment for abnormal penile curvature: Peyronie's disease and congenital deviation by a modified Nesbit plication (tunica shaving and plication). J Urol 1997; 157: 1288–1291

106. Klevmark B, Andersen M, Schultz A, Talseth T. Congenital and acquired curvature of the penis treated surgically by the plication of tunica albuginea. Br J Urol 1994; 74: 501–506

107. Nooter R I, Bosch J L H R, Schrøder F H. Peyronie's disease and penile curvature: long-term results of operative treatment with the plication procedure. Br J Urol 1994; 74: 497–500

108. Sampaio J S, Passarinho A, Olivera A G et al. Surgical correction of severe Peyronie's disease with plaque excision. Eur Urol 1992; 22: 130–133

109. Brock G, Kadioglu A, Lue T F. Peyronie's disease: a modified treatment. Urology 1993; 42: 300–304

110. Faerber G J, Konnak J W. Results of combined Nesbit penile plication with plaque incision and placement of dacron patch in patients with severe Peyronie's disease. J Urol 1993; 149: 1319–1320

111. Moriel E Z, Grinwald A, Rajfer J. Vein grafting of tunical incisions combined with contralateral plication treatment of penile curvature. Urology 1994; 43: 697–701

112. Ganabathi K, Dinochowski R, Zimmera P E, Leach G E. Peyronie's disease: surgical treatment based on penile rigidity. J Urol 1995; 153: 662–666

113. Gelbard M K. Relaxing incisions in the correction of penile deformity due to Peyronie's disease. J Urol 1995; 154: 1457–1460

114. Kim E D, McVany K T. Long-term follow-up of treatment of Peyronie's disease with plaque incision, carbon dioxide laser plaque ablation and placement of a deep dorsal vein patch graft. J Urol 1995; 153: 1543–1546

115. Krishnamurti S. Penile dermal flap for defect reconstruction in Peyronie's disease: operative technique and four years' experience in 17 patients. Int J Impot Res 1995; 7: 195–208

116. Rigaud G, Berger R E. Corrective procedures for penile shortening due to Peyronie's disease. J Urol 1995; 153: 368–370

117. Wilson S K, Delk J R. A new treatment for Peyronie's disease: modelling the penis over an inflatable prosthesis. J Urol 1994; 152: 1121–1123

118. Wilson S K, Cleves M, Delk J R. Long term results with Hydroflex and Dynaflex prostheses: device survival and comparison to multicomponent inflatables. J Urol 1996; 155: 1621–1623

Chapter 46
Priapism

S. Serels and A. Melman

■ INTRODUCTION

Normal physiology of erection

The penile corpora are specialized vascular beds of endothelial-lined sinusoidal spaces supported by a framework of smooth muscle, collagen, nerves and nutritive arterioles and capillaries. Normal erectile function is a complex interaction of both the nervous and vascular systems. In order to understand the vascular component of erections, it is necessary first to understand the vascular anatomy.

The arterial supply to the penis is from the internal pudendal artery, a branch of the internal iliac artery. This artery trifurcates into the dorsal artery, the cavernous arteries and the artery of the bulb/urethra. The cavernous artery enters the hilum of the penis where the two crura merge. The cavernous artery lies close to the septum at the penile base and becomes more centrally located in the mid and distal penis. Throughout the course of the penile portion of the corpora cavernosa, the cavernous arteries give off helicine arterial branches that supply the trabecular erectile tissue and sinusoids. The crural sinusoidal spaces are fed by retrograde flow from the more distal helicine branches. The urethral artery supplies branches to the corpus spongiosum and the glans penis, while the bulbar artery supplies the bulbar urethra as well as the bulbospongiosum muscle. The dorsal artery, which lies under Buck's fascia, also supplies the glans penis.

The venous drainage originates from the small venules that originate inside the trabeculae between the tunica and peripheral sinusoids. The venous blood then exits the tunica albuginea via the emissary veins and returns to the circulation by two main channels — the cavernous vein and the deep dorsal vein. The cavernous veins are primarily responsible for the drainage of the corpus cavernosum. The deep dorsal vein drains the glans penis and the corpus cavernosum. The bulbar vein drains the corpus spongiosum. Subsequently, the deep dorsal, cavernous and bulbar veins drain into the periprostatic plexus. The superficial dorsal vein is another large venous channel, which, unlike the deep dorsal vein, travels above Buck's fascia. This vein drains the prepuce and skin of the penis before emptying into the lesser saphenous vein.

How does the vascular anatomy relate to the vascular and neurological events that occur in the penis? Regarding the vascular component of erection, it can be considered in two parts — one active and one passive. The active vascular component involves relaxation of the smooth muscle, which results in increased compliance of the sinusoids and arterial wall as well as dilatation of the arterioles and arteries. As a result of the arterial engorgement that occurs with smooth muscle dilatation, three passive components occur: (1) trapping of incoming blood by expanding sinusoids; (2) compressing of the subtunical venular plexuses in the trabeculae between the tunica albuginea and the peripheral sinusoids, which reduces venous outflow, and (3) stretching of the tunica albuginea to its capacity, which encloses the emissary veins between the tunical layer and decreases the venous outflow.

Thus, in the flaccid state, the helicine arteries are contracted and tortuous. At this time the blood is shunted to the trabecular framework, and the blood flow to the entire penis is 3–5 ml/min. Only a small fraction of that flow enters the sinusoidal spaces; the remainder percolates through the trabeculae and nourishes its tissues. Furthermore, despite the fact that the metabolic rate of the corporal smooth muscle has not been reported, the penis is an external organ with a lower-than-central body temperature and therefore its energy needs can be met at very low blood flow rates. During sexual excitement, the helicine arteries dilate and straighten, which in turn allows

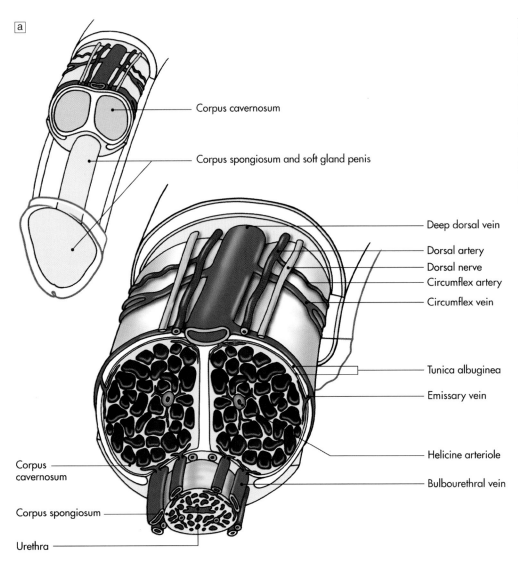

Corpus cavernosum

Corpus spongiosum and soft gland penis

Deep dorsal vein

Dorsal artery

Dorsal nerve

Circumflex artery

Circumflex vein

Tunica albuginea

Emissary vein

Helicine arteriole

Bulbourethral vein

Corpus cavernosum

Corpus spongiosum

Urethra

Figure 46.1. Low- and high-flow priapism models. (a) An example of low-flow priapism (100% rigidity). The emissary veins and circumflex veins are being occluded by the engorged corpus cavernosal tissue while the corpus spongiosum and glans are not involved. The dark blood represents the deoxygenated state.

blood to enter directly into the sinusoidal spaces. At that time, there is a five- to tenfold increase in blood flow to the penis. Blood aspirated by needle from the sinusoidal spaces during normal erection has a PO_2 of approximately 40 mmHg, a PCO_2 of 40 mmHg, and a pH of 7.4.

The innervation to the penis triggers the relaxation of the arterial smooth muscle. The cavernosal nerves arise from the pelvic ganglionic plexus, which is found in the retroperitoneum adjacent to the rectum. The plexus is composed of parasympathetic nerves arising from S2–S4, as well as a sympathetic contribution from the hypogastric plexus. The parasympathetic nerves were historically thought to be responsible for tumescence whereas the sympathetic system facilitated detumescence. However,

there is now known to be involvement of non-adrenergic, non-cholinergic (NANC) nerves, which also are responsible for relaxation of the arterial and cavernosal smooth muscle. These NANC nerves stimulate release of vasodilating neurotransmitters such as nitric oxide, which relaxes smooth muscle via an increase in cyclic guanosine monophosphate (cGMP).[1,2]

Definition and description of priapism

Priapism is a word that was modified from the Greek god Priapus, who was a symbol of bountiful agriculture and hunting. Statues of Priapus always show him in the erect state, which has been transposed to the urologic entity that is described as a prolonged, painful, penile erection

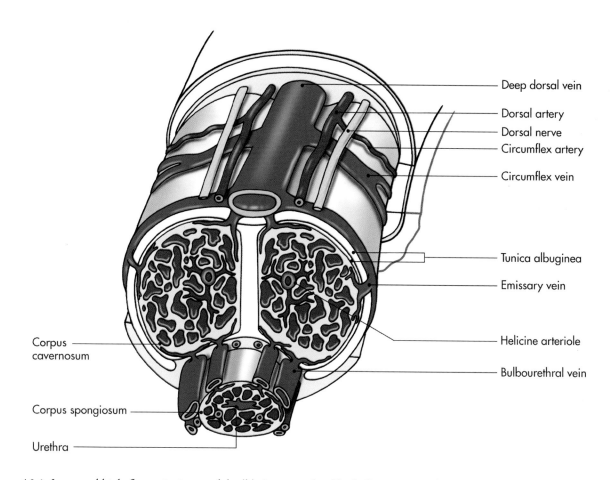

b

Deep dorsal vein

Dorsal artery

Dorsal nerve

Circumflex artery

Circumflex vein

Tunica albuginea

Emissary vein

Helicine arteriole

Bulbourethral vein

Corpus cavernosum

Corpus spongiosum

Urethra

Figure 46.1. Low- and high-flow priapism models. (b) An example of high-flow priapism (<100% rigidity). In this state, the blood flows in and out at extremely high rates. The bright blood filling the sinusoids represents the oxygenated state.

that fails to subside despite orgasm. An erection lasting longer than 4–6 hours is considered to be priapic; nevertheless, pain does not usually ensue until 6–8 hours have elapsed. Priapism is considered to be a failure of the detumescence mechanism, which may be due to excess release of contractile neurotransmitters, obstruction of draining venules, malfunction of the intrinsic detumescence mechanism, or prolonged relaxation of intracavernosal smooth muscle.

There are essentially two main types of priapism — high flow (non-ischaemic) and low flow (ischaemic). Low-flow priapism is the more common form of priapism. It is associated with a decrease in venous outflow and vascular stasis, which, in turn, cause tissue hypoxia and acidosis. This form of priapism is usually quite painful because of tissue ischaemia, and penile blood aspirated from the cavernous spaces appears dark in colour. The causes of low flow are multiple and are discussed below. Low-flow priapism generally affects the corpora cavernosa

with preservation of blood flow in the glans and corpus spongiosum; however, tricorporal priapism has been described in sickle-cell patients.[3,4] Tricorporal priapism is believed to start in a similar manner to bicorporal priapism: the sickle red cells adhere to the endothelial cells lining the vascular bed; however, with time and continued stasis, permanent vaso-occlusion occurs. It is further hypothesized that the urethral/bulbar artery may also become obstructed and in turn lead to corpus spongiosum involvement.

High-flow priapism is usually due to trauma, although on rare occasions it has been idiopathic or due to sickle-cell disease. The hallmark of this type of priapism is an increase in arterial inflow in the setting of a normal venous outflow. Aspirated penile blood is noted to be bright and has a high Po_2. This form of priapism is not usually painful and is non-ischaemic. Figure 46.1 shows diagrammatically the differences between high- and low-flow priapism.

CLASSIFICATION OF LOW-FLOW PRIAPISM

Haematologic/thrombotic causes

Sickle-cell patients commonly have episodes of priapism because of the sickled red blood cells impeding the outflow of penile blood. Two recent retrospective studies showed that 38–42% of men with sickle-cell disease have at least one episode of priapism in their lifetime.[5,6] Approximately 23% of adult cases and as many as 63% of paediatric priapism are a result of sickle-cell disease.[7] However, not all episodes of priapism are severe enough to result in the patient seeking medical attention. Furthermore, though this is normally a low-flow priapism, there have been several reports of high-flow priapism in sickle-cell patients for unknown reasons.[7,8] It has been hypothesized that high-flow sickle priapism may result from a failure of autonomic regulation.[9] Figure 46.2 shows normal cavernosal histology compared with tissue from a man with sickle-cell priapism. In the early phase of sickle-cell priapism, sickled blood cells are seen in the cavernosal sinuses. With continued hypoxia, the endothelial and smooth muscle cells of the corpus cavernosum become hypoxic and eventually die. The corpora cavernosa are then replaced with collagen, as shown in Figure 46.2(e–f).

Leukaemia is the cause of less than 1% of all priapism. This form of priapism is most commonly seen with chronic granulocytic leukaemia. Patients with this type of leukaemia have a 50% chance of having priapism; fortunately, chronic granulocytic leukaemia accounts for only 5% of paediatric leukaemias.[10,11] The aetiology of this type of priapism is not known, but it is hypothesized that leukaemia may result in hyperviscosity and sludging due to the increased number of white blood cells.

Total parenteral nutrition that contains 20% fat emulsion has also been noted to cause priapism. It is thought that this occurs owing to an increase in blood coagulation.[12,14] This increased coagulation may be due to a distortion in erythrocyte morphology, which, in turn, results in an increase in adhesiveness. There are others who believe that priapism in this setting is simply due to embolization of fat.[13,14]

Oral medications

There is a well-known association between certain medications and priapism. The most common medications are antidepressant, antipsychotic and antihypertensive medications. Trazodone is the antidepressant that causes priapism most often. The mechanism is thought to be secondary to alpha-adrenergic blockage. Chlorpromazine (a phenothiazine) and clozapine (an atypical antipsychotic) have been reported to cause priapism.[15] Several antihypertensives, such as hydralazine, prazosin and guanethidine, have been associated with priapism.[7,16,17] Furthermore, heparin and cocaine abuse, although less frequent, have also been reported to cause priapism.[18–20]

Intracavernous injection therapy

Intracavernous injection therapy has been used for the treatment of erectile dysfunction since 1982, when Virag introduced papaverine as a means of inducing erections.[21] Excessive dosage of intracavernous agents can result in priapism, and today it is the most common cause of this problem. The incidence of priapism appears to be less with prostaglandin E1 than with papaverine alone or in combination. The lower incidence of priapism with prostaglandin E1 is thought to be due to the presence of enzymes in the penile tissue that metabolize prostaglandin E1.[22] Lomas and Jarow investigated risk factors that would predispose patients to priapism after using intracavernous therapy. They concluded that patients with neurogenic or psychogenic impotency were at greater risk for priapism than those with vasculogenic impotence; furthermore, those with coronary artery disease were found to have a lower risk of priapism.[23] Nevertheless, all impotent patients are potentially at risk of pharmacologically induced priapism.

Metastatic lesions

Common primary cancers that can metastasize to the penis and result in priapism are those of the bladder (30%), prostate (30%), rectosigmoid (16%), and renal (11%).[24] This phenomenon is believed to be due to an obstruction of the venous outflow by the tumour and should always be considered as a possible cause of priapism in an individual with a history of carcinoma.

Neurological

Individuals who have suffered spinal cord injuries, especially high cord lesions, are also prone to experience priapism.[25] This form of priapism is usually self-limiting and does not require intervention. In addition, Baba and colleagues have reported on several cases of intermittent priapism associated with spinal stenosis.[26,27]

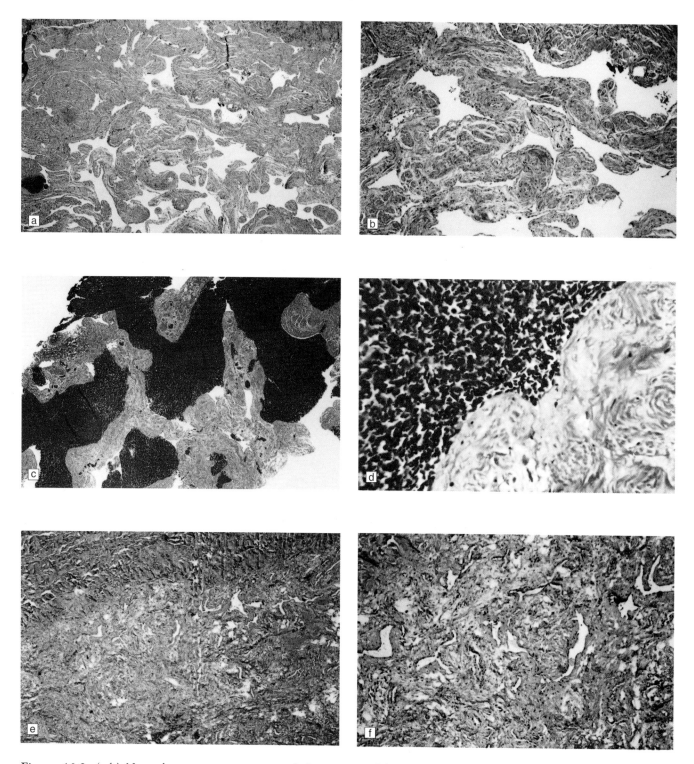

Figure 46.2. (a,b) Normal corpus cavernosum with large sinusoidal spaces (a, ×4 magnification; b, ×10 magnification.); (c,d) sickle-cell corpus cavernosum in acute phase of low-flow priapism. Note the sickle-shaped cells, which engorge the sinusoids. (c, ×4 magnification; d, ×40 magnification.); (e,f) sickle-cell corpus cavernosum after multiple episodes of low-flow priapism. Note the obliteration of the sinusoidal spaces and the replacement of the smooth muscle cells with collagen. (e, ×4 magnification; f, ×10 magnification.)

Idiopathic

Of all priapism events, 30–50% are considered idiopathic.[28] Most of these events are considered to be low flow. Many interesting associations have been described: in two recent case reports, priapism was described to occur in patients who were asplenic;[29,30] in addition, there was a reported case of priapism in a 12-year-old with *Mycoplasma pneumoniae*, which was hypothesized to be due to a hypercoagulable state induced by the infection.[31] Furthermore, there are a number of other diseases that have been associated with priapism but in which no clear aetiology has been identified, and therefore the occurrence of priapism in these settings may be coincidental.[32]

CLASSIFICATION OF HIGH-FLOW PRIAPISM

The most common cause of high-flow priapism is penile or perineal trauma that results in a cavernosal artery to corporal tissue fistula.[33–35] Figure 46.3 shows angiographic examples of cavernous artery fistulae that resulted in high-flow priapism. Furthermore, there are several reports of idiopathic high-flow priapism,[9,36–38] and, as mentioned

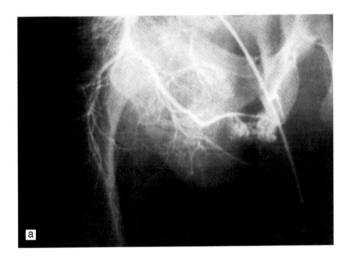

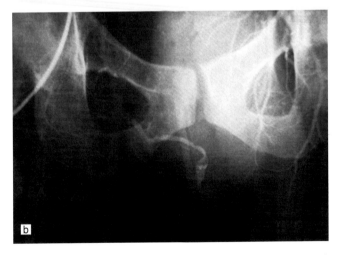

Figure 46.3. (a, b) Angiographic demonstration of cavernosal artery to corporal tissue fistulae resulting in high-flow priapism.

previously, there are a few cases of high flow in association with sickle-cell disease in the absence of trauma. The term high-flow priapism, although identified in case reports as early as the 1960s, was not clearly defined until 1983 by Hauri and colleagues.[9] This entity is due to an increase in arterial flow that is not regulated by the helicine arteries and does not activate the veno-occlusive mechanism; thus, blood flows in and out at extremely fast rates. There is a paucity of reported cases of documented high-flow priapism. Bastuba in 1994 commented that there are only 16 cases of angiographically proven high-flow priapism, which supports the rarity of this entity.[34]

EVALUATION OF PRIAPISM

As with any patient evaluation, a good history is needed to identify any previous conditions, drug use, or recent trauma. The physical examination is also essential. It is through the examination that one may find an abdominal mass, enlarged lymph nodes, or signs of trauma. It is also important to note that, in a low-flow priapism, the glans penis is usually soft whereas the corpora cavernosa are 100% rigid. In contrast, high-flow priapism usually causes 60–100% rigidity.[35] In addition, laboratory tests such as a complete blood count and perhaps a sickle-cell preparation or electrophoresis should be performed where applicable. In order to distinguish high- from low-flow priapism, aspiration of the corpora cavernosa can also be performed and the aspirate sent for blood gas analysis as well as visual inspection. Blood gas values of pH<7.25, Po_2<30, and Pco_2>60 have been suggested to represent ischaemic or low-flow states.[39] Furthermore, Doppler evaluation can be helpful in confirming high-flow priapism by showing increased arterial flow in one or both cavernous arteries.[40,41] In addition, angiography can be performed to establish the diagnosis of high-flow priapism, but is not essential.

THERAPY FOR LOW-FLOW PRIAPISM

In low-flow priapism, it is important to treat the patient expeditiously by increasing the outflow of cavernous blood. In just 24 hours, endothelial and trabecular destruction have occurred, and by 48 hours, widespread smooth muscle necrosis has taken place.[42] The natural sequel of untreated ischaemic priapism is impotence. The treatment of this type of priapism depends on the aetiology. Priapism that is caused by metastatic disease is usually indicative of advanced disease as well as a short life expectancy and is therefore treated expectantly. If leukaemia is the cause of priapism, chemotherapy and/or radiotherapy is recommended.

Sickle-cell priapism is usually treated with medical therapy. The mainstay of therapy is hydration, alkalinization, analgesia and hypertransfusions. The use of hypertransfusion is performed so as to increase the haemoglobin concentration to more than 10 mg/dl and reduce the haemoglobin S to less than 30%. If these conservative measures are ineffective, then corporal aspiration and instillation of alpha-adrenergic agents can be attempted. The use of surgery is considered to be a last resort and is rarely used. Some believe that the conservative measures work better in high-flow states than in low flow because irreversible ischaemia is not occurring. In addition, if tricorporal priapism exists, the type of shunt procedure is severely limited, as is discussed later in this chapter. In a recent review by Miller et al., of 400 paediatric patients with sickle-cell priapism with an age range of 5–19 years, only eight sought medical evaluation for priapism; four of the eight were noted to have low-flow priapism. Two of the four patients had resolution of their priapism with conservative measures, whereas the other two required surgery. Of the four patients with high-flow priapism, three improved with conservative therapy.[43] Virag and colleagues described the use of an oral alpha-adrenergic agent, etilefrine, as a preventive measure in association with intracorporal injection therapy for acute episodes.[44] There is also a case

report of hydralazine being used to treat sickle-cell priapism, although this therapy requires further investigation.[45]

For all other types of low-flow priapism, it is acceptable to try corporal aspiration of blood with irrigation with non-heparinized saline as a first-line therapy. If the priapism still persists, the corpora can be irrigated out with an alpha agonist. Most urologists prefer to use phenylephrine at a dose of 100–200 μg. This dose can be repeated several times at approximately 5 min intervals. Phenylephrine is a relatively pure alpha-1-adrenergic agonist with minimal beta-adrenergic activity. Other agents that can be used are adrenaline, noradrenaline, ephedrine and metaraminol. All these agents should be used with careful patient monitoring, especially if the patient has a previous cardiovascular condition. The use of metaraminol at present has been almost abandoned, owing to a reported death from this agent.[39] Table 46.1 summarizes the preparation of dilutions of alpha-adrenergic agonists that are useful for the treatment of priapism (Table 46.1).

Oral and parenteral medications have been tried to treat low-flow priapism. Terbutaline, a beta-2-adrenergic agonist, has been used to treat priapism.[46,47] Beta-2 agonists normally relax smooth muscle, which would, if anything, perpetuate priapism; thus, terbutaline may have some alpha contractile activity or perhaps some central nervous system activity that enables it to be effective. Alternatively, a recent study by Govier and colleagues[48] failed to show a benefit of terbutaline over placebo, although reports of an earlier study by Lowe and Jarow did show it to be effective.[46] Stilboestrol and gonadotrophin-releasing hormone (GnRH) analogues have been tried for the treatment of sickle-cell priapism.[49,50] Steinberg and Eyre

Table 46.1. Alpha-adrenergic agonists for the treatment of priapism

Drug	Dosage (Intermittent injection)	Alpha-adrenergic activity	Beta 1-adrenergic activity	Beta 2-adrenergic activity
Ephedrine	50–100 mg	+	++	++
Adrenaline	10–20 μg	+++	+++	+++
Metaraminol	2–4 mg	++	+	+
Phenylephrine	100–200 μg (10 dose max.)	+++	–	–
Noradrenaline	10–20 μg	+++	++	++

have reported on the use of adrenaline self-injection therapy in association with monthly intramuscular GnRH to treat sickle-cell priapism.[51] Ironically, GnRH has also been associated with priapism.[52] Glycopyrrolate was reported to reduce intra-operative priapism and may be considered useful when cardiovascular stability is desired, and/or the use of alpha agonists is prohibited.[53] Thus, the exact roles of oral and parenteral drug therapy for priapism have yet to be completely determined, but studies are ongoing.

Surgical therapy is always an option if all attempts at conservative treatment have failed. The goal of surgical therapy is to provide a shunt between the corpus cavernosum and either the glans penis, the corpus spongiosum, or a vein, so as to bypass the obstructed veno-occlusive mechanism. This can be performed by a variety of methods,[54–58] as shown in Table 46.2.

The cavernoglanular shunts are usually the first shunts performed, owing to their technical ease and low morbidity. If these shunts fail, then the Quakles shunt is attempted. This shunt should be performed as proximally as possible, where the corpus spongiosum is thickest, to avoid injuring the urethra. The Grayhack and the cavernopenile dorsal vein shunts are more difficult technically and have been associated with pulmonary emboli; therefore, these two shunts are usually not performed. However; for tricorporal sickle-cell priapism that is refractory to conservative therapy, one of the latter two shunt types might be considered.

The problem with surgical therapy is that there is a high rate of impotence (approx. 50%),[59] and, for this reason, it is used only after conservative methods have failed. Furthermore, if impotence occurs from events of priapism, it is an extremely difficult problem to treat because of the considerable fibrosis that ensues. The patient in this circumstance is best treated with a prosthesis, and even the type of prosthesis is limited by this disease. It has been recommended that semi-rigid non-inflatable prostheses should be used because the fibrotic corpora prohibit proper inflation.[60]

■ THERAPY FOR HIGH-FLOW PRIAPISM

High-flow priapism is not considered an emergency. The penis is not ischaemic, and potency has been maintained, even if priapism exists for months. Therefore, observation has been considered as an option with the hope of spontaneous detumescence. Other forms of conservative therapy, such as ice packs to the perineum and external compression, have been tried but, as of now, have not been shown to be effective.[35] Alpha-adrenergic agonists have been used but result in only temporary detumescence. Methylene blue, which blocks the effect of nitric oxide, has been tried in high-flow states that are not due to cavernosal artery injury, with some success;[38,61,62] however, the use of this agent is discouraged by the possibility of penile necrosis and the formation of necrotic abscesses.[61,62] High-flow priapism in the case of sickle-cell disease is best treated with conservative measures in the same manner as low-flow

Table 46.2. Shunt procedures

Type of shunt	Description
Winter shunt (cavernoglanular shunt)[54]	Percutaneous shunt with Tru-Cut needle from glans to tip of corpus cavernosum
Al-Ghorab (cavernoglanular shunt)[55]	Formal incision at corona and removal of corporal tips → communication between glans and corpora
Quakles (cavernospongiosal shunt)[56]	Formal surgical anastomosis of corpus cavernosum with proximal corpus spongiosum
Grayhack (cavernosaphenous shunt)[57]	Anastomosis of corpus cavernosum with saphenous vein
Cavernopenile dorsal vein shunt[58]	Anastomosis of corpus cavernosum with dorsal vein

sickle-cell priapism. Shunt procedures have also been tried in those patients refractory to conservative therapy.[43] In addition, Ramos and colleagues have reported the successful use of bilateral pudendal artery ligation for this condition.[8]

The more definitive therapy for high-flow priapism, which is due to penile or perineal trauma or in certain cases is idiopathic, is either cavernosal artery ligation or embolization.[33-35,38,63-68] Embolization is usually recommended and surgery is reserved for failures. Autologous clot and absorbable gelatin sponges have been advocated for embolization because they permit rapid return of blood flow after clot lysis and thereby minimize complications.[34,69] In a report by Bastuda and colleagues,[34] six patients were embolized and all recovered erectile function.[34] Nevertheless, all patients undergoing this type of intervention should be aware of the possibility of impotence. Other than impotence, there are few complications reported after selective embolization. There is, however, a report in the literature of a perineal abscess after embolization.[70]

■ CONCLUSION

Priapism can be quite debilitating and result in serious sequelae. There are essentially two broad categories of priapism (i.e. high flow and low flow). Low-flow priapism is much more common and can be caused by haematological disease states, oral medications, intracavernous injection therapy, metastatic disease, and neurological causes. This type of priapism may also occur idiopathically. High-flow priapism, on the other hand, is more likely to be due to trauma, although it can also be idiopathic or associated with sickle-cell disease. Low-flow priapism is considered to be a urologic emergency and should be treated promptly, whereas high-flow treatment is not an emergency. The treatments for all types of priapism are initially conservative, but surgical therapy is available when applicable. The problem with surgical intervention for this disease, which affects so many young sexually active individuals, is that the impotence rates are high. At this time, there is no good oral-parenteral therapy available for all types of priapism. It is the author's hope that, in the future, some form of therapy will be available that will treat priapism effectively, with low morbidity.

■ REFERENCES

1. Kim N, Azadzoi K M, Goldstein I et al. A nitric oxide-like factor mediates nonadrenergic relaxation of penile corpus cavernosum smooth muscle. J Clin Invest 1991; 88: 112–118
2. Bush P A, Aronson W J, Buga G M et al. Nitric oxide is a potent relaxant of human and rabbit corpus cavernosum. J Urol 1992; 147: 1650–1655
3. Hashmat A I, Raju S, Singh I, Macchia R J. ^{99m}Tc penile scan: an investigative modality in priapism. Urol Radiol 1989; 11: 58
4. Sharpsteen J R Jr, Powars D, Johnson C et al. Multisystem damage associated with tricorporeal priapism in sickle cell disease. Am J Med 1993; 94: 289
5. Edmond A M, Holman R, Hayes R J et al. Priapism and impotence on homozygous sickle cell disease. Arch Intern Med 1980; 140: 1434–1437
6. Fowler J E, Koshy M, Strub M et al. Priapism associated with the sickle cell hemoglobinopathies: prevalence, natural history and sequelae. J Urol 1991; 145: 65–68
7. Nelson J H, Winter C C. Priapism: evolution of management in 48 patients in a 22-year series. J Urol 1977; 117: 455–458
8. Ramos C E, Jin P S, Ritchey M L, Benson G. High flow priapism associated with sickle cell disease. J Urol 1995; 153: 1619–1621
9. Hauri D, Spycher M, Bruhlmann W. Erection and priapism: a new physiopathologic concept. Urol Int 1983; 38: 138–145
10. Steinhardt G F, Steinhardt E. Priapism in children with leukemia. Urology 1981; 18: 604–606
11. Schreibman S M, Gee T S, Grabstald H. Management of priapism in patients with chronic granulocytic leukemia. J Urol 1974; 111: 786–788
12. Hebuterone X, Frere A M, Bayle J, Rampal P. Priapism in a patient treated with total parenteral nutrition. J Parenter Enteral Nutr 1993; 16: 171–174
13. Ekstrom B, Olsson A M. Priapism in patients treated with total parenteral nutrition. Br J Urol 1987; 59: 170–171
14. Klein E A, Montague D K, Steiger E. Priapism associated with the use of intravenous fat emulsion: case reports and postulated pathogenesis. J Urol 1985; 133: 857–859
15. Seftel A D, Saenz de Tejada I, Szetela B et al. Clozapine-associated priapism: a case report. J Urol 1992; 147: 146–148
16. Becker L E, Mitchell A D. Priapism. Surg Clin North Am 1965; 45: 1523–1534
17. Bhalla A K, Hoffbrand B I, Phatak P S et al. Prazosin and priapism. Br Med J 1979; 2: 1039
18. Klein L A, Hall R L, Smith R B. Surgical treatment of priapism: with a note on heparin-induced priapism. J Urol 1972; 108: 104–106
19. Fiorelli R L, Manfrey S J, Belkoff L H et al. Priapism associated with intranasal cocaine abuse. J Urol 1990; 143: 584–585
20. Mahler J C, Perry S, Sutton B. Intraurethral cocaine administration. [Letter to the editor.] JAMA 1988; 259: 3126
21. Virag R. Intracavernous injections of papaverine for erectile failure. [Letter to the editor.] Lancet 1982; 2: 938

22. Roy A C, Tan S M, Kottegoda S R et al. Ability of human corpora cavernosal muscle to generate prostaglandins and thromboxanes in vitro. IRCS Med Sci 1984; 12: 608

23. Lomas G M, Jarow J P. Risk factors for papaverine-induced priapism. J Urol 1992; 147: 1280–1281

24. Powell B L, Craig J B, Muss H B. Secondary malignancies of the penis and epididymis: a case report and review of the literature. J Clin Oncol 1985; 3: 110–115

25. Bedbrook G. Medical management. In: The care and management of spinal cord injuries. New York: Springer-Verlag, 1981: 155

26. Baba H, Furusawa N, Tanaka Y et al. Intermittent priapism associated with lumbar spinal stenosis. Int Orthop 1994; 18: 150–153

27. Baba H, Maezawa Y, Furusawa N et al. Lumbar spinal stenosis causing intermittent priapism. Paraplegia 1995; 33: 338–345

28. Pohl J, Pott B, Kleinhans G. Priapism: a three phase concept of management according to aetiology and prognosis. Br J Urol 1986; 58: 113–118

29. Thuret I, Bardakdjian J, Badens C et al. Priapism following splenectomy in an unstable hemoglobin: hemoglobin Olmsted beta 141 (H19) Leu → Arg. Am J Hematol 1996; 51: 133–136

30. Atala A, Amin M, Harty J I et al. Priapism associated with asplenic state. Urology 1992; 40: 371–373

31. Hirshberg S J, Charles R S, Ettinger J B. Pediatric priapism associated with Mycoplasma pneumoniae. Urology 1996; 47: 745–746

32. Bloom D A, Wan J, Key D. Disorders of the male external genitalia and inguinal canal. In: Kelalis P P, King L R, Belman A B (eds) Clinical pediatric urology, 3rd edn. Philadelphia: Saunders, 1992: 1023

33. Ricciardi R Jr, Bhatt G M, Cynamon J et al. Delayed high flow priapism: pathophysiology and management. J Urol 1993; 149: 119–121

34. Bastuba M D, Saenz de Tejada I, Dinlenc C Z et al. Arterial priapism: diagnosis, treatment and long-term follow-up. J Urol 1994; 151: 1231–1237

35. Brock G, Breza J, Lue T F et al. High flow priapism: a spectrum of disease. J Urol 1993; 150: 968–971

36. Lue T F, Hellstrom W J G, McAninch J W et al. Priapism: a refined approach to diagnosis and treatment. J Urol 1986; 136: 104–108

37. Burt F B, Schirmer H K, Scott W W. A new concept in the management of priapism. J Urol 1960; 83: 60–61

38. Steers W D, Selby J B Jr. Use of methylene blue and selective embolization of the pudendal artery for high flow priapism refractory to medical and surgical treatments. J Urol 1991; 146: 1361–1363

39. Broderick G A, Lue T F. Priapism and the physiology of erection. AUA Update Ser 1988; Vol VII, lesson 29.

40. Feldstein V A. Posttraumatic 'high-flow' priapism evaluation with color flow doppler sonography. J Ultrasound Med 1993; 12: 589–593

41. Hakim L S, Kulaksizoglu H, Mulligan R et al. Evolving concepts in the diagnosis and treatment of arterial high flow priapism. J Urol 1996; 155: 541–548

42. Spycher M A, Hauri D. The ultrastructure of the erectile tissue in priapism. J Urol 1986; 135: 142–147

43. Miller S T, Rao S T, Dunn E K, Glassberg K I. Priapism in children with sickle cell disease. J Urol 1995; 154: 844–847

44. Virag R, Bachir D, Lee K, Galacteros F. Preventive treatment of priapism in sickle cell disease with oral and self-administered intracavernous injection of etilefrine. Urology 1996; 47: 777–781

45. Baruchel S, Rees J, Bernstein M L, Goodyer P. Relief of sickle cell priapism by hydralazine. Report of a case. Am J Pediatr Hematol Oncol 1993; 15: 115–116

46. Lowe F C, Jarow J P. Placebo-controlled study of oral terbutaline and pseudoephedrine in management of prostaglandin E1-induced prolonged erections. Urology 1993; 42: 51–54

47. Shantha T R, Finnerty D P, Rodriguez A P. Treatment of persistent penile erection and priapism using terbutaline. J Urol 1989; 141: 1427–1429

48. Govier F E, Jonsson E, Kramer-Levien D. Oral terbutaline for the treatment of priapism. J Urol 1994; 151: 878–879

49. Serjeant G R, de Ceuler K, Maude G H. Stilbestrol and stuttering priapism in homozygous sickle-cell disease. Lancet 1985; 2: 1274–1276

50. Levine L A, Guss S P. Gonadotropin-releasing hormone analogues in the treatment of sickle cell anemia-associated priapism. J Urol 1993; 150: 475–477

51. Steinberg J, Eyre R C. Management of recurrent priapism with epinephrine self-injection and gonadotropin-releasing hormone analogue. J Urol 1995; 153: 152–153

52. Whalen R K, Whitcomb R W, Crowley W F Jr et al. Priapism in hypogonadal males receiving gonadotropin releasing hormone. J Urol 1991; 145: 1051–1052

53. Valley M A, Sang C N. Use of glycopyrrolate to treat intraoperative penile erection. Case report and review of the literature. Reg Anaesth 1994; 19: 423–428

54. Winter C C. Cure of idiopathic priapism: new procedure for creating fistula between glans penis and corpus cavernosum. Urology 1976; 8: 389–391

55. Ercole C J J, Pontes J E, Pierce J M Jr. Changing surgical concepts in the treatment of priapism. J Urol 1981; 125: 210–211

56. Wasmer J M, Carrion H M, Mekras G et al. Evaluation and treatment of priapism. J Urol 1981; 125: 204–207

57. Grayhack J T, McCullough W, O'Connor V J Jr. Venous bypass to control priapism. Invest Urol 1964; 1: 509–513

58. Barry J M. Priapism: treatment with corpus cavernosum to dorsal vein of the penis shunt. J Urol 1976; 116: 754–756

59. Bertram R A, Webster G D, Carson C C III. Priapism: etiology, treatment and results in series of 35 presentations. Urology 1985; 26: 229–232

60. Kabalin J N. Corporeal fibrosis as a result of priapism prohibiting function of self-contained inflatable penile prosthesis. Urology 1994; 43: 401–403

61. Perry P M, Meinhard E. Necrotic subcutaneous abscess following injection of methylene blue. Br J Clin Pract 1974; 28: 289

62. Mejean A, Marc B, Rigot J M et al. Letter to the editor. J Urol 1993; 149: 149

63. Wear J B Jr, Cummy A B, Munson B O. A new approach to the treatment of priapism. J Urol 1977; 117: 252–254

64. Ji M X, He N S, Wang P, Chen G. Use of selective embolization of the bilateral cavernous arteries for posttraumatic arterial priapism. J Urol 1994; 151: 1641–1642

65. Miller S F, Chait P G, Burrows P E et al. Posttraumatic arterial priapism in children: management with embolization. Radiology 1995; 196: 59–62

66. Lazinger M, Beckmann C F, Cossi A, Roth R A. Selective embolization of bilateral arterial cavernous fistulas for posttraumatic penile arterial priapism. Cardiovasc Intervent Radiol 1996; 19: 281–284

67. Numan F, Cakirer S, Islak C et al. Posttraumatic high-flow priapism treated by N-butyl-cyanoacrylate embolization. Cardiovasc Intervent Radiol 1996; 19: 278–280

68. Kim S C, Park S H, Young S H. Treatment of posttraumatic chronic high-flow priapisms by superselective embolization of cavernous artery with autologous clot. J Trauma 1996; 40: 462–465

69. Walker T G, Grant P W, Goldstein I et al. High flow priapism: treatment with superselective transcatheter embolization. Radiology 1990; 174: 1053–1054

70. Sandock D S, Seftel A D, Herbener T E et al. Perineal abscess after embolization for high-flow priapism. Urology 1996; 48: 308–311

Chapter 47
Diabetic impotence

S. Minhas and I. Eardley

INTRODUCTION

Diabetes mellitus is the single most common cause of erectile dysfunction (ED) seen in clinical practice, with up to 28% of men attending an impotence clinic being diabetic.[1] The association between diabetes and impotence was first documented by Rollo in 1798 and, although the mechanisms by which diabetes leads to ED are still unclear, it does seem that a number of factors are involved, of which vascular and neuronal factors are probably the most important.

EPIDEMIOLOGY

Around 50% of diabetic men are impotent.[2–4] In most, the ED develops during the course of the disease but, in a small proportion, it may be the presenting feature. Indeed, in one study of 497 men who had been referred for assessment of their ED, 11.1% were found to suffer from undiagnosed diabetes mellitus while a further 4.2% had impaired glucose tolerance.[1]

Although there is some evidence that patients with diet-controlled diabetes are less likely to become impotent[4] most reports suggest that there is no difference in incidence between those who are treated with oral hypoglycaemics and those who require insulin. In those men who do develop impotence, the onset is associated with increasing age,[4–7] the duration of the diabetes[4,6] and the development of other complications, of which microangiopathy and neuropathy are the most important.[5–7] The most usual clinical indicator of microangiopathy used in these studies was retinopathy, while symptomatic autonomic neuropathy was found to be more closely associated with the development of impotence than was peripheral sensory neuropathy. It has also been suggested that the likelihood of developing ED

is directly related to the degree of glycaemic control;[6,7] for instance, one study demonstrated a definite association between ED and the level of the glycosylated haemoglobin.[7] Other factors that appear to increase the risk of ED in diabetic subjects include alcohol intake[7] and the use of antihypertensive medication.[6]

PATHOPHYSIOLOGY

The roles of neuropathy and vasculopathy in the aetiology of diabetic ED are well recognized and are discussed below. Historically, it was considered that diabetes somehow led to gonadal dysfunction with associated endocrine abnormalities, and that this contributed to the pathophysiology of the condition. Currently, attention is increasingly being focused on the role of the vascular endothelium and the control of smooth muscle tone within the penis. There is increasing evidence that diabetes leads to abnormal endothelial and smooth muscle function throughout the body and that, in the penis, this can lead to ED.

Animal models of diabetic impotence

There are a number of models of diabetic impotence,[8,9] but only four have been used to any extent in the study of diabetic impotence. First, diabetes may be induced by the intravenous or intraperitoneal injection of streptozotocin so that diabetes develops within 8–14 weeks. In the study of diabetic impotence, the streptozotocin has usually been administered to rats with indicators such as weight loss, glycosuria and an increase in the serum blood sugar confirming the developement of diabetes. Similarly, diabetes may also be induced (usually in rabbits) by the intravenous injection of alloxan. Recently, two rat models in which the rat is genetically predisposed to develop diabetes (the BB rat which is insulin dependent and the

BBZ rat which is insulin independent) have also been used to study diabetic impotence.

Although animal models are an imperfect means of understanding any human disease, for the purpose of studying the physiology and pharmacology of erection and the pathophysiology of a condition such as diabetic impotence, they are invaluable. Corporal tissue from both potent men and from diabetic men (both potent and impotent) is often difficult to obtain and the models outlined above at least provide tissue for study in the laboratory. However, there are a number of problems: for instance, some of the animals have uncontrolled and untreated hyperglycaemia, which does not directly relate to the human situation where treatment with insulin or with oral hypoglycaemic agents is usual. Secondly, clinical diabetes is a chronic condition and the animal models are largely acute diabetic models. Currently, it is unclear exactly what effect the duration of the hyperglycaemia has on the results obtained in experimental studies. Finally, the animal models described above are all different, and it is not clear what their relationship is with each other, let alone what their relationship is with human physiology and pathophysiology.

Despite these disadvantages, animal models continue to be integral to the investigation of diabetic impotence and in the future it will be vital that both the similarities and the differences between the different animal models are identified, together with the relevance of the animal models to the human situation.

Neurogenic factors

There is considerable evidence to suggest that the development of neuropathy in men with diabetes might have a role in the subsequent development of ED. The neuropathy seen in diabetes initially affects small unmyelinated fibres which, in turn, can lead to functional abnormalities in a number of organ systems: for instance, there may be postural hypotension and disorders of the gastro-intestinal tract while peripherally there may be disordered thermal sensation and abnormalities of sweating. In the later stages of the disease, larger myelinated fibres are also affected, with the longest fibres usually being affected first. This produces the classical 'glove and stocking' distribution of the peripheral neuropathy.

Morphological evidence from both human tissue and from diabetic animal models has usually demonstrated changes in innervation. In diabetic rats, a reduction in the size of the myelinated nerve fibres, together with accumulation of glycogen in axons and lipid droplets in Schwann cells, has been demonstrated in the dorsal nerve, although no changes were noted within the cavernous nerve.[10] Human studies have provided conflicting evidence: whereas both light microscopy and electron microscopy have demonstrated changes in the nerves of the corpus cavernosum in some groups,[11–13] these changes have not been demonstrated in other groups.[14]

At a cellular level, the bulk of the evidence, both in humans and in animal models, seems to suggest depletion of neurotransmitters. Early qualitative studies in both humans and rats demonstrated both reduced vasoactive intestinal polypeptide (VIP) and acetylcholinesterase immunoreactivity.[15,16] Later studies have usually demonstrated reduced VIP and nitric oxide synthase (NOS) immunoreactivity, both in experimental animals and in humans,[17,18] although two recent reports in the streptozotocin rat have appeared to contradict these findings.[19,20] These differences may simply reflect the different tissues being used and, in particular, the duration of the diabetes. However, it is interesting that, although the levels of VIP were increased in the penis and major pelvic ganglia of the diabetic rat, intracavernous injection of VIP induced erections in control but not in diabetic rats, suggesting an abnormality at the receptor level.[19]

A reduction in noradrenaline levels in the erectile tissue of both animal and human tissue has also been demonstrated,[14,15] suggesting that any neuropathy may affect sympathetic as well as the parasympathetic nerve fibres.

In clinical studies, a number of groups have investigated neurophysiological changes in diabetic patients. The most usual measure has been the latency of the bulbocavernosus reflex (BCR), whereby a response is measured electrically in a muscle of the pelvic floor such as the striated urethral sphincter or the bulbocavernosus muscle itself, following electrical stimulation of the dorsum of the penis or occasionally of the bladder neck. The reflex is known to be polysynaptic, with both somatic afferents (when the dorsal nerve of the penis is stimulated) and efferents (the pudendal nerve). Using this technique, abnormal BCR latencies have been demonstrated in up to 50% of patients.[21–25] However, when taken as a group, some studies have shown no difference from control values[26] and most have concluded that the BCR has little role in the diagnosis of neuropathic impotence in diabetic men.[23,26]

The fundamental problem with the BCR (and other tests of the sacral reflex latency) is that it measures conduction in large myelinated fibres, whereas the autonomic neuropathy of diabetes primarily affects the small unmyelinated nerves and, actually, affects the larger fibres only relatively late in the disease. Accordingly, there will always be a proportion of men with diabetic autonomic neuropathy who will have normal BCR latencies. This means that the BCR has little diagnostic accuracy in this respect and, indeed, is a marker only of relatively severe neuropathy.

A number of approaches have been tried to resolve this problem. One variation of the BCR is to stimulate the vesico-urethral junction with a catheter-mounted stimulating electrode. This approach stimulates small unmyelinated afferent nerves, and an electrical response can be recorded in the pelvic floor. Using this technique it was found that 66% of diabetic subjects with impotence exhibited abnormal responses and, as a group, there was a significant difference from control values.[27] Other groups have tested for thermal threshold (which assesses small unmyelinated cutaneous nerve fibres) either on penile skin[28] or on the sole of the foot,[21] and both have claimed that it is a much more sensitive indicator of neuropathic impotence in diabetic subjects. Studies are still awaited in potent diabetic men before this can be confirmed. Finally, the use of corpus cavernosum electromyography,[24,29] if it really does record cavernosal smooth muscle activity, may also provide evidence about neuropathy and diabetic impotence.

Vascular factors

The penis is a vascular organ. Increased arterial inflow and relaxation of the smooth muscle lining the sinusoidal spaces is fundamental to the process of penile erection. Factors that impede blood flow into the penile helicine vessels and sinusoidal spaces will lead to ED. Diabetes mellitus is associated both with atherosclerosis in large arteries (which appears more frequently and at an earlier age than in non-diabetics) and with a microangiopathy, characterized by increased thickening of the capillary basement membrane.

Arteriography has demonstrated that stenosis of the internal pudendal artery is more common in impotent than in potent diabetics,[30] and duplex ultrasound scanning of the penile arteries has shown that, in impotent men, diabetes is associated with a smaller penile artery diameter and lower peak flow velocities following injection of an intracorporal vasoactive agent.[28,31,32] Morphological studies of diabetic tissue have demonstrated ultrastructural changes within small penile vessels, including endothelial proliferation, subintimal fibrosis and endarteritis obliterans.[33,34] Recently, endothelial injury, as well as morphological changes in the smooth muscle cells, have been documented in diabetic rabbits[35] while, in the same animal model, a direct correlation between smooth muscle fibrosis and the degree of hyperglycaemia has been demonstrated.[36] The fibrosis was thought to be consistent with a vascular lesion.

Clinical studies have clearly demonstrated a close correlation between diabetic ED and other manifestations of diabetic vascular disease — namely, retinopathy, intermittent claudication and the risk of amputation.[4,6,7]

Diabetes is also associated with other conditions that can cause vascular problems. For instance, there is an increased risk of both hypercholesterolaemia and hypercoagulability.[37,38] Hypercholesterolaemia is a risk factor for impotence in its own right and also leads to an increased risk of atherosclerosis.[39] At a cellular level it can lead to increased contractility and impaired endothelium-dependent relaxation of the cavernosal smooth muscle, both of which have been demonstrated in animal models of hypercholesterolaemia.[40,41] The hypercoagulability associated with diabetes is secondary to an increase in coagulation factors such as factor IX (Von Willebrand factor) and tissue plasminogen activator, which in turn can lead to subsequent vessel thrombosis and reduced vascular inflow.

Endothelial and smooth muscle factors

The endothelium lining the lacunar spaces is important in controlling corporal smooth muscle tone. Nitric oxide, constrictor prostanoids and endothelins are all produced by the endothelium[42-44] and act directly on the smooth muscle cell. In diabetes, impaired neurogenic and endothelium-dependent smooth muscle relaxation to acetylcholine has been demonstrated in both animal and human studies of penile erection[45,46] although the mechanism by which this occurs is poorly understood.

As suggested above, the evidence relating to nitric oxide production within the diabetic penis has been conflicting. In one diabetic rat model there was reduced soluble NOS activity in the diabetic penis together with reduced neuronal NOS.[17] In another human study there was reduced NOS immunoreactivity within the nerves of the diabetic penis.[18] However, increased NOS activity has been demonstrated in the corpus cavernosum of another diabetic rat model,[20] whereas increased numbers of NOS-binding sites have been demonstrated in this rat model.[47] With evidence that nitric oxide synthesis is impaired in the penis of the diabetic rabbit,[48] the situation is most confused.

It may be that diabetes can lead to depletion of the neuronal NOS with other effects upon the endothelial NOS; however, the differences outlined above may simply represent differences between different animal models and further work is required in human tissue to clarify whether nitric oxide synthesis is impaired in the diabetic penis. To some extent this is peripheral to the main question, which is why both neuronal and endothelial-dependent relaxation of the cavernosal smooth muscle is impaired.

There are a number of possible explanations for this and, as is often the case, several of them may ultimately prove to be important. It has been suggested that a simple rise in the blood sugar may mediate these changes. Certainly, in vitro experiments in other tissues have demonstrated an augmentation of the contractile response to adrenergic agonists and a reduced relaxation response to nitric oxide upon exposure to hyperglycaemia.[49,50] Initial studies in rabbit corporal tissue have provided similar findings and it may be that some of these effects are due to an increased production of constrictor prostanoids.[51]

Another possibility is that oxygen free radicals (such as the superoxide anion) have a role in producing impaired cavernosal relaxation. It is known that free radicals are able to inactivate nitric oxide and regulate smooth muscle tone in some tissues,[52] and it has been proposed that, in diabetes, increased auto-oxidation of glucose results in overproduction of free-radical species which in turn leads to smooth muscle dysfunction.[53,54] Interestingly, the impaired endothelium-dependent relaxation seen in diabetic vascular tissues is reversed by the addition of superoxide dismutase, which is able to inactivate the superoxide anion.[54]

It may be that the polyol pathway is also involved in the pathogenesis of hyperglycaemic-induced changes of vascular endothelial and smooth muscle function.[50,55,56] In hyperglycaemia, induction of the enzyme aldose reductase leads to an increased production of sorbitol, which in turn causes an increased consumption of NADPH which is an essential cofactor in the production of nitric oxide. Although it has been proved that this is important in the diabetic rat aorta, as yet it has not been confirmed in penile erectile tissue from either experimental animals or humans.

One increasingly popular theory is that advanced glycosylation end-products (AGEs) have an important pathophysiological role in the complications of diabetes mellitus. AGEs are compounds that are formed as a result of non-enzymatic reaction between glucose and the amino groups of long-lived tissue proteins such as collagen.[55,57] They are found to occur in increasing amounts, not only in association with diabetes but also with ageing. Amongst their various pathological effects has been demonstrated an ability to bind (or 'quench') nitric oxide, at least in animal models including corpus cavernosum.[58,59] AGEs have now been demonstrated in both human corpus cavernosum and tunica albuginea and have been found to increase with age.[60]

However, a simple reduction in mediators of smooth muscle relaxation, as would be produced by any of the above explanations, may provide only part of the story. Certainly, one group of investigators[61] have demonstrated an increase in endothelin 1 binding in the diabetic rabbit penis and have suggested that this may represent a possible pathophysiological mechanism of the ED seen in diabetes. Others have demonstrated an increased sensitivity of human diabetic smooth muscle cells to alpha-adrenergic agonists,[62,63] and it may be that, in diabetes, there is heightened contractility as well as decreased relaxation of the corporal smooth muscle. It also seems likely that the vascular and sinusoidal endothelium has a central role in the modulation of this process.

Endocrine factors

Both erectile function and sexual physiology are reliant upon a normal endocrine milieu which is provided by a normally functioning pituitary, hypothalamus, adrenal gland and testis (Chapter 9). The pathophysiological importance of abnormalities in this axis with respect to diabetic impotence is controversial. An early study suggested both that hypogonadism was common in diabetics and that treatment with testosterone was effective.[64] Although subsequent studies have not always confirmed this view, a number have demonstrated that diabetes may be associated with diminished levels of serum testosterone as well as impairment in testicular function. For instance, it was shown that there were decreased serum free testosterone levels in diabetic men with primary organic impotence when compared with both normal men and diabetic men with primary psychogenic impotence.[63] This study also demonstrated increased urinary excretion of luteinizing hormone (LH), although the serum LH was similar in all groups. Those authors also reported improved sexual function, both subjectively and as assessed by nocturnal penile tumescence (NPT) studies following therapy with parenteral testosterone. Finally, studies in diabetic rats demonstrated both a reduced serum testosterone[17,64] and a reduction in size of androgen-sensitive accessory reproductive organs.[64]

Overall, then, there is some evidence of hypogonadism in some men with diabetic impotence and it appears that this is primarily a gonadal abnormality. In the majority of men, however, the abnormality is only mild and is of somewhat secondary importance in the pathogenesis of ED compared with the other factors outlined above.

Psychogenic factors

Although the majority of men with diabetes will probably have primarily an organic component to their impotence, a number may have supplementary psychological factors. In fact, in a number of studies, some of which have used NPT to identify organic impotence, up to 30% of diabetic men with ED have been found to have significant psychogenic problems that contributed to their impotence.[65–67] In the majority of cases these were secondary to the organic problems but in a significant proportion the psychogenic factors were the most important.[66]

Summary

In most patients with diabetic ED there will be a number of pathophysiological mechanisms at work and the relative importance of these factors will vary between individuals. Whereas neuropathy, endocrinopathy and atherosclerosis are undoubtedly important in a proportion, it is becoming increasingly evident that endothelial and smooth muscle function is disordered in diabetes and that this may be the most important factor for the majority of men. Further work is required to explain these abnormalities fully, in the hope that specific therapeutic and preventative treatments can be developed.

■ MANAGEMENT OF DIABETIC IMPOTENCE

Clinical features

The clinical assessment of diabetic men with ED is similar to the assessment of other impotent men. Although impotence is occasionally the presenting symptom of undiagnosed diabetes,[1] in the majority the diabetes has already been diagnosed. It is important not to miss other potentially important aetiological factors, some of which may be associated with diabetes. For instance, if the patient is also hypertensive it may be that some of his antihypertensive medication may be contributing to the ED.

Although the physical examination often contributes very little to patient management, it does provide an opportunity to identify other diabetic complications and to form an opinion about whether there are prominent vascular or neurological components to the pathogenesis of impotence. For instance, diabetic retinopathy appears to correlate directly with the presence of ED,[4,6,7] while evidence of peripheral vascular disease with loss of peripheral pulses and intermittent claudication suggests significant large vessel disease. The neurological examination may identify a peripheral sensory neuropathy, which typically has a glove-and-stocking distribution and which initially affects the small unmyelinated fibres that mediate vibration. Finally, there may be postural hypotension, indicative of an autonomic neuropathy.

It is sensible to assess the quality of diabetic control, by performing a random blood sugar and a glycosylated haemoglobin test, particularly since the quality of the control seems to be a significant risk factor in the development of diabetic impotence.[6,7] Given the possible increased risk of hypogonadism, serum testosterone should be checked, but it is not the authors' practice to perform any other investigations routinely, unless otherwise indicated.

Treatment

Provided that there is no biochemical evidence of hypogonadism, most diabetic men attending the authors' impotence clinic are routinely offered either intracorporal injection therapy or the use of a vacuum erection device (VED) as first-line therapy. The choice between these two treatments is usually left to the patient.

Intracorporal injection therapy

Many diabetic men will respond to intracorporal injection therapy. The authors' standard primary agent is prostaglandin E1 (PGE1), although papaverine is also effective in many men. In men with prominent neuropathy, relatively small doses of both agents are effective, whereas in men with severe vascular disease large doses may be needed and, indeed, combination therapy may be required. PGE1 can usefully be combined with either papaverine or phentolamine or both, although in a small proportion of men there is no response, even at maximal doses.

It can be argued that diabetic patients are likely to comply better with injection therapy than many other patient groups: first, they are often young men who are well motivated; second, a significant proportion will already be self-injecting with insulin. However, it also seems that diabetic patients are less likely to respond to injection therapy. In one study, using PGE1 as monotherapy, only 52% of diabetic men responded successfully to injection therapy;[68] in another study, using papaverine monotherapy, only 61% of men responded.[66] Finally, in a third study, using a papaverine-phentolamine combination, 21 of 33 diabetic patients with ED failed to get a satisfactory response.[69] Interestingly, there was no difference in neurological, vascular or drug-related risk factors between those patients who responded and those who did not. There was, however, a correlation with the age of the patient, in that younger men tended to respond better to injection therapy.

Complications of injection therapy in diabetic patients are similar to those seen in the general impotent population. However, there is potentially an increased risk of infection and occasional rare cases of sepsis have been reported in diabetic patients following injection therapy.[70] In addition, it has recently been reported that pain at the site of injection may be more problematic in diabetic patients and particularly in those who use high doses of PGE1.[71]

Vacuum erection devices (VEDs)

VEDs are the other main form of treatment for diabetic men with ED and a number of studies have confirmed their efficacy in such men. For instance, one study reported that, when given the choice, 44 of 54 men chose vacuum therapy over injection therapy and that 75% of them were able to achieve a satisfactory erection after 2 months.[72] Another group suggested that VEDs might provide an effective alternative in that significant proportion of diabetic men who fail to respond to intracorporal injections.[73]

Other treatments

Although injections and vacuum pumps are the mainstay of treatment in most diabetic men, in a proportion other treatments may be effective. For instance, as has been suggested above, androgen deficiency may have a role in the pathogenesis of diabetic ED. Whereas some authors have demonstrated moderate efficacy for testosterone in the treatment of these patients[63,64] others have not.[74] Although it is obviously important to diagnose and to treat any remediable endocrinological causes for impotence, particularly in the young diabetic patient, in the present authors' experience hypogonadism is uncommon and treatment with testosterone is usually ineffective in this group of patients.

Whereas the oral agent yohimbine is probably ineffective in organic impotence,[75] the recently developed phosphodiesterase inhibitor sildenafil has shown efficacy in clinical trials of diabetic men[76] (Chapter 26). In a randomized crossover study of 21 diabetic men, efficacy as assessed by Rigiscan was reported in up to 52% of men, although the dose of sildenafil used in that study was relatively low. It may well be that greater efficacy will be achieved with larger doses of the compound.

In a number of patients, psychological factors will be important. One group reported the value of initial psychosexual assessment: in 52% of their patients, significant psychosexual factors were identified and, of 24 diabetic men who then went on to receive psychosexual therapy, 60% were successfully treated.[66]

Vascular surgery

Patients with diabetes often have coexistent arteriosclerotic disease and, in some cases, this may be the primary factor in the pathogenesis of the ED. In a few cases, either aorto-iliac reconstruction or angioplasty may theoretically improve the penile circulation but, in the authors' experience, this is rarely indicated or effective. Similarly, reconstructive microvascular surgery is also often unsuccessful, even in the hands of enthusiasts. The current consensus is that, in patients with arteriosclerotic disease, arterio-arterial anastomoses are rarely indicated, although dorsal vein arterialization may be effective in a proportion.[77] The obvious problem with diabetic patients is that even if any reconstructive procedure is technically successful, effective erections may not be possible because of coexistent neuropathy or endothelial dysfunction.

Penile prostheses

If all other treatments have failed or have proved unacceptable, the final therapeutic option remaining is a penile prosthesis. The different types of implant, the selection criteria for surgical implantation and the techniques of surgery have all been outlined elsewhere in this volume (Chapters 37–39) and apply equally well to diabetic patients. However, where the use of implants in diabetic patients does differ from that in other patient groups is in the consideration of the septic complications of surgery. Most importantly, it appears that diabetic patients are probably more prone than the general population to infection of the prosthesis. Certainly, a number of early studies all suggested an increased risk of infection in diabetic patients.[78–80] In a more recent publication, a British group confirmed this increased infective risk in a group of patients operated upon between 1985 and 1990. Interestingly, however, they were able significantly to reduce the risk of prosthesis infection by adherence to a meticulous preoperative, intra-operative and postoperative regime. When they used this protocol on a group of 62 patients, there was only one infected prosthesis, and in the 13 diabetic patients there were no infections at all.[81] Recently, a much larger series has reviewed the results of 1337 implants and has reported no increased risk of prosthesis infection in diabetic patients compared with the general population.[82] A trend towards an increased risk of infection in penile prosthesis revision surgery was reported, although this did not reach statistical significance. The difference between the older results and the more recent reports may simply reflect more meticulous preoperative preparation, better antibiotic prophylaxis and improved surgical technique. However, when infections do occur in diabetic patients the consequences can be severe. A recent report described three cases of gangrene of the penis following implantation of a prosthesis in patients with insulin-dependent diabetes mellitus; in two of the patients, penile amputation was required.[83]

As to the reasons behind this apparent increased risk of periprosthetic infection, there is controversy as to whether poor diabetic control is important. For instance, one recent publication suggested that preoperative glycosylated haemoglobin levels in excess of 11.5%

predisposed to periprosthetic infections,[84] whereas another, more recent, prospective study showed no correlation between the glycosylated haemoglobin and the risk of prosthesis infection: indeed, there were no infected prostheses in the group of patients with poorly controlled diabetes.[85] Further evidence in this area is eagerly awaited.

■ CONCLUSIONS

The aetiology of ED in diabetes mellitus is multifactorial, with neurovascular and endothelial factors playing a prominent role. As the understanding of corporal physiology improves, more therapeutic options will inevitably become available for the treatment of ED in this group of patients. Although this has been reflected recently in the emergence of the oral phosphodiesterase inhibitor sildenafil, it is interesting to note that, in the early studies, only 52% of diabetic men taking sildenafil were able to achieve a satisfactory erection. If these figures are substantiated in future studies, then a considerable number of men will continue to need the more traditional treatments of intracorporal injections, vacuum pumps and penile prostheses. However, for the diabetic patient, it may be just as important (if not more so) in the future to identify ways in which impotence may be prevented. This requires a deep understanding of the natural history of the disease and will, again, require greater knowledge relating to the pathophysiology of the condition.

■ REFERENCES

1. Maatman T J, Montague D K, Martin L M. Erectile dysfunction in men with diabetes mellitus. Urology 1987; 29: 589–592
2. Rubin A, Babott D. Impotence in diabetes mellitus. JAMA 1958; 168: 498–500
3. Kolodny R C, Kahn C B, Goldstein H, Barnett D M. Sexual dysfunction in diabetic men. Diabetes 1973; 23: 306–309
4. McCulloch D K, Campbell I W, Wu F C et al. The prevalence of diabetic impotence. Diabetologia 1980; 18: 279–283
5. Naliboff B D, Rosenthal M. Effects of age on complications in adult onset diabetes. J Am Geriatr Soc 1989; 37: 838–842
6. Klein R, Klein B E, Lee K E et al. Prevalence of self-reported erectile dysfunction in people with long-term IDDM. Diabetes Care 1996; 19: 135–141

7. McCulloch D K, Young R J, Prescott R J et al. The natural history of impotence in diabetic men. Diabetologia 1984; 26: 437–440

8. Gwilliam D J, Bone A J. Animal models of insulin dependent diabetes mellitus. In: Pickup J C, Williams G (eds) Textbook of diabetes. Oxford: Blackwell Science, 1997

9. Bailey C J, Flatt P R. Animal models of non insulin dependent diabetes mellitus. In: Pickup J C, Williams G (eds) Textbook of diabetes. Oxford: Blackwell Science, 1997

10. Italiano G, Petrelli L, Marin A et al. Ultrastructural analysis of the cavernous and dorsal penile nerves in experimental diabetes. Int J Impot Res 1993; 5: 149–160

11. Faerman I, Glocer L, Fox D et al. Impotence and diabetes. Histological studies of the autonomic nervous fibres of the copora cavernosa in impotent diabetic males. Diabetes 1974; 23: 971–976

12. de Tejada I S, Goldstein I. Diabetic penile neuropathy. Urol Clin N America, 1988; 15: 17–22

13. Mersdorf A, Goldsmith P C, Diederichs W et al. Ultrastructural changes in impotent penile tissue: a comparison of 65 patients. J Urol 1991; 145: 749–758

14. Melman A, Henry D P, Felten D L, O'Connor B L. Alteration of the penile corpora in patients with erectile impotence. Invest Urology 1980; 17: 474–477

15. Lincoln J, Crowe R, Blacklay P F et al. Changes in the VIPergic, cholinergic and adrenergic innervation of human penile tissue in diabetic and non-diabetic impotent males. J Urol 1987; 137: 1053–1059

16. Crowe R, Lincoln J, Blacklay P F et al. Vasoactive intestinal polypeptide like immunoreactive nerves in diabetic penis. A comparison between streptozocin treated rats and men. Diabetes 1983; 32: 1075–1077

17. Vernet D, Cai L, Garban H et al. Reduction of penile nitric oxide synthase in diabetic BB/WORdp(type1) and BBZ/WOR dp(type2) rats with erectile dysfunction. Endocrinology 1995; 136: 5709–5717

18. Ehmke H, Junemann K P, Mayer B, Kummer W. Nitric oxide synthase and vasoactive intestinal polypeptide colocalization in neurons innervating the human penile circulation. Int J Impot Res 1995; 7: 147–156

19. Maher E, Bachoo M, Elabbady A A et al. Vasoactive intestinal peptide and impotence in experimental diabetes mellitus. Br J Urol 1996; 77: 271–278

20. Elabbady A A, Gagnon C, Hassouna M M et al. Diabetes mellitus increases nitric oxide synthase in penises but not in major pelvic ganglia of rats. Br J Urol 1995; 76: 196–202

21. Fowler C J, Ali Z, Kirby R S and Pryor J P. The value of testing for unmyelinated fibre, sensory neuropathy in diabetic impotence. Br J Urol 1988; 61: 63–67

22. Parys B T, Evans C M, Parsons K F. Bulbocavernosus reflex latency in the investigation of diabetic impotence. Br J Urol 1988; 61: 59–62

23. Desai K M, Dembny K, Morgan H et al. Neurophysiological investigation of diabetic impotence. Are sacral response studies of value? Br J Urol 1988; 61: 68–73

24. Gertsenberg T C, Nordling J, Hald T, Wagner G. Standardised evaluation of erectile dysfunction in 95 consecutive patients. J Urol 1989; 141: 857–862

25. Vodusek D B, Ravnik-Oblak M, Oblak C. Pudendal versus limb nerve electrophysiological abnormalities in diabetics with erectile dysfunction. Int J Impot Res 1993; 5: 37–42

26. Kaneko S, Bradley W E. Penile electrodiagnosis. Value of bulbocavernosus reflex latency versus nerve conduction velocity of the dorsal nerve of the penis in diagnosis of diabetic impotence. J Urol 1987; 137: 933–935

27. Sarica Y, Karacan I. Bulbocavernosus reflex to somatic and visceral nerve stimulation in normal subjects and in diabetics with erectile impotence. J Urol 1987; 138: 55–58

28. Robinson L Q, Woodcock J P, Stephenson T P. Results of investigation of impotence in patients with overt or probable neuropathy. Br J Urol 1987; 60: 583–587

29. Wagner G, Gerstenberg T, Levin R J. Electrical activity of corpus cavernosum during flaccidity and erection of the human penis: a new diagnostic method? J Urol 1989; 142: 723–725

30. Herman A, Adar R, Rubinstein Z. Vascular lesions associated with impotence in diabetic and nondiabetic arterial occlusive disease. Diabetes 1978; 27: 975–981

31. Lue T F, Mueller S C, Jow Y R, Hwang T I. Functional evaluation of penile arteries with duplex ultrasound in vasodilator induced erection. Urol Clin North Am 1989; 16: 799–807

32. Wang C J, Shen S Y, Wu C C, Chiang C P. Penile blood flow study in diabetic impotence. Urol Int 1993; 50: 209–212

33. Ruzbarsky V, Michal V. Morphologic changes in the arterial bed of the penis with aging. Relationship to the pathogenesis of impotence. Invest Urol 1977; 15: 194–199

34. Jevtich M J, Kass M, Khawand N. Changes in the corpora cavernosa of impotent diabetics: comparing histological with clinical findings. J Urol (Paris) 1985; 91: 281–285

35. Sullivan M, Thompson C, Mikhailidis D, Morgan R. Ultrastructural changes in diabetic rabbit corpus cavernosa. Int J Impot Res 1996; 8: 126 (D16)

36. Gupta S, Moreland R E, Pabby A et al. Diabetes-induced structural changes in rabbit corpus cavernosum. Int J Impot Res 1996; 8: 136 (D55)

37. Conlan M G, Folsom A R, Finch A et al. Associations of factor VIII and von Willebrand factor with age, race, sex and risk factors for atherosclerosis. Thromb Haemost 1993; 70: 380–385

38. Akoi I, Shimoyama K, Aoki N et al. Platelet dependent thrombin generation in patients with diabetes mellitus: effects of glycaemic control on coagulability in diabetes. J Am Coll Cardiol 1996; 27: 560–566

39. Virag R, Bouilly P, Frydman D. Is impotence an arterial disorder? Lancet 1985; i: 181–184

40. Azadzoi K M, de Tejada I S. Hypercholesterolemia impairs endothelium-dependent relaxation of rabbit corpus cavernosum smooth muscle. J Urol 1991; 146: 238–240

41. Kim J H, Klyachkin M L, Svendsen E et al. Experimental hypercholesterolemia in rabbits induces cavernosal

atherosclerosis with endothelial and smooth muscle cell dysfunction. J Urol 1995; 151: 198–205

42. Kim N, Azadzoi K M, Goldstein I, de Tejada I S. A nitric oxide like factor mediates nonadrenergic neurogenic relaxation of penile corpus cavernosum smooth muscle. J Clin Invest 1991; 88: 112–118

43. Andersson K E, Wagner G. Physiology of penile erection. Physiol Rev 1995; 75: 191–236

44. Hedlund H, Andersson K E. Contraction and relaxation induced by some prostanoids in isolated human penile erectile tissue and cavernous artery. J Urol 1985; 134: 1245–1250

45. Azadzoi K M, de Tejada I S. Diabetes mellitus impairs neurogenic and endothelium dependent relaxation of rabbit corpus cavernosum smooth muscle. J Urol 1992; 148: 1587–1591.

46. de Tejada I S, Goldstein I, Azadzoi K et al. Impaired neurogenic and endothelium mediated relaxation of penile smooth muscle from diabetic men with impotence. N Engl J Med 1989; 320: 1025–1030

47. Thompson C S, Dashwood M R, Mikhailidis D P et al. Autoradiographic localisation of nitric oxide synthase in the penis of the long term diabetic rat. Int J Impot Res 1994; 6(suppl): D215

48. Sullivan M E, Thompson C S, Mikhailidis D P et al. Nitric oxide synthesis and guanyl cyclase activity by the penis of the diabetic rabbit. Int J Impot Res 1996; 8: D01

49. Bohlen H G, Lash J M. Topical hyperglycemia rapidly suppresses EDRF-mediated vasodilation of normal rat arterioles. Am J Physiol 1993; 265: H219–225

50. Taylor P D, Poston L. The effect of hyperglycaemia on function of rat isolated mesenteric resistance artery. Br J Pharmacol 1994; 113: 801–808

51. Minhas S, Eardley I, Morrison S. The effect of hyperglycaemia on contraction and relaxation of rabbit corporal smooth muscle. J Physiol 1997; 501: 117–118

52. Katusic Z S. Superoxide anion and endothelial regulation of arterial tone. Free Radic Biol Med 1996; 20: 443–438

53. Chang K C, Chung S Y, Chong W S et al. Possible superoxide radical-induced alteration of vascular reactivity in aortas from streptozotocin-treated rats. J Pharmacol Exp Ther 1993; 266: 992–1000

54. Tesfamariam B, Cohen R A. Free radicals mediate endothelial cell dysfunction caused by elevated glucose. Am J Physiol 1992; 263: H321–326

55. King G L, Shiba T, Oliver J et al. Cellular and molecular abnormalities in the vascular endothelium of diabetes mellitus. Annu Rev Med 1994; 45: 179–188

56. Cameron N E, Cotter M A. Impaired contraction and relaxation in aorta from streptozotocin diabetic rats: role of polyol pathway. Diabetologia 1992; 35: 1011–1019

57. Brownlee M. Glycation and diabetic complications. Diabetes 1994; 43: 836–841

58. Bucala R, Tracey K J, Cerami A. Advanced glycosylation products quench nitric oxide and mediate defective endothelium-dependent vasodilation in experimental diabetes. J Clin Invest 1991; 87: 432–438

59. Allen D, Seftel M D, Krista A et al. AGEs. Int J Impot Res 1996; 8: A08

60. Jiaan D B, Seftel A D, Fogarty J et al. Age-related increase in an advanced glycation end product in penile tissue. World J Urol 1995; 13: 369–375

61. Bell C R, Sullivan M E, Dashwood M R et al. The density and distribution of endothelin 1 and endothelin receptor subtypes in normal and diabetic rat corpus cavernosum. Br J Urol 1995; 76: 203–207

62. Christ G J, Schwartz C B, Stone B A et al. Kinetic characteristics of alpha-1-adrenergic contractions in human corpus cavernosum smooth muscle. Am J Physiol 1992; 263: H15–19

63. Murray F T, Wyss H U, Thomas R G et al. Gonadal dysfunction in diabetic men with organic impotence. J Clin Endocrinol Metab 1987; 65: 127–135

64. Murray F T, Johnson R D, Sciadini M et al. Erectile and copulatory dysfunction in chronically diabetic BB/WOR rats. Am J Physiol 1992; 263: E151–157

65. Bancroft J, Malone N. The clinical assessment of erectile dysfunction: a comparison of nocturnal penile tumescence monitoring and intracavernosal injections. Int J Impot Res 1995; 7: 123–130

66. Veves A, Webster L, Chen T F et al. Aetiopathogenesis and management of impotence in diabetic males: four years experience from a combined clinic. Diabetic Med 1995; 12: 77–82

67. Watkins S E, Williams P, Ryder R E, Bowshier W. Psychometric assessment of diabetic impotence. Br J Psych 1993; 162: 840–842

68. Desvaux P, Mimoun S. Prostaglandin E1 in the treatment of erectile insufficiency. Comparison of efficacy and tolerance based on different etiologies. J Urol (Paris) 1994; 100: 17–22

69. Bell D S, Cutter G R, Hayne V B, Lloyd L K. Factors predicting efficacy of phentolamine–papaverine intracorporeal injection for treatment of erectile dysfunction in the diabetic male. Urology 1992; 40: 36–40

70. Parfitt V J, Wong R, Robbie A et al. Staphylococcal septicaemia complicating intracavernosal autoinjection therapy for impotence in a man with diabetes. Diabetic Med 1992; 9: 947–949

71. Earle C, Chew K, Stuckey G, Keogh E. Pain with intracavernosal therapy. Int J Impot Res 1996; 8: A62

72. Price D E, Cooksey G, Jehu D et al. The management of impotence in diabetic men by vacuum tumescence therapy. Diabetic Med 1991; 8: 964–967

73. Ryder R E, Close C F, Moriarty K T et al. Impotence in diabetes: aetiology, implications for treatment and preferred vacuum device. Diabetic Med 1992; 9: 893–898

74. Ellenberg M. Impotence in diabetes: the neurologic factor. Ann Intern Med 1971; 75: 213–219

75. Morales A, Condra M, Owen J A et al. Is yohimbine effective in the treatment of organic impotence? The results of a controlled trial. J Urol 1987; 137: 1168–1172

76. Boolell M, Pearson J, Gingell J C, Gepi Attee S. Sildenafil is an efficacious therapy in diabetic patients with erectile dysfunction. Int J Impot Res 1996; 8: P14

77. Sharlip I D. Microvascular surgery for vasculogenic impotence. Curr Opin Urol 1993; 3: 496–499

78. Kaufman J J, Lindner A, Raz S. Penile surgery for impotence. J Urol 1982; 128: 1192–1194

79. Wilson S K, Wahman G E, Lange J L. Eleven years experience with the inflatable penile prosthesis. J Urol 1988; 139: 951–952

80. Fallon B, Ghanem H. Infected penile prostheses: incidence and outcomes. Int J Impot Res 1989; 1: 175–181

81. Lynch M J, Scott G M, Inglis J A, Pryor J P. Reducing the loss of implants following penile prosthetic surgery. Br J Urol 1994; 73: 423–427

82. Wilson S K, Delk J R. Inflatable penile implant infection: predisposing factors and treatment suggestions. J Urol 1995; 153: 659–661

83. Bejany D E, Periton P E, Lustgarten M, Rhamy R K. Gangrene of the penis after implantation of penile prostheses: case reports, treatment recommendations and review of the literature. J Urol 1993; 150: 190–193

84. Bishop J R, Moul J M, Sihelnik S A et al. Use of glycosylated haemoglobin to identify diabetics at high risk for penile periprosthetic infections. J Urol 1992; 147: 386–388

85. Wilson S K, Cleves M A, Delk J R. Glycosylated hemoglobin and risk of infection among penile implant patients. Int J Impot Res 1996; 8: A85

Chapter 48
Chronic renal failure and sexual dysfunction

C. C. Carson and R. Krishnan

INTRODUCTION

Chronic renal failure (CRF) and subsequent uraemia are commonly associated with erectile dysfunction (ED), diminished libido and infertility.[1–3] A variety of problems contribute to this overall sexual dysfunction, including uraemia, changes associated with dialysis, medication used to control underlying disease processes, and renal failure-associated conditions, as well as the sequelae of renal transplantation.

PREVALENCE

Abnormalities in male sexual and reproductive function have been widely reported in patients with CRF. Studies in which patients and spouses were interviewed or evaluated by questionnaire have demonstrated impotence in 20–60% of patients surveyed.[4–9] Although both Kinsey et al.[10] and Masters and Johnson[11] reported the incidence of impotence in normal men in their 40s as less than 5%, Sherman[7] identified more than 50% of patients with uraemia on haemodialysis in the same age-group as having significant sexual dysfunction and impotence. Levy and Abram[12] documented decreased erectile function in 38–80% of male CRF patients, with 20–50% of these being completely impotent.

Procci et al.[13] combined questionnaires and nocturnal penile tumescence monitoring (NPT) to evaluate further the incidence of ED in uraemic males (Fig. 48.1). The NPT monitoring technique has been demonstrated by Karacan[14] and others to differentiate organic from psychogenic causes of ED by observing erection during rapid eye movement (REM) sleep. If neurovascular,

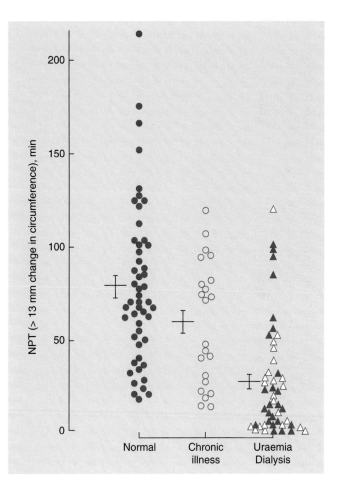

Figure 48.1. Nocturnal penile tumescence (NPT) in normal subjects (●), patients with chronic illness and normal renal function (○), those with advanced renal failure (uraemia; △) and dialysis patients (▲). The vertical bars represent the mean ± SEM. (Reproduced from ref. 13 with permission.)

hormonal or pharmacological factors are responsible for impotence, patients should have altered NPT results; if, however, psychological factors are primarily responsible

551

for ED in uraemia, NPT would be expected to be normal. Procci's results demonstrated a significant abnormality in NPT recordings in 50% of uraemic patients on haemodialysis.[13] Questionnaires quantifying frequency of intercourse correlated with NPT findings in this group of patients. Interestingly, the incidence of depression common in uraemic patients did not correlate with NPT findings or frequency of intercourse. Thus, this study strongly suggests an organic or physiological cause for ED identified in uraemic patients on haemodialysis.

■ AETIOLOGICAL FACTORS IN IMPOTENCE IN URAEMIC MEN

As a result of the multisystem disease processes present in many uraemic men, it is apparent that the pathogenesis of impotence is most probably multifaceted. Uraemic men complain of loss of libido, loss of potency, inadequate or lost ejaculation and decreased penile sensation. Each of these functional changes may be caused by different and separate, although linked, physiological mechanisms.[15,16] Factors to be considered include decreased arterial blood flow, venous occlusive incompetence, altered smooth muscle function, neurogenic abnormalities and hormonal disturbances. These physiological functions may be supplemented by significant psychological stresses and abnormalities resulting from chronic illness and generalized changes in body function (Fig. 48.2).

Arterial abnormalities

In 1923, Leriche described the association of obstructive vascular disease and erectile impotence.[17] The pelvic steal syndrome has long been associated with ED, as have abnormalities in distal, arterial, and vascular obstructive processes.[18] Dalal et al.[19] have reported a haemodialysis patient with penile vascular calcification.

It is well known that patients with uraemia on chronic haemodialysis have accelerated atherosclerosis associated with both large vessel and small vessel occlusive disease. Vasculogenic impotence can be suspected in these patients regardless of age.[20] Kaufman et al.[21] have demonstrated cavernous artery occlusive disease in 78% of impotent patients with CRF. The multifactorial nature of vascular insufficiency in uraemic patients makes specific treatment of these patients difficult. Diabetes mellitus, smoking, hypertension, hyperlipidaemia, and multiple medications are all factors producing arterial insufficiency in these

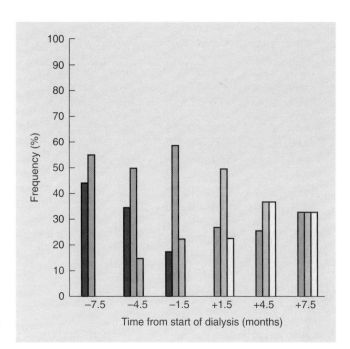

Figure 48.2. Quality of sexual performance (■, very good; ▨, good; ▩, poor; □, very poor) relative to the start of dialysis in 26 uraemic patients during an 18-month follow-up. (Reproduced from ref. 1 with permission.)

patients. Virag et al.[22] have demonstrated these factors as causes for ED in uraemic as well as non-uraemic individuals.[22] Since many dialysis patients have long-term hypertension and as many as 50% require continuous antihypertensive therapy, hypertension and its treatment medications can be strongly suspected as contributing to arterial ED. Since as many as 15% of uraemic patients are diabetic, diabetic vascular changes also can be suspected to contribute to ED.

Additionally, those patients who have undergone renal transplantation may have vascular compromise to their lower extremities and genitalia. These vascular changes can be documented using Doppler sonography and are well reported.[23]

As a result of recent developments in the understanding of the physiology of ED, not only arterial inflow but also venous outflow abnormalities must be considered in the vascular assessment of ED.[24–26] Standard investigation techniques for the abnormality include dynamic infusion pharmacocavernosometry and pharmacocavernosography (DICC). These studies, combined with colour Doppler evaluation of arterial inflow, are necessary to identify specific vascular abnormalities producing ED.[24] Veno-occlusive dysfunction as a cause of erectile problems probably results from a combination of venous vascular abnormalities associated with peripheral smooth muscle function of the corpora cavernosa. Kaufman et al.[21] used pharmacocavernosometry and pharmacocavernosography to demonstrate veno-occlusive dysfunction in 90% of CRF patients. However, veno-occlusive studies have not been performed widely in patients with CRF.[24,25]

Neurogenic impotence

Autonomic control of erectile smooth muscle tissue is critical in the maintenance of erectile function. Penile smooth muscle tone is controlled primarily by adrenergic and cholinergic neurotransmitters and regulates blood flow within the corpora cavernosa.[20] Since autonomic nerve dysfunction is a common problem with uraemic patients on haemodialysis, a significant role for autonomic neuropathy in the impotent haemodialysis patient can be suspected.[27,28] Campese et al.[29] studied the autonomic nervous system in uraemic patients by monitoring the heart rate response to the Valsalva manoeuvre.[29] This technique can, to some extent, measure the integrity of the afferent parasympathetic and efferent sympathetic pathways. They correlated this response with NPT result and intercourse frequency by questionnaire. In the 12 uraemic men studied, there was a significantly abnormal Valsalva ratio that corresponded to significant abnormalities in NPT and a significant decrease in frequency of intercourse. These data suggest that autonomic nervous system dysfunction is an aetiological factor in impotence associated with uraemia. Kersh et al.[30] reported significant vascular instability and hypotension in patients with uraemia, further suggesting autonomic insufficiency in their patients.

Peripheral neuropathy frequently is associated with ED. Peripheral neuropathy that occurs most commonly in patients with diabetes mellitus also can be seen in patients with non-diabetic uraemia. Measured abnormalities in the bulbocavernosus reflex have been demonstrated in this group of patients.[3] Although there are few satisfactory neurophysiological tests to identify patients with neurogenic impotence, clinical neurophysiology can be useful in assessing patients with defects in somatic nervous system pathways to the sacral segments affected by uraemia, diabetes, or other metabolic disease processes. There are, however, no satisfactory direct methods for assessing autonomic nervous system function, and only secondary evidence for autonomic neuropathy is available.[31]

Psychological factors

The psychological impact of uraemia and its treatment and management have a significant role in sexual dysfunction in patients with CRF. Patients with uraemia, especially those on haemodialysis, have a significant incidence of psychiatric and depressive illness compared with the normal population.[8] These psychological abnormalities will certainly add to the already significant physiological abnormalities in these patients. The psychological conditions identified include low self-esteem; lack of a sense of well-being; a significant increase in stress from chronic illness, job loss, and financial concerns; and a documented increase in depression and marital discord. Dunante et al.[32] clearly demonstrated the association between depression, its severity and ED in the Massachusetts Male Aging Study (MMAS). Procci et al.[13] have identified a higher incidence of depressive episodes in patients on haemodialysis in comparison with a normal population.[13] Glass et al.[9] studied the psychological impact of CRF, dialysis and renal transplantation and found that dialysis patients were more likely to be depressed than transplant patients, whereas transplant patients showed a greater level of anxiety. Marital discord rates were higher in all patients with CRF, and they were especially marked in those patients on haemodialysis. The findings of Glass et al.[9] which demonstrated impotence in many patients in whom physiological erectile function could be measured, suggested that psychological stresses and abnormalities were a significant part of uraemic sexual dysfunction.

Pharmacological factors

Because of the underlying conditions that have produced ED in patients with CRF, close attention must be paid to erectile abnormalities associated with medications. Pharmacological treatment of conditions associated with CRF may produce side effects causing or increasing impotence and diminished libido (Table 48.1). Such agents may produce abnormalities in central, neuroendocrine regulation or in the neurovascular control of erectile function either in the corpora cavernosa or at a central level.[33] Agents that increase prolactin or are associated with other central neurological abnormalities are likely to reduce libido. Antihypertensive agents, which are commonly used in patients with CRF, are well-known causes of ED. Impotence has been associated with virtually all available antihypertensive medications.[34–36] These antihypertensive medications, added to the

Table 48.1. Agents frequently used in CRF associated with sexual dysfunction

Antihypertensives
  Sympatholytics
    Methyldopa (Aldomet)
    Clonidine (Catopres)
    Reserpine (Serpasil, Sandril)
    Guanethidine (Ismelin)
  Beta-adrenergic antagonists
    Propranolol (Inderol)
    Pindolol (Vislein)
    Atenolol (Tenormin)
    Metoprolol (Lopressor)
    Labetalol (Trandate, Normadyne)
  Vasodilators
    Hydralazine (Apresoline)
  Diuretics
    Thiazides (Diuril)
    Spironolactone (Aldactone)

Cimetidine (Tagomet)

Digoxin

Clofibrate (Atromid-S)

Metoclopramide (Reglan)

Antidepressants (depress libido)

associated physiological arterial changes noted to occur with atherosclerosis, magnify the problem of ED in these individuals. Although calcium-channel-blocking agents, alpha-adrenergic blocking agents, and angiotensin-converting enzyme (ACE) inhibitors are least likely to impair physiological erectile response, the sympatholytics, beta-adrenergic blocking agents and vasodilators are strongly associated with local effects that overcome the normal physiological response of the smooth muscles of the corpora cavernosa and (locally as well as centrally) inhibit erectile function.[34,35] Patients with hypertension and ED who can be appropriately controlled are best treated with selective alpha-1 blocking agents, such as prazosin, doxazosin and terazosin. Cases of priapism have been reported with alpha-1-adrenergic blocking agents,

such as prazosin.[3,4] Many dialysis patients are treated with sympatholytic medications such as methlydopa and clonidine, beta-blockers such as propranolol, and vasodilators such as hydralazine. Patients treated with these agents can be expected to exhibit physiological ED as a result of the local cavernosal effects of these agents.[35] Alpha-2-adrenergic antagonists, such as clonidine, may produce central cavernosal artery constriction or limit its dilatation potential, decreasing cavernosal perfusion and diminishing erectile function.[37]

Endocrine factors

The kidney plays an integral role in endocrine function. Hormonal effects of the kidney are well known, and the kidney provides significant hormonal metabolism. CRF, therefore, can be expected to produce profound changes in endocrine function and hormone balance that affect many bodily functions, including male sexual activity. Impairment of the hypothalamic–pituitary–testicular axis in men with CRF has been well documented (Fig. 48.3).[38–41] Semen analyses in these patients demonstrate a low or absent sperm count with abnormalities in both morphology and motility.[27] These abnormalities are supported by testicular histological abnormalities on biopsy, including abnormalities in both spermatogenesis and interstitial cell morphology.[42] Interstitial cell abnormalities can be correlated with reduced testosterone secretion.[43–45] Most male patients with CRF on dialysis have low serum testosterone levels, although many may be at the low end of the normal range.[42] Low testosterone levels are most probably caused by decreased testosterone production, but there is evidence for elevated metabolic clearance of testosterone in addition to decreased production.[38,40,42] As a result of normal testicular binding capacity, free testosterone and salivary testosterone levels are low.[38,41,43,46] These abnormalities have been identified in patients despite differing methods of dialysis, including haemodialysis and peritoneal dialysis (continuous ambulatory peritoneal dialysis; CAPD).[44,45] Some dialysis patients have elevated levels of testosterone-binding globulin, and some patients have normal testosterone and free testosterone levels.[47–49] These low free and total testosterone levels remain low despite attempted stimulation with administration of exogenous human chorionic gonadotrophin (HCG).[50] These data strongly suggest that testosterone deficiency is a result of decreased hormone production and secretion. Investigation of patients immediately after initiation of dialysis in early

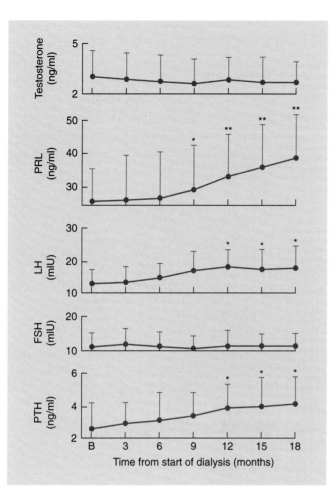

Figure 48.3. Behaviour of serum hormones in males during the 18-month follow-up. *p<0.05; **p<0.001 vs basal [B]. (Reproduced from ref. 1 with permission.)

uraemia demonstrates an initial elevation in testosterone levels, suggesting that circulating toxins may be important in uraemic testicular failure.[40] Unfortunately, however, testicular function is only temporarily restored, and men with CRF on haemodialysis or CAPD fail to experience restoration of hormone production satisfactory to restore fertility or potency. Although the exact level of testosterone synthesis deficiency remains controversial, recent evidence points to abnormalities in the production of dehydroisoandrosterone (DHA) from 17-hydroxy-pregnenolone via the enzyme-catalysed reaction with desmolase C17–20. Nevertheless, restoration of testosterone levels with exogenous testosterone administration in patients with deficient circulating testosterone frequently fails to restore adequate sexual functioning and fertility.[38–50]

Most uraemic males demonstrate abnormalities of pituitary hormone secretion, including changes in luteinizing hormone (LH), follicle-stimulating hormone (FSH) and prolactin. LH levels are characteristically increased in males with uraemia on maintenance dialysis. This increase is caused by both an increase in secretion and reduced metabolic clearance of the hormone.[51,52] It has been estimated that LH levels exceed 20% of normal in many of these patients, probably as a result of decreased testosterone levels caused by hypogonadism. Evaluation of FSH levels similarly demonstrates abnormalities; however, FSH is usually increased only in patients with significantly diminished spermatogenesis.[52] Holdsworth et al.[52] have suggested that the FSH levels in patients with uraemia can be used as prognostic indicators for the return of fertility following renal transplantation. Occasionally, pituitary abnormalities can be suggested by low LH levels despite low testosterone concentration;[53,54] more commonly, however, pituitary response to gonadotrophin-releasing hormone (GnRH) with increased FSH and LH production is quite normal.[49,52,54,55] Rodger et al.[49] have suggested that testosterone secretion is further affected by the loss of pulsatile rhythm of luteinizing hormone-releasing hormone (LHRH), resulting in diminished LH peak levels.[49]

A proposed cause of sexual dysfunction in patients with chronic renal failure is hyperprolactinaemia. Sexual dysfunction is commonly experienced by patients with hyperprolactinaemia caused by pituitary neoplasms or pharmacological abnormalities with normal renal function. Although the mechanism of sexual dysfunction caused by hyperprolactinaemia remains controversial, loss of libido, decreased erectile function and infertility have been widely associated with elevations in prolactin.[56] The cause of sexual dysfunction in those patients with elevated prolactin may be a result of a disordered hypothalamic–pituitary axis or a direct peripheral gonadal effect of prolactin. Hyperprolactinaemia without renal failure usually results in increased levels of LH and hypogonadism. This response differs from the usual low testosterone and low LH associated with the hyperprolactinaemia of CRF.

Hyperprolactinaemia is identified in more than 50% of CRF patients on dialysis.[57,58] There is evidence to suggest that the elevation in prolactin in uraemic men is a result not only of increased secretion but also of reduced degradation of secreted prolactin.[59] Increased prolactin levels also can be a result of medications used in patients with CRF: these medications include methyldopa, digoxin, cimetidine and metoclopramide. There are numerous reports of improvement of ED and fertility when hyperprolactinaemia alone is treated.[57]

Other endocrinological abnormalities can strongly contribute to ED in patients with CRF on dialysis treatment. Most common among these is diabetes mellitus, which is one of the most common causes of ED with or without renal failure. Vascular changes in long-term insulin-dependent diabetic patients are well known and cause corporal arterial insufficiency and veno-occlusive dysfunction. In younger patients with normal vascular function, diabetic renal complications frequently are associated with autonomic peripheral neuropathy and neuropathic dysfunction, resulting in inadequate erectile response. These abnormalities significantly increase the neurological abnormalities associated with ED, previously described.[60,61]

Other hormonal abnormalities that contribute to ED in uraemic men include abnormalities in parathyroid hormone (PTH). Massry et al.[62] have suggested that elevated PTH levels are an integral part of uraemic male ED. They report two impotent dialysis patients in whom sexual function was restored following parathyroidectomy without other changes in CRF management.[62] These investigators have suggested that elevated PTH may result in both peripheral and central nervous system defects that decrease erectile function. Akmal et al.,[63] in a laboratory study using a canine uraemic model, demonstrated significantly decreased serum testosterone levels, which could be prevented by parathyroidectomy before producing experimental uraemia.

Other factors associated with ED

Zinc deficiency and abnormal zinc metabolism in uraemic patients, associated with gonadal dysfunction, have been reported but remain controversial.[64–66] Because of the difficulty in assessing true tissue zinc levels and the effect of these levels on erectile function, it cannot be satisfactorily concluded that serum or tissue zinc levels are directly responsible for ED, and it cannot be concluded that zinc administration could be expected to produce improvement in sexual function, fertility or libido.[67–69]

Hypoxia associated with CRF has also been implicated as a potential cause of ED.[19,70] Two sources of hypoxia in CRF have been identified — pulmonary-associated hypoxia and anaemia-associated hypoxia. Pulmonary-associated hypoxia is due to hypoventilation and pulmonary micro-embolization, whereas anaemia-associated hypoxia is due to diminished erythropoietin production.[19,71] Hypoxia can lead to ED by affecting nitric oxide (NO) synthesis in the corpora cavernosa. Kim et al.[72] showed that, in the presence of hypoxia, NO synthesis was low and smooth muscle tone was increased. Hypoxia has also been shown to increase the release of endothelium-derived contracting factors, further increasing smooth muscle tone.[73] Endogenous nitric oxide synthase (NOS) inhibitors such as asymmetrical dimethyl arginine are normally excreted in the urine. Levels of these inhibitors are increased in CRF patients and may also contribute to ED.[74] Yamamato et al.[75] reported decreased NOS activity in the epididymis during renal failure; NOS activity was restored after renal transplantation.

■ DIAGNOSIS OF URAEMIC IMPOTENCE

It is clear from the foregoing discussion that the causes of ED and infertility in uraemic men can be multifactorial. As a result, a careful history, physical examination and appropriate laboratory studies are necessary to provide specific, tailored and adequate treatment for these individuals. A careful history to identify psychological factors, such as significant depression, must be carried out by a qualified mental health care professional. A careful physical examination, including studies for the identification of peripheral neuropathy and vascular abnormalities, is also helpful. The use of NPT monitoring in patients with marginal ED may be helpful in differentiating those patients with clear organic causes for their ED from those with a significant psychogenic diagnosis. In patients in whom veno-occlusive incompetence or arterial abnormalities are suspected by Doppler screening studies, dynamic infusion pharmaco-cavernosometry and cavernosography, together with colour Doppler arterial response studies may be helpful, especially if surgical intervention is planned.

A hormone profile to include testosterone, LH, prolactin and FSH should be performed. Although provocative studies using LHRH or thyroid-releasing hormone (TRH) may be academically interesting, their importance in treatment programmes remains controversial. Communication with nephrologist and transplant surgeon is essential, as transplantation may reverse many of the previously mentioned abnormalities of uraemia, and initiation of specific impotence treatment modalities may be delayed until after transplantation is carried out in some patients.

■ TREATMENT ALTERNATIVES

Management options for patients with CRF and ED are shown in Figure 48.4.

Medical treatment

Patients with deficient testosterone levels may be treated with testosterone replacement therapy, with benefit in some cases. Most commonly, testosterone replacement therapy improves libido without significant impact on potency or fertility. Although testosterone can be replaced using oral medication, it is usually most effectively administered with sustained-release injectable testosterone preparations[76,77] or with a transdermal testosterone delivery system. Many studies, however, have demonstrated that even the use of 100–200 mg testosterone injected weekly produces only variable improvement in sexual function.[77–79] Other methods of raising serum testosterone have been more effective, including clomiphene (100 mg/day) and HCG (500 IU/week).[80,81]

Pharmacological methods for decreasing hyperprolactinaemia also appear to be effective in some males with uraemia-associated sexual dysfunction. Dopaminergic agonists, such as bromocriptine or lisuride hydrogen maleate, have been effective in some patients.[47,59,82] Bromocriptine can be administered in doses of 1.25–5 mg daily, and lisuride can be given at doses from 0.05 to 0.2 mg daily, with expected decrease in prolactin levels to the low normal range. Subsequent rises in plasma testosterone with expected improvement in sexual function result from these medications. Side effects of bromocriptine, including hypotension, nausea and dizziness, are intolerable to some patients but seem to be less frequent with lisuride.[82]

Zinc therapy with administration of zinc through the dialysate or oral administration remains controversial. Further studies with dialysis and zinc administration are

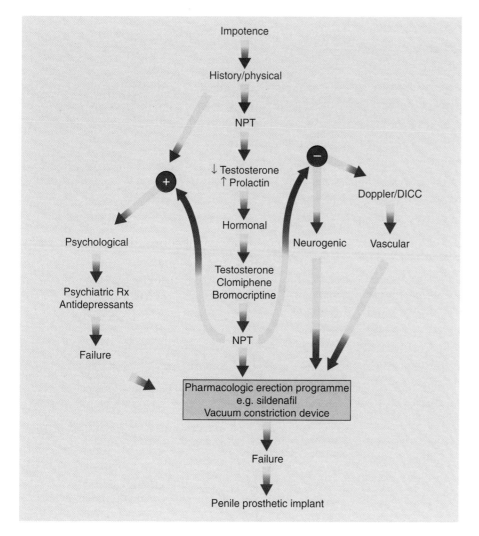

Figure 48.4. Management options for patients with CRF and erectile dysfunction.

necessary before firm conclusions can be drawn about the effectiveness of zinc replacement and restoration of sexual function.[83,84]

CRF and uraemia frequently are associated with profound anaemia, which may result in psychological erectile dysfunction caused by weakness, fatigue and anxiety. The physiological effects of anaemia and hypoxia on erectile function have been described previously in this chapter. The association of anaemia and hormonal abnormalities is also the subject of some controversy.[85] Treatment of anaemia with recombinant human erythropoietin in male uraemic patients has been reported to improve sexual performance and fertility and to increase serum testosterone and FSH levels. Although the studies on recombinant human erythropoietin are preliminary, there appears to be some salutary effect of this method of treatment in some uraemic patients.[86,87] Combining testosterone and erythropoietin has been shown to enhance and restore the erectile response to prostaglandin E (PGE) in a dose-dependent fashion in a feline model of CRF.[88]

Intracavernosal injection of vasoactive agents
Since the majority of uraemic patients on haemodialysis in the younger age-group have adequate vascular supply to their corpora cavernosa, injection of vasoactive agents into the corpora cavernosa can be expected to result in return of erectile function. Some patients with vascular problems, such as diabetic microangiopathy, mild to moderate arteriosclerosis and partial arterial dysplasia, may respond to higher doses of intracavernosal injections. Patients with concomitant veno-occlusive incompetence, however, may not respond to these agents and may require surgical intervention or other therapeutic techniques. As noted in other discussions in this text, treatment with papaverine, papaverine and phento-lamine, PGE1 or combinations of these agents may be effective for long-term treatment of ED, with few complications. Successful injection in older patients has been reported, with expected higher dosage requirements but comparative success rates without increased complications.[89] Long-term use of these intracavernosal vasoactive agents has been demonstrated to be effective with few long-term complications in patients following renal transplantation.[90] No other abnormalities or effect on the transplanted kidney have been identified with this treatment technique, and it can be expected to be safe and effective.

Oral and transurethral corporal drug therapy
Phosphodiesterase enzymes (PDE) type III and V are found in the corporal smooth muscle. These enzymes break down the cyclic nucleotides adenosine and guanine monophosphate (cAMP and cGMP). cGMP is the second messenger responsible for NO-induced smooth muscle relaxation. Inhibition of PDE results in a greater erectile response to NO-mediated cGMP. Sildenafil (Viagra, Pfizer) is an oral type V PDE inhibitor that has been shown to be effective in the treatment of ED.[91] Clinical phase III trials are ongoing in the USA. Although there are no specific data on the use of oral PDE inhibitors in patients with CRF, sildenafil is a possibility for the treatment of ED in CRF.

The recent FDA approval of the Medicated Urethral System for Erection (MUSE, Vivus) provides CRF patients with another treatment option for ED. The system allows for transurethral delivery of alprostadil (PGE1), which is then transferred to the corpora cavernosa by direct venous communications.[92,93] Although the system has not been tested in patients with CRF, it has been effective in the treatment of ED arising from most other causes.

Vacuum constriction devices
Vacuum constriction devices have been widely reported as effective in patients who are impotent from a variety of aetiologies. These devices, which appear to be effective in diabetic males as well as in patients with other causes for ED, are rarely associated with morbidity but are difficult for some patients to use and to tolerate. Vacuum constriction devices, however, can be an alternative for motivated patients who find this method of treatment satisfactory.[94,95]

Surgical treatment of ED
A variety of surgical procedures have been proposed for arterial insufficiency causing ED. Although the success rates of these procedures are variable, their use in patients with CRF before transplantation may be associated with significant morbidity. Because most patients with CRF and uraemia associated with ED have significant large and small vessel disease, adequate response from arterial bypass procedures cannot be expected. In selected patients, however, balloon dilatation of pelvic arteries may be helpful, with low morbidity expected.[18]

Implantation of penile prostheses
Implantation of penile prostheses in these patients may be expected to be successful, with low morbidity. Although there

are few reports of penile prosthesis implantation in haemodialysis patients, penile implants are used commonly in patients with CRF following renal transplantation.[96] These surgical procedures are best restricted to patients who have undergone transplantation, since many patients will find return of sexual function, potency and fertility after reversal of the toxic effects of uraemia by renal transplantation. If, however, underlying disease processes preclude the return of normal erectile function, penile prosthesis implantation can be expected to be successful in many of these men. There is little question, however, that the immunocompromised patient is at increased risk for complications of prosthesis infection. Despite this increased risk, however, successful implantation and function can be expected in the vast majority of patients, with little morbidity.[97,98]

IMPROVEMENT IN SEXUAL FUNCTION AFTER RENAL TRANSPLANTATION

As a result of normalization of metabolic and hormonal function in patients after successful renal transplantation, many patients reported improved sexual function. Within 2–3 months of transplantation, testosterone levels frequently return to a normal range, with a concomitant normalization of LH, FSH and prolactin levels. Lim and Fang reported a return of normal sperm count and motility 9–16 months after transplantation in four of five patients.[53] Gonadal resistance to gonadotrophin stimulation also improves when haemodialysis and renal transplantation are successful. A more normal HCG stimulation with a higher testosterone response is observed in transplanted patients compared with those on haemodialysis. Salvatierra et al.[99] studied a group of patients with CRF: their results demonstrate a 66% potency rate before the onset of CRF, declining to only 22% during dialysis. Following successful renal transplantation, however, 84% of patients with functioning renal allografts resumed their pre-uraemia degree of potency within 3 years. Psychological problems of haemodialysed patients improved after transplantation, although there continued to be some increased anxiety despite decreased depression.[100]

Many patients, however, remain impotent after transplantation. Causes of post-transplant impotence include failure to resolve hormonal abnormalities, underlying disease processes that have resulted in continued ED, and the effects of renal transplant itself.[101] As many as 87% of patients will continue to be impotent

following transplantation.[102,103] The causes of this ED vary: the majority of patients will have restoration of hormone values, and no specific post-transplant diagnosis is consistent with ED. Reports of marked increase in ED following bilateral renal transplantation may be a result of changes in pelvic haemodynamics resulting in decreased penile blood flow, although reports of patients who are potent following interruption of bilateral hypogastric arteries are common. Impotence following sequential bilateral renal transplantation, however, appears to be increased as a result of decreased blood flow associated with ligation of both internal iliac arteries.

Because of the difficulties with underlying vascular disease, multiple surgical interventions and patient risk factors, revascularization may result in higher potential morbidity than the use of penile implant in these complex surgical patients.[23,104,105] Billet et al.,[104] however, reported a successful saphenous vein bypass graft between the external iliac and internal iliac arteries in a patient who was impotent following bilateral renal transplantation. Their patient demonstrated substantial improvement in penile blood flow and reported subjective return of erections and sexual function.

CONCLUSIONS

Patients with CRF, uraemia, haemodialysis and transplantation frequently suffer from loss of libido, ED and infertility. This multifactorial condition results in psychological, hormonal, neurological, vascular, and pharmacological effects, all of which combine to limit sexual activity. Although pharmacological manipulation of hormonal abnormalities may improve libido, ED is more difficult to resolve. Renal transplantation appears to be the most effective method for improving sexual function in the majority of patients. Despite renal transplantation and the resolution of hormonal abnormalities, however, underlying medical problems frequently continue to produce the chronic ED. Treatment alternatives must therefore be directed not only at the CRF but also at the specific causes of ED. Treatment alternatives, in addition to pharmacological manipulation, include intracorporal injection of pharmacoactive agents, vacuum constriction devices, and penile prosthesis implantation. Although re-vascularization after transplantation is an option, it should be considered only in highly selected patients.

■ REFERENCES

1. Di Paolo N, Capotondo L, Gaggiotti E, Rossi P. Sexual function in uremic patients. Contrib Nephrol 1990; 77: 34–44

2. Abram H S, Hester L R, Sheridan W F, Epstein G M. Sexual functioning in patients with chronic renal failure. J Nerv Ment Dis 1975; 160: 220–226

3. Waltzer W C. Sexual and reproductive function in men treated with hemodialysis and renal transplantation. J Urol 1981; 126: 713–718

4. Rodger R S C, Fletcher K, Dewar J H et al. Prevalence and pathogenesis of impotence in 100 uremic men. Uremia Invest 1984; 8: 89–92

5. Massry S G, Goldstein D A, Procci W R, Kletzky O A. On the pathogenesis of sexual dysfunction of the uremic male. Proc Eur Dial Transplant Assoc 1980; 17: 139–148

6. Levy N B. Sexual adjustment and maintenance, hemodialysis and renal transplantation. National survey by questionnaire: preliminary report. Trans Am Soc Artif Intern Organs 1973; 9: 138–146

7. Sherman F P. Impotence in patients with chronic renal failure on dialysis: its frequency and etiology. Fertil Steril 1975; 26: 221–225

8. Procci W R. The study of sexual dysfunction in uremic males: problems for patients and investigators. Clin Exp Dial Apheresis 1983; 7: 289–293

9. Glass C A, Fielding D M, Evans C, Ashcroft J B. Factors related to sexual functioning in male patients undergoing hemodialysis and with kidney transplants. Arch Sex Behav 1987; 16: 189–194

10. Kinsey A C, Pomeroy W B, Martin C E (eds) Sexual behavior in the human male. Philadelphia: Saunders, 1948: 86

11. Masters W H, Johnson V E (eds) Human sexual inadequacy. Boston: Little, Brown, 1970

12. Levy N, Abram H S. Endocrinology of chronic renal failure. In: Massry S G, Sellers D (eds) Clinical aspects of uremia and dialysis. Springfield, IL: Charles C Thomas, 1996: 248–263

13. Procci W R, Goldstein D A, Adelstein J, Massry S G. Sexual dysfunction in the male patient with uremia: a reappraisal. Kidney Int 1981; 19: 317–323

14. Karacan I. NPT/rigidometry. In: Kirby R S, Carson C C, Webster G D (eds) Impotence: diagnosis and management of erectile dysfunction. Boston: Butterworth Heinemann, 1991: 62–71

15. Krumlovsky F A, Madsen J D. Mechanism and therapy of impotence associated with chronic renal failure and chronic dialysis. J Dial 1979; 3: 395–409

16. Pacitti A, Segoloni G P, Gallon E G et al. An outpatient approach to sexual problems in uremic patients. Contrib Nephrol 1990; 77: 45–54

17. Leriche R. Des oblitérations arterielles hautes (oblitération de la termination de l'aorte) comme cause d'insuffisance circulatoire des membres inferieures. Bull Mem Soc Chir Paris 1923; 49: 1404–1409

18. Goldwasser B, Carson C C, Braun S D, McCann R L. Impotence due to the pelvic steal syndrome: treatment by iliac transluminal angioplasty. J Urol 1985; 133: 860–862

19. Dalal S, Gandhi V C, Yu A W et al. Penile calcification in maintenance hemodialysis patients. Urology 1992; 40: 422

20. Lindner A, Charra B, Sherrar D, Scribner B H. Accelerated atherosclerosis and prolonged maintenance hemodialysis. N Engl J Med 1974; 290: 697

21. Kaufman J, Hatzichristou D, Mulhall J et al. Impotence and chronic renal failure: a study of the hemodynamic pathophysiology. Urology 1994; 151: 612–618

22. Virag R, Bouilly R, Frydman D. Is impotence an arterial disorder? Lancet 1985; 1: 181

23. Ngheim D D, Corry R J, Mendez G P, Lee H M. Pelvic hemodynamics and male sexual impotence after renal transplantation. Am Surg 1982; 48: 532

24. Carson C C. Impotence: new diagnostic modalities. Urol Annu 1992; 6: 229

25. Rudnick J, Becker H C. Present state of diagnostic management in venoocclusive dysfunction. Urol Int 1992; 49: 9

26. Saenz de Tejada I. Etiology of impotence. Contemp Urol 1992; 4: 52–68

27. Fraser C L, Arief A I. Nervous system complications in uremia. Ann Intern Med 1988; 109: 143

28. Nogues M A, Starkstein S, Davolas M et al. Cardiovascular reflexes and pudendal evoked responses in chronic hemodialysis patients. Funct Neurol 1991; 6: 359

29. Campese V M, Procci W R, Levitan D et al. Autonomic nervous system dysfunction and impotence in uremia. Am J Nephrol 1982; 2: 140

30. Kersh E S, Kronfield S J, Unger A et al. Autonomic insufficiency in uremia as a cause of hemodialysis induced hypotension. N Engl J Med 1974; 290: 650

31. Eardley I, Kirby R S, Fowler C J. Neurophysiological testing. In: Kirby R S, Carson C C, Webster G D (eds) Impotence: diagnosis and management of male erectile dysfunction. Boston: Butterworth Heinemann, 1991: 109

32. Dunante R, Aroujo A, Feldman H et al. An epidemiologic perspective on the association between depression and erectile dysfunction. J Urol 1997; 157: 360

33. Wein A J, van Arsdalen K N. Drug-induced male sexual dysfunction. Urol Clin North Am 1988; 15: 23

34. Stevenson J G, Umstead G S. Sexual dysfunction due to antihypertensive agents. Drug Intell Clin Pharm 1984; 18: 113

35. Kim J Y, Park H Y, Kerfoot W W et al. Local effects of antihypertensive agents on isolated corpus cavernosum. J Urol 1993; 150: 249–252

36. Jandhyala B S, Clarke D E, Buckley J P. Effects of prolonged administration of certain antihypertensive agents. J Pharm Sci 1974; 63: 1497–1503

37. Hedlund H, Andersson K E. Comparison of the responses to drugs acting on adrenoreceptors and muscarinic receptors in human isolated corpus cavernosum and cavernous artery. J Auton Pharmacol 1985; 5: 81–90

38. Copolla A, Cuomo G. Pituitary testicular evaluation in patients with chronic renal insufficiency in hemodialysis treatment. Minerva Med 1990; 81: 461–469

39. Menchini-Fabris G F, Turchip-Giorgi P M, Canale D. Diagnosis and treatment of sexual dysfunction in patients affected by chronic renal failure on hemodialysis. Contrib Nephrol 1990; 77: 24–32

40. Stewart-Bently M, Gans D, Horton R. Regulation of gonadal function in uremia. Metabolism 1974; 23: 1065–1078

41. Ramirez G, Butcher D, Bruggenmyer C D, Gungangly A. Testicular defect: the primary abnormality in gonadal dysfunction of uremia. South Med J 1987; 80: 698–706

42. Corvol B, Beretagna X, Bedrossian J. Increased steroid metabolic clearance rate in anephric patients. Acta Endocrinol 1974; 75: 756–759

43. DeVries C P, Gooren L J G, Oe P L. Hemodialysis and testicular function. Int J Androl 1984; 7: 97–110

44. Gokal R, Utley L. A collection of problems in CAPD. Adv Perit Dial 1989; 5: 76–81

45. Altman J J. Sex hormones and chronic renal failure of the diabetic. Ann Endocrinol 1988; 49: 412–420

46. Muir J W, Besser G M, Edwards C R W et al. Bromocriptine improves reduced libido and potency in men receiving maintenance hemodialysis. Clin Nephrol 1983; 20: 308–314

47. Bommer J, Kugel M, Schwobel B et al. Improved sexual function during recombinant human erythropoietin therapy. Nephrol Dial Transplant 1990; 5: 204–209

48. Rodger R S C, Morrison L, Dewar J H et al. Loss of pulsatile luteinizing hormone secretion in men with chronic renal failure. Br Med J 1985; 291: 1598–1611

49. Rodger R S C, Dewar J H, Turner S J et al. Anterior pituitary dysfunction in patients with chronic renal failure treated by hemodialysis or continuous peritoneal ambulatory dialysis. Nephron 1986; 43: 169–178

50. Rager K, Bundschu H, Gupta D. The effect of HCG on testicular androgen production in adult men with chronic renal failure. J Reprod Fertil 1915; 42: 113–125

51. Zumoff B, Walter L, Rosenfeld R S. Subnormal plasma adrenal androgen levels in men with uremia. J Clin Endocrinol Metab 1980; 51: 801–809

52. Holdsworth S, Atkins R C, deKretsker D M. The pituitary testicular axis in men with chronic renal failure. N Engl J Med 1977; 296: 1245–1253

53. Lim V S, Fang V S. Gonadal dysfunction in uremic men: a study of hypothalamo–pituitary–testicular axis before and after renal transplantation. Am J Med 1975; 58: 655–665

54. LeRoith D, Danovitz G, Testian S, Spitz J M. Dissociation of pituitary glycoprotein response to releasing hormones in chronic renal failure. Acta Endocrinol 1980; 93: 277–284

55. Distiller L A. Pituitary gonadal function in chronic renal failure: the effect of luteinizing hormone-releasing hormone and the influence of dialysis. Metabolism 1975; 24: 711–719

56. Spark R E. Hyperprolactinemia in males with and without pituitary microadenomas. Lancet 1982; 2: 129–131

57. Sieverstein G D, Lim V S, Nakawates E C. Metabolic clearance and secretion rates of human prolactin in normal subjects and in patients with chronic renal failure. J Clin Endocrinol Metab 1980; 50: 846–854

58. Vircburger M I, Prelevick G M. Testosterone levels after bromocriptine treatment in patients undergoing long-term hemodialysis. J Androl 1985; 6: 113–116

59. Bommer J, del Pozo E, Ritz E, Bommer G. Improved sexual function in male hemodialysis patients on bromocriptine. Lancet 1979; 2: 496–509

60. Saenz de Tejada I, Goldstein I. Diabetic penile neuropathy. Urol Clin North Am 1988; 15: 17–34

61. Brindley G S. Neurophysiology. In: Kirby R S, Carson C C, Webster G D (eds) Impotence: diagnosis and maintenance of erectile dysfunction. Boston: Butterworth Heinemann, 1991; 27–31

62. Massry S G, Goldstein D A, Procci W R, Kletzky O A. Impotence and patients with uremia. A possible role for parathyroid hormone. Nephron 1977; 19: 305–311

63. Akmal M, Goldstein D A, Kletzky O A, Massry S G. Hyperparathyroidism and hypotestosteronemia of acute renal failure. Am J Nephrol 1988; 8: 166–172

64. Rodger R S, Sheldon W L, Watson M J et al. Zinc deficiency and hyperprolacinemia are not reversible causes of sexual dysfunction in uremia. Nephrol Dial Transplant 1989; 4: 888–899

65. Condon C J, Freeman R M. Zinc metabolism in renal failure. Ann Intern Med 1970; 73: 531–536

66. Mahaja S K, Abbasi D A, Prasad A A et al. Effect of oral zinc therapy on gonadal function in hemodialysis patients. Ann Intern Med 1982; 97: 357–364

67. Ritz E, Bommer J. Discussion. Zinc metabolism. Contrib Nephrol 1984; 38: 126–128

68. Sprenger K B, Schmitz J, Hetzel D et al. Zinc and sexual dysfunction. Contrib Nephrol 1984; 38: 119–128

69. Rodger S C, Brook A C, Muirhead N, Kerr D N S. Zinc metabolism does not influence sexual function in chronic renal insufficiency. Contrib Nephrol 1984; 38: 112–118

70. Sobb M, Humid I, Attu M, Refuie A. Effect of erythropoietin on sexual potency in chronic hemodialysis patients. Scand J Urol Nephrol 1992; 26: 181–189

71. DeBroe M, DeBacker W. Pathophysiology of hemodialysis-associated hypoxemia. Adv Nephrol 1989; 18: 297–314

72. Kim N, Vardi Y, Padma-Nathan H et al. Oxygen tension regulates the nitric oxide pathway. J Clin Invest 1993; 91: 437–442

73. Luscher T F, Borelungeri M, Duhi Y, Yang Z. Endothelium-derived contracting factors. Hypertension 1992; 14: 117–122

74. Vallance P, Leone A, Calver A et al. Accumulation of an endogenous inhibitor in nitric oxide synthesis in chronic renal failure. Lancet 1992; 339: 572–577

75. Yamamato Y, Sifikitis N, Ono K et al. Kidney transplantation restores the effects of chronic renal failure on epididymal sperm maturation and nitric oxide synthase activity. J Urol 1995; 153: 322A

76. van Coeverden A, Stolear J C, de Haen E M et al. Effect of chronic oral testosterone on the pituitary testicular axis in hemodialyzed male patients. J Clin Nephrol 1988; 26: 48–56

77. Barton C H, Mirahamadi M K, Vairi N D. Effects of long-term testosterone administration on pituitary testicular axis and end-stage renal failure. Nephron 1982; 31: 61–69

78. Lim V S. Reproductive function in patients with renal insufficiency. Am J Kidney Dis 1987; 4: 363–368

79. Foulks C J, Cushner H M. Sexual function in the male dialysis patient. Pathogenesis, evaluation and therapy. Am J Kidney Dis 1986; 4: 211–219

80. Lim V S, Fang V S. Restoration of plasma testosterone levels in uremic men with clomiphene citrate. J Clin Endocrinol Metab 1976; 43: 1370–1377

81. Canale D. Human chorionic gonadotropin treatment of male sexual inadequacy in patients affected by chronic renal failure. J Androl 1984; 5: 120–125

82. Ruilope L, Garcia-Robles R, Paya C et al. Influence of lisuride and dopaminergic agonists on the sexual function of male patients with chronic renal failure. Am J Kidney Dis 1985; 3: 182–186

83. Brook A C, Johnston D G, Ward M K et al. Absence of therapeutic effect of zinc in sexual dysfunction of hemodialysis patients. Lancet 1980; 2: 618–626

84. Mahajan S K, Handburger R J, Flamenbaum W et al. Effect of zinc supplementation and hyperprolactinemia in uremic men. Lancet 1985; 2: 750–753

85. Campese V M, Liu C L. Sexual dysfunction in uremia. Contrib Nephrol 1990; 77: 1–18

86. Imagawa A, Kawanish Y, Numata A. Is erythropoietin effective for impotence in dialysis patients? Nephron 1990; 54: 95–101

87. Schaefer R M, Kokot F, Wernze H et al. Improved sexual function in hemodialysis patients on recombinant erythropoietin: a possible role for prolactin. Clin Nephrol 1989; 31: 1–12

88. Hellstrom W, Shenassa B, Garrison E et al. Effect of combined erythropoietin and testosterone on the prostaglandin E erectile response in the chronic renal failure feline model. J Urol 1995; 153: 509A

89. Kerfoot W J, Carson C C. Pharmacologically induced erections among geriatric men. J Urol 1991; 146: 1022–1027

90. Rodriguez Antolin A, Morales J M, Andres A et al. Treatment of erectile impotence in renal transplant patients with intracavernosal vasoactive drugs. Transplant Proc 1992; 24: 105–111

91. Boolell M, Allen M J, Ballard S J et al. Sildenafil: an orally active type 5 cyclic GMP-specific phosphodiesterase inhibitor for the treatment of penile erectile dysfunction. Int J Impot Res 1996; 8: 47–52

92. Padma-Nathan H. Corporal pharmacotherapy for erectile dysfunction. Monogr Urol 1996; 17: 4–11

93. Padma-Nathan H, Bennett A, Gesundheit N et al. Treatment of erectile dysfunction by the medicated urethral system for erection. J Urol 1995; 153: 975–984

94. Wiles P G. Successful noninvasive management of erectile impotence in diabetic men. Br Med J 1988; 296: 161–169

95. Whitherington R. External penile appliances for management of impotence. Semin Urol 1990; 8: 124–139

96. Kabalin J N, Kessler R. Successful implantation of penile prostheses in organ transplant patients. Urology 1989; 33: 282–289

97. Walther P J, Andriani R T, Maggio M I, Carson C C. Fournier's gangrene: a complication of penile prosthetic implantation in a renal transplant patient. J Urol 1987; 137: 299–301

98. Carson C C. Infectious complications of genitourinary prostheses. Probl Urol 1993; 7: 368–381

99. Salvatierra O, Fortmann J L, Belzer F O. Sexual function in males before and after renal transplantation. Sobhma Abd el Hamidia At tamg Refaief: Effect of erythropoietin on sexual potency in chronic hemodialysis patients. Scand J Urol Nephrol 1992; 26: 181–217

100. Charmet G P. Sexual function in dialysis patients: psychological aspects. Contrib Nephrol 1990; 77: 15–24

101. Reinberj Y, Baumgardner G L, Aliabadi H. Urological aspects of renal transplantation. J Urol 1990; 143: 1087–1094

102. Dillard F T, Miller B S, Sommer B G et al. Erectile dysfunction post transplant. Transplant Proc 1989; 21: 3961–3969

103. Brannen G E, Peters T G, Hambridge K M et al. Impotence after kidney transplantation. Urology 1980; 15: 138–149

104. Billet A, Dagher F J, Querell A. Surgical correction of vasculogenic impotence in a patient after bilateral renal transplantation. Surgery 1982; 91: 108–114

105. Gittes R F, Waters W B. Sexual impotence: the overlooked complication of a second renal transplant. J Urol 1979; 121: 719–724

Chapter 49
Spinal cord injury

P. J. R. Shah

■ INTRODUCTION

A spinal cord injury (SCI) is devastating and produces profound changes in the lifestyle of the individual and his family. Not only is there the consequence of the loss of limb function but there are also changes in bladder and bowel function that require careful supervised management. Changes in sexual function accompany SCI and will depend upon the level of the injury. However, although concerns about sexual function are strongly present in all these — often young — men, they are not always considered until some time after the injury has occurred and occasionally not at all. Sexual feelings are not affected by injury.[1] These patients thus require early counselling to reduce their anxiety about future sexuality and to be provided with the option to obtain appropriate treatment when they request it.

Spinal cord injured patients are particularly emotionally vulnerable, especially if they have major neurological impairment,[2] and this physical vulnerability overflows into the sexual needs and desires of these patients.

Sexual function has as high a priority after SCI as it did before the injury, particularly in young males.[3] Problems in obtaining a partner or the lack of a regular partner, particularly for those patients with cervical injuries and thus greater degrees of disability, contribute to sexual dissatisfaction. Half of all patients, once rehabilitation has been achieved, appear to indulge in sexual activity once a week or more often.[4]

Althof and Levine[5] have recommended that four aspects of sexual function should be considered, as follows:

1. Sexual equilibrium between two people;
2. Sexual psychology of the individual;
3. Biology of the organically impaired individual;
4. Sexual pathophysiology of the spinal cord deficit.

Each of these factors should be considered during the assessment of the patient with sexual dysfunction after SCI.

■ NEUROPHYSIOLOGY OF ERECTION AND RELATIONSHIP TO ERECTILE DYSFUNCTION

The level of the SCI has a relationship to the nature of the residual erectile function. All patients with lesions high in the spinal cord can be expected to develop reflex erections in association with stimulation to the penis. Psychogenic stimulation, however, will produce erections in 90% of patients with lower lesions.[6] However, this is not to say that these patients do not require assistance with obtaining an erection at an appropriate time. Thus, although patients may report in questionnaires that they are well able to obtain a reflex or psychogenic erection, the erection may not be of sufficient quality or duration to enable sexual intercourse when required; thus, many men will require assistance with erection.[7]

Single-potential analysis of cavernous electrical activity has been shown to be abnormal in SCI.[8]

Self-reporting of sexual arousal is not always reliable in patients with SCI. Kennedy and Over[9] were able to demonstrate penile tumescence during erotic stimulation by film, text and fantasy in male patients who claimed that they were unable to obtain an erection. It would appear that SCI patients experience arousal parallel to that experienced by a non-neurological group.

EVALUATION OF THE PATIENT WITH ERECTILE DYSFUNCTION

The evaluation of the patient with sexual dysfunction requires a knowledge of the particular sexual difficulty and the degree of disability. A knowledge of the relationship with the partner is also necessary and joint consultation may be appropriate. Since difficulties may arise within the sexual act, the provision of an erection without consideration of other factors may not provide a solution to what may be a multifactorial problem with sexual activity.[6]

As both bladder and bowel function are generally altered by SCI, a knowledge of the function of each of these systems is necessary. Bladder dysfunction has a particularly profound effect on the patient's well-being, and effective bladder emptying (preferably without uncontrolled incontinence) acts to reduce the anxiety that accompanies sexual activity. A patient with an acontractile bladder who is managing with clean intermittent self-catheterization (CISC) will be able to empty his bladder before intercourse and will thus not have to worry about the possibility of urinary leakage during intercourse. However, the patient managed by continuous condom drainage cannot easily determine whether the bladder is empty prior to sexual activity, and hyperreflexic contractions may occur during intercourse that cause urinary incontinence and may cause considerable distress. Patients who use continuous condom drainage for bladder management, who do not have a partner, often find that they become socially isolated as a consequence. Thus, when bladder management is being considered, sexual needs should be borne in mind before irreversible surgery is performed.

A basic neurological examination to include an assessment of limb function, and examination of the perineum and perianal sensation and reflexes, should be performed.

PATIENT PERCEPTION OF SEXUAL FUNCTION

A number of studies have been conducted to assess the nature of sexuality after SCI.[10] Questionnaire studies have shown that as many as 95% of patients could develop an erection with stimulation, with 66% stating that erection was sufficient for penetration. Patients below the age of 30 years appear to be more likely to record erectile capabilities.

THE PLACE OF OBJECTIVE EVALUATION OF ERECTILE DYSFUNCTION

It is usually considered that patients with neurological dysfunction affecting erectile capabilities have genuine pathological reasons for erectile failure/dysfunction. Tay et al.[11] performed nocturnal penile tumescence (NPT) monitoring on 30 SCI patients (20 with complete injuries and 10 with incomplete injuries). They discovered that, with incomplete injuries, patients tended to maintain normal erections, whereas there were discrepancies between a patient's perception and the findings from NPT in those patients with complete injuries. They found that psychogenic dysfunction could be present in 10% of patients with SCI.

SEXUAL COMPLICATIONS OF UROLOGICAL TREATMENT

As the majority of patients will require urological treatment of one sort or another, it is important to be aware of the consequences of such treatment on sexual function. The most effective treatment for the dysfunctional bladder is CISC, to enable continence and freedom from appliances. This routine is very successful for the patient with a low injury leading to an acontractile bladder. Patients with detrusor hyperreflexia are also effectively managed with CISC, provided that bladder contractions can be reduced or inhibited with anticholinergic medication or by surgery (augmentation ileocystoplasty). A continent patient without an appliance is more likely to feel confident about sexual function in these circumstances.

The quadriplegic patient managed by continuous condom drainage with or without a sphincter-relaxing procedure may feel anxious about the risk of incontinence during sexual activity due to the reflex bladder emptying that may take place in association with penile stimulation. Wearing a condom for protection can help. If sphincterotomy is to be performed it should be at the 12 o'clock position, which is not likely to be associated with disordered erectile function.[12,13] Sphincter stents[14] do not appear to contribute to erectile dysfunction (ED). Bladder neck incision at the same time as external striated sphincterotomy should not be performed routinely unless bladder neck obstruction has been confirmed by video-urodynamics. If bladder neck incision is performed in young men, and if retrograde ejaculation develops after surgery, later difficulties with fertility may cause significant problems, both physical and psychological.

■ TRANSCUTANEOUS DRUG STIMULATION OF ERECTION (TOPICAL TREATMENT)

Patients who respond to injection therapy with papaverine may respond to transcutaneous nitroglycerine patches.[15] Of 17 men in whom this treatment was attempted, five were able to have sexual activity after application of a patch containing nitroglycerine to the penile shaft. If this treatment is effective, patients prefer it to the use of injections, as would be expected. Minoxidil has been tried as a spray application to the penis for the same indication but with no success.[16] The topical application of a papaverine gel to the penis does produce increases in penile blood flow in SCI males and may have a place in augmenting reflex erections.[17] Prostaglandin E1 (PGE1) applied topically increased peak systolic blood flow to the penis,[18] although clinical erections were noted in only two of nine men.

■ VACUUM THERAPY

The use of a vacuum constriction device to assist erection has been in use for patients with SCI since the late 1980s.[19,20] Although there is early enthusiasm for the use of these non-invasive devices, many patients do not continue to use them in spite of the fact that they initially invested their own funds to purchase one. However, of those patients that obtain their own vacuum aid, 50% may be expected to be using the device for regular sexual activity after 21 months,[21] frequency of coitus being reported to increase in these individuals from 0.3 to 1.5 times per week. Denil et al.[22] later reported a similar experience in their SCI patients, with initial enthusiasm for the device of 93% at 3 months, although this fell to 41% at 6 months. Female satisfaction with the device appeared to be similar to that of the males, i.e. around 40%. Minor sequelae of use,

such as petechiae and skin oedema, were frequent but did not require treatment.

Patients with SCI must be warned of the need to remove the vacuum constriction ring after 15 minutes. Impaired or absent genital sensation makes the patient unaware of the presence of the ring.

■ INJECTION THERAPY

Following the discovery by Brindley,[23] that drugs injected into the corpus cavernosum caused penile erection, the use of this form of treatment for impotence has become widespread. Although patients with injuries above the sacral reflex arc will develop reflex erections, these erections may not be sustained for long enough to enable sexual intercourse to take place, or they may occur at inappropriate times. Injection therapy thus provides an opportunity to create an erection at a time suitable to both patient and partner.

Papaverine has the longest pedigree in the treatment of ED in SCI and was the first agent to be used regularly in SCI patients. Sidi et al.[24] were able to demonstrate, in a controlled study of the use of papaverine, that 37 of 52 (71%) patients who completed the study were able to obtain functional erections. These authors encountered a 4% rate of priapism that required corporal irrigation, with one patient developing a degree of intracorporal scarring. Similar success was achieved by Momose et al.,[25] but prolonged erection was encountered after the injection of 40–60 mg papaverine. It has since been learnt that smaller doses are likely to be just as effective in patients with SCI, and that titration of the dose to the patient is essential if this therapy is to be both effective and free from complications.

Although initial enthusiasm for injection therapy occurs in all series, there tends to be a gradual fallout in use over time such that, after 2 years of use, approximately 50% of patients may have stopped using this injection treatment.[26]

A variety of other agents have been developed over the years, including papaverine/phentolamine, PGE1, moxisylyte, and Trimix (a mixture of all the above).[27]

The agent that has gained the most widespread use is PGE1, which is used in doses varying from 5 to 20 µg. Titration of the dose from a small trial dose of 2–5 µg upwards is necessary in order to avoid prolonged erection.

■ TITRATION OF THE DOSE IN SPINAL CORD INJURED PATIENTS

Smaller doses of injectable agents are often more effective in patients with neurological dysfunction. As a consequence, the starting dose in a spinally injured patient should be small and larger doses used depending upon the efficacy. PGE1 should be started at a dose of 2–3 µg; some patients may be able to produce effective erections with this small dose. Intelligent and motivated patients may be able to monitor the incremental increases in drug dosage on an outpatient basis: however, if there is doubt as to the patient's ability to calculate the correct dosage, trials held in an outpatient clinic of incremental doses over a period of weeks may be necessary.

■ PENILE IMPLANTS

When a patient has failed to respond to all of the conservative methods of management of ED, a penile prosthesis may provide a satisfactory alternative. Penile implants have been available for a number of years, with reports of successful implantation in SCI patients as early as 1979.[28] In this early report, Golji cautions the careful selection of patients in order to provide a successful outcome. Light and Scott[29] were able to report their experience of penile implantation with inflatable prostheses in this group of patients; and produced no greater complication rate than in non-neurologically impaired patients; partner satisfaction was high. Rossier and Fam[30] treated 36 patients with semi-rigid prostheses, both for sexual purposes and to enable the easier use of an external condom drainage appliance. They experienced complications in 16.5% due to extrusion or removal of the device. Other reports of the use of a penile implant for maintaining a condom drainage appliance have been published.[31,32] Infective complications of these devices in SCI patients appear to be higher (9–33%) than in other, non-neurological, patients.[33–36] Absent sensation in this group of patients may also lead to erosion, increasing the risk of complications and requiring further surgery in up to 33%.[34]

The sacral anterior root stimulator implant (SARSI) and erectile function

Those male patients who prefer to obtain as close to normally controlled voiding as possible may seek the implantation of the Brindley Finetech sacral anterior root stimulator implant (SARSI), which provides control of micturition with continence in more than 80% of those patients who have a device implanted. Reflex erections are lost as a consequence of division of the posterior roots prior to the implantation of the nerve electrodes adjacent to the anterior roots of S2–4. Implant-driven erection is reported to occur in 60% of patients, with 13 of 32 patients using full-implant driven erections.[37]

■ EJACULATION AND SCI

The majority of patients are unable to ejaculate after complete SCI. Because the pathways that supply the ejaculatory mechanism are usually interrupted, both orgasm and ejaculation are lost. This has major implications for the management of such a patient: not only is the orgasmic pleasure lost, but also the provision of seminal fluid for fertilization is hindered. Thus, the patient loses sexual pleasure through the loss of penile sensation, the loss of normal orgasm and the loss of ejaculation. The awareness that ejaculation is not possible without medical assistance may have a major effect on the psyche of the patient who is keen to become a father. Early counselling is therefore most important and the patient should be made aware of the potential methods of providing semen for fertilization.

Ejaculation may occur in some patients after SCI. If ejaculation does not occur, owing either to an abnormality of the bladder neck mechanism, which may be altered by neurological bladder dysfunction, or to the neurological condition, semen may be obtained by artificial means.

Ejaculation by vibration
Stimulation of the undersurface of the penis in the region of the frenum using a high-frequency stimulator will produce ejaculation in some patients. Pryor et al.[38] were able to produce ejaculation with vibration in all six men that they studied; pregnancies occurred in five of the six partners. A high-frequency vibrator is usually necessary to achieve this aim. Sonksen et al.[39] were able to demonstrate that a frequency of vibration of 100 MHz with peak-to-peak amplitudes of 2.5 mm would produce ejaculation in 34 of 41 men (83%), irrespective of patient age, level of injury, years since injury and bladder management. Autonomic dysreflexia was not seen in their patients.

Sperm quality appears to be better in patients who undergo vibratory ejaculation than those who undergo electroejaculation.[40] Vibratory ejaculation should be first-line treatment in patients with lesions above T10.[41] Such successfully treated patients may use a vibrator at home to enable ejaculation to take place, and the semen produced may be used for insemination. This technique gives a considerable degree of confidence to the patient and is to be encouraged.

Electro-ejaculation

When vibratory stimulation does not produce ejaculation, electrical stimulation may be effective for those patients with injuries above the sacral reflex arc. Both Brindley and Seager have described techniques of stimulation achieved by transrectal stimulation of the pelvic splanchnic nerves. Unfortunately, this technique is hospital based and is used primarily for obtaining semen for artificial insemination. Careful monitoring of blood pressure is necessary in patients with lesions above T6 because of the risk of hypertensive crises as a consequence of autonomic dysreflexia. Electro-ejaculation using the Seager model can be expected to produce ejaculation in 93% of patients with upper motor neuron lesions and 63.6% of those with lower motor neuron lesions.[42]

■ CONCLUSIONS

ED is a common accompaniment of SCI. There is an increasing awareness that such patients require counselling and reassurance and that help can be provided in order that a satisfactory and enjoyable sexual life may be achieved by appropriate management. Each of the available varieties of current treatment may be used by patients, although vacuum aids and intracavernosal injections currently appear to be the most popular modalities. Failure to ejaculate may be addressed by the use of vibration applied to the penis or by transrectal electrical stimulation.

■ REFERENCES

1. Harrison J, Glass C A, Owens R G, Soni R M. Factors associated with sexual functioning in women following spinal cord injury. Paraplegia 1995; 33: 687–692

2. Levi R, Hultling C, Nash M S, Seiger A. The Stockholm spinal injury study 1. Medical problems in a regional SCI population. Paraplegia 1995; 33: 308–315

3. Sjogren K, Egberg K. The sexual experience in younger males with complete spinal cord injury. Scand J Rehabil Med Suppl 1983; 9: 189–194

4. Kreuter M, Sullivan M, Siosteen A. Sexual adjustment after spinal cord injury (SCI) focussing on partner experiences. Paraplegia 1994; 32: 225–235

5. Althof S E, Levine S B. Clinical approach to the sexuality of patients with spinal cord injury. Urol Clin North Am 1993; 20: 527–534

6. Courtois F J, Charvier K F, Leriche A et al. Clinical approach to erectile dysfunction in spinal injured men: a review of clinical and experimental data. Paraplegia 1995; 33: 628–635

7. Watanabe T, Chancellor M B, Rivas D A et al. Epidemiology of current treatment for sexual dysfunction in spinal cord injured men in the USA model spinal injury centres. J Spinal Cord Med 1996; 19: 186–189

8. Stief C G, Hoppner C, Sauerwein D, Jonas U. Single potential analysis of cavernous electrical activity in spinal cord injury patients. J Urol 1994; 151: 1562–1563

9. Kennedy S, Over R. Psychophysiological assessment of male sexual arousal following spinal cord injury. Arch Sex Behav 1990; 19: 15–27

10. Slot O, Drewes A, Andreason A, Olsson A. Erectile and ejaculatory function of males with spinal cord injury. Int Disabil Stud 1989; 11: 75–77

11. Tay H P, Juma S, Joseph A C. Psychogenic impotence in spinal injury patients. Arch Phys Med Rehabil 1996; 77: 391–393

12. Jameson R M. Division of the external urethral sphincter and potency in spinal cord injury patients. J Urol 1983; 130: 86–87

13. Leriche A. Analysis of 278 sphincterotomies of the urethral sphincter in 232 patients. Ann Urol (Paris) 1985; 19: 193–201

14. Shah P J R, Milroy E J, Timoney E J et al. Permanent external sphincter stents in patients with spinal injuries. Br J Urol 1990; 66: 297–302

15. Sonkson J, Biering-Sorensen F. Transcutaneous nitroglycerin in the treatment of erectile dysfunction in spinal cord injury. Paraplegia 1992; 30: 554–557

16. Chancellor M B, Rivas D A, Panzer D E et al. Prospective comparison of topical minoxidil to vacuum constriction device and intracorporeal papaverine injection in treatment of erectile dysfunction due to spinal cord injury. Urology 1994; 43: 365–369

17. Kim E D, el-Rashidy R, McVary K T. Papaverine topical gel for treatment of erectile dysfunction. J Urol 1995; 53: 361–365

18. Kim E D, McVary K T. Topical prostaglandin E1 for the treatment of erectile dysfunction. J Urol 1995; 153: 1828–1830

19. Lloyd E E, Toth L L, Perkash I. Vacuum tumescence: an option for spinal cord injured males with erectile dysfunction. SCI Nurs 1989; 6: 25–28

20. Zasler N D, Katz P G. Synergist erection system in the management of impotence secondary to spinal cord injury. Arch Phys Med Rehabil 1989; 70: 712–716

21. Heller L, Keren O, Aloni R, Davidoff G. An open trial of vacuum penile tumescence: constriction therapy for neurological impotence. Paraplegia 1992; 30: 550–553

22. Denil J, Ohl D A, Smythe C. Vacuum erection device in spinal cord injured men: patient and partner satisfaction. Arch Phys Med Rehabil 1996; 77: 750–753

23. Brindley G S. Cavernosal blockade: a new technique for investigating and treating erectile impotence. Br J Urol 1983; 143: 332–337

24. Sidi A A, Cameron J S, Dykstra D D et al. Vasoactive intracavernous pharmacotherapy for the treatment of erectile impotence in men with spinal cord injury. J Urol 1987; 138: 539–542

25. Momose H, Natsume O, Yamamoto M et al. Intracavernous injection of papaverine hydrochloride for impotence in patients with spinal cord injury. Hinyokika Kiyo 1987; 33: 1065–1069

26. Bodner D R, Leffler E, Frost F. The role of intracavernous injection of vasoactive medications for the restoration of erection in spinal cord injured males: a three year follow-up. Paraplegia 1992; 30: 118–120

27. Chao R, Clowers D E. Experience with intracavernosal tri-mixture for the management of neurogenic erectile dysfunction. Arch Phys Med Rehabil 1994; 75: 276–278

28. Golji H. Experience with penile prosthesis in spinal cord injury patients. J Urol 1979; 121: 288–289

29. Light J K, Scott F B. Management of neurogenic impotence with inflatable penile prosthesis. Urology 1981; 17: 341–343

30. Rossier A B, Fam B A. Indication and results of semi-rigid penile prostheses in spinal cord injury patients: long-term follow-up. J Urol 1984; 131: 59–62

31. Van-Arsdalen K N, Klein F A, Hackler R H, Brady S M. Penile implants in spinal cord injury patients for maintaining external appliances. J Urol 1981; 126: 331–332

32. Iwatsubo E, Tanaka M, Takahashi K, Ahatsu T. Non-inflatable penile prosthesis for the management of urinary incontinence and sexual disability of patients with spinal cord injury. Paraplegia 1986; 24: 307–310

33. Kabalin J N, Kessler R. Infectious complications of penile prosthesis surgery. J Urol 1988; 139: 953–955

34. Collins K P, Hackler R H. Complications of penile prostheses in spinal cord injured patients. J Urol 1988; 140: 984–985

35. Kimoto Y, Iwatsubo E. Penile prostheses for the management of the neuropathic bladder and sexual dysfunction in spinal cord injury patients: long-term follow-up. Paraplegia 1994; 32: 336–339

36. Wilson S K, Delk J R. Inflatable penile implant infection: predisposing factors and treatment suggestions. J Urol 1995; 153: 659–661

37. Brindley G S, Rushton D N. Long-term follow-up of patients with sacral anterior root stimulator implants. Paraplegia 1990; 28: 469–475

38. Pryor J L, LeRoy S C, Nagel T C, Hensleigh H C. Vibratory stimulation for treatment of anejaculation in quadriplegic men. Arch Phys Med Rehabil 1995; 76: 59–64

39. Sonksen J, Biering-Sorensen F, Kristensen J K. Ejaculation by penile vibratory stimulation in men with spinal cord injuries. Paraplegia 1994; 32: 651–660

40. Brackett N L, Padron O F, Lynne C M. Semen quality of spinal cord injured men is better when obtained by vibratory stimulation versus electroejaculation. J Urol 1997; 157: 151–157

41. Nehra A, Werner M A, Bastuba M et al. Vibratory stimulation and rectal probe electroejaculation as therapy for patients with spinal cord injury: semen parameters and pregnancy rates. J Urol 1996; 155: 554–559

42. Momose H, Hirao Y, Yamamoto M et al. Electroejaculation in patients with spinal cord injury: first report of a large scale experience from Japan. Int J Urol 1995; 2: 326–329

Chapter 50

Causes and treatment of ejaculatory disorders

W. F. Hendry

■ INTRODUCTION

The purpose of ejaculation is the transmission of spermatozoa to impregnate the female partner. It consists of the forcible expulsion of the contents of the ejaculatory ducts and seminal vesicles from the urethra, coincident with the pleasurable sensation known as orgasm. Penile erection usually accompanies ejaculation, but this is not essential: the control mechanisms for the two processes, although coordinated, are in fact quite separate. The anatomy of the prostate, seminal vesicles and ejaculatory ducts is shown in Figure 50.1. The sequence of ejaculation has been studied in detail in man by serial transrectal ultrasound scanning during orgasm.[1] After an initial pre-ejaculatory phase when the bladder neck closes, the contents of the prostate and the ampullary parts of the vasa deferentia are expelled into the prostatic part of the urethra where they appear to be thoroughly mixed, forming an acoustic interface. This is followed by forcible expulsion of the contents of the seminal vesicles with closure of the bladder neck; subsequent rhythmic contraction of the bulbospongiosus muscle expels the ejaculate from the urethra via the external meatus in a series of spurts.

The ejaculate can be split into four to six fractions,[2] and serial biochemical analysis of its component parts confirms that the order of contraction of the various organs normally follows the sequence outlined above. Thus, the first part contains the maximum number of spermatozoa, and subsequent fractions contain sequentially less. Acid phosphatase, citric acid and zinc, emanating from the prostate, are in highest concentration in the first part of the ejaculate, whereas fructose, coming from the seminal vesicles, increases in concentration towards the end of the ejaculatory process. Alteration of

the pH values in successive parts of the split ejaculate indicates how the acid component provided by the prostate is replaced by the more alkaline contribution of the fructose-rich fluid from the seminal vesicles. Approximately 15–30% of the entire ejaculate is contributed by the prostatic and 50–80% by the vesicular secretion; there is, in addition, a small contribution to the first part of the ejaculate from the bulbo-urethral (Cowper's) glands which is rich in enzymes and plasminogen activator.[3]

The entire process of ejaculation is under sympathetic nervous control (Fig. 50.2). The efferent sympathetic nerves emerge from the spinal column at T10–L2 to form the lumbar sympathetic ganglia which encircle the aorta on each side, before combining in the midline to form the hypogastric plexus just below the bifurcation of the aorta (Fig. 50.3). From there the hypogastric nerves pass through the pelvis to terminate as postganglionic fibres on the bladder neck, prostate, vasa deferentia and seminal vesicles.[4] Sympathetic inflow stimulates contraction of the prostate, vesicles and vasa along with partial bladder neck closure producing ejaculation, and division of these nerve fibres leads to loss of ejaculation. Parasympathetic innervation of the corpora cavernosa, prostate, base of bladder and bladder neck is from roots S2–S4 via the pelvic nerves: division or injury of these nerves (for example during radical prostatectomy) leads to loss of erection. The somatic muscles surrounding the urethra, which are innervated via the pudendal nerve, accomplish the final act of ejaculation.

There are many causes of disturbance of the ejaculatory process, leading to partial or complete loss of the ejaculate. Total absence of the ejaculate is termed aspermia, which must be distinguished from azoospermia,

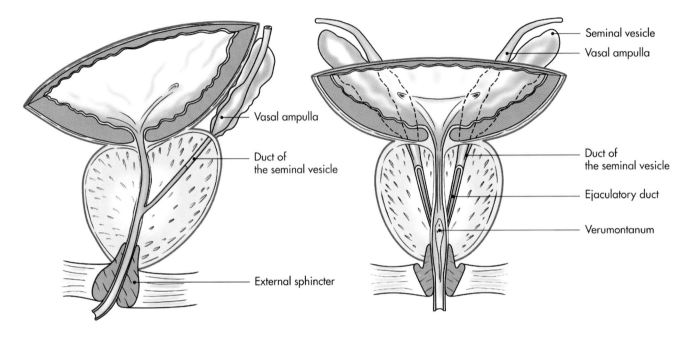

Figure 50.1. Normal anatomy of the prostate with the ejaculatory ducts formed by the confluence of the ampullary parts of the vasa and the seminal vesicles.

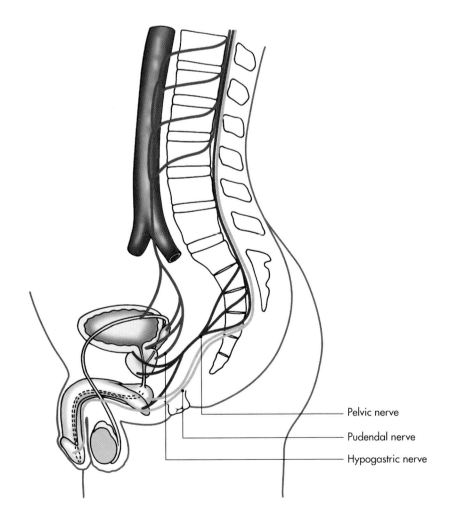

Figure 50.2. Innervation of the male genitalia. (Adapted from ref. 52 with permission.)

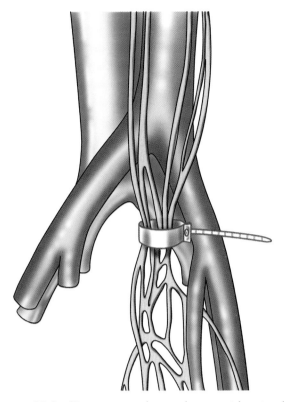

Figure 50.3. Hypogastric plexus shown with stimulator electrode in situ. (From ref. 45 with permission.)

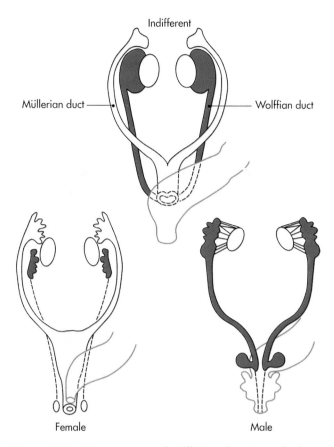

Figure 50.4. Disappearance of müllerian ducts in male foetus under the influence of müllerian inhibitory factor.

indicating absence of spermatozoa from an otherwise normal ejaculate. If there is no ejaculate at all, the first and most important fact to establish is whether there is failure of ejaculation, or whether the ejaculate is slipping back into the bladder owing to incompetence of the bladder neck. The difference can be established easily by examination of centrifuged urine after orgasm: the presence of spermatozoa indicates retrograde ejaculation. Since the management is different, although the causes may be similar, it is important to recognize the true nature of the ejaculatory dysfunction early in the diagnostic workup.

The causes of ejaculatory duct obstruction have been fairly well defined.[5] Functional abnormalities may be behavioural, may follow neurological damage or be induced by drugs. The cause should be defined as accurately as possible before treatment is instituted.

■ CAUSES OF EJACULATORY DYSFUNCTION

Congenital

Embryology

As the male foetus develops, the müllerian ducts normally disappear from above downward (Fig. 50.4) under the influence of müllerian inhibitory factor (MIF), which is produced by the Sertoli cells in the primitive testis. Failure of complete absorption may leave a small müllerian duct remnant at the lower end, which lies between the ejaculatory ducts.

The wolffian (mesonephric) ducts are composed of three distinct areas (Fig. 50.5). The upper part forms the epididymis and distal vas deferens, while the proximal vas deferens, seminal vesicle and ejaculatory duct are derived from the middle area. The most caudal part is the common mesonephric duct, from which the ureteric bud springs at approximately 4 weeks of development to become the ureter, and will induce the metanephric blastema to form the kidney. The lower end of the mesonephric duct is reabsorbed into the urogenital sinus as the trigone is formed. The ureteric orifices are thus separated from the vas deferens, seminal vesicles and ejaculatory ducts. Several complex anomalies may occur in this area, leading to ectopic opening of the vas deferens and sometimes associated with anorectal anomalies.[6] If

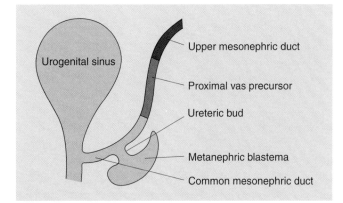

Figure 50.5. Development of ureter and vas deferens from the mesonephric (wolffian) duct: the proximal part of the common mesonephric duct normally disappears.

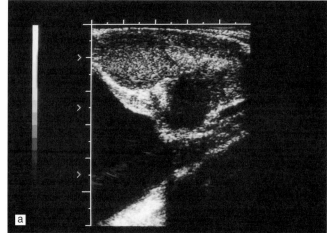

too much of the proximal vas precursor is absorbed, a variable amount of the proximal vas, seminal vesicle and/or ejaculatory duct may be absent. There may be coexisting abnormalities in the ipsilateral kidney or ureter.

Müllerian duct cyst

Persistence of a small remnant of the müllerian duct may lead to formation of a cyst between the ejaculatory ducts, which can become obstructed and cause diminution of the volume of the ejaculate and infertility. Haemospermia is not uncommon in these patients. Seminal analysis shows the changes characteristic of obstruction (see below), and both vasa are palpable; the epididymides usually feel distended. The diagnosis is made by transrectal ultrasound scan (TRUS) (Fig. 50.6a) or vasography (Fig. 50.6b). Alternatively, the lesion can be delineated by percutaneous puncture of the cyst with instillation of radiopaque medium (Fig. 50.6c). The cyst can then be incised or deroofed endoscopically after delineating its extent by injection of blue dye (usually 1% methylene blue). Improvement in ejaculate volume and seminal quality follows in most cases.[7]

Wolffian duct abnormalities

Congenital anomalies may be either sporadic, with a localized defect in the proximal part of the vas deferens (Fig. 50.7), or there may be a more generalized maldevelopment due to a systemic genetic abnormality.[8] The latter is usually bilateral and is often associated with carriage of the cystic fibrosis (*cf*) gene.[9] Unilateral absence of the vas deferens was observed in 5%, and bilateral absence in 18% of 370 azoospermic males with

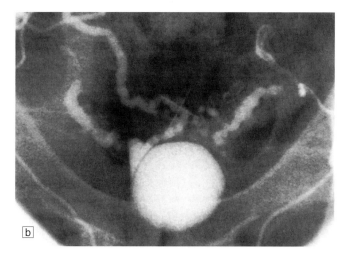

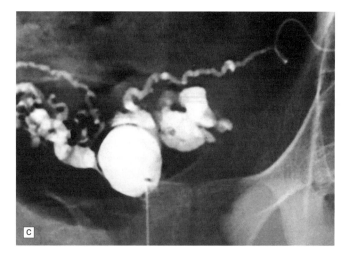

Figure 50.6. Müllerian duct cyst shown by (a) transrectal ultrasound scan, (b) vasogram and (c) percutaneous puncture.

normal serum follicle-stimulating hormone (FSH) levels investigated by the author.[10]

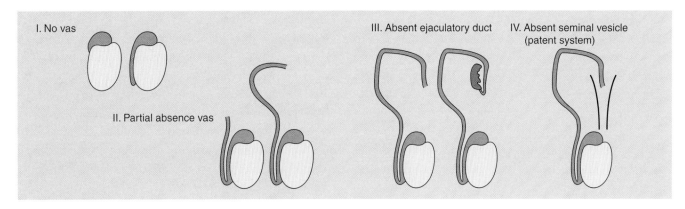

Figure 50.7. Classification of wolffian duct abnormalities.

Local wolffian duct abnormality involves loss of a variable amount of one vas deferens, seminal vesicle and/or ejaculatory duct, and sometimes parts of the ipsilateral urinary system as well. The loss usually appears to commence at the proximal juxta-urethral end and extend laterally (Fig. 50.8). Unilateral absence of the vas deferens with the kidney and ureter may also be associated with maldevelopment of the ipsilateral part of the bladder neck and trigone, which fails to close effectively thus allowing retrograde ejaculation to occur. This anomaly should be recognized on the TRUS scan and may be confirmed at cystoscopy.

Hypospadias/epispadias/bladder exstrophy
Congenital malformation of the penis can deflect the ejaculate and prevent it from emerging at the tip of the penis. Correction of the defect using modern reconstructive techniques can ensure that the semen is deposited high in the vagina at intercourse. After correction of severe epispadias or bladder exstrophy, sexual activity can be good despite a short penis and pregnancies may be produced even after cystectomy and urinary diversion,[11] but artificial insemination may be necessary.

Open bladder neck
Congenital incompetence of bladder neck closure is sometimes associated with unilateral absence of the genitourinary tract, and this can lead to retrograde ejaculation. The man may state that he has never seen a normal emission. The condition is recognized by TRUS or cystoscopy and may be corrected by bladder neck reconstruction. Alternatively, spermatozoa can be retrieved from the urine by centrifugation and used for insemination.[12]

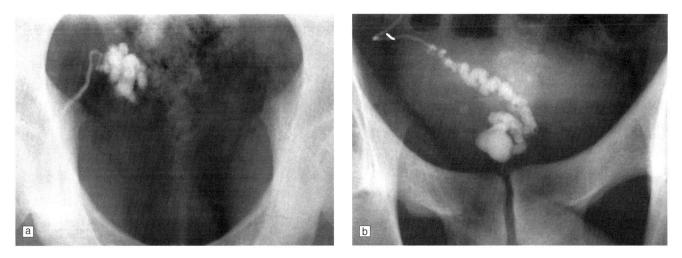

Figure 50.8. Examples of absence of proximal vas deferens: (a) terminating on pelvic side wall and (b) adjacent to urethra suitable for endoscopic incision.

Imperforate anus

Ejaculatory duct obstruction or ejaculatory failure due to pelvic nerve damage may follow correction of imperforate anus. The pull-through procedure passes close to the posterior aspect of the prostate, and damage to the ejaculatory mechanism is most likely if there has been a recto-urethral fistula that required closure. Recent analysis of 20 subfertile males who had repair of imperforate anus in infancy indicated that seven had no ejaculate, 11 were azoospermic, one was severely oligozoospermic and only one had a normal sperm concentration in a very small volume of ejaculate.[13] Investigation revealed that both vasa were blocked in five men and one vas in a further eight, apparently as a result of the original operative procedure.

Acquired causes

Traumatic

Bladder neck incision, prostatectomy, excision of rectum and para-aortic lymphadenectomy are all examples of operative procedures that carry a risk of damage to the ejaculatory mechanism or its nervous control. Loss of ejaculation has an obvious deleterious effect, not only upon the reproductive process but also on sexual relationships. Failure to warn the patient about the possibility of such damage may well be regarded as negligent. It is essential that the effects of any operation that may impact upon a man's sexual function be fully explained before the procedure is carried out. It cannot be assumed, however old the man may be, that he is beyond the age where reproductive function is important. He may well have, or come to have, a female partner of a younger age who wishes to bear children. In a recent survey, informed consent to transurethral prostatectomy was found to include written reference to these facts in only one-third of patients, irrespective of whether the men were married, single or widowed.[14]

Retrograde ejaculation occurs in about 25% of men after transurethral prostatectomy and to a lesser extent after bladder neck incision, owing to failure of bladder neck closure.[14] After radical prostatectomy, ejaculation is bound to be lost, since the seminal vesicles are removed with the prostate gland, and erectile impotence was the rule until detailed anatomical studies showed where the parasympathetic nerves ran behind the prostate gland,[15] and a nerve-sparing operative technique was developed.[16]

Postinfective

Genital infection such as gonorrhoea or non-specific urethritis can produce cicatrization and obstruction anywhere in the male reproductive tract, especially if treatment is delayed. Urinary infection with *Escherichia coli*, especially if complicated by epididymitis, can also produce obstruction that may be situated at ejaculatory duct level. Postinfective ejaculatory duct obstruction may also be seen after prolonged catheterization, for example following a road traffic accident or a spell in intensive care. A history of such an episode should alert the urologist to this possibility. Routine vasography in subfertile men with azoospermia and normal serum FSH levels revealed postinfective vasal blocks in 8% and acquired ejaculatory duct obstruction in 4%.[10] Such blocks are often asymmetrical, so that epididymal obstruction on one side may coexist with a more proximal block on the other side. They are often associated with high titres of antisperm antibodies, initially provoked by the infective process[17] and perpetuated by the obstruction.[18] Recognition of this immunological response to the obstruction is important, as the results of corrective surgery are significantly less successful in the presence of such antibodies.[19]

Schistosomiasis is endemic in large parts of Africa, and is seen with increasing frequency in tourists returning from Africa who have contracted the disease while enjoying water sports: Lake Malawi has acquired an evil reputation in this respect. The disease may present with haemospermia,[20] and fibrosis and calcification may lead to genital obstruction.

Genitourinary tuberculosis can cause great damage to the male reproductive tracts and, as healing occurs with calcification, the lesions may be irreparable, in the author's experience. Plain X-ray will often show the extent of the disease.

Haemospermia is seldom as ominous a symptom as haematuria, but this complaint should not be ignored. Analysis of the findings in 81 patients revealed that an inflammatory cause could be defined in most men under 30 years of age; however, there were a few (8%) with more serious disease including carcinoma of prostate and bladder.[21] It should be remembered, also, that schistosomiasis and tuberculosis could present in this way.

Stone

Routine investigation of haemospermia by TRUS not uncommonly reveals the presence of small stones in the

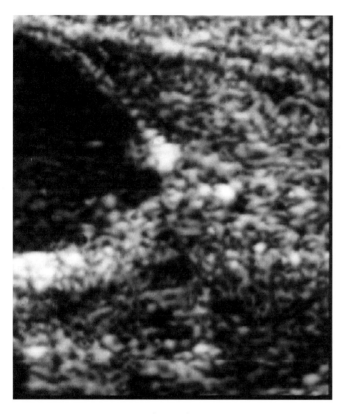

Figure 50.9. Stone in ejaculatory duct.

ejaculatory ducts, which may be associated with obstruction and dilatation of the seminal vesicles (Fig. 50.9). Such stones usually pass spontaneously, although resection of the distal parts of the ducts may occasionally be required if the symptoms are pressing or pain is persistent.

Neuropathic

Paraplegia

A period of spinal shock occurs for some weeks after the injury, during which time erection and ejaculation may be impossible. Once the initial phase is over, damage to the spinal cord at the level of T10–L2 may affect central reflex pathways and lead to permanent loss of ejaculation. Injury above T11 may allow reflex erection and ejaculation, although this may provoke autonomic dysreflexia with marked rise in blood pressure.[22] Many of these couples are keen to produce a family, and investigation and treatment may help them to achieve this aim.[23]

Para-aortic lymphadenectomy

This operation is done to clear lymph node metastases from testicular tumours, usually in young men who may have family and reproductive responsibilities still ahead of them. In the process of removing the para-aortic nodes, the sympathetic nerves and ganglia, which lie alongside the aorta, may be removed, leading to loss of ejaculation. Earlier studies have shown that up to three-quarters of patients will lose antegrade ejaculation after full bilateral retroperitoneal lymph node dissection.[15] As a result of careful anatomical studies, the technique of retroperitoneal lymph node dissection has been modified so that antegrade ejaculation is maintained in 70–90% of patients.[24,25] Some temporary loss of ejaculation is not uncommon but generally recovers over the months following the procedure. Careful prospective studies have shown that this operation is unnecessary in patients with early stage disease, when careful surveillance will detect relapse early enough to treat it effectively;[26] however, some centres do persist in doing this procedure.

One-quarter of the patients who complete chemotherapy for advanced testicular tumour have residual masses in the para-aortic region, or in the chest, or in both sites: when resected, this tissue is found to contain residual undifferentiated malignancy (MTU) in one in five cases.[27] Among 231 consecutive patients undergoing para-aortic lymphadenectomy after chemotherapy at the Royal Marsden Hospital, London, there was MTU in 21%, differentiated teratoma in 57%, and fibrosis/necrosis in 22%.[28] A nerve-sparing operative technique introduced in 1984 led to a significant reduction in ejaculatory dysfunction after para-aortic lymphadenectomy, from 37 to 19% in the author's experience of 186 patients.[29] Loss of ejaculation occurred significantly more often after bilateral (46%) than after unilateral (14%) dissection, and was related to the size of the excised mass (<4 cm, 4%; 4–8 cm, 19%; >8 cm, 60%). The chemotherapy combination used for treatment of metastatic testicular tumours such as bleomycin–etoposide–cisplatinum (BEP) allows recovery of spermatogenesis after a period of 1 to 2 years.[30] It is, therefore, particularly important that patients at high risk of loss of ejaculation should be recognized early in the course of their treatment so that seminal analysis and cryopreservation of semen can be arranged in suitable cases.[31] Excellent results have been reported with artificial insemination using cryopreserved semen.[32]

Functional

Congenital anorgasmia

Congenital anorgasmia is a rare but well-defined cause of total absence of ejaculation,[33] usually ascribed to an over-strict upbringing. The individual is unable to achieve orgasm and hence he never ejaculates. Nocturnal emission may occur, but repression of the normal sexual responses to stimulation prevents the individual from achieving climax and ejaculation. Psychotherapy may help, but orgasm can usually be provided by vibration.

Premature ejaculation

This common complaint is generally ascribed to anxiety. However, recent careful observational studies have indicated that there is hypersensitivity of the penile skin, as evidenced by perception of minute vibratory stimuli in those suffering from this condition compared with controls. Interestingly, the hypersensitivity appeared to be confined to penile skin, and there was no significant difference in skin sensitivity elsewhere, for example on the index finger.[23] Many drugs delay orgasm and ejaculation and this effect can be used in the treatment of premature ejaculation (see below).

Side effects of drug therapy

Many commonly used drugs cause delay or absence of orgasm and ejaculation (see Table 50.1).[34] The prevalence of both impotence and failure of ejaculation is higher in treated hypertensive patients than in matched controls. Methyldopa, for example, leads to loss of libido and delayed ejaculation, as well as erectile difficulty.[35] While psychotropic drugs are also associated with sexual dysfunction in a high proportion of patients, it is not always clear whether this is due to the drugs or to the underlying illness. Nevertheless, it is known that up to 40% of patients taking monoamine oxidase inhibitors experience sexual dysfunction, and the tricyclic antidepressants can cause reduced libido, erectile impotence and delayed ejaculation in up to 20% of patients. Selective serotonin re-uptake inhibitors are less often associated with adverse side effects; however, fluoxetine (Prozac) does cause delay in ejaculation and absence of orgasm in up to 40% of patients. A new drug, mirtazapine (Istrin), which is a noradrenergic and specific serotonergic antidepressant, is claimed not have this undesirable side effect, but does produce drowsiness when first taken, which may diminish interest in sexual activity. These adverse side effects are important, as they may lead to non-compliance in taking the required dose of the drug. On the other hand, these effects can be used therapeutically to treat premature ejaculation (see below).

Other drugs with adrenergic or anticholinergic effects can enhance ejaculation by sensitizing the nerve endings

Table 50.1. Drugs known to be associated with impairment of ejaculation

Alcohol
Amitriptyline
Baclofen
Bethanidine
Chlordiazepoxide
Chlorimipramine
Chlorpromazine
Chlorprothixene
Clomipramine
Epsilon aminocaproic acid
Guanethidine sulphate
Haloperidol
Hexamethonium
Imipramine hydrochloride
Methadone
Naproxen
Pargyline
Perphenazine
Phenelzine sulphate
Phenoxybenzamine hydrochloride
Phentolamine
Prazosin hydrochloride
Reserpine
Thiazides
Thioridazide
Trifluoroperazine hydrochloride

(From ref. 34 with permission.)

Table 50.2. Drugs used to achieve seminal emission

Brompheniramine maleate

Chlorpheniramine

Ephedrine sulphate

Imipramine hydrochloride

Phenylephrine hydrochloride

Phenylpropanolamine

Pseudoephedrine hydrochloride

(From ref. 34 with permission.)

in the seminal vesicles and vasa deferentia, and by encouraging closure of the bladder neck (Table 50.2).[34] Such drugs have been used with limited success to treat retrograde ejaculation, or loss of ejaculation following para-aortic lymphadenectomy (see below).

Megavesicles

Adult polycystic kidney disease has been found in association with pathological dilatation of the seminal vesicles in six patients.[36] TRUS and percutaneous puncture of the seminal vesicles before and after resection of the ejaculatory ducts revealed that the gross dilatation of the seminal vesicles was not caused by obstruction, but appeared to be due to atonicity (megavesicles). These ultrasonic appearances, when described previously, were incorrectly thought to be due to seminal vesicle cysts. Pathological dilatation of the seminal vesicles in the absence of obstruction has been described previously, although the aetiology remains obscure.[37]

■ DIAGNOSIS

Haemospermia requires full investigation. Culture of expressed prostatic secretion and urine will define the nature of an infective process such as prostatitis,[38] and urine cytology and serum prostate-specific antigen should be assayed to exclude bladder or prostatic cancer. Ultrasound scan of the testicles and epididymides should define any local disease. TRUS will demonstrate structural abnormality in the prostate or seminal vesicles,

or may show up a stone in the ejaculatory duct or even a müllerian duct cyst. Cystoscopy is seldom helpful.

If a man has difficulty with ejaculation, or has a small-volume or absent ejaculate, it must first be established whether the problem is congenital or acquired. A careful clinical history should be taken, and physical examination will establish whether the testicles and epididymides are normal, and whether the vasa are present or absent, on each side. Next, it is essential to establish whether there is retrograde or completely absent ejaculation, by examination of a deposit of urine after centrifugation. The presence of spermatozoa indicates retrograde ejaculation. These facts will allow the patient to be placed into one of several broad categories, after which more detailed evaluation can take place.

Patients with ejaculatory duct obstruction usually present with infertility. Seminal analysis may simply be reported as showing azoospermia or oligozoospermia, but the characteristic biochemical changes should be sought. There should be absence of part or all of the component of the ejaculate that comes from the vasa and seminal vesicles via the ejaculatory ducts. The volume is low (usually less than 1.5 ml), the pH is low (less than 7) and the fructose content is either low (less than 120 mg/100 ml) or absent. If both vasa are palpable, a diagnosis of ejaculatory duct obstruction is very likely. The diagnosis should be confirmed by TRUS, and the exact cause ascertained by percutaneous perineal puncture of the distended seminal vesicles (or other cystic structures) to define the anatomy more clearly. Exploration of the scrotum and vasography should not be done until arrangements have been made for definitive treatment of the obstructing lesion (see below).

When there is absence of the vasa, it is important to establish whether the condition is unilateral or bilateral. With unilateral absence of the vas deferens, the urinary system must also be checked by ultrasound scanning, as coexisting renal anomalies may be present.[8] Cystic malformation may occur, which can impede normal ejaculation from the contralateral side. Zinner's syndrome[39] associates this abnormality with ipsilateral absence of the kidney. Unilateral testicular obstruction can lead to production of antisperm antibodies in individuals who are immunologically responsive; this can cause infertility even though the contralateral testis is unobstructed, and can complicate restoration of fertility after reconstruction.[40]

With bilateral absence or malformation of the vasa, it is essential to consider whether the anomaly may be part

577

of a genetic defect associated with carriage of the potentially harmful cystic fibrosis chromosome anomaly.[9] Treatment by assisted reproduction could lead to the birth of an affected child if the female partner carries the *cf* gene as well. Genetic counselling should always precede definitive treatment in such cases.

■ TREATMENT

Reducing penile skin sensitivity with the application of local anaesthetic gel can treat premature ejaculation. By keeping the cream in contact with the skin with a condom for 30 min, significant improvement has been obtained.[41] It is, however, important to wash off the local anaesthetic prior to intercourse if diminution of vaginal sensitivity in the female partner is to be avoided.[42] Clomipramine, a tricyclic antidepressant, has been shown to produce significant delay in time to orgasm with increased satisfaction with sex life in a prospective controlled trial, when given in a dose of 25 mg 12–24 h before intercourse.[43] Fluoxetine (Prozac), given in a dose of 20 mg daily for 1 week and 40 mg daily thereafter, has also been used and produced significant benefit after 4 weeks treatment.[44] The female partners involved in the latter study subjected the effects to careful scrutiny, including verification of intravaginal latency time.

Retrograde ejaculation can be treated with adrenergic drugs such as ephedrine (30–60 mg), or a tricyclic antidepressant with anticholinergic effects such as desipramine (50 mg), taken 1–2 h before sexual activity. One patient with azoospermia and small-volume ejaculate associated with an open bladder neck and unilateral absence of the vas deferens responded well to ephedrine, with normalization of the seminal analysis; subsequently, a pregnancy was produced. Alternatively, spermatozoa can be retrieved from postorgasmic urine by centrifugation after retrograde ejaculation, then resuspended and used for artificial insemination with success: a cumulative pregnancy rate as high as 72% at 6 months has been achieved.[12]

In some paraplegic patients, application of a vibrator to the penis will lead to ejaculation; in others, electroejaculation may be necessary to produce spermatozoa that can be used for insemination. If the spinal reflex arc is intact, a hypogastric plexus stimulator will provoke ejaculation.[45] This method has the advantage that it can be used in the security of the patient's home, and repeated ejaculation can improve the quality of the semen. Alternatively, direct electro-ejaculation by rectal probe may be effective, but this generally requires a general anaesthetic and takes place in hospital.[46] In a recent analysis of 40 paraplegic patients, 22 successfully produced pregnancies by natural insemination or assisted reproductive techniques.[47]

Drug treatment for loss of ejaculation after para-aortic lymphadenectomy is not very successful,[48] but electro-ejaculation can produce spermatozoa for insemination.[49] It is important to anticipate this complication in young men

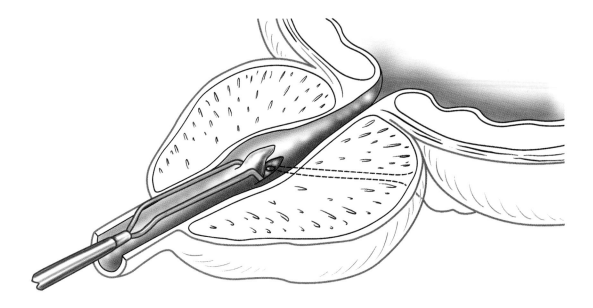

Figure 50.10. Resection of verumontanum to relieve ejaculatory duct obstruction.

with testicular tumours who may need chemotherapy or node dissection, and arrangements should be made for sperm storage at the earliest opportunity before treatment commences. Excellent results can be obtained with artificial insemination using cryopreserved spermatozoa.[32]

Ejaculatory duct obstruction can be treated endoscopically. It is very helpful if the lesion is accurately defined preoperatively by TRUS, so that arrangements can be made in advance. The obstruction should be defined radiologically by vasography or percutaneous puncture, and 5–10 ml 1% methylene blue dye should be instilled to indicate when the ejaculatory system has been entered. The patient should be placed in the lithotomy position and suitable drapes applied to allow access to rectal examination during the procedure. After preliminary cystoscopy, the resectoscope or optical urethrotome is inserted. A müllerian duct cyst may simply be incised, releasing a gush of fluid, but there is a tendency for the incision to heal over and it may be preferable to resect the edges or make a cruciate incision. If the ejaculatory ducts are blocked at their lower ends, it may be simpler to resect the verumontanum, commencing just above it in the prostatic urethra and drawing the loop carefully downwards (Fig. 50.10). The appearance of the ejaculatory ducts is characteristic and

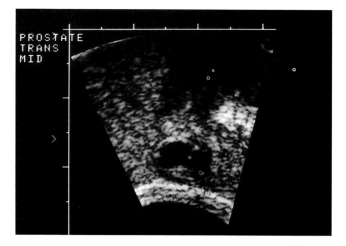

Figure 50.11. Transrectal ultrasound scan showing typical appearance of dilated ejaculatory ducts.

easily recognized, resembling a horse's nostrils (Fig. 50.11). Pressure on the seminal vesicles will produce abundant efflux once the obstruction has been relieved. Analysis of results obtained with 87 patients with ejaculatory duct obstruction is summarized in Table 50.3. It may be seen that incision of müllerian duct cyst was much the most successful procedure, but satisfactory results have been obtained in other patients and have

Table 50.3. Treatment and outcome in 87 patients with ejaculatory duct obstruction of various aetiologies

Aetiology	Total number	Number with follow-up	Postoperative patency	Pregnancies produced
Congenital				
Müllerian duct cyst	17	12	10	5
Wolffian duct abnormalities	19	6	1	1
Acquired				
Traumatic	15	6	2	1
Infective	19	6	4	2
Tuberculous	8			1
Neoplastic	1			
Functional				
Megavesicles	8	1	1	
Total	87	31	18	10

(From ref. 5 with permission.)

continued to be seen since this study was completed. If reconstruction is not possible, sperm can be withdrawn by microscopic epididymal sperm aspiration (MESA) or percutaneously (PESA) and used for in vitro fertilization.[50] Attempts to insert a permanent sperm reservoir had only limited success and this treatment has now been abandoned.[51]

■ REFERENCES

1. Gil-Vernet J M Jr, Alvarez-Vijande R, Gil-Vernet A, Gil-Vernet J M. Ejaculation in men: a dynamic endorectal ultrasonographical study. Br J Urol 1994; 73: 442–448

2. Eliasson R, Lindholmer C. Functions of male accessory genital organs. In: Hafez E S E (ed) Human semen and fertility regulation in men. St Louis: Mosby, 1976: 44–50

3. Mann T, Lutwak-Mann C. Secretory function of the prostate, seminal vesicle, Cowper's gland and other accessory organs of reproduction. In: Male reproductive function and semen. Berlin: Springer-Verlag, 1981: 171–193

4. Thomas A J. Ejaculatory dysfunction. Fertil Steril 1983; 39: 445–454

5. Pryor J P, Hendry W F. Ejaculatory duct obstruction in subfertile males: analysis of 87 patients. Fertil Steril 1991; 56: 725–730

6. Nesbitt J A, King L R. Ectopia of the vas deferens. J Pediatr Surg 1990; 25: 335–338

7. Hendry W F, Pryor J P. Mullerian duct (prostatic utricle) cyst: diagnosis and treatment in subfertile males. Br J Urol 1992; 69: 79–82

8. Schlegel P N, Shin D, Goldstein M. Urogenital anomalies in men with congenital absence of the vas deferens. J Urol 1996; 155: 1644–1648

9. Mickle J, Milunsky A, Amos J A, Oates R D. Congenital unilateral absence of the vas deferens: a heterogeneous disorder with two distinct subpopulations based upon aetiology and mutational status of the cystic fibrosis gene. Hum Reprod 1995; 10: 1728–1735

10. Hendry W F, Levison D A, Parkinson M C et al. Testicular obstruction: clinicopathological studies. Ann R Coll Surg Engl 1990; 72: 396–407

11. Woodhouse C R J, Ransley P G, Williams D I. The patient with exstrophy in adult life. Br J Urol 1983; 55: 632–635

12. Scammell G E, Stedronska-Clark J, Edmonds D K, Hendry W F. Retrograde ejaculation: a successful treatment with artificial insemination. Br J Urol 1989; 63: 198–201

13. Holt B, Pryor J P, Hendry W F. Male infertility following surgery for imperforate anus. J Pediatr Surg 1995; 30: 1677–1679

14. Thorpe A C, Cleary R, Coles J et al. Written consent about sexual function in men undergoing transurethral prostatectomy. Br J Urol 1994; 74: 479–484

15. Walsh P C, Donker P J. Impotence following radical prostatectomy: insight into etiology and prevention. J Urol 1982; 128: 492–497

16. Quinlan D M, Epstein J I, Carter B S, Walsh P C. Sexual function following radical prostatectomy: influence of preservation of neurovascular bundles. J Urol 1991; 145: 998–1002

17. Shahmanesh M, Stedronska J, Hendry W F. Antispermatozoal antibodies in men with urethritis. Fertil Steril 1986; 46: 308–311

18. Hendry W F. The immunological consequences of unilateral and bilateral testicular obstruction. In: Schoysman R (ed) Microsurgery of male infertility. Fondazione per GU studi sulla riproduzione umana, 1994: 101–116

19. Hendry W F. Testicular obstruction: causes, evaluation and the results of surgery. In: Webster G, Kirby R S, Goldwasser B, King L (eds) Reconstructive urology. Oxford: Blackwell, 1993: 1031–1048

20. McKenna G, Schousboe M, Paltridge G. Subjective change in ejaculate as symptom of infection with Schistosoma haematobium in travellers. Br Med J 1997; 315: 1000–1001

21. Fletcher M S, Herzberg Z, Pryor J P. The aetiology and investigation of haemospermia. Br J Urol 1981; 53: 669–671

22. Brindley G S. Neurophysiology. In: Kirby R S, Carson C C, Webster G D (eds) Impotence: diagnosis and management of male erectile dysfunction. London: Butterworth-Heinemann; 1992; 27–31

23. Xin Z C, Chung W S, Choi Y D et al. Penile sensitivity in patients with primary premature ejaculation. J Urol 1996; 156: 979–981

24. Jewett M A S, Kong Y S P, Goldberg S D et al. Retroperitoneal lymphadenectomy for testis tumour with nerve sparing for ejaculation. J Urol 1988; 139: 1220–1224

25. Richie J P. Clinical stage 1 testicular cancer: the role of modified retroperitoneal lymphadenectomy. J Urol 1990; 144: 1160–1163

26. Read G, Stenning S P, Cullen M H et al. Medical Research Council prospective study of surveillance for stage I testicular teratoma. J Clin Oncol 1992; 10: 1762–1768

27. Tait D, Peckham M J, Hendry W F, Goldstraw P. Post-chemotherapy surgery in advanced non-seminomatous germ-cell testicular tumours: the significance of histology with particular reference to differentiated (mature) teratoma. Br J Cancer 1984; 50: 601–609

28. Hendry W F, A'Hern R P, Hetherington J W et al. Para-aortic lymphadenectomy after chemotherapy for metastatic non-seminomatous germ cell tumours: prognostic value and therapeutic benefit. Br J Urol 1993; 71: 208–213

29. Jones D R, Norman A R, Horwich A, Hendry W F. Ejaculatory dysfunction after retroperitoneal lymphadenectomy. Eur Urol 1993; 23: 169–171

30. Dearnaley D P, Horwich A, A'Hern R et al. Combination chemotherapy with bleomycin, etoposide and cisplatin (BEP) for metastatic testicular teratoma: long term follow-up. Eur J Cancer 1991; 27: 684–691

31. Hendry W F, Stedronska J, Jones C R et al. Semen analysis in testicular cancer and Hodgkin's disease: pre- and post-treatment findings and implications for cryopreservation. Br J Urol 1983; 55: 769–773

32. Scammell G E, White N, Stedronska J et al. Cryopreservation of semen in men with testicular tumour or Hodgkin's disease: results of artificial insemination of their partners. Lancet 1985; 2: 31–32

33. Brindley G S. Le syndrome de 'primary anorgasmia' chez l'homme. In: Buvat J, Jouannet P (eds) L'éjaculation et ses perturbations. Lyons: Simep 1984; 79–83

34. Wang R, Monga M, Hellstrom W J G. Ejaculatory dysfunction. In: Comhaire FH (ed) Male infertility: clinical investigation, cause evaluation and treatment. London: Chapman and Hall, 1996; 205–221

35. Beeley L, Chaput de Saintonge D M. The unwanted effects of drugs on the male reproductive system. In: Whitfield H N, Hendry W F, Kirby R S, Duckett J (eds) Textbook of genito-urinary surgery, 2nd edn. Oxford: Blackwell, 1998: in press

36. Hendry W F, Rickards D, Pryor J P, Baker L R I. Seminal megavesicles with adult polycystic kidney disease. Human Reprod 1998: in press

37. Colpi G M, Casella F, Zanollo A et al. Functional voiding disturbances of the ampullo-vesicular seminal tract: a cause of male infertility. Acta Eur Fertil 1987; 18: 165–179

38. Drach G W, Fair W R, Meares E M, Stamey T A. Classification of benign diseases associated with prostatic pain: prostatitis or prostatodynia? J Urol 1978; 120: 266

39. Zinner A. Ein fall von intravesikaler samenblasenzyste. Wien Med Wochenschr 1914; 64: 605–609

40. Hendry W F, Parslow J M, Parkinson M C, Lowe D G. Unilateral testicular obstruction: orchidectomy or reconstruction? Hum Reprod 1994; 9: 463–470

41. Berkovitch M, Keresteci A G, Koren G. Efficacy of prilocaine–lidocaine cream in the treatment of premature ejaculation. J Urol 1995; 154: 1360–1361

42. Sahin H, Bircan M K. Efficacy of prilocaine–lidocaine cream in the treatment of premature ejaculation. J Urol 1996; 156: 1783–1784

43. Haensel S M, Rowland D L, Kallan K T H K, Slob A K. Clomipramine and sexual function in men with premature ejaculation and controls. J Urol 1996; 156: 1310–1315

44. Kara H, Aydin S, Agargun M Y et al. The efficacy of fluoxetine in the treatment of premature ejaculation: a double-blind placebo controlled study. J Urol 1996; 156: 1631–1632

45. Brindley G S, Sauerwein D, Hendry W F. Hypogastric plexus stimulators for obtaining semen from paraplegic men. Br J Urol 1989; 64: 72–77

46. Ohl D A. Electroejaculation. Urol Clin North Am 1993; 20: 181–188

47. Dahlberg A, Ruutu M, Hovatta O. Pregnancy results from a vibrator application, electroejaculation, and a vas aspiration programme in spinal-cord injured men. Hum Reprod 1995; 10: 2305–2307

48. Hendry W F. Treatment for loss of ejaculation after para-aortic lymphadenectomy. In: Jones W G, Harnden P, Appleyard I (eds) Germ cell tumours III. 3rd edn. Oxford: Pergamon, 1994: 353–358

49. Ohl D A, Denil J, Bennett C J et al. Electroejaculation following retroperitoneal lymphadenectomy. J Urol 1991; 145: 980–983

50. Craft I, Tsirigotis M. Simplified recovery, preparation and cryopreservation of testicular spermatozoa. Hum Reprod 1995; 10: 1623–1627

51. Brindley G S, Scott G I, Hendry W F. Vas cannulation with implanted sperm reservoirs for obstructive azoospermia or ejaculatory failure. Br J Urol 1986; 58: 721–723

52. Kedia K R, Markland C. The ejaculatory process. In: Hafez E S E (eds) Human semen and fertility regulation in men, 1st edn. Saint Louis: Mosby, 1976: 497–503

Chapter 51

Premature ejaculation

A. D. Seftel and S. E. Althof

INTRODUCTION

In this era, when male and female sexuality have risen to heightened levels of awareness, premature ejaculation (PE) is being recognized as a common male sexual health problem. Oral pharmacotherapy offers urologists an additional option for managing this problem. This chapter reviews the literature on pharmacotherapy for rapid ejaculation, discusses several other types of therapy available for the urologist and offers guidelines for integrating the psychological and pharmacological approaches to therapy.

The problem
It is anecdotal that, although PE is the most common type of male sexual dysfunction, with a prevalence of 30–40% of adult men, it is the disorder for which men are least likely to seek help.[1,2] The reasons for this are unclear, but probably are an amalgam of man's selfishness as a lover, not defining it as a problem until the partner has repeatedly declared it a serious concern, and man's general avoidance of asking others to help him with any problems.

DEFINITION OF PREMATURE EJACULATION

There is no consensus regarding the criteria for rapid ejaculation. Various studies have defined the dysfunction in terms of time from intromission to ejaculation, number of coital thrusts, partner satisfaction and degree of voluntary control. The most recent set of criteria appearing in the fourth edition of the Diagnostic and Statistical Manual of the American Psychiatric Association[3] delineates three criteria for PE (302.75):

1. Persistent or recurrent ejaculation with minimal stimulation before, on, or shortly after penetration and before the person wishes it. The clinician must take into account factors that affect duration of the excitement phase, such as age, novelty of the sexual partner or situation and recent frequency of sexual activity.
2. The disturbance causes marked distress or interpersonal difficulty.
3. The PE is not due exclusively to the direct effects of a substance (e.g. withdrawal from opioids).[3]

The clinician is required to make three additional specifications: first, whether the dysfunction is lifelong or acquired; second, whether it is of a generalized or specific type; third, whether it is due to psychological or combined factors. Although this criterion set employs a multidimensional definition utilizing time and voluntary control, it provides few quantifiable points of reference: for instance, what is meant by minimal sexual stimulation and what time-lapse after penetration should one consider to be dysfunctional?

NEW CONCEPTS OF THE PATHOPHYSIOLOGICAL AETIOLOGY OF PREMATURE EJACULATION

There are emerging data to suggest that men with PE have hypersensitivity and hyperexcitability of the glans penis and the dorsal nerve. Xin et al.[4,5] studied 34 men with PE and 30 normal controls and found, using somatosensory evoked potentials, a significant decrease in dorsal nerve (1.51 ms) and glans penis (6.80 ms) mean latency versus controls. Thus, there may be an organic basis for some forms of PE.

■ HISTORICAL TREATMENT OPTIONS

Individual, conjoint and group psychotherapy approaches combined with behavioural strategies such as 'stop–start' or 'squeeze' techniques have all been utilized to treat rapid ejaculation.[6–12] It is now known that the initial post-treatment success rates ranging from 60% to 95%[11,13,14] were not sustainable: 3 years after treatment, success rates dwindled to 25%.[15,16] This suggests that clinicians have failed to develop long-term strategies that allow patients to maintain their initial therapeutic gains. It would be interesting to see data on the efficacy of treatment where therapists employ periodic booster or maintenance sessions after the termination of the original treatment.

■ ORAL THERAPY FOR PREMATURE EJACULATION

The psychological/behavioural approach to rapid ejaculation, which has been in ascendancy for over 20 years, became challenged by studies that suggested that ejaculatory latency could be prolonged by clomipramine or the selective serotonin re-uptake inhibitor drugs (SSRIs) — fluoxetine, sertraline and paroxetine — without troublesome side effects.[17–23] These early reports led to a large trial, which is summarized below.

Clomipramine

Several studies have examined the role of clomipramine in the treatment of PE.

Segraves et al.[20] reported on the double-blind comparison of clomipramine and placebo on ejaculatory latency in 20 men complaining of PE. Self-report of ejaculatory latency was utilized, with a partial check of validity being supplied by the partner report of ejaculatory latency in married subjects. Clomipramine significantly increased ejaculatory latency over placebo. Subjects also completed twice a week ratings of quality of libido, quality of ejaculation, satisfaction with ejaculatory timing and overall sexual satisfaction. All indices improved in patients receiving clomipramine. Side effects were minimal and consisted of transient fatigue and nausea in a few subjects.

The authors' group[21] conducted a double-blind, randomized, placebo-controlled study employing strict dosages in a carefully selected population to ascertain if clomipramine was biologically and psychologically efficacious in delaying ejaculation. The results with 15 couples were that 25 mg clomipramine increased ejaculatory latency by 249% while 50 mg of the drug increased time to orgasm by 517%. However, when the men discontinued the medication the improvements vanished and their ejaculatory latencies returned to baseline. Placebo administration (non-significantly) increased ejaculatory latency 30% over baseline. These results were consistent with prior studies conducted by Segraves et al.[20] and Assalian.[17]

Psychosocially, there were significant improvements in male and female sexual satisfaction, male relationship satisfaction and male psychological well-being. Three women partners, who had never achieved coital orgasm, became orgasmic while the man was taking medication. Furthermore, 6 of 10 women who commonly achieved orgasm reported that this occurred with greater frequency when their partners were taking active drug.

Side effects were generally mild and dose related, and tended to diminish with time. Dry mouth, constipation, and feeling 'different' were the longest-lasting effects with 50 mg, but were not generally clinically significant at 25 mg. Nausea, sleep disturbance, fatigue and hot flushes were infrequently observed at 50 mg.

A second open-label study was undertaken to ascertain (1) whether prolonged treatment with clomipramine could lead to continued ejaculatory control upon discontinuation of medication (2) whether men can take the drug on less than a daily basis and (3) the characteristics of those subjects who continue with pharmacological treatment and of those that drop out.

Subjects were placed on various doses of medication for 7 months, at which point they were asked to take a 1 month drug holiday while reporting on ejaculatory latency and sexual satisfaction.

After 7 months, 14 men continued to take medication while 13 dropped out. All 14 stayers reported an improvement of at least 55 seconds. Equal numbers of drop-outs and stayers reported side effects. By 7 months the 14 subjects were distributed among seven medication schedules, as follows (in mg): one subject, 25 qd; two, 25 qod; one, 25 prn; seven, 50 qd; two, 50 qod; one, 50 prn. Only two of the 14 subjects were successful with taking the medication on the day of intercourse: the other 12 required more intensive regimens.

Of the 14 men, 11 went on drug holiday, three by design at 7 months and eight of their own accord at various intervals ranging from 2 to 7 months. None of the four men who went on holiday by design at 7 months was able to maintain the increases in ejaculatory latency: two of the four men returned to baseline; the other two reported losing 25–50% of the ejaculatory gains. All the men that placed themselves on holiday returned to baseline ejaculatory latencies. This open-label trial confirmed the previous findings of the authors' group regarding the efficacy of clomipramine in the treatment of rapid ejaculation: 7 months of treatment was not successful in allowing men to maintain their gains off medication. Only a minority of subjects were able to delay ejaculation on less than a daily dose of medication. This would indicate a lifelong dependency on oral therapy for PE.

The results of the second study should be viewed as preliminary and interpreted with caution because of the small sample size and the lack of control groups, objective timing, or blinding of the investigators or subjects. The authors consider the 48% drop-out rate to be due in part to their failure to monitor the patients' progress closely. They now recommend that, initially, patients should be followed at least monthly. Drop-outs should be expected because some patients unrealistically expect the medication to remedy relationship problems as well as to cure rapid ejaculation.

A note of caution regarding the use of clomipramine. One study[23] reported that a daily regimen of 75 mg clomipramine taken for 3 months in a series of 11 depressed patients resulted in pathological spermiograms in all patients in terms of volume, sperm motility and sperm morphology. This important finding warrants replication and further research into the possible consequences on male fertility of pharmacotherapy with clomipramine and/or other antidepressant medications.

Haensel et al.[24] evaluated clomipramine in a placebo-controlled, double-blind crossover trial. Interestingly, this study included six men with secondary PE (PE most probably due to erectile dysfunction). These authors found that clomipramine increased ejaculatory latency in the eight men with primary PE from 2 to 8 minutes; however, there were no significant effects in the eight control men or in the six men with secondary PE. Interestingly, clomipramine inhibited nocturnal penile tumescence in all subjects; these data were collected using a snap gauge-like device. These data provide further support for the use of clomipramine for men with primary PE.

Sertraline

In a double-blind, randomized placebo-controlled study, Mendels and colleagues[25,26] reported that sertraline produced clinically and statistically significant improvements relative to placebo in time to ejaculation and number of successful attempts at intercourse. The average daily dose was 121 mg. Similarly, in an open-label trial, Swartz[27] reported on ten patients who were prescribed either 25 or 50 mg sertraline. The average ejaculatory delay was 20 minutes. Side effects were infrequent and consisted of transient anorexia and headaches.

Fluoxetine and paroxetine

Lee et al.[28] evaluated fluoxetine in 11 men with primary PE. Patients were started on 20 mg/day for 2 weeks and were then titrated to 60 mg/day, depending on tolerability and response. Fluoxetine resulted in an increased ejaculatory latency time.

Kara et al.[29] evaluated fluoxetine in 17 men with primary PE in a double-blind fashion. Patients were started on 20 mg/day for 1 week and the dose was then increased to 40 mg/day. The placebo group followed a similar schedule. A marked improvement in ejaculatory latency was noted. Side effects reported included nausea, headache and insomnia.

Waldinger et al.[30] studied the effect of paroxetine on ejaculation in a double-blind, placebo-controlled trial in men with PE. The dose of paroxetine was increased from 20 to 40 mg after the first week. Successful outcomes were noted in most patients and side effects were minimal. Currently, there are no double-blind placebo-controlled studies regarding the efficacy of fluoxetine in treating rapid ejaculation, however, several anecdotal reports and the authors' clinical experience suggest that it may also be effective at doses ranging from 20 to 40 mg daily.

■ TOPICAL THERAPY

Two recent studies have examined the effects of topical creams in the treatment of primary PE. Xin et al.[31] examined the effects of topical 'SS' cream on rabbit cavernosal tissue in the organ bath and found that the cream had a vasorelaxant effect on the smooth muscle. These authors have had clinical experience with this cream and have found it effective for PE.[32] Next, Sahin and Bircan.[33] found that topical anaesthesia with prilocaine–lidocaine (lignocaine) was effective in the treatment of PE. This application awaits further study.

CWRU EXPERIENCE WITH CLOMIPRAMINE FOR PREMATURE EJACULATION: THE UROLOGIST'S PERSPECTIVE

As the treatment of erectile dysfunction (ED) has become less surgical, urologists are faced with new challenges in the treatment of male sexual dysfunction. Pharmacotherapy of rapid ejaculation is one such new frontier. The urologist must now become conversant and knowledgeable with diagnosis and management of this dysfunction. A sample questionnaire[34] has been described previously. To this end, an ongoing trial of clomipramine was initiated for those patients with primary, lifelong PE, based upon the above work, and remains in effect. The selection process was a careful one: excluded were those patients who were suspected of secondary or acquired PE or those patients with concomitant ED. Cursory psychosocial screening excluded patients with overt psychopathology. To date, the authors have accrued 15 patients with an average follow-up of 2.5 years. Five of the patients were happily married, and the remaining ten patients had a stable relationship with a solo partner. The subjects sought to improve upon their sexual relationship, and they believed that the dysfunction had not impacted negatively upon their sex lives or relationships. These realistic expectations are central to cure, rather than the belief that the treatment for PE is a substitute for marital harmony. Those seven patients who continue to have a stable relationship all continue to use the therapy and find it helpful and fulfilling. Six treatment 'failures' were either relationship failures, attesting to the need to assess relationship issues, or in men with previously undiagnosed ED. This therapy is not a substitute for marital counselling, should not be used for treatment of ED and should not be offered to men who are contemplating new relationships and are concerned about their possible sexual performance (performance anxiety). The two other failures with clomipramine were in middle-aged men, both married. One man found the clomipramine to be of no help and has been switched to paroxetine. The second man tried oral clomipramine for 2 weeks (25 mg qd for the first week, and 25 mg qod the

second week). However, he could not tolerate the medication, owing to side effects that included headache, nausea and chest flushing; this patient has now been switched to paroxetine. Thus, the authors have seven patients on long-term therapy with good results. Interestingly, two of these men take the drug on the morning of anticipated intercourse, which is now characterized as on a 'prn' basis.

Treatment experience

Initially, these patients were treated with clomipramine (25 mg qd). At an early stage, this regimen produced significant side effects (including headache, hot flushes, nausea, vomiting and fatigue) for many of these patients, which contrasts with some of the data presented above. Subsequently, the oral therapy has been tailored to qod or twice a week — and now most commonly to the day of anticipated intercourse. This has significantly reduced the incidence of side effects and appears to have reasonable efficacy. The urologist currently employs this regimen for all new patients.

Treatment recommendations

The 'lifelong' versus 'acquired' classification of rapid ejaculation may prove to be a useful marker for formulating treatment recommendations. The ideal candidate for drug therapy might be a man with several years of sexual experience, with a lifelong pattern of rapid ejaculation and who is free of substance abuse, depression and psychosis and is capable of developing stable, satisfying non-sexual relationships. Drug therapy can also be considered for those patients who have not profited from a competently conducted psychological treatment. In contrast, acquired rapid ejaculation begs the clinician to be interested in the forces that generated the new symptom. Given a relatively recent onset and some degree of psychological mindedness, these men/couples might, in the long run, do better with a behavioural or psychological intervention.

Sexual experience level

Pharmacological treatment should not be a first-line consideration for the young or inexperienced man who, in his first few sexual encounters, experiences rapid ejaculation. Reassurance and education are likely to be worth-while and it is hoped that, in time, these men will develop increased confidence and learn to control ejaculation.

Quality of the non-sexual relationship

Whether PE is lifelong or acquired, caution is warranted in offering drug therapy alone to men where the symptom clearly reflects intrapsychic or interpersonal conflict. Therapists must not lose sight of the time-honoured dynamic maxim that symptoms exist for reasons. Rapid symptom removal may disrupt the equilibrium of the individual or couple. This caution is not simply a restatement of the psychoanalytic theory of symptom substitution, but is a concern based on the authors' experience, where treatment in a small minority of cases resulted in destructive acting out.

■ REFERENCES

1. Laumann E O, Gagnon J H, Michael R T, Michaels S. The social organization of sexuality. Chicago, IL: University of Chicago Press, 1994

2. Frank E, Anderson C, Rubinstein D. Frequency of sexual dysfunction in 'normal' couples. N Engl J Med 1978; 299: 111

3. APA. Diagnostic and statistical manual of mental disorders, 4th edn, rev. Washington, D.C.: American Psychiatric Association, 1987

4. Xin Z C, Choi Y D, Rha K H, Choi H K. Somatosensory evoked potentials in patients with primary premature ejaculation. J Urol 1997; 158(2): 451–455

5. Xin Z C, Chung W S, Choi Y D et al. Penile sensitivity in patients with primary premature ejaculation. J Urol 1996; 156(3): 979–981

6. Halvorsen J, Metz M. Sexual dysfunction, part I: classification, etiology and pathogenesis. J Am Board Fam Pract 1992; 5: 51–61

7. Kaplan H. Overcoming premature ejaculation. New York: Brunner/Mazel, 1989

8. Levine S. Sexual life: a clinician's guide. New York: Plenum, 1992

9. LoPiccolo J, LoPiccolo L. Handbook of sex therapy. New York: Plenum, 1978

10. McCarthy B. Cognitive–behavioral strategies and techniques in the treatment of early ejaculation. In: Leiblum S R, Rosen R (eds) Principles and practice of sex therapy: update for the 90's. New York: Guilford Press, 1990: 143–167

11. Masters W, Johnson V. Human sexual inadequacy. Boston: Little, Brown, 1970

12. Semans J. Premature ejaculation: a new approach. South Med J 1956; 49: 353–358

13. Hawton K. Erectile dysfunction and premature ejaculation. Br J Hosp Med 1988; 40: 428

14. Hawton K, Catalan J. Prognostic factors in sex therapy. Behav Res Ther 1986; 24: 377–385

15. Bancroft J, Coles L. Three years experience in a sexual problems clinic. Br Med J 1976; 1: 1575–1577

16. DeAmicus L, Goldberg D, LoPiccolo J et al. Clinical follow-up of couples treated for sexual dysfunction. Arch Sex Behav 1985; 14: 467–489

17. Assalian P. Clomipramine in the treatment of premature ejaculation. J Sex Res 1988; 24: 231–251

18. Goodman R. An assessment of clomipramine (Anafranil) in the treatment of premature ejaculation. J Int Med Res 1980; 8: 53–59

19. Goodman R E. Premature ejaculation. Br Med J 1981; 282: 1796

20. Segraves R T, Saran A, Segraves K, Maguire E. Clomipramine versus placebo in the treatment of premature ejaculation: a pilot study. J Sex Marital Ther 1993; 19: 198–200

21. Althof S, Levine S, Corty E et al. Clomipramine as a treatment for rapid ejaculation: a double-blind crossover trial of fifteen couples. J Clin Psychiatry 1995; 56(9): 402–407

22. Kaplan P. The use of serotonergic uptake inhibitors in the treatment of premature ejaculation. J Sex Marital Ther 1995; 20: 321–324

23. Maier U, Koinig G. Andrological findings in young patients under long-term antidepressant therapy with clomipramine. J Clin Pharmacol 1995; 15: 341–346

24. Haensel S M, Rowland D L, Kallan K T. Clomipramine and sexual function in men with premature ejaculation and controls. J Urol 1996; 156(4): 1310-1315

25. Mendels J, Camera A, Sikes C. Sertraline treatment for premature ejaculation. J Clin Psychopharmacol 1995; 15(5): 341–346

26. Mendels J. Sertraline for premature ejaculation. J Clin Psychiatry 1995; 56(12): 591

27. Swartz D. Sertraline hydrochloride for premature ejaculation. Programs and Abstracts of the 89th Annual Meeting of the American Urological Association, San Francisco. Abstract 471. J Urol 1994; 151(Suppl): 345A

28. Lee H S, Song D H, Kim C H, Choi H K. An open clinical trial of fluoxetine in the treatment of premature ejaculation. J Clin Psychopharmacol 1996; 16(5): 379–382

29. Kara H, Aydin S, Yucel M et al. The efficacy of fluoxetine in the treatment of premature ejaculation: a double-blind placebo controlled study. J Urol 1996; 156(5): 1631–1632

30. Waldinger M, Hengeveld M, Zwinderman A. Paroxetine treatment of premature ejaculation: a double-blind randomized placebo-controlled study. Am J Psychiatry 1994; 151: 1377–1379

31. Xin Z C, Choi Y D, Choi H K. The effects of SS-cream and its individual components on rabbit corpus cavernosal muscles. Yonsei Med J 1996; 37: 312–318

32. Xin Z C, Choi Y D, Seong D H, Choi H K. Sensory evoked potential and effect of SS-cream in premature ejaculation. Yonsei Med J 1995; 36: 397–401

33. Sahin H, Bircan M K. Efficacy of prilocaine–lidocaine cream in the treatment of premature ejaculation. J Urol 1996; 156(5): 1783–1784

34. Seftel A D, Althof S E. Premature ejaculation. In: Mulcahy J (ed) Diagnosis and Management of Male Sexual Dysfunction. Chapter 11. New York: Tgaka-Shoin, 1997: 196–204

Chapter 52
Phalloplasty

G. H. Jordan

■ INTRODUCTION

The penis is a unique organ that cannot be replicated exactly. The ideal characteristics of a penis-like organ (i.e. a phallus) include tactile, protective and erogenous sensibility that allow for intercourse; anatomical and aesthetic acceptability, with the neo-urethra ending at the tip of the glans; ability to achieve rigidity adequate for intercourse; and appropriate growth potential, if reconstruction is accomplished in childhood. In addition, the construction should ideally be accomplished using a single-staged procedure that results in an acceptable degree of donor site morbidity. Unfortunately, in most centers, these goals cannot be accomplished in a single-stage procedure, despite employment of state-of-the-art techniques. However, by using microsurgical techniques to borrow distant autologous tissues, an acceptable phallus can be created.

■ NEOPHALLIC FLAP DESIGNS

Phallic construction has undergone a series of evolutionary developments since it was first described in Russia, in 1917.[1-4] The state-of-the-art technique for phallic construction today involves a microsurgical free forearm flap (Fig. 52.1).[5,6]

Chang and Huang (Chinese flap)

The flap design published in 1984, by Chang and Huang,[7] employs a radial forearm flap that incorporates a portion of the flap as a vascularized urethral tube. The neo-urethra is constructed from a skin paddle on the most ulnar aspect of the flap (Fig. 52.1a). The superficial sensory nerves to the forearm tissues (lateral and medial antebrachial cutaneous nerves) are carried in the flap design, allowing for the creation of sensibility. A number of free forearm flap phallic designs have emanated from this design.

Farrow and Boyd

Farrow and Boyd modified the forearm flap, calling it the 'cricket bat' design (Fig. 52.1b).[8,9] The modification involves placement of the neo-urethra and shaft in tandem. Like the Chinese flap, in the 'cricket bat' design sensibility to the neophallus is provided by the lateral and medial antebrachial cutaneous nerves. An advantage of this design is that it allows for easy adjustments to accommodate the length of the urethra and penile stump because the urethra is centred over the vessel. The flap has produced excellent results when used in paediatric cases or for reconstruction of total or subtotal amputations of the penis. However, many transgender patients have complained of the limited phallic length produced when this technique is used for neophallic construction.

Biemer

Biemer further modified the radial forearm flap design, also centring the urethra over the radial artery (Fig. 52.1c).[10] In his original description, the flap also carried a portion of the radial bone on the vessel, and the shaft coverage was separated into two skin islands. With this design, the neo-urethra can extend proximally and distally along the shaft length, making it versatile in cases where the length of the native urethra is variable. Sensibility is provided from the lateral and medial antebrachial cutaneous nerves. There are several disadvantages of this flap design for phallic construction: centering the urethra over the radial pedicle means that the hairiest portion of the forearm is used for the urethra; using two skin paddles to cover the shaft results in two suture lines on the phallus; and using the original design results in a delayed fracture of the radius in some patients.

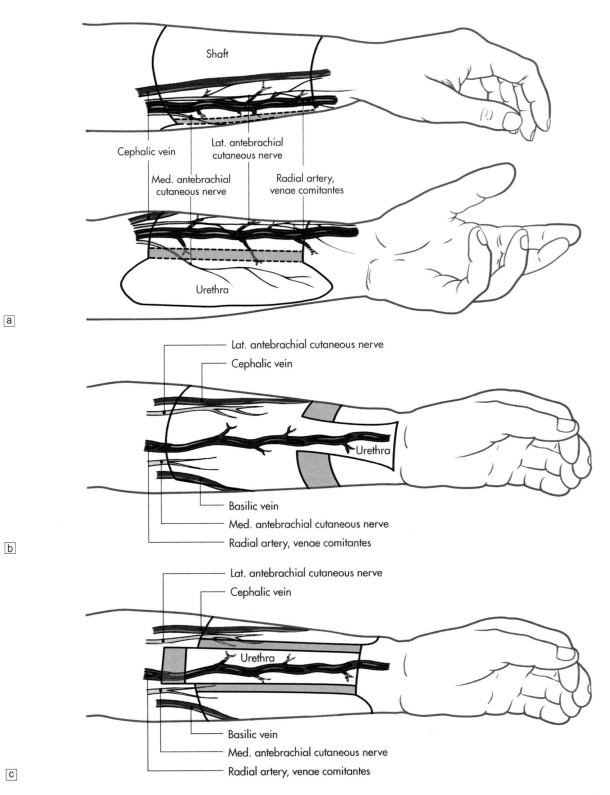

Figure 52.1. Radial forearm flap designs for phallic construction. (a) Flap design after Chang and Huang. Note, the flap has two skin islands separated by a de-epithelialized strip. The urethral portion is on the ulnar aspect of the forearm; the shaft portion overlies the radial portion of the forearm. (b) Flap design after Farrow and Boyd (cricket bat). Note, the urethra is centered over the radial artery; the illustrated de-epithelialized portions add bulk to the glans; the shaft portion is on the proximal forearm. (c) Flap design after that proposed by Biemer. Note, the urethral strip is centered over the radial artery. The shaft coverage is separated by two de-epithelialized strips that are separate islands — one on the radial portion and one on the ulnar portion of the forearm.

Louvie

Louvie described a forearm flap based on the ulnar artery that was originally described for maxillofacial reconstruction.[11] The advantage of the forearm flap in maxillofacial reconstruction (thin, non-hirsute skin) also applies to the forearm flap in penile reconstruction and phallic construction. Sensibility for this flap is also derived from the lateral and medial antebrachial cutaneous nerves.

Puckett

A tubed free groin flap that included an innovative integral glans was designed by Puckett.[12] Early in his series, the flap was transferred in delayed fashion to the area of the penile stump. Later in the series, a microvascular free transfer technique was employed. Although the flap has the disadvantage of being insensible, it is cosmetically acceptable. When used in combination with the forearm fascia cutaneous flap, Puckett's integral glans design is the design preferred by the author for phallic construction and penile reconstruction (Fig. 52.2a,b).

■ SURGICAL TECHNIQUE

Pre-operative assessment

All patients evaluated for a microsurgical tissue transfer procedure must undergo a careful pre-operative assessment. In general, microvascular procedures require patients to be in good health. Smokers, and patients older than 50–55 years of age, are not considered strong candidates for microvascular surgery. Two-vessel patency in the non-dominant upper extremity and an intact palmar arch are evaluated using the Allen's test. If there is doubt about the vascular integrity of either forearm, an upper extremity duplex vascular study and/or angiography is performed.

The flap design incorporates a combination of the original Biemer triple skin paddle design, Puckett's glansplasty (i.e. a distal extension of the central skin island) and Louvie's elevation of the flap on the ulnar artery.[6] The flap dimensions are planned to accommodate the patient's anatomical needs. In prepubertal patients, the growth rate of the phallus during maturation must be accommodated. In all patients, the depth of subcutaneous fat on the forearm must be assessed: patients who will have thicker flaps (greater depth of fat) will require larger paddles for outer shaft coverage. In some cases, these flaps

have been covered with a split-thickness skin graft with excellent cosmetic results.

Flap elevation

Doppler evaluation of the ulnar artery is performed and its course is drawn on the forearm. The flap is then drawn on the forearm and select areas are de-epithelialized (Fig. 52.2a). The flap is elevated, raising the superficial lamina with the flap and leaving the deep lamina intact on the forearm musculature (Fig. 52.2b).

The ulnar artery and its vena comitans are identified and ligated distally, and the radial and ulnar nerves are identified and left undisturbed to preserve the distal sensory branches. Two predictable vascular perforators from the ulnar artery end of the flap are identified within the distal forearm: typically, the largest is usually found at the mid-forearm level and the second is distally located, between the proximal perforator and the wrist.

Numerous veins are encountered in the proximal forearm. Because the diameter is similar to the recipient saphenous vein, the basilic and cephalic veins are preferred for anastomosis. An attempt is also made to anastomose the donor venae comitantes to the recipient inferior epigastric venae comitantes.

The phallus is configured while the flap is perfused on the forearm. The neo-urethra is tubed with a running, absorbable, monofilament suture (Fig. 52.2c,d). The phallic shaft is completed by suturing the lateral flaps to each other in 'clam shell' fashion, using a subcuticular absorbable braided or monofilament suture (Fig. 52.2e). A nylon or Prolene suture is used to approximate the skin. The neoglans is formed by proximal rotation of the glans paddle (Fig. 52.2f), creating an anatomically appropriate, conical glans configuration. The flap's vessels and nerves are carefully marked prior to transfer.

Preparation of flap recipient site

While the flap is being elevated and configured on the forearm, a second surgical team is simultaneously addressing the genitalia to prepare the flap recipient site. When present (i.e. penile reconstruction), the penile base is dissected. In transgender patients, a bipedicle flap is raised in the area where the flap is to be transferred. The flap is transposed to the scrotal aspect of the phallus (Fig. 52.3). In all transgender patients and many penile injury patients, the non-dominant gracilis muscle is elevated and transposed over the urethral anastomosis.

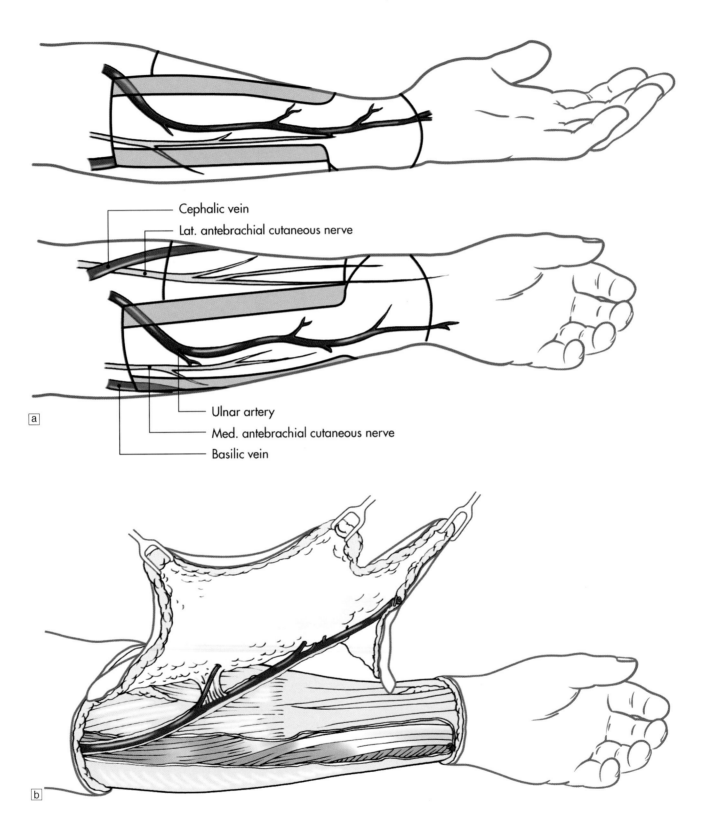

Cephalic vein
Lat. antebrachial cutaneous nerve

Ulnar artery
Med. antebrachial cutaneous nerve
Basilic vein

Figure 52.2. The favored design for phallic construction at the author's center. (a) The urethral portion of the flap is centered over the ulnar artery and separated from the shaft islands. The flap's shape is similar to that proposed by Biemer. The distal extension creates an integral glans after the design proposed by Puckett. (b) Illustration of the flap elevated on the ulnar artery. The superficial lamina of the deep fascia is elevated with the flap; the deep lamina is left intact on the forearm musculature.

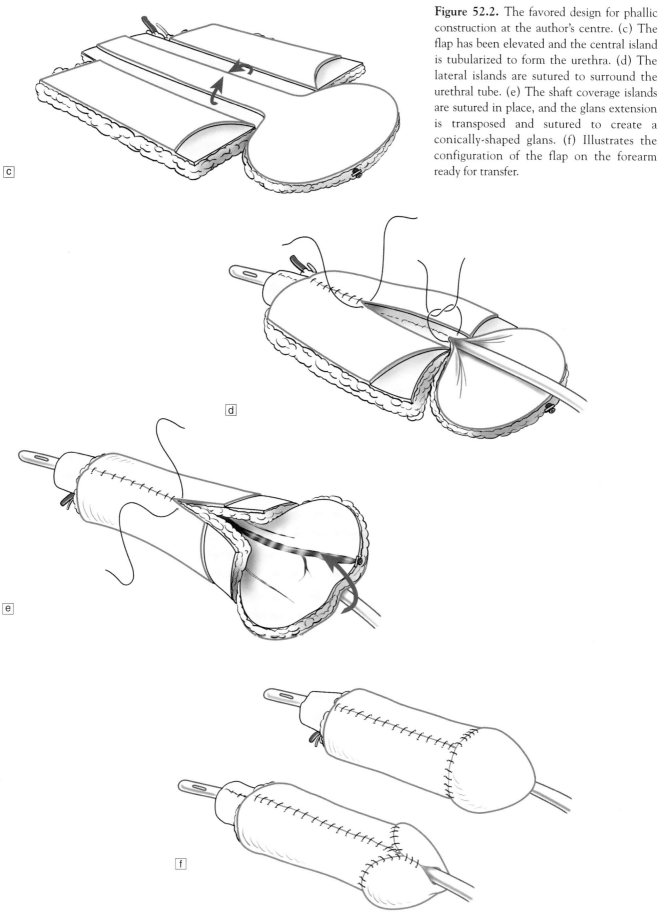

Figure 52.2. The favored design for phallic construction at the author's centre. (c) The flap has been elevated and the central island is tubularized to form the urethra. (d) The lateral islands are sutured to surround the urethral tube. (e) The shaft coverage islands are sutured in place, and the glans extension is transposed and sutured to create a conically-shaped glans. (f) Illustrates the configuration of the flap on the forearm ready for transfer.

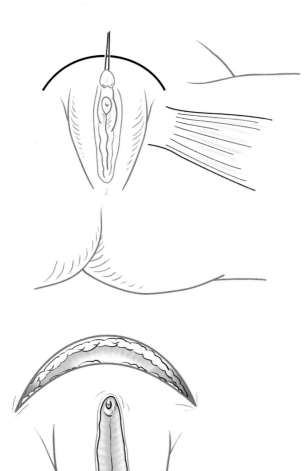

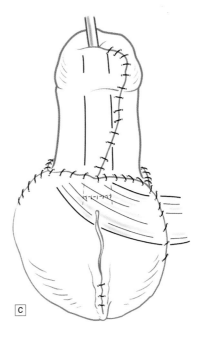

Figure 52.3. Illustration in a trans-sexual patient. (a) A bipedicle flap is outlined at the desired position of the neophallus. (b) The bipedicle flap is elevated and transposed to the scrotal aspect of the phallus. (c) The phallus has been transferred to its perineal position. The bipedicle flap is sutured in place, adding bulk to the area of the scrotum. Note, the gracilis muscle flap is elevated and transposed to cover the urethral anastomosis.

In both situations, the recipient vessels are prepared (Fig. 52.4). Optimally, the recipient vessels include the deep inferior epigastric vascular pedicle and the patient's non-dominant saphenous vein (Fig. 52.4a). The saphenous vein is dissected distally where a natural prominent bifurcation occurs in the thigh. In patients whose deep inferior epigastric vessels are not patent, more extensive dissection of the non-dominant saphenous vein is performed, allowing for a saphenous vein interposition graft to the femoral artery (Fig. 52.4b). In these patients, the interposition graft and the saphenous vein are the recipient vessels.

Flap transfer

Flap transfer involves vascular anastomoses, urethral anastomosis and nerve coaptation. The flap is transferred and the ulnar artery is anastomosed to either the deep inferior epigastric artery or the saphenous vein interposition graft to the femoral artery. The ulnar vena comitans is anastomosed either to the epigastric vena comitans or to the saphenous vein. The basilic and cephalic veins are anastomosed to the saphenous vein.

When the phallus is well perfused, the urethral anastomosis is performed, using monofilament absorbable suture. The gracilis muscle, if elevated, is transposed over the urethral anastomosis, and nerve coaptation is performed (Fig. 52.4b). In the genetic male trauma patient, the medial and/or lateral antebrachial nerves are coapted microsurgically to the proximal penile nerves; in the transsexual patient, they are coapted to the dorsal nerves of the clitoris or, via nerve

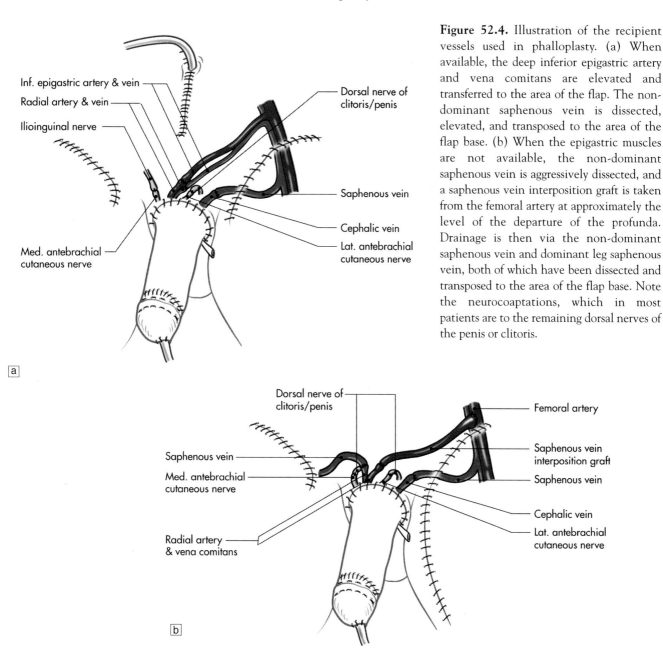

Inf. epigastric artery & vein

Radial artery & vein

Ilioinguinal nerve

Med. antebrachial cutaneous nerve

Dorsal nerve of clitoris/penis

Saphenous vein

Cephalic vein

Lat. antebrachial cutaneous nerve

a

Dorsal nerve of clitoris/penis

Femoral artery

Saphenous vein

Med. antebrachial cutaneous nerve

Saphenous vein interposition graft

Saphenous vein

Cephalic vein

Lat. antebrachial cutaneous nerve

Radial artery & vena comitans

b

Figure 52.4. Illustration of the recipient vessels used in phalloplasty. (a) When available, the deep inferior epigastric artery and vena comitans are elevated and transferred to the area of the flap. The non-dominant saphenous vein is dissected, elevated, and transposed to the area of the flap base. (b) When the epigastric muscles are not available, the non-dominant saphenous vein is aggressively dissected, and a saphenous vein interposition graft is taken from the femoral artery at approximately the level of the departure of the profunda. Drainage is then via the non-dominant saphenous vein and dominant leg saphenous vein, both of which have been dissected and transposed to the area of the flap base. Note the neurocoaptations, which in most patients are to the remaining dorsal nerves of the penis or clitoris.

interposition graft, to the pudendal nerves, giving protective and erogenous sensibility to the neophallus or reconstructed penis.

Closure

The forearm flap donor site is covered with a full-thickness skin graft and the forearm is placed in a splint. Closure with a full-thickness skin graft offers less donor-site morbidity and an improved cosmetic result compared with a split-thickness skin graft. Suprapubic diversion is performed, and a soft silicone catheter is passed to stent the urethral anastomosis. Supportive dressing is constructed for the phallus or reconstructed penis.

Follow-up

A voiding study with contrast is performed at approximately 28 days after surgery and removal of the suprapubic catheter is scheduled. Further assessment is performed at 6 weeks, 3 months, 6 months and a year. Sensibility begins to return at 3 months, and reasonably full sensibility is achieved at 6 months. If a durable result is achieved, the urethra is patent and the patient is free of voiding difficulties and urinary infections, and sensibility is acceptable, prosthetic implantation can be accomplished at 1 year. If no sensation occurs, or if the neophallus was created from an insensate flap, sural nerve interposition grafts are coapted to branches of the pudendal or dorsal nerves and laid into the neophallus to form sensate neuromas (neurotization).

PROSTHETIC IMPLANTATION

Although the radial or ulnar free fasciocutaneous forearm flap allows for creation of an aesthetically pleasing and sensible neophallus that enables the patient to void while standing, adequate rigidity for sexual intercourse is lacking. However, because it does provide protective sensation, decreasing the incidence of extrusion and migration, successful prosthetic implantation is possible with this design.[13,14] Once sensation is present, semi-rigid or hydraulic penile prostheses are the preferred devices. If a patient has poor sensation, a hydraulic penile prosthesis is the implant of choice.

The amount of rigidity and the aesthetic result are greatly improved with the use of two cylinders as implants. Occasionally, however, only one will fit in the neophallus. Controlled-expansion cylinders (American Medical Systems Model 700 CX or CXM) are used. The author has had extensive experience with the Duraphase or Dura II devices, with excellent results.

Surgical technique

The patient is placed in a low lithotomy position. Dissection is performed through a low suprapubic incision carried to the pubic periosteum at the base of the neophallus (Fig. 52.5). A space is created in the neophallus for the implant, using scissors, and dilated with a sound or an Otis urethrotome. Care is taken to avoid the urethra, nerves and vascular pedicle. Because catheterization may hinder the dilatation process and/or increase the chance of injury, a catheter is not placed in the urethra. Several centimeteres of the most distal neophallus are left undisturbed, providing a cushion for the implant.

In most cases, the author prefers to use two cylinders. Through a second incision overlying the ischial

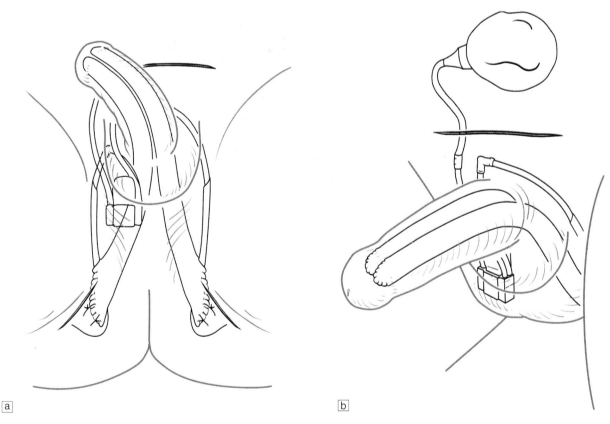

a

b

Figure 52.5. (a) The appearance of a phalloplasty patient with a prosthesis in place. Note, the Gore-Tex sleeve is sutured firmly to the ischial tuberosity. The cylinders are entirely surrounded with Gore-Tex, and the Gore-Tex sleeves are sutured together in the shaft. (b) In trans-sexual patients, the pump mechanism is placed in the neoscrotum on the side of the dominant hand; in genetic male patients, the pump mechanism is placed on the dominant side in the hemiscrotum. When a reservoir is used, it is placed in the normal position in the space of Retzius.

tuberosity, a space is made for proximal fixation of the prosthesis (Fig. 52.5a). Dilatation of the area from the suprapubic incision to the tuberosity is performed while hugging the inferior pubic ramus. A similar dissection is accomplished on the opposite side for placement of the second cylinder.

In the past, proximal and distal implant migration was common, due to the lack of a tunica and corporal bodies. To prevent this from occurring, neocorpora cavernosa have been created from 14 m vascular stretch Gore-Tex (polytetrafluoroethylene) (W.L. Gore Associates, P.O. Box 1800, Flagstaff, AZ 86002, USA). The implant cylinder is placed inside the sleeve of Gore-Tex, enclosing the distal and proximal ends, while strips or struts of Gore-Tex cover the cylinder shaft (Fig. 52.6). This design provides a secure base for the ends of the cylinder, while creating an open system that prevents seroma formation.

The cylinders and Gore-Tex corpora are inserted into the flap using the Furlow device. Several Gore-Tex sutures are used to secure the proximal end of the neotunica to the ischium and periosteum, creating a firm anchor for the implant. The Gore-Tex corpora are also sutured to the pubic symphysis. The entire neotunica is not needed in the genetic male with proximal corporal remnants. In these cases, a circumferential Gore-Tex strip, located proximal to the struts, is sutured to the remaining tunica. An exit is created for the tubing from

an inflatable cylinder through a slit in the neotunica, and the tubing is secured by tightening the Gore-Tex around it. If a multicomponent inflatable implant is used, the reservoir is placed in the space of Retzius. In the genetic male, the pump is inserted into the scrotum; in the transsexual it is inserted into the neoscrotum (Fig. 52.5b).

Placement of TLS drains (Porex Surgical, 4715 Highway, College Park, GA 30349, USA) for 2 days decreases the incidence of postoperative infections and seromas. An aminoglycoside and broad-spectrum antistaphylococcal antibiotic (usually vancomycin) is given preoperatively and continued for 72 hours. Antibiotic coverage is continued with 14 days of oral cephalosporins.

CONCLUSIONS

Microsurgical creation of a sensible neophallus from a forearm free flap allows for successful insertion of an implant, and represents a major step forward with regard to phallic construction and penile reconstruction. The use of a Gore-Tex neotunica with struts allows for implant fixation and stabilization, and the use of pre- and postoperative antibiotics and TLS drains limits the incidence of seromas and infections. Furthermore, modern techniques of dissecting the forearm fascia and closing the site with a full-thickness skin graft have limited donor site morbidity. At the author's institution, experience with microvascular free transfer phallic construction proceeding to prosthetic implantation exceeds over 100 cases. The success rate in that group is approximately 80%. Ongoing modification of these techniques will continue to improve the success rate, more closely approaching the optimal goals of phallic construction and penile reconstruction.

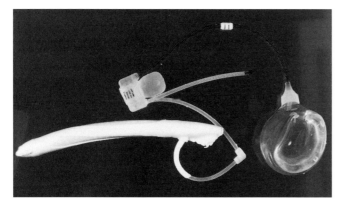

Figure 52.6. Photograph of an AMS-700CX prosthesis with one cylinder to be used. Note, the entire cylinder is housed in a 14 m thin-walled Gore-Tex graft, tailored to fit the cylinder. Large windows are cut in the shaft portion of the Gore-Tex to enhance tissue ingrowth and prevent fluid collections inside the Gore-Tex. In this case, the second cylinder's tubing is plugged with a tubing plug, available from American Medical Systems, Pfizer Hospital Products Group, 11101 1 Bren Road East, Minnetonka, MN 55343, USA.

REFERENCES

1. Filatov V P. Plastike na Kruglom stebl. Vestn Oftalmol 1917; 149: 4–5
2. Granzer H. Weichteilplastik des gesichts bei kieferschussverletzunger. Dtsch Monatsschr Zahnh 1917; 35: 348
3. Gillies H A. The tubed pedicle in plastic surgery. N Y State J Med 1920; 20: 404

4. Bogoraz N A. Plastic restoration of the penis. Soviet Khir 1936; 8: 303–309

5. Horton C E, McCraw J B, Gilbert D A et al. Phallic construction with genital sensation. Presented at International Congress of Plastic Surgery, 1983, Montreal, Canada

6. Gilbert D A, Schlossberg S M, Jordan G H. Ulnar forearm phallic construction and penile reconstruction. Microsurgery 1995; 16: 314–321

7. Chang T S, Huang H Y. Forearm flap in one-stage reconstruction of the penis. Plast Reconstr Surg 1984; 74: 251

8. Semple J L, Boyd J B, Farrow G A, Robinette M A. The 'cricket bat' flap. A one-stage free forearm phalloplasty. Plast Reconstr Surg 1991; 88: 514–519

9. Farrow G A, Boyd J B, Semple J L. Total reconstruction of a penis employing the 'crickp;. et bat flap' single stage forearm free graft. AUA Today 1990; 3

10. Biemer E. Penile construction by the radial arm flap. Clin Plast Surg 1988; 15: 425

11. Louvie M J, Duncan G M, Glasson D W. The ulnar artery forearm flap. Br J Plast Surg 1984; 37: 486

12. Puckett C L, Montie J E. Construction of male genitalia in the transsexual using a tubed groin flap and a hydraulic inflation device. Plast Reconstr Surg 1978; 61: 523–529

13. Jordan G H, Alter G I, Gilbert D A et al. Penile prosthesis implants in total phalloplasty. J Urol 1994; 152: 410–414

14. Alter G J, Gilbert D A, Schlossberg S M, Jordan G H. Prosthetic implantation after phallic construction. Frontiers in microsurgery: urological microsurgery. Microsurgery 1995; 16: 322–324

Chapter 53

Potency-preserving surgery

G. L. Smith and T. J. Christmas

■ INTRODUCTION

Sexual dysfunction is a well-recognized complication of abdominal and pelvic surgery. Radical procedures for pelvic malignancy, vascular operations and transurethral prostatic surgery can all lead to erectile dysfunction (ED). As most of these procedures are performed in elderly patients, there has, in the past, been a tendency to disregard the importance of loss of potency. However, some men now have expectations of unimpaired sexual function well into their seventh or even eighth decades; impotence can, therefore, have a profound effect on their quality of life. Over the past 15 years, major advances in understanding of the mechanisms leading to impotence after surgery have fostered the development of surgical approaches that allow preservation of sexual function. Together with improvements in the treatment of postoperative ED, potency-preserving techniques have significantly improved the outlook for patients undergoing abdominal and pelvic surgery.

■ RADICAL PROSTATECTOMY

As prostatic carcinoma continues to undergo a real increase in incidence,[1] and diagnosis tends to be made at earlier stages than in the past,[2] an increasing number of men are being offered treatment by radical prostatectomy, usually via the retropubic route. Traditionally, impotence was almost inevitable after this procedure; in the early 1980s, however, Patrick Walsh and his colleagues demonstrated that ED after radical prostatectomy was secondary to injury to the branches of the pelvic plexus that innervate the corpora cavernosa.[3] On the basis of their discovery, they proposed alterations in surgical technique to avoid this complication.

Anatomy

Although the importance of the pelvic plexus in erectile processes was well recognized, the branches of the plexus supplying the corpora cavernosa had not been accurately located prior to Walsh's work. Because the cavernous nerves are of small calibre and lie encased within fibrofatty tissue, they are difficult to dissect in the adult cadaver. Walsh and Donker therefore initially traced their course by dissections in male foetuses and stillborn infants.[3] Their findings were later confirmed in adult cadavers.[4]

The pelvic plexus is formed by parasympathetic visceral efferent preganglionic fibres (the nervi erigentes) arising from sacral segments S2, 3 and 4 and postganglionic sympathetic fibres arising from the thoracolumbar region (T11–L2) and travelling to the plexus via the hypogastric nerve. The parasympathetic fibres control erectile function, while the sympathetic fibres play an important role in ejaculation. The plexus is situated retroperitoneally in the sagittal plane on the lateral wall of the rectum, 5–11 cm from the anal verge (Fig. 53.1). It lies lateral and posterior to the seminal vesicle. Because the plexus is surrounded by thick fascia, the seminal vesicle is a useful intra-operative landmark as its tip is opposite the midpoint of the plexus. The cavernous branches travel from the plexus towards the posterolateral aspect of the base of the prostate in association with the capsular arteries and veins of the prostate. As they gradually coalesce towards the gland, the fibres are running in the lateral pelvic fascia outside the prostatic capsule and outside Denonvillier's fascia. This arrangement underlies two important anatomical principles: first, location of the cavernous nerves outside the prostatic capsule and Denonvillier's fascia means that, if cancers are located entirely within the capsule, preservation of potency should be possible without

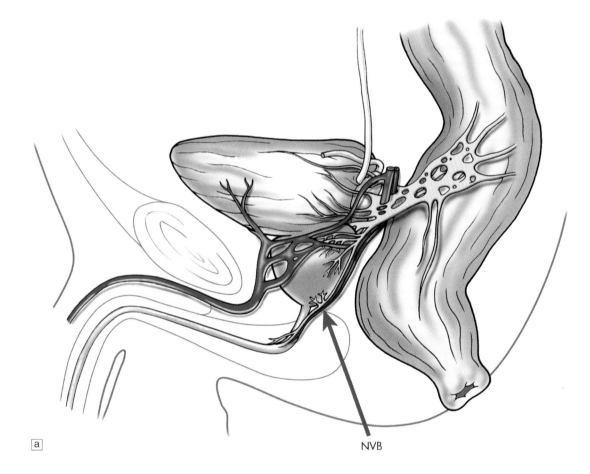

a

NVB

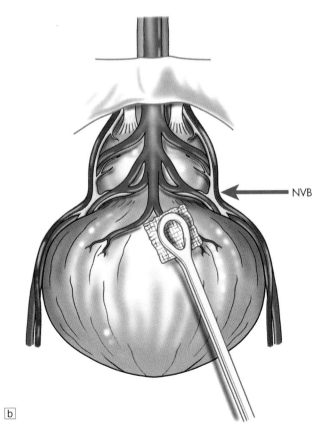

b

NVB

Figure 53.1. Anatomy of the pelvic plexus and cavernous nerves, showing the neurovascular bundles (NVBs) innervating and supplying blood to the corpora cavernosa: (a) lateral view; (b) anteroposterior view at surgery.

compromising excision of organ-confined tumours; secondly, the cavernous nerves are not themselves visible with the naked eye and their association with the capsular vessels of the prostate to constitute the neurovascular bundle therefore provides a macroscopic landmark for these microscopic nerves. From the apex of the prostate, the nerves run posterolateral to the urethra to penetrate the urogenital diaphragm. The fibres then pass behind the dorsal penile artery and nerve before diverging laterally to enter the corpora cavernosa.[3-5]

Surgical technique

Traditional methods of radical prostatectomy have often relied on blind or blunt dissection. Since the importance of the neurovascular bundle in erectile function was not appreciated, no attempts were made to preserve it. Examination of pathological specimens from non-nerve-sparing prostatectomies reveals no evidence that the bundles were actually resected;[6] instead, it appears that they were inadvertently damaged. The cavernous nerves are particularly vulnerable at several points during the procedure, including apical dissection and transection of the urethra, separation of the prostate from the rectum and division of the lateral pedicle.[3,5-7] On the basis of his anatomical studies, Walsh described a new method of radical prostatectomy designed to avoid damage to the cavernous nerves in these areas. His single most important innovation was the application of the neural anatomy described above to facilitate accurate intraoperative identification of the neurovascular bundles. This in turn is critically dependent on a second manoeuvre — namely, control of blood loss from the dorsal venous complex and Santorini's plexus, the anatomy of which was also clarified by Walsh and his colleagues.[8]

The nerve-sparing technique involves initial control of bleeding from the dorsal complex followed by transection of the urethra and separation of the prostate from the rectum in the midline. At this point, the neurovascular bundles are identified, allowing the surgeon to determine whether the bundle can be preserved or whether the extent of the tumour mandates excision. If unilateral neurovascular bundle excision is necessary, it may be possible to preserve the contralateral bundle. When this technique is used, all structures can be visualized and a deliberate decision made as to whether they can be preserved or must be sacrificed for disease control.[5]

Results of nerve-sparing radical prostatectomy
Tumour excision

It is clearly important that preservation of potency is not achieved at the expense of cancer control. Findings on whole-mount specimens from standard blunt dissection radical retropubic and perineal prostatectomies have therefore been compared with nerve-sparing prostatectomy specimens to determine the effect of the nerve-sparing modification on histology of the surgical margins. Although perineal prostatectomy tends to remove less periprostatic tissue and skeletal muscle than either of the retropubic techniques, it appears that all of the approaches allow adequate removal of limited prostatic cancer.[6] In one series of 100 nerve-sparing radical prostatectomies, capsular penetration was present in 41% of cases but only seven patients had positive surgical margins, all of whom had extensive extraprostatic disease.[9] In no case was the margin positive only at the site of the nerve-sparing modification. Further studies have also indicated that patients with positive surgical margins tend to have extensive extracapsular disease, often with seminal vesicle or lymph node involvement.[10,11] It is unlikely that surgery of any type will eradicate these tumours completely.[7,10] In one series of 459 patients, three patients were identified with positive margins only at the site of the nerve-sparing modification.[12] Although margin positivity might have been avoided by excision of the neurovascular bundle, the number of affected patients is small. Furthermore, the long-term significance of these involved margins remains unclear. Current wisdom therefore is that the nerve-sparing technique rarely compromises cancer control. Precise identification of the neurovascular bundle with wide excision when necessary may even allow more extensive resection than blunt dissection in selected cases.[5]

Several major centres have reported the results of large series of nerve-sparing radical retropubic prostatectomies since the introduction of the technique (Table 53.1). The best results are reported by the originator of the technique and his associates with overall potency rates of 68% among men potent preoperatively.[13] On the whole, other groups have found potency rates to be somewhat lower (Table 53.1). For example, Geary and colleagues report potency rates of 13.3% for unilateral nerve-sparing procedures and 31.9% for bilateral nerve-sparing.[12] Therefore, although rates of recovery of erectile

Table 53.1. Prevalence of, and risk factors for, erectile dysfunction following radical prostatectomy

Series	Catalona and Basler[14] 1993	Drago et al.[15] 1992	Geary et al.[12] 1995	Leandri et al.[16] 1992	Quinlan et al.[13] 1991
Mean age (years)	64	64	64	68	59
No. of patients evaluated for potency (total no.)	295 (522)	151 (528)	459 (481)	106 (620)	503 (600)
Postoperative potency	Bilateral 63% Unilateral 41%	66% Non 1.1%	Bilateral 31.2% Unilateral 13.3%	Bilateral 71% Non 0%	Bilateral 76% Unilateral 60%
Factors influencing potency	Age Stage	Age Tumour volume	Age Stage No of nerves spared Frequency of intercourse pre-op Incontinence, stricture	No effect of age	Age Stage No of nerves spared

function are better than with non-nerve-sparing techniques, the morbidity in terms of sexual function is still considerable. Various factors affect the likelihood of impotence following radical prostatectomy.

Number of neurovascular bundles spared
The single most important factor in determining preservation of potency is the number of neurovascular bundles injured. Potency rates are reported as 31.9–76% for bilateral nerve-sparing procedures, 13.3–60% for unilateral nerve-sparing procedures and 0–1.1% for non-nerve-sparing procedures.[12,13]

Stage and tumour volume
Stage and tumour size also influence postoperative potency.[12–15] In one series, a tumour volume of less than 3 cm^3 and the absence of lymph node or seminal vesicle involvement were associated with preservation of potency.[12] However, stage determines the extent of surgery required for tumour excision and therefore the number of neurovascular bundles which can be spared; it is not, therefore, an independent predictor of outcome. For example, in one report, only 9% of patients in whom

a bilateral nerve-sparing procedure was possible presented with clinical stage B2 or C disease compared with 51% of those in whom unilateral excision of the neurovascular bundle was required.[13]

Age
Younger patients tend to fare better in terms of postoperative potency than their older counterparts.[12–15] Men less than 50 years of age tolerate unilateral neurovascular bundle excision with potency rates similar to those of bilateral nerve-sparing procedures (90% potency). In older men, however, excision of one neurovascular bundle significantly reduces the likelihood that potency will be retained.[13] The relatively young average age of patients in Walsh's series (see Quinlan et al.[13] in Table 53.1) may partly explain the excellent overall results achieved in this centre.[13]

Preoperative sexual activity
Patients who are sexually active before surgery are more likely to recover their potency postoperatively, even allowing for the higher incidence of sexual activity in younger men.[12]

Although impotence after radical prostatectomy is primarily neurogenic in most cases, the existence of patients who do not respond to intracavernosal papaverine postoperatively suggests that vascular injury can also contribute to ED.[17] This impression is confirmed by penile Doppler ultrasound studies that reveal evidence of arterial insufficiency in 40% of men after radical prostatectomy.[18] The main blood supply to the corpora cavernosa is from the internal pudendal artery, which is not usually ligated during radical prostatectomy. However, it is likely that there are also collateral sources, and it is thought that loss of these collaterals may lead to vasculogenic impotence. Older patients with atherosclerosis of the internal pudendal vessels may be at particular risk. Likely sources of collateral blood supply to the penis include the arterial branches running beneath the anterior capsule of the prostate, which are visible following division of the dorsal complex. These vessels are not amenable to preservation during radical prostatectomy.[19] There has also been a great deal of interest in the effect of damage to accessory branches to the internal pudendal artery that can arise from the obturator and inferior and superior vesical arteries. One cadaveric study has suggested that accessory arteries are present in 70% of patients.[20] At radical prostatectomy, however, it appears that accessory arteries amenable to preservation are present in only 4% of patients and preservation has no effect on potency rates.[19]

It is also important to recognize that, although most impotence after radical prostatectomy has an organic basis, anxiety is common in men receiving treatment for prostate cancer and psychogenic factors may contribute to ED.[21]

Most patients who regain potency after radical prostatectomy recover within 6–12 months,[12] although improvement can continue for up to 2 years postoperatively. Patients who have undergone excision of one neurovascular bundle lag behind those who have a bilateral nerve-sparing operation.[13]

Although potency rates from large series are impressive, these data should be interpreted with caution. In the literature, potency is generally defined as the ability to achieve an erection sufficient for vaginal penetration and orgasm. Although patients may fit this description, many notice a definite change in the quality of their erections after surgery that can be associated with reduced sexual satisfaction.[12,14] Geary and associates found that less than half of their patients defined as potent on the basis of erections sufficient for vaginal penetration were satisfied with their erections or achieved intercourse at least once a month.[12] Furthermore, potency is only a single aspect of sexual function. Radical prostatectomy may also alter orgasmic sensation, although few studies address this problem. Geary and colleagues noted that only 10% of patients (regardless of potency) reported decreased orgasmic sensation.[12] This is important, in that these patients are likely to respond well to intracavernosal injection therapy, vacuum devices or penile prostheses. In a study from the Netherlands, however, which was based on a semi-structured interview and a self-administered questionnaire, 80% of men experienced weakened orgasmic sensation after surgery. Moreover, 64% suffered involuntary loss of urine at orgasm, although all but one were completely continent at other times; this caused half of these men to avoid sexual contact. Diminished libido was also common.[22] The pathophysiology of these changes in orgasmic sensation is poorly understood but may relate to the unavoidable excision of small nerve fibres surrounding the prostate and seminal vesicles. These statistics illustrate two important principles: first, preservation of erections adequate for penetration does not in itself guarantee satisfactory sexual performance in all patients; secondly, it is becoming clear that, when patients are asked in person about their sexual function, satisfaction rates tend to be lower than those reported by clinicians.[12,23] Allowing for these factors, it is probably unrealistic to offer the average prostate cancer patient a greater than 50% chance of retaining satisfactory sexual function after radical prostatectomy.

■ TRANSURETHRAL PROSTATIC SURGERY

ED is less common following transurethral prostatic surgery but nevertheless affects up to 16% of men undergoing transurethral resection of the prostate (TURP).[24] The aetiology of post-TURP impotence is not absolutely clear; it is, however, likely that the cavernous nerves and arteries are damaged, either by perforation of the prostatic capsule, extravasation of irrigant or injudicious electrocautery of the capsule, particularly at the apices. These events should therefore be avoided if possible. It is also essential to discuss the risk of postoperative impotence with the patient in obtaining informed consent for the procedure.

RADICAL CYSTOPROSTATECTOMY AND URETHRECTOMY

ED is a common complication of radical cystoprostatectomy for bladder carcinoma and the nerve-sparing approach described above can also be applied to this procedure.[25] Proponents of the technique have reported potency rates similar to those achieved following radical prostatectomy (71%).[26]

Understanding of the pelvic neuroanatomy has also been applied to urethrectomy. As described above, the cavernous nerves lie posterolateral to the membranous urethra as they traverse the urogenital diaphragm. Distal to the membranous urethra they diverge laterally into the corpora cavernosa. The nerves are, therefore, most vulnerable during dissection of the membranous urethra. Brendler and colleagues[27] recommend removing only urethral mucosa and smooth muscle during separation of the urethra from the urogenital diaphragm, preserving as much striated muscle as possible; the neurovascular bundles can then be gently pushed away from the posterolateral aspect of the urethra. This technique has allowed preservation of potency in the small number of cases reported.[27]

RECTAL SURGERY

ED is a well-recognized complication of rectal surgery and is usually a result of injury to pelvic autonomic nerves.[28] The incidence after abdominoperineal excision or anterior resection for carcinoma is between 15 and 100%, whereas only 4.7% of men undergoing proctectomy for inflammatory bowel disease are affected. This difference reflects the more extensive resection required when dealing with malignancy: wide excision of perirectal tissues carries a greater risk of neural damage and consequent impotence than techniques such as close rectal dissection and mucosal proctectomy, which can be exploited in benign disease.[29,30] As in prostatectomy and cystectomy, accurate knowledge of the pelvic neuroanatomy is the key to preservation of potency.

The pelvic parasympathetic nerves may be damaged at a number of points during rectal surgery. Excessive

traction on the rectum during posterior mobilization can result in neuropraxia or avulsion of sacral roots 2, 3 and 4.[5] The pelvic plexus itself is most at risk during ligation of the middle haemorrhoidal vessels, to which it is intimately related.[29,30] Neural injury may also occur during perineal dissection of the rectum. After division of the rectourethralis muscle, the neurovascular bundles are visible in association with the lateral prostatic fascia and are vulnerable to trauma by excessive dissection or diathermy anterolateral to the rectum.[5]

As stated, ED following rectal surgery is usually neurogenic in origin. However, ligation of the anterior division or distal branches of the internal iliac artery is sometimes necessary. As a result, patients occasionally develop vasculogenic impotence, particularly if both internal pudendal arteries are ligated.[5]

VASCULAR SURGERY

ED complicates between 30 and 80% of aorto-iliac operations.[31–33] Since pre-existing erectile problems due to atherosclerotic arterial disease or diabetes are also common in this population, sexual dysfunction is a major concern for some patients.[34] The pelvic plexus and cavernous nerves are not at risk during dissection around the bifurcation of the aorta and iliac vessels. The internal iliac artery, however, is commonly occluded during these procedures, leading to a reduction in pelvic visceral blood flow and consequent vasculogenic ED.[35,36] Although restoration of adequate blood flow to the lower limbs or safe resection of aneurysmal disease are the primary aims in aorto-iliac surgery, careful technique can allow preservation of potency in men with normal preoperative sexual function. Internal iliac ligation or embolization of atherosclerotic debris and thrombus into this vessel during flushing manoeuvres should be avoided, if possible.

It is also worth remembering that a number of patients with pre-existing vasculogenic impotence do regain erectile function following aorto-iliac reconstruction.[34,36,37] In one series, for example, sexual function was regained in 30% of patients with preoperative impotence and no normal patients were rendered impotent.[37]

TREATMENT

Because postoperative ED is usually neurogenic in origin, most patients respond well to standard treatments.

Intracavernosal injections and vacuum devices are the most popular modalities, although penile prostheses have also been widely used in selected patients.

It has recently been suggested that early treatment with intracavernosal prostaglandin E1 (PGE1) injections, starting 1 month after surgery, results in an improved potency rate after radical prostatectomy.[38] Although these data are preliminary, it is thought that the use of PGE1 maintains cavernous oxygenation and therefore avoids hypoxia-induced damage to erectile tissue.

One possibility for treatment in the future is intra-operative reconstruction of damaged cavernous nerves using an interposition nerve graft. The genitofemoral nerve has been successfully used in this context to restore erectile function in rats following surgical damage to the neurovascular bundle.[39]

■ CONCLUSIONS

Recent advances in the understanding of pelvic autonomic neuroanatomy have led directly to the development of potency preserving surgical techniques. These new approaches have had a major impact on surgical practice, particularly in urology. As a result, it is now possible to preserve potency in many patients who are undergoing abdominal and pelvic surgery, without compromising disease control.

■ REFERENCES

1. Carter H B, Coffey D S. The prostate: an increasing medical problem. Prostate 1990; 16: 39–48
2. Ohori M, Wheeler T M, Dunn J K et al. Pathologic features and prognosis of prostate cancers detectable with current diagnostic tests. J Urol 1994; 151(suppl): 451A (894) abstr
3. Walsh P C, Donker P J. Impotence following radical prostatectomy: insight into etiology and prevention. J Urol 1982; 128: 492–497
4. Lepor H, Gregerman M, Crosby R et al. Precise localization of the autonomic nerves from the pelvic plexus to the corpora cavernosa: a detailed anatomical study of the adult male pelvis. J Urol 1985; 133: 207–212
5. Walsh P C. Radical pelvic surgery with preservation of sexual function. Ann Surg 1988; 208: 391–400
6. Walsh P C, Lepor H, Egglestone J C. Radical prostatectomy with preservation of sexual function: anatomical and pathological considerations. Prostate 1983; 4: 473–485

7. Walsh P C, Epstein J I, Lowe F. Potency following radical prostatectomy with wide unilateral excision of the neurovascular bundle. J Urol 1987; 138: 823–827
8. Reiner W G, Walsh P C. An anatomical approach to the surgical management of the dorsal vein and Santorini's plexus during radical retropubic surgery. J Urol 1979; 121: 198–200
9. Egglestone J C, Walsh P C. Radical prostatectomy with preservation of sexual function: pathological findings in the first 100 cases. J Urol 1985; 134: 1146–1148
10. Catalona W J, Dresner S M. Nerve-sparing radical prostatectomy: extraprostatic tumour extension and preservation of erectile function. J Urol 1985; 134: 1149–1151
11. Wahle S M, Reznicek M J, Fallon B et al. Incidence of surgical margin involvement with various forms of radical prostatectomies. Urology 1990; 36: 23–26
12. Geary E S, Dendinger T E, Freiha F S, Stamey T A. Nerve sparing radical prostatectomy: a different view. J Urol 1995; 154: 145–149
13. Quinlan D M, Epstein J I, Carter B S, Walsh P C. Sexual function following radical prostatectomy: influence of preservation of neurovascular bundles. J Urol 1991; 145: 998–1002
14. Catalona W J, Basler J W. Return of erections and urinary continence following nerve sparing radical retropubic prostatectomy. J Urol 1993; 150: 905–907
15. Drago J R, Badalement R A, York J P et al. Radical prostatectomy: OSU and affiliated hospitals' experience 1985–1989. Urology 1992; 39: 44–47
16. Leandri P, Rossignol G, Gautier J R, Ramon J. Radical retropubic prostatectomy: morbidity and quality of life with 620 consecutive cases. J Urol 1992; 147: 883–887
17. Bahnson R R, Catalona W J. Papaverine testing of patients following nerve sparing radical prostatectomy. J Urol 1988; 139: 773–774
18. Aboseif S, Shinohara K, Breza J et al. Role of penile vascular injury in erectile dysfunction after radical prostatectomy. Br J Urol 1994; 73: 75–82
19. Polascik T J, Walsh P C. Radical retropubic prostatectomy: the influence of accessory pudendal arteries on the recovery of sexual function. J Urol 1995: 153: 150–152
20. Breza J, Aboseif S R, Orvis B R et al. Detailed anatomy of penile neurovascular structures: surgical significance. J Urol 1989; 141: 437–443
21. Schover L R. Sexual rehabilitation after treatment for prostate cancer. Cancer 1993; 71: 1024–1030
22. Koeman M, van Driel M F, Schultz W C, Mensink H J. Orgasm after radical prostatectomy. Br J Urol 1996; 77: 861–864
23. Fowler F J Jr, Barry M J, Lu-Yao G et al. Patient-reported complications and follow-up treatment after radical prostatectomy. The national Medicare experience: 1988–1990 (updated June 1993). Urology 1993; 42: 622–629
24. Roehrborn C G. Standard surgical interventions: TUIP/TURP/OPSU. In: Kirby R, McConnell J, Fitzpatrick J, Roehrborn C, Boyle P (eds) Textbook of benign prostatic hyperplasia. Oxford: Isis Medical Media, 1996: 341–378

25. Schlegel P N, Walsh P C. Neuroanatomical approach to radical cystectomy with preservation of sexual function. J Urol 1987; 138: 1402–1406

26. Marshall F F, Mostwin J L, Radebaugh L C et al. Ileocolic neobladder post-cystectomy: continence and potency. J Urol 1991; 145: 502–504

27. Brendler C B, Schlegel P N, Walsh P C. Urethrectomy with preservation of potency. J Urol 1990; 144: 270–273

28. Neal D E. The effects on pelvic visceral function of anal sphincter ablating and anal sphincter preserving operations for cancer of the lower part of the rectum and for benign colo-rectal disease. Ann R Coll Surg Engl 1984; 66: 7–13

29. Bauer J J, Gelernt I M, Salky B, Kreel I. Sexual dysfunction following proctocolectomy for benign disease of the colon and rectum. Ann Surg 1983; 197: 363–367

30. Santangelo M L, Romano G, Sassaroli C. Sexual function after resection for rectal cancer. Am J Surg 1987; 154: 502–504

31. May A G, De Weese J A, Rob C G. Changes in sexual function following operation on the abdominal aorta. Surgery 1969; 65: 41–47

32. Sabri S, Cotton L T. Sexual function following aorto-iliac reconstruction. Lancet 1971; 2: 1218–1219

33. Weinstein M H, Machleder H I. Sexual function after aorto-iliac surgery. Ann Surg 1975; 181: 787–790

34. Schwartz T H, Flanigan D P. Repair of abdominal aortic aneurysms in patients with renal, iliac, or distal arterial occlusive disease. Surg Clinic North Am 1989; 69: 845–857

35. Queral L A, Whitehouse W M, Flinn W R et al. Pelvic haemodynamics after aortoiliac reconstruction. Surgery 1979; 86: 799–809

36. Metz P, Frimodt-Moller C, Mathiesen F R. Erectile function before and after reconstructive arterial surgery in men with occlusive arterial leg disease. Scand J Thor Cardiovasc Surg 1983; 17: 45–50

37. Flanigan D P, Schuler J J, Keifer T et al. Elimination of iatrogenic impotence and improvement of sexual function after aorto-iliac revascularization. Arch Surg 1982; 117: 544–550

38. Montorsi F, Guazzoni G, Barbieri L et al. Recovery of spontaneous erectile function after nerve sparing radical prostatectomy with and without early intracavernous injections of prostaglandin E1: results of a prospective randomized trial. J Urol 1996; 155 (suppl): 468A no. 628

39. Quinlan D M, Nelson R J, Walsh P C. Cavernous nerve grafts restore erectile function in denervated rats. J Urol 1991; 145: 380–383

40. Kirby R S, Christmas T J, Brawer M. Prostate cancer. London: Mosby, 1996: 7

Chapter 54

Erectile dysfunction induced by pelvic, perineal and penile injuries

C. G. Stief, J. Hagemann, A. Chavan, T. Pohlemann, R. Raab and U. Jonas

■ INTRODUCTION

By definition, complex pelvic trauma includes fractures of the bony pelvis and additional soft tissue, organ, vascular and/or neural damage. The incidence of urological co-morbidity in complex pelvic trauma is rather high, with 15–25% bladder injury and a similar percentage of urethral injuries.[1–6] The close collaboration of trauma and urological surgeons is mandatory, not only in the acute management of these severely endangered patients but also in their long-term follow-up, where a significant percentage are likely to suffer from chronic erectile dysfunction (ED).[1–6]

Similarly, a larger number of patients undergoing extensive pelvic surgery for oncological indications are at risk of losing their erectile capacity. Thus, up to 100% of patients may develop ED after radical cystectomy for bladder cancer or abdominoperineal extirpation of the rectum for rectal carcinomas.[7,8]

Acute or chronic perineal trauma has been reported to induce both priapism and ED.[1–6,9,10] Penile trauma may also lead to priapism;[9,10] however, in the overwhelming majority of cases, direct penile trauma results in rupture of the tunica albuginea ('penile fracture'), representing a urological emergency that necessitates immediate surgical repair in most cases.[11,12]

■ DIAGNOSTIC WORK-UP

Complex pelvic fractures, extensive radical surgery and perineal or penile trauma not only may damage the organic erectogenic axis but also may cause significant psychogenic co-aetiology of ED.[13] At the authors' institution, therefore, patients are evaluated in close cooperation with the Department of Psychological Medicine. This specific psychogenic evaluation is especially advisable in these patients, since the methods used in modern psychology allow for a subdifferentiation of psychogenic factors, thus rendering treatment options more effective as a result of a better patient selection.[13]

All patients attending the authors' impotence clinic undergo a comprehensive assessment regarding the aetiology of their ED: this includes case history, physical examination, routine haematological tests (including testosterone assay), sexual case history (taken by a psychiatrist),[13] corpus cavernosum electromyography (CC-EMG),[14,15] standardized pharmacotesting[16] and colour coded duplex Doppler ultrasonography of the penile arteries.[17,18]

CC-EMG assessment is conducted according to the guidelines drawn up at the International Consensus Conferences.[19,20] After a resting period of 20 minutes, cavernous electric activity is recorded using two needle electrodes for 30 minutes. The recording is then evaluated by two urologists as well as by a computer-based expert system. Colour-coded duplex Doppler ultrasonography is done using a 10–5 MHz scanner (Ultramark 3 HDI) after intracavernous injection of 5 µg prostaglandin E1 (PGE1) to reduce the risk of prolonged erections, which may occur particularly in patients with ED after pelvic trauma. For arterial evaluation, peak systolic (flow) velocity (PSV) is measured during maximal tumescence after PGE1. As the cavernous arteries are crucial for the erectile mechanism, the PSV of the cavernous arteries determines the arterial status.

When indicated, patients are submitted to further examinations such as cavernosometry and cavernosography, penile angiography or somatomotor and/or autonomic neurological examination.[21]

ERECTILE DYSFUNCTION AFTER COMPLEX PELVIC TRAUMA

The intimate relationship of the bony and visceral pelvic structures and the arteries and nerves supplying the penis is often responsible for their possible involvement in the aetiology of post-traumatic ED (Fig. 54.1). To elucidate demographic data on post-traumatic ED, the authors have undertaken an extensive survey of consecutive patients undergoing complex pelvic fractures. Of 1722 cases of pelvic fracture seen in ten collaborating trauma centres from 1991 to 1993, male patients who had suffered the trauma in 1991 and 1992 were evaluated 2 years after their accident. ED was reported in 11.6% (type A, 11.4%; type B, 8.1%; type C, 20.5%) (Fig. 54.2). Of these, 31 underwent a comprehensive assessment at the authors' centre and 21 normal men with normal erectile function, undergoing the same tests, served as controls. The study was approved by the University Ethical Committee.

No significant abnormalities were detected on physical or laboratory examination. In colour duplex, PSV values were 41.6 ± 12.6 cm/s after PGE1 (Fig. 54.3) and 29.5 ± 17.2 cm/s after linsidomine (SIN-1) injection (significantly above normal values). Four of these patients also underwent selective penile arteriography: in all four the arteriogram showed extensive vascular lesions in the area of the pelvic floor, with complete obliteration without obvious collaterals (Fig. 54.4), similar to observations made by other authors[22,23] and suggesting a high percentage of arterial injury in patients after pelvic fracture. However, duplex sonography of these patients showed supranormal values of the cavernous and dorsal penile arteries, indicating an adequate peripheral cavernous blood supply.

In the evaluation of the autonomic nervous cavernous supply, the CC-EMG showed normal results in two and abnormal in five patients (Fig. 54.5); the remaining had normal as well as abnormal findings (considered as abnormal regarding the clinical interpretation). These observations of a high incidence of autonomic neurogenic lesions as aetiological factors of post-traumatic ED are in accordance with the findings of post-traumatic

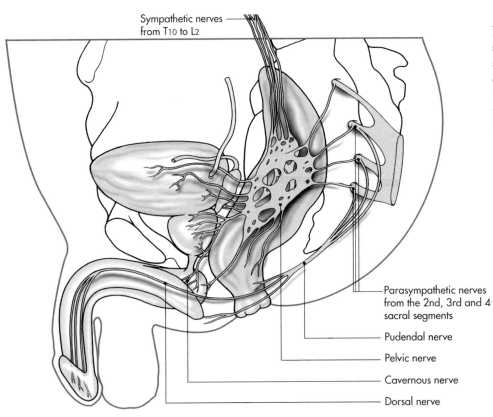

Sympathetic nerves
from T10 to L2

Parasympathetic nerves
from the 2nd, 3rd and 4
sacral segments

Pudendal nerve

Pelvic nerve

Cavernous nerve

Dorsal nerve

Figure 54.1. The nervous supply to the cavernous bodies, arising from the thoracolumbar sympathetic centre (T11–L2) and the sacral parasympathetic centre (S2–4).

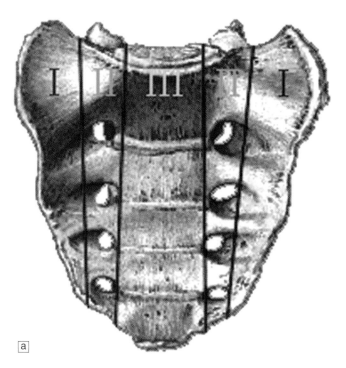

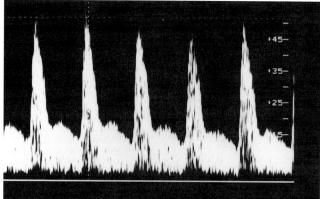

Figure 54.3. Colour-coded duplex Doppler evaluation after 5 μg PGE1 showed a significantly increased peak flow velocity of the cavernous artery in men with ED after pelvic fracture (here 51.2 cm/s) compared with that in normal men (mean 28.7 ± 4 cm/s).

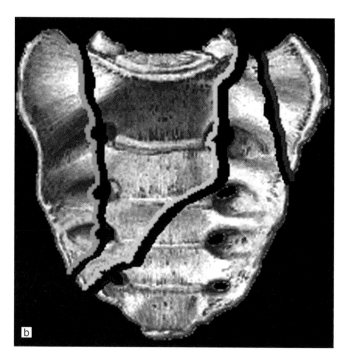

Figure 54.2. Classification of sacral fractures according to Denis et al. The incidence of fractures is decreasing from lateral to medial, whereas the rate of neurological injuries is increasing from lateral to medial. In a study on 377 patients, Pohlemann et al. showed that the grade of instability is the primary predictor for neurological injuries (below 10% after TILE B-type fractures in all regions compared with 33–64% after C-type injuries) and the fracture pattern is only a secondary parameter. (a) Examples of the different fracture lines and their classification; (b) examples of type A, B and C fractures.

micturition disorders. Similarly, a high percentage of neurogenic bladder dysfunctions are detected in urodynamic studies.

In pharmacotesting, patients developed almost full (E4) to full sustained erections (E5) after injection of 5 μg PGE1 or 1 mg SIN-1. These findings indicate that cavernous smooth muscle function is intact, as would be expected in these (mostly) young patients.

These results strongly suggest that the chief cause of ED after (complex) pelvic trauma is damage to the autonomic cavernous supply. These neural lesions may be caused either by fracture of the sacrum, by extensive pelvic haematoma or by disruption at the level of the pelvic floor. Although extensive arterial lesions in the pudendal axis are also found in a large proportion of these patients, in the main these do not appear to cause a significant reduction in cavernous blood supply (at least not after intracavernous application of vasoactive drugs). The reasons for these surprising findings are not yet known, but penile accessory arteries, known to occur in up to 70% of subjects, certainly play an important role. However, in the light of these data, surgical therapeutic options such as penile revascularization procedures should be discussed very carefully with the patients, since the failure rate is likely to be excessively high when significant neurogenic lesions are present. If such neurological lesions are present, local measures such as intracavernous injections,[24,25] intra-urethral applications,[26] vacuum devices[27] or penile prosthesis implantation[28] should be recommended. The potential therapeutic

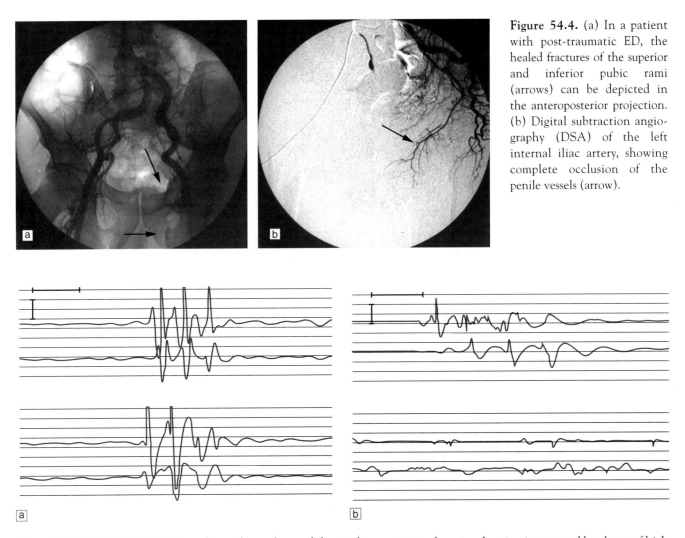

Figure 54.4. (a) In a patient with post-traumatic ED, the healed fractures of the superior and inferior pubic rami (arrows) can be depicted in the anteroposterior projection. (b) Digital subtraction angiography (DSA) of the left internal iliac artery, showing complete occlusion of the penile vessels (arrow).

Figure 54.5. (a) CC-EMG of a normal man shows phases of electrical zero activity of varying duration interrupted by phases of high electrical activity ('potentials'); these are synchronous in both cavernous bodies and comparable to findings in other normal men as well as to electrical activity of other smooth muscle organs. (b) CC-EMG of a patient with ED after pelvic trauma shows no distinct phases of electrical zero activity and no phases of high, synchronous electric activity of distinct shape ('potentials'); only irregular and asynchronous activity was recorded. In both (a) and (b), the horizontal bar represents 5s and the vertical bar represents 100 μV.

benefit of an orally active phosphodiesterase inhibitor (sildenafil)[29] or apomorphine[30] cannot be predicted in these patients as no data are currently available. Surgical revascularization should be reserved for isolated cases of arterial lesions.[31,32]

ERECTILE DYSFUNCTION AFTER PERINEAL TRAUMA

There are reports in the literature that acute perineal trauma in men may cause priapism.[10] Refined diagnostic procedures, such as colour-coded duplex sonography and selective penile arteriography, have revealed traumatic aneurysms or traumatic arteriovenous fistulae as aetiological factors in these patients.[10]

Consequently, treatment of these cases of high-flow priapism involves the (temporary) obstruction of the aneurysm or fistula concerned. Superselective embolization of such traumatic tissue damage has been used successfully.[9,10] In the authors' experience with non-traumatic high-flow priapism, superselective embolization with gelfoam or degradable starch microspheres did not result in adequate detumescence; the same holds true for only unilateral coil-embolization of the penile artery. Only a patient who underwent bilateral micro-coil embolization of the penile arteries responded immediately with detumescence; this patient

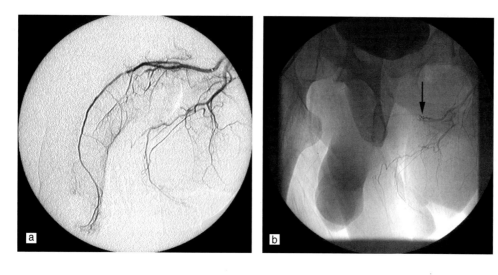

Figure 54.6. (a) DSA of a young patient with a high-flow priapism showed widened penile vessels; (b) superselective embolization of the penile artery (arrow) resulted in immediate detumescence.

recovered his erectile function after 2 months (Fig. 54.6). Although the coils used by the authors are non-absorbable, it is known that collateral supply of distal vessels occurs, thus allowing spontaneous erections to be regained (provided that the cavernous tissue has not undergone irreversible degeneration as a result of the long-lasting ischaemia caused by the priapism before the embolization). In contrast to the authors' experience, however, other authors have reported satisfactory long-term results with the application of absorbable materials.[10]

Chronic perineal trauma, such as that caused by prolonged bicycle riding, has been reported to cause ED. The authors have also seen two professional cyclists who presented with chronic ED: their workup revealed significant neurogenic and arteriogenic damage.

■ PENILE FRACTURE

Penile fracture describes traumatic rupture of the tunica albuginea followed by subsequent subcutaneous haematoma of various degrees. Although the cavernous bodies can sustain suprasystolic pressures, and intracavernous pressures of over 1000 mmH$_2$O can be applied before the tunica albuginea ruptures,[11,12] penile fractures constitute a fairly frequent urological emergency. In most cases, the aetiology remains obscure with the patients reporting 'normal' sexual activity before the rupture. Another fairly constant finding in the case history of patients with penile fractures is the perception of a typical 'cracking' sound, followed by detumescence and rapid development of a haematoma.

The management of penile fracture should be in accordance with the clinical (and possibly diagnostic) findings. In many cases, high-resolution ultrasound can aid the diagnosis and subsequent management, since tunical defects as well as the extent of the haematoma and the cavernous (and possibly spongy) lesions can be precisely determined. The following measures are recommended:

1. In the case of a small and stable haematoma less than 2 cm in diameter, without significant depth and no (or only a minimal) tunical lesion, a conservative approach (such as local application of cold compresses) may be advised, with close supervision of the patient.
2. Larger (and especially increasing) haematomas necessitate formal surgical exploration with evacuation of the haematoma, possibly a débridement and a water-tight closure of the ruptured tunica albuginea.
3. Microscopic or gross haematuria, as well as ventral haematomas, are suggestive of (additional) lesions of the corpus spongiosum. Here, preoperative antibiotics and a retrograde urethrogram are advisable. Owing to the high incidence of urethral stricture formation after conservative management, lesions of the corpus spongiosum should be treated surgically.

In any case, the patient presenting with a penile fracture should be informed about the different treatment modalities and warned that occurrence of ED, although rare, is possible even in small lesions, regardless of the mode of management.

■ REFERENCES

1. Carr L K, Webster G D. Genitourinary trauma. Curr Opin Urol 1996; 6: 140–143

2. Cass A S. Urethral injury in the multiple injured patient. J Trauma 1984; 24: 901–905

3. Goldmann S M, Sandler C M, Corriere J N, McGuire E J. Blunt urethral trauma. J Urol 1997; 157: 85–89

4. Pokorny M, Pontes J E, Pierce J M. Urological injuries associated with pelvic trauma. J Urol 1979; 121: 455–457

5. Mee S L, McAninch J W, Federle M P. Computerized tomography in bladder rupture. J Urol 1985; 137: 207–209

6. Sandler C M, Hall T J, Rodriguez M B, Corriere J N. Bladder injury in blunt pelvic trauma. Radiology 1986; 158: 633–638

7. Walsh P C, Donker P J. Impotence following radical prostatectomy: insight into etiology and prevention. J Urol 1982; 128: 492

8. Marshall F F, Mostwin J L, Radebaugh L C et al. Ileocolic neobladder post-cystectomy. J Urol 1991; 145: 502

9. Wear J B, Crummy A B, Munson B O. A new approach to the treatment of priapism. J Urol 1977; 117: 252

10. Witt M A, Goldstein I, Saenz de Tejada I et al. Traumatic laceration of intracavernosal arteries. J Urol 1990; 143:

11. Özen H A, Erkan I, Alkibai T et al. Fracture of the penis and long term results of surgical treatment. Br J Urol 1986; 58: 551–554

12. Anselmo G, Fandella A, Faggiano L et al. Fractures of the penis. Br J Urol 1991; 67: 509

13. Hartmann U. Psychological subtypes of erectile dysfunction: results of statistical analyses and clinical practice. World J Urol 1997; 15: 56

14. Stief C G, Thon W F, Djamilian M et al. SPACE (single potential analysis of cavernous electric activity)—a possible diagnosis of autonomic impotence? World J Urol 1990; 8: 75

15. Gorek M, Stief C G, Hartung C, Jonas U. Computer-assisted interpretation of electromyograms of the corpora cavernosa using fuzzy logic. World J Urol 1997; 15: 65

16. Stief C G, Bähren W, Gall H, Scherb W. Functional evaluation of penile hemodynamics. J Urol 1988; 139: 734

17. Jevtich M J. Non-invasive vascular and neurologic tests in use for evaluation of angiogenic impotence. Int Angiol 1984; 3: 225

18. Lue T F, Hricak H, Schmidt R A, Tanagho E A. Functional evaluation of penile veins by cavernosography in papaverine-induced erection. J Urol 1986; 135: 479

19. Jünemann K P, Bührle C P, Stief C G. Current trends in corpus cavernosum EMG. Conclusions of the 'First International Workshop on Smooth Muscle EMG Recordings/Leiomyogram' April 15 to 17, 1993 in Mannheim, Germany. Int J Impot Res 1993; 5: 105–108

20. Stief C G, Jünemann K P, Kellner B et al. Consensus and progress in corpus cavernosum-EMG (CC-EMG). Second International Workshop on CC-EMG in Hannover/Germany, February 25 and 26, 1994. Int J Impot Res 1994; 6: 177–183

21. Padma-Nathan H, Goldstein I. Evaluation of the impotent patient. Semin Urol 1986; 4: 225

22. Sharlip I D. Penile arteriography in impotence after pelvic trauma. J Urol 1981; 126: 477

23. Levine F J, Greenfield A J, Goldstein I. Arteriographically determined occlusive disease within the hypogastric–cavernous bed in impotent patients following blunt perineal and pelvic trauma. J Urol 1990; 144: 1147

24. Jünemann K P, Aken P. Pharmacotherapy of erectile dysfunction. Int J Impot Res 1989; 1: 71

25. Truss M, Becker A J, Schultheiss D, Jonas U. Intracavernous pharmacotherapy. World J Urol 1997; 15: 71

26. Gesundheit N, Place V. Transurethral alprostadil for treatment of men with chronic erectile dysfunction. Int J Impot Res 1996; 8: 146

27. Lewis R W, Witherington R. External vacuum therapy for erectile dysfunction. World J Urol 1997; 15: 78

28. Montague D K. Penile prosthesis. An overview. Urol Clin North Am 1989; 16: 7

29. Boolell M, Allen M J, Ballard S A et al. Sildenafil: an orally active type 5 cyclic GMP-specific phosphodiesterase inhibitor for the treatment of penile erectile dysfunction. Int J Impot Res 1996; 8: 47

30. Heaton J P, Adams M A, Morales A et al. Apomorphine SL is effective in the treatment of non-organic erectile dysfunction. Int J Impot Res 1996; 8: 115

31. Levine F J, Gasior B L, Goldstein I. Reconstructive arterial surgery for impotence. Semin Intervent Radiol 1989; 6: 220

32. Goldstein I. Penile revascularisation. Urol Clin North Am 1987; 14: 805

Chapter 55

Sexual function in congenital anomalies

C. R. J. Woodhouse

INTRODUCTION

All of the problems that are commonly seen in an andrology clinic may be the result of major congenital genito-urinary anomalies (Table 55.1). Surprisingly, most affected individuals have a rather better sex life than might be expected. Furthermore, the recent advances in the management of male infertility will be of particular benefit to those whose testes are normal but whose ejaculatory function is compromised by their anomaly or its reconstruction.

Gross as some of these abnormalities are, very few commonly cause erectile failure. The main exception is severe myelomeningocoele. General sexual function may be compromised for six possible reasons:

1. The penis may be grossly malformed (e.g. exstrophy and micropenis).
2. The penis may be a little deformed but the patient's perception may so exaggerate the deformity that sexual function is impaired (e.g. hypospadias).
3. Obstructive lesions of the bladder outlet may cause back pressure on the prostate, leading to ejaculatory failure and seminal abnormalities (e.g. posterior urethral valves).
4. Developmental failure may impair hormonal or ejaculatory function (e.g. prune-belly syndrome).
5. Penile innervation may be incomplete (e.g. spina bifida) or destroyed by pelvic surgery.
6. Embarrassment about some aspect of the general abnormalities may prevent the formation of a partnership in which intercourse can take place (e.g. an external urinary diversion).

Whatever the anomaly, it should always be assumed that erectile function and intercourse are desired and possible until proved otherwise. It is astonishing how severe

handicaps can be overcome and how small a penis is necessary for apparently satisfactory intercourse.

EXSTROPHY AND EPISPADIAS

Reconstructive surgery of the basic bladder condition has progressed so much that patients can now live a normal life and, in the last 15 years, can expect to have a normally working bladder. Although it has always been recognized that the penis required reconstruction as well, a good functional result for sexual intercourse was not always achieved. The exstrophy patient now grows up in normal society and has the same sexual and reproductive aspirations as his more normal peers. The author's clinical impression is that their libido is as high as that of other adolescents. It is a matter of priority to reconstruct the genitalia to allow normal intercourse to take place.[1]

In this section the terms 'exstrophy penis', 'exstrophy pelvis', etc., include the same anomalies in epispadiac patients.

Genital anatomy

The anatomy of the exstrophy pelvis and penis is obviously abnormal. The details have been investigated clinically, by cavernosography, computerized tomography (CT) and magnetic resonance imaging (MRI), by experimental models and by dissection.[2-10]

The visible part of the penis (Fig. 55.1) is short, not (as might be thought) because most of the penis is buried in the perineum but because the corpora are short.[3,11] However, the penis is longer if the divarication of the pubic bones is 3 cm or less and it is shorter if the divarication is 4 cm or more. In the past, surgical apposition of the pubic bones was said not to lengthen the visible penis. Some experimental evidence suggests that the visible penis would be longer if the pelvic ring

Table 55.1. General effects of congenital genito-urinary anomalies on male sexual and reproductive function

Organ	Effect	Example
Adrenal	Precocious puberty Oligozoospermia	Congenital adrenal hyperplasia
Kidney	Poor libido Infrequent erections Priapism	Renal failure Dialysis
Bladder	Retrograde ejaculation	Open bladder neck
Prostate	Slow ejaculation Seminal abnormalities	Exstrophy or posterior valves
Urethra	Slow ejaculation	Epispadias Hypospadias
Penis	Erectile deformity Social ostracism	Epispadias Micropenis
Testes	Infertility	Prune-belly syndrome
Spinal cord	Impotence Ejaculatory failure Inheritance	Spina bifida

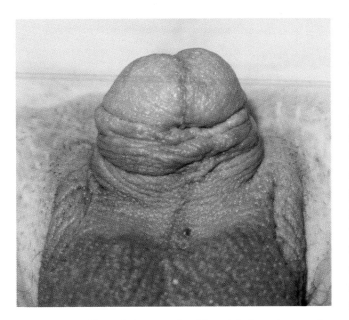

Figure 55.1. Clinical photograph of the adult flaccid exstrophy penis.

were closed. Osteotomies performed in infancy may be more effective in producing a normal penis, at least in childhood.

MRI investigation of the normal and the exstrophy penis has established that, whatever the condition of the pelvic ring, the exstrophy penis is short but broad. The total corporal length was 60% greater in the normals (16.1 cm vs 10.1 cm in exstrophy). Most of this deficiency was in the anterior or exophytic part of the penis (12.3 cm for normals vs 6.9 cm for exstrophy). The posterior penis was much the same length in both (3.9 cm vs 3.2 cm). The corporal diameter was 1.0 cm in normal men and 1.4 cm in men with exstrophy.[11] The abnormalities may be exaggerated by the recession of the suprapubic area (Fig. 55.2), absence of the mons pubis and the normal size of the scrotum.

The prostate is present. In the initial dissection in the neonate it is detached from the penile urethra and

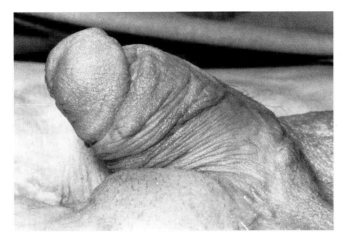

Figure 55.2. Clinical photograph to show the recession of the suprapubic scar commonly seen in exstrophy.

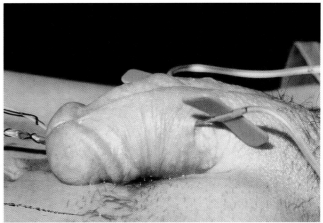

Figure 55.3. Clinical photograph showing an artificial erection with tight dorsal chordee in an exstrophy penis.

remains in its normal relationship to the bladder base. In adult men the prostate is of normal weight for age but lies completely behind the urethra. The verumontanum, which is normally positioned, is a useful landmark for surgery in later life.

The shape of the erect penis depends on the initial reconstruction. In the natural state, the erect epispadiac penis has a tight dorsal chordee (Fig. 55.3). Cavernosography in such cases shows that the site of the maximum curvature is at the point where the corpora emerge from the perineum.[12] Increasing awareness of this problem has modified the reconstruction in infancy, to produce a more normal angle of erection.[9]

The degree of chordee is variable. In some the angle is such that sexual intercourse is possible either in the conventional position or in one that brings the female introitus in more direct apposition to the penis.

A more complex deformity occurs when one or both of the corpora are damaged in the initial surgery so that they fail to fill completely. If one corpus fails to fill on erection it acts as a 'bow-string' on the other and causes lateral deviation in addition to the dorsal chordee (Fig. 55.4).[12]

If both corpora are rudimentary, the visible or exophytic part of the penis is normal except that it is a little higher than usual on the abdomen (Fig. 55.5). On cavernosography, the corpora appear to have no attachment to the pubic rami; erection is very limited and the penis unstable. In one of the author's patients the whole of one corpus and the exophytic part of the other is missing so that there is no visible penis at all.

The evidence suggests that the corpora are of equal size at birth and are damaged at the primary (and

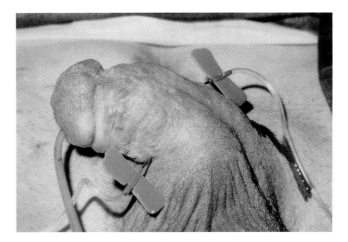

Figure 55.4. Clinical photograph showing an artificial erection with dorsal chordee and deviation to the right.

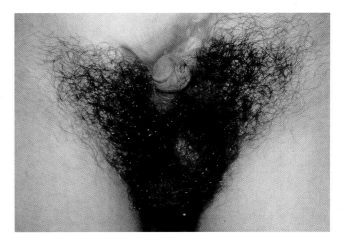

Figure 55.5. Clinical photograph to show a rudimentary exstrophy penis.

revision) reconstructive surgery.[12,13] The distribution of types of erectile deformity currently seen in adult exstrophy patients is shown in Table 55.2.

Awareness of the erectile problems and appropriate reconstruction in infancy may improve the function in adults. Although the techniques reviewed by Snyder[9] have not been in use for long enough to allow adult follow-up, results from the Mayo Clinic suggest that modern techniques of reconstruction do lead to just this situation. A short but normal penis with a normal angle of erection was found in 24 of 44 adults.[14] Perovic et al. have reported that the penis in infants is similar in length to that of normal boys, although slightly different in appearance.[15] Even in adolescents and adults, correction of chordee can be successful and will give a little increase in length.[16]

In adult exstrophy patients at present, the pubic area is nearly always recessed from the uncorrected divarication of the pubic bones. The pubic hair lies on either side of the midline (Fig. 55.6). Many exstrophy patients find the appearance distressing and try to hide it from their partners.

It is most important, either in infancy or in adolescence, to rotate hair bearing flaps of skin and fat to cover the midline defect.

Sexual function

There is no reason, special to exstrophy, why the erections should not be normal. Even where both corpora are rudimentary, penile tumescence occurs. Exstrophy patients presenting with impotence should be investigated in the same manner as other males. The only difference is that there is no cross-circulation between the corpora; therefore, if intracorporal prostaglandin is to be used, each corpus will have to be injected individually.

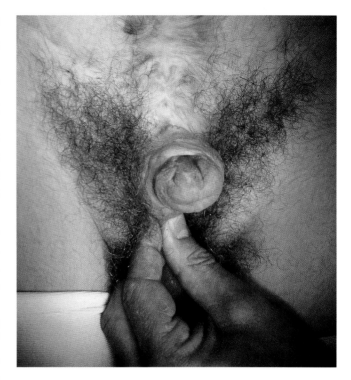

Figure 55.6. Clinical photograph of the distribution of pubic hair.

Orgasm is normal. In an early review of adult patients, all but two of 31 patients ejaculated.[17] In another series, 16 of 25 patients had ejaculation but its quality was not recorded.[14] Silver et al. report that eight of ten men ejaculated normally with a volume of 5 ml.[11] Although poor or absent ejaculation may follow genital reconstruction, complete absence of ejaculation is rare but the emission that does occur may be slow and may continue for several hours after orgasm. Some patients describe a more-or-less continuous urethral discharge of semen-like fluid.

It has been suggested that patients who had early urinary diversion have better ejaculation than those who have been reconstructed (particularly if the reconstruction was unsuccessful). Most authors who have specifically addressed this point have results that appear to support this conclusion. For example, Stein et al. report that all of five patients who had not had reconstruction did have normal ejaculation, whereas 18 of 23 reconstructed patients had only a postorgasmic dribble and the rest had a dry orgasm.[18]

The opposite view is held by the group from Johns Hopkins Hospital in Baltimore: 12 of 16 patients had satisfactory orgasm, although their diversion status was not given. It was suggested that cystectomy might be the

Table 55.2. Distribution of types of erectile deformity in exstrophy and epispadias

Deformity	Percentage
Dorsal chordee	77
Unilateral rudimentary corpus	9
Bilateral rudimentary corpora	14

(From ref. 3 with permission.)

cause of infertility, although supporting figures were not given.[19]

Reviewing the literature as a whole, the author has been unable to support either conclusion. About 75% of patients in both groups have some form of ejaculation. In several papers it is difficult to deduce which patients were diverted and which were not, or to ascertain whether the ejaculation was anything like normal (Table 55.3).

With or without surgical correction, the men appear to have a normal libido. The author's patients report fewer casual sexual partners than would be expected. They appear to form very stable partnerships with normal girls and have normal family life; in Stein's series, 16 of 23 males were cohabiting.[18] Patients reported by Ben-Chaim et al. were said to have random and short-term relationships.[19]

In the author's own series, 33 of 43 patients for whom full information is available have been married or lived with a partner. One patient is known to be homosexual. One epispadiac patient has doubts about his gender identity; he may come to gender reassignment eventually. The remaining patients of all ages do not admit to any sexual contact and for many of them the combination of abnormal genitalia and an external urinary diversion seems to be too overwhelming.[1]

Although complete reconstruction in infancy is desirable, later surgery also produces a satisfactory sexual outcome. Using a variety of techniques, Audry et al. established normal function in seven of 14 adolescents or adults.[20] With the Cantwell–Ransley technique, four of seven adolescents have normal intercourse.[15] Obviously, those who were not having intercourse in these series may yet establish sexual relationships.

Cloacal exstrophy

A case has been made for early gender reassignment for male infants with grossly deficient penis and exstrophy, especially cloacal exstrophy.[14] Cases have been cited where refusal of such advice by the parents has resulted in poorly adjusted adolescents who commit sexual offences.[21] In a series of eight males with cloacal exstrophy, only one achieved successful vaginal intercourse; two were impotent and three required intensive psychiatric counselling.[21] Gender reassignment is particularly recommended if the penis fails to achieve 2 cm of stretched length within 1 month of the administration of 50 mg testosterone i.m.[22]

Male cloacal exstrophy patients can certainly be made into very nice little girls. However, there has been no long-term follow-up of exstrophy patients re-assigned to

Table 55.3. Ejaculation in classical exstrophy patients

First author	Reference	Date	No. of patients	No. with ejaculation	Notes
Hanna	17	1972	31	29	
Mesrobian	14	1986	25	16	All diverted
Audry	20	1991	12	6	
Stein	18	1994	23	18	Reconstructed
			5	5	Diverted
Feitz	70	1994	10	4	All diverted
Mitchell	23	1996	2	2	
Ben-Chaim	19	1996	16	13	
Silver	11	1996	10	8	Reconstructed

Table 55.4. Semen analysis and fertility in male exstrophy and epispadias patients: results of nine series[*]

Semen	Exstrophy		Epispadias	
	Recons.	Diverted	Recons.	Diverted
Azoospermia		3[†]		
	12	17		
Poor		1[†]	4[†]	
Good	3	11	3	6
Paternity		2[†]		
	5	12		

[*]Most of these series give little, if any, information regarding the total number of patients in the review.
[†]Status not defined.

the female gender and it is possible that they will make equally unhappy female adolescents. The trend now is to rear in the genetic sex and to reconstruct the male genitalia as fully as possible.[23]

Fertility

Although the genital tract from the testes to the verumontanum is normal, there is a high incidence of poor or absent sperm. Of the author's own patients and of those reported in the literature, about half the men who wish to do so are able to father children (Table 55.4).

The main causes of infertility appear to be early genital reconstruction and repeated prostatic and bladder infections. Thus, ironically, the boys who underwent early urinary diversion have the best record for fertility.[18,24] In a series in which 70% of the patients were reconstructed, only 12% were fertile, although this might have been due to a mean age of only 24 years.[19]

■ THE SMALL PENIS

It is generally agreed that a small penis must have normal anatomy but be more than 2 or 2.5 standard deviations below the normal stretched length. Thus, it ranges from 1.75 to 2.7 cm at birth.[25,26] Growth curves have been constructed from which the normal penile lengths can be derived at any age.[27]

The andrologist may be asked to see a neonate or adult with a small penis for whom endocrine treatment is impossible or has failed. The questions that then arise are what use will the present organ be, can it be made any bigger and, in an extreme case, should a gender reassignment be made?

Sexual function with a small penis

There is little in the literature on the sexual consequences of a small penis. In some cases this may be because the penile anomaly is a part of a broader syndrome that contributes to sexual failure. Aside from this, the literature that does exist may be contradictory.

Reilly[28] has investigated the male role in 20 patients who had a small penis from a variety of causes (8 pre- and 12 post-pubertal). Patients were included only if their penis, at the time of review, conformed to the standard definition of 'micropenis', even though some had previously had hypospadias. In spite of the very short length of penile shaft, sexual function was satisfactory (Fig. 55.7).

The most surprising feature of these patients was the firmness with which they were established in the male role and the success that they had in sexual relationships. In the adult group all had heterosexual interests, erections and orgasms; 11 of 12 had ejaculates.

Three-quarters had had sexual intercourse. The mean age of sexual debut was 16.4 years (range 13.5–20 years)

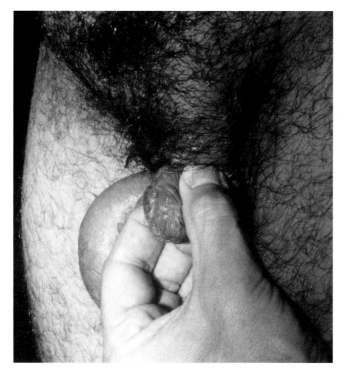

Figure 55.7. Clinical photograph of an adult micropenis.

while the normal is 16.2. All claimed to find intercourse enjoyable, although their partner's views were unknown. One patient had a wife and a mistress. The partnerships were stable and long lasting, a situation that some patients attributed to the extra attention that had to be paid to intercourse because of the short penis. Although vaginal penetration was usual, there was an experimental attitude to positions and methods. One patient was the father of a child.[28]

There is little supportive evidence for these data from other units. However, the pattern is sufficiently consistent that it seems safe to conclude that even the possession of the very small penis illustrated in Figure 55.7 is compatible with a normal male role, especially with proper parental support.

At first sight, the patients reviewed by Money and co-workers were less successful. Their main problem was in voiding and changing in public, which was also noted in some of Reilly's patients. From the sexual point of view they functioned reasonably. Some had problems with gender identity and some were homosexual but, in strictly physical terms, the erectile system did work.[29]

Medical treatment of the small penis
It cannot be emphasized too strongly that a small penis may be the only presenting sign of a specific endocrine anomaly.[30] Correct treatment may restore the child and his penis to normality.

There remains a group of boys with a small penis who are either of undefined diagnosis or who lack definitive treatment.

The role of hormone treatment is uncertain. If there is good volume of erectile tissue and no androgen insensitivity, the penis may grow with testosterone or human chorionic gonadotrophin (HCG) treatment. There is no doubt that early treatment has a role in defining responsiveness of the genitalia to testosterone. The resulting growth encourages the parents to persevere with upbringing in the male gender. From the young boy's point of view, the improved growth usually brings the penis into the normal range of size.

Because of the risk of testosterone causing premature epiphyseal fusion, the use of dihydrotestosterone (DHT) has been explored. When applied as a cream to the penis, the effects appear to be confined to the penis and prostate, both of which show rapid growth. In a series of 22 children, all demonstrated penile growth with a mean increase of length of 53% in the first month and a further 18% in the second month. The group included four boys who had failed to respond to testosterone.[31]

The late results of such treatment are much less clear. The follow-up in most series is short. It would seem from the author's own patients that the position on the penile growth curve is not maintained. Treatment probably achieves only that which puberty would achieve anyway and the adult ends up with a small penis. Indeed, in the experimental rat, early treatment produces the shortest penis in adults, whereas treatment delayed to puberty or adolescence leads to normal adult length.[32] Late treatment of a 12- and a 17-year-old boy have been reported but the responses were poor.[33] In view of the response of testosterone failures to DHT, a trial in adults might be worth while.

Surgical treatment of the small penis
Small penis is not a condition that lends itself to surgical correction. No operation has yet been devised to make the corpora of the truly small penis longer. Theoretically, the techniques used for female-to-male gender reassignment could be used. However, they would certainly not appeal for the infant as the phallus created would not grow; they seem to be also of limited appeal for the adult, who will have his small but sexually sensitive penis replaced by a large but insensitive and inert object.

The male with a small penis can have satisfactory sexual function and surgery should be avoided. Patients may need help to come to terms with the abnormality if they have been badly counselled in childhood.

HYPOSPADIAS

There are few major subjects in paediatric urology that are as difficult to review as the adult sexual consequences of hypospadias. For several decades, large numbers of hypospadias repairs have been done by small numbers of specialist surgeons. Most reviews seem to begin with a section on the shortcomings of earlier surgical methods; there then follows a description of the new method. It is disappointing to find that new methods continue to be described, suggesting that the predecessor must have been found wanting. Well-established techniques are subject to modification, often by the surgeon who first described them.[34,35] There has even been a spirited correspondence in a leading journal on the relative merits of the two-stage repair over the single-stage repair that is supposed to have replaced it.[36]

From all of these data it is difficult to ascertain the long-term results, let alone the sexual consequences. Except in the most severely affected hypospadias cripples, there seems to be no vascular or neurological reason why erections and orgasm should not be normal. In perineal hypospadias, absence of the bulbospongiosus muscle may weaken ejaculation. The remaining question, then, is whether there are hormonal or psychological consequences of hypospadias that may alter sexuality.

It is interesting to note that there does not seem to be a disproportionate number of hypospadiac patients in sexual therapy clinics. For example, in a series of 384 patients assessed for the contribution of various factors to impotence, hypospadias was not noted, although poor self-image (1.1% of cases) and gender identity (0.4%) were found.[37]

Most of the patients who are now adults are likely to have been operated on with techniques that have largely been abandoned, relatively late in childhood and in two or more stages. If sexual function in adult life is dependent on a good cosmetic result, it might be assumed that there will be better results from the current single-stage repairs performed in infancy.

In assessing overall sexual function in hypospadias, a number of factors must be considered, as follows:

1. The original severity of the hypospadias.
2. The success of the surgical repair, though probably not the type of repair.
3. Age at completion of surgery.
4. Whether the observed results are based on all patients in a series or only on those who responded to a specific recall for review.
5. The coincidence of other conditions such as sexual ambiguity or testicular anomalies.

Penetrative intercourse

All series record that most men claim to have normal intercourse. It is not always possible to decipher a precise figure from the published data, or to discover the quality or frequency thereof. Figures range from 77% to 90%. The mean age of sexual debut is given as 16.9 years in Sweden (normal 16.6) and as 17.3 or 18.0 in the UK.[38–41]

Success of the repair

The cosmetic success appears to depend very much on the interests of the assessor. Surgeons reviewing their own cases give impressive results, whereas independent observers paint a less good picture.[40,42] It is interesting to find, however, that in all series intercourse seems to be prevented only by fairly gross surgical failure; the commonest cause is pain from persistent chordee.[39,41,42]

It has been suggested that a delayed cure gives a less satisfactory sexual result. However, Johanson and Avellan describe a group of boys whose 'curative' repair was delayed beyond the age of 12 years. Although the sexual results in this group were less good than in those having an earlier 'cure', 50% had their sexual debut before their final surgery.[40]

Degree of original hypospadias

The worse the original problem, the worse the long-term results. In the case of sexual function this is a fairly universal observation. A poor surgical result is commoner with severe degrees of hypospadias, which leads to sexual difficulties.[39,43]

Both penile hypoplasia and sexual ambiguity are associated with severe hypospadias. The more proximal the original meatus, the shorter the erect length of the adult penis, with coronal cases being normal and penoscrotal cases being about one-third shorter than normal.[39] Both of these problems are associated with poor sexual function.[39,42,43] Conversely, in patients with the meatus on or distal to the shaft, 66% of young males are married even though many have residual penile problems.[44]

In a review of 18 patients (aged 17.6–35.6 years) who had sexual ambiguity at birth with gross hypospadias, Miller and co-workers found poor sexual function. Only 11 had had heterosexual intercourse, of whom four had a regular partner. Surprisingly, the age of sexual debut was normal at 17.0 years.[45]

Ejaculation

The quality of ejaculation is difficult to measure. Few patients have the comparative experience that might be helpful. The first stage of ejaculation is the formation of a bolus of semen in the prostatic urethra. It is expelled by a combination of prostatic and bulbospongiosus muscle contraction. These components should both be normal except in the most severe hypospadias, only seven of 18 intersex patients in Miller's series having normal ejaculation.[45] A patulous or a stenosed distal urethra may be associated with less forceful ejaculation.[42,46]

Most authors report 'normal' ejaculation. However, where specific questions have been asked, Bracka found that 33% had 'dribbling', and 4% had dry ejaculation.[39]

Hormones and fertility

In uncomplicated cases of hypospadias it seems likely that hormonal function is normal. In an unselected series of 213 patients recalled for review, hormonal profiles were measured only in the first 100, because they were always normal.[39] Other series have found hormone abnormalities chiefly when hypospadias was a part of a more complex sexual ambiguity. However, in Gearhart's series of 16 adult patients, the mean levels of follicle-stimulating hormone and luteinizing hormone were higher than in normals but still in the normal range. Five had grossly abnormal androgens, although three were fertile.[44] Low levels of 5-alpha-reductase were reported by Berg et al.[47]

There have been no prospective studies on fertility. It seems probable that otherwise-normal boys with hypospadias have normal fertility. However, one series reported that 50% of unselected patients had abnormal results of semen analysis.[48] When hypospadias is part of a complex of sexual ambiguity, the late outcome is poor but not hopeless.[45] All series include, amongst their least sexually successful patients, those with other developmental problems. In Bracka's series, 25% of patients had 'infertile semen' but most had other anomalies.[39] This point is particularly emphasized by

Marberger, in whose series there were 13 with sexual ambiguity, 11 of whom did not have intercourse and all of whom had azoospermia.[43]

In discussing fertility with patients it is important to remember that hypospadias is a hereditary condition. In a prospective series of 430 patients there was a 21% incidence of hypospadias in another family member.[49]

Psychosexual results

Several authors have suggested that there might be psychosexual consequences from hypospadias or from its treatment. There have been few formal studies of adults.

Summerlad found that 20% of patients appeared to have suffered from their several admissions: 21 of 60 patients avoided changing in public and 31 admitted to anxieties during adolescence, mainly about sexual function and fertility; 43 thought that their penis was abnormal.[42]

Very similar views were expressed by Bracka's patients, 74% of whom felt that they had had 'inadequate guidance' on sexual function; 40% said that it had affected their personal relationships,[39] but this did not stop 77% claiming to have satisfactory intercourse. There were no controls in these series and it may be that they reflect the general adolescent anxiety about sexual development.

At the worst end of the scale, Miller found that 12 of 18 patients had impaired psychological well-being, nine with impaired quality of life and four with severe psychosexual disability.[45]

Two investigations of psychosexual characteristics have been made in hypospadiac patients with normal controls (appendicectomy and hernia patients, respectively). Both investigations revealed quite marked morbidity.

In the older study of 33 hypospadiac patients, they were underachievers compared with the controls. They had reduced capacity for social and emotional relationships, and high castration anxiety. The severity of these abnormalities was not related to the original severity of the hypospadias. They were less secure in their gender identity, had delayed sexual debut and a smaller number of sexual partners.[47,50–54]

In the later study of 73 patients in Holland, the emphasis was on the sexual function. None of the patients was impotent and there were no differences in sexual behaviour or function compared with controls. However, 33% were inhibited in seeking sexual contacts (compared with 13% of controls) and they had a more negative appraisal of their penile appearance. The more severe the original deformity, the greater the number of operations and the later the age at which they were completed, the worse the psychosexual outcome.[55] Similar comments are found in the series of Eberle et al., though without such a detailed protocol.[43]

These studies are open to several criticisms.[56] None the less, they are detailed and important studies and their results cannot be dismissed without proper thought. If patients treated for hypospadias have psychological problems, the reasons should be sought and an attempt made to correct them.

Late surgical problems

The results of surgery may not be perfect but, in general, they are better in the surgeon's eye than in that of the patient.[57] Occasionally, patients have unrealistic expectations.

Even with an imperfect result, the patient may not have sufficient symptoms to request further surgery. In some cases he may develop symptoms many years after a successful repair: up to 50 years has been reported.[58]

Symptoms are usually of stricture or fistula but some patients may have chordee that inhibits intercourse. Although the problem may, at first sight, appear simple, it should be assumed that all have a total inadequacy of the repair until proved otherwise. Many may be described as 'hypospadiac cripples', with a neo-urethra that is too short, too narrow and of poor material. No specific type of primary repair is particularly associated with this disastrous complication.[59]

Chordee may occur with a urethra of normal calibre. Correction of the deformity by excision of the ventral chordee tissue will result in a urethra that is too short and further urethroplasty will be needed. If the penis is of adequate length, the patient may be content with a dorsal Nesbit's procedure rather than risk yet more reconstruction.

The site of chordee may be easy to identify, being opposite the neo-urethra. Occasionally, the author and others have found the deformity to be more proximal (Fig. 55.8).[54] In difficult cases an artificial erection will clarify the problem. This should be achieved either by intracorporal injection of prostaglandin or by the infusion technique. If a tourniquet is put around the penis at scrotal level and saline is injected into the corpora, the chordee may be missed.

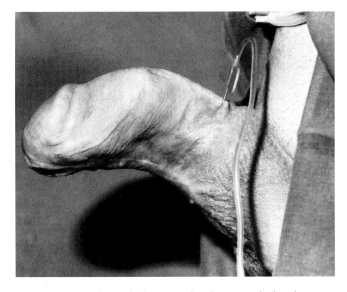

Figure 55.8. Clinical photograph of proximal chordee in a patient born with a distal hypospadias.

■ MYELOMENINGOCOELE

Spinal abnormalities, especially myelomeningocoele, are probably the only strictly physical cause of congenital erectile failure. Even the most crippled spina bifida patient has sexual desires. Normal sexual intercourse is quite possible even when life is spent in a wheelchair.

Those with minimal neurological defect are probably normal. Those who are grossly abnormal are often assumed to be 'asexual', although this may be a cover for unwillingness to tackle a difficult subject.

In investigating sexual function, there is a difference between theory and practice and between findings in adolescents and adults. In practice, sexual activity is more common than would be expected from theory or from investigating the adolescent alone.

Dorner interviewed 63 spina bifida teenagers and their families; 70% of the patients had moderate or severe handicap. It was found that sexual discussion with peers was inhibited; 23% did not know how babies were conceived; few patients understood anything of contraception; only 18 patients had 'dated'.[60]

This lack of education in patients who had grown up in the 1960s, a period of great sexual openness and freedom, is very worrying. It is in contrast to the patients' expressed interests, which were actively sexual in at least 80%.

Not surprisingly, sexual function (but not social success) is related to neurological defect.

In assessing sexual potential, it is important to remember that erections are often reflex and not necessarily a sexual response. Diamond et al.[61] related erections to the neurological defect but pointed out that many observed erections could have been purely reflex in origin. In a series of 52 post-pubertal males, 70% claimed to have erections, in most cases supported by parental observation. Erections occurred in all patients with a positive anocutaneous reflex and in 64% of those with a negative reflex and a sensory level at or below the sympathetic outflow (D10 to L2). Only 14% of males with higher lesions and absent reflex had erections.[61]

With a rather more detailed sexual history, Cass et al.[62] showed that orgasm and ejaculation occurred in seven of nine men with a sensory level at L3 or below. Only three men with higher levels were studied and, although two of them had ejaculations, only one had sexual sensation.[62]

Translating theory into practice is altogether more difficult. In Dorner's series of adolescents, only the males with minimal handicap had dated, none had established a steady relationship and none had had intercourse.[60]

The situation improves as the patients get older. In a review[63] of 49 adults it was found that nine had steady partners and 22 were married. Nine had fathered 23 children. Of the others, ten were under 20 years old, two were mentally handicapped and two had overprotective parents. It could, therefore, be said that 88% of those with realistic prospects were married or had a steady partner. Many of the patients were severely handicapped and incontinent, which seemed to be no bar to their achievements.[63]

Patients who are impotent or do not ejaculate should be investigated along conventional lines. Although there have been no studies specifically on these patients, it is known that patients with spinal cord defects can be managed with intracorporal injections of papaverine and other agents with appropriate dose reductions.[64]

Electro-ejaculation may have a role in a few patients.[65] However, although semen can successfully be collected, it may serve no purpose. It has been shown in one study that all of ten spina bifida males requiring electro-ejaculation were azoospermic and had primary testicular failure on biopsy.[66]

Combined series have shown an increased risk of neural tube defects (NTD) as high as 4% in the offspring of spina bifida patients. The risk is the same whether the affected parent is male or female, but daughters have a 1 in 13 incidence while the risk for sons is only 1 in 50.[63,67] The risk can be reduced by treating the mother with folate supplement for 3 months before pregnancy and continuing to week 12. In a double-blind trial in 1195 high-risk pregnancies using 4 mg folic acid daily versus placebo, there were six offspring with NTD in the treatment group and 21 in the placebo group.[68]

Pregnancies can be monitored for NTD both by foetal ultrasound and by measuring maternal alpha-foetoprotein. A programme of selective termination can largely eliminate spina bifida.[69]

■ REFERENCES

1. Woodhouse C R J. Long-term Paediatric Urology. Oxford: Blackwell Scientific, 1991: 127–150
2. Johnston J H. Lengthening of the congenital or acquired short penis. Br J Urol 1974; 46: 685–687
3. Woodhouse C R J, Kellett M J. Anatomy of the penis and its deformities in exstrophy and epispadias. J Urol 1984; 132: 1122–1124
4. Schillinger J F, Wiley M J. Bladder exstrophy penile lengthening procedure. Urology 1984; 24: 434–437
5. Hurwitz R S, Woodhouse C R J, Ransley P G. The anatomical course of the neurovascular bundles in epispadias. J Urol 1986; 136: 68–70
6. Schlegel P N, Gearhart J P. Neuroanatomy of the pelvis in an infant with cloacal exstrophy: a detailed microdissection with histology. J Urol 1989; 141: 583–585
7. McLorie G A, Bellemore M C, Salter R B. Penile deformity in bladder exstrophy: correlation with closure of the pelvic defect. J Pediatr Surg 1991; 26: 201–203
8. Gearhart J P, Young A, Leonard M P et al. Prostate size and configuration in adults with bladder exstrophy. J Urol 1993; 149: 308–310
9. Snyder H M. Epispadias and exstrophy. In: Whitfield H N (ed) Rob and Smith's Operative Surgery — Genito-Urinary Surgery. Oxford: Butterworth-Heinemann, 1993: 786–813
10. Sponsellar P D, Gearhart J P, Jeffs R D et al. Anatomy of the pelvis in the exstrophy complex. J Bone Joint Surg [Am] 1995; 77: 117–189
11. Silver R I, Yang A, Ben-Chaim J et al. Penile length in men after exstrophy reconstruction. J Urol 1997; 157: 999–1003
12. Woodhouse C R J. The management of erectile deformity in adults with exstrophy and epispadias. J Urol 1986; 135: 932–935
13. Brzezinski A E, Homsy Y L, Laberge I. Orthoplasty in epispadias. J Urol 1986; 136: 259–261
14. Mesrobian H-G J, Kelalis P P, Kramer S A. Long term follow-up of cosmetic appearance and genital function in boys with exstrophy: review of 53 patients. J Urol 1986; 136: 256–258
15. Perovic S, Scepanovic D, Sremcevic D et al. Epispadias surgery — Belgrade experience. Br J Urol 1992; 70: 674–677

16. Woodhouse C R J. Epispadias repair in the adolescent. In: Erlich R M, Alter G J (eds) Reconstructive and plastic surgery of the external genitalia. Orlando: Saunders, 1998: in press

17. Hanna M K, Williams D I. Genital function in males with vesical exstrophy and epispadias. Br J Urol 1974; 44: 169–174

18. Stein R, Stockle M, Fisch M et al. The fate of the adult exstrophy patient. J Urol 1994; 152: 1413–1416

19. Ben-Chaim J, Jeffs R D, Reiner W G, Gearhart J P. The outcome of patients with classic bladder exstrophy in adult life. J Urol 1996; 155: 1251–1252

20. Audry G, Grapin C, Loulidi S et al. Genital prognosis of boys with bladder exstrophy or epispadias with incontinence: apropos of 14 cases. Ann Urol (Paris) 1991; 25: 120–124

21. Husmann D A, McClorie G A, Churchill B M. Phallic reconstruction in cloacal exstrophy. J Urol 1986; 142: 563–564

22. McClorie G A, Khoury A E, Husman D A. Surgery for the small penis in childhood. Dial Ped Urol 1989; 12: 6–7

23. Mitchell M E. Epispadias repair and sexual assignment in the cloacal exstrophy patient. Dial Ped Urol 1995; 18(10): 2–3

24. Lattimer J K, Macfarlane M T, Puchor P J. Male exstrophy patients: a preliminary report on the reproductive capability. Trans Am Assoc Genito-Urinary Surg 1979; 70: 42–46

25. Feldman K W, Smith D W. Fetal phallic growth and penile standards for newborn male infants. J Pediatr 1975; 86: 395–398

26. Flatau E, Josefsberg Z, Reisner S H et al. Penile size in the new born infant. J Pediatr 1975; 87: 663–664

27. Schonfeld W A. Primary and secondary sexual characteristics. Am J Dis Child 1943; 65: 535–549

28. Reilly J M, Woodhouse C R J. Small penis and male sexual role. J Urol 1989; 142: 569–571

29. Money J, Lehne G K, Pierre-Jerome F. Micropenis: gender, erotosexual coping strategy and behavioural health in nine pediatric cases followed to adulthood. Compr Psychiatry 1985; 26: 29

30. Salisbury D M, Leonard J V, Dezateux C A, Savage M O. Micropenis: an important early sign of congenital hypopituitarism. Br Med J 1984; 288: 621–622

31. Choi S K, Han S W, Kim D H, de Lignieres B. Transdermal dihydrotestosterone therapy and its effects on patients with microphallus. J Urol 1993; 150: 657–660

32. McMahon D R, Kramer S A, Husman D A. Micropenis: does early treatment with testosterone do more harm than good? J Urol 1995; 154: 825–829

33. Klugo R C, Cerny J C. Response of the micropenis to topical testosterone and gonadotrophin. J Urol 1978; 119: 667–668

34. Duckett J W. The current hype in hypospadiology. Br J Urol 1995; 76 (suppl3): 1–7

35. Koyanagi T, Nonomura K, Kakizaki H, Yamashita T. Hypospadias repair. In: Thuroff J W, Hohenfellner M (eds) Reconstructive surgery of the lower urinary tract in children. Oxford: Isis Medical Media, 1995: 1–21

36. Correspondence. Br J Urol 1996; 78: 659–661

37. Cole M. Psychological approaches to treatment. In: Gregoire A, Pryor J P (eds) Impotence: an integrated approach to clinical practice. Edinburgh: Churchill Livingstone, 1993

38. Avellan L. Development of puberty, sexual debut and sexual function in hypospadiacs. Scand J Plast Reconstr Surg Hand Surg 1976; 10: 29–34

39. Bracka A. A long term view of hypospadias. Br J Plast Surg 1989; 42: 251–255

40. Johanson B, Avellan L. Hypospadias. A review of 299 cases operated 1957–1969. Scand J Plast Reconstr Surg Hand Surg 1980; 14: 259–267

41. Kenawi M M. Sexual function in hypospadiacs. Br J Urol 1976; 47: 883–890

42. Summerlad B C. A long-term follow-up of hypospadias patients. Br J Plast Surg 1975; 28: 324–330

43. Eberle J, Uberreiter S, Radmayr C. Posterior hypospadias: long term follow-up after reconstructive surgery in the male direction. J Urol 1993; 150: 1474–1477

44. Gearhart J P, Donohue P A, Brown T R et al. Endocrine evaluation of adults with mild hypospadias. J Urol 1990; 144: 274–277

45. Miller M A W, Grant D B. Severe hypospadias with genital ambiguity: outcome after staged hypospadias repair in 18 young men. Br J Urol 1997; 80: 485–488

46. Marberger H, Pauer W. Experience in hypospadias repair. Urol Clin North Am 1981; 8: 403–419

47. Berg R, Berg G. Penile malformation, gender identity and sexual orientation. Acta Psychiatr Scand 1983; 68: 154–166

48. Zubowska J, Jankowska J, Kula K et al. Clinical, hormonal and semiological data in adult men operated in childhood for hypospadias. Endokrynol Pol 1979; 30: 565–573

49. Bauer S B, Retik A B, Colodny A H. Genetic aspects of hypospadias. Urol Clin North Am 1981; 8: 559–565

50. Berg R, Berg G, Svensson J. Penile malformation and mental health. Acta Psychiatr Scand 1982; 66: 398–416

51. Berg G, Berg R. Castration complex, evidence from men operated for hypospadias. Acta Psychiatr Scand 1983; 68: 143–153

52. Berg R, Berg G, Edman G et al. Androgens and personality in normal men and men operated for hypospadias in childhood. Acta Psychiatr Scand 1983; 68: 167–177

53. Berg R, Svensson J, Astrom G et al. Social and sexual adjustment of men operated for hypospadias during childhood: a controlled study. J Urol 1983; 125: 313–317

54. Svensson J, Berg R. Micturition studies and sexual function in operated hypospadiacs. Br J Urol 1983; 55: 422–426

55. Mureau M A, Slijper F M E, van der Meulen J C et al. Psychosexual adjustment of men who underwent hypospadias repair: a norm related study. J Urol 1995; 154: 1351–1355

56. Woodhouse C R J. Hypospadias. In: Woodhouse C R J. Long-term paediatric urology. Oxford: Blackwell Scientific, 1991: 159–166

57. Mureau M A, Slijper F M E, Slob A K et al. Satisfaction with penile appearance after hypospadias surgery: the patient and surgeon view. J Urol 1996; 155: 703–706

58. Flynn J T, Johnston S R, Blandy J P. The late sequelae of hypospadias repair. Br J Urol 1980; 52: 555–559

59. Stecker J F, Horton C E, Devine C J, McCraw J B. Hypospadias cripples. Urol Clin North Am 1981; 8: 539–544

60. Dorner S. Sexual interest and activity in adolescents with spina bifida. J Child Psychol Psychiatry 1977; 18: 229–237

61. Diamond D A, Rickwood A M K, Thomas D G. Penile erections in myelomeningocoele patients. Br J Urol 1986; 58: 434–435

62. Cass A S, Bloom B A, Luxenberg M. Sexual function in adults with myelomeningocoele. J Urol 1986; 136: 425–426

63. Laurence K M, Beresford A. Continence, friends, marriage and children in 51 adults with spina bifida. Dev Med Child Neurol 1975; 17(suppl35): 123–128

64. Lue T F, Tanagho E A. Physiology of erection and pharmacological management of impotence. J Urol 1987; 137: 829–836

65. Brindley G S. Electro ejaculation: its technique, neurological implications and uses. J Neurol Neurosurg Psychiatry 1981; 44: 9–18

66. Reilly J M, Oates R D. Preliminary investigation of the potential fertility status of postpubertal males with myelodysplasia. Paper read at International Paediatric Nephrology Association Meeting, Jerusalem, September 1992

67. Woodhouse C R J. Sexual and reproductive consequences of congenital genitourinary anomalies. J Urol 1994; 152: 645–651

68. MRC Vitamin Study Research Group. Prevention of neural tube defects: results of the Medical Research Council vitamin study. Lancet 1991; 338: 131–133

69. Chan A, Robertson E F, Haan E A et al. Prevalence of neural tube defects in South Australia, 1966–91: effectiveness and impact of prenatal diagnosis. Br Med J 1993; 307: 703–706

70. Feitz F J, van Grunsven E J K J E M, Froeling F M J A, de Vries J D M. Outcome analysis of the psychosexual and socio-economic development of adult patients born with bladder exstrophy. J Urol 1994; 152: 1417–1419

Chapter 56

Female sexual dysfunction

J. R. Berman, J. M. Shuker and I. Goldstein

■ INTRODUCTION

Sexuality is an important aspect of every individual's life. Although it is intuitive that sexual intercourse is a couple's function, there has been limited physiological investigation of female sexual function as its own entity. Female sexuality encompasses multiple components including physiological, psychological, social and emotional factors. The first phase of the female sexual response is mediated by a combination of vasocongestive and neuromuscular events which include increased clitoral length and diameter, as well as increased vaginal lubrication, wall engorgement and luminal diameter.[1-4] A physiological disorder resulting in female sexual dysfunction can ultimately lead to or exacerbate a psychological condition, further complicating the clinical picture. As a result, it is important that female sexual complaints be addressed multidimensionally.

Female sexual dysfunction may be a common medical problem. A woman may have her own psychological or organic conditions that may ultimately result in diminished responses to sexual stimulation. These dysfunctional responses may include disorders of vaginal arousal, engorgement, lubrication, sensation and comfort, as well as clitoral sensation, the ability to achieve orgasm, and sexual desire. Outpatient surveys have estimated that 18–76% of adult females complain of sexual dysfunction during sexual activity. There are numerous women, often partners of male urologic patients, with complaints of vaginal and clitoral function that receive little or no evaluation by their physicians. A preliminary investigation at Boston University found a prevalence of the self-reported vaginal/clitoral complaints exceeding 50% in women who accompanied their men for evaluation of male erectile dysfunction. The female partners of impotent patients completed a questionnaire concerning vaginal and clitoral function. Such information included questions on changes that may have occurred during the course of the relationship in terms of vaginal sensation, vaginal lubrication, time for vaginal arousal, vaginal orgasm, vaginal size, painful vaginal penetration, clitoral sensation and clitoral orgasm. Relationships were found to exist between these complaints of female sexual functioning and age, menopause and vascular risk-factor history.

The National Institutes of Health and other major funding agencies have begun to promote and encourage the investigation into female health issues. The American Foundation of Urologic Diseases has recently conceived the Sexual Health Council with the goal of supporting and promoting education and public awareness in the field of male and female sexual dysfunction. In particular, the field of female sexual dysfunction is in critical need of basic science and precise clinical investigation. Whereas there has been a virtual focus on the physiology of erection and the pathophysiology of impotence, there has been little scientific evaluation of the mechanisms involved in female sexual function and the pathologies thereof, especially with respect to the vagina and clitoris. For example, the existing physiological information concerning characterization of the mechanisms modulating clitoral and vaginal smooth muscle contractility is limited. Such mechanisms regulate the pelvic vasocongestive phase of the female sexual response; therefore, proposed studies in that direction should have important clinical significance. There is optimism, and a certain amount of expectancy, that future diagnostic and therapeutic strategies such as duplex ultrasonography and oral vasodilating agents, respectively, will emerge from the information provided by these and other studies concerning the physiology of clitoral and vaginal smooth muscle and the pathophysiology of vaginal engorgement and clitoral erectile insufficiencies. Ultimately, sexual relationships and the problems that arise from them need to be expressed within the context of the couple. The best management of sexual problems will result from the team of physicians that coordinate the treatment of male and female urological problems.

It is foreseen that there will be additional Food and Drug Administration approvals for newer intra-urethral and intracavernosal vasoactive agents as well as new oral, sublingual and topical vasoactive substances that promote corpus cavernosum smooth muscle relaxation. These latter convenient, on-demand oral, sublingual and topical pharmaceutical medications may be used in the future for women with complaints of vaginal and clitoral dysfunctions associated with pelvic organ vasocongestion, clitoral erection and vaginal engorgement. The future availability of convenient on-demand vasoactive agents for men may, for the first time, provide convenient on-demand non-hormonal, non-mechanical approaches to enhance blood flow to the female pelvic organs during the pelvic vasocongestive phase of the female sexual response. If this is imminently so, these new vasoactive therapies will lead to increased numbers of women seeking treatment for psychological and physiological conditions that have resulted in diminished pelvic vasocongestive responses to sexual stimulation. Physicians will be obliged to direct new attention to the diagnosis and treatment of women with physiological sexual dysfunctions of the vagina and clitoris. Encouragement, support and the promotion of research into the understanding of the physiology and pathophysiology of the female sexual response will inevitably become increasingly important.

Future studies will have wide clinical significance. The arousal phase of the female sexual response involves pelvic vasocongestion and there is, at present, only limited understanding of the various local regulatory mechanisms that modulate tone in the clitoral erectile tissue and the vaginal muscularis smooth muscle. Since such mechanisms regulate this second phase of the female sexual response, it is anticipated that knowledge gleaned in the next few years will lead to the development of future diagnostic and therapeutic strategies to care for female urologic patients with complaints of vaginal and clitoral function during sexual activity.

This chapter focuses on female sexual dysfunction. The functional anatomy of the vagina and clitoris,

relevant physiology of arousal, animal model studies, potential diagnosis and treatment options are reviewed.

■ VAGINAL AND CLITORAL ANATOMY

A thorough understanding of female pelvic anatomy is fundamental to the evaluation and treatment of physiological conditions adversely affecting normal female sexual function.

Vagina

The vagina is the canal that connects the uterus with the external genital organs; its design is such that it easily accommodates penetration of a rigid penile erection. At the posterior end the rounded neck of the uterus, the cervix, projects into the space known as the fornix or vaginal vault. Anteriorly, two pleats of sensitive tissue, the labia minora, surround the opening of the vagina and are further protected by larger folds known as the labia majora.[5–8]

The walls of the vagina consist of three layers: these are an inner aglandular mucous membrane epithelium, an intermediary richly supplied vascular muscularis layer, and an outer supportive fibrous mesh. The vaginal mucosa is a mucous-type stratified squamous cell epithelium that undergoes hormone-related cyclical changes, such as slight keratinization of the superficial cells during the menstrual cycle. The muscularis portion is known to be highly infiltrated with smooth muscle and an extensive tree of blood vessels, which may swell during intercourse. The surrounding fibrous layer provides structural support to the vagina; this layer consists of elastin and collagen fibres that allow for expansion of the vaginal vault during sexual arousal or childbirth. Large blood vessels run within the mucosa, and nerve plexuses exist within muscular and adventitial layers. The vagina has many rugae or folds that are necessary for the distensibility of the organ; just how elastic it can become is exemplified during childbirth. Still smaller ridges lend to the frictional tension that exists during intercourse.[5–8]

The arterial supply to the vagina is derived from an extensive network of branching vessels, surrounding it from all sides. The anterior branch of the internal iliac artery continually bifurcates as it descends through the pelvis with a series of the newly generated vessels, each supplying the vagina to some degree. After giving off an obturator artery branch, the umbilical and the middle rectal arteries diverge to supply a superior and inferior vesical artery, respectively. Between the umbilical and the mid-rectal branches there is generation of a uterine artery, which further bifurcates to give the vaginal artery. The internal pudendal and accessory pudendal arteries also send branches. Finally, the common clitoral artery sends a branch to the vaginal muscularis.[5–8]

The neurological innervation of the vagina originates from two separate plexuses, the superior hypogastric plexus and the sacral plexus. The hypogastric nerve plexus descends on the great vessels, spreading into an inferior hypogastric plexus, which systematically branches further into a uterovaginal nerve. The somatic pudendal nerve originates off the pelvic splanchnic branches from the sacral plexus. Pudendal branching innervates the vagina towards the opening of the introitus as the perineal and posterior labial nerves.[5–8]

Immunohistochemistry studies have been used to increase understanding of the innervation of the human vaginal mucosa. In a study by Hilliges et al.[9] using protein gene product 9.5, more distal areas of the vagina had significantly more nerve fibres than the more proximal parts, and the anterior wall showed a denser innervation than the posterior wall. Graf et al.[10] studied the distribution patterns and the occurrence of helospectin and pituitary adenylate cyclase-activating polypeptide (PACAP) immunoreactivity: they confirmed a dense network of vasoactive intestinal peptide (VIP) immunoreactive nerve fibres showing subpopulations of helospectin and LI-type PACAP. Nerve fibres of the vagina had previously been shown to be active in association with specific peptides which include VIP, peptide histidine methionine (PHM), calcitonin gene-related peptide (CGRP), and galanin. Genital vasodilatation and subsequent increase in vaginal blood flow and lubrication have been observed upon exposure of vessels to VIP. VIP has been implicated as the neurotransmitter for mediating vaginal vasodilatation and the formation of lubricating fluid during sexual arousal. Helospectin and PACAP, a potent vasodilator, belong to the same peptide family as VIP and PHM, and recent observations have been made to the effect that distributions and co-localizations of helospectin and VIP as well as PACAP and VIP have been reported in the mammalian gastrointestinal tract.[9–16]

The canal is lubricated primarily from a transudate originating from the subepithelial vascular bed and passively transported through the interepithelial spaces, sometimes referred to as intercellular channels. Additional moistening during intercourse comes from secretion of the paired greater vestibular or Bartholin's glands, although some believe these to have a more primal function of emitting an odiferous fluid to attract the male.[5–8,11,12]

The effects of oestrogen on the maintenance and function of female genitalia have been well documented in studies. Oestrogen receptors have been shown to exist throughout the vaginal epithelium, in stromal cells, and in the smooth muscle fibres in the muscularis. Weaker conformations of oestrogen such as oestriol appear more effective in stimulating the vagina as opposed to the uterus. Thickness and rugae of the vaginal wall, as well as vaginal lubrication, have been shown to be oestrogen dependent. Although this fluid production has been shown to be hormone dependent, both in the resting state and during sexual excitement, quantitative changes apparently do not occur during the menstrual cycle. An insufficient amount of oestrogen will result in thin vaginal walls more easily susceptible to trauma and with a decreased ability to heal, as well as a drier and less acidic vaginal environment that is more vulnerable to infection. Vaginal dryness is associated with ovarian failure and is effectively controlled by oestrogen replacement therapy. Some women who are not sexually active may not notice the extent of vaginal atrophy but, when coitus does resume, pain and discomfort from intercourse can be considerable.[17–20]

Clitoris

The clitoris is the homologue of the penis, arising from the embryological genital tubercle. The clitoris consists of a cylindrical, erectile organ composed of three parts — the outermost glans or head, the middle corpus or body, and the innermost crura. The glans of the clitoris is visualized as it emerges from the labia minora, which bifurcate to form the upper prepuce anteriorly and the lower frenulum posteriorly. The body of the clitoris consists of two paired corpora cavernosa of length about 2.5 cm and lacks a corpus spongiosum. The body extends under the skin at the corona to the crura. The two crura of the clitoris, formed from the separation of the most proximal portions of the corpora in the perineum, attach bilaterally to the undersurface of the symphysis pubis at the ischiopubic rami.[2–4,11–14]

A fibrous tunica albuginea ensheathes each corporal body made up of lacunar space sinusoids surrounded by trabeculae of vascular smooth muscle and collagen connective tissue. No retractor clitoridis muscle exists in humans as it does in other animals such as cattle and sheep; however, a supporting suspensory ligament does hold the clitoris in the introital region.[2–4,11–14]

The main arterial supply to the clitoris is from the iliohypogastric–pudendal arterial bed. The internal pudendal artery is the last anterior branch off the internal iliac artery. Distally, the internal pudendal artery traverses Alcock's canal, formed from the obturator fascia, and lies on the inner side in apposition to the ischiopubic ramus. In this latter location, the artery is susceptible to blunt perineal trauma. The internal pudendal artery terminates as it supplies the inferior rectal and perineal arteries, which supply the labia. The common clitoral artery continues to the clitoris. This artery bifurcates into a dorsal clitoral artery and a cavernosal clitoral artery.[2–4,11–14]

Autonomic efferent innervation of the clitoris passes from the pelvic and hypogastric nerves to the clitoris through the urogenital diaphragm. Pelvic nerve stimulation results in clitoral smooth muscle relaxation and arterial smooth muscle dilatation. There is a rise in clitoral cavernosal artery inflow and an increase in clitoral intracavernous pressure which lead to tumescence and extrusion of the glans clitoris.[2–4,11–14,21]

Using pseudorabies virus injected into the clitoris of the female rat, neurons that may be involved in regulating the autonomic and somatic reflexes seen in sexual behaviour have been identified by immunohistochemical assay.[22] Major input to the clitoris was seen in spinal segments L5–S1, and to a lesser extent in T12–L4 as well as S2–S4. Virus-labelled cells were found in the brain in multiple locations including the nucleus paragigantocellularis, raphe pallidus, raphe magnus, Barrington's nucleus, ventrolateral central grey, hypothalamus, and the medial pre-optic region. This implies that a multisynaptic circuit of neurons may be involved in clitoral neurological control rather than just a simple somatic reflex connection. Morphological studies have been performed using wheat germ agglutinin conjugated with horseradish peroxidase (WGA-HRP) injected into the clitoris of the female cat to compare afferent pathways to the entire population of pudendal nerve afferents.[23] Central projections of the clitoral afferents were identified in the L7–S3 segments, with the most prominent labelling in S1–S2. In the same study, electrophysiological analysis of the clitoris performed under constant mechanical pressure stimulation indicated both phasic and tonic discharges in L7–S2, but most prominently in S1. In contrast, electrical stimulation of the clitoris evoked discharges at S1 only. The neurotransmitters mediating clitoral and arterial smooth muscle dilatation remain undetermined; however, preliminary studies suggest that nitric oxide is involved. Histochemical studies have revealed VIP and neuropeptide Y (NPY) immunoreactive nerves in the clitoral erectile tissues.[24]

Somatic sensory pathways originate from the clitoral skin. There exists a dense collection of Pacinian corpuscles innervated by rapidly adapting myelinated afferents, as well as Meissner's corpuscles, Merckel tactile discs, and free nerve endings. These sensory afferents pass from the dorsal clitoral nerve to the pudendal nerve.[2–4,11–14]

■ PHYSIOLOGY OF FEMALE SEXUAL AROUSAL

The female sexual response phase of arousal is not easily distinguished from the phase of desire until physiological changes begin to take place in the vagina and clitoris as well as other sexual organs. Sexual excitement and pleasure are accompanied by pelvic vasocongestion and swelling of the external genitalia including vaginal engorgement and clitoral erection.[3,4,8,11–14]

Vaginal engorgement enables a process of plasma transudation to occur, allowing a flow through the epithelium and onto the vaginal surface. Plasma transudation results from the rising pressure in the vaginal capillary bed during the arousal state. In addition there is an increase in vaginal length and luminal diameter, especially in the distal two-thirds of the vaginal canal.[3,4,8,11–14]

Central nervous system areas primarily implicated in sexual arousal, based on animal research, include the medial pre-optic, anterior hypothalamic region and related limbic–hippocampal structures. Cognitive effects have been investigated and, although not the focus of this report, at least one study is worth mentioning. Laan et al.[25–28] suggest that the greatest contribution to sexual arousal in the female results from cognitive processing of stimulus content and meaning, and not from peripheral vasocongestive feedback. There does not appear to be a relation between menstrual phases and physiological arousability. Meuwissen and Over[29] have found that neither film-induced nor fantasy-induced levels of sexual arousal varied significantly throughout the menstrual cycle. There are conflicting reports as well as to the habituation of the female sexual response. Some claim that levels of subjective and physiological sexual arousal decrease over repeated exposure to sexual stimuli; others could not elucidate similar results even after 21 trials, yet both concur that the subsequent presentation of a novel stimulus will increase the female sexual response. The desire for increased sexual performance on sexual arousal in functional women has been found to facilitate genital responses, most prominently with the stimulus of erotic fantasy as opposed to erotic film. Interestingly, masturbation frequency had no effect on genital responses despite its significance on subjective reports of arousal.[25-30]

Clinicians and researchers have assumed that sexual arousal is inhibited by the sympathetic nervous system, whereas facilitation and maintenance are through the parasympathetic nervous system. Meston and Gorzalka have offered a pair of studies that investigate and challenge these notions in women. First, they found that intense exercise, consisting of 20-minute bicycle-riding sessions, increased physiological sexual arousal measured by photoplethysmography.[31] This challenged the notion that sympathetic nervous system stimulation inhibited sexual arousal in women and further provided evidence that sexual arousal was actually facilitated by the sympathetic nervous system. Another study examined the temporal effect of sympathetic activation through acute exercise on immediate, delayed, and residual sexual arousal.[32] Sexual arousal was objectively assessed by plethysmography. A relationship between sympathetic nervous system activation and sexual arousal was found, such that sexual arousability was inhibited 5 minutes after exercise, facilitated 15 minutes after exercise, and only marginally increased 30 minutes after exercise. The two studies suggest that sympathetic nerve stimulation activation plays an important facilitatory role in the early stages of sexual arousal.[31,32]

What is the role of the clitoris in sexual arousal? The clitoris may play a major role during sexual activity in that it is not only part of what makes the sexual act enjoyable for the woman but also enhances her response to coitus upon clitoral stimulation. Clitoral stimulation may induce local autonomic and somatic reflexes causing vaginal vasocongestion, engorgement and subsequent transudation, lubricating the introital canal and making the sexual act easier, more comfortable, and more pleasurable. The more stimulation, the higher the level of arousal and the easier it is to further increase stimulation.[33]

■ VASCULOGENIC FEMALE SEXUAL DYSFUNCTION

Female sexual dysfunction has traditionally included disorders of desire/libido, disorders of arousal, pelvic pain disorders and inhibited orgasm. Patient surveys estimate that 18–76% of adult women have such complaints during sexual activity.[34]

Female sexual dysfunction that may have its origin in abnormal arterial circulation into the vagina or clitoris during sexual stimulation, usually from atherosclerotic vascular disease, may be considered a disorder of arousal. This vasculogenic female sexual dysfunction may include such clinical symptoms as delayed vaginal engorgement, diminished vaginal lubrication, pain or discomfort with intercourse, diminished vaginal sensation, diminished vaginal orgasm, diminished clitoral sensation or diminished clitoral orgasm. Traumatic injury to the iliohypogastric–pudendal arterial bed from pelvic fractures or blunt perineal trauma may also result in diminished vaginal/clitoral blood flow following sexual stimulation and fall into this vasculogenic category.

■ ANIMAL MODEL STUDIES

In a female New Zealand White rabbit model, direct recording of vaginal and clitoral haemodynamic responses followed vaginal and clitoral nerve stimulation. Laser Doppler flow probes were placed within the vaginal muscularis and clitoral erectile tissues to record vaginal and clitoral blood flow, respectively. A series of animals were studied in which arteriograms were performed to confirm normal iliohypogastric–pudendal arterial beds. In such control animals, pelvic nerve stimulation resulted in increased vaginal and clitoral blood inflow, as well as increased vaginal wall pressure, vaginal length and clitoral intracavernosal pressure.[35]

The same animal model was used to examine haemodynamic function in the presence of pelvic atherosclerotic vascular disease of the iliohypogastric–pudendal arterial bed. This was induced by repeated aortofemoral balloon de-endothelialization followed by placing the animal on a 16-week high-cholesterol diet. Arterial occlusive pathology was confirmed by arteriography and histomorphological examination of the arterial walls of the iliohypogastric–pudendal arteries, including the clitoral cavernosal artery. In addition, diffuse vaginal and clitoral fibrosis was observed. In those with pelvic atherosclerosis, significant diminution of nerve-stimulated vaginal and clitoral blood flow was observed, together with reduced vaginal wall pressure and changes in vaginal length. The haemodynamic alteration in vaginal and clitoral physiological function secondary to pelvic atherosclerotic pathology in the iliohypogastric–pudendal arterial bed was termed vaginal engorgement and clitoral erectile insufficiency, respectively.[35]

In summary, using pelvic nerve stimulation in normal and atherosclerotic New Zealand White female rabbits, it was determined that both vaginal engorgement and clitoral erection depend on increased blood flow. Furthermore, nerve-stimulated changes in blood flow were found to be significantly less in the atherosclerotic group than in the control group. Such altered blood flow responses were also associated with other diminished physiological changes in vaginal wall pressure, vaginal length and clitoral intracavernosal pressure.

■ NON-INVASIVE DIAGNOSTIC STUDIES OF VASCULOGENIC FEMALE SEXUAL DYSFUNCTION

Pulsed-wave Doppler ultrasonography can provide a non-invasive means of detecting blood flow changes in the vaginal and clitoral arteries. Lavoisier et al.[36] reported on the use of Doppler ultrasonography to measure blood velocity in the clitoral cavernosal artery and to record changes in flow associated with intravaginal pressure changes. They found that vaginal pressure stimulation along the lower or outer third of the vagina greatly increased blood velocity in the clitoral arteries by up to 11 times the prestimulation baseline levels. It is anticipated that duplex Doppler ultrasonography will be widely used as the diagnostic study of choice to assess clitoral cavernosal and vaginal artery integrity in women suspected of having vasculogenic female sexual dysfunction.[36]

Vaginal photoplethysmography is another non-invasive technique that provides a quantitative record of the extent vasocongestion has occurred in vaginal capillaries. When positioned within the vagina, the tampon-shaped, infrared-light-emitting probe has a photosensitive receiving sensor that detects light reflected back from the mucosa. Less infrared light is reflected back to the photosensitive sensor with increasing vaginal mucosal engorgement. Vaginal pulse amplitudes are recorded from the AC signal and relate minute short-term changes in vaginal mucosal engorgement; vaginal blood volumes are recorded from the DC signal, and record slowly developing pooling of blood in the vaginal tissue. Both measures are good indicators of sexual function in the arousal phase of the sexual response. Until duplex Doppler studies are developed, vaginal plethysmography will be used clinically to assess vaginal engorgement capabilities.[37–41]

Vaginal thermal clearance techniques are based on the principle that vaginal blood flow changes can be recorded by measuring the heat transfer away from an intravaginal probe kept at constant temperature (usually slightly above core body temperature). As vaginal blood flow increases, more heat is transferred away from the heated device; thus more electrical power in milliwatts is needed to maintain the electrode at the fixed temperature. Higher amounts of energy indicate higher levels of blood flow. Fisher et al. were able to use a vaginal thermistor to measure nocturnal patterns of vaginal blood flow, similar to nocturnal penile tumescence measurements in the male.[42]

■ FEMALE SEXUAL DYSFUNCTION AND OTHER MEDICAL CONDITIONS

Sexual dysfunctions often accompany or arise as a result of other diseases, conditions or syndromes. For example, epilepsy may be associated with diminutions in sexual desire/arousal and with a lack of social and sexual confidence. Morrell et al.[43] studied the sexual response in men and women with partial temporal lobe epilepsy by measuring genital blood flow during sexual arousal.[43] Female genital blood flow was measured as vaginal pulse amplitudes using the AC signal from a vaginal photoplethysmograph in response to alternating segments of sexually neutral and erotic videotape. Both women with temporal lobe epilepsy and subjects without temporal lobe epilepsy showed an increase in genital blood flow when viewing the erotic videotape, but temporal lobe epilepsy subjects showed significantly lower differential scores from baseline than the control group. Although the investigators did demonstrate decreased genital vasocongestion in response to sexually arousing stimuli in women with temporal lobe epilepsy, they did not probe more deeply into the degree to which the sexual dysfunction was attributable to epilepsy itself. However, in addition to suggesting functional and structural disruptions to the cortical regions mediating sexual behaviour, they also implicated anti-epileptic medications as possible contributors to sexual dysfunction by direct action on the cerebral cortex and through hormones involved in sexual physiology.

Women with spinal cord injuries provide an interesting opportunity to study the mechanism of sexual function. A case study reported by Levin and Macdonaugh[44] shows increasing genital blood flow induced by implant electrical stimulation of the anterior sacral roots S2 and S3 in a conscious paraplegic woman. The presumption is made that released VIP relaxes the blood vessel walls, creating vasodilatation, elevated vaginal blood flow and increased vaginal blood volume. Sipski et al.[45] showed that spinal cord injured subjects with complete transection at T6 and above, despite reporting subjective sexual arousal, had no vasocongestive response to isolated audiovisual erotic stimulation. Able-bodied subjects consistently recorded increasing vaginal pulse amplitudes to audiovisual erotic stimulation. The addition of manual clitoral stimulation, however, did indicate similar positive vaginal pulse amplitude responses in both groups regardless of the lack of reported sexual arousal in the spinal cord injured group. Therefore, Sipski has shown that women with complete spinal cord injury do elicit a reflex genital vasocongestion to tactile clitoral stimulation despite the inability to respond to audiovisual stimulation. A subsequent study by the same investigators observed the effect of performance of a self-distracting task, in the form of the Stroop test, on manual clitoral stimulation.[46] No change in vaginal pulse amplitude was observed in spinal cord injured women, indicating a lack of reflex vaginal vasocongestion, whereas increased vaginal pulse amplitude was seen in able-bodied subjects under similar conditions. Removal of the self-distracting task increased vaginal pulse amplitude in the normal subjects but had no effect on the spinal cord injured subjects. This was not surprising in women with no direct connection from the central nervous system to the peripheral sexual organs. It was suggested

that, perhaps, the spinal cord injured women in this particular study were not able adequately to perform manual clitoral stimulation, and that thus these subjects did not provide significant increases in vaginal blood flow. There is some evidence that spinal cord transection need not totally abolish a woman's subjective arousability upon manual stimulation alone. Although not confirmed to date in the human, research performed by Komisaruk et al.[47] has shown indirectly in rats that the vagus nerve provides a functional sensory pathway from the reproductive tract directly to the medulla oblongata of the brain, bypassing the spinal cord. These results provide an explanation for responses to vaginal self-stimulation including analgesia, menstrual cramping and even orgasm, in women diagnosed with complete spinal cord injury.

What happens to female organs following irradiation for pelvic malignancies? The rapid cell-renewal system of the epithelia of the pelvic organs that normally allows for natural exfoliation (vagina) and monthly sloughing (uterus) makes them susceptible to the effects of radiation. The uterus, for example, demonstrates a decrease in size, more prominent in women of reproductive age than in premenarchal or postmenopausal women: the myometrium undergoes a diffuse decrease in size, the endometrium undergoes atrophy as well as decreases in width, and the zonal anatomical differentiation between the two is lost. The mechanism for this atrophy of the uterus is twofold — a direct radiation effect on the uterine tissue and a radiation-induced ovarian hypofunction that causes reduced hormonal stimulation of the uterus.[48] Changes in the irradiated uterus appear to be caused by the effects of radiation on the small blood vessels, resulting in endarteritis (inflammation of the intimal layer) and increased endothelial permeability, which can persist into a chronic phase. Ovaries become smaller. The vagina demonstrates changes that vary, based on time after radiation: in the acute phase there are probably oedematous and hypervascular inflammatory changes, whereas chronically the vaginal tissue becomes atrophic. Abitbol and Davenport[49] examined patients with gynaecological cancers who were disease-free at least a year after completing treatment,[49] and found that all women who received radiation therapy had at least one of the three following effects: obliteration or narrowing of at least two-thirds of the vagina; moderate to massive pelvic fibrosis; or pain and discomfort during pelvic examination; surgical subjects reported the same effects in only 32% of cases. Yet more important is the fact that surgery results in less change to the vagina and subsequently in lower rates of sexual dysfunction. Women treated surgically for cervical carcinoma demonstrate up to 88% return to previous sexual enjoyment, whereas as many as 50% of women treated with radiation for the same condition do not achieve that same result.[50] In a separate study, ten women who had undergone pelvic surgery even reported an increase in orgasm frequency.[51] The majority of the irradiated patients showed shortening and/or stenosis of the vaginal canal. It should be noted that vaginal anatomy, as measured by vaginal calibre (diameter), length and vulvovaginal atrophy, has not correlated well with symptoms of sexual function such as dyspareunia (vaginal pain or discomfort) or vaginal dryness in at least one study.[52] What may have benefited those patients seeking better post-treatment comfort during intercourse includes the use of synthetic vaginal lubricants and alternative positioning, among other techniques.[53] Abitbol and Davenport, in an earlier study,[54] have also suggested that, by continuing sexual activity or by regular vaginal dilatation, subsequent sexual dysfunction may be preventable.

Although priapism, a prolonged erection of the corpora cavernosa not associated with sexual stimulation, is most commonly known as a condition of the penis, it can occur in the clitoris as well. Priapism of the clitoral corpora is most commonly reported in association with erectile tissue malignancies.[55] Pescatori et al.[56] reported a clinical case that persisted for 24 hours, and that was believed to be pathophysiologically related to persistent drug-induced clitoral corporal smooth muscle relaxation. Introital changes such as tenderness, firmness, and clitoral engorgement defined the priapistic state. This result followed administration of the oral psychotropic drug trazodone, which is well known to cause penile priapism.[57] Trazodone is a triazolopyridine antidepressant with serotonergic and alpha-adrenoreceptor-blocking properties, suspected to enhance penile erection through a mechanism proposed to be related to interference in the sympathetic control of detumescence. Psychotropic medications can influence sexual functioning by four mechanisms:[58] (1) non-specific central nervous system effects may lead to a global change in sexual interest and functioning; (2) specific central nervous system effects (medication altering neurotransmitter function, for example) may increase or decrease some aspect of sexual function; (3) specific peripheral effects may alter neurotransmitter effects at local end-organ sites; and (4) medications may affect levels of hormones known to modulate sexual functioning, such as prolactin in men. At least one case of clitoral priapism has also been reported with buproprion treatment, an atypical antidepressant.[59] Priapistic-type symptoms have been observed in the clitoris following the use of other pharmacological drugs. For example, bromocriptine, a dopamine-receptor agonist that slows turnover of the neurotransmitter, may induce recurrent clitoral tumescent episodes of several minutes in duration.[60] Fluoxetine (Prozac), a bicyclic propylamine antidepressant that inhibits serotonin re-uptake, also may induce short-duration recurrent clitoral engorgement episodes in association with yawning and multiple spontaneously occurring orgasms.[61] To complicate the issue further, buproprion has also been shown (in a separate case) to reverse sexual dysfunctions including erectile impotence and delayed orgasm brought on by fluoxetine.[62]

There is good reason to suspect that, like antipsychotic drugs, antihypertensive drugs are likely to affect sexual functioning adversely in women, as they are known to do so in men.[63] Drug effects on sexual function are often predictable on the basis of the known pharmacology of the drug, and are usually dose dependent.[64] Adverse effects of drugs on sexual function can be divided into those affecting fertility, libido, lubrication and orgasm. There are minimal scientific data concerning sexual dysfunction in females on antihypertensive drug regimens.[65] A study by Poloniecki and Hamilton[66] reported that 16% of women being treated pharmacologically for mild hypertension also had some impairment of sexual functioning, a value that increased to 23% when sexually inactive women were excluded from the analysis. Unfortunately, the extensive section in a review by Duncan and Bateman[67] of the literature on female sexual dysfunction and antihypertensive drugs either lacks control groups or is merely anecdotal. Nevertheless, some of the key points are worth mentioning. Sympatholytics such as clonidine and methyldopa are alpha-adrenergic agonists that cause anorgasmia and decreases in libido. Nadolol, a beta-adrenergic-blocking agent, has been reported to induce non-specific sexual dysfunction in a limited number of hypertensive patients. Diuretics may cause alterations in vaginal lubrication and a decrease in libido. It should be mentioned that, in addition to negative side effects from antihypertensive agents, some of the drugs — such as calcium antagonists, angiotensin-converting enzyme inhibitor, and vasodilators — can have positive effects on sexual functioning, including a decrease in dysfunction symptoms due to increased circulation following vascular smooth muscle relaxation.

TREATMENT

Treatment of female sexual dysfunction is gradually evolving as more clinical and basic science studies are dedicated to the investigation of this medical problem. Female sexual complaints are not all psychological in pathophysiology, especially for those individuals who may have a component of vasculogenic dysfunction contributing to the overall female sexual complaint. Apart from hormone replacement therapy, medical management of female sexual dysfunction remains in the early phases of development. All non-hormonal medications listed below are undergoing safety and efficacy testing for the treatment of male erectile dysfunction. Use of these agents in women with female sexual health issues should at this time be considered experimental.

Oestrogen replacement therapy

This treatment is indicated in menopausal women (either spontaneous or surgical) for the treatment of hot flushes, prevention of osteoporosis and reduction of risk of heart disease. Oestrogen replacement results in improved clitoral sensitivity, increased libido and decreased pain/burning during intercourse.[68,69] Local or topical oestrogen application relieves symptoms of vaginal dryness, burning, urinary frequency and urgency. No clinical evidence exists, so far, that the use of topical oestrogen cream results in relief of sexual complaints other than local vaginal pain or vaginal dryness.[70]

Methyl testosterone

Methyl testosterone may be used in combination with oestrogen in menopausal women for symptoms of inhibited desire, dyspareunia or lack of vaginal lubrication. Topical vaginal testosterone is used for treatment of vaginal lichen planus. These women, usually elderly, are noted to have clitoral enlargement, increased facial hair and increased sexual appetite. There are conflicting reports regarding the benefit of methyl testosterone for treatment of inhibited desire and/or

vaginismus in premenopausal women;[71] in such women, before prescribing methyl testosterone, it is advisable to obtain a psychological and gynaecological evaluation.

Prostaglandin E1

In men, topical application of prostaglandin E1 (PGE1) combined with a skin enhancer such as soft enhancement of percutaneous absorption (SEPA), is currently showing initial success in pilot phase II clinical trials. Clinical studies are necessary to determine the safety and efficacy of this medication used as a topical, vaginally administered, vasoactive agent in the treatment of vasculogenic female sexual dysfunction. One study has demonstrated increased clitoral blood flow and clitoral erection following local PGE1 injection into clitoral corporal erectile tissue.[72]

Sildenafil

Functioning as a selective type V (c-GMP-specific) phosphodiesterase inhibitor, this medication decreases the metabolism of c-GMP, the second messenger in nitric-oxide mediated relaxation of clitoral and vaginal smooth muscle.[73] This oral medication has proved to be safe and effective in improving erectile duration and rigidity.[74,75] In females, nitric oxide/NOS (nitric oxide synthase) exists in human vaginal and clitoral tissue. Sildenafil may prove useful alone, or possibly in combination with other vasoactive agents for treatment of vasculogenic female sexual dysfunction. Clinical studies to evaluate the efficacy of this medication in women are currently in progress. Preliminary reports suggest that this medication will benefit women with organic sexual dysfunction.

Phentolamine

Phentolamine is currently available in an oral preparation with rapid absorption and metabolism. Its mechanism of action, inducing vascular smooth muscle relaxation, occurs via alpha-adrenergic blockade as well as by direct smooth muscle relaxation. Studies are currently in progress using this medication in women with sexual dysfunction.

Apomorphine

This short-acting dopamine agonist facilitates erectile responses via central mechanisms. A new sublingual delivery form of the medication is being tested in men with psychogenic erectile dysfunction and in those with mild organic impotence. Data suggest that dopamine mediates both sexual desire and arousal. Clinical studies in women with sexual dysfunction are needed to evalute the safety and efficacy of this medication.

CONCLUSIONS

Clinical research is expanding with regard to the management of female sexual dysfunction. Female patients with complaints of sexual dysfunction may, in selected cases, undergo diagnostic studies including duplex Doppler imaging of vaginal and clitoral arteries, and assessment of pudendal nerve latencies and of clitoral vibratory thresholds and sensory-pressure thresholds. Laboratory studies include blood chemistry as well as hormonal profiles. Such evaluations may result in a growing body of evidence that women with sexual dysfunction will commonly have physiological abnormalities, such as vasculogenic female sexual dysfunction, contributing to their overall sexual health problems. Such physiological abnormalities will probably benefit from medical therapies such as oral and/or topical vasodilators. The ideal approach to the management of women with sexual health problems is a collaborative effort between psychologists, therapists and physicians.

REFERENCES

1. Masters W H, Johnson V E. Human sexual response. Boston: Little, Brown, 1996

2. Wagner G. Aspects of genital physiology and pathology. Semin Neurol 1992; 12: 87

3. Levin R J. The mechanisms of human female sexual arousal. Annu Rev Sex Res 1992; 3: 1

4. Levin R J. The physiology of sexual function in women. Clin Obstet Gynecol 1980; 7: 213

5. Weber A M, Walters M D, Schover L R, Mitchinson A. Vaginal anatomy and sexual function. Obstet Gynecol 1995; 86: 946

6. Huffman J. The gynecology of childhood and adolescence. Philadelphia: Saunders, 1969: 68

7. Burgos M H, Roig de Vargas-Linares C E. Ultrastructure of the vaginal mucosa. In: Hafez E S E, Evans E T (eds) The human vagina. Amsterdam: Elsevier, 1978

8. Sjoberg I. The vagina: morphological, functional and ecological aspects. Acta Obstet Gynecol Scand 1992; 71: 84

9. Hilliges M, Falconer C, Ekman-Ordeberg G, Johanson O. Innervation of the human vaginal mucosa as revealed by PGP 9.5 immunohistochemistry. Acta Anat (Basel) 1995; 153: 119

10. Graf A-H, Schiechl A, Hacker G W et al. Helospectin and pituitary adenylate cyclase activating polypeptide in the human vagina. Regul Pept 1995; 55: 277

11. Levin R J. The mechanisms of human female sexual arousal. Annu Rev Sex Res 1992; 3: 1

12. Schiavi R C, Segraves R T. The biology of sexual function. Psychiatr Clin North Am 1995; 18: 7

13. Levin R J. VIP, vagina, clitoral and periurethral glans: an update on female genital arousal. Exp Clin Endocrinol 1991; 98: 61

14. Ottesen B. Vasoactive intestinal peptide as a neurotransmitter in the female genital tract. Am J Obstet Gynecol 1983; 147: 203

15. Uddman R, Luts A, Absood A et al. PACAP, a VIP-like peptide in neurons of the esophagus. Regulatory Peptides 1991; 36: 415

16. Desai H, Uddman R, Malina J, Sundler F. Helospectin-like immunoreactivity in the esophagus. Regulatory Peptides 1992; 40: 363

17. Gould S F, Shannon J M, Cunha G R. The autoradiographic demonstration of estrogen binding in normal human cervix and vagina during the menstrual cycle, pregnancy, and the menopause. Am J Anat 1983; 168: 229

18. MacLean A B, Nicol L A, Hodgins M B. Immunohistochemical localization of estrogen receptors in the vulva and vagina. J Reprod Med 1990; 35: 1015

19. Press M F, Nousek-Goebl N A, Bur M. Estrogen receptor localisation in the female genital tract. Am J Pathol 1986; 123: 280

20. Forsberg J-G. A morphologist's approach to the vagina: age-related changes and estrogen sensitivity. Maturitas 1995; (suppl) 22: S7

21. Diederichs W, Lue T, Tanagho E A. Clitoral responses to central nervous stimulation in dogs. Int J Impot Res 1991; 3: 7

22. Marson L. Central nervous system neurons identified after injection of pseudorabies virus in the rat clitoris. Neurosci Lett 1995; 190: 41

23. Kawatani M, Tanowitz M, de Groat W C. Morphological and electrophysiological analysis of the peripheral and central afferent pathways from the clitoris of the cat. Brain Res 1994; 646: 26

24. Cocchia D, Rende M, Tiesca A et al. Immunohistochemical study of neuropeptide Y-containing nerve fibers in the human clitoris and penis. Cell Biol Int Rep 1990; 14: 865

25. Laan E, Everaerd W, van der Velde J, Geer J H. Determinants of subjective experience of sexual arousal in women: feedback from genital arousal and erotic stimulus content. Psychophysiology 1995; 32: 444

26. Laan E, Everaerd W, van Aanhold M-T, Rebel M. Performance demand and sexual arousal in women. Behav Res Ther 1993; 31: 25

27. Laan E, Everaerd W, van Bellen G, Hanewald G. Women's sexual and emotional responses to male- and female-produced erotica. Arch Sex Behav 1994; 23: 153

28. Laan E, Everaerd W. Habituation of female sexual arousal to slides and film. Arch Sex Behav 1995; 24: 517

29. Meuwissen I, Over R. Sexual arousal across phases of the human menstrual cycle. Arch Sex Behav 1992; 21: 101

30. Meuwissen I, Over R. Habituation and dishabituation of female sexual arousal. Behav Res Ther 1990; 28: 217

31. Meston C M, Gorzalka B B. The effects of sympathetic activation on physiological and subjective sexual arousal in women. Behav Res Ther 1995; 33: 651

32. Meston C M, Gorzalka B B. The effects of immediate, delayed, and residual sympathetic activation on sexual arousal in women. Behav Res Ther 1996; 34: 143

33. Verkauf B S, von Thorn J, O'Brien W F. Clitoral size in normal women. Obstet Gynecol 1992; 80: 41

34. World Health Organization: The ICD-10 Classification of Mental and Behavioral Disorders: clinical descriptions and diagnostic guidelines. Geneva: WHO, 1992

35. Park K, Goldstein I, Andry C et al. Vasculogenic female sexual dysfunction: the hemodynamic basis for vaginal engorgement insufficiency and clitoral erectile insufficiency. Int J Impot Res 1997; 9: 27

36. Lavoisier P, Aloui R, Schmidt M H, Watrelot A. Clitoral blood flow increases following vaginal pressure stimulation. Arch Sex Behav 1995; 24: 37

37. Novelly A, Berone P J, Ax A F. Photoplethysmography: system calibration and light history effects. Psychophysiology 1973; 10: 67

38. Geer J H, Morokoff P, Greenwood P. Sexual arousal in women: the development of a measurement device for vaginal blood volume. Arch Sex Behav 1974; 3: 559

39. Sintchak G, Geer J H. A vaginal photoplethysmograph system. Psychophysiology 1975; 12: 113

40. Hoon P W, Wincze J P, Hoon E F. Physiological assessment of sexual arousal in women. Psychophysiology 1976; 13: 196

41. Geer J H, Morokoff P, Greenwood P. Sexual arousal in women: the development of a measurement device for vaginal blood volume. Arch Sex Behav 1974; 3: 559

42. Fisher C, Cohen H D, Schiavi R C et al. Patterns of female sexual arousal during sleep and waking: vaginal thermo-conductance studies. Arch Sex Behav 1983; 12: 97

43. Morrell M J, Sperling M R, Stecker M, Dichter M A. Sexual dysfunction in partial epilepsy: a deficit in physiological sexual arousal. Neurology 1994; 44: 243

44. Levin R J, Macdonaugh R P. Increased vaginal blood flow induced by implant electrical stimulation of sacral anterior roots in the conscious woman: a case study. Arch Sex Behav 1993; 22: 471

45. Sipski M L, Alexander C J, Rosen R C. Physiological parameters associated with psychogenic sexual arousal in women with complete spinal cord injuries. Arch Phys Med Rehabil 1995; 76: 811

46. Sipski M L, Rosen R C, Alexander C J. Physiological parameters associated with the performance of a distracting task and genital self-stimulation in women with complete spinal cord injuries. Arch Phys Med Rehabil 1996; 77: 419

47. Komisaruk B R, Bianca R, Sansone Gomez L E et al. Brain mediated responses to vaginocervical stimulation in spinal cord-transected rats: role of the vagus nerves. Brain Res 1996; 708: 128

48. Hricak H. Magnetic resonance imaging evaluation of the irradiated female pelvis. Semin Roentgenol 1994; 29: 70

49. Abitbol M M, Davenport J H. The irradiated vagina. Obstet Gynecol 1974; 44: 250

50. Seibel M S, Freeman M G, Graves W L. Carcinoma of the cervix and sexual function. Obstet Gynecol 1980; 55: 484

51. Poad D, Arnold E P. Sexual function after pelvic surgery in women. Aust N Z J Obstet Gynaecol 1994; 34: 471

52. Weber A M, Walters M D, Schover L R, Mitchinson A. Vaginal anatomy and sexual function. Obstet Gynecol 1995; 86: 946

53. Tharnov I, Klee M. Sexuality among gynecologic cancer patients — a cross-sectional study. Gynecol Oncol 1994; 52: 14

54. Abitbol M M, Davenport J H. Sexual function after therapy for cervical carcinoma. Am J Obstet Gynecol 1974; 119: 181

55. Slavin R E, Christie J D, Swedo J, Powell L C. Locally aggressive granular cell tumor causing priapism of the crus of the clitoris. A light and ultrastructural study, with observations concerning pathogenesis of fibrosis of the corpus cavernosum in priapism. Am J Surg Pathol 1986; 10: 497

56. Pescatori E S, Engelman J C, Davis G, Goldstein I. Priapism of the clitoris: a case report following trazodone use. J Urol 1993; 149: 1557

57. Saenz de Tejada I, Moroukian P, Tessier J et al. Trabecular smooth muscle modulates the capacitor function of the penis. Studies on a rabbit model. Am J Physiol 1991; 260: H1590

58. Gitlin M J. Psychotropic medications and their effects on sexual function: diagnosis, biology and treatment approaches. J Clin Psychol 1994; 55: 406

59. Levenson J L. Priapism associated with buproprion treatment (letter). Am J Psychiatry 1995; 152: 813

60. Blin O, Schwertschlag U S, Serratrice G. Painful clitoral tumescence during bromocriptine therapy (letter). Lancet 1991; 337: 1231

61. Modell J G. Repeated observation of yawning, clitoral engorgement, and orgasm associated with fluoxetine administration (letter). J Clin Psychopharmacol 1989; 9: 63

62. Labbate L A, Pollack M H. Treatment of fluoxetine-induced sexual dysfunction with buproprion: a case report. Ann Clin Psychiatry 1994; 6: 13

63. Bateman D N. Drugs and sexual function. Adverse Drug React Bull 1980; 80: 308

64. Beely L. Drug-induced sexual dysfunction and infertility. Adverse Drug React Acute Poisoning Rev 1984; 3: 23

65. Moss H B, Procci W R. Sexual dysfunction associated with oral antihypertensive medication: a critical survey of the literature. Gen Hosp Psychiatry 1982; 4: 121

66. Poloniecki J, Hamilton M. Subjective costs of antihypertensive treatment. Hum Toxicol 1985; 4: 287

67. Duncan L, Bateman D N. Sexual function in women: do antihypertensive drugs have an impact? Drug Safety 1993; 8: 225

68. Pearce M J, Hawton K. Psychological and sexual aspects of menopause and HRT. Baillieres Clin Obstet Gynaecol 1996; 10(3): 385–399

69. Collins A, Landgren B M. Reproductive health, use of estrogen and experience of symptoms in perimenopausal women: a population based study. Maturitas 1994; 20(2): 101–111

70. Ayton R A, Darling G M, Murkies A L et al. A comparative study of safety and efficacy of continuous low dose oestradiol released from a vaginal ring compared with conjugated equine oestrogen vaginal cream in the treatment of postmenopausal vaginal atrophy. Br J Obstet Gynaecol 1996; 103: 351–358

71. Pearce M J, Hawton K. Psychological and sexual aspects of menopause and HRT. Baillières Clin Obstet Gynecol 1996; 10: 385–399

72. Akus E, Carrier S, Turzan C et al. Duplex ultrasonography after prostaglandin E1 injection of the clitoris in a case of hyperreaction luteinalis. J Urol 1995; 153(4): 1237–1238

73. Park K, Goldstein I, Andry C et al. Vasculogenic female sexual dysfunction: the hemodynamic basis for vaginal engorgement insufficiency and clitoral erectile insufficiency. Int J Impot Res 1997; 9: 99–111

74. Weiner D N, Rosen R C. Medications and their impact. In: Sexual function in people with disability and chronic illness. 85–114

75. Boolell M, Allen M J, Ballard S A et al. Sildenafil: an orally active type 5 cyclic GMP-specific phosphodiesterase inhibitor for the treatment of penile erectile dysfunction. Int J Impot Res 1996; 8: 47–52

Chapter 57

Sexual dysfunction and prostate cancer therapy

J. M. Fitzpatrick, R. S. Kirby, R. J. Krane, J. Adolfsson, D. W. W. Newling and I. Goldstein

■ INTRODUCTION

The management of prostate cancer focuses on effective methods of cure and palliation. The complications associated with radical surgery for localized disease, such as urinary incontinence and erectile dysfunction (ED), have been greatly reduced with the development of the nerve-sparing radical prostatectomy technique.[1] In advanced disease, palliation of pain and prevention of additional complications of prostate cancer are the main treatment objectives.

With the diagnosis of prostate cancer shifting to younger patients than was the case 10 years ago, and the availability of effective treatment of localized disease, attention has shifted to issues of quality of life. Factors affecting patients' lifestyles are being considered, sexuality in particular. Physicians should consider how a patient will feel when given treatment options that might deprive him of his sexual function. For all patients, seemingly irrespective of age, sexual dysfunction is still an important element in their perceived quality of life and must be discussed fully when planning any therapeutic strategy.

■ CAUSES OF ERECTILE DYSFUNCTION IN PROSTATE CANCER

ED in prostate cancer patients has a number of causes (Table 57.1). Psychologically, some patients fear that sexual activity may cause pain, may stimulate the cancer or, indeed, cause the cancer to spread to their partner. Depression itself is an important cause of ED and loss of libido. Patients may also put up a psychological barrier to

Table 57.1. The main causes of erectile dysfunction (ED) in prostate cancer patients

- Neurological
- Psychological
- Arterial
- Hormonal
- Veno-occlusive dysfunction
- Geometric

sexual activity because they feel less attractive to their partners. These issues must be taken into consideration when discussing sexual potency with prostate cancer patients. Pain from metastatic disease and lack of muscle strength are two important physical problems that can lead to ED. Painful gynaecomastia may also limit sexual activity in some patients.

Treatment for prostate cancer can, in itself, cause a considerable degree of dysfunction (Table 57.2).[2] Tissue fibrosis resulting in veno-occlusive ED can be caused in a variety of ways (Table 57.3). Absence of erections can lead to decreased blood flow to the corpora cavernosa. The concomitant reduction in oxygen supply to the tissues produces tissue fibrosis, which in turn leads to veno-occlusive dysfunction. The fibrosis is probably due to increased local deposition and activation of transforming growth factor beta 1, resulting from the ischaemia.

Androgen withdrawal

Patients with advanced prostate cancer who are receiving androgen withdrawal therapy may be unable to develop

Table 57.2. Mean percentage of patients developing ED following a particular treatment[2]

Treatment	ED (%)
Medical/surgical castration	100
Radical prostatectomy	98
Nerve-sparing radical prostatectomy	30–75
Radiation therapy	50
Brachytherapy	25
Watchful waiting	0

Table 57.3. Causes of veno-occlusive ED

■ Arterial injury; prolonged tissue ischaemia; tissue fibrosis; veno-occlusive dysfunction

■ Radiation injury to tissues; tissue fibrosis; veno-occlusive dysfunction

■ Nerve injury; loss of nocturnal erections; tissue fibrosis; veno-occlusive dysfunction

erections and, in addition, may experience a loss of libido. Tiredness, reduced levels of concentration and hot flushes are also serious side effects, which may result in withdrawal from working life and an inability to enjoy hobbies. Androgen withdrawal can also produce a change in body image, with the development of a more female form; some men may fear the development of osteoporosis.

Radiation therapy

Radiation therapy (external beam), conformal beam radiotherapy and brachytherapy can cause ED in 50, 35 and 25% of cases, respectively. Goldstein and co-workers evaluated radiation-induced alterations to penile haemodynamics using history, physical examination and dynamic infusion pharmacocavernosometry and cavernosography (DICC).[3] The cause of ED was found to be arterial insufficiency, which has a higher incidence in smokers, older patients and those with pre-existing vascular conditions, such as hypertension and diabetes.

Both proximal corporal veno-occlusive dysfunction and cavernosal arterial insufficiency were present in all patients. Cavernosography indicated that, in the majority of cases, site-specific venous leakage was crucial; proximal spongiosal, cavernosal and dorsal venous leaks were far less frequent.

Surgery

Non-nerve-sparing radical prostatectomy can result in impotence rates as high as 98%. If preservation of the neurovascular bundles is achieved, the rate drops to between 30% and 75%, depending on whether the bundles are preserved bilaterally or unilaterally and on the patient's age. ED following nerve-sparing prostatectomy may be due to removal of an accessory pudendal artery that had been acting as the main cavernosal artery.[4] The prevalence of this phenomenon is thought to be approximately 35%, with the origin of the artery occurring from the left side in 50% of cases and from the right side or bilaterally in 25% of cases each. In the majority of cases, the accessory pudendal artery arises from the internal pudendal or the obturator artery.

■ MANAGEMENT OF ERECTILE DYSFUNCTION

Normal sexual activity for a patient's own age-group is an important consideration for urologists treating patients with prostate cancer. Older patients may be satisfied with less sexual activity and tolerate more complications than younger patients. Consequently, it is important to establish baseline values for sexual activity.

Patient expectations of treatment depend on a number of factors, such as age and disease stage. For instance, the expectations of a 40-year-old patient with localized disease who had full sexual function before therapy and is now left with no erectile function will certainly differ from those of a 75-year-old patient with metastatic cancer. Patient counselling is essential in order to clarify the likelihood of developing ED following treatment. Patients should be made fully aware of the risk of dysfunction in order to avoid subsequent frustration, which in itself can lead to decreased potency. It is interesting to observe that, statistically, of the approximately 17 million men with ED of various aetiologies in the USA, only 10% will seek treatment and even fewer will adjust to the subsequent therapy.[5]

It is important to maintain sexual desire when treating patients with prostate cancer as, in most patients with an intact vascular system, loss of potency can be treated by injection therapy, vacuum pump devices or a penile prosthesis. Loss of libido cannot be treated unless patients are given androgen replacement, and this is a separate but important issue. Injection therapy, if selected, should be started at an early stage, owing to the risk of tissue anoxia and corporal fibrosis associated with lack of erections. Injection therapy and vacuum devices appear to be acceptable therapeutic options from the patient's perspective, although neither is without drawbacks. A penile prosthesis is another option that is sometimes requested at the same time as surgery for the cancer itself. Caution should be exercised in these circumstances, as it is not clear which patients will actually become impotent. The possibility of penile shortening following radical prostatectomy is a serious concern to patients. An assessment of penile length pre- and postoperatively in the erect state should be carried out to judge the effects of surgery accurately. The patient's anger and frustration over this problem may be avoided with the use of a penile prosthesis at the time of radical prostatectomy.

■ QUALITY OF LIFE

Treatment choices for prostate cancer are frequently based on the evaluation of possible benefits balanced against side effects of treatment. Owing to a lack of information, little regard is paid to quality-of-life issues. Previous assessments of quality of life are unsatisfactory, as they measured sexual function and not how the patient felt towards potency or lack of it. These assessments dealt only with figures, functions and scales. Understandably, it may mean very little to the patient that he has a score of 10.7 on a 'health and quality of life' scale. Physicians should be aware that this assessment does not truly reflect the patient's quality of life. For example, there are major differences between the patient's and the physician's appreciation of quality-of-life issues in endocrine treatment of prostate cancer. Physicians tend to overestimate patients' quality of life with respect to sexual activity and hot flushes, and underestimate their psychological distress.[6] A validated instrument is essential in order that the physician knows what should be, and is being, measured.

■ QUALITY-OF-LIFE INSTRUMENTS

A psychometric scale is the most commonly used method for evaluating quality of life. Each symptom experienced by the patient is given a value and the total score is analysed statistically. Such symptom-based assessment can be carried out in a number of ways: pain, fatigue and general symptoms can be evaluated in a health-related quality-of-life questionnaire; alternatively, symptoms prevalent in a selected group of patients can be identified, e.g. characterization of symptoms related to localized or advanced prostate cancer in order to evaluate sexual dysfunction.

Physicians need to devise methods of evaluating their patients' symptoms in the absence of a validated questionnaire. The actual development of a formal questionnaire is a long and laborious process. Initially, in-depth interviews with a number of patients are conducted, followed by re-testing of the questions on a similar patient group. Validation should ideally be carried out against a 'gold standard' instrument of assessment, which unfortunately is not available in the area of sexual function. Test–retest reliability is measured by asking the same question of the same group of patients after a specific time interval. It should be noted that the resulting questionnaire is specific only for the condition for which it was designed.

A questionnaire for assessing sexual function in patients with prostate cancer has been developed in Sweden by Helgason.[7] A three-level approach was involved, with patients first being asked how frequently a particular dysfunction occurred; verbal categories of numbers were used to represent the answers (1–7). The next question asked was: 'If you were to live with this problem for the rest of your life, how much distress would you get from it?' Four categories of answer were provided: none; a little; a moderate amount; and a lot. The third question, to which an answer on a scale of 1–7 was requested, was: 'How would this affect your overall well-being, either psychological or physical?' In this way, the questionnaire assessed three aspects of quality of life: function, inconvenience and overall well-being, resulting in a scale specific to prostate cancer patients. Elements of the questionnaire were validated against objective measurements and found to have a very high reliability (90%).[8] For example, three different aspects of erection were assessed with regard to nocturnal tumescence. The observation was made that all patients who said that they

Table 57.4. Proportion of men reporting decrease in sexual function compared with their youth; prostate cancer therapy indicated

Aspects assessed	Men without prostate cancer (n = 314)	Men with prostate cancer (n = 342)	Endocrine treatment/ castration (n = 109)	Radical prostatectomy (n = 22)	External radiation (n = 37)	Mixed group (n = 35)	Other cases (n = 139)
Sexual desire/ thoughts	156/305 (51%)	240/321 (75%)	82/99 (83%)	16/22 (73%)	27/37 (73%)	24/33 (73%)	91/130 (70%)
Erection capacity	235/304 (77%)	286/318 (90%)	93/97 (96%)	19/22 (86%)	35/37 (95%)	34/34 (100%)	105/128 (82%)
Orgasm pleasure	209/305 (69%)	252/302 (83%)	81/93 (87%)	14/20 (70%)	32/37 (86%)	26/31 (84%)	99/121 (82%)
Ejaculate volume	232/298 (78%)	256/287 (89%)	78/89 (87%)	18/21 (86%)	31/33 (94%)	25/28 (89%)	104/116 (90%)

*Variations in denominators of 'n' are caused by different response rates for individual questions.

were impotent had no erections on the Rigiscan device, compared with evidence of nocturnal tumescence in the 80% who said that they were potent.

The questionnaire was tested in men with and without prostate cancer, including 342 patients diagnosed in 1992 in Stockholm.[9] An equivalent sample of healthy men from the general population was investigated. The assessment looked at the prevalence of decreased sexual function by comparing current function with that experienced in a patient's youth. This also provided a 'maximum' function reference for each of the men studied.

One interesting observation was that there was a high prevalence of decreased desire and erections among the group of healthy men: 77% reported decreased function compared with that experienced in their youth (Table 57.4).[10] The study indicated that the relative risk of experiencing ED and a decreased sexual desire in prostate cancer patients in general was almost double that in the controls.

■ PATIENT PREFERENCE SURVEY

A survey was conducted in 400 patients with prostate cancer in four countries — USA, Germany, Italy and the UK. The objectives of the study were to investigate the patients' understanding of the treatment options they received, to explore the importance of patient–doctor communication in the treatment of prostate cancer and to determine the effect of treatment on patients' sexual

function. Concomitant conditions such as hypertension, heart disease and psychological illness, therapy for which may have influenced erectile function, were not recorded.

The majority of the patients were interviewed within 5 years of being diagnosed. Radical prostatectomy had been performed in 44.7% of patients, while 8.8% had received hormone therapy and 3.5% had undergone bilateral orchiectomy (Fig. 57.1). Patients were asked

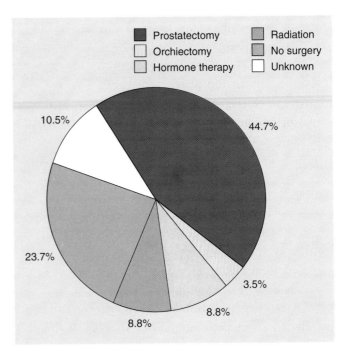

Figure 57.1. Patient profile by treatment status.

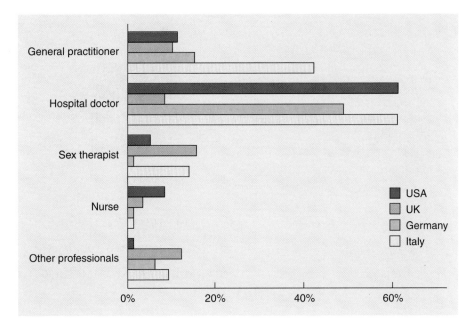

Figure 57.2. Patients given advice by different medical professionals according to country.

whether they were given sexual advice or help after diagnosis or treatment. Overall, of the five categories of healthcare professional about which enquiry was made, hospital doctors were cited as giving advice by 46% of patients, general practitioners by 21%, sex therapists by 9%, other professionals by 7% and nurses by 3%. On a country basis, the hospital doctor was more likely to give advice in the USA, Germany and Italy, whereas in the UK this advice was more likely to have been given by a sex therapist (Fig. 57.2). With regard to patients who would find sex counselling helpful to themselves or their partner, 46% of all patients said that they would.

A comparison was made of patients' sexual activity before diagnosis, 3 months after diagnosis and in the previous month, and what the patient would prefer the activity to be (Fig. 57.3). Clearly, patients in each of the countries studied would prefer their sexual activity to be the same as it was before diagnosis, or even greater.

Patients' preferences for the mode and frequency of delivery of hormonal treatment were studied and interesting differences according to country were observed. In the UK, patients preferred to take one to three tablets daily, whereas in Italy, patients were more willing to have monthly injections (Fig. 57.4). From a pyschological viewpoint, seeing a patient on a monthly basis makes a significant difference.

The survey also showed a tendency for patients to discontinue certain hobbies and activities — an important aspect in terms of diminished quality of life. Almost one-third of patients gave up sporting activities,

which (although this was not determined) could be because of pain or weakness caused by hormonal therapy.

In conclusion, this survey raised a number of important issues. Sexual dysfunction following therapy for prostate cancer should be assessed. Large multicentre, prospective, controlled studies into the incidence of ED after radical prostatectomy are needed. With regard to hormonal therapy, the effect on sexuality should be assessed prospectively through questionnaires and

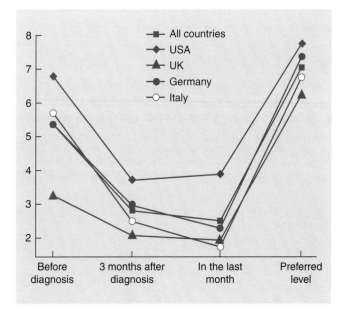

Figure 57.3. Comparison of patients' preferred level of sexual activity with levels before and after diagnosis and current levels.

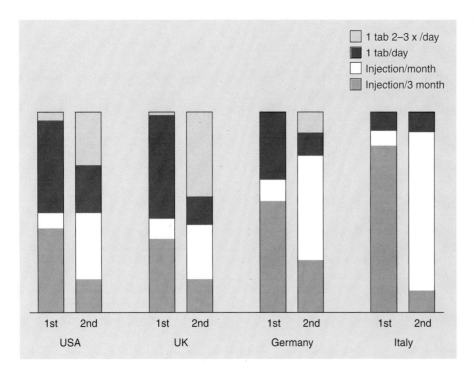

Figure 57.4. Patients' preferences for mode and frequency of delivery of hormonal therapy by country.

objective methods. The problem must be quantified, with definition of the number of patients suffering from sexual dysfunction and the ways in which they are affected; the effects on patient/partner relationships should be evaluated. Studies are also needed on what is considered to be the normal level of sexual activity in different age-groups. In general, a universally accepted method of quantification of sexual dysfunction is urgently required, as this is an area that will be increasingly important to urologists involved in the management of prostate cancer.

■ REFERENCES

1. Walsh P C, Lepor H, Eggleston J C. Radical prostatectomy with preservation of sexual function: anatomical and pathological considerations. Prostate 1983; 4: 473–485

2. Meuleman E J, Diemont W L. Investigation of erectile dysfunction. Diagnostic testing for vascular factors in erectile dysfunction. Urol Clin North Am 1995; 22: 803–819

3. Goldstein I, Feldman M, Deckers P J, Krane R J. Radiation associated impotence — a clinical study of its mechanism. JAMA 1984; 1251: 9031

4. Nehra A, Ramakumar S, McKusick M A et al. Pharmaco-angiographic prevalence of accessory pudendal arteries: role of maintaining sexual function following radical retropubic prostectomy. J Urol 1997; 157: 357 (abstr 1396)

5. Feldman H A, Goldstein I, Hatzichristou D G et al. Impotence and its medical and psychosocial correlates: results of the Massachusetts Male Aging Study. J Urol 1994; 151: 54–57

6. Fossa S D, Woehre H, Kurth K H et al. Influence of urological morbidity on quality of life in patients with prostate cancer. Eur Urol 1997; 31(suppl3): 3–80

7. Helgason A R. Prostate cancer treatment and quality of life — a three level epidemiological approach. Thesis, University of Stockholm, 1997

8. Helgason A R, Aldolfsson J, Dickman P et al. Factors associated with waning sexual function among elderly men and prostate cancer patients. J Urol 1997; 158: 155–159

9. Helgason A R, Aldolfsson J, Dickman P et al. Waning sexual function — the most important disease-specific distress for patients with prostate cancer. Br J Cancer 1996; 72: 1417–1421

10. Helgason A R, Adolfsson J, Dickman P et al. Sexual desire, erection, orgasm and ejaculatory functions and their importance to elderly Swedish men: a population-based study. Age Ageing 1996; 25: 285–291

Index

V

U